Surgical Care for the Elderly

Second Edition

Editors

R. Benton Adkins, Jr., M.D.
Professor of Surgery and Cell Biology
Department of General Surgery
Vanderbilt University School of Medicine
Nashville, Tennessee

H. William Scott, Jr., M.D.
Professor of Surgery, Emeritus
Vanderbilt University School of Medicine
Nashville, Tennessee

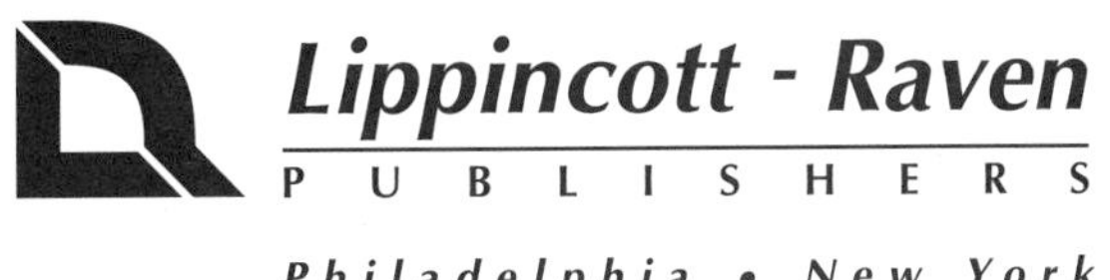

Acquisitions Editor: Lisa McAllister
Developmental Editor: Rhoda Dunn
Manufacturing Manager: Dennis Teston
Associate Managing Editor: Kathleen Bubbeo
Production Editor: Jenn Nagaj
Cover Designer: Jill Wood
Indexer: Ann Blum
Compositor: Lisa Cunningham
Printer: Maple Press

Printed in the United States of America

9 8 7 6 5 4 3 2 1

Library of Congress Cataloging-in-Publication Data

Surgical care for the elderly / edited by R. Benton Adkins, Jr. and H. William Scott, Jr. -- 2nd ed.
p. cm.
Includes bibliographical references and index.
ISBN 0-7817-1450-8
1. Aged--Surgery. I. Adkins, R. Benton. II. Scott, H. William (Henry William), 1916-
[DNLM: 1. Surgery, Operative--in old age. WO 950 S959 1997]
RD145. S92 1997
617. 9'7--dc21
DNLM/DLC
for Library of Congress 97-23283
CIP

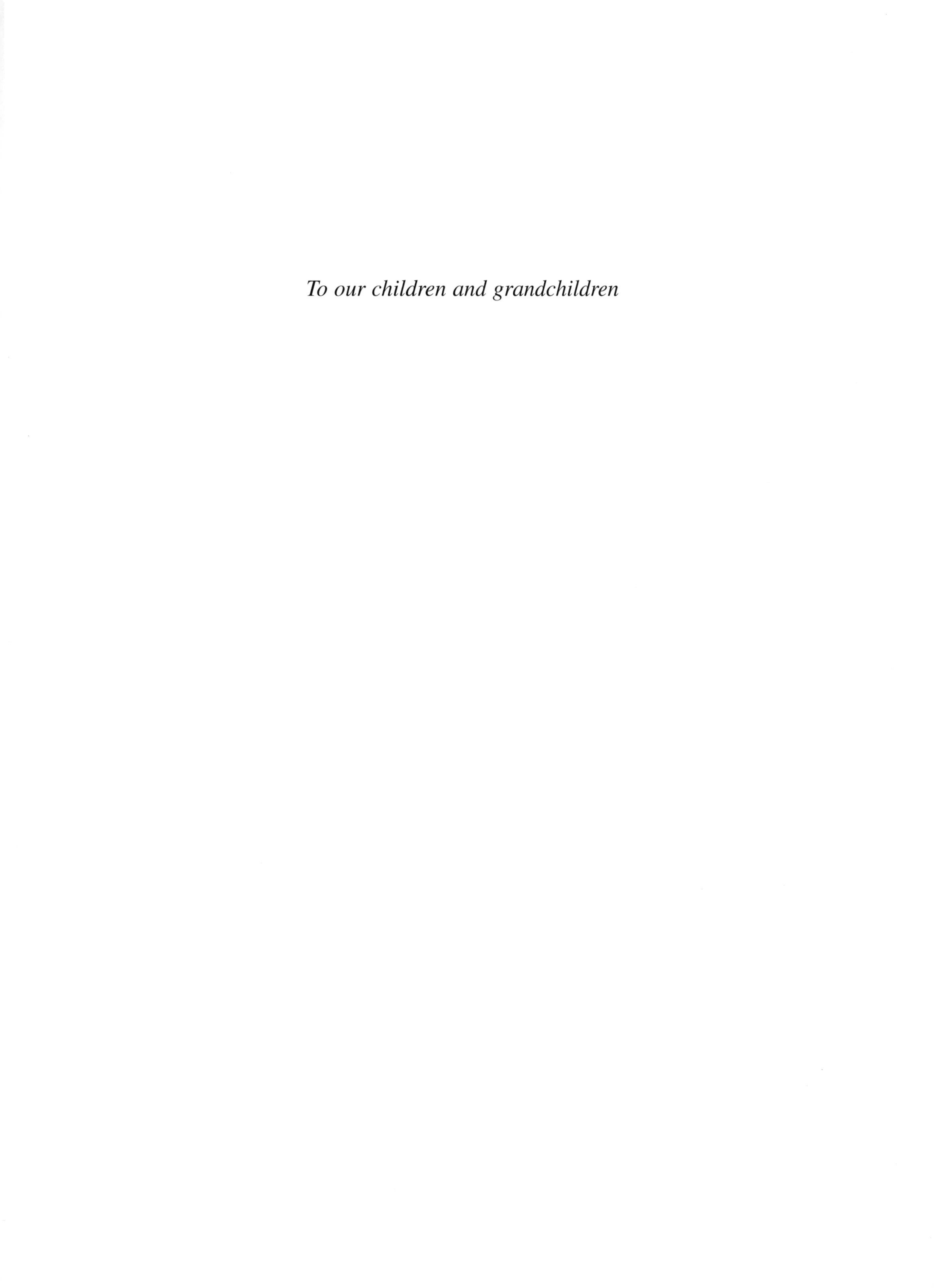

To our children and grandchildren

Contents

Contributors

R. Benton Adkins, Jr., M.D.
Professor of Surgery and Cell Biology
Department of General Surgery
Vanderbilt University School of Medicine
206 Medical Center South
2100 Pierce Avenue
Nashville, Tennessee 37232-2730

John A. Aucar, M.D.
Assistant Professor of Surgery
Baylor College of Medicine
Ben Taub General Hospital
Department of Surgery
One Baylor Plaza
Houston, Texas 77030

George R. Avant, M.D.
Associate Professor of Medicine
Department of Gastroenterology
Vanderbilt University School of Medicine
1414 The Vanderbilt Clinic
Nashville, Tennessee 37232-5280

Oliver H. Beahrs, M.D.
Professor of Surgery, Emeritus
Mayo Clinic
200 First Street, Southwest
Rochester, Minnesota 55905

F. Tremaine Billings, Jr., M.D., D.H.L.
Professor of Medicine, Emeritus
Vanderbilt University School of Medicine
2553 The Vanderbilt Clinic
Nashville, Tennessee 37232

Pamela S. Bohrer, M.D.
Department of Head and Neck Surgery
Kaiser Hospital
401 Bicentennial Way
Santa Rosa, California 95405

Lonnie S. Burnett, M.D.
The Frances and John C. Burch Professor of Obstetrics and Gynecology
Vanderbilt University School of Medicine
B1100 Medical Center North
Nashville, Tennessee 37232

John L. Cameron, M.D.
Professor and Chairman, Department of Surgery
Johns Hopkins University School of Medicine
720 Rutland Avenue, Ross 759
Baltimore, Maryland 21205

John M. Castle, M.D.
Department of Surgery
Memorial Hospital
67 Belmont Street
Worcester, Massachusetts 01605

Michael L. Cheatham, M.D.
Associate Director, Department of Surgical Education
Orlando Regional Medical System
86 West Underwood Street
Orlando, Florida 32806

David L. Crosby, M.B., B.Ch. (Wales)
Honorary Consulting Surgeon
University Hospital of Wales
15 Pencisely Road
Cardiff, CF 51DG
United Kingdom

Anh H. Dao, M.D.
Associate Professor of Pathology
Vanderbilt University School of Medicine
21st Avenue at Garland
Nashville, Tennessee 37232

James G. Drougas, M.D.
Department of Vascular Surgery
Emory University School of Medicine
1364 Clifton Road, Northeast
Atlanta, Georgia 30322

Richard Eller, M.D.
Resident in General Surgery
Fellow in Laparoscopic General Surgery
Columbia Medical Center of Plano
3901 West 15th Street
Plano, Texas 75075

James H. Elliott, M.D.
Professor of Ophthalmology and Visual Sciences
Vanderbilt University School of Medicine
8000 Medical Center East, Vanderbilt Eye Center
Nashville, Tennessee 37232-8808

Stephen S. Feman, M.D.
Professor of Ophthalmology
Department of Ophthalmology and Visual Sciences
Vanderbilt University School of Medicine
8011 Medical Center East
Nashville, Tennessee 37232-8808

D. Scott Fortune, M.D.
Resident in Otolaryngology–Head and Neck Surgery
Vanderbilt University Medical Center
S-2100 Medical Center North
Nashville, Tennessee 37232-2559

Mark Fox, M.D., Ph.D.
Assistant and Resident in Medicine and Pediatrics
Strong Memorial Hospital
University of Rochester School of Medicine
601 Elmwood Avenue, Box 702
Rochester, New York 14642

Giorgio Gaggiotti, M.D.
Surgeon
Clinica di Semeiotica Chirurgica
Università degli Studi di Ancona–INRCA
Via Della Montagnola 166
Ancona, 60100
Italy

Roberto Ghiselli
Researcher
Clinica di Semeiotica Chirurgica
Università degli Studi di Ancona–INRCA
Via Della Montagnola 166
Ancona, 60100
Italy

Claudia Giammarchi
Researcher
Dipartimento Ricerche Gerontologiche e Geriatriche
Università degli Studi di Ancona–INRCA
Via S. Margherita 5
Ancona, 60124
Italy

Michael E. Glasscock, III, M.D.
Clinical Professor of Otology and Neurotology
Department of Otolaryngology
Vanderbilt University School of Medicine
4410 Medical Drive, Suite 340
Nashville, Tennessee 37232

Richard Goldstein, M.D., Ph.D.
Associate Professor of Surgery
Department of General Surgery
Vanderbilt University School of Medicine
A-2219 Medical Center North
Nashville, Tennessee 37232

Clive S. Grant, M.D.
Professor of Surgery
Mayo Clinic
200 First Street, Southwest
Rochester, Minnesota 55905

Lazar J. Greenfield, M.D.
Frederick A. Coller Professor and Chairman, Department of Surgery
University of Michigan Medical School
1500 East Medical Center Drive
2101TC Box 0346
Ann Arbor, Michigan 48109-0346

Thomas E. Groomes, M.D.
Assistant Professor Orthopaedics and Rehabilitation
Vanderbilt University Medical Center
2201 Capers Avenue
Nashville, Tennessee 37212

John D. Hainsworth, M.D.
Director of Clinical Research
Sarah Cannon Cancer Center
Centennial Medical Center
250 25th Avenue, North
Suite 412
Nashville, Tennessee 37203

David T. Harrington, M.D.
Chief, Burn Study Branch
U.S. Army Institute of Surgical Research
3400 Rawley E. Chambers Avenue
Fort Sam Houston, Texas 78234

David S. Haynes, M.D.
Assistant Professor of Otolaryngology
Vanderbilt University School of Medicine
S-2100 Medical Center North
Nashville, Tennessee 37232

Howard W. Jones, III, M.D.
Professor of Obstetrics and Gynecology
Director of Gynecologic Oncology
Vanderbilt University School of Medicine
B-1100 Medical Center North
Nashville, Tennessee 37232-2516

Kim U. Kahng, M.D.
Associate Professor of Surgery
Allegheny University of the Health Sciences
Medical College of Pennsylvania and Hahnemann School of Medicine
3300 Henry Avenue
Philadelphia, Pennsylvania 19129

Joseph A. Kwentus, M.D.
Assistant Professor of Psychiatry
Vanderbilt University School of Medicine
1500 21st Avenue, South
Suite 2200
Nashville, Tennessee 37212

J.K. Ladipo, M.D.
Surgical Fellow, Department of Surgery
Vanderbilt University Medical Center
Senior Lecturer, Department of Surgery
University College Hospital, Ibadan, Nigeria
3661 The Vanderbilt Clinic
23rd Avenue South at Pierce
Nashville, Tennessee 37232-5732

Giovanni Lamura, Ph.D.
Dipartimento Ricerche Gerontologiche e Geriatriche
Università degli Studi di Ancona–INRCA
Via S. Margherita 5
Ancona, 60124
Italy

Keith D. Lillemoe, M.D.
Professor of Surgery
Johns Hopkins University School of Medicine
600 North Wolfe Street
Blalock 603
Baltimore, Maryland 21287-4603

John B. Lynch, M.D.
Professor of Plastic Surgery
Vanderbilt University School of Medicine
2100 Pierce Avenue
230 Medical Center South
Nashville, Tennessee 37232-3631

Richard A. Margolin, M.D.
Director, Geriatric Psychiatry
Vanderbilt Medical Center
2200 VAV
1500 21st Avenue, South
Nashville, Tennessee 37232-8646

James B.D. Mark, M.D.
Professor of Cardiothoracic Surgery, Emeritus
Stanford University School of Medicine
CVRB 207
Stanford, California 94305

Bess Adkins Marshall, M.D.
Assistant Professor of Pediatrics
Division of Endocrinology and Metabolism
St. Louis Children's Hospital
Washington University School of Medicine
One Children's Place
St. Louis, Missouri 63110

Kenneth L. Mattox, M.D.
Professor of Surgery
Baylor College of Medicine
One Baylor Plaza
Houston, Texas 77030

Wanda G. McKnight, A.R.T.
President
Seminars, Training, & Association Resources, Inc.
200 Burgundy Hill Road
Nashville, Tennessee 37211

William F. Meacham, M.D.
Professor of Neurologic Surgery, Emeritus
Vanderbilt University School of Medicine
21st Avenue South
Nashville, Tennessee 37232

Massimo Mengani
Researcher
Dipartimento Ricerche Gerontologiche e Geriatriche
Università degli Studi di Ancona–INRCA
Via S. Margherita 5
Ancona, 60124
Italy

Walter H. Merrill, M.D.
Professor of Surgery
Department of Cardiac and Thoracic Surgery
Vanderbilt University School of Medicine
2986 The Vanderbilt Clinic
1301 22nd Avenue South
Nashville, Tennessee 37232

James L. Netterville, M.D.
Associate Professor and Director, Head and Neck Oncologic Surgery
Department of Otolaryngology
Vanderbilt University School of Medicine
S-2100 Medical Center North
24th Avenue South
Nashville, Tennessee 37232-2559

Lloyd M. Nyhus, M.D.
Warren H. Cole Professor, Emeritus
Department of Surgery
University of Illinois College of Medicine
840 South Wood Street
Chicago, Illinois 60612-7322

Pat O'Donnell, M.D.
3187 Katherine Avenue
Fayetteville, Arkansas 72703

C. Keith Ozaki, M.D.
Fellow in Vascular Surgery
University of Michigan Medical School
1500 East Medical Center Drive, 2210 THCC
Ann Arbor, Michigan 48109-0329

Benjamin B. Peeler, M.D.
Chief Resident in General Surgery
Vanderbilt University School of Medicine
D-4309 Medical Center North
Nashville, Tennessee 37232

Richard M. Peters, M.D.
Professor of Surgery, Emeritus
University of California, San Diego, School of Medicine
550 Everett Court
Palo Alto, California 94301

Richard N. Pierson, III, M.D.
Assistant Professor of Surgery
Department of Cardiac and Thoracic Surgery
Vanderbilt University School of Medicine
2986 The Vanderbilt Clinic
Nashville, Tennessee 37232-5734

C. Wright Pinson, M.D., M.B.A.
Professor and Vice Chairman, Department of Surgery
Chief, Division of Hepatobiliary Surgery and Liver Transplantation
Vanderbilt University School of Medicine
1313 21st Avenue South
Nashville, Tennessee 37232-4753

Raymond Pollak, M.B., B.Ch.
Professor of Surgery
Chief, Division of Transplantation
University of Illinois College of Medicine
840 South Wood Street, Room 402
Chicago, Illinois 60612

James S. Powers, M.D.
Associate Professor of Medicine
Vanderbilt University School of Medicine
7155 Medical Center East
Nashville, Tennessee 37232

Mary C. Proctor, M.S.
Clinical Trialist
Department of Surgery
University of Michigan Medical Center
2101 Taubman Center, Box 0346
Ann Arbor, Michigan 48109-0346

Basil A. Pruitt, Jr., M.D.
Professor of Surgery
University of Texas Health Science Center at San Antonio
7703 Floyd Curl Drive
San Antonio, Texas 78284-7842

Riley Rees, M.D.
Professor of Surgery
Department of Plastic and Reconstructive Surgery
University of Michigan Medical Center
2130 Taubman Health Center
1500 East Medical Center Drive
Ann Arbor, Michigan 48109-0340

Robert E. Richie, M.D.
Professor of Surgery
Department of General Surgery, Renal Transplantation Division
Vanderbilt University School of Medicine
Nashville, Tennessee 37232

D. Michael Rose, M.D.
Chief Resident in General Surgery
Vanderbilt University Medical Center
21st Avenue and Garland
Nashville, Tennessee 37232

Ronald E. Rosenthal, M.D.
Associate Professor of Orthopaedic Surgery
Albert Einstein College of Medicine of Yeshiva University
Long Island Jewish Medical Center
270-05 76th Avenue
New Hyde Park, New York 11040

Joel J. Roslyn, M.D.
Alma Dea Morani Professor and Chairman
Department of Surgery
Allegheny University of the Health Sciences
Medical College of Pennsylvania and Hahnemann School of Medicine
3300 Henry Avenue
Philadelphia, Pennsylvania 19129

Vittorio Saba
Professor of Surgery
Clinica di Semeiotica e Metodologia Chirurgica
Università degli Studi di Ancona–INRCA
Via Della Montagnola 164
Ancona, 60100
Italy

John L. Sawyers, M.D.
Professor of Surgery, Emeritus
Department of General Surgery
Vanderbilt University School of Medicine
1001 Oxford House
Nashville, Tennessee 37232-4730

H. William Scott, Jr., M.D.
Professor of Surgery, Emeritus
Vanderbilt University Medical Center
206 Medical Center South
2100 Pierce Avenue
Nashville, Tennessee 37232-2730

R. Bruce Shack, M.D.
Professor and Chairman, Department of Plastic Surgery
Vanderbilt University School of Medicine
230 Medical Center South
2100 Pierce Avenue
Nashville, Tennessee 37232-3631

Bradley E. Smith, M.D.
Professor of Anesthesiology
Vanderbilt University School of Medicine
21st and Garland
Nashville, Tennessee 37232

Ian S. Storper, M.D.
Director of Neurotology and Neurotologic Skull Base Surgery
Department of Otolaryngology
Columbia University College of Physicians and Surgeons
161 Fort Washington Avenue, #511
New York, New York 10032

Geoffrey B. Thompson, M.D.
Associate Professor of Surgery
Mayo Clinic and Mayo Foundation
200 First Street, Southwest
Rochester, Minnesota 55905

Jon A. van Heerden, M.B., Ch.B., M.S.
Fred C. Andersen Professor of Surgery
Mayo Clinic and Mayo Foundation
200 First Street, Southwest
Rochester, Minnesota 55905

Horace E. Watson, M.D.
Assistant Professor of Orthopaedics
Vanderbilt University School of Medicine
1739 The Vanderbilt Clinic
Nashville, Tennessee 37232

Sarah J. White, B.S.N., M.S.N.
Gerontologic Nurse Practitioner
Department of Patient Care Services
Vanderbilt University Medical Center
AAA 1200 Medical Center North
Nashville, Tennessee 37232

Byron Young, M.D.
Chairman, Department of Surgery
University of Kentucky College of Medicine
800 Rose Street
Lexington, Kentucky 40536-0084

Robert W. Youngblood, M.D.
Professor of Surgery
East Carolina University School of Medicine
Moye Boulevard
Greenville, North Carolina 27858

Foreword

At the end of the twentieth century, we can look back on a succession of remarkable medical advances that have lengthened life expectancy in most parts of the world. The consequences of this achievement are predictable and the progressively enlarging aging population will exert increasing sociologic and economic pressures well into the next century. In healthcare, we are accustomed to thinking of this impact in terms of the management of illness and disability, which this book is designed to address. In this scenario, we would consider it a favorable outcome to return a patient to the home environment. As more seniors are recovering and aging at home, however, they are relying on their children and grandchildren for assistance instead of formal nursing care. The current estimate is that more than 14 million U.S. workers are providing such care to elderly family members at an estimated cost to business of more than $29 billion per year in lost productivity from absenteeism, job turnover, and workday interruptions. Therefore, the perspective of industry is changing to include not only the direct costs of elderly care but also the indirect costs that affect productivity. This increases the need for effective case management, referral services, and training courses as an important component of elderly healthcare management. Drs. R. Benton Adkins, Jr., and H. William Scott, Jr., have anticipated these issues in their assembly of experts from different countries to contribute to this second edition of *Surgical Care for the Elderly*. The result is a comprehensive and eminently readable collection of the views of experienced physicians and nurses.

Because aging is a universal human experience, the same physicians and nurses are not immune to its effects. The end of mandatory retirement and any restriction of activity based on age alone has introduced concern for the performances of the aging healthcare provider. In terms of assessing the effects of aging on cognitive performance, we remain in the infancy of a rapidly developing field. As information technology and computer imaging continue to demonstrate remarkable progress, we will undoubtedly become more dependent on these more objective determinants of both cognitive and physical performance. Although it is disconcerting to consider this ability to document the consequences of aging on ourselves, on the positive side, such quantitation will allow the testing of interventions that should forestall—even reverse—some of the changes. Until that happens, we are fortunate to have the experience of this remarkable collection of essayists to guide us in the practice of surgical care for the elderly.

Lazar J. Greenfield, M.D.

Preface to the First Edition

The intention of this book is to provide an overview of the challenges, risks, and rewards involved in providing surgical care to the elderly. Older persons constitute a rapidly growing segment of our society, and they are beginning to receive more and more of the medical resources of this country. They will, by necessity, require a larger share of the health care dollar, occupy more space in hospitals and other health facilities, and claim more professional attention for the solutions to their special needs.

Because of the growing realization that there is an increasing number of Americans who are age 65 and older, because of the cost involved in their health care, and because of the volatile ethical questions that arise in the course of their medical and surgical management, media and political interest in this subject has been intense. Simultaneous with the growth in numbers of the elderly segment of the population, increased government surveillance and cost-saving measures have been instituted in the Medicare program. The current effects of the trend of accountability are discussed briefly in this book and will likely be an issue of importance for many years to come. The circumstances now demand that health care providers be aware of these issues.

The subjects of these chapters were selected and designed to allow the reader to use this book as a reference source for his or her specific areas of interest. A few chapters address the general problems distinctive to the care of the elderly. Most chapters are devoted to specific organ systems with special emphasis on the particular problems of each of these systems where the surgical care of the elderly is involved. Other chapters deal with the issues of interest to allied health professionals. Bibliographies are selected to serve as a ready source of reference for nurses, dietitians, social service personnel, physical therapists, respiratory therapists, occupational therapists, home health care providers, nursing home personnel, psychology specialists, and those interested in gerontology in general.

Our intention is that this book would allow the practicing physician, house officer, medical student, and allied health professional easy access to advice and counsel for the specific problems that arise in the day-to-day care of the surgical diseases of the older patient. It is our hope that this text will serve as an especially valuable source of information and advice for the practitioners of all of the surgical specialties involved in the care of the elderly.

In virtually every chapter, examples are given of common disease processes that require special attention when they occur in the elderly. Whatever the disease process, the elderly patient's symptoms are often subtle. Complaints of the aged patient sometimes border on those of functional disorders and they may mimic many "normal" age-related problems. It is when these early signs and symptoms of a subtle nature are thoroughly investigated that many disease processes are detected at a time when they are curable and when life-threatening complications can be avoided. In an older patient, failure to investigate subtle symptoms, some of which will not lead to a firm diagnosis of organic disease, may result in the neglect of conditions until they have progressed to the point of an irretrievable pathologic state.

The theme of this book has developed into a surprisingly optimistic message for those involved with the surgical care of the elderly. This encouraging theme appears repeatedly where contributors report results of surgical treatment for many of the life-threatening and debilitating diseases in the elderly that are shown to be amazingly good. This is especially true of elective surgical treatment for most conditions.

It is our hope that this effort will stimulate further interest in research and study for the solution of those special problems that are encountered when the treatment of the elderly is undertaken. If the elderly patient needing surgical care can be treated in the appropriate manner and can be afforded the proper care, and if readers of this book can find information that might acquaint them with the many problems that are peculiar to the care of the elderly, and if those providing medical and supportive care for the elderly can find here a ready reference for many of the medical needs for these special individuals, our efforts will have been well rewarded.

Preface to the Second Edition

Since the publication of the first edition of *Surgical Care for the Elderly* in 1988, the number of elderly persons has increased globally, and with it our awareness of the unique worldwide health care problems this presents. In July 1990, we were invited by the renowned Italian surgeon Nino Massera of Milan to participate in a full-day session at the World Congress of Surgery dedicated to surgical problems of the elderly. During a subsequent two-day retreat and symposium in Ancona, Italy, surgeons from Europe, Asia, and North and South America learned in dramatic fashion how the surgical profession in different societies and governments is responding to the problems associated with the increasing number of elderly patients with surgical illnesses. Each country is handling this issue with slightly different approaches. In the second edition, chapters by surgeons from Italy and England point out how two European countries are working toward solutions to some of these problems. Clearly, all surgeons are challenged to provide the best care—from preoperative assessment to convalescence—regardless of the technological, economic, and political climates of the societies in which they practice. It is in this spirit of improvement through shared knowledge that these chapters on comparative experience and other chapters dedicated to patient selection, methods, and outcomes are included in the second edition.

Surgical care for the elderly must improve. If our best treatment methods are to keep pace with the increasing number of surgical candidates, they must become an integral part of our surgical training programs. In October 1996, we were invited by Dr. Walter Pores, the past chairman of the Association of Program Directors for General Surgery Residency Training, to participate in a symposium dedicated to expanding the geriatric component in surgical training programs throughout the United States. Dr. Ben Eisman of Colorado, Dr. Lloyd Nyhus of Chicago, Dr. Brad Aust of San Antonio, Dr. Pores, and I discussed the problems and some solutions associated with the growing interest in geriatric surgery. We recommended that, within the curriculum for surgical residents, special attention be focused on the various aspects of surgical care for the elderly patient. The completed version of this curriculum requirement was made available to program directors in July 1997.

It is our belief that more innovations and improvements of older concepts of caring for the elderly surgical patient will be facilitated by synthesizing the components of that care. It is the goal of each chapter of this second edition to contribute to that synthesis. Geriatric surgery is now a rapidly expanding field, and as such, many improvements are on the way. One has only to peruse the chapters on anesthesia, nutrition, and nursing care to realize that vast changes in concepts and techniques have recently evolved and will increase the speed at which other innovations occur.

Despite the magnitude of the effort required to furnish the care for what seems to be an endless supply of elderly surgical candidates in the future, most contributors to the second edition are optimistic. Spurred on by the surprisingly good results attained with most recent elderly patients, older individuals are now successfully undergoing procedures for which they would not have been considered only a few years ago. It has become commonplace to hear that age alone is no longer a contraindication for aortic valve replacement, renal transplant, coronary artery bypass, and total hip replacement. The list of procedures available to the elderly is long and is growing for each surgical specialty.

It remains our hope that this optimism is not misplaced and that this attitude is deserved. If further interest in research and study of the elderly surgical patient is stimulated in the reader of this edition, our efforts will be handsomely rewarded.

R. Benton Adkins, Jr., M.D.

Acknowledgments

We wish to express our sincere gratitude to each contributor and his or her assistants for making this second edition a comprehensive review. We are also indebted to Nancy Chorpenning, formerly of Little, Brown and Company, for her persistence in securing our copyright for this book and to Lisa McAllister and Rhoda Dunn of Lippincott–Raven for so ably bringing to completion a project they inherited. Finally, we thank Joel Vaughn, our coordinating editor, for staying in touch with the contributors, keeping track of their submissions, and maintaining close contact with our publisher.

SECTION I

Background Information

Surgical Care for the Elderly, 2nd ed., edited by
R. Benton Adkins, Jr., and H. William Scott, Jr.
Lippincott–Raven Publishers, Philadelphia © 1998.

CHAPTER 1

History and Philosophy

R. Benton Adkins, Jr., and Wanda G. McKnight

The "graying" of America has become an issue of concern to citizens and policy makers in the United States. Life expectancy in this country has increased from 47.3 years at the turn of the century to 75.7 years in 1991 [1]. Because of this phenomenon, there has been an increasing acceptance among internists and general practitioners of the concept of elective surgical care in the elderly. Biliary tract disease, peptic ulcer disease, hernia, and vascular diseases are excellent examples of disorders for which surgical consultations are now being requested earlier in the disease process [2]. Correctable conditions that require relatively major surgical procedures are being successfully managed in older and older people. When performed under well-controlled elective conditions, the results are very good [3,4]. Even in urgent and emergency settings, the situation is not always hopeless. In this book, we have undertaken the task of documenting the current status of and recommendations for surgical treatment of the elderly.

The surgical care of older persons is not a new concept for the medical profession. Physicians have always devoted what may appear to be a disproportionate share of their time to the care of the elderly. The number of elderly persons in our society is steadily increasing, to the point that many medical doctors now choose to devote their entire practice to the care of older patients. It has been estimated that 40% to 50% of the time of most nonpediatric physicians and more than 30% of all health care dollars are currently devoted to the diagnosis, treatment, and long-term care of older persons [5]. Approximately 130.5 million office visits were made to nonfederal office-based physicians in the United States from 1985 to 1986 by persons ≥65 years of age. From 1980 to 1985, this group increased the number of office visits by 60.6 million [1]. The population of elderly persons is growing steadily in numbers and in age level, and their medical needs are gradually changing. The special problem of the surgical care for these older, more active, generally healthy members of American society is now of even greater interest to most political, business, industrial, medical, and social groups than at the time of the first edition of *Surgical Care for the Elderly* [6].

The medical advances of the nineteenth century have enabled people in our society to live and remain healthy longer. The discovery of anesthesia, a better understanding of the relationship between microorganisms and disease, the concept of antisepsis, the inadvertent discovery of antimicrobial agents, and a better understanding of the physiologic basis of many metabolic diseases have led to more effective life-saving and life-prolonging medical care [7]. The twentieth century has brought with it a refinement and elaboration of the discoveries of the previous 100 years.

In recent years, epidemics have been rare. The only current epidemic of any magnitude is the acquired immunodeficiency syndrome. Thus far, it has had little impact on the aging population. Infections, which were lethal only a few years ago, are now either nonexistent or readily treated by the use of the appropriate antibiotic. Surgical techniques are continually refined, and the more recent use of surgical mechanical devices, grafts, and organ transplantation has allowed persons who, just a few years ago, would have died of their diseases to return to healthy, productive lives. The electron microscope, invented in the late 1930s, has led to medical advances in the fields of oncology and virology. The culture and study of viruses resulted in control of poliomyelitis and other viral diseases. Public health and sanitation have continued to improve [7]. Appendicitis was first recognized as a surgical entity in the late 1890s. Consider that a person born in 1900 has seen during his or her adult years the discovery of major red blood cell types, the discovery of penicillin, the advances of roentgenography, the discovery of insulin, internal fixation of fractures, the evolution of kidney dialysis and organ transplantation, and major advances in cardiovascular procedures. Advances in the care of trauma and cancer victims in the last 50 years have resulted both in the saving and prolonging of many additional lives. The rapidly developing fields of computerized body scanning, immunologic genotyping, and cancer chemotherapy are having an incalculable influence on longevity. The benefactors of these scientific and medical phenomena are now adding to the population pool of elderly Americans at the most dramatic rate in the

TABLE 1-1. *Life expectancy*

Age	Years expected
65	16.6
70	13.4
75	10.6
80	8.4
85	6.7[a]
90	4.4
95	3.3
100	2.7
105	2.4
110	2.2[b]

[a] Modified from Expectation of Life at Single Years of Age, by Race and Sex, United States, 1979, Vital Statistics of the United States. Washington, DC: U.S. Department of Health and Human Services, Public Health Service, National Care for Health Statistics, 1979.

[b] Modified from U.S. Life Tables: 1969–1971. Washington, DC: Department of Health, Education and Welfare Publication No. HRA 75-1150, Public Health Service, National Center for Health Statistics, 1975.

history of our country. As the reader of other chapters in this book will learn, this is a worldwide phenomenon [8].

IMPACTS OF AGING AND DEMOGRAPHIC TRENDS

Population

We are now living in what has been called "the century of old age" [5]. The increase in average life expectancy realized in this century almost equals the total increase of the previous 5,000 years. Even at age 100, one is expected to live almost 3 more years (Table 1-1). It has been estimated that by the year 2030 there will be 55 million people in the United States who are ≥65 years of age as compared with only 9 million in 1940 [5]. From 1960 to 1986, the death rate for those 65 years and older decreased by 16.3% [1]. Persons born in the 1980s can expect to see the proportion of elderly persons *double* in their lifetimes. Seven of 10 newborns today can expect to reach age 65 [5]. Over the course of a decade, 60% of the older population is replaced by other individuals who become 65 years of age and older [5]. This rapid turnover of membership in the club of the elderly may become less rapid as our medical successes complicate the equation. Some authors have subdivided the population of older persons into two groups: young-old (55 to 75 years) and old-old (>75 years). Surprisingly, the >75-year group is now growing proportionally faster than the elderly population as a whole. It is estimated that by the year 2040, there will be 8 million persons over age 85 (14.5% of all elderly persons) [5]. The percentage of older persons will continue to be greater in the white population than it is among blacks.

Socioeconomic Trends

Increased incidence and prevalence of disease and disability in older persons obviously result in an increased need for medical care. The current financial impact of health care for increasing numbers of older persons is substantial, and the future impact can be anticipated based on current statistics. Even now, 30% of all health care costs are associated with persons over 65 years of age. In 1987, health care spending for the older populations totaled $162 billion. In 1986, there were 29 million enrollees in the Medicare program. Most of these (two-thirds) have private insurance in addition to Medicare [1]. Forty percent of our Medicaid dollars are now being spent for nursing home care. There are some 20,000 long-term care facilities in this country housing approximately 1.4 million older Americans, or only 5% of our elderly population, at any given time. However, in the group of persons 85 years of age and older, a greater percentage (22%) are living in nursing homes [5]. The demands for the medical community to respond more effectively and efficiently to older patients' medical needs will increase dramatically in the next few years. Currently, this group costs hospitals more, and Medicare has made the decision to eliminate older age (≥70 years) as a Diagnosis Related Group criterion for classifying an illness for prospective payment [9].

As greater demands are placed on the medical community, there is a simultaneous demand to lower the cost of health care. The federally supported and private insurers have initiated programs designed to encourage physicians and hospitals to hospitalize fewer patients for shorter periods and use the absolute minimum of resources for each patient. These efforts could potentially lower the quality of care for all patients, especially for the most costly—the elderly. The inclusion of patient age in prospective payment formulas may make hospital reimbursement for the elderly more equitable and more attractive to hospitals [10]. Immediate, expedient treatment is obviously less costly than long-term treatment for a condition that could be corrected. This issue receives more attention in later chapters.

Although they use a substantial percentage of health care dollars, many elderly citizens are not financially secure. However, the economic disadvantage that has generally been associated with the elderly population has lessened in recent years. In 1959, 35.2% of elderly persons lived below the poverty level; in 1974 the percentage had decreased to only 14.6% [5]. Of those elderly persons living alone, however, 27% were poor in 1977. Only 8% of those living with their own families were classified as poor [5]. This trend continues today as social programs and retirement benefits have improved.

Social and Cultural Trends

In addition to the ever increasing numbers of older Americans, the characteristics of the population of older people are constantly changing as well. As new individuals enter the older age group each year, they bring with them slightly different values, ideals, expectations, and life experiences. They are becoming a group of well-informed, "modern" individuals.

In the past, there was a considerable educational disadvantage among the elderly. Today, slightly more than 40% of our elderly have only an elementary school education. This percentage will decrease to 20% in the next few years [5]. Before many years, a substantial percentage will be college graduates.

Other social and cultural aspects of aging have also changed dramatically in the last century. In eighteenth-century America, older citizens were highly respected and venerated. In that mostly agrarian culture, they controlled most of the wealth and land, served as role models, and were the keepers of traditions and history within the society. Most historians suggest that the bias began to shift toward the young in the mid-nineteenth century with gradually increasing urbanization and industrialization. Many young adults broke the bonds of clan and family dependence and became self-reliant in the industrial arena. This bias toward the young is consistent with the findings of many cross-cultural researchers who maintain that the status of elderly persons varies directly with the control that they have over the valued resources of the family [11]. The mid-twentieth century brought with it forced retirement, a degree of family abandonment, increased poverty among the elderly, and a correspondingly diminished social status of some of the aged members of society.

Nevertheless, the financial and social status of most older persons has significantly improved since World War II, due in part to government social programs, which resulted from widespread revival of sensitivity to the plight of the elderly. Evidence of increased sensitivity to the needs of the elderly can be found in the large number of social programs now in existence. Many of the first gerontologic researchers had assumed that the public's view of the elderly was basically negative, but the opposite was actually found to be true [11]. In fact, elderly persons in this country are not generally the victims of social prejudice. Due in part to widespread news media coverage, Americans are taught to overestimate the dismal plight of the elderly today. We tend to have an inflated perception of the percentage of older persons living in institutions or below the poverty line. There is no statistical evidence to support the notion that a large percentage of older persons are neglected by their children or are left alone to die in nursing homes. Conversely, 81% of older Americans have caring, loving, living children, and in one study, more than 80% of the older persons surveyed had seen one of their children in the preceding week [11]. In a similar study, 55% of those surveyed had seen at least one of their children within the past 24 hours [11]. This is not to belittle or underestimate the serious disadvantage that a few elderly people do experience both financially and socially when little or no family support is available.

We can realistically expect that the social status of America's elderly will continue to improve in the coming years. Evidence of our increased awareness of the importance of the elderly is growing in this country. For instance, the highly influential advertising agencies now recognize the >50 group as a large and desirable segment of consumers [12]. This is a radical change from the youth-oriented attitude of advertising in the recent past. In movies and television shows, more and more older Americans are being featured in positive, attractive roles. The list of much older Americans in politics, business, and the entertainment industry continues to grow and, in fact, has become lengthy and impressive. These Americans are setting the pace for the average older American and are helping to change the attitudes of all Americans toward older people. The elderly are also in a position to know what is available medically, will expect to benefit from it, and will continue to demand consideration for more and more aggressive medical and surgical treatments.

Health Status and Medical Care

The general public tends to underestimate the good health status of most older Americans. Although only approximately one-half of America's elderly are limited at all in their daily living activities, it is true that over 80% of older persons report having one or more chronic medical conditions [13]. The incidence of acute disease in the elderly is relatively low; the treatment of chronic illness therefore constitutes the major health care problem and cost for older Americans. Despite this high incidence of a variety of chronic medical conditions, most older persons do not actually consider themselves to be seriously handicapped by their age or these conditions. When questioned, the overwhelming majority of older persons rate their health as "good" or "excellent" and, when asked to compare their health status with that of others in their own age group, rate it as better [13].

The major causes of death in persons 65 years of age and older are heart disease, malignant tumors, and cerebrovascular disease. As mentioned previously, this older group of our population now accounts for almost one-third of the nation's health care expenditures, generally requires more frequent hospital visits and more physician time, and consumes about one-fourth of all legal drugs purchased in the United States [13].

In spite of the few well-publicized and dramatic incidences of fraud and abuse, there are actually few inadequacies in the vast health care system in this country. It is true that the few service gaps that do exist generally tend to affect older patients, especially those with lower incomes, more than younger patients. Delivery systems for home health care, long-term care, rehabilitation, and preventive services are not as efficient, well defined, or as intensely monitored as are other more traditional health care delivery systems. Attention to these areas is increasing at the time of this writing and is addressed in subsequent chapters. The special health needs of the elderly are becoming a top priority for health care planners.

In addition to improving the health care system for all of those who need medical care in this country, attention is now being focused on promoting healthy life-styles. This will undoubtedly have a positive effect on the health status of the future elderly and also on longevity itself. Decreased pollution exposure, better exercise habits, improved nutrition, reduction of smoking, and modification of drinking habits will significantly affect the health status of all age groups. The beneficial effect of these efforts is already being reflected in the numbers of healthy, well-educated Americans reaching more advanced age groups each year. They will expect and demand the same health care offered to younger age groups.

IMPACT OF CHRONIC DISEASE IN THE AGED

Chronic disease is the major health factor among the elderly. In the population group aged 45 to 64, approximately 72% have one or more chronic illnesses. The percentage increases to 86% for persons 65 years of age and older. Additionally, the incidence of *multiple* chronic conditions also increases. The most common of these are reported to be arthritis (38%), hearing impairments (29%), vision impairments (20%), hypertension (20%), and heart conditions (29%) [13]. The incidence of arthritis and hypertension is higher among women, but they demonstrate a lower incidence of hearing impairments. Heart conditions occur with similar frequency in men and women. All chronic conditions except for peptic ulcer disease are found to occur more frequently among those elderly who are classified as "poor" [13].

The impact of chronic disease on the daily living activities of the elderly is statistically substantial in spite of the fact that most individuals in this age group do not consider themselves to be seriously handicapped by their conditions. Most older persons do not experience serious activity limitations, but almost half of all elderly persons are limited to some degree in carrying out the activities of daily living. The conditions that are most limiting are heart conditions (52%), diabetes (34%), asthma (27%), and arthritis (23%) [13].

In terms of general mobility, most elderly persons (approximately 82%) are not seriously restricted. Women are more likely to have some degree of mobility limitation than men. The major causes of mobility limitation are arthritis, rheumatism, lower-extremity disorders, heart conditions, and cerebrovascular disease. It is interesting to note that if the major cardiovascular and renal diseases (i.e., heart disease, stroke, hypertension, and so forth) were eliminated, an extra 11.4 years would be added to life expectancy after age 65. These are the illnesses that are and should be most heavily researched at this time [13]. As mentioned previously, most of the health care costs for the elderly are attributed to these chronic conditions. They also consume the largest amount of time and support given by family members and health care providers to elderly patients. Surprisingly, the chronic illnesses do not affect results of surgical care of older patients to the degree that one might expect.

IMPACT OF DELAYED TREATMENT IN THE ELDERLY

In spite of the prevalence of chronic disease among the elderly, America's elderly are amazingly resilient. Several investigators have found little correlation between the presence of chronic disease and operative mortality. In many studies, urgent and emergency operations rather than chronic disease have proved to be the greatest risk factor in operative mortality of elderly patients who require surgical treatment [3,4,14–16]. Emergency procedures have been shown to increase the risk of operative mortality twofold to threefold [17–19]. The operative mortality in the elderly varies from a low of 0.85% [14] for elective procedures to a high of 45% [4] for emergency operations. When surgical disease states are recognized and corrected in a timely manner under careful, controlled, elective conditions, older patients have been found to tolerate even the most major surgical procedures and recover remarkably well. However, the elderly patient's tolerance for delay, technical mistakes, or errors in judgment is lower than that in younger patients. Accurate preoperative appraisal of the elderly patient and *early*, careful attention to the surgical needs of the patient are essential in producing a good outcome. The use of the American Society of Anesthesiologists' Physical Status Scale with the addition of invasive evaluation in very high-risk patients has been suggested [15]. This type of aggressive evaluation allows us to choose more intelligently the proper surgical candidates from all age groups.

As more of the care of elderly patients is occurring in the emergency departments of many hospitals, this issue has come into focus. There is some evidence and much concern that the problem may be reaching a crisis situation in some emergency departments [6]. Because we and others have shown that the surgical management of diseases is safer if handled on an elective basis and less safe when performed in an emergency situation, it is critical that emergency departments are equipped and trained for these special patients.

As patients are living longer, most physicians are seeing that when surgical problems are left unattended, an emergency situation is likely to arise. In an earlier report of 75 patients aged 90 years or more who had 85 major surgical procedures, we found strong evidence to support the notion that elective operations are tolerated well in the elderly [4]. In 42 elective cases, postoperative mortality was only 2.3% compared with 45% in the group of patients whose situations required emergency procedures (Fig. 1-1). Even under urgent and emergency conditions, the results were not overwhelmingly disastrous in these very old patients.

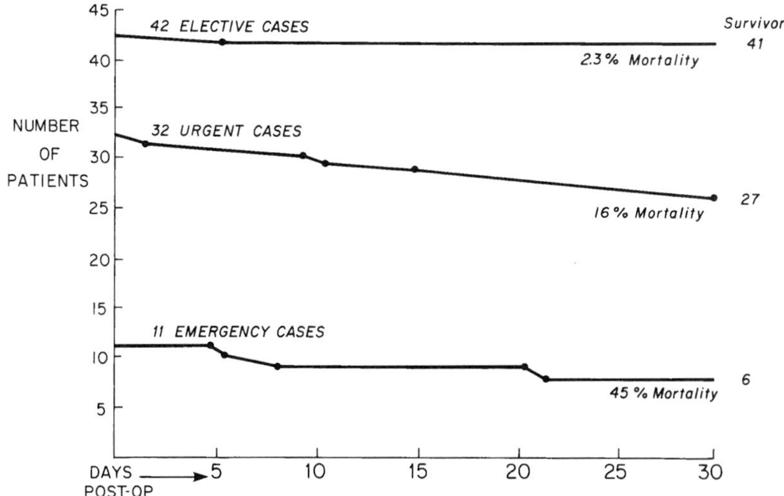

FIG. 1-1. Postoperative deaths related to original exigency of operative procedure. Elective operations were those for which indications allowed ample time for preparation of the patient. Urgent operations were done after short planning and preparation time for potentially life-threatening conditions. Emergency procedures were those done for progressive, life-threatening conditions. (Reprinted with permission from Adkins RB, Scott HW. Surgical procedures in patients aged 90 years and older. South Med J 1984;77:1357–1364.)

SPECIAL SURGICAL CONSIDERATIONS FOR THE ELDERLY

The special needs and problems of elderly patients should receive personalized attention before any significant operation is considered. This, of course, is not always possible in some urgent and in most true emergency situations. In cases of planned, elective procedures, however, the surgeon would do well to consider all of the special needs of his or her elderly patient (see Chapters 4 and 5).

The patient's home or extended care environment should also be evaluated. Will the patient be returning to a safe atmosphere for recovery after the operation? If it seems unlikely that the patient will be able to return home, efforts must be initiated early to find placement in an extended care facility where rehabilitation, return to independence, and return to a home environment can be pursued. A close relationship with the patient's family and the social services department of the hospital can expedite these procedures. The economic impact of the operative procedure and recovery period on the patient, family, community, and public resources that will be required should be considered, but these factors should not outweigh the purely medical and surgical needs of the patient in the decision-making process. Elderly patients themselves may be able to assist in these deliberations, and their wishes must always be considered.

Another special concern that must be remembered in the surgical care of the elderly is the patient's feelings about hospitals and attitude toward doctors in general. Consider that many of an elderly person's peers have died in hospitals and that he or she may fear the same fate. Although most older people continue to have a great reverence for doctors in general, their previous experience with hospitals may have been before many of the new technological advances were available. Moreover, because older persons have probably seen many of their counterparts become disabled and helpless over the years, their fear of disability and dependence is usually greater than in the young. Other authors have described this situation [18].

An honest appraisal of the elderly patient's prognosis and expectations should be communicated to him or her and the family. The surgeon and the referring doctor must do this in a straightforward manner. The fact that patients are older is not necessarily an indication that they cannot understand their disorders. They can usually make their own intelligent decisions about their future. As in dealing with any surgical patient, the necessary emotional support should be provided, using all available and necessary resources. Geriatric nurses are specially trained to meet the needs of older patients (see Chapter 11).

More than any other group of physicians, American doctors must be aware of the special cultural characteristics of our many ethnic groups. Such characteristics as those seen in some ethnic groups with a strong matriarchal structure and in many Eastern cultures where there is an adoration of the parents must be recognized. The fatalistic approach of some religious groups, and the stoicism of others (such as Native Americans), become important when doctors and families plan operative, postoperative, and rehabilitative care for elderly patients.

Problems that are known to be more common in the postoperative period for the older patient should be anticipated and avoided by appropriate measures taken in the preoperative and perioperative periods. Pulmonary function, renal function, and nutritional status should be carefully evaluated preoperatively, and corrective steps should be taken whenever possible in an attempt to avoid postoperative complications. The widespread use of corticosteroids and antihypertensive agents in the elderly should be remembered and documented. Their effect should be recognized and their continued use monitored. If possible, corticosteroids should be tapered and discontinued during the preoperative period [18]. Special attention to these and other specific medical conditions are addressed in subsequent chapters.

WHEN ENOUGH IS ENOUGH

In the course of events associated with any terminal disease or condition, there arrives a time, regardless of the patient's age, when the hope of reasonable success is unlikely. To press forward with heroic measures beyond this point becomes an exercise in prolonging death rather than prolonging life. Before this point is reached, we, like Wagner [20] and others, suggest that some understanding of the patient's wishes be discussed. This must always be considered when the propriety of withholding or offering cardiopulmonary resuscitation in the elderly is at issue. As Levinson [21] has so eloquently stated, there comes a time when "death is the best life has to offer." Obviously, advanced age alone must not be equated arbitrarily with universally hopeless situations [22,23]. It is our office to distinguish that which is appropriate, advise that which should be done, and administer the correct decision in these circumstances.

TROUBLING TRENDS

Since there has been a progressive increase in the numbers of elderly individuals living for longer periods of time and needing more medical, surgical, and long-term care, the cost of keeping the elderly alive and healthy has become an issue of great social importance. The Health Care Financing Administration (HCFA) has placed a priority on cutting Medicare costs. In 1982, the Tax Equity Fiscal Responsibility Act (TEFRA—PL 97.248) was passed, which established a prospective payment system and appointed professional review organizations (PROs) to reduce the federal expenditures in the Medicare program.

The Inspector General of the HCFA once vowed to seek out the "criminal element" in the medical profession perceived as the culprit in increasing costs [24]. PROs were given specific guidelines regarding the amount of money to recover each year by denying hospital payment for medical care. Immediate review of cases and eventually sanctions against physicians and hospitals for perceived inappropriate care were determined based on a generic screening process. These so-called quality screens included situations that often occur in the course of treatment through the fault of no one, as the result of uncontrollable circumstances. These generic screens are outlined in Table 1-2. Although they are modified frequently, the authors believe that the screens warrant mention because of the impact the screening process may have on surgical care. The screens are generally effective retroactively.

TABLE 1-2. *Generic quality screens*

1. Admission following inadequate outpatient management and/or complication of outpatient procedure.
2. Unplanned transfer from general care unit to special care unit (intensive care unit/critical care unit).
3. Inappropriate transfer to another acute care facility.
4. Unapproved transfer to another acute care facility.
5. Blood administration incident/error (*not* life-threatening complications).
6. Operation for perforation, laceration, tear, or injury of an organ incurred during an invasive procedure.
7. Unnecessary invasive procedure.
8. Inappropriate invasive procedure.
9. Cancellation of or repeat diagnostic procedure because of improper preparation of patient, technician error, or equipment failure.
10. Myocardial infarction during or within 48 hours of a surgical procedure on this admission.
11. Neurologic deficit or footdrop present at discharge which was not present upon admission.
12. Cardiac or respiratory arrest (not resulting in death).
13. Adverse reaction and/or complication resulting from respiratory therapy.
14. Delay in administration of services.
15. Repeated laboratory test due to error in obtaining, handling, or storage of laboratory samples.
16. History and physical examination, discharge summary, operative reports, etc. not dictated on a timely basis as defined.
17. No chest x-ray to validate primary diagnosis of pneumonia.
18. No smear and culture of sputum and/or bronchial secretions to validate primary diagnosis of pneumonia.
19. No culture and sensitivity and/or appropriate bacterial investigation prior to initiating antibiotic for pneumonia.
20. Pathology report does not match preoperative diagnosis.
21. Unexpected specimen received by pathology department.
22. Patient ordered NPO, but received diet despite the order.
23. Diet not given to the patient as ordered.
24. Reaction to x-ray dye during cardiac catheterization or radiologic procedures (*not* life-threatening complications).
25. Attempted or unsuccessful radiologic or angiographic procedure.
26. Attempted or unsuccessful cardiac catheterization.
27. Attempted or unsuccessful percutaneous transluminal coronary angioplasty procedure.
28. Hematoma as a result of an invasive procedure (*no* major treatment necessary).
29. Surgical backup not documented prior to percutaneous transluminal coronary angioplasty procedure.
30. Barium administered without physician's orders.
31. Other complications *or* quality of care concerns not classifiable in any of the previously mentioned elements.

Source: With permission from Chumbly P. Mid-South Foundation for Medical Care, Inc., Memphis, TN.

When the PRO determines that a provider or practitioner has violated Medicare guidelines, notice is given to the affected party. An opportunity for informal discussion and formal appeal follows. The final PRO determination is reported to the Office of the Inspector General, who then reviews the PRO recommendation. If the final determination is that a violation of guidelines did occur, notice of such determination is given to the practitioner or provider, the local and regional PROs, state licensing bodies, state Medicaid agencies, hospitals, skilled nursing facilities and health maintenance organizations where the practitioner has privileges, medical societies and other professional organizations, fiscal intermediaries, and local newspapers. The effect of the sanction is financial assessment or invalidation of

Medicare assignments. The affected practitioner or provider has the right to judicial review *after* the sanction has been imposed and publicized.

The PROs have been charged with reducing the number of hospital admissions and thereby saving federal dollars spent through the Medicare program. In actuality, the great reduction has been in *reimbursed* hospitalizations; most physicians and hospitals have continued to admit and treat the elderly sick as indicated, regardless of the patient's financial status or the threat of sanction.

It seems inevitable that most of the physician contributors to this text, because of their love for and interest in the medical and surgical care of elderly citizens in this country, will have their names listed among those against whom sanctions have been levied by the HCFA. It is ironic that those of us who have the strongest interest in the elderly and indeed who love them most are liable to be excluded from participating in their care by these punitive and arbitrary rules. We have, it seems, returned to the code of Hammurabi [25], wherein failure to cure, a perception of inefficient care, or the unavoidable trap of a catch-22 situation imposed by the sanctioning process will result in the "cutting off" of the hand that cares for the aged. Examples that horrify and frustrate the medical profession are already abundant. In a few instances, the medical care in rural communities has been seriously hampered by sanctions against all of the few available providers and practitioners in that area [26].

The recent report of the large settlement of an audit of the faculty of the University of Pennsylvania for $30 million for "inadequate documentation" of Medicare billings is alarming. June Gibbs Brown, Inspector General of Health and Human Services, congratulated the U.S. Attorney's office for their work and promised to pursue investigation of other institutions [27]. This appears to be a new focus of the HCFA in its effort to trim the cost of care for the elderly.

PROSPECTS FOR THE FUTURE

The emergence of geriatric medicine as a viable treatment and research specialty is evidence of the growing concern of the profession for the medical care of the elderly in our country. The premise of geriatric medicine is that aging itself is a clinical phenomenon worthy of some clinicians' full attention. This is not to say that only gerontologists are qualified to care for older patients. As noted previously, America's physicians have always spent a large percentage of their time caring for the elderly. As is appropriate with all special patient populations, the medical community must commit itself to providing the best possible care for and meeting the health needs of the older patient. We must work toward developing improved attitudes, efficient and effective service organizations, sufficient monetary funds, and an accurate appreciation of the importance of the elderly person's role in our society and within our professions. It is obvious to all of us that each year a larger percentage of our population is entering the older decades of life. It behooves the medical profession, which is at least partially responsible for creating this situation, to prepare for the challenge of dealing with the medical and surgical care of more and more of these not-so-fragile survivors of the game of life. The issues uppermost in the minds of all of those involved are the economic and ethical solutions that must be addressed.

REFERENCES

1. Vital and Health Statistics. Health Data of Older Americans: United States, 1992. Hyattsville, MD: U.S. Department of Health and Human Services, January 1993.
2. Glenn F. Surgical Principles for the Aged Patient. In Reichel W (ed), Clinical Aspects of Aging. Baltimore: Williams & Wilkins, 1983; 453–468.
3. Harbrecht PH, Garrison RN, Fry DE. Surgery in elderly patients. South Med J 1981;74:594–598.
4. Adkins RB, Scott HW. Surgical procedures in patients aged 90 years and older. South Med J 1984;77:1357–1364.
5. Watts D, McCally M. Demographic Perspectives. In Cassel DK, Walsh JR (eds), Geriatric Medicine. New York: Springer, 1984;3–15.
6. Adkins RB, Scott HW (eds). Surgical Care for the Elderly (1st ed). Baltimore: Williams & Wilkins, 1988;12.
7. Lyons AS, Petrucelli RJ. Medicine, An Illustrated History. New York: Abrams, 1978.
8. Steele K, Maggie S. Ageing as a global issue. Age Ageing 1993;22: 237–239.
9. Rosenthal GE, Landefeld CS. Do older Medicare patients cost hospitals more? Arch Intern Med 1993;153:89–96.
10. Sanders AB. Care of the elderly in emergency departments: conclusions and recommendations. Ann Emerg Med 1992;21:830–834.
11. Schulz R, Manson S. Social Perspectives. In Cassel DK, Walsh JR (eds), Geriatric Medicine. New York: Springer, 1984;16–27.
12. Hoyt MF. The new prime time. USA Weekend December 13–15, 1985;4–5.
13. Fact Book on Aging. Washington, DC: National Council on the Aging, 1978.
14. Greenburg AG, Saik RP, Farris JM, Peskin GW. Operative mortality in general surgery. Am J Surg 1982;144:22–28.
15. Linn BS, Linn MW, Wallen N. Evaluation of results of surgical procedures in the elderly. Ann Surg 1982;195:90–96.
16. Kohn P, Zekert F, Vormittag E, Grabner H. Risks of operation in patients over 80. Geriatrics 1973;28:100–105.
17. Greenburg AG, Saik RP, Coyle JJ, Peskin GW. Mortality and gastrointestinal surgery in the aged: elective vs emergency procedures. Arch Surg 1981;116:788–791.
18. Robins RE, Budden MK. Major abdominal surgery in patients over 70 years of age. Results during 1962 to 1966 compared with those during 1950 to 1959. Can J Surg 1972;15:1–6.
19. Mohr DN. Estimation of surgical risk in the elderly, a correlative review. J Am Geriatr Soc 1983;31:99–102.
20. Wagner A. Cardiopulmonary resuscitation in the aged. N Engl J Med 1984;310:1129–1130.
21. Levinson AJR. Termination of life support systems in the elderly: ethical issues. J Geriatr Psych 1981;14:71–85.
22. DeBard ML. Cardiopulmonary resuscitation: analysis of six years' experience and review of the literature. Ann Emerg Med 1981;10:408–416.
23. Gulati RS, Bhan GL, Horan MA. Cardiopulmonary resuscitation of old people. Lancet 1983;2:267–269.
24. Hostetler D. AHA meeting focuses on federal budget: "the only game in town." J Am Med Rec Assoc 1987;58(3):42–44.
25. Lyons AS, Petrucelli RJ. Medicine, An Illustrated History. New York: Abrams, 1978;59–69.
26. Scheier RL. Rural areas face MD shortages, hospital closures. Am Med News 1987;53(25):15.
27. Uhlman M, Ditzen LS, FitzGerald S. U.S. assesses Penn doctors $30 million. Philadelphia Inquirer December 13, 1995;A1.

Surgical Care for the Elderly, 2nd ed., edited by
R. Benton Adkins, Jr., and H. William Scott, Jr.
Lippincott–Raven Publishers, Philadelphia © 1998.

CHAPTER 2

Anatomic and Physiologic Aspects of Aging

R. Benton Adkins, Jr., and Bess Adkins Marshall

All organ systems are affected by the aging process. Some tissues and organ systems respond to the wear and tear of daily existence at a different rate from that of others. The most important effects of aging, which alter the physician's approach to aggressive medical and surgical care, are those that materially diminish the quality of life or that by their changes would exert undue risk if surgical procedures were needed. Some of these changes are irreversible by any medical or surgical intervention. It is the purpose of this chapter to address those aspects of aging within each organ system that significantly alter the physician's approach to the care of the elderly and that alter the methods of care that may be necessary for success in their management.

The cause of aging has been attributed to an incredible variety of factors, including the existence of a finite and immutable maximum number of doublings for a given cell population (the Hayflick principle) [1], cumulative cellular damage from free radicals and radiations [2], errors in protein synthesis [3], alterations in the immune system [4], deleterious effects of endogenous steroid hormones [5], and the cross-linkage theory [6].

The Hayflick principle deserves special consideration because it is supported by solid laboratory observations. According to this principle, aging is based on a genetic clock, and species-specific numbers of cell doublings can occur before all the cells from that parent organism die and will not divide further [7]. If true, the known life span, like that of all species, is genetically fixed at a finite maximum length. For humans, senescence is reached after approximately 50 population doublings [8].

Factors that affect the genetic influence on aging include alterations in DNA synthesis during an individual's life. Telomeres, the genetic elements at the end of linear chromosomes, are necessary components of proper chromosome structure and affect chromosomal functions. These terminal fragments of DNA are not all fully replicated during DNA synthesis. An RNA primer in telomerase uses its own DNA sequence as a template as it extends the chromosome end to replenish the lost telomeres during replication [9]. Because telomeres perform such an important role in chromosome structure and its stability, the genetic fate of a cell and its function may depend upon the dynamics of telomere loss and reacquisition [10]. The implications of telomere loss and chromosome alterations by telomerase activation and replication likely contribute to many aspects of cell life. Aging, cancer, age-related diseases, and the possibility of designing drugs and genetic tools to alter the process are all exciting areas under current study [11].

The immune-autoimmune theory proposes that the cells of successive generations of divisions begin to produce defective proteins within the DNA and RNA phases of replication during cellular growth. These proteins then act as antigens to the immune system, which then begins to attack and damage all the tissues that have developed this histo-incompatible state. As the organism ages, more antigens are formed and more tissues are affected and eliminated by the immune response.

The cross-linkage theory of aging assumes that the constant bonding of two or more molecules in a side-to-side arrangement takes place within all cells. Age-dependent changes result in damage to the tissues, such as loss of elasticity in the connective tissue, reduced "swelling" capacity of all cells, increased molecular weight of critical nuclear molecules, and a brittleness of the tissues. Bjorksten has published an excellent discussion of this concept of aging [6].

Only severe calorie restriction in certain rats and mice has been found consistently to prolong the life span [12], although exercise begun early in life may also extend the life span of mice [13]. The claims of persons living to be as old as 170 years in the Georgia Republic of the former Soviet Union, the village of Vilcabamba in the Ecuador Andes, and the Hunza region in Pakistan have been found to be greatly exaggerated. The uncertainty of the true age of these people is due to the illiteracy of those involved and the desire for political gain for the leaders of the region and for other economic reasons [14–16]. As yet, no data exist to confirm or refute the effectiveness of any intervention aimed at extending the human life span [17]. Thus, although eliminating various diseases has increased human life expectancy, allowing a greater proportion of the population to approach the maximum life span, nothing has been shown to alter that maximum age to which one individual may aspire, which is, presumably, determined by normal physiologic aging [14].

It is sometimes confusing to the laity and even to some members of the medical profession when the normal processes of aging and some unrelated true pathologic processes begin to overlap. We have tried to separate those true pathologic situations that are apt to occur in the elderly from those processes that are most likely due to the normal processes of aging. This chapter deals with the latter, while the former are covered in many of the subsequent chapters that include topics on specific diseases of each organ system in the elderly.

CARDIOVASCULAR SYSTEM

A major consideration to remember when discussing the aging cardiovascular system is the issue of atherosclerosis, which is thought by most of the medical profession to be a pathologic condition rather than a normal process of aging. In this country, it is nonetheless so prevalent and so parallel to aging that it confuses many human studies aimed at examining the normal changes of aging. This discussion deals primarily with the anatomic and physiologic changes associated with aging that are expected to occur regardless of the presence or absence of atherosclerosis.

Vasculature

Histologic studies reveal intimal hyperplasia and thickening that progress with age, beginning early in life [18] with fragmentation of the internal elastic lamina in the arteries, especially those of the lower extremities. Medial sclerosis with calcification is seen in the lower extremity arteries from most persons greater than 50 years old [15]. Upper extremity arteries show these changes in much milder forms with progressing age, suggesting that the greater hydrostatic pressure present in the legs contributes to these changes. In the same study, intimal hyperplasia was found in the aorta of patients of all ages [15].

Pulmonary vessels demonstrate a decrease in medial collagen content of approximately 1% per decade, and the walls of pulmonary arteries show a decrease in elastin content and an increase in muscle content with progressive age. The total wall thickness of the arteries and veins changes little with age, but the intima thickens with age in the arteries [19] and may demonstrate fibrosis after the fourth decade [20].

Physiologically, age changes of the vasculature include increased stiffness and decreased compliance of the pulmonary arteries, but not of the veins [21], and decreased distensibility and increased stiffness of the systemic arteries [22,23]. Presumably as a result of these changes, the maximum systolic blood pressure increases significantly with age, with no increase in mean blood pressure [24].

The elderly vascular system responds and recovers as well as that of the young when a sudden tilt from the supine to the erect position is made, although the older person apparently requires a larger increase in vasopressin and possibly also in sympathetic drive to effect a similar response [25] (see Chapter 19).

Heart

Anatomically, there are few changes in the heart specifically associated with normal aging, and according to Pomerance, "its appearance in an octerarian may be indistinguishable from that in a patient half a century younger" [26]. The size and weight of the heart in a population without ischemic heart disease or hypertension is proportional to body weight [27]. Microscopically, the old myocardium shows a decrease in muscle mass and an increase in collagen, elastic tissue, and fat [23]. The endocardium of the atrium and the valve edges continue to thicken until about age 60 [28], with changes similar to the intimal thickening seen in systemic arteries. Echocardiographic studies demonstrate a decrease in the ejection fraction slope of the anterior mitral valve leaflet of older subjects [29], a parameter usually considered proportional to early diastolic left ventricular filling. The age-related decrease in the slope could indicate a decrease in left ventricular filling due, for example, to delayed ventricular relaxation, which has been reported [30], or perhaps to increased myocardial stiffness. The change in the slope could also reflect age-related changes in the valve [29]. The echocardiogram also showed an increase with age in the left ventricular wall thickness. This change is proportional to the meter squared of body surface area but bears no apparent change or relationship to left ventricular cavity size [29]. The aortic root's diastolic diameter increases with age, which, Gerstenblith and colleagues suggest, occurs to compensate for the aorta's increased stiffness. The larger volume of blood in the aorta during diastole would present the heart with a greater inertial load against which to pump and thus would be expected to cause the observed thickening of the left ventricular wall [29].

The physiologic alterations in cardiac function found to be associated with aging are, like the anatomic changes, difficult to separate from the changes associated with atherosclerotic changes and from other diseases. The apparently healthy elderly myocardium has a prolonged relaxation time, which means the old heart will not function as well as a young heart during periods of tachycardia [30]. Perhaps because of this change, the heart rate of patients over 50 years old is not significantly different from that of younger patients at rest but increases significantly less than that of younger patients in response to equivalent exercise [31]. Similarly, there is a decreased response of heart rate to an increase in blood pressure. This may not be due to the heart itself, but it could be due to the decreased distensibility of the arteries, which would then obviously prevent an accurate stimulation of the baroreceptor mechanism [32]. Reports on changes in stroke volume with age do not give consistent results, but at least one reliable source says that there is a decline of approximately 1% per year in cardiac output, which Landowne and colleagues attribute almost entirely to an increase of similar degree in peripheral vascular resistance [24].

Studies of the heart's rhythm in the apparently healthy elderly (65 and older) allow us to conclude that supraventricular ectopic contractions, premature ventricular contractions, and sinus tachycardia or other types of tachycardias due to atrial arrhythmia are not uncommon, but sinus pauses, atrioventricular block, and bradycardias are extremely uncommon [33,34].

In summary, the major changes with aging in the cardiovascular system are related to a stiffening and decreased distensibility of the pulmonary and systemic arteries and of the heart wall itself. This change is due to changes in collagen and elastic tissue. Under normal conditions, these changes do not adversely affect the functioning of the system, but when the aged cardiovascular system is overstressed, the old heart may not perform as well as the young heart due to slowed filling in diastole. The reduced distensibility of the aorta and systemic arteries contributes to a higher systolic blood pressure in the aged despite a normal mean pressure, and if extrapolated to a stressed heart, this could impair coronary perfusion to the myocardium and lead to myocardial ischemia and damage.

RESPIRATORY SYSTEM

There are three major effects of aging on the respiratory system that account for changes in pulmonary function. They are loss of elastic recoil of lung tissue, fixation and stiffening of the chest wall, and atrophy and weakening of respiratory muscles [35,36].

The alveolar ducts and bronchioles are supported by a helical arrangement of elastin and collagen fibers. The elastic behavior and recoil of the lung result from an enfolding of this complex structure, rather than the lengthening of each individual fiber. This recoil ability is lost, elastic recoil fails, and lung compliance decreases when the lung's elastic quality changes. There is evidence that with age the size of the alveolar ducts increases, the resting size of the lung's elastic components increases, and airway conductance may remain static or become increased [37]. This results in the so-called senile emphysema common in the elderly. The loss of elastic recoil is responsible for an increase in residual volume, a decrease in compliance, and an increase in closing volume [35]. *Closing volume* is the lung volume at which small airways start to close and increasing intrapleural pressure is unable to reopen the small airways. This results in air trapping and in uneven distribution of ventilation and perfusion [36].

The anteroposterior diameter of the chest increases and the chest wall stiffens as a result of calcification of the costal cartilages. The intervertebral disk spaces decrease, kyphoscoliosis develops, and a barrel chest deformity becomes the hallmark of old age. The physiologic results of these changes are increased lung volume, reduced rib cage excursion, shortening of diaphragmatic excursion, and increasing abdominal wall involvement with respiratory movement [38]. Total lung capacity is not appreciably changed.

A perceived effect of decreased respiratory muscle strength that occurs with aging might very well be due to the reduced compliance of the chest wall. For forced expiration, limitation of movement results from a rounded, stiffened, fixed rib cage and vertebral mechanism covering an inelastic lung with altered closing pressures. These factors would pose formidable obstacles even for young, healthy muscles to overcome.

The increased anteroposterior diameter and flaring of the lateral margins of the barrel chest increase the span of peripheral attachments of the diaphragm and contribute to the flattening of the dome effect of the fibromuscular structure. This increased circumference has the added effect of shortening the effective excursion length of the diaphragmatic muscle. This compounds the effects of increased lung volume, which occurs secondary to the senile emphysema [38,39]. Deep inspiration is affected most by these changes, which also decrease the excursion distance of the diaphragm in its ascent and descent, requiring more assistance by the abdominal muscles for this respiratory activity.

Age-related changes in the pulmonary blood vessels are mostly due to intimal fibrosis and loss of elasticity of both pulmonary arteries and veins. These changes are less pronounced than the changes of aging usually seen in peripheral vessels [40]. The actual pulmonary function appears to be unaffected by these pulmonary vascular changes. However, when combined with several pathologic states such as cor pulmonale and other forms of pulmonary hypertension, they may become quite important.

GASTROINTESTINAL TRACT

Changes in the aging gastrointestinal tract decrease its motility, secretions, and perhaps absorptive ability. There is altered distensibility and thinning of perivascular channels due to muscular and collagen weakness.

Esophagus

Deglutition is the result of a complex coordination of reflexes that is dependent on neuromuscular interplay and is easily affected by any changes in the neuromuscular pathways. Muscular weakness in specific sites may lead to abnormal contraction patterns. This may result in diverticular formation, diffuse spasm, chalasia, achalasia, and gastroesophageal reflux.

The changes in swallowing patterns in the elderly usually indicate a degree of neuromuscular degeneration that can mimic true disorders of the esophagus such as those caused by diffuse spasm and gastroesophageal reflux. The subtle differences between the effects of the normal process of aging and the true pathologic situation related to spasm and reflux must be recognized when interpreting esophageal motility patterns in the elderly [41].

Motility pattern changes normal in the aging esophagus are similar to those seen in true neuromuscular disorders of the esophagus. Presbyesophagus may be associated with a mild form of spasm due to age-related changes that, when advanced to a severe degree, represent a pathologic situation. Motility disorders of the pharyngoesophageal region at the level of the cricopharyngeus muscle and the upper esophageal sphincter are not uncommon in the elderly. Disturbances of contraction in this area may produce a misdirection of food and liquids during swallowing and lead to aspiration, Zenker's diverticulum, and dysphagia [42].

It may be difficult to separate problems related to primary esophageal disorders from those caused by some central nervous system (CNS) disturbance. Changes in neural reflexes secondary to cerebrovascular accidents and other conditions related to aging of the CNS must be ruled out in each circumstance. In the elderly, neurologic conditions arise that may affect the complex series of events necessary for the control of normal swallowing. These neurologic conditions should be ruled out before swallowing difficulties are attributed to a primary upper esophageal disorder.

The response of the lower esophageal segment to the normal progression of relaxation and contractions necessary for normal swallowing may be completely absent or markedly altered in the elderly. The elderly experience a universal decrease in amplitude of contraction in the lower esophageal segment, with a weakening of peristaltic waves and slowing of their progress. These changes suggest a degree of neuromuscular inadequacy and simulate those findings seen in well-known pathologic conditions of achalasia, hiatal hernia, and reflux esophagitis. Spontaneous gastroesophageal reflux can occur as a result of an inadequate resting pressure of the lower esophageal segment, and this may then lead to an associated true pathologic condition.

Stomach

The major effects of aging on the stomach predominantly relate to changes in gastric emptying; neuromuscular degenerative changes; and diminished acid secretion, pepsin secretion, mucosal atrophy, and muscular strength.

The stomach is another organ for which the changes that may be due to aging are difficult to separate from the effects of various degrees of disease states. Because many of these conditions increase in frequency with longevity, it is not uncommon to attribute symptoms from some true pathologic condition to an "old stomach" [43,44].

There is some evidence that gastric emptying is prolonged or delayed with advancing age. The ill effects of this delay are difficult to demonstrate and evaluate. Sophisticated studies designed to compare gastric emptying in the young with the elderly have failed to show any associated significant digestive aberrations [45–47]. It is tempting to attribute many of the dyspepsias of aging to poor gastric emptying, but no hard scientific evidence supports this notion.

The gastric mucosa gradually becomes atrophic as age progresses, but histologic studies have been inconsistent in relating advancing age to specific changes such as chronic atrophic gastritis, gastric atrophy, and mucosal aberrations [48–50]. Gastric acid output declines gradually with age [48] and tends to be reflected by a decrease in both basal and peak acid output. This is apt to be more marked among women than men, but in neither is frank achlorhydria or serious hypochlorhydria a common problem. When these conditions exist, a true pathologic explanation must always be sought.

Pepsin secretion tends to be decreased in those cases in which mucosal atrophy is significant and pepsin secretory levels tend to mirror the histologic picture [51]. As previously stated, it is difficult to attribute much significance to this relationship between mucosal atrophy and aging.

Chronic gastritis, atrophic gastritis, and acute gastritis, which may be more common in the elderly than in the young, should all be considered true disease processes and not the natural consequences of aging.

Small Bowel

A reduction in the height of the villi of the small intestinal mucosa begins to develop around age 60 in most individuals [52]. These changes lead to a reduction in the mucosal surface area, the result of which is a decrease in absorption of D-xylose, carbohydrates, and calcium. The amount of decrease in absorption of these substances varies markedly, does not usually become significant until age 70 or older, and may not be clinically important even at those advanced ages [53,54]. Histologic evidence of aging in the small bowel has also been noticed as early as age 40. In these instances, the parenchyma of the mucosa and some of the healthy smooth muscles of the intestinal wall are all replaced in part by fibrous connective tissue [55] (see Chapter 25).

Colon

The aging colon shows a consistent abnormality of the muscularis propria. The thickness of the colon wall and the amount of elastin it contains normally increase with age [56]. These changes, along with a weakness of the muscularis propria at the site of arterial and venous passageways through the muscle layers, allow the expression of diverticular disease.

Diverticulosis is the most common disorder of the colon attributable to the aging process [57]. Drummond first described the mechanism whereby intestinal and colonic diverticula develop [58]. In his description, colonic or intestinal mucosa and submucosa herniate alongside the neurovascular bundle, penetrating the bowel's muscular wall in a manner not unlike the hernia sac when it passes alongside the spermatic cord in an indirect hernia. Increased intraluminal pressure, motility disorders, and thickening of the tinea coli have all been implicated as etiologic contributors to the development of diverticular disease in the aging colon [59].

The mucosa of the aging colon may show a variety of changes, none of which appear to affect the absorptive ability of the large bowel. Microscopic evidence indicates that the muscle layers increase in thickness throughout life. The greatest increase occurs in the last trimester of fetal development and the first 3 months after birth [56].

A slow increase in muscular thickness continues to occur until approximately the sixth decade of life. Then the process becomes more rapid, involves both circular and longitudinal muscles, is associated with an increase in fibrosis, and is characterized by a slight increase in elastin. The elastin increase appears to occur more in the longitudinal layer (tinea coli) than in the circular layer [57]. Many of the bowel complaints associated with aging (i.e., constipation, hard stool, fecal impaction, megacolon, sigmoid volvulus, and abuse of laxatives) can in part be related to these muscular changes [60].

The familiar allegation that the aging colon becomes atrophic and the musculature becomes thin and atonic is a myth. Manometric studies of the aging colon and anorectal pressures in the elderly fail to show such an age-related abnormality [61].

Liver

At or near age 50, the liver accounts for approximately 2.5% of total body weight [62,63]. From that point on, it gradually decreases both in relative and absolute size until at age 90 it represents only 1.6% of total body weight. Blood flow to and from the liver may show a corresponding decrease as the relative liver size changes [64]. Microscopic and morphologic changes relate to an increased mean volume in liver cells and decreased number of hepatocytes associated with the atrophy of aging. Liver cell nuclei increase in size from age 30 onward, and mitochondria decrease in number but increase in volume, as do isosomes. This suggests that fewer cells are doing the work in old age that many cells did some years before. This may be due to the decreased ability to grow new hepatocytes by cell division [65]. A mild ductal proliferation associated with minimal inflammatory response may be seen in biopsies from aging livers [66]. The results of most conventional liver function tests are not altered by increased age. Some sophisticated liver clearance tests (Bromsulphalein [sulfobromophthalein sodium; BSP], antipyrine) may be altered by the aging liver's decreased capacity for storage. There is a marked decrease in BSP stored in cells that have increased nuclear DNA (i.e., the old large liver cells). Ethanol elimination is not affected by age [67].

Detoxification, demethylation, conjugation, and hepatic extraction of most compounds do not appear to be affected by increased age. Synthesis of body proteins and clotting factors may be decreased because of reduced protein binding capacity in the aged liver. This is usually not a problem under normal conditions, and homeostasis is not generally affected. In times of stress, however, enzymes in the aging liver cannot increase their activities much beyond that necessary to maintain normal function [68]. Poor nutrition also seems to exert an undue influence on the aged liver's ability to respond to stress, disease, and increased metabolic demands [64].

Gallbladder and Bile Ducts

The incidence of gallstones increases with age in most Western societies. In Britain and the United States, over 30% of women and 20% of men over age 80 will have gallstones [69]. In 1978, Valdivieso et al. concluded that aging modifies the proportion of biliary lipids and cholesterol [70]. This leads to the situation in which lipids supersaturate the bile to a lithogenic level at some point during the aging process. There is no evidence that the gallbladder contractibility, absorptive abilities, or any mucosal function is altered by aging to a degree that gallstone formation would be more likely. The mechanism by which more cholesterol-saturated bile is produced with increased age is unclear.

Pancreas

There appears to be little change in the size of the pancreas as age progresses, although some report that dilatation, ectasia, and the overall increased size of the main pancreatic duct and its major branches are seen in normal elderly individuals [71]. Concomitant with this ductal change, the gland generally declines in weight beginning around age 70. A small percentage of elderly individuals will have an incomplete stenosis of the pancreatic duct that causes no symptoms and reflects no underlying pathology. Therefore, pancreatography in elderly patients should be interpreted with caution [72]. No microscopic picture that could be called typical evidence of senile changes has been described, although perilobular fibrosis may occur and lead to some atrophy of the entire gland [72,73]. There may be a slight decrease in lipase, amylase, and trypsin measured in the pancreatic juice of the elderly individual following infusion of pancreozymin [74]. The absorption of fat sometimes seen in elderly individuals may be slightly impaired due to a slight decrease in pancreatic lipase [75]. The addition of lipase to the fat meal in elderly subjects seems to abolish this defect [76]. Others have failed to show a difference between fat absorption in healthy older and healthy younger individuals [77].

HEMATOPOIETIC SYSTEM

Spleen

The weight of the human spleen decreases with old age due to involution, fibrosis, and possibly multiple small infarcted areas. A slight hypofunction of the spleen in the elderly can be measured by the increased percentage of pitted erythrocytes seen in the peripheral blood and the ability of the spleen to remove heat-damaged erythrocytes from circulation. This evidence of hypofunction is thought to be caused by a reduction of splenic tissue volume [78]. It may also have some effect on the elderly patient's decreased ability to deal with pneumococcal and similar infections.

Hematology

There seems to be a definite relationship between loss of telomeric DNA with age and the changes seen in hematopoietic functions. The ability of the bone marrow stem cell to remain proliferative is dependent on the sequential loss of telomeric DNA from the chromosomes with each cell division until a critical point is reached. At some point the change in DNA becomes great enough to cause senescence of the stem cell, and hematopoietic function is altered. This has been likened to a mitotic time clock for bone marrow function [79]. This concept is supportive of the Hayflick limit postulated in the 1960s [80].

The major effects of aging in the hematopoietic system are related to the degranulation and reduced chemotaxis of the peripheral blood granulocytes. There is some evidence to suggest that these changes are due to a reduced ability for the production of cyclic adenosine monophosphate by the marrow cells of elderly patients [81]. This may affect the ability of the granulocytes and the monocytes to phagocytize bacteria, fungi, and other foreign material [82]. It has been previously recognized that the monocytes and other phagocytes decrease in number after age 70. Additional evidence for a decreased ability of these leukocytes to perform in a normal manner is now being gathered. Also after age 70, the bone marrow demonstrates a decline in the actual production of myelocytes, platelets, and perhaps granulocytes. Red blood cells continue to be produced with normal functional ability but also in slightly fewer numbers. Anemia is not thought to be a normal feature of aging. The fact that nonanemic elderly patients show some reduction in hematopoiesis suggests that age will likely contribute to the defect of anemia when some other underlying pathologic condition exists [83]. When anemia occurs in the elderly, another pathologic condition should always be sought. Iron deficiency and the anemia of chronic disease are the two most frequent underlying causes for anemia in the elderly [84].

Lymphocytes appear to remain in normal numbers in the peripheral circulation of elderly patients, and the results of their laboratory reports are not significantly different from the counts reported from young controls or from lymphocyte counts from elderly anemic individuals. Neutrophil counts in the anemic elderly were markedly decreased when compared with that of young controls and were slightly decreased in nonanemic elderly [83].

IMMUNOLOGY

Many changes occur in the immune system as age progresses. The most dramatic of these is the involution of the thymus gland and a concomitant decrease in the ratio of suppressor T-cell lymphocytes and an increase in helper T-cell lymphocytes. This results in a functional impairment of T cell–mediated immunity and an increased susceptibility to infections such as pneumococcus, influenza, tetanus, and so forth.

Lymphocytes arise from the thymus gland, which undergoes a gradual secondary involution beginning at approximately age 40. This adult involutional change may be a major cause of immunosenescence. By age 60, mature T-lymphocyte populations actually begin to decline [85].

As a result of decreased numbers of thymocytes, which are known to differentiate into mature T lymphocytes, the gradual involution of the thymus gland materially affects humorally mediated immune response. Pneumococcal pneumonia and tetanus infections are materially affected by this aspect of immunosenescence [85].

An associated increase in autoimmune activity is often noticed with increased age. This latter factor has been suggested as an explanation for pernicious anemia, susceptibility to neoplasms, and an acceleration of the aging process itself [86]. T cells have also been noticed to have an impaired proliferative response to interleukin-2. Interleukin-2 is a T-lymphocyte growth factor that possesses an immune-enhancing property. Its actual production is decreased in the elderly, which causes a decrease in cellular immunity in these individuals [85,86].

The total number of B-cell lymphocytes produced by the bone marrow and the total amount of immunoglobulin produced by the elderly hematopoietic system remain unchanged, but there must be a defect in immunoglobulin production. An apparent paradox in antibody production in the elderly exists. Studies show a decreased production of antibodies to foreign antigens and increased production of autoantibody. Weksler suggests that this may be due to increased activity of most suppressor T cells, which regulate antibody production to foreign antigens and a concomitant decrease in activity of a subpopulation of suppressor T cells that regulate autoantibody production [87].

Several agents have been demonstrated to improve the immune responses in the elderly. They include vitamin C, isoprinosine, immucytal, tuftsin, and interleukin-2, as mentioned previously. All of these have been tested in studies that are encouraging, although clear evidence of consistent clinical benefits remains to be shown.

GENITOURINARY TRACT

There is a gradual loss in mass, weight, and size of the kidney after age 50. From birth to maturation, the combined weight of the two kidneys increases from approximately 45 to 50 g to 250 to 270 g by the age of 40 to 50 years [88]. The combined weight of both kidneys gradually declines until at age 90 and older, the usual weight is 180 to 185 g. Dunnill and Halley have shown that this loss after age 50 is due to an absolute volume loss and that it is due primarily to cortical tissue loss with relative sparing of the renal medulla [89]. The cortical loss is due to two main changes of the arteriolar glomerular apparatus. One of these senescent changes is a collapse of the glomerular tuft and the obliteration of the preglomerular arteriole. The other is the development of a shunt around the sclerotic glomerulus between the afferent and efferent arterioles [90]. This maintains good perfusion of the medulla and the collecting system parenchyma [91].

Renal function changes related to aging are mostly due to decreased renal blood flow, glomerular filtration rate, ability to consume sodium, and ability to concentrate urine [91,92]. These altered abilities of the elderly patient's kidney to concentrate urine and conserve water are due primarily to decreased glomerular filtration rate and an age-related impairment in solute conservation. These deficiencies are likely due to a defect in the transport of Na^+, Cl^-, urea, and water from tubular lumen to the medullary interstitial space [93]. It remains unclear what role the aging adrenal cortex and a declining level of aldosterone in the elderly may play in this process [94].

As is noted in subsequent chapters, fluid balance, electrolyte balance, drug dosage, and the use of diuretics all become important when the intrepid surgeon treads on the thin ice of surgical management of the elderly. Preoperative preparation, intraoperative speed and gentleness, and vigilant postoperative care are all necessary components of avoiding renal failure in the ill elderly patient who requires a major surgical procedure.

INTEGUMENT

The organization of the collagen fibers in the dermis changes gradually with aging. In the young dermis, discrete bundles of coiled interlaced and contorted collagen fibers are seen in the relaxed skin. These coils straighten as the skin is stretched and recoil as the skin is relaxed. In the dermis of older subjects, the collagen is in sheets and no longer in individual bundles, and the collagen fibrils are mostly straight, even in the relaxed state. A baby's skin will stretch 40% to 60% more than its resting length, but by age 65, it can be stretched only 15% to 20% more than its resting length. It has lost its elastic properties as it has aged [95].

The delicate architecture of the connective tissue of the dermis degenerates in a dramatic way with aging. Both collagenous and elastic components display a loss of integrity, which allows the characteristic changes of sagging and wrinkling synonymous with aging. After 50 to 100 doublings, fibroblasts have been shown to cease replicating and become senescent. This is also being blamed on DNA damage due to telomeric changes of the genome as aging occurs [96].

Skin regrowth is measured by the ability of the epidermis to regrow dermal-epidermal skin ridges of the fingers and finger pads. When the ridges were abraded from fingerprints and the regrowth measured, it was found that the elderly regrowth potential is the same as in all healthy subjects from every age group after childhood.

The thinning of the skin in the elderly is common and is due to a similar process as is seen in younger individuals on corticosteroid therapy [97–99]. This thinning has been shown to be due to actual loss of primary collagen and also possibly to a loss of ability of fibroblasts to produce new collagen.

Collagen and elastin in the dermis are both affected by age. Soluble collagen decreases and insoluble collagen increases. Elastin increases, but the elastic quality of the elastin fibers decreases with age. As the body ages, collagenous structures undergo maturation and polymerization, with markedly increased numbers and types of covalent cross links. This cross-link theory of aging is one that appears on many lists of hypotheses designed to explain the limitations imposed on the human organism by the changing molecular structures within the aging body [6]. This concept is described earlier in this chapter.

The adnexal structures also begin to show evidence of aging after age 65, with thinning of scalp, axillary, and pubic hair and a decreased ability to secrete oil and sweat from the appropriate glands.

CENTRAL NERVOUS SYSTEM

The most striking and widely known change that occurs within the CNS as a result of aging is a loss of brain weight [100]. There is a concomitant decrease in volume, with widening of sulci, deepening of sulci, narrowing of gyri, and a steady increase in the size of the ventricles with age. It is not surprising that the microscopic and morphologic correlates to those findings are that of cortical cell loss [101]. Cortical thickness decreases, neuronal cells in the cortex are lost at random, and glial cells increase in number, along with the size of their processes. The cerebellum, basal ganglia, brain stem, thalamus, spinal cord, and cranial nerves have all been studied, and the consensus remains that there is a general, overall CNS-wide loss of neurons with advancing age [102]. It is generally agreed that the constant cell loss begins at an early age and continues throughout life [100].

The normal process of aging in the CNS is clinically productive of subtle changes and functional losses that make findings associated with aging more difficult to separate from true pathologic processes than in other systems (see Chapter 31).

The actual counting of cell loss is difficult. There is a noticeable lack of dependable methods and a recognized difficulty in interpretation of the findings due to our inability to study the same individual over a long time. A loss of extracellular substance is often seen with aging, along with a concomitant, spurious increase in cell counts. Poor correlation has been shown between the actual or even in the calculated cell loss and the measurable functional aspects of aging.

Atrophy of the cortical gyri is common in old age and is seen especially in senile demented individuals. Correlated functional losses, which can be shown in these individuals, are in short-term memory, emotional expression, and intellectual capacity. Histochemically and cytologically there is cytoplasmic shrinkage of nerve cells with a deposition of brown lipofuscin pigment. Most of the studies have been done with the cerebral cortex (especially in the two granular layers), the basal ganglia, the brain stem nuclei such as locus ceruleus, cerebellar nuclei such as dentate, all three cortical layers, and the inferior olive of the medulla. Functional deficits are as expected from the anatomic sites: higher function in the cortex, emotionalism and so forth in the hypothalamus, abnormal motor activity in the basal ganglia, sleepiness in the locus ceruleus, and ataxia in the cerebellar system and olive. Fe^{++} changes are noted to occur with aging in the spinal cord and the white tracts and spinal ganglia. Proprioception is not markedly diminished, nor is tactile sense [103].

Blood flow is altered in aging in proportion to changes in the vessels. When reduced, it may be correlated with psychological functional deficits. Senile dementia and Alzheimer's disease are pathologic and always associated with severe cell loss.

In one excellent review of the subject by Samorajski, many of the morphologic changes seen in the old adult human brain are correlated to disease entities such as Alzheimer's disease, atherosclerosis, and senile dementias [104]. The control of aging by the hypothalamus as proposed by Dilman [105] and refined by Everitt [106] is covered by Samorajski's fine review.

As noted in subsequent chapters, many of the uncorrectable effects of aging, some of the age-related dementias, and the tendency of the general public and many physicians to expect all old people to have CNS changes may lull us into a failure to recognize, diagnose, and treat correctable lesions, such as tumors, aneurysms, and extracranial vascular problems in otherwise healthy elderly patients.

AUTONOMIC NERVOUS SYSTEM

Not much is known about age changes of the parasympathetic and sympathetic nervous system. As is seen in the CNS, progressive cell loss occurs. Pfeifer and coworkers reviewed 103 normal men and found an age-related increase of cardiovascular sympathetic nervous system activity and a decrease of activity of the cardiac parasympathetic nervous system [107]. These changes in response to adrenergic stimulation and to blocking drugs suggest that the increase in cardiovascular sympathetic activity may occur as compensation for an age-related decrease in baroreceptor sensitivity. Neuroendocrine changes also occur. Metabolic changes in the liver may account for many of these findings because of alterations in drug responsiveness and to toxic synergy.

PERIPHERAL NERVOUS SYSTEM

Age-related changes in proprioception have been the subject of relatively little study. Changes are reported in tactile and proprioceptive sensation in elderly individuals [108,109]. In a study of 29 subjects of all ages with normal knee joints, Skinner and colleagues found that aging is associated with a decline in joint-position sense, but they could not determine whether these deficiencies were actually the result of the aging process. Kokmen and coworkers found a decrease in joint motion sensation in normal elderly subjects. No significant changes in nerve fiber numbers have been reported, but reflex time is diminished with age [103].

ENDOCRINOLOGY

Many age-related changes in various types of hormone levels have been reported, but the physiologic consequences of these changes are not well defined in many cases. The subjects used for many of the well-known endocrinologic studies on aging are hospitalized patients or those categorized as "apparently" or "fairly" healthy. In many cases, there is no way to identify those elderly patients who may have mild or unrecognized, significant, pathologic endocrine conditions. Therefore, some of the reported endocrine changes that have been attributed to senility may be due not to the truly normal process of aging but to prevalent pathologic conditions.

Endocrine Pancreas

The nondiabetic elderly person will show signs of impaired glucose tolerance much more often than the young; in fact, one study reported nine out of 20 elderly patients (mean age, 80 years) had abnormal oral glucose tolerance test results as opposed to no abnormal test results in 20 patients in their 20s [110]. This relative glucose intolerance that appears with aging is independent of obesity [111] and gender [110] and is not related to a deficiency of endogenous insulin. This can be shown by elderly patients who do not have deficient insulin secretion [110,112] but actually have increased arterial insulin levels [113]. The elderly individuals can be shown to have a degree of insulin resistance that is not due to altered insulin binding to cell membrane receptors, but is in part due to a "reduction in the capacity of the glucose uptake system" [110]. This may involve and be the result of a reduction in the number of glucose transporters or metabolic systems [112]. One study suggests that a diet that eliminates sugar and is moderately calorie restricting may delay the onset or reduce the degree of age-related glucose intolerance [114].

The endocrine response to mild hypoglycemia appears to be preserved in the elderly. Both glucagon and adrenal hormones respond normally to moderate insulin-induced hypoglycemia [115]. Likewise, basal arterial levels of glucagon do not change with age, but the elderly respond to glucagon with greater glucose production than do the young [116].

Thyroid

The aged thyroid shows some degree of atrophy, fibrosis, increased nodularity, decreased follicle size, an increased amount of interfollicular connective tissue, and a reduction in total gland weight [117]. By the eighth decade of life, 20% of apparently healthy subjects in one study showed increased levels of antithyroglobulin and antimicrosomal antibody, which are both associated with autoimmune hypothyroidism [117]. The elderly have a lower serum level of the thyroid hormone thyroxine (T_4) and free T_4 index than the young; but triiodothyronine (T_3) and free T_3 are not decreased significantly until after age 60 in men and age 80 in women [118]. The decrease in T_3 level, when it finally occurs, is believed to be due to declining peripheral conversion of T_4 to T_3 [119]. A significant number of healthy elderly patients show elevated thyroid-stimulating hormone levels [118,119]. It is not clear from current data whether these changes in hormone levels have physiologic consequences in the elderly [120] or represent a forerunner or predisposition to true hypothyroidism [118].

The parathyroid glands and calcitonin-producing cells are of particular interest in the elderly because osteoporosis is such a widespread problem in this segment of the population. Berlyne et al. hypothesized that a decreasing glomerular filtration rate, which is found in the healthy elderly, could lead to a decrease in the serum calcium level [121]. This may be due to phosphorus retention or to a decreased renal production of active vitamin D. This would in turn increase the secretion of parathyroid hormone and thereby lead to osteoporosis [121]. Other work has shown that total serum calcium does decrease with age, but it is not clear whether the parathyroid hormone levels actually increase with age when the variable glomerular filtration rates of the elderly are controlled [122,123]. The hypothesis of Berlyne et al. has not been confirmed. Serum calcitonin, the coregulator of calcium homeostasis seems to increase with age [124].

Male Reproductive Endocrine System

The major age-related change in the male reproductive hormone system is a decrease in testosterone levels both in serum and the tissue of the testis. This gradual decrease of testosterone production begins at age 40 despite increasing luteinizing hormone and follicle-stimulating hormone levels and a decrease in metabolic clearance of testosterone [125]. Takahashi et al. and Baker et al. suggest the etiology is a primary decline in function of the testis [125,126]. They believe that there is evidence to show that the problem is caused by a reduced supply of mitochondrial steroid precursors in Leydig's cells [125,126]. Estradiol levels decrease in aging men despite an increase in conversion of testosterone to estradiol. The sex hormone–binding globulin level also increases [125]. Kinsey and colleagues reported that 75% of 80-year-old men were impotent, but this figure likely includes a large proportion of men impotent due to causes other than normal aging [127] (see Chapter 28).

Female Reproductive Endocrine System

With the onset of menopause, women experience a marked decline in serum estrogen levels as both the ovary and the adrenal gland diminish and then stop secreting estrogens. Only the conversion of androstenedione to estrogen, which occurs primarily in fat tissue, provides estrogen to the elderly postmenopausal woman. Circulating levels of luteinizing hormone and follicle-stimulating hormone from the pituitary are elevated in the postmenopausal woman. This is thought to be because of the greatly reduced estrogen level and the loss of the usual feed-lock inhibition on the pituitary for the secretion of luteinizing and follicle-stimulating hormones [128].

Pituitary System

There are interesting similarities between pituitary responses in the aged and the depressed patient. Both the diurnal cortisol nadir and the maximum peak occur earlier in the day in the aged. This correlates with the frequently reported earlier bedtime and early awakening time in the elderly. These "sleep disturbances" are also frequently reported in patients with endogenous depression [129]. The sensitivity of the hypothalamic-pituitary complex to inhibition by dexamethasone increases in the elderly. This is also seen in patients with endogenous depression, stress, atherosclerosis, and endometrial and prostate carcinoma [130].

There appears to be no difference in prolactin secretion [131] or number of prolactin-secreting cells [132] in the pituitary gland of the elderly. Likewise, the elderly show no difference in basal beta-endorphin levels or the response of this hormone to a cold pressor test (immersion of a hand in 40°C water) [133]. There is, however, a decreased response of growth hormone to synthetic growth hormone–releasing factor in the elderly [124]. As is the case with many of the endocrine alterations and nonalterations seen in aging, the physiologic significance of these pituitary changes is not entirely clear.

Renin-Aldosterone System

Aldosterone levels are lower in the aged both before and after sodium depletion [134,135], but the difference is much greater when a patient is upright than when recumbent [136]. This report agrees with the cardiovascular literature findings discussed previously in this chapter. Renin levels decrease with aging, possibly due to decreased conversion of inactive to active renin [135].

Plasma noradrenaline levels in the elderly are higher than in the young, and the elderly show a greater increase in noradrenaline in response to stress [137]. This may be due to diminished adrenergic receptor sensitivity, because the elderly have been found to have a diminished response to beta blockade [138]. Increased noradrenaline levels in the aged can confuse the diagnosis of hypertension, and the possible diminution of adrenergic receptor sensitivity would affect the reaction of the elderly to the many adrenergic agonist and antagonist drugs [137].

EYE AND VISUAL SYSTEM

In the eye itself there are changes in all parts: increased opacity of the cornea, increased rigidity of the lens, delayed pupillary reflex time, reduced removal time of aqueous humor, and an increase in the incidence of glaucoma. Changes in vitreous humor (e.g., floaters) become troublesome. The most important retinal changes are those of vascular origin, and macular degeneration often occurs, which may be idiopathic or related to hypertension. Optic nerve fibers are reduced significantly with age. Several subjective changes that are universally reported include hypermetropia, decreased acuity, and reduction of visual fields, especially in the upper half and peripherally [139].

The changes in the cornea that are most characteristic of aging are arcus senilis and corneal opacity. The former is an annular lipid deposit near the limbus, and the latter is a centralized loss of corneal clarity. The cornea becomes more fragile and less sensitive with age and leaves the eye more susceptible to injury without the patient's awareness of its occurrence [140].

The anterior chamber becomes shallow as the aging lens gradually enlarges. It has been shown that an 80-year-old lens is three times the size of a newborn lens [141]. As the anterior chamber becomes more shallow, the chamber angle becomes narrow and closes, causing acute closed-angle glaucoma, a condition rare in patients under age 60.

Senile cataracts are present when the crystalline lens loses its normal transparency with age, and there is alteration of the passage of light through the lens. Other causes of cataracts are genetic, congenital, metabolic, traumatic, toxic, and unknown [142]. The diagnosis of senile cataract is made in persons over 45 to 50 years of age when other causes are ruled out. Cataracts account for approximately 9% of all blindness and are the third leading cause of blindness in the United States. Senile changes and senile cataracts affect 10% and 1% of people aged 55 to 59 years and 37% and 45% of people aged 75 to 79 years [143]. Factors that increase the risk and incidence are demographic, geographic, and disease related. Nutritional deficiency, diabetes, hypertension, increased serum phospholipids, and decreased hand grip strength were all found in the Framingham Eye Study to bear a positive relationship to cataracts [144]. Ionizing and infrared radiation and possibly ultraviolet and microwave radiation are thought to be high-risk factors [145].

Senile macular degeneration of the retina accounts for most forms of blindness in the United States, with a peak age incidence of 50 to 70 years [146]. Subretinal deposits of pigment excreted from the retina and picked up in choriocapillaries are associated with neovascular changes that occur beneath the retina. An opaque membrane is then found beneath the retinal pigment epithelium. These neovascular membranes may be cauterized with the argon laser. If treated before the fovea is involved, blindness may be avoided.

The number of optic nerve fibers are reduced significantly by age 70 (estimated loss of approximately 400,000 fibers during 70 years) [147]. Optic radiation, however, is not affected. Cosmetic defects of the lids, including increased laxity, loss of elasticity, dermatochalasis, entropion, ectropion, dry eye pterygium, xanthelasma, and skin neoplasms, increase with age [141] (see Chapter 15).

EAR

External Ear

Changes in the external ear are largely the result of aging skin and cartilage. Atrophy and itching may occur in the external auditory canal, and these changes are exacerbated by the effects of aging on the sebaceous glands and ceruminal gland [148]. Biopsies have shown a decrease in the number of ceruminal glands in the ear canals of older persons [149]. Tragi, the large hairs found in the external auditory canals of most men, become coarser and longer as early as the fourth decade of life.

Middle Ear

Middle ear changes are mostly in the incudomalleal and incudostapedial joints of the ossicles. Etholm and Belal studied the joint changes that occur during the human life span and found that the earliest changes were fraying, fibrillation, and vacuolation in the articular cartilages [150]. These were followed by hyalinization of the joint capsule, cartilaginous thinning and calcification, and occasionally, narrowing of the joint space. All subjects over 70 years of age showed moderate-to-severe arthritic changes in these joints. Surprisingly, these changes were not found to affect sound transmission. The earlier reports of *conductive* hearing losses associated with aging [151,152] are now in question and are believed to have been inaccurate because of the faulty testing equipment and techniques [148].

Inner Ear

Inner ear changes associated with aging are largely responsible for the gradual hearing loss experienced by more than 25 million people in the United States over the age of 65 years [148]. Many of these individuals have one of the four major types of presbycusis. This aging disorder involves loss of speech processing and discrimination as well as loss of perception of pure tones. Sensory presbycusis involves atrophy of the organ of Corti, especially in the basal coil where high tones are recorded and in the auditory nerve where there is loss of fibers. Neural presbycusis results from a loss of the cochlear neurons and may begin at any age. Strial presbycusis usually begins in middle to older age. With strial presbycusis, spotty atrophy of the strict vascularis occurs. In cases of documented hearing loss for which adequate explanatory degenerative changes cannot be found, a category called *cochlear conductive presbycusis* has been established [148].

Vestibular changes are also common in the aged and result in dizziness, loss of balance, and vertigo. Less is known about the effects of aging on the vestibular portion of the inner ear than is known about the cochlea. It is known, however, that in individuals older than 74 years a 40% decrease in the number of myelinated vestibular nerve fibers should be expected [153]. Similarly, Rosenhall found a 20% to 40% decrease in the number of hair cells in the cristae and maculae in older individuals [154] (see Chapter 14).

MUSCLE

A loss of muscle strength is associated with aging. This is due, in part, to altered nutrition and physical activities in older individuals, rather than a direct effect of aging. In a report by Moller, the muscles of apparently healthy, elderly individuals were studied and compared with subjects 30 to 40 years younger [155]. The elderly muscles were found to have elevated levels of sodium, chloride, and extracellular water. Total concentrations of essential amino acids were lower in elderly women and higher in elderly men than found in their younger counterparts. A 5% decrease in total adenine nucleotides and phosphocreatine was observed in the elderly group, whereas the concentrations of creatinine and myoglobin were increased. After a 6-week period of physical training, a percentage of the elderly subjects was studied again and showed a decrease in creatinine, an increase in adenosine triphosphate to adenosine diphosphate and phosphocreatine to total creatinine ratios, and unchanged concentrations of myoglobin. Moller concluded that the changes in skeletal muscle associated with aging could in part be due to physical inactivity. He found more advanced muscle deterioration in elderly subjects with lung disease and liver cirrhosis.

There is also evidence that muscle fiber areas decrease with age [156]. This decrease appears to be more prominent in women than in men [157]. Inokuchi and colleagues found that the proportion and cross-sectional area of type II fibers were significantly diminished in elderly men compared with younger subjects [158]. Only minor enzymatic changes were identified in these subjects, and these were thought to be reflective of the change in type II fibers. Isometric and dynamic strength in the knee extensor muscles declined with increasing age and correlated with the loss of type II fibers. An increase in total reflex time was also apparent.

BONE

All parameters of bone strength are altered with aging and disuse. Torsion, tension, and fracture resistance are all reduced. Fractures are more common in the elderly because a decrease in tensile energy absorption accompanies aging [159]. The bone changes related to aging are no different between elderly men and women except in the postmenopausal woman with advanced osteoporosis.

With aging, the metabolism of osteoblasts and osteoclasts is diminished [160]. Compact bone tends to become spongy, the cortex is thinned, and the marrow cavity enlarged. There is less red marrow and more yellow marrow. Red marrow persists until very old age in the skull, ribs, vertebrae, pelvic bones, and proximal long bones. This accounts for the prevalence of and preference for these areas as sites of metastasis for certain tumors. Loss of bone mass from the fourth to the fifth decade is estimated to be 20% [161] and is associated with an age-related increase in parathyroid activity [162]. The increase in parathyroid activity may occur in response to an age-related decrease in calcium absorption. Loss of teeth and absorption of alveolar bone are common in the elderly.

Osteoporosis is a common degenerative condition associated with aging. This disorder involves a general loss of vertebral bone substance and a greater loss of horizontal trabecular components, resulting in reduced capability of the vertebral bodies to bear weight [163]. The severity of this disorder and the rate at which it progresses are both greater in elderly women than in elderly men. Tsai and coworkers have hypothesized that elderly women have abnormal vitamin D metabolism, which results in decreased calcium absorption that in turn stimulates increased parathyroid hormone secretion [162]. The parathyroid hormone stimulates increased bone turnover that, because of diminished bone formation in the elderly, results in a loss of bone mass. Their study was directed toward senile osteoporosis and excluded consideration of postmenopausal osteoporosis.

SUMMARY

Each organ system that is affected by particular changes as a result of aging is discussed in subsequent chapters. We have attempted here to introduce the concept of aging, and we have also made an effort to mention those areas in each organ system that are most vulnerable to the passage of time. It will be the intent of the contributors of the chapters that follow to relate the changes of aging to the practice of the art and science of surgery.

Much exciting research is under way at this time on the mechanism of aging. Favorite subjects are somatic mutations with brain aging [164], mutations of mitochondrial DNA [165], apoptosis [166], programmed cell death [167] and the ever popular telomerase [168], and DNA repair systems [169].

At this writing it seems that workers in this field may be on the verge of unraveling a mystery that has been the subject of interest to humans since the beginning of recorded history. It is intriguing to speculate that the answer to this riddle might indeed be near.

REFERENCES

1. Hayflick L, Moorehead PS. The serial cultivation of human diploid cell strains. Exp Cell Res 1961;25:585–621.
2. Harmon D. Aging: a theory based on free radical and radiation chemistry. J Gerontol 1956;11:298–300.
3. Orgel L. The maintenance of accuracy of protein synthesis and its relevance to aging. Proc Natl Acad Sci U S A 1963;49:517–521.
4. Burnet FM. An immunologic approach to aging. Lancet 1970;2: 358–360.
5. Landfield PW, Baskin RK, Pitler TA. Brain aging correlates: retardation by hormonal-pharmacological treatments. Science 1981;214: 581–584.
6. Bjorksten J. The cross linkage theory of aging. J Am Geriatr Soc 1968;16:408–427.
7. Hayflick L. Aging under glass. Exp Gerontol 1970;5:291–303.
8. Hayflick L. The biology of human aging. Am Med Sci 1973;265: 432–445.
9. Greider C, Blackburn E. A telomeric sequence in the RNA of *Tetrahymena* telomerase required for telomere repeat synthesis. Nature 1989;337:331–337.
10. Harley Calvin B, Villeponteau B. Telomeres and telomerase in aging and cancer. Curr Opin Genet Dev 1995;5:249–255.
11. Marx J. Chromosome ends catch fire. Science 1994;265:1656–1658.
12. McCay CM, Crowell MF, Maynard LA. The effect of retarded growth upon length of lifespan and upon ultimate body size. J Nutr 1935;10:63–79.
13. Goodrick CL. The effects of exercise on longevity and behavior of hybrid mice which differ in coat color. J Gerontol 1974;29:129–133.
14. Hayflick L. The biology of human aging. Plast Reconstr Surg 1981; 64:536–550.
15. Mazess RB. Health and longevity in Vilcabomba, Ecuador. JAMA 1978;240:1781.
16. Medvedev ZA. Caucasus and Altay longevity: a biologic or social problem. Gerontologist 1974;14:381–387.
17. Schneider EL, Reed JD. Life extension. N Engl J Med 1985;312: 1159–1167.
18. Lidman D. Histopathology of human extremital arteries throughout life including measurements of systolic pressures in ankle and arm. Acta Chir Scand 1982;148:575–580.
19. Mackay EH, Banks J, Sykes B, Lee G. Structural basis for the changing physical properties of human pulmonary vessels with age. Thorax 1978;33:335–344.
20. Warnock ML, Kunzmann A. Changes with age in muscular pulmonary arteries. Arch Pathol Lab Med 1977;101:175–179.
21. Banks J, Booth FVML, MacKay EH, et al. The physical behavior of human pulmonary arteries and veins. Clin Sci 1978;55:477–484.
22. Roach MR, Burton AC. The effect of age on the elasticity of human iliac arteries. Can J Biochem Physiol 1959;37:557–570.
23. Newman DL, Lallewood RC. The effect of age on the distensibility of the abdominal aorta of man. Surg Gynecol Obstet 1978;147:211–214.
24. Landowne M, Brondfoneuener M, Shock N. The relation of age to certain measures of performance of the heart and the circulation. Circulation 1955;12:567–576.
25. Vargas E, Lye M, Faragher EB, et al. Cardiovascular hemodynamics and the response of vasopressin, aldosterone, plasma renin activity and plasma catecholamines to head-up tilt in young and old healthy subjects. Age Ageing 1986;15:17–28.
26. Pomerance A. Cardiac Pathology in the Elderly. In Nobley RJ, Rothbaun DH (eds), Geriatric Cardiology, Cardiovascular Clinics (Vol 12). Philadelphia: Davis, 1981;9–54.
27. Reiner L, Mazzoleni A, Rodriguez FL, Freudenthal RR. The weight of the human heart. I. Normal cases. Arch Pathol 1959;68:58–73.
28. McMillan JB, Len M. The aging heart. I. Endocardium. J Gerontol 1959;14:268–283.
29. Gerstenblith G, Frederiksen J, Yin FCP, et al. Echocardiographic assessment of a normal adult aging population. Circulation 1977;56:273–278.
30. Harrison TR, Dixon K, Russell RO, et al. The relation of age to the duration of contraction, ejection, and relaxation of the normal human heart. Am Heart J 1964;67:190–191.
31. Petrofsky JS, Lind AR. Aging, isometric strength and endurance, and cardiovascular responses to static effort. J Appl Physiol 1975;38: 91–95.
32. Gribbin B, Pickering T, Sleight P, Peto R. Effect of age and high blood pressure on baroreflex sensitivity in man. Circ Res 1971;29:424–431.
33. Camm AJ, Evans KE, Ward DE, Martin A. The rhythm of the heart in active elderly subjects. Am Heart J 1980;99:598–603.
34. Kantelip JP, Sage E, Duchene-Marulloz P. Findings on ambulatory electrocardiographic monitoring in subjects older than 80 years. Am J Cardiol 1986;57:398–401.
35. Wahba WM. Influence of aging on lung function—clinical significance of changes from age twenty. Anesth Analg 1983;62:764–776.
36. Dhar S, Shastri SR, Lenora RAK. Aging and the respiratory system. Med Clin North Am 1976;60:1121–1139.
37. Pelzer AM, Thomson ML. Effect of age, sex, stature, and smoking habits on human airway conductance. J Appl Physiol 1966;21: 469–476.
38. Fowler RW. Ageing and lung function. Age Ageing 1985;14: 209–215.
39. Thurlbeck WM, Angus GE. Growth and aging of the normal human lung. Chest 1975;67:3S–7S.
40. Smith P, Heath D. The ultrastructure of age-associated intimal fibrosis in pulmonary blood vessels. J Pathol 1980;130:247–253.
41. Khan TA, Shragge BW, Crispin JS, Lind JF. Esophageal motility in the elderly. Digest Dis 1977;22:1049–1054.
42. Pelemans W, Vantrappen G. Esophageal disease in the elderly. Clin Gastroenterol 1985;14:635–656.
43. James OFW. Gastrointestinal and liver function in old age. Clin Gastroenterol 1983;12:671–691.
44. Steinheber FU. Ageing and the stomach. Clin Gastroenterol 1985;14: 657–688.
45. Webster SGP, Leeming JT. Assessment of small bowel function in the elderly using a modified xylose tolerance test. Gut 1975;16:109–113.
46. Evans MA, Triggs EJ, Cheung M. Gastric emptying rate in the elderly. Implications for drug therapy. J Am Geriatr Soc 1981;29: 201–205.
47. Kramer PA, Chapron DJ, Benson J, Mercik SA. Tetracycline absorption in elderly patients with achlorhydria. Clin Pharmacol Ther 1978;23:467–472.
48. Andrews GR, Haneman B, Arnold BJ, et al. Atrophic gastritis in the aged. Aust Ann Med 1967;16:230–235.
49. Bird T, Hall MRP, Schade ROK. Gastric histology and its relation to anaemia in the elderly. Gerontology 1977;23:309–321.
50. Giacosa A, Cheli R. Corrélations anatomo-sécrétories gastriques en fonction de l'âge chez des sujets ayant une muqueuse fundique normale. Gastroenterol Clin Biol 1979;3:647–650.

51. Bock OAA, Arapakis G, Witts LJ, Richards CD. The serum pepsinogen level with special reference to the histology of the gastric mucosa. Gut 1963;4:106–111.
52. Montgomery RD, Hainey MR, Ross IN, et al. The ageing gut: a study of intestinal absorption in relation to nutrition in the elderly. QJM 1978;47:197–211.
53. Feibusch J, Holt PR. Impaired absorptive capacity for carbohydrates in the elderly. Am J Clin Nutr 1979;32:942.
54. Holt PR. The small intestine. Clin Gastroenterol 1985;14:689–723.
55. Schuster MM. Disorders of the aging GI system. Hosp Prac 1976; 11:95–103.
56. Pace JL. A detailed study of musculature of the human large intestine [PhD thesis]. University of London, 1966.
57. Whiteway J, Morson BC. Pathology of the ageing—diverticular disease. Clin Gastroenterol 1985;14:829–846.
58. Drummond H. Sacculi of the large intestine with special reference to their relations to the blood vessels of the bowel wall. Br J Surg 1916;4:407–413.
59. Hodgson J. Transverse taeniamyotomy for diverticular disease. Dis Colon Rectum 1973;16:283–289.
60. Brocklehurst JC. Colonic disease in the elderly. Clin Gastroenterol 1985;14:725–747.
61. Loening-Baucke V, Anuras S. Effects of age and sex on anorectal manometry. Am J Gastroenterol 1985;80:50–53.
62. Calloway NO, Foley CF, Lagerbloom P. Uncertainties in geriatric data II: organ size. J Am Geriatr Soc 1965;13:20–28.
63. Thompson EN, Williams R. Effect of age on liver function with particular reference to bromsulfophthalein excretion. Gut 1965;6: 266–269.
64. Skauni V, Hulek P, Martinkova J. Changes in Kinetics of Exogenous Dyes in the Aging Process. In Kitani K (ed), Liver and Ageing. Amsterdam: Elsevier, 1978;115–130.
65. Tauchi H, Sato T. Hepatic Cells of the Aged. In Kitani K (ed), Liver and Ageing. Amsterdam: Elsevier, 1978;3–19.
66. Schaffner F, Popper H. Non-specific reactive hepatitis in aged and infirm people. Am J Digest Dis 1959;4:389–399.
67. Vestal RE, McGuire FA, Tobin JD, et al. Ageing and ethanol metabolism. Clin Pharmacol Ther 1977;21:343–354.
68. Salem SAM, Rajjayal Nun P, Shepherd AM, Stevenson IH. Reduced induction of drug metabolism in the elderly. Age Ageing 1978;7: 68–73.
69. Bateson MC, Bouchier IAD. Prevalence of gallstones in Dundee: a necropsy study. BMJ 1975;4:427–430.
70. Valdivieso V, Palma R, Wunkaus R, et al. Effect of ageing on biliary lipid composition and bile acid metabolism in normal Chilean women. Gastroenterology 1978;74:871–874.
71. Weill-Bousson M, Bushcer P, Geisler F. Pancreas du sujet age. Aspects anatomopathologiques. Ann Gastroenterol Hepatol 1979;15: 568–573.
72. Walters MNI. Studies on the pancreas I. Non-specific pancreatic ductular ectasia. Am J Pathol 1964;19:973–981.
73. Schmitz-Moormann P, Himmelmann G, Brandes HJ, et al. Quantitative Assessment of Pancreatitis-Like Lesions in Humans Without Pancreatic Disease. In Gyr KE, Singer MV, Sarles H (eds), Pancreatitis Concepts and Classification. Amsterdam: Elsevier, 1984;67–70.
74. Moessner J, Pusch HJ, Koch W. Die Exkretorische pankreas funktion altersveranderungen Ja oder Nein? Aktuelle Gerontol 1982; 12:40–43.
75. Laugier R, Sarles H. The pancreas. Clin Gastroenterol 1985;14: 749–756.
76. Citi S, Salvini L. The intestinal absorption of 131-labelled olein and triolein, of 58 Co vitamin B and 59 Fe, in aged subjects. J Gerontol 1961;12:123–126.
77. McEvoy A. Investigation of Intestinal Malabsorption in the Elderly. In Evans JG, Caird FE (eds), Advanced Geriatric Medicine 2. London: Pitman, 1982;100–110.
78. Zago MA, Figueiredo MA, Covas DT, Bottura C. Aspects of splenic hypofunction in old age. Klin Wochenschr 1985;63:590–592.
79. Vaziri H, Dragowska W, Allsopp RC, et al. Evidence for a mitotic clock in human hematopoietic stem cells: loss of telomeric DNA with age. Proc Natl Acad Sci U S A 1994;91:9857–9860.
80. Macieria-Coelho A. The implications of the 'Hayflick limit' for aging of the organism have been misunderstood by many gerontologists. Gerontology 1995;41:94–97.
81. McLaughlin B, O'Malley K, Cotter TG. Age-related differences in granulocyte chemotaxis and degranulation. Clin Sci 1986;70:59–62.
82. Nielsen H, Blom J, Larsen SO. Human blood monocyte function in relation to age. Acta Pathol Microbiol Immunol Scand 1984;92: 5–10.
83. Lipschitz DA, Udupa KB, Milton KY, Thompson CO. Effect of age on hematopoiesis in men. Blood 1984;63:502–509.
84. Lewis R. Anemia—a common but never a normal concomitant of aging. Geriatrics 1976;31:53–60.
85. Delafuente JC. Immunosenescence. Clinical and pharmacologic considerations. Med Clin North Am 1985;69:475–486.
86. Busby J, Caranasos GJ. Immune function, autoimmunity, and selective immunoprophylaxis in the aged. Med Clin North Am 1985; 69:465–474.
87. Weksler MD. Senescence of the immune system. Med Clin North Am 1983;67:263–272.
88. Roessle R, Roulet F. Nieren. In Mass und Zahl in der Pathologie. Berlin: Springer, 1932;63–66.
89. Dunnill MS, Halley W. Some observations on the quantitative anatomy of the kidney. J Pathol 1973;110:113–121.
90. Takazakura E, Sawabu K, Hande A, et al. Intrarenal vascular changes with age and disease. Kidney Int 1972;2:224–230.
91. Epstein M. Effects of aging on the kidney. Fed Proc 1979;38:168–172.
92. Shock NW. Current trends in research on the physiological aspects of aging. J Am Geriatr Soc 1967;15:995–1000.
93. Rowe JW, Shock NW, DeFronzo RA. The influence of age on the renal response to water deprivation in man. Nephron 1976;17:270–278.
94. Weidmann P, De-Myttenaere-Bursztein S, Maxwell MH, DeLima J. Effect of aging on plasma renin and aldosterone in normal man. Kidney Int 1975;8:325–333.
95. Millington PF, Wilkinson R. Changes in skin with age. Scand J Clin Lab Invest 1973;34(Suppl 141):52–53.
96. West MD. The cellular and molecular biology of skin aging. Arch Dermatol 1994;130:87–95.
97. McConkey B, Fraser GM, Thigh AS, Whiteley H. Transparent skin and osteoporosis. Lancet 1963;1:693–695.
98. Shuster S, Bottoms E. Senile degeneration of skin collagen. Clin Sci 1963;25:487–491.
99. Ryckwaert A, Parot S, Tamisier S. Variations, sélon l'âge et le sexe, de l'épaisseur du pli cutane mésure du dos de la main. Rev Fr Etud Biol 1967;12:803–806.
100. Long DM. Aging in the nervous system. Neurosurgery 1985;17: 348–354.
101. Brizzee KR. Gross morphometric analyses and quantitative histology of the aging brain. Adv Behav Biol 1975;16:401–423.
102. Kaack B, Ordy JM, Trapp B. Changes in limbic, neuroendocrine and autonomic systems, adaptation, and homeostasis during aging. Adv Behav Biol 1975;16:209–231.
103. Kokmen E, Bossemeyer RW, Barney J, Williams WJ. Neurological manifestations of aging. J Gerontol 1977;32:411–419.
104. Samorajski T. How the human brain responds to aging. J Am Geriatr Soc 1976;24:4–11.
105. Dilman VM. Age-associated elevation of hypothalamic threshold to feedback control and its role in development, ageing, and disease. Lancet 1971;1:1211–1219.
106. Everitt AV. The hypothalamic-pituitary control of ageing and age related pathology. Exp Gerontol 1973;8:265–277.
107. Pfeifer MA, Weinberg CR, Cook D, et al. Differential changes of autonomic nervous system function with age in man. Am J Med 1983;75:249–258.
108. Kaplan FS, Nixon JE, Reitz M, et al. Age-related changes in proprioception and sensation of joint position. Acta Orthop Scand 1985;56:72–74.
109. Skinner HB, Barrack RL, Cook SD. Age-related decline in proprioception. Clin Orthop 1984;184:208–211.
110. McConnell JG, Buchanon KD, Ardill J, Stout RW. Glucose tolerance in the elderly: the role of insulin and its receptor. Euro J Clin Invest 1982;12:55–61.
111. Chen M, Bergman RN, Pacini G, Porte D. Pathogenesis of age-related glucose intolerance in man: insulin resistance and decreased B-cell function. J Clin Endocrinol Metab 1985;60:13–20.
112. Fink RL, Wallace P, Olefsky JM. Effects of aging on glucose-mediated glucose disposal and glucose transport. J Clin Invest 1986;77:2034–2041.

113. Fink RI, Revers RR, Koherman OG, Olefsky JM. The metabolic clearance of insulin and the feedback inhibition of insulin secretion are altered with aging. Diabetes 1985;34:275–280.
114. Grobin W. Progressive deterioration of glucose transport in the aged. J Am Geriatr Soc 1975;23:31–37.
115. Meneilly GS, Miraker KL, Young JB, Landsberg L. Induced glucose reduction in the elderly. J Clin Endocrinol Metab 1985;61:178–182.
116. Simonson DC, DeGronzo RA. Glucagon physiology and aging: evidence for enhanced hepatic sensitivity. Diabetologia 1983;25:1–7.
117. Sirota DK. Thyroid function and dysfunction in the elderly: a brief review. Mt Sinai J Med 1980;47:126–131.
118. Sawin CT, Chopra D, Azizi F, et al. The aging thyroid: increased prevalence of elevated serum thyrotropin levels in the elderly. JAMA 1979;242:247–250.
119. Harmon SM, Wehmann RE, Blackman MR. Pituitary-thyroid hormone economy in healthy aging men: basal indices of thyroid function and thyrotropin responses to constant infusions of thyrotropin-releasing hormone. J Clin Endocrinol Metab 1984;58:320–326.
120. Ingbar SH. Effect of aging on thyroid economy in man. J Am Geriatr Soc 1976;24:49–53.
121. Berlyne GM, BenAri J, Kucheleusky A, et al. The etiology of senile osteoporosis: secondary hyperparathyroidism due to renal failure. QJM 1975;44:501–521.
122. Marcus R, Madriug P, Young G. Age-related changes in parathyroid hormone and parathyroid hormone action in normal humans. J Clin Endocrinol Metab 1984;58:223–230.
123. Gallagher JC, Riggs BL, Jerpbok CM, Arnaud CD. The effect of age on serum immunoreactive parathyroid hormone in normal and osteoporotic women. J Lab Clin Med 1980;95:373–385.
124. Roos BA, Bergeron G, Guggenheim K, Deftos LJ. Maturational increases in plasma calcitonin related to gastrointestinal function. Clin Res 1977;25:398A.
125. Baker HWG, Bwger HG, de Hretser DM, et al. Changes in the pituitary-testicular system with age. Clin Endocrinol 1976;5:349–372.
126. Takahashi J, Higashi Y, LaNasa JA, et al. Studies of the human testis. XVIII. Simultaneous measurement of nine intratesticular steroids: evidence for reduced mitochondrial function in testis of elderly men. J Clin Endocrinol Metab 1983;56:1178–1187.
127. Kinsey AC, Pomeroy WB, Martin CE. Sexual Behavior in the Human Male. Philadelphia: Saunders, 1948.
128. Monroe SE, Menon KMJ. Changes in reproductive hormone secretion during the climacteric and postmenopausal periods. Clin Obstet Gynecol 1977;20:113–122.
129. Sherman B, Wysham C, Pfohl B. Age-related changes in the circadian rhythm of plasma cortisol in man. J Clin Endocrinol Metab 1985; 61:439–443.
130. Dilman VM, Ostroumova MN, Tsyrlina EV. Hypothalamic mechanisms of ageing and of specific age pathology. II. On the sensitivity threshold of hypothalamo-pituitary complex to homeostatic stimuli in adaptive homeostasis. Exp Gerontol 1978;14:175–181.
131. Mongioi A, Vicari E, D'Agata R. The prolactin-secreting system in relation to aging. J Endocrinol Invest 1985;8(Suppl 2):33–39.
132. Kovacs K, Ryan N, Horrath E, et al. Prolactin cells of the human pituitary gland in old age. J Gerontol 1977;32:534–540.
133. Casale G, Pecorini M, Cuzzoni G, deNicola P. Beta-endorphin and cold pressor test in the aged. Gerontology 1985;31:101–105.
134. Shibasaki T, Shizume K, Nakahara M, et al. Age-related changes in plasma growth hormone response to growth hormone-releasing factor in man. J Clin Endocrinol Metab 1984;58:212–214.
135. Tsunoda K, Abe K, Goto T, et al. Effect of age on the renin-angiotensin-aldosterone system in normal subjects: simultaneous measurement of active and inactive renin, renin-substrate and aldosterone in plasma. J Clin Endocrinol Metab 1986;62:384–389.
136. Hegstad R, Brown R, Jiang NS, et al. Aging and aldosterone. Am J Med 1983;74:442–448.
137. Ziegler MG, Lake CR, Kopin IJ. Plasma noradrenaline increases with age. Nature 1976;261:333–335.
138. Conway J, Wheeler R, Sunnerstedt R. Sympathetic nervous activity during exercise in relation to age. Cardiovasc Res 1971;5:577–581.
139. Haas A, Flammer J, Schneider U. Influence of age on the visual fields of normal subjects. Am J Ophthalmol 1986;101:199–203.
140. Millodot M, Owens H. The influence of age on the fragility of the cornea. Acta Ophthalmol 1984;62:819–824.
141. Wuest FC, Sayther KD, Carlson CA, Wicklund PE. The aging eye. Minn Med 1976;59:540–546.
142. Leske MC, Sperduto RD. The epidemiology of senile cataracts: a review. Am J Epidemiol 1983;118:152–165.
143. Podgor MJ, Leske MC, Ederer F. Incidence estimates for lens changes, macular changes, open-angle glaucoma and diabetic retinopathy. Am J Epidemiol 1983;118:206–212.
144. Kahn HA, Leibowitz HM, Ganley JP, et al. The Framingham Eye Study. II. Association of ophthalmic pathology with variables previously measured in the Framingham Heart Study. Am J Epidemiol 1977;106:33–41.
145. Taylor HR. The environment and the lens. Br J Ophthalmol 1980;64: 303–310.
146. Weingeist TA. Macular degeneration associated with aging. J Iowa Med Soc 1983;73:502–505.
147. Balazsi AG, Rootman J, Drance SM, et al. The effect of age on the nerve fiber population of the human optic nerve. Am J Ophthalmol 1984;97:760–766.
148. Anderson RG, Meyerhoff WL. Otologic manifestations of aging. Otolaryngol Clin North Am 1982;15:353–369.
149. Perry ET. The Human Ear Canal. Springfield, IL: Thomas, 1957;57–70.
150. Etholm B, Belal A. Senile changes in the middle ear joints. Ann Otol 1974;83:49–54.
151. Glorig A, Davis H. Age, noise, and hearing loss. Ann Otol 1961;70: 556–571.
152. Rosen S. Presbycusis study of a relatively noise-free population in Sudan. Ann Otol 1962;71:727–743.
153. Bergstrom B. Morphology of the vestibular nerve. Acta Otolaryngol 1973;76:173–179.
154. Rosenhall U. Degenerative patterns in the aging human vestibular neuro-epithelia. Acta Otolaryngol 1973;76:208–220.
155. Moller P. Skeletal muscle adaptation to aging and to respiratory and liver failure. Acta Medica Scand 1981;654:1–40.
156. Grimby G, Saltin B. Mini-review. The ageing muscle. Clin Physiol 1983;3:209–218.
157. Essen-Gustavsson B, Borges O. Histochemical and metabolic characteristics of human skeletal muscle in relation to age. Acta Physiol Scand 1986;126:107–114.
158. Inokuchi S, Ishikawa H, Iwamoto S, Kimura T. Age-related changes in the histological composition of the rectus abdominis muscle of the adult human. Hum Biol 1975;47:231–249.
159. Burnstein AH, Reilly DT, Martens M. Aging of bone tissue: mechanical properties. J Bone Joint Surg Am 1976;58:82–86.
160. Schmidt UJ, Kalbe I, Sielaff F. Bone aging. Adv Exp Med Biol 1975;53:371–374.
161. Sharpe WD. Age changes in human bone: an overview. Bull N Y Acad Med 1979;55:757–773.
162. Tsai KS, Heath H, Kumar R, Riggs BL. Impaired vitamin D metabolism with aging in women. J Clin Invest 1984;73:1668–1672.
163. Twomey L, Taylor J, Furriss B. Age changes in the bone density and structure of the lumbar vertebral column. J Anat 1983;136:15–25.
164. Evans DAP, Burbach JPH, van Leeuwen FW. Somatic mutations in the brain: relationship to aging? Mutat Res 1995;338:173–182.
165. Kadenbach B, Munscher C, Frank V. Human aging is associated with stochastic somatic mutations of mitochondrion DNA. Mutat Res 1995;338:161–172.
166. Kerr JFR, Wyllie AH, Currie AR. Apoptosis: a basic biological phenomenon with wide-ranging implications in tissue kinetics. Br J Cancer 1972;26:239.
167. Kroemer G, Petit P, Zamzami N. The biochemistry of programmed cell death. FASEB J 1995;9:1277–1287.
168. Blackburn EH. Telomerases. Annu Rev Biochem 1992;61:113–129.
169. Sancar A. DNA repairs in humans. Annu Rev Genet 1995;29: 69–105.

Surgical Care for the Elderly, 2nd ed., edited by
R. Benton Adkins, Jr., and H. William Scott, Jr.
Lippincott–Raven Publishers, Philadelphia © 1998.

CHAPTER 3

Age and the Surgeon

Mary C. Proctor and Lazar J. Greenfield

To see youth as the preferred stage of life is a dangerous perception that may result in untold pain for those who have passed this milestone. An essayist tells us how to avoid this state of mind: "Remember that youth does not last and that by keeping thoughts to the future, we might never grieve for the past" [1]. For many, the advancing years are seen in negative terms, a time of loss and minimization, rather than as points along a continuum. In other cultures, age is equated with wisdom. The Japanese celebrate Respect for the Aged Day as a means of demonstrating their reverence for those who have successfully negotiated the obstacles of youth and middle age and are able to share their hard-won knowledge.

To ensure a satisfying later life, it is helpful to develop an accurate understanding of the aging process—biological, psychological, and social—and to dispel any misconceptions [2]. Physicians experience the changes associated with aging no differently from their age-mates. The material presented in the foregoing chapters describes these changes in detail. Armed with this knowledge, surgeons can adapt their practice to account for the age of their patients and begin to plan for that time when they are ready to move on to the next phase of their careers. With good fortune, the transition will be self-selected and smooth, but regardless, it will take place.

By 2030, when the "baby boomers" approach early old age, 20% of Americans will be older than 60 years of age. This will severely challenge the resources of the medical community. The vast number of individuals requiring care with all the associated economic implications will tax the already stretched Medicare system. From another perspective, the number of physicians who are as old or older than their patients will challenge the ingenuity of the medical establishment. Failure to deal with these realities will doom physicians to a disappointing and unfulfilling later life.

In this chapter we address the ways in which the changes associated with aging affect physician performance. The economic factors affecting both the surgeon and the practice setting are discussed, as well as factors leading to a rewarding retirement. Finally, the ethical concerns facing the patient, surgeon, and society are explored.

PHYSIOLOGY OF AGING AND PHYSICIAN PERFORMANCE

Youth can be distinguished from old age by both physiologic and pathologic characteristics. The effects of aging can be recognized in decreased strength and stability, stiffness, reduced reaction time, impaired memory, and overall decline [3]. One of the problems is a lack of age-specific norms for the customary evaluation tests. The Baltimore Longitudinal study is currently attempting to establish norms of physiologic functioning for those in the middle years and older [4]. People age at various rates, and within individuals, one system may age more rapidly than others. These differences are due to both genetic and environmental factors. To try to characterize individuals solely by a chronological measure leads to serious errors. To evaluate the effects of aging, it is necessary to study individuals system by system using physical examination, laboratory tests, tests of functional ability, and self-reports.

The physiologic effects of age are detailed throughout this text, and the reader is referred to the appropriate chapters. There is little reason to believe that the surgeon should be spared these effects. We have selected a few systems for additional review, with special attention to the effects they may have on the performance of the surgeon.

Among the problems that age imposes on the cardiovascular system is a decrease in systolic pressure and ejection volume. The consequences may be a decline in physical reserve. Surgery is a discipline that requires significant stamina, and loss of this reserve may limit the types of procedures that a surgeon is willing to undertake.

Age also results in loss of static visual acuity, which limits the ability to discriminate fine, high-contrast details. There is reduction of the visual field, and the frightening fact is that less than half of those with this condition are aware of it. Depth perception is reduced. There is hardening of the lens, reducing the light admitted to the retina and limiting the ability to focus on near objects. In addition, the ability to dilate the pupil decreases. Problems with color perception, especially blue and green, develop as the lens yellows. Cataracts and glaucoma are eight times more common among those >65 years of age, and these limit the ability to focus on both static and moving items. Any of these changes can affect the performance of a surgeon.

Hearing also changes with time. Nearly 24% of those aged 65 to 74 develop hearing impairment. This may be more significant for surgeons because the constant background noise in the operating room may interfere with communication. For those with moderate hearing loss, lip reading may provide additional information, but the use of a surgical mask, precludes this assistance in the operating room.

Arthritis presents a major limitation to motion in 40% of those between 65 and 74 years. The dexterity required for psychomotor functions declines with age, and these activities require longer to perform. The dropped instrument or cramped fingers may become a more frequent experience.

Cognition involves attention, stimulus recognition, and response. Age may limit the ability to focus attention and interfere with selectively attending to the most important stimulus [5]. The ability to process information slows, which may be associated with declines in performance of complex multifactor tasks. As these limitations increase, organic brain syndrome may be suspected. Typical signs include loss of interest in appearance and environment, overprescribing, forgetfulness (missing meetings or appointments), loss of concentration, tremulousness, and confusion. With respect to intelligence testing, losses on performance scales are greater than those on verbal scales. Overall, intelligence tests show a deleterious association between deviations from ideal health and test scores [4].

The psychological effects of aging are unavoidable. Changes in hair color, texture, and quantity; skin tone; wrinkles; and weight distribution may have a profound psychological impact. The slowed pace that may be imposed by age places one out of synchrony with the rest of the world and may cause conflict and psychological discomfort.

One of the more encouraging findings is that creativity and scientific output do not suffer the ill effects of aging. For many, the natural slowing related to age provides time for increased creative expression.

EFFECTS OF AGING ON PERFORMANCE

The physical and psychological changes associated with the aging process may cause difficulty in daily practice. Three areas are vulnerable to the limitations: patient assessment, manual dexterity, and the need to keep up with scientific advances.

The ability to accurately assess a patient is essential to providing quality care. Clinicians who are demonstrating the effects of aging with respect to vision may find it difficult to accurately assess a patient, perceive subtle changes in a wound, or read a monitor. Loss of visual field and depth perception may lead to errors during surgical procedures or result in undetected problems.

Among those experiencing cognitive difficulties, errors in diagnosis may be made as a result of failing to make the proper associations or to appreciate the significance of a patient's complaint. The inability to sustain concentration may seriously impair the ability to complete long procedures. Surgical errors may occur as a result of the combination of visual and information-processing limitations.

Manual dexterity can be problematic. With age, motor response time increases: This can impose serious limitations in the operating room. Years of repetitive practice can offset some of the decline but, ultimately, performance is negatively affected. Problems with dexterity may be associated with the stiffness caused by arthritis as well as gross motor activities such as rotating the upper torso. As many as 12.6% of those between 65 and 74 years of age report problems conducting activities of daily living, and the number approaches 25% in those between 75 and 84 years of age. These limitations carry over to the operating room.

To remain effective, the surgeon must keep up with changes in technology. Concerns regarding the ability to keep current and remain competent are voiced by many aged surgeons. They fear the rejection and disrespect of younger colleagues if they are found to be outdated. They may also find that the time required to master new techniques is not warranted by the relatively short period they will remain in practice.

The use of laser techniques has significantly simplified many surgical interventions. The public's awareness of the benefits of laparoscopic procedures is increasing the demand for this less invasive surgical approach. These new techniques require excellent hand-eye coordination and the ability to operate by visual cues from a television monitor, rather than by touch. This may be an impossible transition for those already experiencing limitations in visual acuity and manual dexterity.

All surgeons are challenged to remain current in their knowledge, but the aged find it increasingly more difficult to adapt. Routine cases can normally be carried out successfully by the surgeon experiencing the effects of age, but if the case becomes more complex and problem solving requires more steps, the surgeon may lose up to 30% of the speed and efficiency necessary to bring the case to a successful conclusion [5].

There is a need to identify the visual, cognitive, and psychomotor impairments associated with increasing surgical risk. There may also be unidentified characteristics associated with surgical risk. Research needs to be aimed at learning how attentiveness, information processing, and problem-solving ability are distributed across the full age range of surgeons so that we can better understand the effects of age and their implications [5].

ECONOMIC IMPLICATIONS

Financial concerns often keep surgeons operating beyond their prime. For those in private practice, there may be no

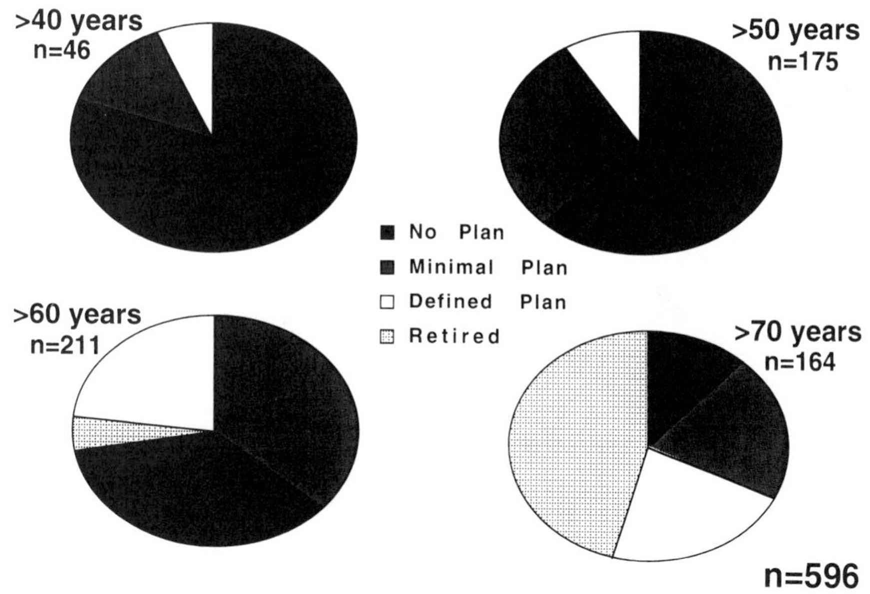

FIG. 3-1. Extent of plan for retirement by age group. Extent of planning for retirement varied significantly (P <0.001) among age groups as shown. The respondents who indicated that they already had retired also are shown. (With permission from Greenfield LJ, Proctor MC. Attitudes toward retirement. A survey of the American Surgical Association. Ann Surg 1994;220:382–390.)

safety net of a funded retirement policy. Many have yielded to the temptation to live for today and let the future sort itself out. For others, there are the economic burdens of a second marriage and the costs of educating additional children.

Few surgeons have taken the time to determine the style of life they wish to assume during retirement and to make adequate provisions for health care. In a recent survey of the American Surgical Association members [6], we found that only a small percentage of surgeons under 70 had a well-defined plan for future finances (Fig. 3-1). Those who planned to work on a reduced schedule often find that the cost of malpractice insurance wipes out any potential financial gain.

Surgeons who remain in practice beyond their ability inflict economic loss on themselves in that they tend to run down the value of their practice so that when it is time to sell, the return is far less than anticipated. Not only their patients but also their referring physicians are aging and the practice size declines. Peers who have referred patients leave practice and younger practitioners tend to refer their patients to contemporaries. Other physicians who observe the effects of age or reports of surgical mishaps may change their referral pattern.

The effects of aging also have implications for the practice group. For the surgeon who recognizes his limitations and begins to reduce his total number of cases or refuses to accept the more difficult cases, there is an associated decrease in revenue, which affects all of the partners. In addition, these older surgeons are at the high end of the pay scale, which drains the group resources if they cannot generate expected revenue. A surgical mishap resulting in a lost malpractice suit can have significant impact on the financial status of the practice. Finally, when the senior surgeon refuses to step aside, the group is prevented from recruiting younger surgeons due to the salary overhead.

RETIREMENT

While the economic effects of aging are significant, the larger question of retirement is a major turning point for surgeons because it significantly affects their self-image. For most individuals, work is their self-defining activity, and retirement is traumatic because it deprives them of membership in adult society [4]. For the surgeon, retirement is even more traumatic because it represents the loss of identification as a physician [7,8]. Several excuses are given for not retiring—economics, job satisfaction, or contribution to society—but the real reason is that surgeons know little outside of medicine and often cannot conceive of life beyond surgery. Many have formed a jaundiced attitude about retirement because the majority of retired persons they come in contact with are ill and seeking medical care [9]. Many surgeons want to die with scalpel in hand, but if the blade becomes dull, the result is disastrous [10].

Attitude is far more significant to postretirement adjustment than the circumstances that led to retirement [4]. It is necessary to develop a philosophy that separates self-esteem from productivity and allows one to accept the changes related to age. Failure to plan for retirement is a serious mistake, as one cannot withdraw from something without moving toward something else [11]. Planning for successful retirement should take place over 1 to 2 years. Various sources indicate the importance of the participation of a life partner in the planning for life after medicine and suggest that the selection of a companionable mate is an essential component [3,11]. Some type of second career is almost essential to a satisfying old age. Without a plan, retirement will be plagued by anxiety, discontent, unhappiness, and even illness [3,12].

Several medical-related avenues are open to surgeons (Fig. 3-2). They can remain active in teaching and research

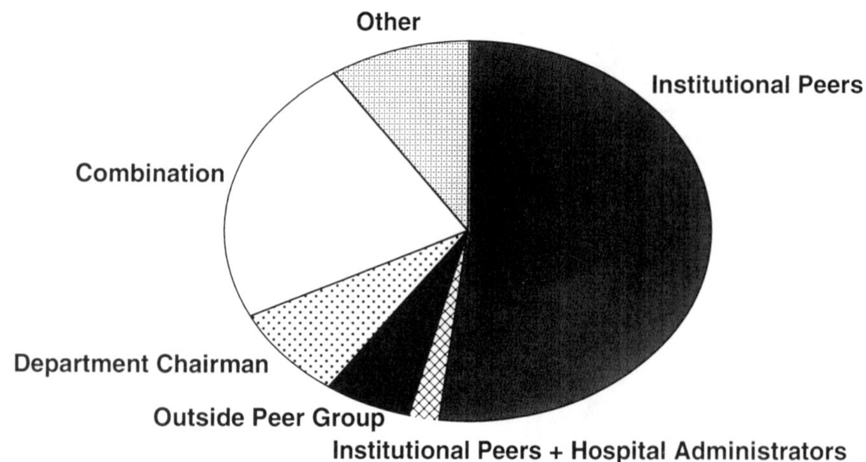

FIG. 3-2. Method of peer review. Further response on peer review showed a majority in favor of institutional peers as opposed to outside group or department chair. (With permission from Greenfield LJ, Proctor MC. Attitudes toward retirement. A survey of the American Surgical Association. Ann Surg 1994;220:382–390.)

or can move into administrative areas. Others devote time to volunteer work among the poor or in government programs. Writing is also a viable alternative. Some of these activities may be new because few physicians have sufficient time to devote to volunteer work during their working years. A series of articles written years ago in the *Bulletin of the New York Academy of Medicine* profiles the activities and attitudes of a number of physicians [1,3,10–12]. It provides useful insights into the roles they assumed in retirement and demonstrates how they were able to accentuate the positive aspects of age while avoiding the negative outcomes of practicing beyond their time. These reflections include both medical as well as unrelated retirement pursuits.

Those whose retirement plans are foreign to their previous work may have difficulty adjusting, but many surgeons have unfulfilled creative potential that can be developed during retirement, providing both personal satisfaction and economic reward.

ETHICAL CONCERNS

In determining when a surgeon should consider retirement, the needs of the patients and of society at large also need to be taken into account. The impact of age on memory and judgment may develop so slowly that neither the physician nor his or her colleagues are aware of the impairment. However, this may place the welfare of the patient at risk. It may breach the public trust placed in the profession and destroy the reputation of the physician. As a general rule, the surgeon must retire before the point at which age becomes a factor that must be calculated into the risk-to-benefit equation for the patient.

Age has frequently been used as a public policy criterion in areas such as social security, tax benefits, voting privileges, and so forth. Before the Age Discrimination Act of 1975, many institutions forced retirement at age 65. This process was thought to protect the patient as well as the surgeon because no stigma was associated with mandatory retirement. When age could no longer be used as the objective standard, it became extremely difficult to determine when a surgeon should step aside. The additional risk associated with the age of the surgeon results from several different performance characteristics for which there are no established objective tests. There is a need to determine how attentiveness, information processing, and problem solving are distributed across the full age distribution of surgeons [5]. A battery of neuropsychological tests has been developed by Powell et al. that may provide a means of determining the effects of age [13]. Norms have been determined for physicians in general but not for surgeons in particular. Attempts to conduct a pilot study at the authors' own institution have proved difficult due to the hesitancy of the faculty to be evaluated, which highlights the reluctance with which surgeons approach this issue. When surveyed, most surgeons believed that a body of peers provided the best guide for determining when a colleague ought to retire, but that they were the best judge of their own ability to continue working [6] (see Fig. 3-2).

Many questions remain to be addressed, such as: Who should bear the responsibility for deciding when a surgeon should step down? What type of physical and mental testing is appropriate? What is the responsibility owed to patients and referring physicians?

A way must be found to assure society that the older surgeon has the physical and mental stamina, coordination, reaction time, and quick judgment to provide appropriate care [14]. Individuals age at different rates and, within individuals, systems age differently, making mandatory retirement an inappropriate standard. The Age Discrimination Act prohibits

its use except in situations when age can critically affect the individual's ability to perform [6]. We have not reached the point at which we are able to determine when the effects of age of the surgeon become a risk to the patient. We must find methods to measure visual, cognitive, and psychomotor impairments associated with increasing the risk of surgery and to determine when the deficits become significant [14].

The patient and society, as well as the surgeon, deserve to be protected from the changes in performance brought on by increasing age. We must discover tests to measure the point at which these changes affect surgical outcome and finally to find means of preparing the aging surgeon to move into a new career phase that will allow him or her to continue to be a contributing member to both the medical and larger worlds for as long as he or she is able.

REFERENCES

1. Berry FB. Preface to symposium: introduction to old age. Bull N Y Acad Med 1971;47:1245–1247.
2. Portnoi VA. The natural history of retirement. Mainly good news. JAMA 1981;245:1752–1754.
3. Cole WH. Problems and opportunities for the aged. Bull N Y Acad Med 1971;47:1318–1330.
4. Belsky J. The Psychology of Aging Theory, Research, and Practice. Monterey, CA: Brooks & Cole, 1984.
5. Committee for the Study on Improving Mobility and Safety for Older Persons. Transportation in an Aging Society. Washington, DC: National Research Council, 1988.
6. Greenfield LJ, Proctor MC. Attitudes toward retirement. A survey of the American Surgical Association. Ann Surg 1994;220:382–390.
7. Grauer H, Campbell NM. The aging physician and retirement. Can J Psychiatry 1983;28:552–554.
8. Virshup B, Coombs RH. Physicians' adjustment to retirement. West J Med 1993;158:142–144.
9. Vincent MO. Free to retire? Can Med Assoc J 1979;120:1001–1002, 1022.
10. Maynard EP Jr. Should we die with our boots on? Bull N Y Acad Med 1971;47:1350–1354.
11. Sulzberger MB. Age and retirement. Bull N Y Acad Med 1971;47: 1311–1317.
12. Garland J. The shortened step. Bull N Y Acad Med 1971;47: 1276–1280.
13. Powell DH. Profiles in Cognitive Aging. Cambridge, MA: Harvard University Press, 1994.
14. Schmitz RL. The elderly surgeon. Proc Inst Med Chgo 1988;41:134.

SECTION II

Fundamentals of Surgical Care for the Elderly

Surgical Care for the Elderly, 2nd ed., edited by
R. Benton Adkins, Jr., and H. William Scott, Jr.
Lippincott–Raven Publishers, Philadelphia © 1998.

CHAPTER 4

Management of Perioperative Problems in the Aged

James S. Powers and F. Tremaine Billings, Jr.

PREVALENCE OF SURGERY IN THE AGED

Persons over age 65 are increasing both in absolute numbers and in relative proportion of the American population. In 1900, 3 million individuals, or 4% of the population, were over age 65. In 1990, 56 million, or 13% of the population were over age 65, and there are now approximately 100,000 individuals aged 100 years. Population projections estimate that 25% of the American population will be over age 65 by the early part of the twenty-first century. Indeed, individuals over the age of 85 are the fastest growing segment of the population [1,2].

There were 100 million surgical procedures performed in 1990. Patients over age 65 account for 20% to 40% of surgical procedures, 50% of emergency procedures, and 75% of surgical mortality [3]. Surgical procedures are being performed with increased frequency in older patients (Table 4-1).

Age itself, however, accounts for little of the excessive mortality in surgical procedures; rather, the presence of coexisting disease processes is the most important determinant of operative risk. All evidence indicates that major surgical procedures can be performed without excessive morbidity and mortality in selected patients, and that the operative risk of these procedures has decreased in recent years due to improved surgical techniques, safer anesthetic agents, and improved perioperative care. The provision of surgical care that may reverse or retard disease processes is an important therapeutic modality that should not be denied a patient solely on the basis of age (Table 4-2).

OPERATIVE RISKS ASSOCIATED WITH AGING

Perioperative deaths are divided into three categories. Approximately 10% to 15% of perioperative mortality occurs during induction of anesthesia, 30% to 40% occurs in the operating room, and 50% to 60% occurs within 48 hours postoperatively [4].

Cardiovascular complications are the most important cause of mortality, making up 3% to 5% of perioperative mortality in older patients. The risk of postoperative myocardial infarction is 1% to 4%, and the risk of congestive heart failure (CHF) is 4% to 10%. Respiratory complications are the most common cause of postoperative morbidity in older persons, affecting approximately 15% to 45%, due to pneumonia in half the cases. Postoperative delirium occurs in 10% to 15% of elderly patients [5]. Approximately 10% to 50% of all elderly surgical patients develop deep vein thromboses [6].

The high prevalence of risk associated with surgical treatment of the older individual should encourage careful selection of appropriate surgical candidates, with objective weighing of the risks and benefits associated with the proposed procedure. An aggressive effort to optimize preoperative status in the older patient will maximize postoperative outcome. The perioperative mortality of urgent cases is approximately eight times that of elective cases, and the mortality associated with emergency cases may be as high as 15 times that of elective cases [7].

The higher risks of surgical care associated with aging should not preclude operating on any older patients. Age as an independent risk factor is not the most important parameter in assessing the operative risk in the older individual. Analyses of the characteristics of elderly patients who sustain operative complications have identified numerous physiologic parameters with clear implications for decreasing operative risk by improving clinical management [8].

SUPPORT SERVICES

Multidisciplinary Care Needs

The care of the older patient is characterized by a multitude of needs representing many different domains. Just as the medical and surgical problems affecting the older patient

TABLE 4-1. *Surgical procedures in the elderly*

Procedure	Number of procedures per year, by age*	
	65–74 years	>75 years
Cardiac catheterization	296	150
Prostatectomy	158	138
Coronary artery bypass graft	146	60
Cholecystectomy	107	77
Pacemaker	85	160
Partial colon resection	67	72
Wound debridement	58	79
Open reduction of fracture	50	120

*Numbers of procedures performed in thousands.

Source: National Center for Health Statistics. Detailed diagnosis and procedures, National Hospital Discharge Survey, 1990. DHHS Publication No. (PHS) 92-1773. Hyattsville, MD: U.S. Department of Health and Human Services, 1992.

TABLE 4-2. *Perioperative concerns in older patients*

Decision to operate
Medical considerations
Ethical considerations
Effects of acute illness
Associated diseases
Anesthesia
Surgical procedures
Adequacy of postsurgical follow-up
In hospital
Postdischarge

Source: Modified from Keating HJ, Lubin MF. Perioperative responsibilities of the physician/geriatrician. Clin Geriatr Med 1990;6:459–467.

can cross many disciplines and require a coordinated approach among medical and surgical consultants, the older patient often has multiple additional needs in the social, psychological, economic, rehabilitative, and nursing spheres. It is important to anticipate, identify, and address these potential issues early during hospitalization to maximize success.

When treating particularly complicated disease processes in older patients, many centers have found that using a multidisciplinary geriatric team often helps to coordinate the many care needs and services required by the older surgical patient. The expertise of health professionals in the fields of nutrition, social work, nursing, pharmacy, medical ethics, mental health, rehabilitation, and geriatric medicine can offer valuable contributions to the ultimate benefit and successful outcome in treating the older surgical patient [9–11]. Informing the patient and family of anticipated postoperative needs should begin in the preoperative period. The social worker, family members, nurses, and rehabilitation therapists need direction from the attending surgeon on the prognosis and expected outcome. In most cases, a conference involving family members and health care personnel may be the most efficient way to coordinate the patient's care needs and to acquire the appropriate support services.

Nutrition

The contribution of protein calorie malnutrition to increased morbidity and mortality in geriatric populations is not well recognized. Clinical indicators of malnutrition include low body mass index, a history of weight loss, and low serum levels of proteins, cholesterol, and hemoglobin. Approximately 10% of community-dwelling elderly and 25% or more of hospitalized elderly are, by these criteria, malnourished [12–14].

Early identification and correction of malnutrition are extremely important in the treatment of the elderly surgical patient. Among the frail elderly, diseases of undernutrition, including protein calorie malnutrition and specific vitamin and mineral deficiencies, are much more prevalent than diseases of overnutrition, such as obesity and hypercholesterolemia. Older patients have a reduced ability to taste and smell and to sense thirst and are therefore more prone to inadequate oral intake. Drugs can also modify nutrient needs and metabolism among older patients. Diuretics cause urinary loss of minerals, broad-spectrum antibiotics decrease intestinal bacterial production of vitamin K, antacids impair iron absorption, and digoxin and theophylline, even at therapeutic levels, can cause anorexia.

Nutritional status can have a profound influence on disease processes in older patients [15]. Operative risk and wound healing are heavily dependent on protein status. Dehydration is a frequent complication of fever, gastrointestinal disorders, and altered mental status. Vitamin and mineral deficiencies contribute to poor wound healing and skin breakdown.

A dietitian with expertise in the care of the elderly is a valuable resource for promoting optimal nutritional status in elderly surgical patients. Older patients have reduced muscle mass associated with a reduced basal metabolic rate and caloric requirement. Their glucose tolerance and renal excretory function are impaired, and their total body water may be reduced to approximately 55% of total body weight. Nutritional requirements have to be individualized and consist of a basal caloric requirement multiplied by an activity factor and an injury factor as appropriate. Basal energy expenditure (BEE) may be approximated using the following formulas:

$$\text{Ideal body weight} = 50 \text{ kg} + 2.3 \text{ (kg/in. over 5 ft)}$$

$$\text{BEE} = 30 \text{ kcal/d} \times \text{ideal body weight (kg)}$$

$$\text{Protein requirement} = 1 \text{ g/kg ideal body weight}$$

BEE and protein requirement may be modified by the presence of diseases, stress of acute illness, and patient tolerance.

Activity factors range from 1.2 for bedfast patients to 1.5 for ambulatory patients. Injury factors are estimated at 1.2 for mild illness to 1.6 for sepsis and 2.0 for burns [16]. The protein component should be approximately 1 g per kilogram of ideal body weight multiplied by a stress factor of 1.5 to 2.0, depending on patient needs. If an older individual is significantly below ideal body weight, then a target weight midpoint between actual and ideal body weight is used for calculations so as not to compromise gastrointestinal and renal reserve.

Albumin, the most common laboratory parameter used to assess nutritional status, has a half-life of approximately 20 days. In acute states of negative nitrogen balance and early during nutritional repletion, serum albumin levels remain static and do not accurately reflect protein status. The measurement of visceral proteins with faster turnover rates, such as prealbumin and transferrin, may provide earlier indications of the status of protein nutriture [17].

At times, both nutritional supplements and specialized feedings—enteral and parenteral—may be required. Even a few days of nutritional support preoperatively may greatly improve the surgical outcome in a malnourished individual [18]. Tube feeding with either a small-bore nasogastric tube or gastrostomy tube may be indicated in certain patients (Table 4-3). Nutritional formulas vary widely in composition and clinical indications. Elderly patients generally have better tolerance for iso-osmolar formulas with low fat content. Tube feedings should be started at low rates, increasing gradually in volume to allow accommodation of the gastrointestinal tract, particularly in individuals who have not been fed enterally for some time. Additional free water is often required by those on tube feedings. Gastric residuals should be checked and must remain less than the hourly flow rate of the feeding solution.

Tube feeding has potential complications. Diarrhea and malabsorption may occur and require changes in feeding formulas. Aspiration is a potential complication that can be minimized by elevating the head of the bed and checking for gastric residuals. Gastrostomy tubes and replacement tubes must be anchored securely to the abdomen to prevent migration of the inner bulb to the pylorus, with resultant gastric outlet obstruction.

Feeding by the enteral route generally carries less risk of complication and is less expensive than feeding by vein; however, total parenteral nutrition (TPN) may be required when gastrointestinal function is inadequate. Peripheral TPN is a temporizing measure providing approximately 800 calories per day. The higher concentration of nutrients provided through a central line can support nutrition indefinitely. However, the elderly are more prone to the complications of TPN such as CHF, glucose intolerance, infection, and fatty liver. Many hospitals have a nutrition support team composed of a physician, nurse, pharmacist, and dietitian skilled in TPN therapy.

TABLE 4-3. *Caveats on the use of enteral tubes*

Nasogastric tubes
For short-term use
May be misplaced into lung
Require patient cooperation
Gastrostomy tubes
Maximum patient acceptance and comfort
Require adequate gastric anatomy
Inner bulb and outer flange required to prevent migration
Permit bolus feeding
Jejunostomy tubes
Frequent leakage around tube site
Require external fixation device
All enteral tubes
Potential for aspiration of feedings

Pharmaceuticals

Elderly patients frequently suffer from multiple chronic diseases that involve several organ systems. As our aging population yields increasing numbers of chronic diseases, more and more drugs are prescribed. People aged 25 to 44 years fill an average of slightly more than five prescriptions per person per year, whereas those over 65 years old fill an average of 12 prescriptions per person per year. The number of adverse reactions to drugs increases in direct proportion to the number of drugs taken: 4% when one to five drugs are taken, 7% when five to 11 drugs are taken, and 24% when 11 to 15 medications are taken concurrently [19].

The activity of a drug in the body, whether therapeutic or toxic, depends on the plasma concentration of that drug. The plasma concentration depends on the size of the dose and its frequency of administration, the absorption rate, the volume in which the drug is distributed, and the rate of clearance from the body. The factors that govern the pharmacodynamics of drugs are altered by the aging process. The proportion of body fat increases, and lean body mass and total body water tend to decrease as persons age. These changes alter the distribution of certain drugs. For example, fat-soluble drugs (e.g., benzodiazepines and phenothiazines) have a delayed onset of action in the elderly, but their effect may be prolonged because they are accumulated and then released from relatively increased amounts of body fat [20–22].

Blood perfusion to most organs declines with increasing age. Because drugs are eliminated from the body primarily through renal excretion or by hepatic metabolic action, decreased perfusion through these organs can lead to increased plasma drug levels. Decreased perfusion and changes in acid-base concentrations in the stomach and intestine can also lead to unpredictable absorption rates of orally administered drugs [23].

All of these potential problems are exaggerated and become unpredictable before, during, and after surgical procedures as intravenous (IV) fluids (with possible changes in electrolyte levels) and blood products are administered. Changes in blood pressure occur intraoperatively, thus altering organ perfusion. Deprivation of food occurs postoperatively (often compounded by nasogastric suctioning), which has the potential for producing malnutrition over varying periods of time. Under these circumstances, it is important to monitor carefully drug use perioperatively by clinical observation for toxic effects, by plasma levels when indicated and possible, and by the electrocardiographic changes when such monitoring is appropriate [24].

Because of the vulnerability of the aged patient to adverse drug reactions and the increased frequency with which they occur, the following suggestions are made to reduce the risk of these problems [22,25,26]:

1. Periodically (daily) review the medication regimen that the elderly patient is receiving while in the hospital.
2. After careful clinical assessment, consider whether any unnecessary drug is being prescribed or whether any additional medication is indicated. At this point, take into account any factors that might alter the patient's responsiveness to the drug.
3. Simplify the dose and drug regimen as much as possible. Start with the lowest effective dose possible; it is easier to build up to a therapeutic dose in the elderly patient than it is to remove a drug and deal with an adverse reaction due to overtreatment.
4. Consider nonpharmacologic forms of therapy whenever possible—for example, sodium restriction as the first intervention, rather than a drug, when it is deemed necessary to lower the patient's blood pressure.
5. Avoid inappropriate or overenergetic therapy when the patient's physical and mental disabilities indicate the possibility that a less active therapeutic role would be effective.

A hospital pharmacist can be an important resource to the attending surgeon and other members of the treatment team. The pharmacist assists in the treatment of patients with complicated drug histories by suggesting less costly alternatives with more convenient dosing schedules and by assessing the potential for drug-to-drug and drug-to-nutrient interactions. Pharmacists can educate patients and caregivers regarding medications and assist in achieving compliance. For unusual or new medications, they may provide the treatment team with drug information and assist with obtaining needed nonformulary items and approval for restricted medications and biologicals.

Ethical Decisions and Support

The decision to submit an elderly patient to a surgical procedure is never made lightly. Surgeons and patients alike carefully weigh the risks and benefits of any procedure. For the patient, the acceptance of a surgical procedure is an emotionally laden process. Proper preparation of the patient and family is essential. Careful attention to patient autonomy, informed consent, and respect for patient wishes and advanced directives remain the standard of care [27].

Preoperative teaching by members of the treatment team, supported by the attending surgeon, will assist the older patient in preparation for an operation. At times, spiritual counseling and medical ethics consultation may be appropriate for particularly difficult decisions or for times when patients and their surrogate decision-makers face dilemmas concerning the appropriate treatment strategy. At times, patients may be unable to articulate a choice reflecting their own values and goals. In these instances, the family surrogate decision-makers may need tremendous support to arrive at an appropriate decision promoting the best interest of the patient.

Iatrogenic Problems

With increasing age and functional disability, the potential for iatrogenic complications increases. The wise surgeon carefully includes this factor in any discussion of the benefits and risks of surgical procedures on elderly patients. Iatrogenic risks may be minimized by careful selection of patients with a higher potential for a good outcome and by avoiding unnecessary medications and therapies. Attempting less risky and less invasive treatments first, when appropriate, may also be in the best interest of the individual patient. Whenever possible, preoperative evaluation and preparation with the inclusion of medical specialists, nursing personnel, dietitians, and rehabilitation specialists may improve outcome and reduce postoperative complications. Elective procedures have the best outcomes and are preferred when possible. Timing procedures to coincide with the optimal functional and physiologic status of the patient also improves outcome. Invariably, operating early rather than late in the disease process provides the best opportunity for a successful outcome for the older surgical patient.

GERIATRIC SYNDROMES AND AGING ORGAN SYSTEMS

Functional Assessment

Realistically, approximately 20% of individuals over age 65 and 40% of individuals over age 75 have some functional disability limiting their capability for self-care [2]. Functional ability is strongly correlated with numerous outcome measures, including length of stay in the hospital, severity of disease processes, mortality, morbidity, and physiologic reserve. Measurement of function is also an important indicator of overall progress during treatment.

The activities of daily living (ADL) scale of Katz et al. [28,29] is frequently used to determine the degree of independence or need for assistance in bathing, dressing, toileting, transfer ability, continence, and feeding. Problems with continence and feeding, especially, make it less likely that the patient can return to independent living and more likely that he or she will represent a heavy burden to family caregivers. The Lawton Instrumental Activities of Daily Living Scale [30] assesses the patient's ability to perform higher-order functions such as using the telephone, preparing meals, and managing finances. When deficiencies in instrumental ADL are present, these higher-level functions may be individually addressed to aid in the return to independent living.

A focus on functional abilities rather than exclusively on disease entities fosters a team-oriented approach to patient care, addressing real issues of major concern to patients and family caregivers.

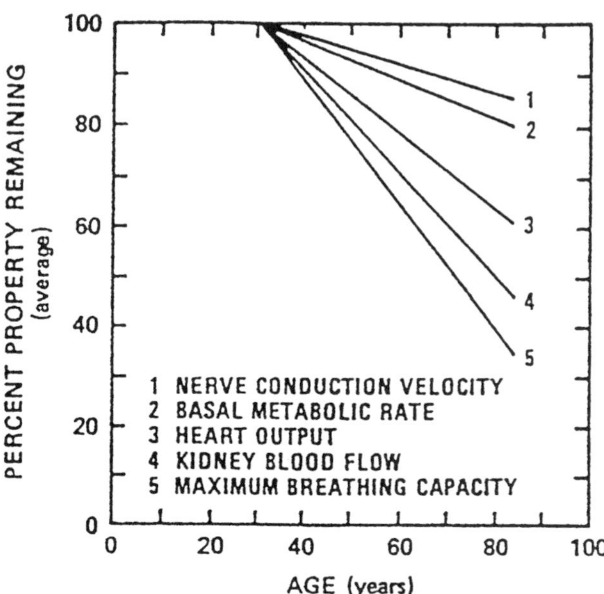

FIG. 4-1. The decline of organ reserve with age. (Reprinted with permission from Shock NW. Discussion on Mortality and Measurement of Aging. In Strehler BC, Ebert SB, Glass HB, et al. [eds], The Biology of Aging: A Symposium. Washington, DC: American Institute of Biological Sciences, 1960; and Fires JF, Crapo LM. Vitality and Aging. San Francisco: Freeman, 1981. Copyright 1960, American Institute of Biological Sciences.)

Biomarkers of Aging

Differentiating between the effects of physiologic aging and disease processes can be difficult. Many diseases seen with increased prevalence in older individuals do not equate to an aging effect, and the rate of physiologic aging is not uniform among all individuals. Additionally, aging effects can vary between different organ systems, as for example, the 50-year-old patient with presenile dementia who may have the cognitive function of an elderly demented individual, but normal cardiac and renal function.

A biomarker estimating the biological and functional age of an individual as distinct from the chronologic age is an interesting concept that, if available, could be used to predict the biological age of an individual. This would assist in making treatment decisions, allowing more accurate assessment of the risks and benefits of the treatment intervention. It is the biological age and functional organ reserve and not the chronologic age of a person that are the strongest predictors of outcome in clinical situations.

Human survival curves have shown an increased survival at all ages in the U.S. population, but no change in the maximum potential life span of approximately 85 to 100 years [31]. This phenomenon has been attributed to a decrease in the random death rate, due to improved nutrition, sanitation, and control of many infectious diseases. Although aging and maximum life span have remained unchanged, a greater proportion of individuals will approach the maximum human life span in the next few years.

Many theories of aging have been proposed; however, none fully accounts for the phenomenon of aging. A genetic program modulating the rate of human aging seems plausible. Women outlive men, and different cell lines from different organs all seem to have a finite limit to life span and finite capacity for cell division. The effects of environmental factors are difficult to separate from genetic influences when factors producing aging effects are studied. With time, cellular and extracellular proteins become glycosylated, producing molecular cross-linking with resultant decreased compliance in many organs. Ionizing radiation produces free radicals that can alter the DNA to produce somatic mutations, and it can also damage mitochondria within cells. Errors in protein synthesis or cellular organelle repair can accumulate over time, approximating aging changes. Antioxidant chemicals can retard some of the effects of ionizing radiation and may be important in modulating the rate of aging. Hormonal influences have far-reaching effects on many organ systems and obviously also contribute to aging changes. Aging can be characterized by an ever-decreasing ability to restore homeostasis in the face of physiologic insult. In other words, there is a decreasing biological reserve inherent in aging organ systems (Fig. 4-1, Table 4-4).

Closely related to the concept of biomarkers in aging, the measurement of severity of illness is important to consider in the planning of treatment programs, in the estimation of risk, and for prognostic purposes. Severity indices span many domains including medical and functional domains. Organ-specific scales such as the New York Heart Association Functional Classification [32] and Child's Classification of Hepatic Cirrhosis [33] are well known. Disease staging for many solid tissue and hematologic malignancies [34] and host response to malignancy

TABLE 4-4. *Physiologic changes associated with aging*

Body composition
Decreased weight and height
Decreased muscle and bone mass
Cardiovascular
Decreased maximum heart rate and stroke volume
Increased systolic blood pressure
Pulmonary
Decreased forced expiratory volume and vital capacity
Increased residual volume
Decreased Pao_2
Renal
Decreased renal blood flow
Decreased creatinine clearance
Decreased urinary concentrating ability
Endocrine
Decreased levels of androgens and estrogens
Decreased glucose tolerance
Decreased growth factors
Immune function
Decreased T-cell function
Decreased antibody production

TABLE 4-5. *Diagnostic criteria for delirium*

Altered consciousness
Altered cognition
Recent onset of symptoms, with fluctuations
Evidence for etiology from history, physical examination, or laboratory evaluation

Source: Modified from Diagnostic and Statistic Manual of Mental Disorders (4th ed). Washington, DC: American Psychiatric Association, 1994.

[35] are also in common use. Other scales exist for affective [36] and cognitive dysfunction [37] and have been adapted to the geriatric population. More global physiologic scales such as the physical status scale of the American Society of Anesthesiologists [38], Acute Physiology and Chronic Health Evaluation (APACHE II) system [39], and functional activity, including the ADL [28], Instrumental ADL [30], and physical performance testing scales [40] are also available to the clinician. It is important, however, to select the scale appropriate to the clinical situation. In this way, the clinician will maximize the sensitivity and specificity of the tool and obtain more appropriate information to enhance the surgical care of the older patient.

Central Nervous System

Despite the fact that the central nervous system (CNS) in the older adult has been extensively studied, many questions still remain regarding age-related changes and the proper management of CNS disorders. With age, brain weight and blood flow decrease, and decreased enzymatic activity can be demonstrated in individual neurons and regions of the brain, referable to many CNS pathways. The density of dendritic synapses decreases. With these anatomic and physiologic changes, functional alterations are also apparent. Central processing and response times slow. Abstract reasoning and short-term memory are also impaired. The ability to cope emotionally under conditions of stress decreases. However, there appears to be a remarkable preservation of long-term memory and overall knowledge and a surprising ability to respond to problems and situations requiring experiential knowledge.

The preoperative assessment of the CNS includes documentation of mental status and any focal neurologic deficits. A history of transient ischemic events indicates the patient should be evaluated for critical carotid occlusive disease or ulcerated atherosclerotic carotid plaques. Patients taking anticoagulant agents should have blood levels carefully checked, and those taking sedating medications should be considered for dose reduction or cessation preoperatively. Alcohol consumption should be documented, and individuals at risk for withdrawal symptoms should be observed closely in the perioperative period. Lithium carbonate can produce metabolic and hematopoietic abnormalities. A complete blood cell count, thyroid profile, and serum chemistry evaluations are always indicated preoperatively.

Fully 10% to 15% of elderly surgical patients undergoing any significant procedure, and up to 50% of older individuals undergoing total hip replacement experience delirium in the hospital. The delirium may take up to 1 week to resolve [41]. Delirium is defined as a disorganization and disorientation of recent onset that fluctuates and includes perceptual changes and disturbances of the sleep and wake cycles [42] (Table 4-5). This is to be differentiated from the more chronic memory, personality, and cognitive changes of dementia. Postoperative delirium is a multifactorial disorder more common in individuals with underlying cognitive impairment. It may be precipitated by electrolyte imbalance, acute sensory changes and deprivation, environmental alterations, pain, and medications, particularly narcotics and anticholinergic agents as well as withdrawal of habitual sedatives including benzodiazepines and alcohol. Delirium is managed by detecting and treating the underlying physiologic precipitants and by environmental manipulation including gentle reassurance, reorientation of the patient, posting of schedules and the use of calendars and clocks, normalizing the waking and sleeping schedule, and most importantly by enlisting the support of family and friends [43]. The temporary use of psychotropic agents and short-acting tranquilizers and the judicious application of restraints to prevent injury may be indicated.

Postoperative stroke is a complication of hypotension, hypovolemia, and cerebral embolism. It is more prevalent in individuals with underlying atrial fibrillation, atherosclerosis, and hypoxia. The presence of a new stroke should be suspected in any postoperative patient with a new onset of swallowing difficulties, motor deficits, or persistence of lethargy or delirium. Brain imaging with computed tomography or magnetic resonance imaging may not be sensitive enough to indicate the presence of early tissue edema related to the infarct, and a follow-up scan in 48 hours should be performed if clinically indicated. The management of stroke includes early attention to rehabilitation, the prevention of aspiration with elevation of the head and evaluation of swallowing function, and initiation of antiplatelet agents in the absence of any contraindications.

Infection

Thermal regulation is impaired in older patients, and infections often present nonspecific findings such as confusion and weakness. When elevated body temperature is present, it may be indicative of a serious infection in the older patient. Urinary tract infections are the most common infections in the elderly and the most frequent cause of bacteremia. Urinary tract infections are increased in frequency among individuals with concomitant diseases including benign prostatic hypertrophy and diabetes. Infections are also common with many neurologic disorders. Pneumonias are the second most common cause of infection in the elderly. Postoperative pneumonia usually can be prevented with careful attention to pulmonary toilet and early mobilization of the patient.

Mortality due to infectious disease is greater among older patients because of the increased prevalence of coexistent disease processes and reduced organ reserve. The mortality related to sepsis may be >50% in older populations. Immunosuppressed elderly patients are at particularly high risk for postoperative infectious complications.

Initial therapy for presumed infectious diseases in the postoperative patient is based on the likely organism responsible. Treatment must be initiated empirically before receiving laboratory culture and sensitivity data. Surveillance cultures are rarely helpful because flora producing the symptoms are constantly changing. The presumed site of infection helps determine the choice of empiric antibiotics. Gram-positive organisms are more common with cutaneous lesions and wound infections, gram-negative organisms with genitourinary sites, gram-positive and gram-negative organisms with pulmonary infection, and gram-negative and other unusual organisms in diabetic and immunosuppressed individuals. Other factors, including prolonged hospitalization, stress, nutritional deprivation, previous infection, and the prolonged use of suppressive antibiotics (which may select for resistant organisms), also influence the choice of empiric therapy.

Colonization with organisms of different virulence is now being repeatedly documented. More sensitive bacteria such as *Escherichia coli*, *Streptococcus pneumoniae*, and *Haemophilus influenzae* are more commonly associated with community-acquired infections. *Klebsiella* and *Enterobacter* are more usual in patients presenting from long-term care facilities. More resistant and virulent organisms such as enterococcus, methicillin-resistant staphylococcus, and *Pseudomonas* are now being seen more often in hospital-acquired infections.

Antibiotics are chosen to cover potential causative organisms and are selected with careful attention to avoid iatrogenic complications. The smallest necessary antibiotic coverage is used for the suspected pathogen. Clinical response and follow-up culture data then dictate appropriate changes in antibiotic therapy, with reduction of the most potentially toxic agent when at all possible. Because of the high propensity for iatrogenic complications in older patients, the use of the antibiotic agent with the narrowest spectrum of activity appropriate to the infection under treatment is an important therapeutic principle. This philosophy is not in conflict with but supports the need for aggressive and early identification of potential infection in this frail population.

Sensory Deficits

Altered sensation is common in elderly individuals. Over 20% of patients over the age of 65 have reduced hearing ability, which increases to 50% in those over age 80 [44]. Up to 30% of older individuals have cataracts and need increased light intensity for visual acuity [45]. The ability to taste and smell is decreased, which interferes with nutrition and the enjoyment of eating. Occasionally, this can produce dietary noncompliance such as the inability to taste the amount of salt applied to food. The sensation of touch is decreased and the sense of position is decreased, which affects balance and mobility. The decrease in hearing acuity is particularly noted in high-frequency tones, and decreased discrimination between sounds also interferes with proper hearing.

Attention to disorders of sensation should attune the surgical team to patient comfort and potential complications related to sensory alteration.

Sexual Function

Older individuals continue to enjoy sexual function, although concurrent disease processes, age-related changes in tissues, and the aging neurologic system may slow or interfere with normal sexual function. Estrogen receptors are present in vaginal tissue, and thinning of the mucosa as well as dryness may be improved with the addition of estrogen cremes and lubrication. Orgasm requires approximately 4 to 6 METS (multiple of the resting metabolism $\dot{V}O_2$) of energy expenditure, and older postsurgical as well as cardiac patients may have concerns regarding their ability to return to sexual intercourse. Reassurance from the physician, even to the point of providing exercise tolerance test results, may greatly help in counseling the patient.

Osteoarthritis of the hip interferes with sexual intercourse in 50% of individuals. Patients undergoing prostate surgery

TABLE 4-6. *Child's prognostic classification for cirrhotic liver disease*

Factor	Class A (minimal)	Class B (moderate)	Class C (advanced)
Bilirubin (mg/dl)	<2.0	2.0–3.0	>3.0
Serum albumin (g/dl)	>3.5	3.0–3.5	<3.0
Ascites	None	Controlled	Poorly controlled
Encephalopathy	None	Minimal	Coma
Nutrition	Excellent	Good	Poor

Source: Modified from Child CG, Turcotte JG. The Liver and Portal Hypertension. Philadelphia: Saunders, 1964.

are frequently concerned about postoperative impotence. However, with transurethral resection, impotence is uncommon and erectile capacity is maintained. Retrograde ejaculation, however, is a frequent occurrence. Even radical prostatectomy has an incidence of impotence of <5%. Women undergoing mastectomies often fear rejection and mutilation. Preoperative counseling by sensitive personnel can help reduce this fear.

Nursing home patients also have sexual desires, and sexual activity between consenting adults is frequent. Attention to privacy and respecting personal choices are important management techniques.

Terminal Care

Experienced physicians realize that not all operations and medical care can be for cure. Many times, care for a chronic condition and palliation in terminal situations remain the appropriate goal of treatment. These situations require adequate counseling and education. Patients and their families progress through various stages of acceptance [46]:

- Denial and isolation
- Anger
- Bargaining
- Depression
- Acceptance

Patients progress through these stages at different rates and may never achieve a final acceptance and peaceful internal resolution. Nevertheless, it is important to respect patient autonomy. In offering treatment alternatives, the overriding principle should be to relieve pain and suffering and to prepare the patient and caregiver for death. Futile treatments should be avoided. Careful discharge planning and involvement of nursing and social work will go far to ease the burden of terminal care for patients and families. In many communities, hospice home care is available to help carry out the palliative treatment program following hospital discharge. Simplifying the treatment plan and discontinuing unnecessary medications, tests, and procedures greatly facilitate palliative care. Bereavement counseling and group therapy for loss may also be available, and selected patients should be referred to appropriate caregivers for these services.

Hepatic and Gastrointestinal Changes

Blood flow to the liver decreases with age. In individuals over age 60, hepatic circulation is approximately 40% of that in those aged 25. Although baseline liver metabolism is preserved, the functional reserve decreases. Albumin levels are slightly decreased with age, although they remain above the clinically accepted lower limits of normal. Likewise, liver enzymes measured by serum chemistry are within the normal limits. However, the stress of major surgical procedures, anesthetic agents, and the use of other potentially hepatotoxic medications place the elderly patient at increased risk of iatrogenic complications.

Older patients with preexisting liver disease are at risk for intraoperative and postoperative complications. The classification scheme of Child is the best accepted method of predicting prognosis based on evaluation of prothrombin time, albumin levels, presence of ascites, and encephalopathy [33] (Table 4-6). This classification, based on studies of large numbers of patients with cirrhosis, accurately estimates prognosis in patients undergoing portosystemic shunting, but may not be directly applicable to other procedures or patients with other types of liver disease.

In the presence of preexisting liver disease, meticulous fluid management, provision of vitamin K, and administration of fresh frozen plasma for acute correction of clotting deficiencies are often necessary. Careful attention to nutrition, particularly protein nutrition, and maintenance of normal glucose levels are also important. Potentially hepatotoxic drugs should be avoided, whenever possible, to optimize care of the older individual with liver disease. This is most critical in the postoperative period.

The gastrointestinal system also has predictable age-related changes. The coordination of the swallowing reflex, termed *presbyesophagus*, is decreased, as is a resting tone in the lower esophageal sphincter, increasing the potential for gastroesophageal reflux. Forty percent of older patients are edentulous. Parietal cells in the gastric mucosa are lost, producing a tendency for achlorhydria. These factors may affect intake and digestion of some food groups and absorption of certain medications dependent on an acid environment. Colonic motility is also impaired, and a third of individuals over age 65 have

TABLE 4-7. *Perioperative sodium balance*

	Hyponatremia	Hypernatremia
Definition	Serum Na^+ <135 mEq/liter	Serum Na^+ >145 mEq/liter
Associated diagnoses/agents		
Renal (urine Na^+ >20 mEq/liter)	Diuretics Osmotic agents Syndrome of inappropriate antidiuretic hormone Renal failure (acute, BUN/creatinine >20; chronic, BUN/creatinine <20)	Diuretics Osmotic agents Diabetes insipidus
Extra renal (urine Na^+ <10 mEq/liter)	Fluid loss Congestive heart failure Cirrhosis	Free H_2O loss Dehydration Na^+ administration
Management		
Edematous states	Fluid restriction	Free H_2O replacement
Volume loss states	Saline administration	

BUN = blood urea nitrogen.

diverticula. Pancreatic function is preserved at baseline; however, there is some evidence that under stress functional reserve may also be reduced, with a potential for both endocrine and exocrine dysfunction. Postoperative return of gastrointestinal motility is slower in older individuals, and careful attention to preventing aspiration events and postoperative ileus is crucial. Maintenance of normal electrolyte balance and hydration status, the provision of an adequate bowel regimen when using pain medications, and early ambulation of the patient are all important factors in the management of the elderly postoperative patient. Routine use of H_2 antagonists is unnecessary in the prevention of stress ulcers in elderly surgical patients unless there is a history of peptic ulcer or if corticosteroids or nonsteroidal anti-inflammatory agents are being administered. H_2 antagonists can adversely affect mental status and impair the absorption and metabolism of many drugs.

Renal Changes

With increasing age, many changes in renal anatomy and physiology can be documented. There is a 50% decrease in cortical blood flow and a 25% reduction in renal mass corresponding to a gradual loss of glomeruli with time. This translates to a reduced glomerular filtration rate with reduced sodium conservation and urine-concentrating abilities. Interstitial fibrous changes increase, and tubular cell basement membranes thicken, producing alterations in the secretory and resorptive function of the renal tubules. These processes can be accelerated with diseases including hypertension, diabetes, and atherosclerosis. The glomerular filtration rate reduces by approximately 1 ml per minute per year over age 40.

The following formula may be used as an estimation to predict glomerular function and to assist with fluid management and adjustment of drug dosages that are dependent on renal clearance.

Renal function:

$$\text{Creatinine (ml/min)} = \frac{[140 \times \text{age (yrs)}] \times [\text{weight (kg)}]}{72 \times [\text{Serum creatinine (mg/dl)}]}$$

Creatinine-based estimates of renal function are dependent on muscle mass. With the reduced muscle mass seen in malnourished or cachectic patients, the measured serum creatinine level is lower and therefore the calculated creatinine clearance artificially elevated. This additional consideration must be estimated in predicting renal function in many older patients.

Urine-concentrating ability remains adequate under resting conditions in the older surgical patient. A urine residual of over 500 ml and urinary sodium concentration of <20 mEq/liter are indicative of preserved renal function. The older patient is more sensitive to hypotension and volume deficits, which may precipitate prerenal azotemia, or even acute tubular necrosis. The concomitant use of nephrotoxic drugs can further impair renal function. Prerenal azotemia is often reversed with adequate hydration and maintenance of normal blood pressure and is characterized by a blood urea nitrogen–to-creatinine ratio of <20. Acute tubular necrosis, however, is characterized by a disproportionately elevated creatinine, reduced urine osmolality, and increased urinary sodium concentrations (Table 4-7). Acute tubular necrosis, with rapidly increasing blood urea nitrogen and creatinine levels may require temporary hemodialysis support with possible spontaneous return of renal function over time.

Patients with chronic renal insufficiency who undergo surgical procedures require careful management of fluid balance. Volume deficits may be calculated by the following formula:

$$\text{Volume (liters)} = 0.6 \times \text{kg body weight} \left(1 - \frac{140}{[\text{NA}]\ \text{serum}}\right)$$

IV fluid volumes and rates should be less than those normally administered to younger patients to avoid fluid overload.

Intraoperative maintenance of blood pressure at usual levels for the patient is also important in the proper management of the renally impaired patient. Chronic renal insufficiency may produce coagulopathies with increased tendency for clot formation due to depressed levels of antithrombin 3. Paradoxically, renal patients may also have a tendency for bleeding because of decreased platelet function. They are also at risk for poor wound healing. In general, any surgical procedure to be performed on chronic renal failure patients should be undertaken after dialysis so that electrolyte balance and fluid status may be optimized before the procedure.

Urologic Care

Postoperative urologic complications fall into four major categories: bleeding, obstruction, infection, and incontinence. There is an additional risk of water intoxication from excessive bladder irrigation during urologic procedures. This risk may be minimized by monitoring fluid and electrolyte balance.

Bleeding

The occurrence of bleeding is common following surgical procedures on the prostate and is related to the release of prostate-derived fibrinolytics. When the bleeding persists longer than 2 days or when transfusions are required, the use of amino caproic acid, an inhibitor of fibrinolysis, is indicated. Patients treated with amino caproic acid must be observed for potential coronary and cerebral vascular occlusive events, and individuals with compromised coronary and cerebral circulation have relative contraindications for the use of this agent. Placing a Foley catheter under tension may also help tamponade bleeding tissue around the trigone of the bladder.

Obstructive Symptoms

Intraoperative use of catheters to monitor urinary output, the administration of medications with anticholinergic effects, and the associated conditions of neurogenic bladder syndromes secondary to diseases such as Parkinson's, stroke, and diabetes can produce obstructive and pseudo-obstructive urinary symptoms. Secondary to catheter-induced inflammation, spasm of the urethral sphincter may be seen after removal of indwelling urinary catheters. A simple in-and-out catheterization schedule every 6 to 8 hours until the residual volume is <100 ml may be sufficient to resolve this complication. In men with benign prostatic hyperplasia, catheter trauma may precipitate obstructive symptoms sufficient to require surgical management. Reduction in dose or substitution of medications with strong anticholinergic effects, ruling out infection, and providing a frequent toileting schedule are useful adjunct therapies.

In individuals with urogenic bladders secondary to other disease processes, a maintenance intermittent catheterization schedule may be required. This treatment is increasingly difficult to provide if the patient is incapable of self-catheterization or does not have a supportive or capable caregiver. Most nursing care facilities are currently not able to provide chronic intermittent catheterization services. Chronic indwelling catheters may be required when obstructive and pseudo-obstructive symptoms cannot be relieved by other methods. In no case should patients be allowed to retain residual volumes >200 ml because this predisposes to infection and worsens bladder and renal dysfunction.

Infections

Urinary tract infections remain the most common type of infection in elderly patients. Postoperative urinary tract infections due to catheterization are frequent and require a high index of clinical suspicion for early diagnosis. Urine analysis, culture, and sensitivity and empiric antibiotic therapy to cover common gram-negative and gram-positive pathogens are usually indicated.

Judicious use of indwelling catheters will reduce the frequency of urinary tract infections. Indwelling urinary catheters produce bacterial colonization of the urinary tract within several days. In most cases, colonization is asymptomatic; however, surveillance cultures have shown that the microbiologic flora changes constantly and is reflective of the environmental pathogens. Hospital-acquired pathogens are likely to be more virulent and antibiotic-resistant organisms. The use of external catheters in men causes a similar rate of colonization and may be associated with balanitis, pressure sores, and tissue sloughing.

Urinary catheters, however, may be required chronically in the presence of sacral decubitus and to relieve obstructive symptoms. When used, urinary catheters should be free of obstruction and tension and allow for continuous gravity drainage of urine. Collection bags should be emptied frequently. Indwelling catheters should be changed when the urine becomes cloudy, thick, or foul smelling, and at least every 2 to 4 weeks, as well as at the first sign of infective symptoms, such as pain, bleeding, or fever. Indwelling catheters that remain in place for too long cause excessive inflammation and leakage around the catheter, and they may become occluded with debris. The use of an indwelling catheter with a 5-ml inner bulb is recommended because larger bulbs produce urinary stasis and may promote infection.

Little is known about the specific factors precipitating infection in patients with chronic urinary catheters. The use of prophylactic suppressive antibiotics does not reduce the incidence of urinary tract infection in catheterized patients; moreover, it selects for multidrug-resistant organisms. Bladder irrigations with 0.25% acetic acid may be useful in reducing the number of urinary tract infections in individuals prone to repeated infections. When infection is sus-

TABLE 4-8. *Urinary incontinence*

Classification	Stress	Urge	Overflow	Functional
Description	Involuntary loss of urine with cough, etc.	Leakage due to sensation of bladder fullness	Leakage from overdistension	Cognitive, emotional, physical, or environmental barriers to toilet
Associated pathology	Weakness of pelvic muscles, sphincter	Dementia, stroke, cystitis	Obstruction, neurogenic bladder	Dementia, depression, inaccessible toilets
Management	Kegel exercises, alpha agonists, estrogens, surgery	Training, anticholinergics, estrogens	Intermittent or chronic catheterization, surgery	Training, environmental changes, incontinence pads, external collection devices

Source: Adapted from Ouslander JG. Diagnostic evaluation of geriatric urinary incontinence. Clin Geriatr Med 1986;2:715–730.

pected, the catheter should be changed and appropriate cultures obtained. Antibiotics should be administered for 7 to 10 days. A single-dose antibiotic regimen frequently recommended for younger patients with simple cystitis has not proven effective in the treatment of older patients with urinary tract infections.

Incontinence

Urinary incontinence is another category of bladder dysfunction in elderly surgical patients. Incontinence may be classified in four different categories [47] (Table 4-8). A simple history, medication review, urinalysis, and catheterization for residual volume are frequently all that is required to diagnose the cause of the urinary incontinence. Appropriate treatment strategies are indicated in Table 4-8.

Particular attention to the causes of functional incontinence is helpful for elderly postoperative patients. Minimizing the use of sedating medications and diuretics and encouraging normal daytime toileting activities are important principles. Avoiding barriers and restraints, the provision of bedside commodes, and frequent toileting are helpful measures in achieving urinary independence. When this fails, diapering is preferred to the use of indwelling catheters, except when sacral decubitus are also present.

Pulmonary Changes

With increasing age, there is a decrease in the elasticity of pulmonary tissue, resulting in increased closing volumes and airway collapse. This produces a decrease in vital capacity of approximately 20 ml per year after age 20. This well-known ventilation-profusion mismatch occurs along with a resultant decrease in arterial oxygen tension. Arterial oxygen tension may be predicted by the following formula:

$$Pao_2 = 109 \text{ mm Hg} - 0.43 \text{ age (years)}$$

Underlying pulmonary disease always exacerbates age-related changes. There is also a neurogenic-medicated decrease in the cough reflex such that aspiration is more likely. The cough reflex may be further suppressed by the presence of comorbid neurologic disorders, the influence of sedating medications, and the presence of feeding tubes.

Postoperative hypoventilation, atelectasis, and pneumonia occur in approximately 20% to 40% of elderly surgical patients. Those with pre-existing illnesses are obviously at increased risk for postoperative pulmonary problems. Especially at risk are those patients with neurologic diseases, chronic obstructive lung disease, obesity, smoking history, underlying abnormal chest radiographs, and pulmonary infections. This is especially true for the elderly patient undergoing upper abdominal and thoracic surgery.

The preoperative identification and treatment of individuals at higher risk for pulmonary complications can dramatically reduce postoperative problems. It is possible to predict outcome and postoperative lung function in a reliable way. Spirometric measurements help stratify individuals with pre-existing pulmonary disease. They identify individuals with forced expiratory volume in 1 second (FEV_1) of 1 liter, which places a patient at 50% risk for significant postoperative pulmonary complications. An FEV_1 of 0.5 liter is predictive of serious postoperative morbidity and mortality [48]. When pulmonary resection is considered, a preoperative xenon ventilation scan can estimate percentage of split lung function. Additional information obtained from spirometry can then predict the percentage of functioning lung remaining after lobectomy.

In individuals with chronic obstructive lung disease, a program of smoking cessation preoperatively, aggressive pulmonary toilet, and inhaled bronchodilators can reduce postoperative complications by as much as 50%. In patients prone to bronchospasm or who have corticosteroid-dependent pulmonary disease, preoperative and postoperative corticosteroid administration at stress doses is indicated.

Postoperative pulmonary toilet, inhaled bronchodilators as indicated, avoidance of excessive pain and sedating medications, and early ambulation are all important in maximizing pulmonary function and preventing postoperative respiratory problems. High-risk elderly patients should be monitored with transcutaneous oxygen saturation measurements. At the first indication of purulent sputum production, fever, or altered mental status, a chest radiograph and sputum culture should be obtained. Empiric antibiotics to cover hospital-acquired flora may be indicated, pending culture results, to minimize the risk of complications from infection.

Cardiovascular Complications

Cardiovascular complications remain the most frequent cause of serious postoperative morbidity and mortality in the elderly because of the high prevalence of underlying coronary atherosclerotic disease. The aging cardiovascular system is characterized by decreased cardiac compliance and increased arterial stiffening, resulting in elevated total peripheral resistance and a high systolic blood pressure. The aging neurologic system contributes to cardiac dysfunction by a reduced responsiveness to stimuli and altered receptor affinities and postreceptor activation. Maximum heart rates, therefore, are usually reduced in older individuals. The age-related maximum heart rate, and its influence on the cardiac output, may be predicted by the following formulas:

$$\text{Maximum heart rate} = 200 - \text{age (years)}$$

$$\text{Cardiac output} = \text{Heart rate} \times \text{stroke volume}$$

With reduced maximum heart rate, the achievable cardiac output is reduced in older patients. With aging, any increase in cardiac output depends increasingly on a larger stroke volume. Because of reduced cardiac compliance, however, the older individual is more prone to heart failure as cardiac output increases under conditions of stress, infection, or fluid overload.

CHF and myocardial infarction constitute the majority of cardiovascular complications associated with major surgical procedures in older individuals. Approximately 20% of complications occur on the day of the operation, with the remainder occurring during the next 4 postoperative days [4]. Approximately 50% of postoperative myocardial infarctions are painless and are manifested by hypotension, arrhythmias, CHF, and altered mental status. Serial electrocardiograms and creatine phosphokinase determinations are mandatory for monitoring these high-risk individuals. CHF may be precipitated early in the postoperative period by the combined overzealous administration of intraoperative IV fluids and the rapid withdrawal of positive pressure ventilation as anesthesia is reversed.

The high risk of cardiovascular complications in older surgical patients has prompted the identification of predictors of outcome and more accurate classification systems [49–51] (Table 4-9). Predisposing factors for major postoperative cardiovascular complications include myocardial infarction within the past 6 months, preexisting arrhythmias, left ventricular hypertrophy, CHF, and the presence of critical aortic stenosis. Thoracic surgery and emergency, intraperitoneal, and aortic procedures are associated with the highest cardiovascular complication rates when compared with other surgical procedures. Significant coronary artery disease is present in approximately 60% of the vascular surgery population. An emergency surgical procedure doubles the risk of cardiac complications in predisposed individuals. Preoperative control of CHF, angina, serious arrhythmias, and hypertension is critical in minimizing cardiac risk.

CHF etiology can be assessed by echocardiography. Segmental and global dysfunction due to ischemia and cardiomyopathies can often be improved by diuretics, vasodilators, and angiotensin-converting enzyme inhibitors. Diastolic dysfunction, frequently seen in hypertensive heart disease, may be improved by calcium channel blockers. Control of rapid atrial fibrillation may often improve cardiac output as well. Individuals with severe cardiac dysfunction require the preoperative placement of a central venous and pulmonary artery catheter to monitor cardiac output and pulmonary capillary wedge pressure and to assess fluid requirements.

Atherosclerotic coronary artery disease may require preoperative evaluation if symptoms exist or evidence of coronary vascular disease is present. Asymptomatic individuals with normal exercise tolerance testing undergoing noncardiac procedures have low complication rates. In individuals with angina pectoris or a strong history for atherosclerotic cardiovascular disease, preoperative evaluation is important. If an exercise thallium test result is negative, then the complication rate is low. If the patient cannot exercise, then a dipyridamole (Persantine) thallium stress test, pharmacologically mimicking a physiologic stress test, is indicated. Strongly positive test results may indicate a need to proceed with coronary arteriography and potential coronary revascularization before an elective noncardiac procedure.

Individuals taking nitrates, calcium channel antagonists, and beta blockers should continue their medication up to the time of surgery. Nitrates can be administered transcutaneously before the patient is able to resume oral medications in the early postoperative period. Long-acting beta blockers have sufficient duration of action so that under normal circumstances the patient can resume oral administration in the early postoperative period without the need to administer IV preparations. The abrupt withdrawal of high doses of short-acting beta blockers, however, is associated with an increased instance of myocardial ischemia and should be avoided. These medications can be tapered, or the patient switched to a long-acting beta blocker, depending on the clinical indications.

Serious arrhythmias that need evaluation before a surgical procedure include rapid atrial fibrillation and other forms of

TABLE 4-9. *Cardiac risk factors for noncardiac surgery*

Risk index	Clinical variable (points)
High (10–20 points)	Myocardial infarction ≤6 mos (10) Emergency operation (10) Acute pulmonary edema (10) Presence of S_3 (11) Jugular venous distention (11) Angina, 1–2 blocks (10) Angina, minimal activity (20) Critical aortic stenosis (20)
Medium (7 points)	Rhythm other than sinus, or atrial ectopy >5 premature ventricular contractions per minute
Low (3–5 points)	Age >70 yrs History of congestive heart failure History of myocardial infarction >6 mos Poor medical status Thoracic, aortic, intraperitoneal procedure Po_2 <60 mm Hg, Pco_2 >50 mm Hg Blood urea nitrogen >50 mg/dl, creatinine >3 mg/dl Potassium <3 mEq/liter, bicarbonate <20mEq/liter
Cardiac risk index class	Percentage of surgical complications*
I (0–5 points)	1
II (6–12 points)	4
III (13–25 points)	14
IV (>26 points)	51

*Tabulation of percentage risk is based on study of Goldman et al.; however, Detsky et al. include additional factors (pulmonary edema, critical aortic stenosis, remote myocardial infarction, and congestive heart failure) and indicate a higher point risk for emergency surgery (10 vs. 4). Additional reported clinical experience indicates that this index is an approximate guide to estimating risk, and that the strongest predictor of low operative risk is the demonstration of moderate exercise capacity and adequate left ventricular function.

Sources: Modified from Goldman L, Caldera D, Nussbaum SR, et al. Multifactorial index of cardiac risk in non-cardiac surgical procedures. N Engl J Med 1977;297:845–850; and Detsky AS, Abrams HB, Forbath N, et al. Cardiac assessment for patients undergoing non-cardiac surgery: a multifactorial clinical risk index. Arch Intern Med 1986;146:2131–2134.

supraventricular tachycardia, frequent premature ventricular ectopy, bradycardia, and sinus pauses. A thorough review of potentially interfering medications and treatment of underlying metabolic and medical problems are crucial to preventing postoperative complications. Cardiac monitoring, control of heart rate, and the institution of antiarrhythmic agents or cardiac pacing all may be appropriate preoperative considerations. In individuals treated with antiarrhythmic drugs, obtaining a preoperative serum drug level is important in optimizing management and avoiding both undertreatment and drug toxicity.

In individuals who are taking anticoagulant agents because of atrial fibrillation, underlying valve disease, or severe cardiomyopathy, the maintenance of safe anticoagulation is important. Approximately 5 days before an elective surgical procedure, heparin may be substituted for warfarin, with the partial thromboplastin time noted to ensure adequate anticoagulation. Heparin may be discontinued the morning of the operation and reinstituted in the early postoperative period, simultaneous with administration of warfarin until therapeutic prothrombin times are achieved.

Patients with known valvular disorders or valvular prostheses require prophylactic antibiotic administration before any surgical procedure [52]. These individuals are at higher risk for arrhythmias and heart failure, and they should be monitored expectantly for these conditions during the perioperative period.

Hypertension is prevalent in the older population, and many elderly surgical candidates take antihypertensive medications. The incidence of myocardial infarction, CHF, and stroke is greatly reduced in individuals with controlled hypertension. Older patients are particularly prone to systolic hypertension, which is believed to be related to stiffening of the arteriolar walls. The multitude of antihypertensive agents available make it mandatory that the surgeon be familiar with these medications. Medications should be continued through the surgical period and diuretics individualized according to the patient's volume status. In most instances, administration of oral medications up to the time of the operation, with resumption of oral medication in the early postoperative period, is sufficient to control the majority of hypertensive patients. The abrupt cessation of short-acting beta blockers or clonidine may result in a hypertensive withdrawal syndrome, which is characterized by severe hypertension, agitation, arrhythmias, angina, and potential heart failure. Stroke may occur if this is not controlled. Approximately 25% of individuals with underlying hypertension experience an increase in blood pressure in the early postoperative period. This is related to pain, volume administration during the procedure, and the physiologic stress of the operation. These may be treated with a variety of different agents administered sublingually, transdermally, or intravenously, but therapy must be individualized. It is important not to overtreat hypertension because hypotension results in hypoperfusion with resultant cardiac, renal, and CNS disturbances. Maintenance of a blood pressure above 140/90 is recommended in the hypertensive elderly surgical patient.

Endocrine Changes

A number of endocrine changes occur with increasing age. The fasting blood sugar level rises gradually, and tissues are less sensitive to the effects of insulin. Tissue response to thyroid hormone stimulation decreases, as well as production of androgens and estrogens in both sexes.

Cyclic adenosine monophosphate is an intracellular mediator of many hormones, and its production is decreased in response to hormonal receptor activation in the tissues from elderly patients. The adrenal gland, however, maintains great functional reserve and is able to respond with a 2- to 7-mg/ml increase in the normal 30- to 100-mg/ml plasma cortisol level under periods of stress.

Diabetes

Maintenance of near normal glycemia intraoperatively maximizes fluid and metabolic homeostasis. Patients taking oral agents should ordinarily stop these agents 1 day preoperatively and be placed on a regimen of regular insulin according to a sliding scale and based on every-6-hour finger-stick glucose checks. Patients taking chlorpropamide have an increased risk for the syndrome of inappropriate antidiuretic hormone secretion, and this agent should be stopped several days preoperatively and serum sodium levels evaluated. Insulin-requiring diabetics should continue their usual dose of insulin up to the day before the operation. The morning of the operation, they should receive 50% of the usual dose, and IV fluids should contain dextrose. A sliding scale, regular insulin schedule should be administered based on every-6-hour glucose checks. For difficult-to-control diabetes, an intraoperative IV insulin administration of 0.1 U/kg per hour may be used. The avoidance of hypoglycemia is important, and glucose levels should be targeted between 100 and 250 mg/dl. Sudden hyperglycemia may be an indication of infection or a response to concomitantly administered corticosteroids. Less commonly, it may be related to the stress of anesthesia and the operation.

Adrenal Gland Function

Patients taking corticosteroids regularly within 1 year of a surgical procedure should be presumed to be adrenally insufficient and covered with exogenous corticosteroids intraoperatively. The preoperative measurement of baseline and stimulated cortisol levels is unnecessary. Physiologic replacement doses of corticosteroids include 20 mg of a hydrocortisone equivalent in the morning and 10 mg in the late afternoon, corresponding to the circadian rhythmic adrenal function. Administration of an approximately 400-mg equivalent of hydrocortisone, corresponding to the output of the adrenal gland under stress, constitutes sufficient treatment to avoid an adrenal crisis. This medical emergency consists of hypotension, hypothermia, and altered mental status. Patients receiving higher doses of therapeutic corticosteroids may be given their usual doses. Postoperatively, steroid-dependent patients should receive approximately half of the preoperative stress dose and be placed on their usual corticosteroid dose over the next 1 to 3 days of the early postoperative period.

Thyroid Gland

Hypothyroidism is more prevalent as age increases. The most common age-associated cause of hypothyroidism is related to autoimmune Hashimoto's thyroiditis. Most cases are mild and diagnosed by elevated thyroid-stimulating hormone and low free thyroxine levels. An increased requirement for thyroid replacement is noted over time as the gland involutes. In more severe hypothyroid cases, CHF, hypotension, and mental status changes can occur. Patients taking thyroid hormone replacement should continue their medication up to the time of any surgical procedure and resume oral medication in the early postoperative period. Patients under treatment may safely undergo procedures despite the fact that thyroid hormones have not completely returned to normal levels.

Hyperthyroid patients, however, are at increased risk for arrhythmias and CHF and should be made euthyroid before undergoing any surgical procedure. Treatment of thyroid storm is an endocrinologic emergency and requires administration of 40 mg propranolol, 1 g propylthiouracil, and 100 mg hydrocortisone every 6 hours.

Water Balance and Posterior Pituitary Function

The posterior pituitary produces antidiuretic hormone (ADH; vasopressin) in response to stress and altered fluid balance. ADH produces increased water resorption by renal tubular cells. Surgical stress, head trauma and CNS infections, CHF, ascites, and the action of chlorpropamide may produce an inappropriate increase in the secretion of ADH with resultant hyponatremia. Certain neoplasms such as small cell and squamous cell carcinoma of the lung are also known to produce ADH exogenously. The condition may be diagnosed by a decrease in urine osmolality compared with serum osmolality and a high urine sodium concentration (see Table 4-7). The condition often responds to free water restriction of 1,500 ml per day, administration of normal saline intravenously, and treatment of the underlying condition. In some instances, additional administration of demeclocycline for long-term treatment may be indicated. In situations where the serum sodium drops below 120 mEq/liter or when seizures occur, administration of IV 3% saline and IV furosemide to promote water diuresis may be indicated.

Inadequate production of vasopressin, termed *diabetes insipidus*, is uncommon, but it may be seen in head injury, brain tumors, and after operations on the CNS. Urinary osmolality is low relative to plasma, and urine sodium concentration is low. Initial therapy includes careful fluid management, and replacement with arginine vasopressin may be indicated.

Hematologic Changes

The hematologic system is altered with age. The total number of white blood cells remains constant; however, there are decreased numbers of T cells. White blood cell function shows a reduced response to cytosine stimulation and a decreased sensitivity of macrophages to pathogens. B cells have a reduced antibody response to stimulation; however, neutrophils appear to maintain normal function. Anemia, although commonly seen in older patients, is not part of the normal aging process but may be related to malnutrition, undiagnosed bleeding, medication reactions, and underproduction of red blood cells secondary to chronic disease processes.

Preoperative transfusion requirements for anemia depend on clinical status. Patients at risk for cerebrovascular and cardiovascular events and those with heart failure may require hematocrits of approximately 30%. Because of the inherent risks in transfusion, including infection, volume overload, and transfusion reactions, hematocrits as low as 25% are acceptable for elderly patients in otherwise stable medical condition. Similar indications for transfusion apply to postoperative bleeding. In general, transfusions are withheld until 2 U is required.

Spontaneous bleeding is rare with platelet counts >20,000, and most surgical procedures can be safely performed with platelet counts between 20,000 and 50,000. Platelet counts >50,000 are preferable for more extensive procedures and platelet counts >100,000 are preferred for cardiac and neurosurgical procedures. When required, pooled platelets are transfused in 6- to 10-U lots. Post-transfusion platelet counts are necessary to ensure achievement of an adequate platelet level. The maintenance of post-transfusion platelet counts may be only several hours. Patients maintained on nonsteroidal anti-inflammatory agents should discontinue these medications 2 days preoperatively, and those on aspirin should stop 1 to 3 weeks preoperatively, particularly before cardiovascular and neurosurgical procedures, because of the inhibitory effects of these agents on platelet function.

Clotting function is usually well preserved in elderly individuals. The coexistence of other disease processes, however, may make elderly patients more prone to postoperative thromboembolism, with a prevalence of 10% to 50%, depending on the procedure. Postoperative prophylaxis and early mobilization of the patient for the prevention of thrombosis is indicated [53,54].

Warfarin anticoagulation therapy should be stopped 3 days preoperatively. Those at high risk for thrombosis should be anticoagulated with heparin at doses sufficient to raise partial thromboplastin times to 50 to 80 seconds. Heparin may be stopped 1 hour before the operation and resumed in the early postoperative period. Alternatively, a low-molecular-weight heparin such as enoxaprin, 30 mg subcutaneously every 12 hours, may be given beginning 24 hours postoperatively. Patients at lower risk for thrombosis may be given 5,000 U of subcutaneous heparin every 12 hours through the perioperative period. Patients with elevated prothrombin times due to nutritional and liver diseases may improve their coagulation status by the administration of vitamin K and acutely by fresh frozen plasma. Patients who are anticoagulated with warfarin and are at high risk for thrombosis, however, should not have this corrected with vitamin K because it will antagonize the effects of warfarin for a prolonged period postoperatively.

TABLE 4-10. *Preoperative testing for elderly patients undergoing major surgical procedures*

Geriatric recommendations
Chest radiography
Electrocardiography
Serum chemistries (electrolytes, renal and hepatic function)
Serum albumin level
Complete blood count and platelet count
Prothrombin and partial thromboplastin times
Therapeutic drug monitoring (digoxin, antiarrhythmics, anticonvulsants)
Body weight
Mental status evaluation
Functional assessment
Recommendations for higher risk patients (chronic pulmonary disease, congestive heart failure, thoracic and upper abdominal procedures, morbid obesity)
Forced expiratory volume in 1 second
Arterial blood gas or oxygen saturation

Preoperative Testing

Selective preoperative testing is indicated to screen for medical problems and to document baseline physiologic function in order to plan surgical procedures more safely and to monitor and anticipate medical problems in the perioperative period. Because of the increased prevalence of disease processes in older surgical patients and the reduced physiologic reserve of many organs, preoperative assessment of renal, cardiac, pulmonary, hematologic, and metabolic function is indicated [55,56] (Table 4-10). Repeating recently performed laboratory testing preoperatively is unnecessary; however, preoperative documentation of baseline weight, nutritional status, functional assessment, mental status, and neurologic examination is extremely helpful.

Signs and Symptoms

Physicians are familiar with the usual physical findings and symptoms of most disease processes. They must also be aware that the physiologic response to many of the stresses of illness are altered in the elderly. The experienced clinician should not be dissuaded by the absence of a fever or localizing signs when common disease entities are suspected. Rather, a strong clinical suspicion and constant vigilance are important to optimize patient care in this population [57]. The discussions of aging organ systems' physiologic reserve and geriatric syndromes elsewhere in this chapter provide more information on the presentation of specific disease processes in older patients.

Prophylactic Treatment

Prophylactic antibiotic therapy is appropriate preoperatively in many different situations [52,58,59] (Table 4-11). Controlled studies of many procedures have shown improved results postoperatively, with fewer infectious complications

TABLE 4-11. *Antimicrobial prophylaxis in surgery**

Procedure	Likely pathogens	Recommended drugs	Intravenous prophylactic dose
Cardiac	Gram positive	Cephalosporin or vancomycin	1 g
Endocarditis prophylaxis	Gram positive	Ampicillin	2 g preoperatively, 1 g 8 hrs postoperatively
		or vancomycin	1 g preoperatively
Vascular	Gram positive	Ampicillin or vancomycin	1 g
Orthopedics	Gram positive	Ampicillin or vancomycin	600 mg
Neurosurgery	Gram positive	Ampicillin or vancomycin	1 g
Head and neck	Gram positive, anaerobes	Cephalosporin	1 g
		or clindamycin	600 mg
Gastrointestinal	Gram negative	Cephalosporin	1 g
Ruptured viscus	Gram negative, anaerobes	Cephalosporin and aminoglycoside	1 g and 1.5 mg/kg, respectively
		or clindamycin	600 mg
Genitourinary	Gram negative	Cephalosporin	1 g
Trauma	Gram positive	Cephalosporin	1 g

*Antimicrobial prophylaxis can decrease the incidence of infection after certain operations. Prophylaxis for clean surgery is not necessary unless it involves implantation of prosthetic material. A single dose of a parenteral antibiotic within 30 minutes of surgery provides adequate tissue concentrations for several hours. Postoperative prophylactic doses are generally not necessary.

Sources: Modified from Antimicrobial prophylaxis in surgery. Med Lett 1992;34:5–8; Kaiser AB. Antimicrobial prophylaxis in surgery. N Engl J Med 1986;315:1129–1138; and Dajani AS, Bisno AL, Chung KJ, et al. Prevention of bacterial endocarditis. Recommendations by the American Heart Association. JAMA 1990;264:2919–2922.

when prophylactic antibiotics are judiciously used for selected elderly patients with underlying disease processes.

Pain Management

Relief of suffering is always an important goal in medical and surgical care. Pain is frequently a component of disease processes and an object of postoperative care. It can be measured on a Likert scale (0 = no pain, 5 = excruciating pain). Quantifying pain is a useful construct when discussing its management with patients. By its very nature, pain is subjective and during the first assessment, the patient's reports should be accepted as accurate.

The more chronic the pain, the more the patient questions its meaning and necessity. Chronic pain involves changes in personality, life-style, and family interaction and has important social and environmental effects. Careful attention on the part of the treating physician is crucial in pain management in order for the patient to understand and accept short-term pain and to develop an appropriate treatment strategy for chronic pain.

General principles of pain therapy apply to most treatment situations. The provision of pain medication on a frequent basis with the dosing interval designed to prevent the return of pain is more effective than an as-needed schedule because the patient experiences pain and must ask for additional medication. This delays pain relief while subsequent doses of medications take effect. Constipation always accompanies narcotic use, and the provision of laxatives and stool softeners is especially important and necessary with any narcotic prescription for elderly patients.

Opiates have at least four different CNS receptors (Table 4-12). Different opiates such as pentazocine, butorphanol (Stadol), and the meperidine (Demerol) metabolite normeperidine preferentially stimulate the sigma receptor, producing dysphoria and confusion. This is a major problem for the elderly. Short-acting opiates preferentially stimulate the mu receptor, producing euphoria and contributing to habituation. All opiates stimulate the kappa or analgesic receptor. However, partial opiate agonists have a limited benefit: Increasing doses cannot achieve greater analgesia compared with that of the other opiates. Dose equivalence for opiates is presented in Table 4-13.

TABLE 4-12. *Opioid receptors*

Receptors	Effects
Mu	Euphoria, analgesia
Delta	Modulates mu-receptor activity
Kappa	Analgesia, sedation
Sigma	Dysphoria

Chronic pain management is important in terminal conditions, amputations, and following certain types of trauma such as crush injuries. Combination therapy and multimodality treatment are important management techniques [60,61]. The combination of analgesics with antidepressants, scheduled acetaminophen doses, or nonsteroidal anti-inflammatory drugs may be effective in many cases. Use of an analgesic ladder, progressing in intensity of pain medication from nonopiates to weak then strong opiates with adjuvant drugs at each step, may be an appropriate treatment strategy. Long-acting morphine and, for patients unable to tolerate oral medications, fentanyl transdermal patches can provide long-lasting relief with a minimum of side effects. Consultation with a pain therapy service, clinical psychologist, psychiatrist, and physical therapist may be useful adjuncts. Biofeedback, transcutaneous electrical

TABLE 4-13. *Analgesic dose comparisons*

Nonsteroidal agents

Drug	Analgesic dose (mg)	Maximum daily dose (mg)	Dose interval (hrs)
Aspirin	500–1,000	4,000	4–6
Acetaminophen	500–1,000	4,000	4–6
Ibuprofen	200–400	2,400	4–6
Salsalate	1,000	6,000	8–12

Narcotics

Drug	Equivalent dose (mg)	Starting dose (mg)	Dose interval (hrs)
Morphine (PO)	30	20–30	3–4
Morphine (SC, IV)	2	2–4	2–3
Codeine	60	30–60	3–4
Oxycodone	5	5	3–4
Fentanyl transdermal	0.025	0.025	72

Source: Modified from American Pain Society. Principles of Analgesic Use in the Treatment of Acute Pain and Chronic Cancer: A Concise Guide to Medical Practice (2nd ed). Skokie, IL: American Pain Society, 1989.

nerve stimulator units, and neural blockade injections may be indicated in certain circumstances.

Older individuals usually have decreased tolerance to the sedating effects of narcotics and antianxiety agents. Careful observation of the clinical response and gradual escalation of the dose are important considerations. Avoiding opiates with preferential sigma receptor affinity and using shorter-acting tranquilizers and antidepressants with lower anticholinergic potential are recommended for the elderly patient.

CONCLUSION

The older patient population is an enlarging consumer force in the American health care system. More and more elderly patients will require surgical care. Major surgical procedures can be performed without excessive morbidity and mortality in selected elderly patients. Age itself is less important than the influence of concomitant disease processes and physiologic parameters in predicting surgical outcome. Emergency procedures greatly decrease the chances of a favorable outcome. Older patients have decreased physiologic reserve in all organ systems; careful attention to this factor is important in the preoperative, intraoperative, and postoperative management of the older surgical patient. A well-targeted medical and surgical approach with clearly outlined postoperative goals and care plans is crucial in optimizing outcome in the older surgical patient. Careful attention to maximizing the preoperative physiologic status will improve outcome.

Attention to postoperative care, functional ability, and disposition is of critical importance and must be part of the treatment plan. A vigorous rehabilitation and restorative approach to maximizing functional abilities and supporting the patient's caregivers enhances surgical outcome. A multidisciplinary approach involving all health care professionals concerned with the patient and including the patient and family are important parts of the care of every elderly surgical patient. The rewards of seeing very elderly patients tolerate, survive, and recover from well-planned surgical procedures are great and are becoming one of the highest measures of our profession's success.

REFERENCES

1. United States Senate Special Committee on Aging, American Association of Retired Persons, Federal Council on the Aging, and United States Administration on Aging. Aging America, Trends and Projections. FCA 91-28001. Washington, DC: U.S. Department of Health and Human Services, 1991.
2. Coroni-Huntley J, Brock DB, Ostfeld AM, et al. Established Populations for Epidemiologic Studies of the Elderly: Resource Data Book. NIH 86-2443. Washington, DC: U.S. Department of Health and Human Services, 1986.
3. National Center for Health Statistics. Detailed Diagnosis and Procedures, National Hospital Discharge Survey, 1990. Vital and Health Statistics, Series 13, No. 112. DHHS (PHS) 92-1773. Hyattsville, MD: U.S. Department Health and Human Services, 1992.
4. Feigal DW, Blaisdell FW. The estimation of surgical risk. Med Clin North Am 1979;63:1131–1143.
5. Seymour DG, Vaz FG. A prospective study of elderly surgical patients: II. postoperative complications. Age Ageing 1989;18:316–325.
6. Merli GJ. Prophylaxis for deep vein thrombosis and pulmonary embolism in the geriatric patient undergoing surgery. Clin Geriatr Med 1990;6:531–542.
7. Adkins RB, Scott HW. Surgical procedures in patients aged 90 years and older. South Med J 1984;77:1357–1364.
8. Hosking MP, Warner MA, Lobdell CM, et al. Outcomes of surgery in patients 90 years of age and older. JAMA 1989;261:1909–1915.
9. MacPherson DA, Parenti C, Nee JN, et al. An internist joins the surgery service: does co-management make a difference? J Gen Intern Med 1994;9:440–444.
10. Lichtenstein H, Winograd CH. Geriatric consultation: a functional approach. J Am Geriatr Soc 1985;32:356–361.
11. Naylor M, Brooten D, Jones R, et al. Comprehensive discharge planning for the hospitalized elderly: a randomized clinical trial. Ann Intern Med 1994;120:999–1006.
12. U.S. Department of Health, Education, and Welfare. Preliminary Findings of the First Health and Nutrition Examination Survey, United States 1971–72. Dietary Intake and Biochemical Findings. DHEW HRA 74-1219-1. Washington, DC: U.S. Department of Health, Education, and Welfare, 1974.
13. Roubenoff R, Roubenoff RA, Preto J, Balke CW. Malnutrition among hospitalized patients: a problem of physician awareness. Arch Intern Med 1987;174:1462–1465.
14. Baker JP, Detsky AS, Wesson DE, et al. Nutritional assessment: a comparison of clinical judgment and objective measurements. N Engl J Med 1982;306:969–972.
15. Sullivan DH, Patch GA, Walls RC, Lipschitz DA. Impact of nutrition status on morbidity and mortality in a select population of geriatric rehabilitation patients. Am J Clin Nutr 1990;51:749–758.
16. Michel L, Serrano A, Malt RA. Nutritional support of hospitalized patients. N Engl J Med 1981;304:1147–1152.
17. Shetty PS, Watrasiewicz KE, Jung RT, et al. Rapid-turnover transport proteins: an index of subclinical protein-energy malnutrition. Lancet 1979;2:230–232.
18. Mullen JL, Buzby GP, Matthews DC, et al. Reduction of operative mortality and morbidity by combined preoperative and postoperative nutrition support. Ann Surg 1980;192:604–613.

19. Cluff LE, Thornton EF, Seidl LG. Studies on the epidemiology of adverse drug reactions. JAMA 1964;188:976–983.
20. Greenblatt DJ, Sellers EM, Shader RI. Drug disposition in old age. N Engl J Med 1982;37:51–55.
21. Sloan RW. How to minimize side effects of psychoactive drugs. Geriatrics 1982;306:1081–1088.
22. Everitt DE, Avorn J. Drug prescribing for the elderly. Arch Intern Med 1986;146:2393–2396.
23. Ouslander JF. Drug therapy in the elderly. Ann Intern Med 1981;95:711–722.
24. Berardi L. Geriatric medicine. Med Clin North Am 1983;67:315–332.
25. Working Party on Medication in the Elderly: medication for the elderly. J Royal Col Phys (London) 1984;18:7–17.
26. Beers MH, Ouslander JG. Risk factors in geriatric drug prescribing: a practical guide to avoiding problems. Drugs 1989;37:105–112.
27. American College of Physicians. American college of physicians ethics manual. Ann Intern Med 1989;111:245–252, 327–335.
28. Katz S, Downs TD, Cash HR, et al. Progress in the development of the index of ADL. Gerontologist 1970;10:20–30.
29. Katz S. Assessing self-maintenance: activities of daily living, mobility, and instrumental activities of daily living. J Am Geriatr Soc 1983;31:721–727.
30. Lawton MD, Brody EM. Assessment of older people: self-maintaining and instrumental activities of daily living. Gerontologist 1969;9:179–185.
31. Fries JF, Crapo LM. Vitality and Aging. San Francisco: Freeman, 1981.
32. Criteria Committee of the New York Heart Association, Inc. Disease of the Heart and Blood Vessels (6th ed). Boston: Little, Brown, 1964.
33. Child CG, Turcotte JG. The Liver and Portal Hypertension. Philadelphia: Saunders, 1964.
34. American Joint Committee on Cancer. Manual of Staging of Cancer (4th ed). Chicago: American Joint Committee on Cancer, 1992.
35. Karnofsky DA, Abelmann WH, Craver LF, Burchenal JH. The use of nitrogen mustards in the palliative treatment of carcinoma. Cancer 1948;1:634–656.
36. Sheilch JI, Yesavage JA. Geriatric depression scale: recent evidence and development of a shorter version. Clin Geriatr Med 1986;5:165–172.
37. Folstein MF, Folstein S, McHugh PR. Mini mental state: a practical method of grading the cognitive state of patients for the clinician. J Psychiatr Res 1975;12:189–198.
38. Owens WD, Felts JA, Spitznagel EL. ASA physical status classifications: a study of consistency of ratings. Anesthesiology 1978;49: 239–243.
39. Knaus WA, Zimmerman JE, Wagner DP, et al. APACHE—acute physiology and chronic health evaluation: a physiologically based classification system. Crit Care Med 1981;9:591–597.
40. Winograd CH, Lemsky CM, Nevitt MC. Development of a physical performance and mobility examination. J Am Geriatr Soc 1994;42: 743–749.
41. Gustafson Y, Berggren D, Brannstrom B, et al. Acute confusional states in elderly patients treated for femoral neck fracture. J Am Geriatr Soc 1988;36:525–530.
42. American Psychiatric Association. Diagnostic and Statistical Manual of Mental Disorders (4th ed). Washington, DC: American Psychiatric Association, 1994.
43. The treatment of sleep disorders in older people. Consensus Statement 1990;8:1–22.
44. Cooper JC, Gates GA. Hearing in the elderly—the Framingham cohort, 1983–1985: part II. Prevalence of central auditory processing disorders. Ear Hearing 1991;1215:304–311.
45. Sommer A. Cataracts as an epidemiologic problem. Am J Ophthalmol 1977;83:334–339.
46. Kübler-Ross E. On Death and Dying. New York: Macmillan, 1969.
47. Ouslander JG. Diagnostic evaluation of geriatric urinary incontinence. Clin Geriatr Med 1986;2:715–730.
48. Crapo RO. Pulmonary function testing. N Engl J Med 1994;331:25–30.
49. Detsky AS, Abrams HB, McLaughlin JR, et al. Predicting cardiac complications in patients undergoing non-cardiac surgery. J Gen Intern Med 1986;1:211–219.
50. Goldman L, Caldera D, Nussbaum SR, et al. Multifactorial index of cardiac risk in non-cardiac surgical procedures. N Engl J Med 1977;297:845–850.
51. Detsky AS, Abrams HB, Forbath N, et al. Cardiac assessment for patients undergoing non-cardiac surgery: a multifactorial clinical risk index. Arch Intern Med 1986;146:2131–2134.
52. Dajani AS, Bisno AL, Chung KJ, et al. Prevention of bacterial endocarditis: recommendations by the American Heart Association. JAMA 1990;264:2919–2922.
53. National Institutes of Health Consensus Development. Prevention of venous thrombosis and pulmonary embolism. JAMA 1986;256: 744–749.
54. Moser KM. Venous thromboembolism. Am Rev Respir Dis 1990; 144:235–249.
55. Berg C, Charpak Y, Szatan M, et al. Evaluation of a protocol for selective ordering of preoperative tests. Lancet 1986;1:139–141.
56. Roizen M. Preoperative patient evaluation. Can J Anaesth 1989;36: S13–S19.
57. Hodkinson HM. Nonspecific presentation of illness. BMJ 1973;4:94–96.
58. Antimicrobial prophylaxis in surgery. Med Lett 1992;34:5–8.
59. Kaiser AB. Antimicrobial prophylaxis in surgery. N Engl J Med 1986;315:1129–1138.
60. American Pain Society. Principles of Analgesic Use in the Treatment of Acute Pain and Chronic Cancer: A Concise Guide to Medical Practice (2nd ed). Skokie, IL: American Pain Society, 1989.
61. Jacox A, Carr DB, Payne R, et al. Management of Cancer Pain. Clinical Practice Guideline No. 9. AHCPR Publication No. 94-0592. Rockville, MD: Agency for Health Care Policy and Research, U.S. Department of Health and Human Services, 1994.

Surgical Care for the Elderly, 2nd ed., edited by
R. Benton Adkins, Jr., and H. William Scott, Jr.
Lippincott–Raven Publishers, Philadelphia © 1998.

CHAPTER 5

Anesthetic Considerations in Elderly Patients

Bradley E. Smith

BASIC CONSIDERATIONS OF ANESTHESIA FOR THE ELDERLY

Demography: Morbidity and Mortality

The twenty-first century may become known as "the century of the centenarian." In 1900 only one in 25 Americans was aged 65 or greater and 1% were 85 or more. The number of centenarians doubled between 1980 and 1996 [1]. Since 1900 the U.S. population under age 65 has tripled, but those aged 65 and older have increased 11-fold. In 1996, one in eight Americans was aged 65 or greater. By the year 2020, a further increase of approximately 50% is expected, indicating that approximately 53 million Americans will be aged 65 or older in 2020 [1].

Currently, approximately 25% of all surgical procedures in the United States involve patients over the age of 65. Approximately 50% of people aged 50 years and older will require a surgical procedure at least once during the balance of their lives [2]. As recently as 1960, overall perioperative and postoperative surgical mortality was reported to be 19% in elderly patients, dropping to 13% in 1972 and 6% in 1983 [3]. Other authors estimated that perioperative mortality doubled for similar procedures between the fourth and seventh decades of life [4]. The chance of a life-threatening complication developing in relation to surgery was approximately 12% in the group aged 65 to 74 and 33% in the surgical patient older than 75 years. Life-threatening complications are over three times more frequent in elderly patients after emergency procedures (35%) than after nonemergency procedures (11%) in similar elder age groups [3]. Therefore, not only now, but increasingly in the future, anesthesiologists must be aware of the altered clinical pharmacology of anesthesia in the elderly and factors pertinent to the choice and management of anesthesia in elderly patients [5–7].

Pathophysiologic Alterations in the Elderly

Body Compartment Composition

Intracellular water gradually decreases with age, along with a gradual increase of approximately 10% in body fat [8]. Thus, elderly patients often store a greater proportion of inhaled or intravenous (IV) anesthetics because of the proportionate increase of the fat reservoir to which these highly lipid-soluble substances are attached [9]. This can lead both to prolonged somnolence in some cases and to the production of an increased percentage of secondary metabolic breakdown products of the anesthetic drugs, which are at times toxic.

Protein Binding

Serum albumin concentration decreases progressively with age, but $alpha_1$ acid glycoprotein may be normal or even elevated [10]. Drugs that are particularly bound to $alpha_1$ acid glycoprotein include propranolol and local anesthetics such as lidocaine and others. Therefore, in the elderly with elevated $alpha_1$ glycoprotein, concentration of the free active form of these drugs in the plasma may be inadequate after "normal" doses, due to increased binding to $alpha_1$-glycoprotein [10,11]. Plasma protein binding is 92% with sufentanil, 92% with alfentanil, and 84% with fentanyl. Thus, the decrease in serum albumin in old age would allow more unbound active drug to be available for binding in opiate receptors [12].

Lower albumin levels may lead to greater concentrations of circulating unbound, active thiopental in the elderly [13–15], although binding of propofol to protein (97% to 99%) has been reported as similar in elderly and young patients [16]. There is a markedly decreased affinity for the binding of etomidate to plasma proteins in the elderly, thus leading to a higher effective plasma concentration of free etomidate [17]. Meperidine also binds strongly to plasma albumin. Therefore, in a typical elderly patient with low serum albumin, the administration of meperidine at unreduced doses will result in markedly greater free (active) plasma drug concentration than in younger patients. This may account for increased sensitivity to respiratory depression from meperidine in elderly patients [18,19].

Neurologic System

Cerebral blood flow is reduced by approximately 20% in the elderly, and in disease states may be even more decreased both globally and regionally [20]. Chronic active hyperventilation and resulting hypocapnia under general anesthesia were found to have no more prolonged or depressive effect in elderly than in young patients [21]. Most inhalation and IV anesthetics, sedatives, and narcotics appear to share an increased effect in the aged [22–24]. This may result from reduction in the numbers of surviving neuronal cells, reduction in the insulating qualities of the neurons [25], relative decreases in some neurotransmitter substances [26], or a change in the quantity or sensitivity of various receptors [27,28]. The latter may be the case with alpha- and beta-adrenergic receptors in brain, substantia gelatinosa, and end receptors in cardiovascular sites [29].

Protective autonomic reflexes of the trachea, pharynx, larynx, and airway are well known to be progressively less effective as age advances, thus leading to far more frequent aspiration of vomitus, secretions, or foreign substances and decreased vigor in clearing the upper airways by coughing [30,31].

There is some evidence that the blood-brain barrier is less efficient in the elderly. A classic example is the more frequent appearance of scopolamine "psychosis" in elderly patients than in younger ones. This may be due to achievement of higher active drug levels in the brain substance of the elderly (see following section on postanesthetic delirium) [32]. Neuromuscular receptor sensitivity has not been thought to be altered until after age 75 [33,34]. Decreased sensitivity of the neuromuscular junction is a possible explanation for the commonly reported reduced steady-state dose requirements and extended recovery time after the use of several nondepolarizing relaxants in the elderly [35].

Cardiovascular System

Cardiac index decreases approximately 1% per year over age 30, but a larger proportion of the output is routed to the brain and less to liver and kidneys. Left ventricular ejection fraction (LVEF) is a good predictor of cardiac-related mortality. Despite observed indications of decrease in other cardiac functions proportionate to age, it has been demonstrated that there is no decrease in LVEF in proportion to age in the absence of cardiac disease. Average resting LVEF remains between 55% and 76% from age 62 to age 98. Baseline peak left ventricular filling rate is reduced in the elderly by approximately 40% [36].

In healthy elderly patients there is some increased atrial contribution to diastolic filling, but the decreased rate of left ventricular diastolic filling appears to relate to increased interstitial tissue in the heart or deterioration of the active process of actin-myosin secondary to impaired calcium transport by the sarcoplasmic reticulum [37]. Resting stroke volume ordinarily is little changed with aging, although cardiovascular response to stress may be reduced. Unlike young patients, who typically increase the ejection and stroke volume under cardiovascular stress, elderly patients are less able to respond in this fashion [38]. Heart rate in the elderly is frequently reduced. In fact, the tachycardiac response to atropine and similar drugs is much attenuated in the elderly. The expected responses to sudden changes in posture or intrathoracic pressure are often not seen at all in the elderly due to the marked decrease in baroreceptor and other homeostatic reflex responses [39].

The effects of aging on the human sympathetic nervous system is still a matter of some controversy. It has been postulated that dysfunction of the postsynaptic adrenergic responsiveness in the heart of the elderly might account for the genesis of ventricular tachyarrhythmias or sudden cardiac death, which is a significant cause of cardiovascular mortality in the elderly (see previous discussion) [40]. Resting sympathetic nervous activity increases progressively with age, and exercise leads to a greater increase in blood pressure, but a lesser increase in heart rate response [40].

There is a well-documented reduction in vagal, particularly cardiac vagal, function with advancing age, which often removes the normal opposing force for sympathetic stimulation of the heart and leads to cardiac acceleration during stress [41]. Furthermore, older patients respond to the isoproterenol-stimulated tilt table test with less frequent development of syncope, and are less likely to develop relative bradycardia during the test [42].

Low-frequency heart rate variability has been said to be an indicator of cardiac sympathetic tone and has been used as a further assessment of cardiac autonomic function. In the elderly, reduced heart rate variability in postinfarction patients has been reported to predict risk for subsequent mortality. It also appears that reduced heart rate variability found on screening electrocardiographs in elderly patients may have some predictive capability for mortality from cardiac events. Therefore, encountering decreased heart rate variability on preoperative evaluation might be considered an increased cardiac risk factor for anesthesia and surgery [43].

Respiratory System

The elderly frequently exhibit progressive decreases in maximum breathing capacity, total lung capacity, and vital capacity consistent with the progressive loss of elasticity of cartilaginous structures and decrease in muscularity of the diaphragm and intercostal muscles. In addition, respiratory rate, tidal volume, minute volume, and maximum diffusing capacity of the lung for oxygen are all decreased progressively with age. Anatomic dead space, residual volume, functional residual capacity, and total lung capacity increase progressively with age, often mimicking or actually involving emphysema [44]. Central control of respiration is even more impaired by narcotics and inhalational anesthetics than in younger patients [45]. Therefore, the aged are less able to respond successfully to hypercarbia and hypoxia in the presence of many anesthetics, analgesics, and sedatives [46].

Lung closing volume and resulting intrapulmonary shunting increases progressively with age due to functional deterioration of terminal lung architecture. The resting arterial oxygen values often gradually decline. Furthermore, there may be less efficient compensation for this increased pulmonary shunting in the elderly due to their less efficient hypoxic pulmonary vasoconstrictor reflex mechanisms [47]. These changes would tend to slow induction of anesthesia by inhalational agents.

Hepatic Function

In the elderly, most liver function test values remain similar to those of younger patients. However, liver blood flow at age 65 is reduced to approximately 40% less than liver blood flow in the same patient at age 30. In addition, the mass of the liver is decreased by approximately 20% in old age [8,16,48,49]. Aging is associated with a loss in the functioning mass of hepatocytes in the liver, and the frequently observed decreased hepatic clearance of many drugs in the elderly is directly related to the loss of hepatocytes and total liver volume [50]. The conversion by the liver of lipid-soluble drugs to water-soluble metabolites by conjugation is therefore hindered. This may lead to an increased duration of action for many lipid-soluble drugs, including some anesthetics and sedatives [51,52]. Despite other changes, acetylation activity and alcohol dehydrogenase enzymes are preserved at near normal levels in the elderly liver. Fentanyl, sufentanil, and alfentanil all depend almost exclusively on phase 1 drug metabolism in the liver (*N*-demethylation, hydroxylation, or both—a process that is greatly decreased in direct proportion to age) [53]. Liver microsomal enzymes, which are important in oxidizing many anesthetic drugs, are less active in older patients, and enzyme induction and glucuronidation are also impaired.

Renal Function

The serum creatinine level in the elderly usually remains normal even though there is reduced renal excretion of creatinine, because there is also relatively less skeletal muscle mass, which produces creatinine, resulting in a net normal serum level [51]. Renal blood flow and glomerular filtration rate decline approximately 1.5% per year past the age of 30, thus resulting in a hindrance to excretion of some drugs and their detoxification breakdown products. Decreased renal function in the elderly can also lead to accumulation of drug metabolites that may have secondary toxic or depressing effects in the body. The accumulation of active drug metabolites may be clinically important in the case of methyldopa, morphine, triamterene, spironolactone, levodopa, and acetylated sulfonamides [18]. Reduced renal clearance in elderly patients affects some anesthetic drugs. Although proximal tubular function may remain essentially unchanged, concentrating ability and other distal tubular functions are progressively impaired, particularly resulting in a decreased ability to excrete acid. Therefore, a greater urinary volume is necessary when an acid-solute load is expected.

Pharmacokinetic Alterations Related to Anesthesia in the Elderly

Pharmacokinetics is the term used to describe the processes of drug uptake, distribution, and elimination and, therefore, explains much of the clinical picture of drug effects. In anesthesia uptake, routes are usually IV or intramuscular but also include prominently respiratory uptake and elimination. Because of the many alterations and impairments of body composition, physiology, and pathology incident to advancing age, most of the altered actions of drugs in the elderly can be described as pharmacokinetic changes. However, a few of the changes in clinical pharmacology of drugs in the elderly are due to changes in the number or sensitivity of the receptor sites or changes in effector pathways or effector sites. Such alterations, although few in number, are known as pharmacodynamic alterations.

Volume of Distribution

Volume of distribution (Vd) refers to the concept that if plasma is sampled for its concentration of a drug and the concentration is divided by the known total dose of the drug already administered at that point in time, the result describes a theoretic volume in which the drug would be diluted if all compartments had the same solubility as plasma and mixing was even [54]. Of course, all organs and spaces are not equally mixed, because some organs have greater solubility for many drugs than does plasma, and blood flow and mass are quite variable in the various organs. Therefore, the Vd may be greater than the real volume of the body.

Central Compartment

The apparent volume of plasma is calculated when the plasma concentration of drug is measured during a period of straight line decline during the distribution phase, and this concentration is divided by the total dose of drug administered; this is often called the *central volume* (V_1). V_1 is characteristically reduced with both lipophilic and hydrophilic drugs in elderly patients because cardiac output and vessel-rich organ blood flow is often reduced, therefore delaying the exit of injected drugs from the central plasma pool and yielding a higher than predicted plasma concentration of the injected drug [55].

Peripheral Compartment

Peripheral compartment (Vd_{SS}) is the apparent volume of plasma calculated from plasma drug concentration divided by drug dose during a period of straight time decline in the drug elimination phase [54]. As mentioned, there is a direct decrease in lean body mass and an increase in fat body mass with increasing age that has been said to predict an increase in Vd_{SS} for lipophilic drugs [8]. If drug clearance is unchanged (see discussion of clearance), this increase in Vd_{SS} will lead to a prolonged elimination half-life. Vd_{SS} for both thiopentone [15] and fentanyl is increased in elderly patients [55]. In contrast to lipophilic agents, the Vd_{SS} of water-soluble compounds is generally *decreased* with age.

If drug clearance is unchanged, a diminished Vd_{SS} will lead to a decreased elimination half-life (accelerated elimination) and also generally to higher plasma levels. Because pharmacologic response is related to plasma drug concentration, a decrease in Vd_{SS} may often produce exaggerated drug effects as well as an increased incidence of adverse drug reactions, but might shorten the total half-life of the drug. Ethanol is a frequently cited example of this effect in the elderly. Since body water is usually diminished in older patients, Vd_{SS} of ethyl alcohol (water soluble) is diminished, and consequently blood alcohol levels are frequently higher in older men after ingestion of similar doses of alcohol than in younger men. However, the rate of metabolism and excretion of alcohol is relatively normal and alcohol dehydrogenase retains normal activity [56].

Clearance

Clearance (Cl) is the volume of plasma from which drug is completely removed in a unit of time, usually minutes or hours. It is a mathematical concept only, because in the body no aliquot of plasma actually has all its drug removed at any one time [54].

Hepatic Clearance

Hepatic Cl (Cl_H) of many drugs decreases with age because of age-related decreases in hepatic blood flow, hepatic mass, and enzymatic activity. Propofol, which is largely eliminated by the liver [16], and etomidate [17] appear to have slightly decreased Cl in the elderly, consistent with a similar decrease in liver blood flow [8], but thiopental does not [13], probably because its liver degradation is rate limited [16].

Half-Life

Half-life ($t_{1/2}$)($t_{1/2\alpha}$)($t_{1/2\beta}$)($t_{1/2E}$) is used to describe the time in minutes or hours required for the plasma drug concentration to decrease to one-half the concentration at any arbitrary starting point. The term $t_{1/2\alpha}$ usually describes the half-life of the distribution phase, $t_{1/2\beta}$ describes the elimination phase, and $t_{1/2E}$ describes the half-life of total elimination of the drug. It is calculated as a function of Vd_{SS} multiplied by a constant, divided by Cl [57].

Benzodiazepines

Many benzodiazepines (BZDs) exhibit a more profound effect and longer duration of effect in elderly patients [58]. There is increasing evidence that this sensitivity is due both to pharmacokinetic and pharmacodynamic changes in the elderly [59–68]. Animal studies indicate that the brain concentration of BZDs does not decrease parallel to decreasing plasma concentration [64]. Both decreased Cl and extended $t_{1/2E}$ have been reported in direct relation to age with a number of BZDs [69–71]. The metabolic clearance of most BZDs is initiated by microsomal oxidation in the liver, a process that is impaired in the elderly [69].

Diazepam

Cl of diazepam (Valium) from the plasma is unchanged in the elderly. However, Vd_{SS} of diazepam is doubled, partly because of the relative increase in body fat, and partly because of decreased protein binding, which leads to greater and more rapid distribution to the tissues. This increase in Vd_{SS} in turn causes a dramatic fourfold increase in $t_{1/2E}$ from 22 hours at age 20 to approximately 70 hours at age 80 [9]. In contrast, oxazepam and lorazepam are two commonly used BZDs that are far more hydrophilic than diazepam. Not surprisingly, the pharmacologic disposition of these two agents has been shown to be very similar in elderly and younger patients [9,72]. Diazepam is increasingly depressive as age advances, even at low doses, especially to cognitive function, but to neuromotor skills to a lesser degree as well, and this effect is shared by alprazolam, triazolam, and most BZDs [24,73].

Midazolam

Anesthesia induction times are reported to be faster with midazolam (Versed) in direct proportion to advancing age due to a slight reduction in protein binding and reduction in V_1 [74–77]. However, Vd_{SS} is expanded and Cl is reduced by nearly half. Therefore, $t_{1/2E}$ is more than doubled, greatly extending the duration of somnolence in the elderly after midazolam use compared with the action in younger patients [74,76]. Furthermore, good evidence now shows that at approximately age 70 there is an acceleration in sensitivity to midazolam that probably represents a deterioration of some pharmacodynamic factor in its action [68]. It has been alleged that diazepam does not share this added danger after age 70 [66]. Flumazenil is quite effective in reversing most of the BZDs' effects even in the elderly; however, disorientation and excitement are frequent side effects of reversal [78–80].

Lorazepam

The pharmacokinetics of lorazepam (Atwan) are little different in elderly and young adult patients [81]. Lorazepam in oral doses of 1 to 2 mg has little effect on the respiratory or cardiovascular system of the elderly [82,83]. In addition, even at very low doses it has a useful ability to totally inhibit memory and does so to a quantitatively greater degree in the aged (65 to 80 years) compared with younger (18 to 30 years) patients [82]. However, the effects of lorazepam are not disproportionate in patients with Alzheimer's disease compared with "normal" patients of the same age [84]. Because the liver is the site of conjugation of lorazepam and because excretion of conjugated lorazepam (glucuronide) is a renal function, this drug is not recommended for use in patients with advanced hepatic or renal failure [9,81].

Flurazepam and Triazolam

Flurazepam (Dalmane) and triazolam (Halcion) are two more BZDs that, although not used intraoperatively by the anesthesiologist, have frequently been prescribed as premedicant drugs. Flurazepam is biotransformed into a cascade of metabolites, one of which has a very long $t_{1/2E}$. Therefore, considerable accumulation of this compound may occur with repeated dosages [85]. However, administration of 0.25 mg orally caused deterioration of psychomotor coordination to a critical level. It was postulated that these effects were due to the achievement of higher peak plasma concentrations of unbound, active triazolam, possibly due to reduced central volume [86]. Triazolam has a shorter $t_{1/2E}$ in the range of 2 to 5 hours. It has no clinically active metabolites and has not been accused of lingering sedation after repeated doses in the elderly [85].

It has been confirmed that elderly patients demonstrate impaired cognitive performance following repeated treatment with flurazepam but not with triazolam; however, abrupt discontinuation of triazolam, unlike flurazepam, may cause post-treatment rebound sleep disorders [85]. A more recent study, however, although confirming the psychomotor effects in elderly patients, reported that the higher plasma drug concentrations achieved in the elderly were due to reduced Cl of the drug both with 0.125-mg and 0.25-mg oral doses of triazolam. These authors recommend that the dosage of triazolam in elderly patients should be reduced on average by 50% [71].

Narcotics

Morphine

In the elderly patient the pharmacology of the classic narcotic, morphine, has many similarities to some of the newer narcotics, but there are also many differences. Morphine clearly leads to greater respiratory depression in the elderly compared with the effects of similar doses in younger adults [45,87,88]. Whether this more profound and longer effect is due to pharmacodynamic changes brought on by aging or the pharmacokinetic alterations of aging has been disputed for decades [89]. On the other hand, narcotics in general are well tolerated by the cardiovascular system of the elderly, with the exception of occasional hypotension due to histamine release caused by morphine, but not the newer narcotics [88,90].

Fentanyl

Early reports on fentanyl (Sublimaze) in elderly patients stated that Cl and $t_{1/2\beta}$ were both reduced fourfold in the elderly [91]. However, a later report showed no differences at all in the pharmacokinetics of fentanyl in elderly versus young adults [92]. Yet later investigators found that Cl is similar in both groups, but V_1 and Vd_{SS} are reported to be significantly smaller in elderly patients and initial plasma concentrations are much higher in the elderly, probably consistent with the restricted central volume [55]. Fentanyl is one of the few anesthetic-related drugs that display a shorter plasma life in the elderly. In the case of fentanyl, this is due to maintenance of a normal Cl combined with a greatly restricted Vd_{SS} [55].

Sufentanil

V_1 has recently been reported to be restricted by nearly 40% with sufentanil (Sufenta) in elderly patients, which may account for its more profound initial effects. One author reports Cl and $t_{1/2E}$ to be similar in elderly and younger patients [53]. However, another report indicates $t_{1/2\beta}$ to be nearly quadrupled in older patients versus young patients [93]. The confusion may be related to the fact that the older studies were carried out in patients undergoing abdominal aortic surgery, which might severely reduce liver blood flow, thereby inhibiting liver clearance of sufentanil, whereas the more recent reports were in general surgical patients [53,93]. Differences in protein binding of sufentanil in elderly patients were deemed not responsible for the increased sensitivity [53]. Nonetheless, there are multiple documentations that sufentanil produces more profound and longer lasting clinical effects in the elderly than can be explained by the pharmacokinetic findings. It has been postulated that this represents evidence of as yet unidentified pharmacodynamic changes (i.e., decreased receptor density, increased receptor sensitivity, etc.) due to aging [53].

Alfentanil

There has also been some controversy concerning the pharmacology of alfentanil (Alfenta) in the aged. There is total agreement among authors that alfentanil produces more profound and prolonged effects in elderly compared with younger adults. Furthermore, respiratory muscle rigidity, hypotension, and bradycardia are found when young adult doses are administered to the elderly [94]. The alfentanil plasma concentration required to shift electroencephalogram spectral edge measurements have been found to decrease with aging, suggesting that elderly patients are more susceptible to alfentanil [95].

However, another study used indirect measurements of analgesic depth and duration and stated that plasma alfentanil concentration-effect curves for perioperative stimuli are identical in older and younger female patients. These authors agreed that the alfentanil dose required to achieve plasma concentrations of alfentanil is significantly lower in older than in younger patients and believe they have demonstrated pharmacokinetic factors causing this phenomenon [96]. V_1 for alfentanil appears to decrease with increasing age [97]. Vd_{SS} has been reported to be slightly expanded in one study [98], and slightly reduced in another report [97]. Most authors have reported that Cl of alfentanil is reduced by approximately one-third. Furthermore, $t_{1/2\beta}$ is prolonged by nearly two-thirds in elderly patients compared with young patients [97–101]. More recently, it has been shown that Cl data derived from single bolus injections of alfentanil greatly underestimate the actual reduction of Cl of alfentanil in the elderly. Cl of alfentanil in the elderly may approximate a 50% reduced rate [102].

Although alfentanil has previously been used exclusively as an IV drug, one recent report suggests that 12.5 μg/kg of alfentanil delivered into the deltoid (but not the gluteal) muscle can deliver complication-free analgesia and sedation lasting approximately 30 minutes in very elderly patients with few side effects [103].

Meperidine

Meperidine (Demerol) binds strongly to plasma albumin. Therefore, administration of meperidine in the elderly also results in a markedly greater free (active) plasma drug concentration than in younger patients [18]. Thus, although measured total blood levels of the combination of bound and unbound meperidine in the elderly are similar to those in young adults, the plasma concentration of the active unbound portion is greater in the elderly due to reduced protein binding. This results in greater respiratory depression in elderly patients [19].

Anesthetic Induction Agents

Thiopental and Methohexital

Loss of lid reflex with thiopental (Pentothal) is often achieved with only 70% of the dose required in younger patients [104]. This effect is probably due to a decreased V_1 of thiopental and not due to decreased Cl or increased drug sensitivity [105]. Thiopental, too, is highly bound to albumin, and, therefore, low plasma albumin levels in elderly patients allow higher plasma levels of active, unbound thiopental. This form penetrates the blood-brain barrier more effectively than albumin-bound thiopental [13,106]. Both reduced protein binding and high lipophilicity contribute to a greatly expanded Vd_{SS} of thiopental in elderly patients. Therefore, because Cl of thiopental remains unchanged, $t_{1/2E}$ is greatly prolonged [13,107]. Although there is some disagreement with these findings [106], corroborative information from the use of slow constant infusions of thiopental reinforces their general accuracy [105], as well as demonstrating the feasibility of anesthetic induction at a lower total dose and therefore a reduction in the incidence of side effects [108]. Thus, in the elderly, IV injection of a dose of thiopental calculated for young adults will usually result in both more profound and more immediate effect and a prolonged duration of somnolence. Based on limited data, it appears that these thiopental pharmacokinetics are shared by methohexital (Brevital) in the elderly [109].

Propofol

Propofol (Diprivan) is a newer induction agent that is becoming popular due to its quick recovery characteristics and reduced tendency for postoperative nausea and emesis. However, it can cause serious hypotension in some situations [110]. Slowing the induction infusion rate has been advocated to reduce the hypotensive effects of propofol in the elderly [111]. After doses similar to younger patients, the elderly achieve higher plasma propofol concentrations during the induction phase [112]. This is probably related to an observed reduction in V_1 [113,114]. In younger patients, Cl of propofol approximates total hepatic blood flow, and little or no Cl is accomplished by the kidney [114]. Cl is only slightly reduced in comparison with young patients. Therefore, it seems reasonable to assume that the slight decrease in Cl of propofol in the elderly may be largely due to an age-related relative decrease in hepatic blood flow and cardiac output in elderly patients [16]. In elderly patients $t_{1/2\beta}$ is prolonged by approximately 33% and $t_{1/2E}$ is extended by approximately 24% [16]. Plasma protein binding of propofol (approximately 99%) is similar in elder and younger patient groups [16,115]. By the use of a reduced rate of infusion, a clear increased sensitivity to propofol in the elderly can be demonstrated. This allows reduction of propofol induction doses by approximately 56% of that required in young adults, without prolongation of effect [116]. Others have confirmed that slower rates of injection of propofol delay induction in elderly patients, but induction occurs at lower doses and with a reduced incidence of hypotension [108].

Etomidate

The primary site of degradation of etomidate (Amidate) is the liver. Therefore, Cl of etomidate is very efficient in younger patients, being approximately one-half the hepatic blood flow. Earlier reports anticipated that the reduced hepatic blood flow commonly found in the elderly might cause decreased Cl of etomidate. However, etomidate Cl has now been demonstrated to be only slightly reduced in the elderly [17]. There is a markedly decreased affinity for the binding of etomidate to plasma proteins in the elderly, thus leading to a reduced calculated V_1 and a much higher effective plasma concentration of free drug in the elderly. This necessitates smaller induction doses of etomidate in the elderly. Reduced protein binding also contributes to an expanded Vd_{SS}, and in turn, a prolonged $t_{1/2E}$ [17]. Reduced injection rate in the elderly leads to delayed induction with etomidate, but induction occurs at a lower infused dose [108].

Ketamine

Ketamine (Ketalar, Ketaject) is a useful induction agent in children, but is rarely used in young adults and almost never in elder patients due to a tendency to cause unpleasant dreams or even hallucinations. These may be seen with the highest frequency in aged patients [117]. Ketamine is notable for its support of blood pressure and sympatheticomimetic effects and therefore is occasionally used in very small doses, along with reduced doses of BZDs. In these small doses and in the presence of BZDs, hallucinations are rarely if ever reported, even in the elderly [117].

Muscle Relaxants

Curare and Metocurine

Similar doses of nondepolarizing muscle relaxants cause much elevated plasma concentrations in elderly compared with younger patients. This is due to a reduced V_1 and Cl, along with reduced Vd_{SS} for these drugs in the elderly [34]. Vd_{SS} with both metocurine (Metubine) and curare (D-tubocurarine) is approximately one-half that of young adults. The reduction of Cl predominates, causing the duration of action to be greatly extended. In fact, $t_{1/2E}$ with metocurine is twice as long in elderly as in young patients, and $t_{1/2E}$ of D-tubocurarine is prolonged nearly as much [34].

Atracurium

The pharmacokinetics of atracurium (Tracrium) were originally reported to be similar in elderly and young adult patients [118], but more recent reports disagree. Because both liver and renal blood flow are reduced in the elderly and the liver and kidney combined are responsible for their clearance, most nondepolarizing relaxants exhibit prolonged duration and need for reduced dosage in the elderly. However, a process largely carried out in circulating blood termed *Hoffman hydrolysis and elimination* is responsible for elimination of atracurium. This process is actually more active in the elderly. Nonetheless, two authors have reported Vd_{SS} to be greater in the elderly, resulting in an extended $t_{1/2E}$ (22 vs. 16 minutes) [119,120]. However, another author reported clearance to be progressively decreased with age, while Vd_{SS} was unchanged, also resulting in an increased $t_{1/2E}$ and extended duration of action. Most recently, both dose requirement and duration of action were demonstrated to be similar in elderly and younger patients [121].

Pancuronium

The pharmacokinetics of pancuronium (Pavulon) in the elderly remain the subject of some controversy. An early study reported a distinct age-related decrease in Cl [122] and this seemed to be verified by clinical evidence of prolonged effect in the elderly [33]. However, more recent reports indicate that elderly patients as a group display only an approximately 25% reduction in Cl, and Vd_{SS} is unchanged from younger adults, resulting in only a 16% extension of $t_{1/2\beta}$ [123]. Further research may clarify this disagreement.

Vecuronium

Early reports showed no differences in dose, onset, or duration of vecuronium (Norcuron) in the elderly [124]. $t_{1/2}$ has been reported to be hastened in the elderly by one group, who postulated that a sharp reduction in Vd_{SS} overrides the 40% reduction of Cl resulting in a decrease in $t_{1/2\beta}$ [123]. More recently, onset of action was reported to be similar in young and elderly patients, but duration was

50% longer in young adults [125]. Yet another report indicates that the elderly have a doubling of $t_{1/2E}$ resulting from a more than 50% reduction in Cl while Vd_{SS} remains unchanged [126]. Finally, the most recent report agrees that dose should be lower because the duration of action in the elderly is markedly longer with vecuronium [121]. In view of this conflicting information, it is clear that in clinical practice, neuromuscular transmission should be carefully monitored during the use of vecuronium in elderly patients, and subsequent doses should be based on the observed response.

Doxacurium

Doxacurium (Nuromax) has also been said to offer the advantage of reduced cardiovascular side effects in the elderly. An earlier study of limited numbers of patients reported $t_{1/2\beta}$ to be extended by approximately 12%, Vd_{SS} to be extended by nearly 50%, and Cl to be slightly improved. Clinical findings in the same study indicated delay in onset by nearly 50% compared with younger patients. In addition, recovery time in the elderly was 150% to 175% of that of younger patients. In this study, $t_{1/2E}$ and Cl were not thought to be significantly different from that of younger patients, but volume of distribution was 150% of that of younger patients. However, their conclusion, that doxacurium can be given in similar doses to young and elderly patients, does not seem justified by their own findings [127]. A more recent report states that recovery from block with doxacurium requires twice as long in the elderly, probably largely due to both reduced renal Cl and liver Cl [128].

Miscellaneous Newer Muscle Relaxants

Rocuronium

Although onset of block with rocuronium (Zemuron) in the elderly is similar or slightly delayed compared with younger patients, the duration of clinical blockade is about half again longer in elderly patients. However, $t_{1/2E}$ is only slightly greater and Vd_{SS} is one-third smaller. Cl (probably largely by the liver, and much less by the kidney) is reduced by one-third [129,130].

Pipecuronium

Pipecuronium (Arduan) and pancuronium are similar in duration of action and chemical structure. However, pipecuronium is said to have minimal cardiovascular side effects in the elderly and might therefore be attractive for use in this patient population. Although Cl is predominately renal, two independent studies have found duration and dose requirement to be unchanged in the elderly [131,132].

Cisatracurium

Cisatracurium (Nimbex) has many characteristics in common with atracurium. In particular, it is broken down by Hoffman elimination, like atracurium, and is therefore ideal in elderly patients with decreased liver and kidney function. It has little effect on blood pressure, and unlike atracurium, releases little histamine [133]. A comparative study of pharmacokinetics in younger versus elderly patients revealed $t_{1/2\beta}$ of 28 minutes in younger and 36 minutes in elderly patients; Vd_{SS} of 10 ml/kg in younger versus 13 ml/kg in elderly patients, and similar plasma Cl in young and elderly patients. Clinical experience thus far is favorable in elderly patients, with similar dose requirements, onset, and duration in younger patients, as with atracurium, but with fewer cardiovascular effects [134].

Anticholinesterases

Anticholinesterases are used to reverse nondepolarizing muscle blockade by increasing the concentration of acetylcholine at the neuromuscular junction.

Edrophonium

Edrophonium (Tensilon) has been reported to display markedly reduced V_1 in the elderly, while Vd_{SS} remains similar to young adults. Therefore, the $t_{1/2E}$ is extended to approximately 50% longer in elderly compared with younger patients [135]. The case of edrophonium well illustrates that pharmacokinetics does not always explain clinical characteristics: the clinical action of edrophonium and the duration of effect in the elderly remain similar to young adults despite the previously mentioned alterations of pharmacokinetics. Concentrations of edrophonium in plasma are indeed elevated, as expected because of its altered pharmacokinetics. However, the clinical response in the elderly seems similar to that of younger patients with much lower plasma edrophonium concentrations, indicating some deterioration of an unspecified process in the elderly or, in other words, a pharmacodynamic change in the elderly [135].

Neostigmine and Pyridostigmine

In contrast to edrophonium, the duration of action of both neostigmine (Prostigmin) and pyridostigmine (Regonol, Mestinon) is doubled or tripled in duration. These differences are probably due to different mechanisms of action of edrophonium compared with neostigmine and pyridostigmine. Whereas edrophonium binds to acetylcholinesterase in a quickly reversible fashion, both neostigmine and pyridostigmine bind to their target much more firmly, thereby inhibiting acetylcholinesterase for longer periods [135,136]. As further demonstration, approximately 25% less neostigmine is required to reverse doxacurium in elderly patients compared with younger patients [128].

Miscellaneous Drugs

Local Anesthetics

Little information concerning use of local anesthetics in the elderly is available except for that related to lidocaine, but information on the use of lidocaine (Xylocaine) is probably roughly applicable to many of the amide local anesthetics. At similar doses, lidocaine achieves lower plasma concentrations in the elderly than in young adults because of an apparent increased Vd_{SS}, but the Cl is essentially unchanged. The $t_{1/2\beta}$ of lidocaine is 75% prolonged in the elderly adults [137]. In clinical use, reduction of doses and volumes to establish epidural block in the elderly is reduced by approximately one-third to one-half [138]. Lidocaine by IV single bolus is often used by anesthesiologists to suppress cough and elevation of pulse and blood pressure during tracheal intubation. The elderly appear to be resistant to this action and may require up to twice the dose that is effective in young adults [139].

Antihypertensive Drugs

Intraoperative hypertension occurs far more frequently in elderly than in young patients and can assume disturbing proportions. Treatment of this hypertension by some potent vasodilator drugs (e.g., nitroprusside) not only may require invasive monitoring but can also elicit reflex tachycardia. Both hypotension and tachycardia can be quite dangerous in the elderly. Tachycardia in the elderly patient with ischemic heart disease may produce infarction.

Propranolol

Propranolol (Inderal), a beta-adrenergic blocking drug, was frequently used by anesthesiologists for over two decades to control intraoperative hypertension and tachycardia despite its prolonged action, largely because of a lack of suitable alternatives. Oral administration of propranolol may result in much higher blood levels in elderly patients than in young adults (150% to 300% of the younger patient's plasma concentration) due to decreased first-pass metabolism in the elderly patient because of decreased liver blood flow. However, starting from this elevated plasma level, further distribution and elimination processes are no different than in younger adults [140]. Curiously, elderly patients also demonstrate reduced sensitivity to the blocking effects of propranolol, possibly on a pharmacodynamic basis [141]. Blood levels achieved by IV administration of propranolol during the maintenance of anesthesia are similar to those achieved in young adults, although similar blood levels may be more effective due to a decreased population of beta-receptors in the aged and due to decreased protein binding [141]. Age, inhalational anesthesia, and fentanyl anesthesia all reduce liver blood flow, and during their use concurrent concentrations of propranolol may remain elevated longer in the elderly due to a secondary decrease in propranolol Cl [142].

Esmolol

Esmolol (Brevibloc) has almost completely replaced propranolol in intraoperative use and is an ultra short-acting cardiovascular beta blocker. The $t_{1/2E}$ of esmolol is only approximately 9 minutes, which allows it to be used for acute episodes of hypertension without prolonged depression of myocardial contractility. If bradycardia or hypotension develops, cessation of administration of the drug allows normal heart rate to return quickly [143].

Labetalol

Labetalol (Normodyne, Trandate), on the other hand, has the mixed pharmacology of both beta-adrenergic blockade and a variable degree of alpha-adrenergic blockade [144]. The $t_{1/2E}$ of labetalol is measured in hours, and therefore, side effects tend to persist. One group reported that in elderly patients when perioperative hypertension of >200 mm Hg systolic or >100 mm Hg diastolic was treated with either a bolus of 500 μg/kg of esmolol (approximately 35 mg) followed by an infusion of 0.3 mg/kg, or labetalol in 5-mg bolus increments to a maximum of 1 mg/kg, both were effective within 10 minutes and lasted at least 2 hours. However, esmolol use was accompanied with bradycardia to <50 beats per minute, which frequently required discontinuation of the drug. This was not true of labetalol [143].

Nitroglycerin

The cardiovascular effects of IV nitroglycerin (Nitro-Bid, Nitrostat) are quite variable even in young adult populations and appear to be exaggerated in elderly patients [144]. Furthermore, the standard of care in most circumstances recommends intra-arterial monitoring of blood pressure when these drugs are required under anesthesia in doses intended to reduce blood pressure. Controlled studies demonstrate that nitroglycerin much more commonly causes unpredicted and excessive hypotension in elderly patients compared with younger patients. This effect has been identified with doses as small as 0.5 μg/kg per minute, and frequently a twofold greater decrease in systolic arterial pressure is seen than even would be predicted in patients in their sixth decade. Unfortunately, trials of nitroglycerin infusion before induction of general anesthesia are not predictable of the effects when combined with the state of general anesthesia [145].

Although evidence exists that administration of nitroglycerin during myocardial ischemia or after acute myocardial infarction reduces the size of the infarct and the incidence of left ventricular failure and death, it is not clear that similar results might not be achieved when blood pressure and particularly heart rate are reduced by other means [145]. For example, 43% of patients >70 years became acutely hypotensive during intra-anesthetic infusion of nitroglycerin (mean arterial pressure averaged 66) whereas only 18% of younger patients did so. When electing to treat anesthetized elderly patients with IV nitroglycerin, it is recommended that intra-arterial monitoring be carried out and dosage rates should be extremely cautious [145].

Clonidine

Clonidine (Catapres) is an alpha$_2$-adrenoceptor agonist and has significant efficacy as an antihypertensive agent. In recent years, administration of clonidine for premedication before surgery has become popular due to its sedative, anxiolytic, analgesic, and antihypertensive effects in elderly patients. In doses from 2.5 to 5 μg/kg, clonidine also significantly reduces intraoperative requirements for narcotics and volatile anesthetics [146]. Its beneficial effects on the cardiovascular system are due to a reduction of sympathetic outflow, simultaneous stimulation of parasympathetic tone of central origin, and a depressive effect on neurons that receive baroreceptor-activating stimuli [147]. The $t_{1/2}$ of oral clonidine is 8.5 hours [147].

The effectiveness of 0.3 mg of clonidine given orally 120 minutes before surgery has been compared with the effectiveness of oral diazepam at 0.15 mg/kg (approximately 10 mg) used as an oral premedicant. It was found to offer more sedation in this dose and less subjective anxiety than diazepam, along with a significant reduction in systolic and diastolic blood pressure and heart rate in the clonidine group but not the diazepam group. The patients given diazepam required more additional IV sedation just before induction of anesthesia than did the clonidine group [147]. Furthermore, the incidence of intraoperative hypertension and tachycardia was significantly greater with diazepam than with clonidine. The clonidine group appeared to recover faster from the effects of anesthesia. Doses of clonidine approaching 5 μg/kg were found to be associated with a 30% incidence of hypotension, along with a small incidence of bradycardia. As might be expected, patients receiving 5 μg/kg were more sedated than those receiving 2.5 μg/kg, and this sedation tended to persist for >6 hours postoperatively. Requirements for narcotic and inhalation anesthetics were also reduced [146]. These patients also experienced a significant decrease in intraocular pressure at the time of surgery as well as better control of cardiovascular variables [147].

Intrathecal clonidine has been proposed as a substitute for local anesthetics or as a sparing agent for local anesthetics and intrathecal or epidural narcotics to provide anesthesia for hip surgery in the elderly [148]. However, two independent studies have failed to demonstrate any advantages to these methods. In addition, twice as many patients in the epidural group required postoperative urethral catheterization compared to the intrathecal anesthetic group [149,150].

Verapamil

Verapamil (Calan) selectively enhances left ventricular diastolic filling and causes a trend toward lowering of systolic, diastolic, and mean blood pressure, along with slowing of the pulse rate in elderly patients compared with young adults, but without affecting systolic function. Improvement in systolic function in healthy elderly patients on therapeutic doses of verapamil may be as great as 50% improvement in filling rate [37].

Inhalational Anesthetics

The term *mean alveolar concentration* (MAC) is used as an index of inhalational anesthetic potency and is defined as the alveolar concentration of the anesthetic at which one-half of patients are adequately anesthetized [151]. MAC is reduced in the elderly [152]. This increased sensitivity of the elderly is parallel to decreases known to take place in cerebral oxygen consumption, cerebral blood flow, and neuronal density [153]. Elderly patients with emphysema, congestive heart failure, renal failure, or other pathologic conditions may exhibit dangerous acceleration of induction by inhalational anesthetic agents because of the reduced MAC, cardiac output, and myocardial reserve of the elderly. This may lead to a decreased transit rate of blood through the pulmonary circulation, leading in turn to enhanced diffusion of the soluble inhalational anesthetics into the blood, and eventually to a higher anesthetic content in the blood ejected from the left heart bound for the brain [154]. This reinforces the concept that reduced concentrations for induction and maintenance of inhalational anesthesia should be used in elderly patients and that cardiovascular depression may be expected more frequently if this caution is not observed, especially in the case of isoflurane.

One group has attempted to describe the classic pharmacokinetic parameters of inhalational anesthetics in *healthy* elderly versus healthy young patients. They were unable to demonstrate differences in V_1, but Cl was reduced slightly, and Vd_{SS} was expanded by approximately 60% [155]. However, another group has demonstrated that wash-in rates for all the current inhalation anesthetics are slightly decreased in the elderly [156]. A comparison of cardiovascular effects of halothane and isoflurane in elderly and young adult patients showed that reduction of heart rate and cardiac index occurred with equal frequency in elderly and young patients with both agents. However, isoflurane caused more profound and more frequent depression of blood pressure in the elderly than did halothane [157]. Total recovery time is more rapid with desflurane than isoflurane in elderly patients due to distributional differences, probably secondary to the different cardiovascular pharmacology of isoflurane and desflurane [158].

Intense interest has been shown in the new inhalational agent sevoflurane, which appears to combine rapid induction, relatively rapid awakening, and greatly reduced depression of the cardiovascular system. Desflurane, which is even more rapid, has demonstrated some stimulation of the cardiovascular functions that are not yet fully understood [158]. As with older inhalational agents, the MAC of sevoflurane is reduced from the young adult concentration of 2.5% to only 1.48% in elderly patients [153]. Measurement of a more recent concept, "MAC awake," or the alveolar anesthetic concentration at which patients awaken from inhalational anesthesia, was shown to be much reduced, or 0.5% in elderly, versus 0.7% in young adults [159].

CLINICAL ASPECTS OF ANESTHESIA IN THE ELDERLY

Preoperative Evaluation of the Elderly

As in younger patients, accurate assignment of the American Society of Anesthesiologists Physical Status Scale (ASA-PS) aids in anticipating an elevated risk of morbidity and mortality [160]. ASA-PS I is defined as those patients without significant abnormalities. ASA-PS II indicates the presence of significant abnormalities that are not an immediate threat to life. ASA-PS III indicates the presence of abnormalities that are an immediate threat, but death is not anticipated. ASA-PS IV indicates a patient in whom immediate risk of death is present. ASA-PS V indicates immediate death is anticipated unless the proposed surgery is carried out [161]. Extensive experience has shown that risk of mortality and morbidity increases in direct relation to higher ASA-PS numbers.

One study demonstrated that 86.5% of elderly patients who had been cleared for anesthesia and surgery by usual evaluations suffered from demonstrated pathologic hemodynamic, respiratory, or oxygen transport mechanisms. For example, 44% were found to have abnormally low blood oxygen levels and 8% of those (previously "cleared for surgery") exhibited Pao_2 <50 mm Hg. Left ventricular function was studied in this same group of cleared patients, demonstrating that 22.3% had poor left ventricular function evidenced by assessing left ventricular stroke work index versus pulmonary capillary wedge pressure. Only 24% had normal myocardial contractility, whereas another 22.3% had demonstrably poor left ventricular function [162].

Another study of 1,000 elderly patients admitted for surgery found that hypertension was noted in 47%, renal disease in 31%, atherosclerosis in 27%, pulmonary disease in 28%, cardiomegaly in 14%, and congestive heart failure, angina, cerebrovascular accidents, diabetes, and liver disease each in from 6% to 9% of these patients [163]. Hypertensive disease in the elderly is more frequently associated with myocardial hypertrophy and infarction than in younger patients [164]. Hypertrophic cardiomyopathy is present in 70% of randomly chosen 85-year-old patients and 43% of all patients aged 70 and over, but in only 10% of adults aged 40 and under [165]. Hypertrophic cardiomyopathy in the elderly is associated with dynamic subaortic obstruction in 77% of elderly patients with hypertrophic cardiomyopathy, thus severely limiting their ability to increase cardiac output in response to stress [166].

A prospective study of 1,886 patients aged 62 years or greater showed that coronary disease developed in 47% during longitudinal study, 29% developed peripheral arterial disease, and 29% experienced brain infarctions. In all groups, coronary disease was somewhat more frequent in men than in women [167]. Prolonged ST interval was found in 16% of elderly women but only 9% of elderly men. It directly correlates with higher blood pressure, larger left ventricular mass, and more severe cardiac infarction injury in response to insult [168]. In octogenarians, the causes of death included cardiac death in 53% and peripheral vascular decrease in 13%. The etiology of cardiac death included atherosclerosis in 65%, acute myocardial infarction in 69%, sudden cardiac arrest in 15%, and congestive heart failure in 12% [169].

A prospective preoperative evaluation by invasive monitoring of 100 elderly patients indicated that 13% of patients who otherwise would have been accepted for surgery required postponement or cancellation of the surgery by the results of preoperative testing. For example, cardiac index was <2.2 liters per minute per m^2 in 11% of patients. Preoperative mean renal clearance (Cl_R) was 50 ml per minute or less in 19%. Mean blood pressure was at least 120 mm in 15%, and intrapulmonary shunting was at least 15% in 10% of the tested patients. Of six patients whose operations were canceled as a result of testing, three died. Another three patients who had indications of chronic vascular disease but who were submitted for surgery for the vascular lesions also died [170].

Cardiopulmonary exercise testing can be a helpful preoperative evaluation tool. When 187 elderly presurgical patients were so evaluated, it was found that the overall surgical mortality was 7.5%. However, if the anaerobic threshold was found to be <11 ml per minute per kg (55 patients), the mortality was 18%. In those whose anaerobic threshold was >11 ml per minute per kg [132], the mortality was only 0.8%. A death rate of 42% was associated with a finding of ischemia by electrocardiogram with low anaerobic threshold, but only 4% with a high anaerobic threshold [171].

Evaluation of anesthetic risk in elderly patients with cardiac or vascular disease can be aided by use of the cardiac risk index proposed by Goldman et al. [172,173]. Factors contributing to increased perioperative mortality include myocardial infarction within the previous 6 months and examination displaying myocardial dysfunction evidenced by jugular venous distention (elevated central venous pressure), or presence of cardiac arrhythmia and age >70 years. Evidence indicates that older patients suffering non–Q-wave acute myocardial infarction are more likely to develop several complications than younger patients. These complications include atrial fibrillation (23% vs. 8%) and congestive heart failure (53% vs. 30%). In the same report, in-hospital mortality was similar in both elderly and younger patients, but the overall 1-year mortality was 36% in the elderly and only 16% in younger patients [172,173].

Myocardial infarction associated with general anesthesia and surgery carries a much higher mortality than for patients admitted through the emergency room with myocardial infarction. Certainly all authors agree that elective surgery should be postponed until 6 months after the last myocardial infarction. Several studies agree that assiduous monitoring of elderly patients with a history of myocardial infarction or other vascular disease, and alert reaction to developing symptoms can markedly reduce severity and incidence of reinfarction in the immediate postoperative period. Elderly patients with Q-wave acute myocardial infarction had more in-hospital complications and a death rate of 25%. Overall, elderly patients with non–Q-wave acute myocardial infarction accounted for 62% of all deaths occurring during the first year after discharge and presented a relative risk factor of 2.6 times that of younger patients with similar findings. These observations suggest that an aggressive diagnostic and therapeutic approach may be of particular benefit in such patients when identified in the course of anesthetic evaluation [174].

Premedication

In general summary, it can be said that elderly patients exhibit far more unwanted side effects of premedication of all types than young adults. In general, they are far more susceptible to the respiratory depressant effects of all drugs (especially narcotics), as well as hypotension and even cardiac arrhythmias. In general, premedicant doses should be smaller (often on the order of one-third to one-half the dose for a young adult) with, of course, much variation between individual drugs. These cautions extend especially to patients sedated under major regional blocks.

Although older information indicated that intramuscular administration of BZDs was ineffective, more recent publications have demonstrated that they are, in fact, effective by this route, particularly when delivered into the deltoid muscle [65,67,175]. Diazepam (and probably most other BZDs as well) increases heart rate variability in elderly patients at a dose of 0.06 mg/kg (approximately 4 mg intramuscularly in a 70-kg person) but not in younger patients [175]. In adults aged 60 to 69 years, midazolam (2 to 3 mg in the deltoid muscle) is effective in providing sedation and anxiolysis without excessive drowsiness. However, in patients aged 70 or greater, dangerous excessive drowsiness may occur, even with doses as low as 1 mg of midazolam intramuscularly [67]. Another report confirms this problem with midazolam but suggests that diazepam does not share this added danger beyond the age of 70, and these authors recommend the use of diazepam in eldest patients [66].

It should be recalled that in case of unwanted drowsiness, respiratory depression, or hypotension with the use of the BZDs as premedication or sedation for surgery, an antagonist (flumazenil) is available. However, great caution should be exercised in elderly patients and its use should be reserved only for those in serious respiratory or cardiovascular depression. Although flumazenil is very successful in achieving complete and rapid reversal of sedation in the elderly, there is almost universal disorientation and lack of cooperation in elderly patients after its use. Its effectiveness in the elderly was demonstrated by reversal of the midazolam, 0.05 mg/kg IV (approximately 5 mg), with a dose of flumazenil of 0.01 mg/kg (approximately 0.7 to 1.0 mg) [80].

In elderly patients with chronic hypertension (even under treatment) intravascular volume is usually decreased, thus potentially synergizing with the tendency of many anesthetic agents to cause hypotension. Despite conflicting practices in former times, most anesthesiologists today continue most types of antihypertensive medication at routine doses until the day of operation and return to them as soon as possible after the operation. However, most agree that it is best to thoroughly diagnose the cause of hypertension and bring it under satisfactory control by medication before elective surgery is attempted. In those patients receiving various diuretics, punctilious attention should be paid to replacement of any depleted total body potassium stores.

Most modern anesthesiologists also recommend continuing the patient's accustomed level of beta-block and calcium-block medications up to the day of surgery. Although the beta blockers exhibit little interference with narcotic-based general anesthesia, they synergize somewhat with the inhalational anesthetics in depression of the myocardium [176]. However, extensive recent research has demonstrated the prominent potentiation of myocardial depressant effects from the combination of most current inhalational anesthetics (but not of narcotic-based general anesthesia) and a wide variety of modern calcium channel blockers.

It has been frequently recommended that in elderly patients, anticholinergic drugs including scopolamine, promethazine, and meperidine, as well as longer-acting BZDs such as diazepam, midazolam, and flurazepam, be avoided whenever possible in the preoperative and postoperative care of elderly patients. The clinician should be aware that other frequent etiologic factors of postanesthetic delirium include impaired cerebral oxygen supplies, deranged metabolism, cerebrovascular disease, and withdrawal from chronic drug therapy, including alcohol and BZDs, particularly triazolam. Sleep deprivation and such specific causes as the aftereffect of reduced cerebral perfusion during cardiopulmonary bypass are some additional causes of delirium in the elderly [177].

Monitoring During Anesthesia in the Elderly

In general, current standards of care indicate that monitoring of all patients, regardless of their age, undergoing anesthetic care of any category should be extensive and appropriate to the procedure and status of the patient [178]. These include monitoring of the inspired oxygen concentration, along with the patient's actual second-to-second blood oxygenation (pulse oximeter). Extensive documentation indicates that continuous pulse oximetry is associated with a lower overall rate of complications, specifically, potential myocardial infarctions in all patients [160]. Various methods to estimate the adequacy of ventilation should be in use, and when an endotracheal tube is in use, end-tidal carbon dioxide concentration and end-tidal oxygen concentration should be monitored. When ventilation is controlled by mechanical ventilator, devices should be used to detect inadvertent disconnection or inadvertent overinflation of the system. Circulation should be monitored at least by frequent blood pressure and pulse estimation, and when indicated by more specific methods as well. A continuing evaluation of the pulse by electrocardiography or other appropriate methods is recommended. Body temperature should be estimated in an appropriate manner [178].

In the case of elderly patients, the consequences of hypothermia are directly related to an increased incidence of postoperative complications, and therefore, monitoring of central body temperature is of even greater importance than in younger patients (see discussion of hypothermia). Some incidence of local hematoma, arteritis, and other complications of radial pulse pressure monitoring can be expected, but the greater risk to elderly patients of serious cardiovascular-related complications in any but the most minor anesthetic and surgical procedures probably justifies more frequent intra-arterial monitoring of pressure in the elderly. In addition, this provides the added benefit of frequent blood gas and acid-base balance monitoring in these patients.

Serious complications of pulmonary artery catheter monitoring such as infection, mediastinal hematoma, mediastinal infection, pneumothorax, hemothorax, internal carotid artery stroke, and other complications can be expected. However, the increased risk of serious cardiovascular complications in elderly patients (see discussion of morbidity and mortality) probably indicates the need for more liberal use of pulmonary artery catheter monitoring than in younger patients [179–182].

Elderly patients with uncompensated or unstable congestive heart failure frequently require invasive monitoring to avoid sudden deterioration under anesthesia. The weakening effects of inhalational anesthetics on the myocardium of the patient with congestive failure are pronounced and may be deadly. Even with the use of narcotic anesthesia, which spares the myocardium to a great extent, alterations in preload or afterload to the heart due to the surgical procedure or pain or surgical stress may quickly worsen the cardiac failure. Therefore, constant monitoring of pulmonary artery pressures and pulmonary artery occluded (wedge) pressures, along with cardiac output, are almost indispensable during all but the briefest anesthesia and surgery in such patients [180–182].

General Anesthesia

Previously described pharmacologic sensitivities to the induction agents and the inhalational anesthetics predicate a much slower, more careful induction of any type of general anesthesia in the aged, using smaller doses and concentrations and careful monitoring of the physiology during slow induction. Blood volume is frequently decreased in the elderly. In addition, due to eating habits, disease, and frequently "nothing by mouth" orders since the previous night, these patients are quite commonly additionally hypovolemic. Many anesthesiologists advocate prophylactic acute IV hydration with 5 to 10 mg of balanced salt solution per kilogram of body weight just before induction of anesthesia.

The choice of general anesthesia for elderly patients depends on the type of surgery and the particular physiologic condition of the specific patient. Although nitrous oxide–narcotic-tranquilizer–muscle relaxant techniques have perhaps the least depressant effect on the myocardium, they do not offer the advantage of decreasing the workload on the heart by reducing peripheral vascular resistance as is the case with some inhalational anesthetics, such as isoflurane. In addition, isoflurane stabilizes the heart against arrhythmias, unlike narcotic-based anesthesia.

Induction of anesthesia with inhalational anesthetics is often dangerously accelerated because of lower cardiac output and lower myocardial reserve. This leads to a decreased transit rate of blood through the pulmonary circulation, leading in turn to enhanced diffusion of soluble inhalational anesthetics into the blood and eventually to a higher anesthetic content in the blood ejected from the left heart and bound for the brain. This increased speed of inhalational induction can, of course, be circumvented by intentional limiting of the inhalational anesthetic concentration during the induction phase in elderly patients [154,156]. Because MAC is reduced in the elderly, inhalational anesthetic maintenance requirements are usually somewhat lower in elderly than in younger adult patients. Frequently, a combination of low-dose narcotics and reduced concentration inhalational anesthetics are used to receive the benefits and minimize the side effects of both [183].

Regional Anesthesia

The general desirability of major regional anesthesia such as subarachnoid (spinal) block and epidural block in comparison with modern endotracheal general anesthesia has been debated vigorously for several decades [184–189]. Assumptions in support of the use of regional block include assumed lower perioperative mortality, less postoperative hypoxemia, and a lower incidence of both thromboembolism and mental changes after surgical procedures. However, these assumptions [190] have not been clearly supported by objective criteria. In fact, overall morbidity and mortality is similar with general or regional anesthesia in the elderly [191–194]. Another point, that of earlier ambulation after use of regional anesthesia, is also not supported by prospective findings [191–194] when regional anesthesia is used solely in the operative period. When postoperative use of epidural analgesia is used, there is clearly earlier ambulation in patients who have undergone lower abdominal and lower extremity surgery, but this early ambulation is not clearly associated with an improvement in final outcome indicators [194,195]. Many operations are not in regions easily conducive to major regional anesthesia care or postsurgical continuous epidural analgesia. On the other hand, use of these continuous postoperative regional analgesic techniques can introduce serious iatrogenic complications and are quite expensive, bringing into question their cost-benefit value. Transurethral resection of the prostate is a typical example of an excellent application of subarachnoid anesthesia. It little disturbs the patient's physiology, ability to respond to the minimal blood loss of the operation, or respiratory, cardiac, and brain function. However, use of sedation may complicate the postoperative care of elderly patients [196].

During the use of major regional anesthesia in elderly patients, extensive sympathetic block may lead to difficulty in maintenance of blood pressure. Elderly patients experience a decrease in systemic vascular resistance and systolic pressure of, on the average, 25%, but cardiac index is unaffected by intrathecal block. In one study of elderly patients, treatment of systolic pressure decreased >25% with infusion of 8 ml/kg of colloid solution resulted in restoration of blood pressure in one-half of the patients, but another half required additional vasopressor therapy to restore systemic vascular resistance and systolic blood pressure to baseline values. Thus, fully 69% of elderly patients in this study required treatment for hypotension after intrathecal blocks. Elderly orthopedic trauma patients were even more likely than others to experience decreases in blood pressure [197].

Reduction in doses and volumes of local anesthetic drug by approximately one-third is a common clinical practice in establishing intrathecal block. In addition, many anesthesiologists preclude the use of epinephrine in intrathecal block for elderly patients, because of the fear of induction of ischemia in spinal arteries nourishing the spinal cord, which might lead to neuropathy or paraplegia. Elderly patients who receive intrathecal anesthesia experience a reduced, but still significant rate of spinal headache, and this complication can even occur in approximately 1% of epidural blocks. Spinal headaches were found in 11% of elderly patients after 20-gauge needle puncture of the dura versus 28% in young adults, and only 8% after 25-gauge needle puncture versus 13% in young adults [198].

During epidural anesthesia in the elderly, there is a reduced response to the tilt test, and the heart rate and catecholamine response to hypotension are impaired more than in younger patients [199]. Technical factors are extremely important both in the success and safety of extradural anesthesia and analgesia. For example, the dose requirement in the elderly for extradural block has been shown to be at least 40% smaller than that of younger adults, yet no absolute dividing line indicates when to restrict the dose in an individual patient's life history, thereby exposing some older adults to overdose situations [200,201].

The ventilatory response to hypercapnia in elderly patients under the influence of uncomplicated epidural blockade without narcotic is similar to that of young adults [202]. However, elderly adults are far more susceptible to the respiratory depressive effects of small amounts of narcotic in the cerebrospinal fluid secondary to both intrathecal and epidural narcotic analgesia techniques [203].

Regional Anesthesia Versus General Anesthesia in the Elderly

A recent study has reviewed all randomized controlled clinical trials in the English language since 1966 that made comparisons between regional and general anesthesia and included over 5,000 patients experiencing surgery below the umbilicus. These authors found no statistically significant differences in overall mortality, cardiac morbidity, postoperative pulmonary complications, or pulmonary emboli between general and regional anesthesia. There was, however, a greater incidence of deep vein thrombosis in patients after hip surgery who received general anesthesia without prophylactic therapy for deep vein thrombosis [204].

A careful prospective study observed patients who received general anesthesia, general anesthesia plus epidural anesthesia ending with the end of surgery, or epidural anesthesia alone followed by patient-controlled administration of a mixture of local anesthesia and narcotic in the epidural catheter in the postoperative period. These authors demonstrated that lesser postoperative analgesic doses were required in the group who received intraoperative epidural anesthesia when compared with both the epidural general group and the general anesthetic group. However, significantly, there was no difference in the incidence of postoperative neurologic, cardiovascular, or pulmonary complications among the three groups [205].

Postoperative Pain Control with Intrathecal or Epidural Administration of Narcotics or Patient-Controlled Administration of Analgesia

Prolonged analgesia can be obtained by the intrathecal or epidural administration of narcotics and alpha-adrenergic receptor agonists. These benefits had originally been thought to be without risk of respiratory depression, significant syncope or hypotension due to sympathetic blockade, or lingering motor neuroparalysis, thereby allowing earlier return to normal orientation, alimentation, and ambulation. A major school of thought has even proposed that complete blockade of afferent signals to the central nervous system is fundamental in preventing and decreasing stress response and postoperative pain (so-called preemptive analgesia) [205]. Disadvantages of these new methods include major additional costs, additional risk of neurologic complications on establishment of epidural block, including the risk of epidural or subdural hematoma and consequent paraplegia, the risk of headache incident to puncture of the dura with the spinal or epidural needle, and particularly, the insidious low but extremely dangerous incidence of delayed respiratory depression or apnea due to the unique pharmacology of intrathecal and epidural instillation of narcotic drugs [203]. Other disadvantages include pruritus and nausea [202,206–208].

When introduced intrathecally or epidurally, the dose of narcotic necessary to produce prolonged analgesia is greatly reduced in the elderly, and the resulting systemic concentration is usually too low to cause sedation, disorientation, or respiratory depression. However, in elderly patients, even more than in the young, severe respiratory depression or apnea may occur either early after administration, due to venous injection or rapid absorption into venous blood, or late, due to the slow cephalad migration of drug carried by cerebrospinal fluid to the medullary respiratory centers.

Unfortunately, this danger persists for as long as 12 hours with fentanyl and up to 24 hours with morphine. It has been shown that even a single dose of epidural fentanyl administered in the proper place (there is also some incidence of inadvertent improper administration of the drug, which can be more dangerous) produces changes in respiratory frequency as well as end-tidal carbon dioxide within minutes after administration [203]. Research indicates that elderly patients subjected to uncomplicated continuous epidural narcotic analgesia after hip or knee replacement, but also monitored constantly with end-tidal carbon dioxide and oxygen saturation monitors, developed readings that indicated serious levels of clinically significant respiratory depression in 27% of cases [209].

Almost all patients can be shown to demonstrate decreased sensitivity to the stimulation of the medullary respiratory center by carbon dioxide during routine clinical use of either intrathecal or epidural methods with all of these drugs, but, fortunately, clinically dangerous depression occurs in as few as 3% of younger patients given the proper dose in the correct location. However, abundant evidence exists to show that elderly patients may be at least twice as susceptible to the respiratory depressant effects and that the doses that are common for younger patients should be reduced as much as one-half or even to one-third [203]. It has been recommended that whenever intrathecal or epidural narcotics are used for analgesia in elderly patients, the patients should be monitored as closely as possible for signs of respiratory depression. Minimum monitoring should include a peripheral oxygen saturation monitor set to alarm loudly, preferably to a central location, when an oxygen desaturation level preset to the individual patient's requirements is reached [209].

Postoperative pain control with epidural narcotics has become popular in the treatment of patients undergoing abdominal operations, gynecologic procedures, urologic procedures such as radical prostatectomy, vascular procedures such as abdominal aortic aneurysmectomy, peripheral vascular procedures, and major orthopedic procedures such as femoral neck fracture repairs and hip and knee arthroplasties [202,205,210,211].

Unfortunately, after nearly 15 years of controversy, there is no consensus concerning the accuracy of the assumptions that these methods of regional anesthesia are significantly preferable to other methods of postoperative pain relief such as patient-controlled administration of IV narcotic analgesics [191,193–195,205,208].

One study, for example, compared narcotic demand when the patient-controlled analgesia route for the same narcotic was administered by IV or via an epidural indwelling catheter. All patients experienced radical retropubic prostatectomy, and all received appropriate dosages of keterolac for 72 hours postsurgery. Postoperative consumption of narcotic by the patient-controlled IV route was nearly twice as great as when the same opioid was administered by patient-controlled analgesia via the indwelling epidural catheter route, but there were no other differences in pain scores or patient satisfaction. Epidural administration of the narcotic resulted in a far greater incidence of pruritus, and there were no other significant complications. There was no evidence of improvement in postoperative analgesia, patient satisfaction, early discharge, or reduction in postsurgical complications [208]. These results demonstrated that continuous epidural narcotic and patient-controlled analgesia were equally effective in pain control and comfort and call into question (because of the added expense and exposure to additional serious technical complications such as paraplegia and spinal headache) the cost-benefit ratio of postsurgical epidural narcotic analgesia compared with patient-controlled administration of IV narcotic analgesics.

SPECIAL AREAS OF IMPORTANCE IN CLINICAL MANAGEMENT OF ANESTHESIA IN THE ELDERLY

Perioperative Hypothermia in the Elderly

Hypothermia in the elderly may be due to a variety of causes including decreased heat production, increased heat loss, and derangement of the central heat regulatory mechanism [212]. Several factors in the operating suite lead to hypothermia in elderly patients already deprived of intrinsic heat preservation mechanisms. These include the habitual cold air conditioning and rapid air turnover of operating rooms and the use of unheated, dry anesthetic gases in the breathing circuit. Neurologic disease, including diabetic retinopathy or damage due to cerebral vascular accident may impair transmission from skin thermal receptors. Older estimates that a 300% to 400% increase in oxygen consumption may be elicited during shivering in an attempt to correct body core hypothermia have been re-examined and found to be exaggerated. Elderly patients do increase oxygen consumption in response to hypothermia, but consumption is only approximately 38% greater in patients who shiver than those who do not [213].

Furthermore, the responses of the elderly to hypothermia are often delayed and less efficient than those of younger patients, and these handicaps continue to accentuate with progressive age past 80 years. The heat-producing response of shivering is inhibited more in elderly patients by general anesthesia than in younger patients, and in spinal anesthesia the threshold to begin shivering is lower in elderly than in younger patients [214].

Several studies indicate that elderly patients routinely drop their temperatures to 90°F and below, particularly when undergoing intraperitoneal procedures. During the recovery period, attempts by the patient's physiology to increase body heat frequently lead to excessive use of oxygen, hypertension, tachycardia, increased cardiac output, and severe evidences of stress. Furthermore, postoperative complications including myocardial ischemia, wound infection, and prolonged drug actions are more frequent in elderly patients with hypothermia [214]. In fact, one group documented that hypothermia <35°C is associated with a two- to threefold increase in the incidence of early operative myocardia ischemia [215], as well as increases in norepinephrine concentration of 100% to 500%, peripheral vasoconstriction, and hypertension [216]. Furthermore, there is a higher incidence of thromboembolism when operations are performed under cold ambient conditions. It is strongly advocated that heated anesthetic gases and body-warming devices such as air or warm water blankets be used for all elderly patients undergoing general anesthesia for more than short periods [213,217].

Hypothermia can also be accentuated by various drug actions. For example, neuromuscular blocking agents may reduce heat production by reducing the ability to shiver. Beta-adrenergic agonists and inhalational anesthetics may actively cause skin vasodilatation leading to extra heat radiation. Additional factors include the additional depression of the brain thermostatic center by general anesthetics, blocking of peripheral autonomic vasoconstriction to conserve heat, and active dilation of skin vasculature caused by several anesthetic agents. The administration of cold blood and fluids also contributes to heat loss.

Postanesthetic Delirium in Elderly Patients

Delirium, excitement, and disorientation are much more frequent after anesthesia and surgery in elderly people than is often appreciated. The existence of this syndrome may not only have importance in the discomfort of the patient, but may also result in increased morbidity, delayed recovery, and prolonged hospital stay, and may adversely affect health care costs. Prospective studies have indicated that in elderly surgical patients, the incidence of postanesthetic delirium may be 7% to 14% during short-term recovery or as great as 40% in patients requiring postsurgical critical care for extended periods [218]. It may occur in as many as 50% of liver and lung transplant recipients, 25% of heart transplant recipients, and 10% of renal transplant recipients [177] and has been reported in 28% to 61% of elderly orthopedic surgery patients [26]. Postoperative delirium states in the elderly may commonly last 6 to 12 days, but as long as 6 weeks in 5% of elderly patients [26].

Causes of the condition are many, including metabolic disturbances, preexisting neurologic deterioration, and preoperative and postoperative drug therapy not directly related to anesthetic management [219]. The etiologic significance of the central cholinergic nervous system in the etiology of ambulatory geriatric depression has been reported. Significant cognitive and behavioral effects after the use of several types of anticholinergic drugs exemplified by scopolamine and promethazine have been extensively reported [84]. When oxidative metabolism in the brain of elderly patients decreases, levels of neurotransmitters such as acetylcholine may decline and may be the source of mental dysfunction [26]. Other etiologic factors such as increased serum cortisol levels from the stress of surgery or reduced availability of tryptophan after events such as cardiopulmonary bypass have also been postulated as causes of postanesthetic delirium in the elderly [26].

Elderly patients with depression are known to exhibit inhibition in serotonergic and noradrenergic transmitter systems that may predispose them to delirium. One report states that the incidence of an acute confusional state after surgery in patients with preoperative depression is 88% [220]. Lingering affects of long-acting BZDs have also been implicated (see previous discussion). Deficits caused by anticholinergics include affects on new learning, access to semantic memory, vigilance, and performance of repetitive acts. Behavior may include restlessness and anxiety, as well as disorientation. A brief clinical evaluation scale has been suggested for the nonpsychiatrist to categorize these patients quickly [221].

A prospective study of elderly patients receiving spinal or general anesthesia found that all patients in all groups experienced a short decline in mental function in the postanesthetic period, and, in fact, the incidence was similar after all types of anesthesia, including spinal and general. The decline in postoperative mental function and subjective sense of well-being was most pronounced in patients with compromise of the cardiovascular or respiratory systems before surgery. Most of the temporary mental and physical decline was found in the first few days and returned to preoperative levels by the fifth day after surgery. Four weeks after surgery there were no signs of mental deterioration, but the subjective sense of physical well-being still had not returned in all patients [219]. Patients 60 years of age and greater undergoing transurethral resection of the prostate or pelvic floor repair were subjected to intrathecal anesthesia or general anesthesia, and psychiatric and mental testing were carried out postoperatively at 6 hours, 1 day, 3 days, 5 days, and 1 month. The cognitive skills of the elderly patients who received spinal anesthesia were better than those who received general anesthesia at 6 hours but not at 1 day or thereafter [196]. Another author showed that delirium was significantly associated with postoperative exposure to meperidine (because of its anticholinergic effects) whether administered intramuscularly or via epidural or IV patient-controlled analgesia methods [218] but not with other narcotics. Meperidine and BZD deliriums were persistent over the first 24 hours postoperatively [218].

In addition to its anticholinergic activity, another possible etiology for the delirium caused by meperidine is its primary metabolite. Normeperidine is active, has a long $t_{1/2}$, and is metabolized by the liver, allowing its accumulation to toxic levels in patients receiving continuous meperidine (particularly with reduced kidney function as in many elderly patients) [218]. These findings support the suggestion that biological rather than calendar age influences the degree of postoperative mental decline after anesthesia and surgery [196,218,219].

Pharmacologic treatment of drug-induced postanesthetic delirium in the elderly rests on identification of the etiologic agent. Neuroleptic medications including haloperidol may be useful for their sedative effect in agitated patients. In the case of identifiable BZD-withdrawal syndrome, small doses of lorazepam have been used with good success. Caution against midazolam, which has a very long $t_{1/2}$ in the elderly, should be noted [177]. In cases where anticholinergic etiology of the delirium is suspected, very slow infusion of 0.5 to 1.0 mg physostigmine sometimes elicits startling beneficial effects. However, this effect sometimes is delayed for as much as 20 minutes and patience is counseled [177]. A rapid, although short-lived reversal of many BZD-induced delirium states may be effected with the slow infusion of 2.5 to 5.0 mg IV flumazenil. Caution should be exercised in that there may be reactivation of the delirium state when the flumazenil redistributes in the elderly patients [80].

When an anticholinergic agent is needed for cardiovascular reasons or for use with an anticholinesterase in the reversal of muscle relaxation in elderly patients, glycopyrrolate is recommended because it does not cross the blood-brain barrier and is not known to cause central nervous system effects as are atropine and scopolamine [26].

Anesthetic Management of the Elderly Diabetic Patient

Elderly diabetic patients present a variety of perioperative problems of interest to the anesthesiologist [222]. These include diabetic ketoacidosis, hyperosmolar syndrome, lactic acidosis, and hypoglycemia. Elderly diabetics must be carefully examined preoperatively for evidence of diabetic retinopathy, diabetic nephropathy, peripheral neuropathies, cardiac and particularly peripheral vascular disease, and chronic hypertension. Risk of cardiac and cerebral infarction is greater in patients with diabetic vascular disease, and they tolerate hypotension less successfully than nondiabetic patients. Survival from infarction is decreased in diabetics. An interesting and fortunately rare syndrome includes sudden cardiac arrest due to diabetic neuropathy of the autonomic nervous system. Because of these conditions, the patient should be carefully evaluated for the status of the heart and peripheral circulation before anesthesia [223].

The impression that diabetes is a serious risk factor for coronary artery bypass grafting (CABG) in the elderly was recently confirmed in 317 diabetic patients found to have a 57% greater risk of death than matched patients without diabetes. However, the relative survival benefits of submitting diabetic patients to CABG versus medical therapy was comparable in diabetic and nondiabetic patients, and in fact, surgical therapy can further reduce mortality by 44% [224].

Blood glucose concentration is the most obvious concern in diabetic patients. Hyperglycemia can be regulated to relatively low normal levels by the frequent intraoperative use of blood glucose estimations. The availability of easy-to-use semiquantitative bedside devices makes it practical for the anesthesiologist to evaluate resulting blood glucose levels frequently during anesthesia.

Extreme hypoglycemia can be a consequence of residual insulin activity from previously administered long-acting preparations. Patients often become symptomatic when blood glucose levels decrease to <50 mg/dl. When this occurs during anesthesia, there are frequently few warning signs. Increased blood pressure, sweating, and tachycardia sometimes give warning, but in elderly patients, these are quite unreliable during general anesthesia. Therefore, constant infusion of small amounts of dextrose throughout surgery is important in elderly diabetic patients and frequent monitoring of blood glucose levels is important even in elderly patients thought to present with only mild diabetes.

To prevent this important complication, many anesthesiologists advocate removing the most severe diabetic patients from long-acting insulin preparations 2 days before major surgery and replacing the insulin with multiple-dose crystalline insulin and the use of a sliding urinary scale for dose regulation. However, at a minimum, most recommend reduction in the preoperative dose of long-acting insulin preparations followed by frequent blood glucose analysis during surgery and in the immediate postoperative period with appropriate treatment for high or low readings.

Patients with diabetic ketoacidosis should, whenever possible, be slowly resuscitated with insulin, adequate systemic fluids, and when necessary, antacid therapy such as bicarbonate. Treatment of diabetic ketoacidosis consists of IV insulin infusion with extremely careful monitoring of blood glucose levels, followed by titrated increments of 1 to 10 U of IV insulin per hour. Meanwhile, careful attention should be given to maintenance and restoration of serum potassium levels. When emergency surgery is necessary in patients exhibiting diabetic ketoacidosis, frequent arterial blood gas measurements and aggressive use of carefully monitored incremental doses of IV insulin and fluid therapy are highly recommended.

Hyperglycemia should be assiduously avoided to prevent hyperosmolar syndrome. This complex leads to dehydration of the brain and severe neurologic symptoms and hypovolemia. The mortality for nonketotic hyperosmolar syndrome may be as great as 50% [225]. Initial treatment with 2 liters of rapidly administered half normal saline is often recommended. This is usually followed by hypotonic saline at the rate of 1 liter every 2 hours while carefully monitoring central venous pressure and blood glucose. This syndrome may be further accelerated by the concurrent administration of corticosteroids, diuretics, the presence of infection, during cerebral vascular accidents, or during total parenteral alimentation. Serum bicarbonate levels may be found to be decreased, but blood urea nitrogen is usually elevated because of hypovolemia and prerenal azotemia. Serum osmolarity is usually >320 mOsm/liter. Blood glucose levels often exceed 600 mg/dl [223].

Some anesthesiologists prefer major regional anesthesia where applicable in diabetic patients because they believe that re-establishment of preoperative maintenance plans is easier, and some believe that the hyperglycemic stress response after intraperitoneal surgery may be reduced by intrathecal or epidural anesthesia [226]. However, many are concerned about preexisting neuropathy, which may later be confused with possible neurologic complications of the regional block. Furthermore, possible diabetic vascular inadequacy of the posterior spinal artery might make elderly diabetic patients more susceptible to occlusion by the irritation of the subarachnoid medication. Even temporary impairment of these vessels might lead to further enhancement of present neuropathy or even disastrous spinal cord ischemia and resulting paraplegia.

When general anesthesia is required, rapid sequence tracheal intubation has been advocated by some who believe that aspiration of gastric contents may be more frequent in elderly diabetics due to manifestations of autonomic neuropathy [226]. Formerly, the use of diethyl ether frequently led to hyperglycemia in diabetics, but there is no current evidence for a particular preference between modern inhalational anesthetics. However, whether narcotic-based IV anesthesia or inhalational anesthesia is chosen, sufficient doses, concentrations, and anesthetic depths are advisable to reduce stress reaction and cortisol and catecholamine release and therefore secondary disturbances in the glucose and insulin levels [226].

Major Vascular Procedures

In addition to the usual range of diseases found in other elderly patients, nearly one-half of patients presenting for abdominal aortic aneurysm surgery have a history of previous myocardial infarction, one-half also exhibit chronic obstructive pulmonary disease, and nearly 70% are chronic smokers. Five percent to 10% of these patients may exhibit symptoms of congestive heart failure, and such patients have been said to account for a fourfold increase in cardiac complications [227]. Routine coronary angiography in a group of patients about to receive vascular surgery showed that up to 30% had significant coronary disease despite a normal resting electrocardiogram. Patients with myocardial infarction account for approximately 50% of early postoperative deaths in vascular surgery and the mortality of reinfarction during this period is as high as 70% [228,229]. Thus, both anesthetic and postoperative management of the patient must consider and minimize the effects of these conditions.

Evaluation of cardiac function in patients with other suspect symptoms is advocated, and it has been noted that an ejection fraction of <35% is associated with a fourfold increase in the incidence of postoperative myocardial infarction. Renal function is frequently depressed in aneurysm patients, due to vascular embarrassment, but in the elderly it may also be evidence of concurrent diabetes, hypertension, or other vascular diseases. Renal dysfunction may be accentuated by various diagnostic tests, bowel preparation, and fluid restriction leading to further restriction of urine flow. Intraoperative renal vascular compromise may be superimposed on this condition. Careful peripheral neurologic evaluation should be carried out as soon as feasible in the postoperative period to gauge potential effects of spinal artery ischemia during crossclamping of the aorta as well as to monitor the rare but potentially disastrous development of epidural or subdural hematoma at the site of an epidural or intrathecal anesthetic needle puncture.

Peripheral Vascular Surgery

Perioperative myocardial infarction is reported to occur in up to 15% of patients undergoing peripheral vascular surgery, and it accounts for >50% of perioperative mortality in these patients. Choice of anesthesia includes major regional block such as intrathecal (spinal), extradural (peridural or epidural), and general anesthesia. The advantages of general anesthesia are quick onset, reliability in providing adequate anesthesia, control of the patient's airway, and avoidance of oversedation or restlessness in an awake patient during surgery, which is common during major regional anesthesia. The disadvantages of general anesthesia include variable success in suppression of neuroendocrine stress response and the potential for adverse hemodynamic events during induction and emergence, such as tachycardia, hypertension, or hypotension.

The desired advantages of major regional anesthesia for peripheral vascular surgery are reduction of neuroendocrine stress response when the block is sufficiently high and a presumed reduction in postoperative pulmonary complications. Disadvantages of regional anesthesia include sympathetic blockade and hypotension, assertions that myocardial wall motion may be abnormal under major regional block, the longer time consumed in establishing regional blocks, and the greater incidence of failure of the block. Minor complications such as postspinal headache occur even with epidural block, and nightmare complications such as paraplegia from epidural or subdural hematoma are a rare but undeniable occurrence, even today.

Nowhere in anesthesia care is there any greater current controversy than over the choice of anesthesia for peripheral vascular surgery in elderly patients. It has been alleged that use of general anesthesia for aortobifemoral or lower-extremity grafting and revascularization procedures results in greater cardiac morbidity, ventricular dysfunction, mortality, and a higher incidence of early graft thrombosis than when regional anesthetic techniques are used [230–233], and that this difference holds true also in emergency major vascular surgery [195]. However, dissidents hold that there have been major flaws in the methodology of each of these studies and deny the conclusions. In one of these studies, opponents of regional anesthesia point out that the general anesthesia group received very large doses of intraoperative narcotic and required prolonged postoperative ventilation, which might have been responsible for some of the findings [232].

Another study compared patients who received either surgical epidural anesthesia and postoperative epidural analgesia with others who received general anesthesia followed by postoperative IV patient-controlled analgesia. This study failed to display any significant difference in the incidence of myocardial ischemia between the two groups on the day of operation or the following day, but when either the patient-controlled analgesia or the epidural analgesia was discontinued, the ischemia rate increased significantly in both groups [232]. Opponents note that none of the studies favorable to regional anesthesia used standardized intraoperative monitoring, anesthetic management, or postoperative analgesia. Furthermore, they object that no attempt was made in any of these studies to compare regional anesthesia groups with general anesthesia groups where postsurgical pain management was comparable with that received by the patients receiving regional anesthesia [194,231,232]. Another equally impressive study found no evidence that combined general anesthesia plus epidural anesthesia techniques are superior to general anesthesia alone nor that there is a significant reduction in the incidence of postoperative pulmonary complications after major abdominal surgery with regional anesthesia or regional combined with general anesthesia [234,235].

A large independent prospective study of intrathecal versus general or epidural versus general anesthesia in revascularization procedures of the lower extremity found no difference in the incidence of perioperative myocardial incidents or mortality [194]. The authors reported no significant differences in cardiac morbidity, mortality, or length of hospital stay among the three different anesthetic techniques. In this experience, the overall incidence of perioperative myocardial infarction and death was actually *greater in the regional anesthesia group (4.5%) than in the general anesthesia group (2.6%),* although this difference did not reach statistical significance [194].

Although it has been asserted that early graft thrombosis rates in peripheral vascular surgery are lesser with regional anesthesia than with general anesthesia, no consensus has been achieved concerning the validity of this position. Reports from supporters of regional anesthesia of patients undergoing major aortic or lower-extremity vascular surgery state their patients who received general anesthesia alone suffered a 20% incidence of early graft thrombosis, compared with only 2.5% in patients receiving combined general plus regional anesthesia [233]. However, in this report the incidence of graft thrombosis in patients receiving general anesthesia is so high as to be remarkably unlike the cumulative incidence of early graft thrombosis in other large studies and is, therefore, somewhat suspect [194]. A conflicting study described the outcome of similar procedures in 307 patients in another institution. These were randomized to receive intrathecal, epidural, or general anesthesia. In this report, the overall incidence of in-hospital graft thrombosis was only 1.6% and did not vary significantly among the three anesthesia groups, thus illustrating that factors other than the choice of anesthesia may have been active in previous series that appeared to favor regional anesthesia [194].

The choice of general anesthesia, epidural anesthesia, or general combined with epidural and postsurgical epidural analgesia for revascularization surgery is clearly not easy to make. All three techniques have the inherent possibility of causing serious complications. Furthermore, epidural anesthesia with postsurgical continuous epidural analgesia is a great deal more expensive than either of the other choices. In the absence of heparinization, continuous epidural anesthesia provides a pathway for continued postoperative analgesia via the epidural catheter by the use of either a low concentration of local anesthetic or small doses of narcotics. Such treatment provides excellent pain relief. However, the use of intrathecal or epidural narcotics by the anesthesiologist may on rare occasion lead to profound delayed central nervous system respiratory depression. Patients so treated should be carefully monitored for respiratory adequacy.

During aortic crossclamping, considerable myocardial ischemia can develop due to increased work and afterload [236]. Therefore, vasodilators are often infused, such as sodium nitroprusside during crossclamping to reduce ischemia. Some also advocate routine prophylactic use of bicarbonate to counteract lactic acid return from the periphery just after unclamping, and some also recommend prophylactic fluid or blood boluses just before unclamping the aorta. At any rate, crossclamp time must be monitored carefully, and the surgeon must be ready to return the cross clamp to complete or partial clamping if the systemic pressure nourishing the coronary and brain vessels decreases uncontrollably. Minimal incremental doses of potent alpha vasoconstrictor drugs are sometimes used to promote vascular tone in the legs immediately after crossclamping, but under no circumstances should these drugs be continued chronically.

Coronary Artery Bypass

In recent years, more aged and more medically complicated patients are being routinely submitted to coronary artery bypass surgery. In a 10-year period, from 1982 to 1992, the incidence of diabetes in CABG patients increased from 2% to 19%, hypertension increased from 42% to 53%, and the incidence of valvular involvement decreased from 19% to 7%, while the overall surgical mortality in the elderly decreased from 4.6% to 2.3%, indicating more effective anesthetic, surgical, and postoperative management. The incidence of three vessel disease in elderly CABG patients increased from 25% to 41%. In later years, failed percutaneous transluminal coronary angioplasty now accounts for nearly 1% of CABG patients, and in itself it presents an emergency for both anesthesiologists and surgeons [237–239]. Surgical mortality in CABG in elderly patients has been reported to be from 1.6% to 10.5%, but in groups over age 70, a 3.6% surgical mortality may be achievable today [239,240].

Overall, surgical mortality in elderly patients undergoing internal mammary artery grafting has been reported to be 7.6% versus 2% in patients <70 years [241]. Preoperative mortality risk factors in descending order or importance included history of previous myocardial infarction, age advancing past 70, left main artery disease, and history of smoking. The causes of death in the patients who died included cardiac factors in 38%, pulmonary in 21%, and infection in 10% [241]. Another group reported that in the elderly, surgical mortality for CABG with left internal mammary artery graft was 6%, but in CABG with saphenous vein graft it was 9.96%, and mortality was 21% when bilateral internal mammary artery grafts were attempted [241].

Cardiac transplantation in patients >60 years of age has not routinely been practiced. A recent report found that in 156 patients aged 59 and younger, 1-year survival was 89% versus only 61% in patients aged 61 to 67 years. Five-year survival was 76% in the younger patients, but only 36% in the elderly group [242]. Anesthesia care in elderly transplant patients features amnesic drugs such as 1 mg IV lorazepam once or 25 mg IV ketamine every 30 minutes, and restricted doses of fentanyl, with occasional short use of sevoflurane to control episodes of hypertension. Postoperative sedation should have the goal of preventing delirium and disorientation as well as immediate discomfort.

Anesthetic management of CABG, whether with saphenous vein or internal mammary artery grafting, more frequently requires pulmonary artery catheter monitoring due to the high incidence of congestive heart failure and valvular and myocardial pathology. Although some reports have called into question the cost, efficacy, and safety of pulmonary artery catheters, they are properly frequently used in delicate elderly patients [182,243]. So-called fast-track anesthesia techniques emphasizing early arousal and extubation of the trachea are not in favor for these patients. Narcotic-based techniques including fentanyl, sufentanil, or alfentanil are currently popular. Muscle paralysis is provided by vecuronium most commonly, due to its benign effects on the cardiovascular system. However, newer relaxants are becoming popular as well. Constant awareness of the alterations in drug pharmacology caused by aging is advised. In practice, this often translates into using lorazepam, etomidate, fentanyl, and vecuronium (Norcuron) techniques, often given at a roughly 50% dosage reduction compared with younger adults [240]. Preparation for anesthesia and amnesic effects are frequently provided with diazepam, midazolam, or small doses (1 mg) of lorazepam, despite earlier hesitancy about the use of lorazepam in elderly patients. Etomidate or a BZD, and in very robust patients, even thiopental, are sometimes used for induction of anesthesia.

Orthopedic Procedures

Elderly patients undergo a wide variety of orthopedic procedures, but by far the greatest current interest is focused on lower-extremity fractures and arthroplasty. Anesthesia for arm operations is particularly appropriate to various types of regional anesthesia including interscalene blocks, supraclavicular brachial blocks, and axillary blocks. IV local block of the arm, hand, lower leg, or foot (Bier blocks) are appropriate in the elderly with care to restrict doses of IV local anesthetic [244]. In approaching the brachial plexus by the neck, particular caution must be taken against inadvertent induction of pneumothorax during the block procedure, because a high percentage of elderly patients may have compromised pulmonary and cardiovascular function, thus tolerating pneumothorax less easily. As previously mentioned, many of the local anesthetic agents exhibit longer durations of systemic activity in the elderly and this extends to some extent to their local actions. Acute confusional states after femoral neck fractures are seen frequently in elderly patients, but are frequently due to the postoperative use of anticholinergic agents such as promethazine or meperidine, or longer-acting BZDs (see also the section on delirium) [228].

The choice between regional and general anesthesia techniques for surgical fixation of hip fractures is another unsolved controversy of many years' duration. Despite these opinions, no significant advantage from regional or general anesthesia by retrospective studies [245] or prospective studies has been shown [191–193]. Variations in mortality ranging from 3.6% to 35% have been reported by various institutions [193]. Although the incidence of thromboembolic complications after intrathecal anesthesia appears to be lower than after general anesthesia [246], the overall mortality is similar following general or regional anesthesia [193,246].

Recently, 1,333 elderly patients with proximal femoral neck fractures were studied prospectively and administered either general anesthesia alone or regional anesthesia without intrathecal or epidural narcotics. Mortality was almost identical between the two groups of patients, nor were there any differences in the incidence of postsurgical pulmonary embolus or length of hospital stay. Surprisingly, the incidence of deep vein thrombosis was actually higher in the regional anesthesia group, although this incidence did not apparently contribute to an increase in mortality or increased hospital stay. The 30-day mortality rate was 8.8% in the general anesthesia group and 9.4% in the intrathecal anesthesia group, and 1-year mortality was 32.6% in the general anesthesia group versus 36.9% in the intrathecal anesthesia group [193].

Surgical mortality for hip arthroplasty in the 1970s was said to be between 1% and 2% and is stated to have declined to an average of 0.72% by 1988. These rates are similar to those reported in Britain. Less information is available concerning mortality after total knee arthroplasty, but it is estimated to have been approximately 0.45% in Medicare patients in 1988 [211]. Over the two decades studied, nonanesthetic changes in patient care for these procedures included changes in antibiotic use, common use of angiotensin-converting enzyme inhibitors, widespread use of beta blockers, increased use of autologous blood transfusions, improvements in perioperative nursing, improved diagnosis and increased surveillance of deep vein thrombosis, as well as advancing surgical techniques. In the 1970s, 1% of patients died of pulmonary embolus after total hip arthroplasty [211]. This incidence has been markedly reduced by the routine use of thromboprophylaxis. Furthermore, more aggressive, extensive, and invasive intraoperative monitoring of the patient's condition is routine now compared with the 1970s [211].

There has also been some controversy concerning which is preferable for hip arthroplasty: general, intrathecal, or extradural anesthesia. The incidence of intraoperative hypotension, intraoperative blood loss, and postoperative blood loss was not significantly different between intrathecal and epidural anesthetics [210,247]. Similar findings were reported by another group in a larger study of intrathecal versus epidural anesthesia in elderly patients [248].

Most patients in the lateral position during certain hip operations require sedation because of the discomfort of the prolonged pressure on the unanesthetized portions of the upper body and from the psychological strain of the position. In addition, in this position, ventilation is often impaired even in the awake state. When sedation is added to the major regional anesthesia, hypoventilation is frequent, if not the rule, often leading to oxygen desaturation. The addition of narcotic accentuates this tendency. On the other hand, the same problem may be solved under general anesthesia by increasing ventilation from the ventilator.

Cardiopulmonary Resuscitation

There has been some degree of concern among both medical professionals and the lay public that the elderly are more likely to suffer an unfavorable outcome from cardiac arrest and in particular that neurologic sequelae are much more frequent. Because of this impression, elderly patients about to undergo anesthesia and surgery have a considerable degree of discomfort and fear. As evidence of this concern, a study of patients from 70 to 97 years of age demonstrated that most desired that cardiopulmonary resuscitation be instituted in their own case if necessary, but in nearly one-half of the patients, the wish to be treated declined as anticipated quality of life or chances of recovery were perceived by the patient to be less. Forty percent of patients believed that somehow they could make the decision about the institution of artificial ventilation themselves, and 24% demonstrated their wish to create some form of advanced legal directive concerning this issue [249].

Two multicenter studies, including 24 acute care hospitals in nine countries, studied 774 patients who were initially comatose after successful resuscitation from cardiac arrest. Unfortunately, the 6-month mortality rate for the entire group was 81%, and mortality was 94% in the patients >80 years of age compared with only 68% in the patients <45 years of age. In addition to age, other independent predictors of mortality were diabetes, cardiac arrest time >5 minutes before cardiopulmonary resuscitation, a history of congestive heart failure, and cardiopulmonary resuscitation time >20 minutes. However, of the 774 patients, 27% recovered good neurologic function. Furthermore, 86% of 6-month survivors had good neurologic outcome, and there was no correlation of bad neurologic outcome with age. Poor neurologic outcome after cardiac arrest is no more likely simply because of the age of the patient, although it may be associated with factors that are more frequently found in the aged patients. Emergency cardiac resuscitation attempts in the elderly age groups are certainly appropriate if they would be also appropriate for a younger patient [250].

SUMMARY

Anesthesia in elderly patients presents a range of difficult problems. These include unusual responses to anesthesia caused by alterations in the physiology of elderly patients and the prevalence of pathologic conditions other than the surgical condition, which in combination with the anesthetic require special precautions and aftercare. Both normal aging processes and pathologic conditions alter pharmacologic responses to many of the anesthetic drugs. In many cases, different kinds of response are predicated by altered neurologic tissue composition and depression of receptor sensitivity. More commonly, the duration of action and the magnitude of dose response in the elderly may simply be altered by body compartment variations from those of young adults or from depressed organ blood flow or excretion functions. In addition, elderly patients have a distinctly different psychology, and many anesthetic procedures and techniques that might be used in younger patients are not acceptable to some elderly patients.

Anesthesia for the elderly patient must be attempted only after careful evaluation of the health and physical and psychological needs of the patient as well as the special requirements of the surgical procedure. Perioperative mortality and morbidity rates related to anesthesia and surgery are declining at an encouragingly rapid rate because of new knowledge of the differences between the elderly and younger adults and the continuing development of new and more appropriate drugs. It can be anticipated that in the near future necessary surgical procedures can be offered to patients of unlimited age with confidence.

REFERENCES

1. U.S. Bureau of the Census. Sixty-Five Plus in the U.S. National Institute on Aging: DOC #1039. Washington, DC: U.S. Bureau of the Census, May 4, 1996.
2. Brody JA. Toward quantifying the health of the elderly. Am J Public Health 1989;79:685–686.
3. Seymour DG, Pringle R. Post-operative complications in the elderly surgical patient. Gerontology 1983;29:262–270.
4. Marx GF, Matteo CV, Orkin L. Computer analysis of post anesthetic deaths. Anesthesiology 1983;59:54–58.
5. Craig DB, McLeskey CH, Mitenko PA, et al. Geriatric anesthesia: anatomical and physiological changes of aging. Can J Anaesth 1987;34:156–167.
6. Katz SM, Fagraeus L. Anesthetic considerations in geriatric patients. Clin Geriatr Med 1990;6:499–510.
7. Ward RM, Hutton P. Factors modifying the use of anaesthetic drugs in the elderly. Br Med Bull 1990;46:156–168.
8. Ouslander JG. Drug therapy in the elderly. Ann Intern Med 1981; 95:711–722.
9. Greenblatt DJ, Sellers EM, Shader PI. Drug disposition in old age. N Engl J Med 1982;306:1081–1088.
10. Wood M. Plasma drug binding implications for anesthesiologists. Anesth Analg 1986;65:786–804.
11. Borga O, Piafsky KM, Nilsen OG. Plasma protein binding of basic drugs. I. Selective displacement from A_1 acid glycoprotein by this (2-butoxyethyl) phosphate. Clin Pharmacol Ther 1977;22:539–544.
12. Matteo RS, Orstein E. Pharmacokinetics and pharmacodynamics of injected drugs in the elderly. Adv Anesthesia 1988;5:25–52.
13. Christensen JH, Andreasen F, Jansen JA. Thiopentone sensitivity in young and elderly women. Br J Anaesth 1983;55:33–40.
14. Sear JW, Cooper GM, Kumar V. The effect of age on recovery. A comparison of the kinetics of thiopentone and althesin. Anaesthesia 1983;38:1158–1161.
15. Homer TD, Stanski DR. The effect of increasing age on thiopental disposition and anesthetic requirement. Anesthesiology 1985;62: 714–724.
16. Kirkpatrick T, Cockshott ID, Douglas EJ, Nimmo WS. Pharmacokinetics of propofol (Diprivan) in elderly patients. Br J Anaesth 1988;60:146–150.
17. Arden JR, Holley FO, Stanski DR. Increased sensitivity to etomidate in the elderly. Initial distribution versus altered brain response. Anesthesiology 1986;65:19–27.
18. Caradoc-Davies TH. Opiate toxicity in elderly patients. BMJ 1981; 283:905–906.
19. Herman RJ, McAllister CB, Branch RA, Wilkinson GR. Effects of age on meperidine disposition. Clin Pharmacol Ther 1985;37:19–24.
20. Naritomi H, Meyer JS, Sakai F, et al. Effects of advancing age on regional cerebral blood flow. Studies in normal subjects and subjects with risk factors for atherothrombic stroke. Arch Neurol 1979;36:410–416.
21. Jhaveri RM. The effects of hypocapnic ventilation on mental function in elderly patients undergoing cataract surgery. Anaesthesia 1989;44:635–640.
22. Munson ES, Hoffman JC, Eger EI II. Use of cyclopropane to test generality of anesthetic requirement in the elderly. Anesth Analg 1984; 63:998–1000.
23. Loss GE, Seifen E, Kennedy RH, Seifen AB. Aging: effects on minimum alveolar concentration (MAC) for halothane in Fisher-344 rats. Anesth Analg 1989;68:359–362.
24. Nikaido AM, Ellinwood EH, Heatherly DG, Gupta SK. Age-related increase in CNS sensitivity to benzodiazepines as assessed by task difficulty. Psychopharmacology 1990;100:90–97.
25. Earnst MP, Heaton RK, Wilkinson WE, Manke WR. Cortical atrophy, ventricular enlargement and intellectual impairment in the aged. Neurology 1979;24:1138–1143.
26. Parikh SS, Chung F. Postoperative delirium in the elderly. Anesth Analg 1995;80:123–132.
27. Dax EM. Receptors and associated membrane events in aging. Rev Biol Res Aging 1985;2:315–336.
28. Roizen MF, Koblin DD, Johnson BH, et al. Mechanism of age-related and nitrous oxide–associated anesthetic sensitivity: the role of brain catecholamines. Anesthesiology 1988;69:716–720.
29. Feldman RD, Limbird LE, Nadeau J, et al. Alterations in leukocyte beta-receptor affinity with aging. A potential explanation for altered beta-adrenergic sensitivity in the elderly. N Engl J Med 1984;310:815–819.
30. Pfeifer MA, Weinberg CR, Cook D, et al. Differential changes of autonomic nervous system function with age in man. Am J Med 1983;75:249–257.
31. Erskine RJ, Murphy PJ, Langton JA, Smith G. Effects of age on the sensitivity of upper airway reflexes. Br J Anaesth 1993;70:574–575.
32. Virtanen R, Kanto J, Iisalo E, et al. Pharmacokinetic studies on atropine with special reference to age. Acta Anaesthesiol Scand 1982;26:297–300.
33. Duvaldestin P, Saada J, Berger JL, et al. Pharmacokinetics, pharmacodynamics, and dose-response relationships of pancuronium in control and elderly subjects. Anesthesiology 1982;56:36–40.
34. Matteo RS, Backus WW, McDaniel DD, et al. Pharmacokinetics and pharmacodynamics of D-tubocurarine and metocurine in the elderly. Anesth Analg 1985;64:23–29.
35. Tasch MD. Neuromuscular blocking agents in geriatric anesthesia. Int Anesthesiol Clin 1988;26:152–155.
36. Aronow WS. New coronary events at four-year follow-up in elderly patients with recognized or unrecognized myocardial infarction. Am J Cardiol 1989;63:621–622.
37. Arrighi JA, Dilsizian V, Perrone-Filardi P, et al. Improvement of the age-related impairment in left ventricular diastolic filling with verapamil in the normal human heart. Circulation 1994;90:213–219.
38. Leithe ME, Hermiller JB, Magorien RD, et al. The effect of age on central and regional haemodynamics. Gerontology 1984;30:240–246.
39. Abernathy, DR. Altered pharmacodynamics of cardiovascular drugs and their relation to altered pharmacokinetics in elderly patients. Clin Geriatr Med 1190;6:285–292.
40. Esler MD, Thompson JM, Kaye MM, et al. Effects of aging on the responsiveness of the human cardiac sympathetic nerves to stressors. Circulation 1995;91:351–357.
41. Folkow B, Svamborg A. Physiology of cardiovascular aging. Physiol Rev 1993;73:725–764.
42. Sheldon R. Effects of aging on responses to isoproterenol tilt-table testing in patients with syncope. Am J Cardiol 1994;74:459–463.
43. Tsuji H, Venditti FJ, Manders ES, et al. Reduced heart rate variability and mortality risk in an elderly cohort. Circulation 1994;90:878–883.
44. Fowler RW. Ageing and lung function. Age Ageing 1985;14:209–215.
45. Daykin AP, Bowen DJ, Saunders DA, Norman J. Respiratory depression after morphine in the elderly. A comparison with younger subjects. Anaesthesia 1986;41:910–914.
46. Brischetto MJ, Millman RP, Peterson DD, et al. Effect of aging on ventilatory response to exercise and CO_2. J Appl Physiol 1984;56: 1143–1150.
47. Wahba WM. Influence of aging on lung-function—clinical significance of changes from age twenty. Anesth Analg 1983;62:764–776.
48. Van Hamme MJ. Pharmacokinetics of etomidate, a new intravenous anesthetic. Anesthesiology 1978;49:274–277.
49. George CF. Drug kinetics and hepatic blood flow. Clin Pharmacokinet 1979;4:433-448.
50. Schnegg M, Lauterburg BH. Quantitative liver function in the elderly assessed by galactose elimination capacity, aminopyrine demethylation and caffeine clearance. J Hepatol 1986;3:164–171.
51. Rowe JW, Andres R, Tobin JD, et al. The effect of age on creatinine clearance in man—a cross sectional and longitudinal study. J Gerontol 1976;31:155–163.
52. Richey DP, Bender AD. Pharmacokinetic consequences of aging. Annu Rev Pharmacol Toxicol 1977;17:49–65.

53. Matteo RS, Schwartz AE, Ornstein E, et al. Pharmacokinetics of sufentanil in the elderly surgical patient. Can J Anaesth 1990;37: 852–856.
54. Smith BE. Pharmacokinetics without calculus—an introduction. Int Anesthesiol Clin 1995;33:11–28.
55. Singleton MA, Rosen JI, Fisher DM. Pharmacokinetics of fentanyl in the elderly. Br J Anaesth 1988;60:619–622.
56. Klotz U, Avant GR, Hoyumpa A, et al. The effects of age and liver disease on the disposition and elimination of diazepam in adult man. J Clin Invest 1975;55:347–359.
57. Wood M, Wood AJJ. General Pharmacological Principles: Drug Disposition and Pharmacokinetics. In Wood M, Wood AJJ (eds), Drugs and Anesthesia: Pharmacology for Anesthesiologists (2nd ed). Baltimore: Williams & Wilkins, 1990;6–9.
58. Hinrichs JV, Ghoneim MM. Diazepam, behavior, and aging: increased sensitivity or lower baseline performance? Psychopharmacology 1987;92:100–105.
59. Kochman RL, Sepulveda CK. Aging does not alter the sensitivity of benzodiazepine receptors to GABA modulation. Neurobiol Aging 1986;7:363–365.
60. Guthrie S, Cooper RL, Thurman R, Linnoila M. Pharmacodynamics and pharmacokinetics of ethanol, diazepam and pentobarbital in young and aged rats. Pharmacol Toxicol 1987;61:308–312.
61. Komiskey HL. Aging: effect on ex-vivo benzodiazepine binding after a diazepam injection. Neurochem Res 1987;12:745–749.
62. Möhler H, Richards JG. The benzodiazepine receptor: a pharmacologic control element of brain function. Eur J Anaesthiol Suppl 1988;2:15–24.
63. Komiskey HL, Rahman A, Mundinger KL. Aging: changes in a passive-avoidance response with brain levels of temazepam. Pharmacol Biochem Behav 1989;31:611–615.
64. Barnhill JG, Greenblatt DJ, Miller LG, et al. Kinetic and dynamic components of increased benzodiazepine sensitivity in aging animals. J Pharmacol Exp Ther 1990;253:1153–1161.
65. Holazo AA, Winkler MB, Patel IH. Effects of age, gender and oral contraceptives on intramuscular midazolam pharmacokinetics. J Clin Pharmacol 1988;28:1040–1045.
66. Scholer SG, Schafer DF, Potter JF. The effects of age on the relative potency of midazolam and diazepam for sedation in upper gastrointestinal endoscopy. J Clin Gastroenterol 1990;12:145–147.
67. Wong HY, Fragen RJ, Dunn K. Dose-finding study of intramuscular midazolam preanesthetic medication in the elderly. Anesthesiology 1991;74:675–679.
68. Jacobs JR, Reves JG, Marty J, et al. Aging increases pharmacodynamic sensitivity to the hypnotic effects of midazolam. Anesth Analg 1995;80:143–148.
69. Greenblatt DJ, Shader RI, Harmantz JS. Implications of altered drug disposition in the elderly: studies on benzodiazepines. J Clin Pharmacol 1989;29:866–872.
70. Montamat SC, Cusack BJ, Vestal RE. Management of drug therapy in the elderly. N Engl J Med 1989;321:303–309.
71. Greenblatt DJ, Harmatz JS, Shapiro L, et al. Sensitivity to triazolam in the elderly. N Engl J Med 1991;324:1691–1698.
72. Swift CG, Ewen JM, Clarke P, Stevenson IH. Responsiveness to oral diazepam in the elderly: relationship to total and free plasma concentrations. Br J Clin Pharmacol 1985;20:111–118.
73. Nikaido AM, Ellinwood EH, Heatherly DG, Dubow D. Differential CNS effects of diazepam in elderly adults. Pharmacol Biochem Behav 1987;27:273–281.
74. Greenblatt DJ, Abernethy DR, Locniskar A, et al. Effect of age, gender, and obesity on midazolam kinetics. Anesthesiology 1984;61:27–35.
75. Dundee JW, Halliday NJ, Loughran PG, Harper KW. The influence of age on the onset of anaesthesia with midazolam. Anaesthesia 1985;40:441–443.
76. Kanto J, Aaltonen L, Himberg J-J, Hovi-Viander M. Midazolam as an intravenous induction agent in the elderly: a clinical and pharmacokinetic study. Anesth Analg 1986;65:15–20.
77. Servin F, Enriquez I, Fournet M, et al. Pharmacokinetics of midazolam used as an intravenous induction agent for patients over 80 years of age. Eur J Anaesthesiol 1987;4:1–7.
78. Klotz U, Kanto J. Pharmacokinetics and clinical use of flumazenil (Ro 15-1788). Clin Pharmacokinet 1988;14:1–12.
79. Servin F, Bougeois B, Farinotti R, Desmonts JM. Does flumazenil improve recovery after midazolam anesthesia in patients over 80 years? Anesthesiology 1989;71:A299.
80. Sibai AN, Sibai AN, Baraka A. Comparison of flumazenil with aminophylline to antagonize midazolam in elderly patients. Br J Anaesth 1991;66:591–595.
81. Meyer BR. Benzodiazepines in the elderly. Med Clin North Am 1982;66:1017–1035.
82. Satzger W, Engel RR, Ferguson E, et al. Effects of single doses of alpidem, lorazepam, and placebo on memory and attention in healthy young and elderly volunteers. Pharmacopsychiatry 1990;23:114–119.
83. Munoz HR, Dagnino JA, Rufs JA, Bugedo GJ. Benzodiazepine premedication causes hypoxemia during spinal anesthesia in geriatric patients. Reg Anesth 1992;17:139–142.
84. Sunderland T, Weingartner H, Cohen RM, et al. Low-dose oral lorazepam administration in Alzheimer subjects and age-matched controls. Psychopharmacology 1989;99:129–133.
85. Woo E, Proulx SM, Greenblatt DJ. Differential side effect profile of triazolam versus flurazepam in elderly patients undergoing rehabilitation therapy. J Clin Pharmacol 1991;31:168–73.
86. Fisch HU, Baktir G, Karlaganis G, et al. Excessive motor impairment two hours after triazolam in the elderly. Eur J Clin Pharmacol 1990;38:229–232.
87. Arunsalam K, Davenport HT, Painter S, Jones JG. Ventilatory response to morphine in young and old subjects. Anaesthesia 1983; 38:529–533.
88. Hertzka RE, Gauntlett IS, Fisher DM, Spellman MJ. Fentanyl-induced ventilatory depression: effects of age. Anesthesiology 1989; 70:213–218.
89. Bellville JW, Forrest W Jr, Miller E, et al. Influence of age on pain from analgesics. JAMA 1971;217:1835–1841.
90. Lemmens HJM, Bovill JG, Hennis PJ, Burm AGL. Age has no effect on the pharmacodynamics of alfentanil. Anesth Analg 1988;67:956–960.
91. Bentley JB, Borel JD, Nenad RE Jr, Gillespie TJ. Age and fentanyl pharmacokinetics. Anesth Analg 1982;61:968–971.
92. Scott JC, Stanski DR. Decreased fentanyl and alfentanil dose requirements with increasing age. A simultaneous pharmacokinetic and pharmacodynamic evaluation. J Pharmacol Exp Ther 1987;240:159–166.
93. Hudson RJ, Bergstrom RG, Thomson IR, et al. Pharmacokinetics of sufentanil in patients undergoing abdominal aortic surgery. Anesthesiology 1989;70:426–431.
94. Lemmens HJM, Bovill JG, Burm AG, Hennis PJ. Alfentanil infusion in the elderly. Prolonged computer-assisted infusion of alfentanil in the elderly surgical patient. Anaesth 1988;43:850–856.
95. Scott JC, Stanski DR. Decreased fentanyl and alfentanil dose requirements with increasing age. A pharmacodynamic basis. Anesthesiology 1985;63:A374.
96. Lemmens HJM, Bovill JG, Hennis PJ, Burm AG. Age has no effect on the pharmacodynamics of alfentanil. Anesth Analg 1988;67:956–960.
97. Sitar DS, Duke PC, Benthuysen JL, et al. Aging and alfentanil disposition in healthy volunteers and surgical patients. Can J Anaesth 1989;36:149–154.
98. Helmers H, Van Peer A, Woestenborghs R, et al. Alfentanil kinetics in the elderly. Clin Pharmacol Ther 1984;36:239–243.
99. Maitre PO, Vozeh S, Heykants J, et al. Population pharmacokinetics of alfentanil: the average dose-plasma concentration relationship and inter-individual variability in patients. Anesthesiology 1987;66:3–12.
100. Kent AP, Dodson ME, Bower S. The pharmacokinetics and clinical effects of a low dose of alfentanil in elderly patients. Acta Anaesthesiol Belg 1988;39:25–33.
101. Raeder JC, Nilsen OG, Hole A. Pharmacokinetics of midazolam and alfentanil in outpatient general anesthesia: a study with concomitant thiopentone, flumazenil or placebo administration. Acta Anaesthesiol Scand 1988;32:467–472.
102. Barvais L, D'Hollander A, Schmartz D, et al. Predictive accuracy of alfentanil infusion in coronary artery surgery: a prebypass study in middle-aged and elderly patients. J Cardiothorac Vasc Anesth 1994;8:278–283.
103. Virkkila M, Ali-Melikkila T, Soini H, Kanto J. Pharmacokinetics and effects of IM alfentanil as premedication for day-case ophthalmic surgery in elderly patients. Br J Anaesth 1993;71:507–511.
104. Muravchick S. Effect of age and premedication on thiopental sleep dose. Anesthesiology 1984;61:333–336.
105. Stanski DR, Maitre PO. Population pharmacokinetics and pharmacodynamics of thiopental: the effect of age revisited. Anesthesiology 1990;72:412–422.
106. Avram MJ, Krejcie TC, Henthorn TK. The relationship of age to the

pharmacokinetics of early drug distribution: the concurrent disposition of thiopental and iodocyanine green. Anesthesiology 1990;72:403–411.
107. Jung D, Mayersohn M, Perrier D, et al. Thiopental disposition as a function of age in female patients undergoing surgery. Anesthesiology 1982;56:263–268.
108. Berthoud MC, McLaughlan GA, Broome IJ, et al. Comparison of infusion rates of three IV anaesthetic agents for induction in elderly patients. Br J Anaesth 1993;70:423–427.
109. Ghoneim MM, Chiang CK, Schoenwald RD, et al. The pharmacokinetics of methohexital in young and elderly subjects. Acta Anaesthesiol Scand 1985;29:480–482.
110. White PF. Propofol: pharmacokinetics and pharmacodynamics: Semin Anesth 1988;7:4–20.
111. Peacock JE, Lewis RP, Reilly CS, Nimmo WS. Effects of different rates of infusion of propofol for induction of anaesthesia in elderly patients. Br J Anaesth 1990;65:346–352.
112. Scheepstra GL, Booij LHDJ, Rutten CLG, Coenen LGJ. Propofol for induction and maintenance of anaesthesia: comparison between younger and older patients. Br J Anaesth 1989;62:54–60.
113. Dundee JW, Robinson FP, McCollum JSC, Patterson CC. Sensitivity to propofol in the aged. Anaesthesia 1986;41:482–485.
114. Kanto J, Gepts E. Pharmacokinetic implications for the clinical use of propofol. Clin Pharmacokinet 1989;17:308–326.
115. Mather LE, Selby DG, Runciman WB, McLean CF. Propofol: assay and regional mass balance in the sheep. Xenobiotica 1989;19:1337–1347.
116. Peacock JE, Spiers SPW, McLauchlan GA, et al. Infusion of propofol to identify smallest effective doses for induction of anaesthesia in young and elderly patients. Br J Anaesth 1992;69:363–367.
117. Edwards ND, Fletcher A, Cole JR, Peacock JE. Combined infusions of morphine and ketamine for postoperative pain in elderly patients. Anaesthesia 1993;48:124–127.
118. D'Hollander AA, Luyckx C, Barvais L, De Ville A. Clinical evaluation of atracurium besylate requirement for stable muscle relaxation during surgery: lack of age-related effects. Anesthesiology 1983;59:237–240.
119. Kent AP, Parker CJR, Hunter JM. Pharmacokinetics and atracurium and laudanosine in the elderly. Br J Anaesth 1989;63:661–666.
120. Kitts JB, Fisher DM, Canfell PC, et al. Pharmacokinetics and pharmacodynamics of atracurium in the elderly. Anesthesiology 1990;72:272–275.
121. Slavov V, Khalil M, Merle JC, et al. Comparison of duration of neuromuscular blocking effect of atracurium and vecuronium in young and elderly patients. Br J Anaesth 1995;74:709–711.
122. McLeod K, Hull CJ, Watson MJ. Effects of aging on the pharmacokinetics of pancuronium. Br J Anaesth 1979;51:435–438.
123. Rupp SM, Castagnoli KP, Fisher DM, Miller RD. Pancuronium and vecuronium pharmacokinetics and pharmacodynamics in younger and elderly adults. Anesthesiology 1987;67:45–49.
124. O'Hara DA, Fragen RJ, Shank CA. The effects of age on the dose-response curves for vecuronium in adults. Anesthesiology 1985;63: 542–544.
125. McCarthy G, Elliot P, Mirakhur RK, et al. Onset and duration of action of vecuronium in the elderly: comparison with adults. Acta Anaesthesiol Scand 1992;36:383–386.
126. Lien CA, Matteo RS, Ornstein E, et al. Distribution, elimination, and action of vecuronium in the elderly. Anesth Analg 1991;73:39–42.
127. Dresner DL, Basta SJ, Ali HH, et al. Pharmacokinetics and pharmacodynamics of doxacurium in young and elderly patients during isoflurane anesthesia. Anesth Analg 1990;71:498–502.
128. Koscielniak-Nielsen ZJ, Law-Min JC, Donati F, et al. Dose-response relations of doxacurium and its reversal with neostigmine in young adults and healthy elderly patients. Anesth Analg 1992;74:845–850.
129. Bevan DR, Fiset P, Balendran P, et al. Pharmacodynamic behaviour of rocuronium in the elderly. Can J Anaesth 1993;40:127–132.
130. Matteo RS, Ornstein E, Schwartz AE, et al. Pharmacokinetics and pharmacodynamics of rocuronium (Org 9426) in elderly surgical patients. Anesth Analg 1993;77:1193–1197.
131. Azad SS, Larijani GE, Goldberg ME, et al. A dose-response evaluation of pipecuronium bromide in elderly patients under balanced anesthesia. J Clin Pharmacol 1989;29:657–659.
132. Ornstein E, Matteo RS, Schwartz AE, et al. Pharmacokinetics and pharmacodynamics of pipecuronium bromide (Arduan) in elderly surgical patients. Anesth Analg 1992;74:841–844.
133. Lien CA, Belmont MR, Abalos A, et al. The cardiovascular effects and histamine releasing properties of 51W89 in patients receiving nitrous oxide/opioid/barbiturate anesthesia. Anesthesiology 1995;82: 1131–1183.
134. Sorooshian SS, Stafford MA, Eastwood NB, et al. Pharmacokinetics and pharmacodynamics of cisatracurium in young and elderly adult patients. Anesthesiology 1996;84:1083–1091.
135. Matteo RS, Young WL, Ornstein E, et al. Pharmacokinetics and pharmacodynamics of edrophonium in elderly surgical patients. Anesth Analg 1990;71:334–339.
136. Young WL, Matteo RS, Ornstein E. Duration of action of neostigmine and pyridostigmine in the elderly. Anesth Analg 1988;67:775–778.
137. Nation RL, Triggs EJ. Lignocaine kinetics in cardiac patients and aged subjects. Br J Clin Pharmacol 1977;4:439–448.
138. Finucane BT, Hammonds WD, Welch MB. Influence of age on vascular absorption of lidocaine from the epidural space. Anesth Analg 1987;66:843–846.
139. Yukioka H, Hayashi M, Terai T, Fujimori M. Intravenous lidocaine as a suppressant of coughing during tracheal intubation in elderly patients. Anesth Analg 1993;77:309–312.
140. Vestal RE, Wood AJJ, Branch RA, et al. Effects of age and cigarette smoking on propranolol disposition. Clin Pharmacol Ther 1979;26:8–15.
141. Zhou H, Whelan E, Wood AJJ. Lack of effect of ageing on the steriochemical disposition of propranolol. Br J Clin Pharmicol 1992;33: 121–123.
142. Reilly CS, Merrell J, Wood AJJ, et al. Comparison of the effects of isoflurane or fentanyl–nitrous oxide anaesthesia on propranolol disposition in dogs. Br J Anaesth 1988;60:791–796.
143. Singh PP, Dimich I, Sampson I, Sonnenklar N. A comparison of esmolol and labetalol for the treatment of perioperative hypertension in geriatric ambulatory surgical pateints. Can J Anaesth 1992;39:559–562.
144. Cressman M, Vidth D, Gifford R. Intravenous labetalol in the management of severe hypertension and hypertensive emergencies. Am Heart J 1987;101:980–985.
145. Cahalan MK, Hashimoto Y, Aizawa K, et al. Elderly, conscious patients have an accentuated hypotensive response to nitroglycerin. Anesthesiology 1992;77:646–655.
146. Filos KS, Patroni O, Goudas LC, et al. A dose-response study of orally administered clonidine as premedication in the elderly: evaluating hemodynamic safety. Anesth Analg 1993;77:1185–1192.
147. Kumar A, Bose S, Bhattacharya A, et al. Oral clonidine premedication for elderly patients undergoing intraocular surgery. Acta Anaesthesiol Scand 1992;36:159–164.
148. Racle JP, Benkhadra A, Poy JY, Bleizal B. Prolongation of isobaric spinal anesthesia with epinephrine and clonidine for hip surgery in the elderly. Anesth Analg 1987;66:442–446.
149. Fogarty DJ, Carabine UA, Milligan KR. Comparison of the analgesic effects of intrathecal clonidine and intrathecal morphine after spinal anaesthesia in patients undergoing total hip replacement. Br J Anaesth 1993;71:661–664.
150. Grace D, Miligan KR, Mollow BJ, Fee JPH. Co-administration of pethidine and clonidine: a spinal anaesthetic technique for total hip replacement. Br J Anaesth 1994;73:628–633.
151. Eger EI II, Saidman LJ, Brandstoter B. Minimum alveolar concentration: a standard of anesthetic potency. Anesthesiology 1965;26:756–763.
152. Gregory GA, Eger EI II, Munson ES. The relationship between age and halothane requirement in man. Anesthesiology 1969;30:488–491.
153. Nakajima R, Nakajima Y, Ikeda K. Minimum alveolar concentration of sevoflurane in elderly patients. Br J Anaesth 1993;70:273–275.
154. Dwyer R, Fee JPH, Clarke RSJ. End-tidal concentrations of halothane and isoflurane during induction of anaesthesia in young and elderly patients. Br J Anaesth 1990;64:36–41.
155. Strum DP, Eger EI, Unadkat JD, et al. Age affects the pharmacokinetics of inhaled anesthetics in humans. Anesth Analg 1991;73:310–318.
156. Dwyer RC, Fee JPH, Howard PJ, Clarke RSJ. Arterial wash-in of halothane and isoflurane in young and elderly adult patients. Br J Anaesth 1991;66:572–579.
157. McKinney MS, Fee JPH, Clark RSJ. Cardiovascular effects of isoflurane and halothane in young and elderly adult patients. Br J Anaesth 1993;71:696–701.
158. Bennett JA, Lingaraju N, Horrow JC, et al. Elderly patients recover more rapidly from desflurane than from isoflurane. Anesthesia 1992;4:378–381.
159. Katoh T, Suguro Y, Ikeda T, et al. Influence of age on awakening concentrations of sevoflurane and isoflurane. Anesth Analg 1993;76: 348–352.

160. Cullen DJ, Nemeskal AR, Cooper JB, et al. Effect of pulse oximetry, age, and ASA physical status on the frequency of patients admitted unexpectedly to a postoperative intensive care unit and the severity of their anesthesia-related complications. Anesth Analg 1992;74:181–188.
161. American Society of Anesthesiologists. New classification of physical status. Anesthesiology 1961;24:111.
162. Del Guercio LRM, Cohn JD. Monitoring operative risk in the elderly. JAMA 1980;243:1350–1355.
163 Stephen CR, Assaf RAE. Risk Factors and Outcome in Elderly Patients: An Epidemiologic Study. In Stephen CR (ed), Geriatric Anesthesia. Boston: Butterworth–Heinemann,1986;345–362.
164. Mulrow CD, Cornell JA, Herrera CR, et al. Hypertension in the elderly. JAMA 1994;272:1932–1938.
165. Lindroos M, Kupari M, Heikklia J, Tilvis R. Echocardiographic evidence of left ventricular hypertrophy in a general aged population. Am J Cardiol 1994;74:385–390.
166. Lewis JF, Maron BJ. Clinical and morphologic expression of hypertrophic cardiomyopathy in patients >65 years of age. Am J Cardiol 1994;73:1105–1111.
167. Aronow WS, Ahn C. Prevalence of coexistence of coronary artery disease, peripheral arterial disease, and atherothrombotic brain infarction in men and women >62 years of age. Am J Cardiol 1994;74:64–65.
168. Rautaharju PM, Manolio TA, Psaty BM, et al. Correlates of QT prolongation in older adults (the Cardiovascular Health Study). Am J Cardiol 1994;73:999–1002.
169. Shirani J, Yousfi J, Roberts WC. Major cardiac findings of necropsy in 366 American octogenarians. Am J Cardiol 1995;75:151–156.
170. Older P, Smith R. Experience with the preoperative invasive measurement of haemodynamic respiratory and renal function in 100 elderly patients scheduled for major abdominal surgery. Anaesth Intensive Care 1988;16:389–395.
171. Older P, Smith R, Courtney P, Hone R. Preoperative evaluation of cardiac failure and ischemia in elderly patients by cardiopulmonary exercise testing. Chest 1993;104:701–704.
172. Goldman L, Caldera DL, Nussbaum SR, et al. Multifactorial index of cardiac risk in noncardiac surgical procedures. N Engl J Med 1977;297:845–850.
173. Goldman L, Caldera DL. Risks of general anesthesia and elective surgery in the hypertensive patient. Anesthesiology 1979;50: 285–292.
174. Chung MK, Bosner MS, McKenzie JP, et al. Prognosis of patients >70 years of age with non–Q-wave acute myocardial infarction compared with younger patients with similar infarcts and with patients >70 years of age with Q-wave acute myocardial infarction. Am J Cardiol 1995;75:18–22.
175. Ikeda T, Doi M, Morita K, Ikeda K. Effects of midazolam and diazepam as premedication on heart rate variability in surgical patients. Br J Anaesth 1994;73:479–483.
176. Slogoff S, Keats AS, Hibbs CW, et al. Failure of general anesthesia to potentiate propranolol activity. Anesthesiology 1977;47:504–508.
177. O'Keeffe ST, Ni Chinchubhair A. Postoperative delirium in the elderly. Br J Anaesth 1994;73:673–687.
178. American Society of Anesthesiologists Task Force on Pulmonary Artery Catheterization. Practice guidelines for pulmonary artery catheterization. Anesthesiology 1993;78:380–394.
179. Tuman KJ, McCarthy RJ, Speiss BD, et al. Effect of pulmonary artery catheterization on outcome in patients undergoing coronary artery surgery. Anesthesiology 1989;70:199–206.
180. Wu AW, Rubin HR, Rosen MJ. Are elderly people less responsive to intensive care? J Am Geriatr Soc 1990;38:621–627.
181. American Society of Anesthesiologists. American Society of Anesthesiologists Guidelines. Park Ridge, IL: American Society of Anesthesiologists, 1993;291–298.
182. Connors AF, Speroff T, Dawson NV, et al. The effectiveness of right heart catheterization in the intial care of critically ill patients. JAMA 1996;276:889–897.
183. Sebel PS, Glass PSA, Fletcher JE, et al. Reduction of the MAC of desflurane with fentanyl. Anesthesiology 1992;76:52–59.
184. Hole A, Terjesen T, Breivik H. Epidural versus general anaesthesia for total hip arthroplasty in elderly patients. Acta Anaesthesiol Scand 1980;24:279–287.
185. Davis FM, Laurenson VG. Spinal anaesthesia or general anaesthesia for emergency hip surgery in elderly patients. Anaesth Intensive Care 1981;9:352–356.
186. Mann RAM, Bisset WIK. Anaesthesia for lower limb amputation: a comparison of spinal analgesia and general anaesthesia in the elderly. Anaesthesia 1983;38:1185–1191.
187. Modig J, Borg T, Karlstrom G. Thromboembolism after total hip replacement: role of epidural and general anesthesia. Anesth Analg; 1983;62:174–180.
188. Riis J, Lomholt B, Haxholdt O, et al. Immediate and long-term mental recovery from general versus epidural anesthesia in elderly patients. Acta Anaesthesiol Scand 1983;27:44–49.
189. Bigler D, Adelhoj B, Petring OU, et al. Mental function and morbidity after acute hip surgery during spinal and general anaesthesia. Anaesthesia 1985;40:672–676.
190. McKenzie PF, Wishart HY, Smith O. Long term outcome after repair of fractured neck of femur. Br J Anaesth 1984;56:581–584.
191. Valentin N, Lomholt B, Jesen JS, et al. Spinal or general anaesthesia for surgery of the fractured hip? Br J Anaesth 1986;58:284–291.
192. Davis FM, Woolner DF, Frampton C, et al. Prospective multicentre trial of mortality following general spinal anaesthesia for hip fracture surgery in the elderly. Br J Anaesth 1987;59:1080–1088.
193. Sutcliffe AJ, Parker M. Mortality after spinal and general anaesthesia for surgical fixation of hip fractures. Anaesthesia 1994;49:237–240.
194. Bode RH, Lewis KP. Con: regional anesthesia is not better than general anesthesia for lower extremity revascularization. J Cardiothorac Vasc Anesth 1994;8:118–121.
195. Tuman KJ, Ivankovich AD. Regional anesthesia is better than general anesthesia for lower extremity revascularization. J Cardiothorac Vasc Anesth 1994;8:114–117.
196. Chung F, Meier R, Lautenschlager E, et al. General or spinal anesthesia: which is better in the elderly? Anesthesiology 1987;67: 422–427.
197. Critchley LAH, Stuart JC, Short TG, Gin T. Haemodynamic effects of subarachnoid block in elderly patients. Br J Anaesth 1994;73: 464–470.
198. Rasmussen BS, Blum L, Hansen P, Mikkelsen SS. Postspinal headache in young and elderly patients: two randomized, double-blind studies that compare 20- and 25-gauge needles. Anaesthesia 1989;44:571–573.
199. Ecoffey C, Edouard A, Pruszczynski W, et al. Effects of epidural anesthesia on catecholamines, renin activity, and vasopressin changes induced by tilt in elderly men. Anesthesiology 1985;62:294–297.
200. Andersen S, Cold GE. Dose response studies in elderly patients subjected to epidural analgesia. Acta Anaesthesiol Scand 1981;25:279–281.
201. Hirabayashi Y, Shimizu R. Effect of age on extradural requirements in thoracic epidural anaesthesia. Br J Anaesth 1993;71:445–446.
202. Sakura S, Saito Y, Kosaka Y. Effect of lumbar epidural anesthesia on ventilatory response to hypercapnia in young and elderly patients. J Clin Anesth 1993;5:109–113.
203. Varrassi G, Celleno D, Capogna G, et al. Ventilatory effects of subarachnoidal fentanyl in the elderly. Anaesthesia 1992;47:558–562.
204. Sorensen RM, Pace NL. Mortality and morbidity of regional versus general anesthesia: a meta analysis. Anesthesiology 1991;75:A1053.
205. Shir Y, Raja SN, Frank SM. The effects of epidural versus general anesthesia on postoperative pain and analgesic requirements in patients undergoing radical prostatectomy. Anesthesiology 1994;80:49–56.
206. Wolf CJ, Chong MS. Preemptive anesthesia treating postoperative pain by preventing the establishment of central sensitization. Anesth Analg 1993;77:362–379.
207. Liu S, Carpenter RL, Weal JM. Epidural anesthesia and analgesia: their role in postoperative outcome. Anesthesiology 1995;82:1474–1506.
208. Liu S, Carpenter RL, Mulroy MF, et al. Intravenous versus epidural administration of hydromorphone. Anesthesiology 1995;82:682–688.
209. Flanagan JF, Patel NP, King PH, Smith BE. Automated end tidal CO_2 monitoring in postoperative patients. Submitted for publication, 1997.
210. Davis S, Erskine R, James MFM. A comparison of spinal and epidural anaesthesia for hip arthroplasty. Can J Anaesth 1992;39:551–554.
211. Sharrock NE, Cazan MG, Hargett MJL, et al. Changes in mortality after total hip and knee arthroplasty over a ten-year period. Anesth Analg 1995;80:242–248.
212. Kurtz A, Plattner O, Sessler DI, et al. The threshold for thermoregulatory vasoconstriction during nitrous oxide/isoflurane anesthesia is lower in elderly than in young patients. Anesthesiology 1993;79:465–469.
213. Frank SM, Fleisher LA, Olson KF, et al. Multivariate determinants of early postoperative oxygen consumption in elderly patients. Anesthesiology 1995;83:241–249.

214. Vassilieff N, Rosencher N, Sessler DI, Conseiller C. Shivering threshold during spinal anesthesia is reduced in elderly patients. Anesthesiology 1995;83:1162–1166.
215. Frank SM, Beattie C, Christopherson R, et al. Unintentional hypothermia is associated with post-operative myocardial ischemia. Anesthesiology 1993;78:468–476.
216. Frank SM, Higgins MS, Breslow MJ, et al. The catecholamine cortisol and hemodynamic responses to mild perioperative hypothermia: a randomized clinical trial. Anesthesiology 1995;82:83–93.
217. Frank SM, Shir Y, Raja SN, et al. Core hypothermia and skin-surface temperature gradients. Anesthesiology 1994;80:502–508.
218. Marcantonio ER, Juarez G, Goldman L, et al. The relationship of postoperative delirium with psychoactive medications. JAMA 1994; 272:1518–1522.
219. Crul BJP, Hulstijn W, Burger IC. Influence of the type of anaesthesia on postoperative subjective physical well-being and mental function in elderly patients. Acta Anaesthesiol Scand 1992;36:615–620.
220. Gustaffson Y, Berggren D, Brannstrom B, et al. Acute confusional states in elderly patients treated for femoral neck fracture. J Am Geriatr Soc 1988;36:325–330.
221. Ni Chonchubhair A, Valacio R, Kelly J, O'Keeffe S. Use of the abbreviated mental test to detect postoperative delirium in elderly people. Br J Anaesth 1995;75:481–482.
222. Gallina DL, Mordes JP, Rossini AA. Surgery in the diabetic patient. Compr Ther 1983;9:8–16.
223. Lipson LG. Diabetes in the elderly: a multifaceted problem. Am J Med 1986;80(Suppl 5A):1–2.
224. Barzilay JI, Kronmal RA, Bittner V, et al. Coronary artery disease and coronary bypass grafting in diabetic patients aged >65 years (report from the Coronary Artery Surgery Study [CASS] registry). Am J Cardiol 1994;74:334–339.
225. Podolsky S. Hyperosmolar nonketotic coma in the elderly diabetic. Med Clin North Am 1978;62:815–828.
226. Brown EM, Brown M. Management of the elderly diabetic patient during anesthesia. Clin Anesthesiol 1986;4:881–898.
227. Goldman L. Cardiac risks and complications of non-cardiac surgery. Ann Surg 1983;198:780–791.
228. Rao TKL, Jacobs KH, El-Etr AA. Reinfarction following anesthesia in patients with myocardial infarction. Anesthesiology 1983;59:499–505.
229. Davison JK. Anesthesia for major vascular procedures in the elderly. Clin Anesthesiol 1986;4:931–957.
230. Diebel LN, Lange MP, Schneider F, et al. Cardiopulmonary complications after major surgery: a role for epidural analgesia? Surgery 1987;102:660–666.
231. Yeager MP, Glass DD, Neff RK, Brinck-Johnsen T. Epidural anesthesia and analgesia in high risk surgical patients. Anesthesiology 1987;66:729–736.
232. Tuman KJ, McCarthy RJ, March RJ, et al. Effects of epidural anesthesia and analgesia on coagulation and outcome after major vascular surgery. Anesth Analg 1991;73:696–704.
233. Christopherson R, Beattie C, Frank SM, et al. Perioperative morbidity in patients randomized to epidural or general anesthesia for lower extremity vascular surgery. Anesthesiology 1993;79:422–434.
234. Baron JF, Bertrand M, Barre E, et al. Combined epidural and general anesthesia versus general anesthesia for abdominal aortic surgery. Anesthesiology 1991;75:611–618.
235. Jayr C, Thomas H, Rey A, et al. Postoperative pulmonary complications. Epidural analgesia using bupivacaine and opioids versus parenteral opioids. Anesthesiology 1993;78:666–676.
236. Attia RR, Murphy JD, Snider M, et al. Myocardial ischemia due to infra-renal aortic crossclamping during aortic surgery in patients with severe coronary artery disease. Circulation 1976;53:961–965.
237. Merrill W, Stewart J, First W, et al. Cardiac surgery in patients age 80 years or older. Ann Surg 1990;211:772–776.
238. Antoniou F, Siminelakis S, Lalos S, et al. The changing profile of coronary artery bypass patients. Implications for different management. J Cardiothorac Vasc Anesth 1994;8:91.
239. Tuman KJ, McCarthy RJ, Najofi H, et al. Differential effects of advanced age on neurologic and cardiac risks of coronary artery operations. J Thorac Cardiovasc Surg 1992;104:1510–1517.
240. McIntyre AB, Ballenger JF, King AT. Coronary artery bypass surgery in the elderly. J S C Med Assoc 1990;86:435–439.
241. He GW, Acuff TE, Ryan WH, Mack MJ. Risk factors for operative mortality in elderly patients undergoing internal mammary artery grafting. Ann Thorac Surg 1994;57:1453–1461.
242. Robin J, Ninet J, Tronc F, et al. Long-term results of heart transplantation deteriorate more rapidly in patients over 60 years of age. Eur J Cardiothorac Surg 1996;10:259–263.
243. Shoemaker WC, Kram HB, Appel PL, et al. The efficacy of central venous and pulmonary artery catheters and therapy based upon them in reducing mortality and morbidity. Arch Surg 1990;125: 1332–1337.
244. Smith BE. Intravenous Regional Anesthesia. In Rogers MC (ed), Current Practice in Anesthesiology. St. Louis: Mosby–Year Book, 1990; 414–420.
245. White IWC, Chappell WA. Anaesthesia for surgical correction of fractured femoral neck. Anaesthesia 1980;35:1107–1110.
246. Covert CR, Fox GS. Anaesthesia for hip surgery in the elderly. Can J Anaesth 1989;36:311–319.
247. Wildsmith JAW. Intrathecal or extradural: which approach for surgery? Br J Anaesth 1987;59:397–398.
248. Sutter PA, Gamulin Z, Forster A. Comparison of continuous spinal and continuous epidural anesthesia for lower limb surgery in elderly patients. A retrospective study. Anaesthesia 1989;44:47–50.
249. Heap MJ, Munglani R, Klinck JR, Males AG. Elderly patients' preferences concerning life-support treatment. Anesthesia 1993;48:1027–1033.
250. Rogrove HJ, Safer P, Sutton-Tyrrell K, Abramson NS. Old age does not negate good cerebral outcome after cardiopulmonary resuscitation: analyses from the brain resuscitation clinical trials. Crit Care Med 1995;23:18–25.

Surgical Care for the Elderly, 2nd ed., edited by
R. Benton Adkins, Jr., and H. William Scott, Jr.
Lippincott–Raven Publishers, Philadelphia © 1998.

CHAPTER 6

Sarcomas, Lymphomas, and Melanomas

R. Benton Adkins, Jr., and Anh H. Dao

SOFT-TISSUE SARCOMAS

The term *soft tissue* refers to the extraskeletal connective tissue of the body that connects, supports, and surrounds other discrete anatomic structures. This includes muscle, fibrous tissue, fat, fascia, and tendon. Despite the ubiquitous presence of soft tissue in every region of the body, malignant soft tissue tumors are rare, representing <1% of all adult malignancies [1]. In 1995, it was estimated that 6,000 new cases of soft-tissue sarcomas (STSs) were diagnosed in the United States and 3,300 deaths occurred from this disease [1]. STSs are relatively more common in children and make up 6.5% of all cancers in children [1].

STSs can arise almost anywhere, but in adults almost two thirds of STSs arise in the extremities, followed in frequency by sarcomas of the trunk and retroperitoneum [2]. In another study, 1,215 patients with sarcomas were reviewed with the following frequencies: 40% of the tumors occurred in the lower extremities, 32% in the trunk, 15% in the head and neck, and 13% in the upper extremities [3]. Many of the primary sites often seen in children, such as the orbit, paratesticular region, and prostate, are virtually never observed in adults.

Classification of Soft-Tissue Sarcomas

Earlier classifications of STSs based largely on the cellular configuration, with such descriptive terms as *round cell* or *spindle cell sarcomas*, have been abandoned. More recent classifications are based primarily on the line of differentiation of the tumor, that is, the type of tissue formed by the tumor, rather than the type of tissue from which the tumor arose. In 1957, Stout presented the first such classification [4], which was later revised by Lattes [5]. The first universally accepted classification for STS was proposed by the World Health Organization in 1969 [6]. Since then, several changes have been made, and the most recent and widely used classification is that of Enzinger and Weiss [7]. This classification is based mainly on the proliferating cell type, a simplified version of which is presented in Table 6-1, addressing STSs of adults and the elderly.

STSs can be divided into three large categories [8]:

1. Sarcomas with a clear line of differentiation and well-defined proliferating cell type, such as liposarcoma, leiomyosarcoma, synoviosarcoma, and rhabdomyosarcoma. Approximately 50% of STSs belong in this category.
2. Sarcomas with a debatable line of differentiation and proliferating cell type, such as malignant fibrous histiocytoma (MFH), fibrosarcoma, and undifferentiated sarcoma. Approximately 40% of STSs fall into this category.
3. Sarcomas of particular types, often of uncertain size, such as alveolar soft part sarcoma, epithelioid sarcoma, and clear cell sarcoma. These tumors make up approximately 5% of all adult STSs.

Relative Incidence of Soft-Tissue Sarcomas

The incidence of different types of STS varies from series to series. This is due in part to the disagreement between pathologists as to the exact histogenesis of a particular tumor. In addition, changes in classification with recognition of new tumor entities give rise to fluctuations in incidence.

MFH and liposarcoma are the two most common STSs of adults; together, they account for 35% to 45% of all sarcomas [7]. Table 6-2 shows relative incidences as tabulated by Hashimoto et al. [9] on review of 1,116 sarcomas.

Staging and Grading of Soft-Tissue Sarcomas

The American Joint Committee on Cancer (AJCC) staging system is widely accepted and has proved useful [10]. It is based on grade and size of the tumor and evidence of dissemination. Details of this system are presented in Table 6-3.

The grade of a tumor is determined by assessing several histologic parameters: degree of cellularity, nuclear atypia, mitotic activities, and necrosis. The AJCC system has three

TABLE 6-1. *Classification of soft-tissue sarcomas of adult patients*

Proliferating cell type	Corresponding sarcoma
Fibrous	Fibrosarcoma
Fibrohistiocytic	Malignant fibrous histiocytoma
Lipomatous	Liposarcoma
Smooth muscle	Leiomyosarcoma
Striated muscle	Rhabdomyosarcoma
Blood vessel	Angiosarcoma
Lymphatic	Lymphangiosarcoma
Synovial	Synoviosarcoma
Mesothelial	Malignant mesothelioma
Neural	Malignant schwannoma
Osseous	Extraskeletal osteosarcoma
Cartilaginous	Extraskeletal chondrosarcoma
Mesenchymal	Malignant mesenchymoma
Uncertain cell type	Alveolar soft part sarcoma
	Epithelioid sarcoma
	Clear cell sarcoma

Source: Adapted from Enzinger FM, Weiss SW. Soft Tissue Tumors (3rd ed). St. Louis: Mosby, 1995;7–10.

TABLE 6-2. *Relative incidence of soft-tissue sarcomas in the elderly*

Sarcoma type	Percentage
Malignant fibrous histiocytoma	25.1
Liposarcoma	11.6
Rhabdomyosarcoma	9.7
Leiomyosarcoma	9.1
Synoviosarcoma	6.5
Malignant schwannoma	5.9
Fibrosarcoma	5.2

Source: Adapted from Hashimoto H, Daimaru Y, Takeshita S, et al. Prognostic significance of histologic parameters of soft tissue sarcomas. Cancer 1992;70:2816–2822.

TABLE 6-3. *American Joint Committee on Cancer Staging of Soft-Tissue Sarcomas*

Stage I	Grade 1 tumor, localized disease
Stage II	Grade 2 tumor, localized disease
Stage III	Grade 3 tumor, localized disease.
Stages I–III are further classified on the basis of tumor size:	
A	Tumor <5 cm in greatest dimension
B	Tumor >5 cm in greatest dimension
Stage IVA	Tumor of any grade or size with regional lymph node metastasis
Stage IVB	Tumor of any grade or size with distant metastasis

Source: Adapted from Beahrs OH, Henson DE, Hutter RVP, et al. Manual for Staging of Cancer, American Joint Committee on Cancer (4th ed). Philadelphia: Lippincott, 1992;131–133.

grades, but in other systems the number varies from two to four. In grading sarcomas, one must take into account the fact that the significance of different histologic parameters varies with the type of tumor. For example, the number of mitoses is important for grading leiomyosarcoma and fibrosarcoma, but much less so for MFH. Nuclear pleomorphism is minimal in highly malignant tumors such as neuroblastoma and alveolar rhabdomyosarcoma. In addition, sarcomas may vary in morphologic appearance, with well-differentiated areas mixed with poorly differentiated foci. In this case, the grade should be determined by the least differentiated areas.

Prognosis of Soft-Tissue Sarcomas

The single most important prognostic factor in the AJCC staging system is the histologic grade of the primary tumor. There is a definite correlation between grade and survival rate. In a recent study, Costa et al. analyzed 163 sarcomas and found 5-year survival rates of 100% for grade 1, 73% for grade 2, and 46% for grade 3 tumors [11].

Size of the tumor and the presence or absence of lymph node involvement are the next prognostic parameters. Tumors measuring 5 cm or less in diameter have a better prognosis than those measuring >5 cm, and tumors with no lymph node metastasis do better than those with nodal metastasis [12]. Other less important and less well-established prognostic parameters include location and DNA ploidy of the tumor. Extremity sarcomas have a better prognosis than sarcomas of the trunk or head and neck. At least with high-grade sarcomas, diploidy tends to be associated with a better prognosis than aneuploidy [13].

Pathology of Soft-Tissue Sarcomas

The frequently encountered histologic subtypes of STSs in the elderly are listed in Table 6-2. The two most common subtypes, MFH and liposarcoma, are discussed in this chapter. Other subtypes include leiomyosarcoma, rhabdomyosarcoma, synoviosarcoma, malignant schwannoma, and fibrosarcoma. In earlier publications, fibrosarcoma was the most commonly diagnosed sarcoma, accounting for up to 43% of all sarcomas, whereas MFH was hardly even mentioned [14]. Following tissue culture study and better defined histologic criteria, MFH has replaced fibrosarcoma as the most frequently encountered sarcoma in the elderly [15].

Differences in the characteristics, other than histologic appearances, are noted between certain sarcoma subtypes, demonstrated by the different growth rates as well as the capability to spread via hematogenous or lymphatic routes. For example, liposarcoma is well known for its slow growth rate and its improbability of spreading to regional lymph nodes. By contrast, other sarcomas such as synovial sarcoma, MFH, and epithelioid sarcoma are much more prone to invade regional nodes [12]. Malignant schwannoma tends to spread along nerve trunks. Alveolar soft part sarcoma has a tendency to show long-delayed metastases. However, because there are sufficient similarities between the subtypes, and given the small number of STSs, it is clinically convenient to consider STSs as a group of locally aggressive tumors, capable of local recurrence and distant metastases [16].

Malignant Fibrous Histiocytoma

MFH is the most common soft-tissue tumor of late adult life, typically occurring between 50 and 70 years of age [17]. It usually presents as a painless, enlarging mass, most often of the lower extremities. Grossly, the tumor appears as fleshy, multilobulated masses located within skeletal muscles (Fig. 6-1). Spreading along fascial planes is common, accounting for the high rate of local recurrence when it is incompletely excised. Microscopically, several subtypes are described, including the pleomorphic, myxoid, giant-cell, and inflammatory MFH. The inflammatory subtype is more often seen in the retroperitoneum of younger patients.

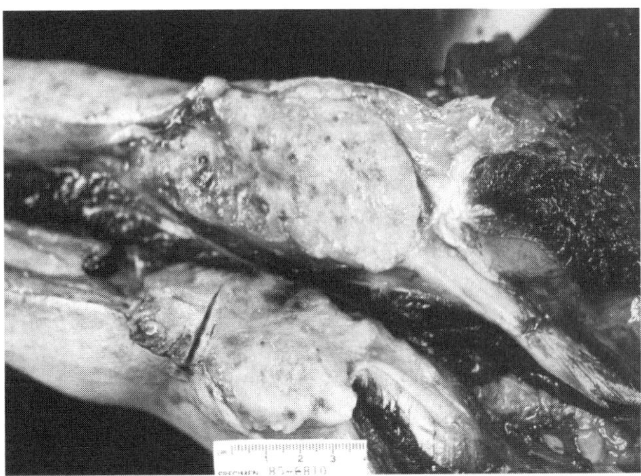

FIG. 6-1. Malignant fibrous histiocytoma, present for 3 months, on the left shoulder of a 79-year-old man. The lesion, bisected, shows a slightly lobulated cut surface that is yellow, with areas of hemorrhage. Note the general fusiform shape of the lesion, which appears to be confined to a single muscular unit.

Liposarcoma

A common soft-tissue tumor of adults, liposarcoma shows a peak incidence between 40 and 60 years of age. It has been observed, however, frequently in persons aged 70 and over, but is virtually unknown in children. It is most frequently found in the thigh and retroperitoneum, where it may reach a very large size [7].

Grossly, the tumor appears well circumscribed with a lobulated surface (Fig. 6-2). The cut surface varies from a pale yellow in well-differentiated tumor to a myxoid or gelatinous appearance in other forms. Areas of hemorrhage and necrosis are frequently present. Microscopically, four different subtypes of liposarcoma are described: well-differentiated, myxoid, round cell, and pleomorphic. Myxoid liposarcoma is the most commonly seen subtype, accounting for up to 55% of all liposarcomas [7].

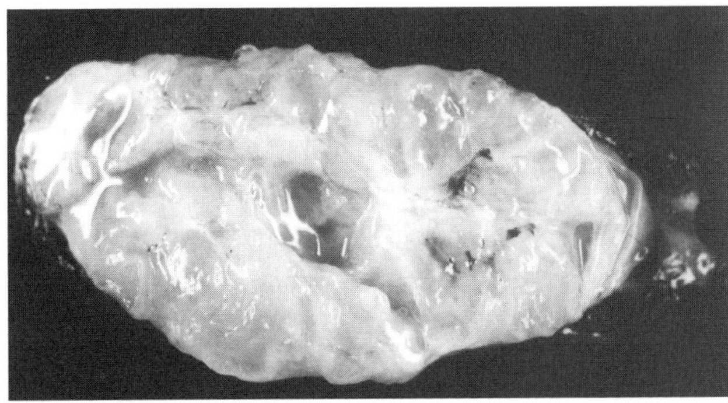

FIG. 6-2. Myxoid liposarcoma from the thigh. The lesion is well circumscribed, with a multilobular cut surface and a gelatinous appearance.

Leiomyosarcoma

Leiomyosarcomas account for between 5% and 10% of STSs (see Table 6-2). They are less common than leiomyosarcomas of the uterus and gastrointestinal tract and can be divided into three groups: leiomyosarcomas of deep soft tissue, especially the retroperitoneum, are the most common group; leiomyosarcomas of the skin and subcutaneous tissue usually have a better prognosis because of their superficial location; and leiomyosarcomas of vascular origin are found in association with large veins.

Treatment of Sarcomas

The treatment of STSs in the elderly should not differ from that offered to younger patients. If they are diagnosed and not adequately treated, most elderly patients will die of that disease before natural causes claim them. The current trend in treating younger patients is toward preserving limb and limb function, with the emphasis on returning the sarcoma patient to a high level of activity. In our opinion this approach should be reserved for the very vigorous and active elderly patient in whom rapid cure and recovery times are expected. This aggressive approach may also be considered when the multimodal approach of surgical resection, radiation, and chemotherapy is being considered. Exceptions to this approach in individual cases must always be considered. It is our experience that elderly patients can tolerate one large curative resection better than they can tolerate lesser resections and prolonged adjuvant treatment and associated secondary reconstructive procedures. For those lesions located within the body cavities, on the chest wall, abdominal wall, and back, some compromise in total resection for cure may be necessary. This is frequently the case for lesions located in the retroperitoneal area.

Extremity Sarcomas

Radical local resection or amputation of those sarcomas occurring in the extremity offers the best chance for cure with the least amount of trauma and usually obviates the necessity for adjuvant irradiation or chemotherapy [18]. There are several reasons to use aggressive radical excision of extremity sarcomas in older patients in whom maintenance of limb function may not be critical. First, recurrence rates after a radical local resection of the tissue within the involved compartment or member without amputation range from 10% to 20%; this improves to a rate as low as 5% after amputation. By contrast, the limb-saving operations are associated with local recurrence rates as high as 50%, thereby necessitating the use of radiation or chemotherapy [19]. These adjuvant therapeutic measures are less well tolerated in older patients than in young age groups and are not very effective in treating STSs. Second, elaborate muscle group, segmental bone, and extended function-saving resections are more traumatic and are associated with a higher morbidity and mortality than extended wide local excisions or amputations. The need for agility is less critical, and the tolerance for reconstructive procedures, adjuvant therapy, and prolonged rehabilitation programs is somewhat diminished in the elderly.

Truncal Sarcomas

For tumors of the thoracic or abdominal wall and back, wide radical excision with prosthetic material and flap reconstruction are well tolerated by the elderly. The unique situation of sarcomas of the retroperitoneal area offers a serious challenge to patient and surgeon alike [20–23].

In most elderly patients, we would not recommend extensive retroperitoneal dissection including kidneys and other abdominal organs for the removal of retroperitoneal sarcomas. Rather, a generous debulking of the tumor followed by postoperative radiation seems most appropriate.

Gastrointestinal Sarcomas

Gastrointestinal tract sarcomas account for the second largest group of malignancies in the stomach and small bowel. These lesions should be treated surgically in all age groups because, unlike primary gastrointestinal tumors, they are not likely to be as responsive to radiation and chemotherapy (see Chapters 22 and 25). Primary pulmonary sarcomas, although rare, do occur and should be treated surgically whenever possible (see Chapter 20).

Leiomyosarcomas of the gastrointestinal tract, although not STSs, are discussed briefly here because of their high recurrence rate. These are typically slow-growing tumors that remain localized for long periods of time without metastasis. Because symptoms are not present in the early course of the disease, these tumors can reach a large size before being detected and treated. The 5-year survival rate is good.

As we have shown, sarcomas of the gastrointestinal tract are usually leiomyosarcomas and can occur in any age group, but especially in the elderly (see Chapter 22). If detected easily and treated adequately by 8- to 10-cm margins of resection, we have observed excellent results (see Chapter 22). In the elderly patient with a gastric lesion, it is especially important that diagnosis and surgical resection be considered. Even in the case of large digestive sarcomas, the prognosis for cure with adequate 10-cm margins in the resection specimen is much better than for gastric carcinoma (see Chapter 22).

CUTANEOUS MELANOMAS

In 1995, approximately 34,000 new cases of cutaneous melanoma were diagnosed in the United States, with an estimated 7,200 deaths as a result of this disease [1]. These are preventable deaths, since virtually all cutaneous melanoma can be cured if detected early enough.

Two important points emerge from the epidemiologic studies of melanomas. First, there is a striking difference in the overall incidence of melanoma among ethnic groups: among whites, it is 11.7 per 100,000, whereas among blacks, it is 0.8 per 100,000 [24]. In some parts of the southwestern United States, this incidence can be as high as 30 per 100,000 among whites. Second, the incidence of melanoma is increasing at the rate of 4% per year [24]. The reason for this increase is unclear and cannot be accounted for by improved methods of diagnosis and reporting because there is also a parallel increase in mortality. This rate of increase, however, appears to be slowing down from a high of 7% per year reported in the 1970s [25].

Within the general population, the incidence of melanoma increases with age: the age-specific incidence for the group aged 50 to 54 is 21.1 per 100,000, whereas that for the group aged 80 to 84 is 31.9 per 100,000 [24].

Clinical Staging of Melanoma

Several staging systems for cutaneous melanomas have been developed, including the MD Anderson Cancer Center system [26], the Union Internationale Centre de Cancer (UICC) system [27], and the AJCC system [28]. None of these systems, however, are accepted or used widely in everyday practice. This lack of a standardized approach to staging led to the TNM system published jointly by the AJCC/UICC in 1988 [29]. This system is based primarily on the pathologic staging of the primary tumor and is gaining acceptance from users worldwide.

Pathologic Staging of Melanoma

Microscopic staging of cutaneous melanoma includes evaluation of the level of invasion and measurement of the tumor thickness. In 1967, Clark proposed a histologic approach to assess the depth of invasion by relating this to standard landmarks of the skin: the dermoepidermal junction, the papillary and reticular dermis, and the subcutaneous fat [30]. There are five levels of invasion. This approach remains practical and has value in assessing prognosis. There are, however, problems in some cases. First, the skin thickness varies according to anatomic site and from person to person. The papillary and reticular dermis are difficult to identify in some areas such as the acral areas. Furthermore, Clark level cannot be determined with certainty for nodular melanoma, or for a mucosal lesion where anatomic landmarks are nonexistent.

Clark's approach has been partly replaced by the microscopic assessment of tumor thickness described by Breslow [31]. Tumor thickness is measured from the top of the granular layer of the overlying epidermis to the base of the tumor and is quantified to the nearest tenth of a millimeter with an ocular micrometer.

Both level of invasion and tumor thickness show good correlation with survival [32]. Tumor thickness, however, has several important advantages that can directly influence the therapeutic approach, such as the risk of local recurrence and distant metastases, which can be accurately predicted from the tumor thickness of the primary lesion [32]. For that reason, it is important to include both Clark level and tumor thickness in the final report.

Pathology of Cutaneous Melanoma

The four major histologic forms of melanoma include superficial spreading melanoma (SSM), nodular melanoma (NM), lentigo maligna melanoma (LMM), and acral lentiginous melanoma (ALM) [33]. SSM, NM, and ALM usually evolve from an initial slowly growing, plaquelike radial growth phase (RGP) to a rapidly growing, expansive vertical growth phase (VGP). NM starts with an expansive VGP only, with no preexisting RGP. Histologic recognition of RGP and VGP forms is important because melanoma with RGP only is clinically benign and can be cured by surgical excision. VGP melanoma, on the other hand, carries the risk of metastasis despite complete removal [34].

Superficial Spreading Melanoma

SSM is the largest group of melanomas, constituting approximately 70% of all cutaneous melanomas [35]. It has no age predilection and in approximately 30% of cases develops from a preexisting nevus. SSM occurs on the trunk and extremities of light-skinned individuals. Typically, it shows a variegated surface, with colors ranging from jet black to grayish white. The borders are irregular with notching and indentation. A thin rim of pink skin is often present at the periphery, denoting host reaction to the lesion. Although most cases remain in a plaque-like state for months to years, the rapid onset of an invasive nodule signals the beginning of the VGP (Fig. 6-3).

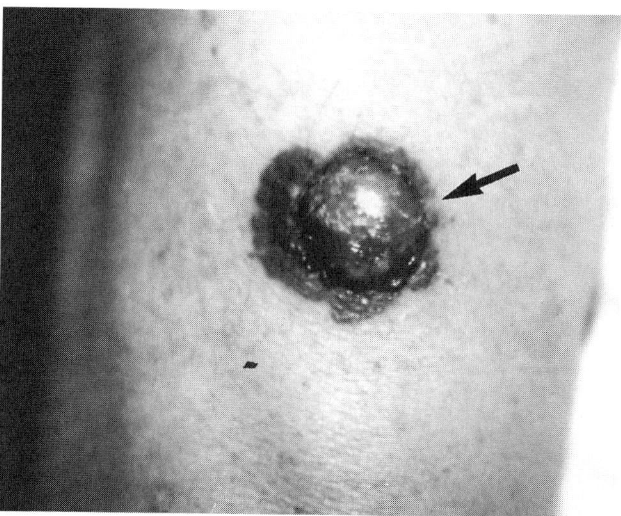

FIG. 6-3. Superficial spreading melanoma with vertical growth phase. The lesion has an irregular border with indentations. The nodular appearance in the left half of the lesion *(arrow)* is characteristic of the vertical growth phase.

Microscopically, the RGP of SSM displays the pagetoid infiltration of the dermoepidermal junction by large, atypical melanocytes. The VGP is characterized by melanocytes streaming into the dermis and spreading upward in the epidermis. The melanocytes of SSM can be spindle or epithelioid. Usually one cell type predominates. The amount of melanin present varies from abundant to almost nonexistent. There is often a chronic inflammatory reaction in the adjacent stroma, consisting of mostly lymphocytes and mononuclear cells.

Nodular Melanoma

NM is the second most common type of melanoma, making up approximately 30% of cases [35]. NM usually arises *de novo* without any preexisting nevi. It is more common in middle-aged patients and tends to be more aggressive than SSM. Clinically, NM is a fast-growing, raised, dome-shaped, blue-black lesion. A small number of NM are amelanotic and show a fleshy appearance. The borders are sharply demarcated. Larger lesions tend to ulcerate and bleed.

Microscopically, only the VGP is present. There is downward growth of tumor cells that tends to form rounded nests or nodules. Cytology is variable, but in most cases, the tumor cells show large vesicular nuclei with prominent nucleoli and an amphophilic cytoplasm containing dusky pigment. Inflammation is minimal unless there is ulceration of the epidermis.

Lentigo Maligna Melanoma

LMM constitutes only a small proportion of malignant melanoma, usually 4% to 10% [35]. Clinically, these are

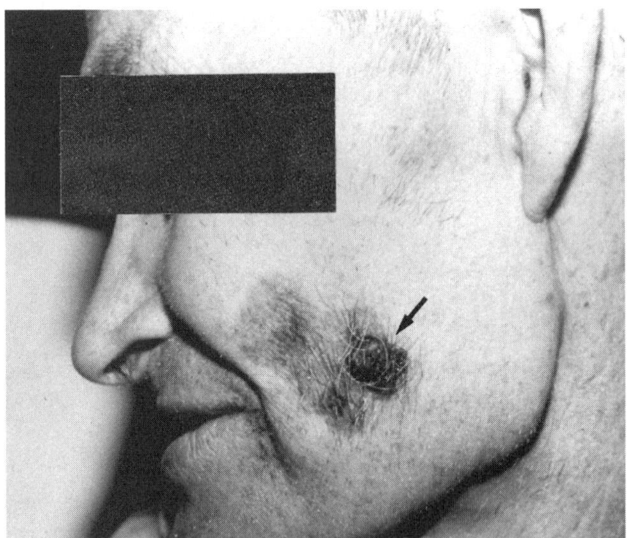

FIG. 6-4. Lentigo maligna melanoma. The patient, a 57-year-old man, had a pigmented lesion on the cheek for several years. It had recently enlarged and showed a nodule near the posterior margin *(arrow)*. (Courtesy of David L. Page, M.D., Department of Pathology, Vanderbilt University, Nashville, TN.)

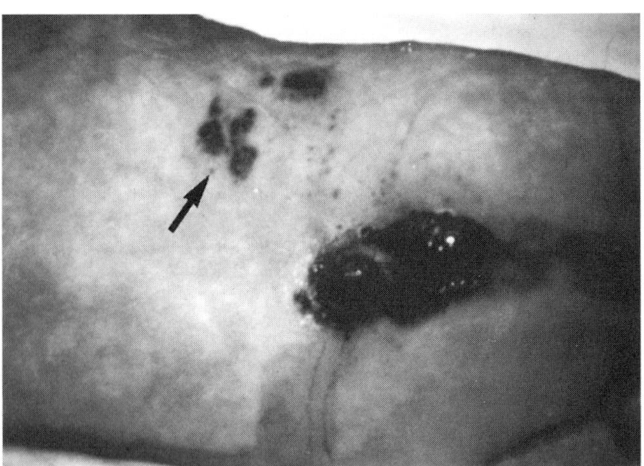

FIG. 6-5. Acral lentiginous melanoma on the plantar, present for 2 years, is ulcerated and nodular. Satellite lesions are present *(arrow)*.

flat, pigmented lesions with irregular borders, located primarily on the face and neck of elderly patients (Hutchinson's freckle) (Fig. 6-4). Characteristically, a long period of growth is observed, with most of the lesions present for 5 to 15 years. As the lesion becomes malignant, a portion of it may show a nodular surface. LMM, however, does not have the same propensity for metastasis as NM or SSM [36].

Microscopically, LMM is characterized by the proliferation of atypical melanocytes at the basal layers of the epidermis. The melanocytes are distributed singly or in nests and exhibit retraction of the cytoplasm as a prominent feature. Nuclear atypia is mild to moderate. There is upward invasion of the epidermis and downward streaming of the melanocytes into the upper dermis. The latter also shows actinic degeneration and contains a band-like inflammatory infiltrate of lymphocytes and monocytes. The NM that develops from a Hutchinson's freckle is often of the spindle-cell type and exhibits limited aggressiveness [36]. Another type of melanoma that may follow Hutchinson's freckle is the desmoplastic melanoma, so called because of the extensive fibrosis in the stroma.

Acral Lentiginous Melanoma

ALM is rare in whites but is the most common form of melanoma reported in blacks, Hispanics, and Asians, with a peak incidence in the sixth decade [37]. It typically occurs on the palm or sole or beneath the nail bed of a toe. Fingers are rarely involved. At the early stage, ALM appears as a densely pigmented macule with irregular borders. The surface is hyperkeratotic, which may give the lesion a less ominous appearance than other melanoma. The biological course of ALM is probably not significantly different from the course of SSM, but because of the hidden location of many ALM, these lesions tend to be more advanced at the time of diagnosis (Fig. 6-5).

Microscopically, ALM exhibits a typical RGP phase with atypical melanocytes at the dermoepidermal border as well as in the epidermis, including the cornified layers. There is a tendency for nest formation, but large pagetoid nests are rare. The VGP consists of spindle cells mostly, accompanied by inflammation and epidermal ulceration.

Treatment of Melanomas

The hallmark of surgical treatment for all cutaneous malignant melanomas is wide local excision of the primary site and regional lymph node dissection for all melanomas beyond Clark's level III or for all those primary lesions that have a tumor thickness >1.5 mm. We perform regional node dissections for all acral lentiginous lesions no matter their thickness. This recommended therapeutic approach should be followed in all age groups. If regional nodes are palpable, we perform a regional node dissection regardless of Clark's level or Breslow's thickness of the primary tumor. In the elderly, only those most severe medical conditions that cannot be corrected or improved should be reason for deviation from this recommendation.

Notably, melanomas of the acral lentiginous variety require an extremely aggressive primary surgical approach, including digital amputation, Ray's amputation of fingers and toes, and sometimes much more extensive amputation of upper and lower extremities with regional lymph node dissection. Again, the age of the patient should not alter the surgical approach for these particular lesions.

Chemotherapy and irradiation for metastatic or unresectable melanoma should be considered palliative only. Although there are sporadic reports of long-term disease-free intervals, systemic chemotherapy, radiation treatment, hormonal therapy, and immunotherapy have failed to show encouraging results. When an otherwise healthy elderly patient who has melanoma beyond the bounds of surgical resection presents for therapy, he or she should be considered a candidate for all forms of adjuvant therapy. Chemotherapy, radiation therapy, and secondary surgical procedures that would be offered to a younger individual should be considered in the elderly. See Chapter 8 for the usual guidelines for the use of chemotherapy and radiation therapy in the elderly.

LYMPHOMAS

Traditionally, lymphomas have been divided into two broad groups: Hodgkin's disease (HD) and non-Hodgkin's lymphoma (NHL). This arbitrary division has been helpful both in clinical management and understanding the biology of lymphomas, because the NHLs comprise a variety of entities that differ from HD in terms of their biology, pathology, and treatment.

Approximately 50,900 cases of NHL and 7,800 cases of HD were seen in patients of all ages in the United States in 1995 [1]. Lymphomas that occur in the elderly are generally considered to have a poor prognosis because patients of this age group often present with advanced disease. Coexisting medical problems make aggressive management difficult and complicated. In addition, chemotherapy is usually less well tolerated. Certain anatomic sites, such as the upper airways and digestive tract, are predilection sites for the relatively frequent occurrence of primary lymphomas in the elderly [38].

Hodgkin's Disease

HD has a characteristic bimodal age distribution with one peak in early adult life (15 to 35 years) and a second peak at 50 years of age or older [39]. The younger age group has an equal male-to-female ratio, with the predominance of the nodular sclerosis HD type and a more favorable clinical course. The older age group shows a higher male-to-female ratio, with a greater incidence of mixed cellularity HD type and a more aggressive course [40].

In the United States, the incidence of HD is 3.5 to 5 per 100,000. The incidence is declining in older patients, whereas in the younger population, there has been a persistent increase, especially of the nodular sclerosis HD [41]. Part of the decrease in older patients may be due to overdiagnosis of mixed cellularity HD and underdiagnosis of NHL.

Histopathologic Classification of Hodgkin's Disease

The histologic classification of HD proposed by Lukes and Butler in 1966 and subsequently modified by the Rye conference is currently in use [42]. Basically, four histologic subtypes are recognized: lymphocytic predominance, nodular sclerosis, mixed cellularity, and lymphocytic depletion. The diagnosis of HD depends on the finding of the characteristic Reed-Sternberg (RS) cell. In its classic form, the RS cell shows a large, polylobulated nucleus with a prominent, inclusion-like nucleolus (Fig. 6-6). There is parachromatin clearing, resulting in a perinucleolar halo. The cytoplasm is abundant and eosinophilic. Occasionally, the cell is binucleated and resembles an owl's eye. It should be pointed out that presence of the RS cell by itself is not pathognomonic of HD. Cells resembling RS cells have been found in other conditions, such as mononucleosis, transformed cell lymphoma, and some poorly differentiated carcinomas.

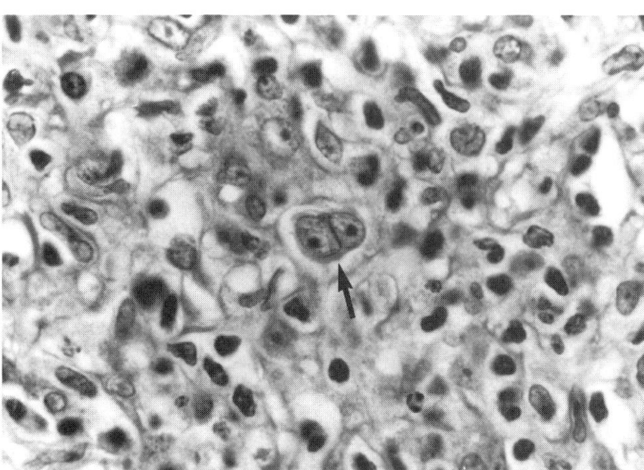

FIG. 6-6. A binucleated Reed-Sternberg cell in a case of lymphocyte-depleted Hodgkin's disease *(arrow)*. The nucleoli are large, and the cytoplasm shows perinuclear clearing. (Hematoxylin and eosin, ×400.)

Lymphocytic predominance HD (LPHD) is characterized by an abundance of small lymphocytes. The involved lymph node architecture may be only partially destroyed. Typical RS cells are hard to find, and those present are usually of the lymphocyte and histocyte variant. Lymphocyte and histocyte variant cells are large polyploid cells with folded, convoluted nuclei, inapparent nucleoli, and a variable amount of cytoplasm. LPHD is usually seen in middle-aged male patients and has the most favorable prognosis of all subtypes. LPHD has recently generated considerable interest with the demonstration that it expresses B-cell lineage characteristics, different than the other subtypes of HD [43]. This finding has led to the proposal that LPHD, especially the nodular type, is a follicular center lymphoma.

Nodular sclerosis HD is so called because of the presence of orderly bands of dense collagenous tissue dividing the involved node into nodules. The RS cells are abundant in this subtype and belong to the lacunar variant: The cell appears to be located in a lacuna, a phenomenon observed only in formalin-fixed tissue, indicative of cytoplasmic

TABLE 6-4. *Ann Arbor Staging Classification of Hodgkin's disease*

Stage I	Involvement of a single lymph node region or lymphoid structure
Stage II	Involvement of two or more lymph node regions on the same side of the diaphragm
Stage III	Involvement of lymph node regions or structures on both sides of the diaphragm
For stages I to III	
Substage E	Involvement of a single, extranodal site contiguous or proximal to known nodal site
Stage IV	Involvement of extranodal site(s) beyond that designated E
For all stages	
A	No symptoms
B	Fever, drenching sweats, weight loss of >10% of body weight

Source: Adapted from Carbone PP, Kaplan HS, Musshoff K, et al. Report of the committee on Hodgkin's disease staging classification. Cancer Res 1971;31:1860–1861.

retraction after fixation. Nodular sclerosis HD is the most common subtype, making up more than 60% of all cases. It most commonly afflicts young female patients and has an excellent prognosis.

Mixed cellularity HD is characterized by a mixed cellular background with a variable proportion of plasma cells, eosinophils, lymphocytes, and histiocytes. RS cells are found in moderate numbers and are of either classical or mononuclear variants. Mixed cellularity HD follows nodular sclerosis HD in frequency. It frequently involves subdiaphragmatic organs and is often associated with systemic symptoms. It has an intermediate prognosis between LPHD and lymphocytic depletion HD.

Lymphocytic depletion HD is found in <5% of cases of HD. It characteristically displays a general depletion of cellular elements with an increase in the reticular framework. Two subtypes have been described: reticular and diffuse fibrosis. The RS cells predominate the histologic picture with numerous anaplastic or sarcomatous forms. Lymphocytic depletion HD is the most aggressive form of HD, affecting mainly an older age group of patients who are frequently symptomatic with lymphadenopathy, hepatosplenomegaly, and bone marrow involvement.

Staging of Hodgkin's Disease

The first useful staging system for HD was proposed by Peters in 1950 [44]. This system was later modified at the Ann Arbor Staging Conference in 1971 [45] (Table 6-4). This system divides HD into four stages depending on the extent of nodal and extranodal involvement. It is almost universally accepted. Recent recommendations to revise the system to accommodate computed tomographic findings and response to therapy have been made [46].

In patients more than 50 years of age, HD should be more carefully evaluated, not only because these patients have a higher proportion of lymphocytic depletion but also because they tend to have more advanced disease at the time of diagnosis, frequent extranodal involvement, poor response to therapy, and a lower tolerance for radiotherapy and chemotherapy [47].

Treatment of Hodgkin's Disease

The surgeon's role in the treatment of localized HD of the gastrointestinal tract, other abdominal viscera, mediastinum, and regional lymph nodes is traditionally reserved for diagnosis, debulking, and palliation. Staging of all forms of HD and removing or debulking those tumor sites that cause symptoms or represent a large mass of tumor cell population should be done in patients of all age groups to offer relief of symptoms and palliation. As mentioned in Chapter 8, HD in the second bimodal age peak tends to have slightly worse prognostic features and should possibly be approached more aggressively than would be required in a similarly staged disease in a younger age group.

Non-Hodgkin's Lymphoma

The term *non-Hodgkin's lymphoma* is used to designate a variety of different types of lymphomas for which we do not have a universally accepted classification. Until the 1960s, NHLs were divided into three large groups: lymphosarcoma, reticulum-cell sarcoma, and giant follicle lymphoma. In 1966, Rappaport proposed a classification that was later modified by other authors [48,49]. The Rappaport classification was widely accepted by oncologists who found it useful in providing guidelines for prognosis and therapy. With the advances made in immunology and immunohistochemistry, other classifications were proposed. The Lukes and Collins classification, based on the immunologic subtypes, was used mainly in the United States [50]. The Kiel classification, proposed by Lennert, is primarily a morphologic scheme and is favored in Europe [51]. An international study, undertaken by the National Cancer Institute in 1976, culminated in the Working Formulation for Clinical Usage [52] (Table 6-5). This was regarded as a common language for investigators to move from one classification to another and is required by the National Cancer Institute for their protocol studies. During the past 10 years, the Working Formulation has become more popular.

Staging of Non-Hodgkin's Lymphoma

There is no optimal staging system for NHL. The standard staging system for NHL is the same as that proposed for HD

TABLE 6-5. *Working formulation of non-Hodgkin's lymphoma for clinical usage*

Low grade
A. Malignant lymphoma, small lymphocytic consistent with chronic lymphocytic leukemia
B. Malignant lymphoma, follicular, predominantly small cleaved cell
Diffuse areas
Sclerosis
C. Malignant lymphoma, follicular mixed, small cleaved and large cell
Diffuse areas
Sclerosis
Intermediate grade
D. Malignant lymphoma follicular, predominantly large cell
Diffuse areas
Sclerosis
E. Malignant lymphoma, diffuse, small cleaved cell
F. Malignant lymphoma, diffuse, mixed small and large cell
Sclerosis
Epithelioid cell component
G. Malignant lymphoma, diffuse
Large cell
Cleaved cell
Noncleaved cell
Sclerosis
High grade
H. Malignant lymphoma, large cell, immunoblastic
Plasmacytoid
Clear cell
Polymorphous
Epithelioid cell component
I. Malignant lymphoma, lymphoblastic
Convoluted cell
Nonconvoluted cell
J. Malignant lymphoma, small noncleaved cell
Burkitt's
Follicular areas

Source: Modified from Rosenberg SA, Berard CW, Brown BW, et al. NCI sponsored study of classification of non-Hodgkin's lymphoma: summary and description of a working formulation for clinical usage. Cancer 1982;49:2112–2135.

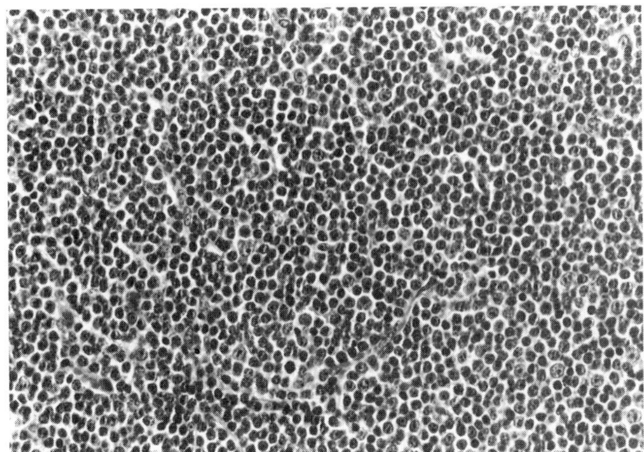

FIG. 6-7. Malignant lymphoma, diffuse, small cells, non-cleaved type; the cells are small with scanty cytoplasm. The nuclei are round with dense chromatin and indistinct nucleoli. (Hematoxylin and eosin, ×400.)

at the Ann Arbor Conference in 1971 [45]. HD spreads by contiguity from lymph node areas, rather than hematogenously as does NHL. For this reason, more than 80% of patients with low-grade lymphoma and more than 50% of patients with intermediate- or high-grade lymphoma present with stage III or IV disease [53]. In addition, the prognosis of NHL is dependent not so much on stage as on the histologic subtype, secondarily influenced by other clinical parameters such as tumor bulk and serum lactic dehydrogenase, and so forth. Proposals for inclusion of these clinical parameters into the staging system have been made [54].

Pathology of Non-Hodgkin's Lymphoma

A. Low-grade malignant lymphomas

1. Malignant lymphoma, small lymphocytic: This group of lymphomas occurs primarily in middle-aged and older patients, with a peak incidence in the sixth to eighth decades. It is relatively rare, making up approximately 5% of all lymphomas. Morphologically, the malignant cells are identical to that of chronic lymphocytic leukemia, and the two entities are thought to represent manifestations of the same disease [55]. Clinically, patients often present with generalized lymphadenopathy. They usually have an indolent course with few symptoms. Microscopically, the lymph node architecture is effaced by a diffuse proliferation of small lymphocytes with round nuclei, clumped chromatin, and scanty cytoplasm (Fig. 6-7). A nodular growth pattern is not observed. The neoplastic cells may exhibit plasmacytic differentiation and become immunosecretory. In these cases, monoclonal protein spikes are observed, often of the IgM kappa type.
2. Malignant lymphoma, follicular, small cleaved cell: This is the most common form of lymphoma in the elderly, making up 30% to 40% of all lymphomas. Peak incidence is in the fifth to sixth decades. Patients usually have stage III or IV disease at time of diagnosis. Involvement of spleen, liver, and bone marrow is common. Some patients present with or develop leukemia. Histologically, the involved node shows a prominent follicular pattern. The follicles or nodules are composed of small cleaved lymphocytes with irregular, indented nuclei (Fig. 6-8). Following a prolonged and indolent course, progression to a diffuse form or a higher grade lymphoma is not uncommon. Immunologically, follicular, small cleaved cell lymphomas are neoplasms of B lymphocytes. Its molecular hallmark is the t(14;18) (q32;q21) chromosomal translocation, which is present in over 95% of cases [56]. In this abnormality, the *bcl*-2 proto-oncogene on chromosome 18 is translocated to the joining region of the immunoglobulin heavy chain gene on chromosome 14.

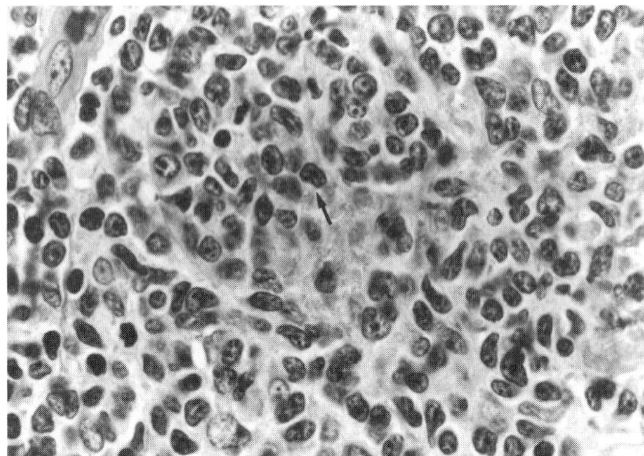

FIG. 6-8. Malignant lymphoma, nodular, small cleaved cells. The neoplastic cells are slightly larger than normal lymphocytes with scanty cytoplasm. The nuclei show characteristic indentation and in-foldings *(arrow)*. (Hematoxylin and eosin, ×1,000.)

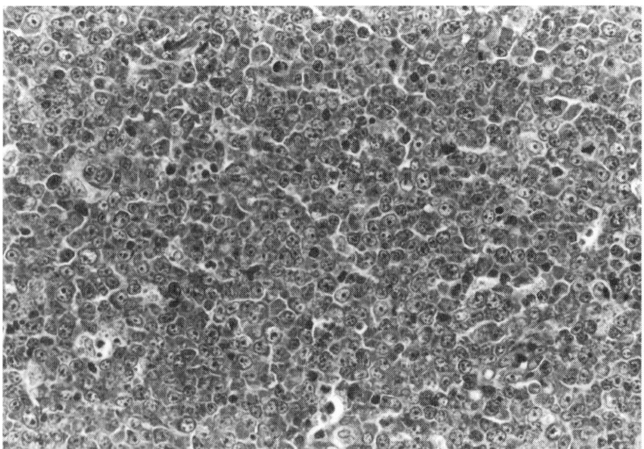

FIG. 6-9. Malignant lymphoma, diffuse, large cell, noncleaved type. The neoplastic cells are large with round to oval nuclei exhibiting sharp nuclear membrane and one to four nucleoli. (Hematoxylin and eosin, ×400.)

3. Low-grade B-cell lymphoma of mucosa-associated lymphoid tissue: Malignant lymphomas arising in mucosa-associated lymphoid tissue have recently been recognized as a distinct clinical entity. They can be of either low or high grade, and of B- or T-cell origin. Low-grade B-cell lymphoma of mucosa-associated lymphoid tissue is one subgroup that is better categorized both clinically and histologically [57]. The disease involves primarily the gastrointestinal tract, but cases involving the lung, salivary gland, thyroid, and thymus have been described [58]. Patients are of the adult or late adult age group, who often have an associated autoimmune disease. They often present with a protracted history of clinical symptoms and signs that may be confused with an inflammatory process.

   Clinically, low-grade B-cell mucosa-associated lymphoid tissue lymphomas tend to remain localized for a prolonged period, thus enhancing the efficacy of local therapy, for example, surgical excision. Dissemination occurs rarely and late, with a predilection for other mucosa-associated extranodal sites. Bone marrow and peripheral blood involvement are not observed in most cases [58]. Histologically, the neoplastic cells can run a spectrum from small lymphocyte-like to monocytoid to small cleaved appearance. Plasmacytic differentiation is often present. Mixed with the lymphocytes are lymphoepithelial lesions, which represent mucosal glands invaded by neoplastic lymphocytes. Large lymphoid follicles with reactive germinal centers are frequently found, especially in the low-grade lesions.

B. Intermediate and high-grade malignant lymphomas

1. Malignant lymphoma, follicular, predominantly large cell: Follicular, predominantly large cell NHL has a more aggressive course than that of other follicular lymphomas. Patients often have advanced stage disease at the time of diagnosis. Peripheral blood involvement is unusual. Follicular, predominantly large cell NHL tends to progress to a diffuse large cell lymphoma more often than the low-grade lymphomas. Immunologically, follicular, predominantly large cell NHL are neoplasms of B lymphocytes. However, a relatively high number of cases do not express surface immunoglobulins.
2. Malignant lymphoma, diffuse mixed, small and large cell: Diffuse mixed, small and large cell NHL are composed of neoplastic lymphocytes that exhibit a spectrum of cell sizes. They can be of either B- or T-cell origin. Diffuse mixed, small and large cell NHL of T-cell origin tend to occur in elderly patients who present with generalized adenopathy. Skin, liver, and spleen are often involved. In many cases, tumor cells are admixed with clusters or cords of epithelioid cells (Lennert's lymphoma).
3. Malignant lymphoma, diffuse large cell: Diffuse large cell NHL are clinically high-grade lymphomas that respond well to combination chemotherapy. They are found mostly in adults, but 15% to 20% can be seen in children. Histologically, diffuse large cell NHL are composed predominantly of large cells with cleaved or noncleaved nuclei and abundant cytoplasm (Fig. 6-9). Mitoses are frequently seen. Immunologically, the tumor cells exhibit either B- or T-cell phenotype, even though the majority of cases are phenotypically B-cell tumor. Rearrangements of the *bcl*-2 gene have been demonstrated in some cases, indicating that these tumors represent progression from follicular lymphomas.
4. Malignant lymphoma large cell, immunoblastic: Large cell, immunoblastic NHLs are clinically high-grade lymphomas that often present in an extranodal location. They respond well to combination chemotherapy. Histo-

logically, large cell, immunoblastic NHLs are characterized by the presence of large numbers of immunoblasts and can be further subdivided into four categories: plasmacytoid, polymorphous, epithelioid, and clear cell. The plasmacytoid subtype shows B-cell phenotype whereas the other subtypes are of T-cell lineage.

Treatment of Non-Hodgkin's Lymphoma

When primary lymphomas of the lung, gastrointestinal tract, mediastinum, or retroperitoneum occur in the elderly, they should be treated surgically using the same indications that have been recommended for all persons with these types of tumors. For disseminated forms of lymphoma, radiation therapy and chemotherapy now offer dramatic and encouraging responses that have resulted in extremely long disease-free intervals and complete remissions or cure in many instances. See Chapter 8 for a detailed discussion of these forms of treatment.

SUMMARY

The occurrence of these special types of tumors in the elderly patient is becoming more and more apparent. As more of our population reaches an advanced age, more of these tumors appear. As we have pointed out, sarcomas, lymphomas, and melanomas tend to appear in slightly different types and in slightly selected forms in the elderly. The fact that some of these tumors are actually more aggressive in the elderly may be somewhat more surprising to those who have the mistaken idea that all tumors grow more slowly and behave in a more benign manner in elderly patients than they do in younger individuals. The surgical, radiotherapeutic, and chemotherapeutic approach to elderly patients with these special types of tumors must at times be more aggressive than the approach to a similar tumor in a younger patient. The intent of this chapter has been to point out those special incidences and situations in which the elderly patient's treatment should be carefully considered and those even more special situations in which the treatment should perhaps be different.

REFERENCES

1. Wingo PA, Tong T, Bolden S. Cancer statistics 1995. CA Cancer J Clin 1995;45:8–30.
2. Lawrence W, Donegan WL, Natarajan N, et al. Adult soft tissue sarcomas: a pattern of care survey of the American College of Surgeons. Ann Surg 1987;205:349–359.
3. Russell WO, Cohen J, Enzinger FM, et al. A clinical and pathological staging system for soft tissue sarcomas. Cancer 1977;40:1562–1570.
4. Stout AP. Tumors of the Soft Tissues. In Atlas of Tumor Pathology (Series 1, Fascicle 5). Washington, DC: Armed Forces Institute of Pathology, 1957.
5. Stout AP, Lattes R. Tumors of the Soft Tissues. In Atlas of Tumor Pathology (Series 2, Fascicle 1). Washington, DC: Armed Forces Institute of Pathology, 1967.
6. Enzinger FM, Lattes R, Tortoni R. Histological Typing of Soft Tissue Tumors. In International Histological Classification of Tumors (Vol. 3). Geneva: World Health Organization, 1969.
7. Enzinger FM, Weiss SW. Soft Tissue Tumors (3rd ed). St. Louis: Mosby, 1995;7–10.
8. Coindre JM. Pathology and Grading of Soft Tissue Tumors. In Verweij J, Pinedo HM, Suit HD (eds), Multidisciplinary Treatment of Soft Tissue Sarcomas. Boston: Kluwer Academic, 1993;1–22.
9. Hashimoto H, Daimaru Y, Takeshita S, et al. Prognostic significance of histologic parameters of soft tissue sarcomas. Cancer 1992;70: 2816–2822.
10. Beahrs OH, Henson DE, Hutter RVP, et al. Manual for Staging of Cancer, American Joint Committee on Cancer (4th ed). Philadelphia: Lippincott, 1992.
11. Costa J, Wesley RA, Glatstein E, et al. The grading of soft tissue sarcomas: results of a clinico-histopathological correlation in a series of 163 cases. Cancer 1984;53:530–541.
12. Weingrad DN, Rosenberg SA. Early lymphatic spread of osteogenic and soft tissue sarcomas. Surgery 1978;84:231–240.
13. Alvegard TA, Berg NO, Baldertorp B, et al. Cellular DNA content and prognosis of high-grade soft tissue sarcomas: the Scandinavian Sarcoma Group experience. J Clin Oncol 1990;8:538–547.
14. Hare HF, Cerny MF. Soft tissue sarcoma: a review of 200 cases. Cancer 1963;16:1332–1337.
15. Potter DA, Glen J, Knisella T, et al. Patterns of recurrence in patients with high grade soft tissue sarcomas. J Clin Oncol 1985;3:353–366.
16. Karakousis CP, Perez RP. Soft tissue sarcomas in adults. CA Cancer J Clin 1994;44:200–210.
17. Weiss SW. Malignant fibrous histiocytoma. A reaffirmation. Am J Surg Pathol 1982;6:773–784.
18. Simon MA, Enneking WF. The management of soft-tissue sarcomas of the extremities. J Bone Joint Surg 1976;58:317–327.
19. Rosenberg SA, Suit HD, Baker LH, Rosen G. Sarcomas of the Soft Tissue and Bone. In DeVita VT (ed), Cancer: Principles and Practice of Oncology. Philadelphia: Lippincott, 1982;1039–1040.
20. Karakousis CP, Velez AF, Emrich LJ. Management of retroperitoneal sarcomas and patient survival. Am J Surg 1985;150:376–380.
21. Binder SC, Katz B, Sheridan B. Retroperitoneal liposarcoma. Ann Surg 1978;187:257–261.
22. Kinne DW, Chu FCH, Huvos AG, et al. Treatment of primary and recurrent retroperitoneal liposarcoma. Cancer 1973;31:53–64.
23. Braasch JW, Mon AB. Primary retroperitoneal tumors. Surg Clin North Am 1967;47:663–678.
24. Miller BA, Ries LAG, Hankey BF, et al. Cancer Statistics Review 1973–1989. NIH 92-2789. Washington, DC: National Institutes of Health, 1992.
25. Sober AJ, Fitzpatrick TB. Melanoma fact sheets. Cancer 1979;29: 276–279.
26. Smith JL. Histopathology and Biological Behavior of Melanoma. In Neoplasms of the Skin and Malignant Melanomas. Chicago: Year Book, 1976;293–330.
27. International Union Against Cancer. TNM Classification of Malignant Melanoma (2nd ed). Geneva: International Union Against Cancer, 1978.
28. American Joint Committee on Cancer. Manual for Staging of Cancer (2nd ed). Philadelphia: Lippincott, 1983;117–118.
29. American Joint Committee on Cancer. Manual for Staging of Cancer (3rd ed). Philadelphia: Lippincott, 1988;143–144.
30. Clark WH. A Classification of Malignant Melanoma in Man Correlated with Histogenesis and Biologic Behavior. In Montagna W, Hu F (eds), Advances in Biology of the Skin: The Pigmentary System, Vol. 8. London: Pergamon, 1967;621–645.
31. Breslow A. Thickness, cross-sectional areas and depth of invasion in the prognosis of cutaneous melanoma. Ann Surg 1970;172:902–908.
32. Balch CM, Soong SJ, Shaw HM, et al. An Analysis of Prognostic Factors in 8500 Patients with Cutaneous Melanoma. In Balch CM, Houghton AN (eds), Cutaneous Melanoma (2nd ed). Philadelphia: Lippincott, 1991;165–185.
33. Elder DE, Jucovy PM, Tuthill RJ, et al. The classification of malignant melanoma. Am J Dermatopathol 1980;2:315–320.
34. Elder DE, Guerry D, Epstein MN, et al. Invasive malignant melanomas lacking competence for metastasis. Am J Dermatopathol 1984;6 (Suppl):55–61.

35. Clark WH, From L, Bernardino EA, et al. The histogenesis and biologic behavior of primary human malignant melanoma of the skin. Cancer Res 1969;29:705–727.
36. McGovern VJ, Shaw HM, Milton GW, et al. Is malignant melanoma arising in a Hutchinson's melanotic freckle a separate disease entity? Histopathology 1980;4:235–242.
37. Arrington JH, Reed RJ, Ichinose H, et al. Plantar lentiginous melanoma. A distinct variant of human cutaneous malignant melanoma. Am J Surg Pathol 1977;1:131–143.
38. Cobleigh MA, Kennedy JL. Non-Hodgkin's lymphomas of the upper aerodigestive tract and salivary gland. Otolaryngol Clin North Am 1986;19:685–710.
39. MacMahon B. Epidemiology of Hodgkin's disease. Cancer Res 1966;26:1189–1200.
40. Newell GR, Cole SR, Meittinen OS, et al. Age differences in the histology of Hodgkin's disease. J Natl Cancer Inst 1970;45:311–317.
41. Glaser SL, Swartz WG. Time trends in Hodgkin's disease incidence: the role of diagnostic accuracy. Cancer 1990;66:2196–2204.
42. Lukes RJ, Craver LF, Hall TC, et al. Report of the Nomenclature Committee. Cancer Res 1966;26:1311.
43. Pinkus GS, Said JW. Hodgkin's disease, lymphocyte predominance type, further evidence for a B-cell derivation. Am J Pathol 1988;133:211–217.
44. Peters MV. A study of survivals in Hodgkin's disease treated radiologically. AJR Am J Roentgenol 1950;63:299–311.
45. Carbone PP, Kaplan HS, Musshoff K, et al. Report of the committee on Hodgkin's disease staging classification. Cancer Res 1971;31: 1860–1861.
46. Lister TA, Crowther D, Sutcliffe SB, et al. Report of a committee convened to discuss the evaluation and staging of patients with Hodgkin's disease: Costwald meeting. J Clin Oncol 1989;7:1630–1636. J Clin Oncol (Erratum) 1990;8:1602.
47. Lokich JJ, Pinkus GS, Moloney WC. Hodgkin's disease in the elderly. Oncology 1974;19:484–500.
48. Rappaport H. Tumors of the Hematopoietic System. In Atlas of Tumor Pathology, (Section III, Fascicle 8). Washington, DC: Armed Forces Institute of Pathology, 1966;97–161.
49. Berard CW, Dorfman RF. Histopathology of malignant lymphomas. Clin Hematol 1974;3:39–76.
50. Lukes RJ, Collins RD. Immunological characterization of human malignant lymphomas. Cancer 1974;34:1488–1503.
51. Gerard-Marchant R, Hamlin I, Lennert K, et al. Classification of non-Hodgkin's lymphoma. Lancet 1974;2:405–408.
52. Rosenberg SA, Berard CW, Brown BW, et al. NCI sponsored study of classification of non-Hodgkin's lymphoma: summary and description of a working formulation for clinical usage. Cancer 1982;49: 2112–2135.
53. Foon KA, Fisher RI. Lymphomas. In Beutler E, Lichtman MH, Coller BS, et al. (eds), Hematology (5th ed). New York: McGraw-Hill, 1995;1076–1085.
54. Moormeier JA, Williams SF, Golomb HM. The staging of non-Hodgkin's lymphomas. Semin Oncol 1990;17:43–50.
55. Pangalis GA, Nathwani BN, Rappaport H. Malignant lymphoma, well differentiated lymphocytic: its relationship with chronic lymphocytic leukemia and macroglobulinemia of Waldenström. Cancer 1977;39:999–1010.
56. Tsujimoto Y, Cossman J, Jaffe ES, et al. Involvement of the bcl-2 gene in human follicular lymphoma. Science 1985;228:1440–1443.
57. Medeiros LJ, Jaffe ES. Pathology of Non-Hodgkin's Lymphoma. In Pangalis GA, Polliack A (eds), Benign and Malignant Lymphadenopathies. Switzerland: Harwood Academic, 1993;187–225.
58. Isaacson PG. Lymphoma of mucosa-associated lymphoid tissue. Histopathology 1990;16:617–619.

Surgical Care for the Elderly, 2nd ed., edited by
R. Benton Adkins, Jr., and H. William Scott, Jr.
Lippincott–Raven Publishers, Philadelphia © 1998.

CHAPTER 7

Endoscopy and Laparoscopic Surgery

R. Benton Adkins, Jr., George R. Avant, Richard Eller, and J.K. Ladipo

The development of flexible endoscopic techniques has been closely linked to the development of laparoscopic surgical techniques. Diagnostic endoscopy often leads to treatment by laparoscopic surgery, while laparoscopic surgical techniques often require intraoperative endoscopy or endoscopic follow-up. The benefits of these two closely related technologies are significant in the elderly population.

ENDOSCOPY IN THE ELDERLY

Endoscopic examinations performed in the elderly may be diagnostic and lead to elective, corrective action before an emergency situation develops; provide treatment that will obviate the need for a larger procedure; and generally benefit the patient's care. The techniques of examination are the same as those performed in younger patients; nonetheless, more attention should be directed toward avoiding complications that might arise from the patient's fragile condition or coexisting diseases. In general, the amount of sedation required for endoscopic procedures in the elderly is considerably less than the doses required for younger patients. In many cases, only pharyngeal anesthesia is required; in other cases, only small amounts of narcotics or benzodiazepines are needed. The exact dose of medication is difficult to determine in any given individual, and the dose should be titrated to minimize adverse effects. Adjustments are required for patients with coexisting cardiac, pulmonary, or hepatic diseases. We have tended to monitor elderly patients very closely during these procedures, and when risk factors are great, the anesthesiology service may manage both medication and monitoring throughout the procedure.

Upper Gastrointestinal Endoscopy

Upper gastrointestinal (GI) endoscopy is perhaps the easiest of the endoscopic procedures in the elderly. This procedure in many cases is simpler and may be more helpful in making the diagnosis than an upper GI series. Certainly, the results of directly visualizing the mucosa of the upper GI tract are more efficacious than a barium meal.

Many elderly patients complain of dysphagia. This may be a reflection of an esophageal motility disorder or a structural abnormality of the esophagus. Carcinoma of the esophagus can be easily diagnosed by endoscopy with direct biopsies or cytologic brushings of the lesion. Cancer of the esophagus in a markedly debilitated patient in whom there is little hope of a cure may occasionally be treated with various types of palliation, as mentioned in Chapter 21. Obstructing tumors may be dilated for transient relief of symptoms, and placement of esophageal stents, including wall stents, may offer short-term palliation. Another option for palliation is laser-induced photo destruction of bleeding and obstructing tumors as described by Nath and coworkers in 1973 and modified and improved especially since 1983 [1–3]. We recommend these procedures as a palliative effort for elderly debilitated patients whenever other types of treatment are unsafe.

Lower esophageal strictures can be easily diagnosed and dilated under direct vision with the endoscope. Dilatation is frequently successful in offering significant relief of symptoms of dysphagia. Some elderly patients may develop dysphagia related either to a distal esophageal ring or to esophageal strictures due to the presence of poorly masticated food, usually secondary to ill-fitting or absent dentures. The acute food impaction that occurs in this setting can easily be relieved by endoscopic treatment. Flexible endoscopy is usually successful for treatment of acute esophageal food impaction and rigid endoscopy is required only rarely.

Symptomatic treatment of dysphagia related to achalasia in the elderly person who is at risk for operative therapy or pneumatic balloon dilatation and who has a moderate risk of esophageal perforation may be achieved by endoscopic botulinum toxin injection directly into the hypertensive lower esophageal sphincter. Local botulinum toxin injection leads to decreased lower esophageal sphincter pressures and may afford short-term relief of symptoms [4]. Gastric lesions can be directly visualized and biopsied. Gastric ulcerations can be better characterized as either benign or malignant by visualization and biopsy. In the elderly patient, there is the special tendency to develop proximally located gastric ulcers, giant gastric ulcers, lymphomas, sarcomas, and various types of gastritis. Repeated endoscopy and biopsy of all suspicious, unhealed, hypertrophic, ulcerated, nodular, or otherwise unusual areas is especially productive in surgically treatable pathologic conditions in the elderly patient. The usual delay in diagnosis of many of these upper GI tract problems in the elderly can be significantly reduced and avoided if an aggressive approach toward repeated endoscopy, visualization, and biopsy of all possible abnormal areas is vigorously pursued.

Many elderly patients now receive nonsteroidal antiinflammatory drugs that cause symptoms of dyspepsia and in fact can lead to both gastric and duodenal ulceration and associated GI bleeding. These lesions can be best defined by endoscopic examination. Other elderly patients with a history of recurrent or active ulcer disease should be evaluated for the presence of *Helicobacter pylori* infection by biopsy for histopathology and culture. If the investigation provides evidence of ongoing infection with *H. pylori*, appropriate antibiotic therapy should be administered.

Upper GI bleeding in the elderly patient can be an event associated with major mortality. The mortality depends on repetitive and uncontrolled blood loss, as well as on the presence of underlying pulmonary or cardiac disease. Endoscopic evaluation early in the acute upper GI tract bleeding episode helps differentiate between bleeding esophageal varices and mucosal lesions, such as Mallory-Weiss tears, gastric or duodenal ulcerations, or vascular lesions. Endoscopy early in the course of bleeding in the elderly patient is beneficial for both diagnosis and therapy. Sclerotherapy or banding of esophageal varices performed by flexible instruments has been shown to be moderately effective for acutely bleeding varices [5]. This may be followed by repetitive sclerotherapy for obliteration of the varices in the elderly cirrhotic patient. Visualization of a bleeding site in the stomach or duodenum has some predictive value: Lesions with a visible vessel suggest that the patient will continue to bleed or have a recurrent bleeding episode. Thermal or injection hemostatic therapy of active bleeding sites and visible vessels has been successful in controlling active and recurrent bleeding and should be considered initial therapy [5].

It is our policy to be very aggressive with elderly patients with upper GI bleeding, especially those with cardiac or pulmonary disease. If there is any evidence of unrelenting or recurrent uncontrolled bleeding or if the patient exhibits cardiovascular instability, an operative procedure may be necessary for the early control of the bleeding site before the situation becomes irreversible. The indications for surgical control of upper GI bleeding from the stomach and duodenum are outlined in Chapter 22, where the volume of bleeding per given episode is shown to be related to the prognosis in the elderly patient.

Endoscopic Retrograde Cholangiopancreatography

Diseases of both the biliary tree and the pancreas occur more frequently in the elderly. Endoscopic examination of the second portion of the duodenum with contrast injection into the biliary system and the pancreatic ductal system is a relatively noninvasive method of radiographic diagnosis. Certainly, endoscopic retrograde pancreatography is the only convenient method of outlining the pancreatic duct. Endoscopic pancreatography may be useful in the patient in whom carcinoma of the pancreas is suspected. If this suspicion is based on clinical evidence and the results of imaging modalities, the diagnosis may be supported by finding such characteristic changes as abrupt ductal obstruction or irregularity of the pancreatic duct. Pancreatography is also helpful in defining the exact location of a malignancy in the pancreatic gland itself. In the elderly patient with known chronic pancreatitis, pancreatography provides information regarding dilatation of the pancreatic duct, thereby allowing critical decisions to be made regarding operability.

Evaluation of jaundice and cholestasis in the elderly is first achieved by noninvasive measures, such as ultrasonography and computed tomographic scanning. Depending on the results of these imaging modalities in conjunction with the remainder of the evaluation, direct visualization of the papilla and endoscopic cholangiography may be most helpful. Carcinoma of the ampulla of Vater can be easily diagnosed by endoscopic visualization of the area with appropriate biopsies. Because carcinoma of the papilla is a malignant tumor that can be cured by resection if diagnosed early, it is important to take special measures to rule out this disease.

Diagnostic cholangiography can be most productive. A normal cholangiogram in the jaundiced patient suggests intrahepatic cholestasis possibly due to a drug. In this case no operative intervention is required. An abnormal cholangiogram result is helpful in planning an operative procedure should one be required. Some biliary tract diseases can be treated with therapeutic endoscopy. The elderly patient found to have common bile duct stones, whether or not a previous cholecystectomy has been performed, can undergo endoscopic sphincterotomy with common duct stone extraction. This technique has low morbidity and mortality and affords relief of obstruction and potential sepsis. Bile duct leaks occurring after laparoscopic cholecystectomy can be treated with stents placed across the ampulla or sphincterotomy. Strictures of the bile duct can be successfully dilated with hydrostatic balloons and obstructions relieved with stenting. Patency of obstructing malignant lesions can also be guaranteed by insertion of stents.

Lower Gastrointestinal Endoscopy

Flexible sigmoidoscopy and colonoscopy have increased our ability to visualize the anus, rectum, and colon in a way that was impossible with rigid anoscopes and sigmoidoscopes. However, the anoscope and rigid sigmoidoscope may still be used to advantage in certain situations and may complement the findings of a digital examination. These rigid instruments allow visualization of the anus, lower rectum, and anal canal in a way that can never be achieved with flexible instruments because of the direct view that is afforded the examiner in the area where fissures, fistulae, hemorrhoids, and condyloma occur. Many of these conditions, which are common in the elderly, can be treated in a definitive manner using the rigid endoscope.

The flexible fiberoptic sigmoidoscope is more expensive, causes less discomfort, allows the examiner to see well beyond the area of the rigid sigmoidoscope, and should be clearly indicated for use in the diagnosis, surveillance, and treatment of problems above the level of view of the rigid sigmoidoscope. We agree, however, with Marks [6] that the need for total colonoscopy should never be preempted by the exclusive use of flexible fiberoptic sigmoidoscopy. The complete examination of the entire colon and rectum can be done only by using the full-length colonoscope.

Lesions within reach of the flexible fiberoptic sigmoidoscope and those above that area within reach of the flexible colonoscope include polyps, carcinoma, inflammatory lesions, intussusception, volvulus, diverticula, and other conditions that can be diagnosed and sometimes treated in a definitive manner by the use of these fiberoptic instruments. In the aging individual in whom the avoidance of excessive anesthesia and surgical intervention may be desirable, these instruments are of great value.

The diagnosis of lower GI tract bleeding, the removal of benign and malignant growths, the diagnosis of inflammatory and neoplastic conditions, the relief of areas of obstruction and pseudo-obstruction, and the surveillance for residual or recurrent disease make these instruments a necessary part of the armamentarium of all surgeons and gastroenterologists involved in the care of elderly individuals.

Special Considerations in Endoscopy in the Elderly

We have tended to perform upper and lower GI endoscopy in the high-risk elderly individual under conditions that are carefully monitored and in some instances attended by nurse anesthetists or anesthesiologists. Occasionally, this has been helpful and perhaps lifesaving. When arrhythmias, respiratory changes, unusual complaints, and the rare incidence of perforation are encountered, careful monitoring has been especially valuable. In the elderly individual who is receiving chronic corticosteroid therapy for pulmonary or musculoskeletal disorders, special caution is necessary. In our experience, endoscopic polypectomy with electrocautery has occasionally been associated with delayed perforation at the site of the polypectomy. These problems can be recognized quickly and solved expeditiously without mortality. When monitoring of this magnitude is not available for the elderly patient undergoing prolonged and difficult endoscopy, it is advised that close attention be paid to any signs of distress occurring during the procedure, which might require the procedure to be aborted early to avoid complications. Most well-equipped endoscopy laboratories have sufficient modern monitoring devices to satisfy these requirements for most elderly patients.

Bronchoscopy

The rigid bronchoscope is used primarily by thoracic surgeons to diagnose pulmonary and bronchial disorders. The fiberoptic bronchoscope has a wide variety of uses, and flexible bronchoscopy is now used by many other medical specialists.

In the postoperative patient, flexible bronchoscopy is useful in cases of respiratory failure to clear secretions from the airway or to treat atelectasis. Frequent bronchoscopy in burn patients or in those who have suffered smoke inhalation is an effective means of irrigation, suction, and removal of desquamated epithelium.

Aspiration of gastric contents is not uncommon in the elderly patient. Flexible bronchoscopy should always be used immediately to clear the bronchi of aspirated contents; in some situations, rigid bronchoscopy may be necessary for a more thorough washing and cleansing of the tracheobronchial tree.

As with other types of endoscopic procedures, careful monitoring of the high-risk elderly patient is essential during the procedure. Cardiac arrhythmias may occur as a result of hypoxia or vagal stimulation. For this reason, many surgeons choose to perform most of the diagnostic endoscopies on the surgical service in the operating room under local anesthesia with full monitoring and attendance by anesthesiologists. Therapeutic endoscopy can be done easily in the intensive care suite with full monitoring as required.

As with obstructing lesions of the esophagus, occasionally it is appropriate to use the laser, multiple biopsies, the cautery, and other instruments for the dilatation and clearing of the airway in the elderly individual who has obstructing strictures and tumors of the bronchi and trachea. With a cooperative effort between the endoscopists and the anesthesiologists, major airway-obstructing tumors can also be handled in elderly individuals using the neodymium:yttrium-aluminum-garnet laser technique [7,8].

Choledochoscopy

The incidence of retained stones in the elderly patient following cholecystectomy and exploration of the common bile duct is at least as high as the usual reported incidence of this occurrence in the general population, and it is our impression that it may be higher. Reports of 5% to 10% are usually given, but the true incidence is never known, obviously, because some retained stones never manifest clinically. When instances of retained stones in elderly individuals arise and a second laparotomy is necessary, most surgeons prefer the rigid endoscope with a right angle viewing arm that is similar to the nephroscope used for kidney stones. An excellent description of the use of this instrument including its indications can be found in Cuschieri's text [9] and subsequently discussed by Berci [10]. We prefer the flexible fiberoptic choledochoscope, which can be used both intraoperatively and postoperatively through a well-established T-tube drainage tract. Our experience with the use of this instrument both during the initial duct exploration and in the postoperative examination has been most gratifying. This instrument is especially useful in elderly individuals in whom a formal second surgical procedure can be successfully avoided.

Summary

Perhaps more than in any other age group, endoscopy can be used in the elderly patients to great benefit. Both the diagnostic and therapeutic uses of these instruments are especially suited to the elderly patient who needs careful surveillance and ultrasafe nonoperative therapy whenever possible. These techniques should not, however, take the place of more definitive procedures when they are indicated for the appropriate treatment of elderly patients.

LAPAROSCOPIC SURGERY

Laparoscopic general surgery is a rapidly expanding field. Many elective and acute surgical conditions are being corrected using advanced laparoscopic techniques. Although some of these laparoscopic techniques are still in various phases of development, it is clear that many will become widely accepted. It is our belief that these procedures will be of great benefit to elderly patients as long as the patients are carefully evaluated for their ability to withstand laparoscopic procedures and are properly prepared.

Benefits of Laparoscopic Surgery

Laparoscopic surgery in geriatric patients has many benefits. Clinical and experimental studies to identify and explain these benefits have been performed largely in animals and young patients; however, the benefits appear to apply equally well to geriatric patients in most circumstances. Procedure for procedure, when compared with more traditional open surgical approaches, laparoscopic surgery results in a shorter hospital stay with an earlier return to preoperative activity levels, decreased metabolic stress, less immunosuppression, less postoperative pulmonary dysfunction, earlier return to regular diet, decreased analgesic requirements, and improved cosmesis. These are all issues central to the care of elderly patients and are discussed individually.

Across the spectrum of surgical procedures with a laparoscopic surgical option, there is a marked decrease in the length of hospitalization with an earlier return to physical activity when a laparoscopic technique is selected. This is a significant advantage for elderly patients. In younger patients, early return to physical activity is largely an advantage seen in an early return to work or to the care of small children. In elderly patients, avoiding long periods of postoperative physical restriction translates into less deterioration of muscle function and coordination, which has been demonstrated to increase the chances for the elderly patient to return to independent mobility [11,12]. Also, better mobility at the time of discharge has been shown to decrease the chances of a fall after returning home [13]. Decreased postoperative complications and less confusion and depression, both more prevalent with long hospital stays and impaired mobility [14–17], are expected benefits. These advantages may be the difference between sending elderly patients home after a brief hospital stay and transferring them to a rehabilitation facility after a prolonged admission. The cost of placement of elderly patients in rehabilitation facilities after hospitalization is not the only expense to be considered. The unfamiliar surroundings are known to lead to an increased risk of falls and fall-related injuries [18].

All operations are associated with metabolic responses much like those well characterized for traumatic injury and shock. The many profound metabolic and physiologic changes are the subjects of current investigations, and individual discussions of these changes are beyond the scope of this chapter. In brief, postoperative metabolism is characterized by low insulin levels and an elevated glucagon level. This leads to hepatic gluconeogenesis and glycogenolysis. There is a rapid increase in catecholamine levels, and this, too, leads to increased gluconeogenesis and glycogenolysis as well as increased lipolysis. Cortisol levels become elevated, contributing to net skeletal muscle proteolysis. Cytokine release at the operative site, although primarily inciting a local response, has systemic metabolic effects as well. Cytokine release stimulates acute phase protein synthesis and the redistribution of trace elements. In sum, these metabolic changes lead to a catabolic state characterized by hyperglycemia and a negative nitrogen balance.

There appears to be a direct relationship between the magnitude of the injury and the degree of metabolic stress placed on the patient [19,20]. Laparoscopic surgery is performed through small puncture wounds as opposed to larger incisions. By decreasing the size of the soft-tissue wound created, there is a decrease in the physiologic stress. Laboratory and clinical studies are broadly divergent in their findings of the exact metabolic changes caused by laparoscopic surgical techniques when compared with open surgical techniques.

There is no agreement in the literature about which physiologic parameters to measure and at what time points during and after surgery these parameters should be assessed. This makes direct comparison of published findings difficult. Several studies, however, point the way. Schauer and Sirinek [21], in a study of 12 laparoscopic cholecystectomy patients and 11 open cholecystectomy patients, showed significantly lower serum epinephrine, norepinephrine, dopamine, cortisol, and glucose levels after the laparoscopic procedure. Glaser et al. [19], also in a study comparing laparoscopic with open cholecystectomy, found similar results for serum epinephrine, norepinephrine, and glucose levels when the patients were examined at 1 and 2 days postoperatively. Mealy et al. [22], looking at erythrocyte sedimentation rates and C-reactive protein, concluded that laparoscopic cholecystectomy incited less of an acute phase response than open cholecystectomy. However, they noted an increased vanillylmandelic acid level in the urine of the laparoscopic cholecystectomy patients and no significant difference in urinary cortisol, metanephrine, or nitrogen excretion when compared with the open procedure. This would suggest a greater adrenergic response and increased catabolism in the laparoscopic surgery patients. These findings are contrary to the findings published by Bolufer et al. [23], who found the 24-hour urinary cortisol and catecholamine levels to be greater in their open surgical patients. Similar findings were reported by Senagore et al. [24] when examining nitrogen balance after laparoscopic and open colectomy. Their finding of an earlier return to a positive nitrogen balance in the patients undergoing a laparoscopic procedure was largely attributable to an earlier return to enteral nutrition. However, decreased metabolic demand may have played a role. The majority of these studies points to decreased physiologic stress on patients undergoing laparoscopic surgical procedures when compared with the stress experienced by patients undergoing open surgical techniques; however, more study is needed to clarify and quantify this observation.

A decrease in the metabolic stress response to surgery would be especially beneficial to elderly patients. Minimizing the postoperative lipolysis, proteolysis, and hyperglycemia as well as an early return to enteral nutrition would decrease the metabolic impact of surgery on the elderly. An earlier return to anabolic metabolism would provide for rapid wound healing and a shortened recuperative period.

The immunologic responses to laparoscopic surgery are closely related to the metabolic changes due to surgical stress. As previously stated, cytokines are released in response to surgical injury. The immunologic alterations caused by the release of interleukin (IL)-1β and IL-6 are compounded in elderly patients due to an impaired T-cell response to and decreased production of IL-2 [25]. This leads to an overall decrease in cellular immunity. Depression of lymphocyte counts as well as suppressed T-cell proliferation occurs with surgical trauma. This has an additive effect with the decline in mature T-cell populations seen as a natural part of aging [26]. Glaser et al. [19] looked at IL-1 and IL-6 response during and immediately after laparoscopic and open cholecystectomy. They found the systemic levels of these two cytokines to be significantly higher in the patients undergoing open cholecystectomy. Redmond et al. [27], in a randomized study, measured various inflammatory mediators after laparoscopic and open cholecystectomy. They found significant increases in monocyte release of tumor necrosis factor and O_2^-, neutrophil release of O_2^-, and neutrophil chemotaxis. These immunologic alterations could explain the higher number of septic complications seen by these authors and others in patients undergoing open cholecystectomy when compared with those undergoing laparoscopic cholecystectomy. This would be of great benefit to the elderly population, which not only has an already impaired immune response, but is less able to tolerate complications should they occur.

The effect of abdominal surgery on pulmonary function has been widely studied. Upper abdominal incisions have been shown to effect decreases in pulmonary function in excess of 50% [28–30]. The physiologic mechanisms by which these changes in pulmonary function are mediated are complex; however, incisional pain and respiratory muscular dysfunction seem to be leading causes. Other factors such as pleural effusions and altered diaphragm function may contribute to the observed impairment of postoperative respiratory function. Because of the changes in pulmonary function that are part of normal aging, it is a logical conclusion that elderly patients will suffer more from these respiratory insults. Use of the abdominal wall musculature for breathing increases with age [31]. Abdominal muscle function is altered and impaired by abdominal surgical procedures, amplifying the effect of abdominal surgical procedures on an elderly patient's respirations. Epidural analgesia has reduced postoperative pulmonary dysfunction by reducing incisional pain [32]. However, epidural analgesia is not possible in all patients, particularly the elderly, due to degenerative changes in the vertebral column.

Numerous studies have reported less postoperative pulmonary dysfunction in laparoscopic surgical patients when compared with patients undergoing equivalent open surgical procedures [22,23,33,34]. Although patients benefit from less postoperative pulmonary dysfunction with laparoscopic techniques, patients must be carefully examined and tested preoperatively to determine which patients are at risk for very high P_{ACO_2} levels and the resulting acidosis when a pneumoperitoneum is established. Preoperative pulmonary function testing is essential in elderly patients with questionable pulmonary function. Age, preoperative blood gas analysis, and the length of the surgical procedure have not been found to be reliable predictors of the development of severe intraoperative acidosis (pH <7.35) [35,36]. Preoperative forced expiratory volumes <70% of predicted values and diffusion defects <80% of predicted values do have predictive value in identifying patients at risk for severe hypercarbia and intraoperative acidosis [35].

As a general rule, laparoscopic procedures allow for an earlier return to a regular diet and earlier discharge home than the equivalent open procedure [37–40]. The advent of laparoscopic surgery and the economic pressures of current managed care systems have pushed surgeons to advance patients rapidly to enteral feeding and early discharge home after all types of surgery. This has resulted in very aggressive early enteral feeding of open surgical patients as well as laparoscopic surgical patients [41,42]. It is apparent, however, that laparoscopic abdominal procedures result in less postoperative ileus than when a large incision is made and the bowel is handled. The exact physiology of this is not clear, but the observation seems nonetheless valid. This early return to a full diet, although a convenience for a healthy young adult, is much more important in an elderly patient who does not have the same nutritional reserve. Avoidance of postoperative dietary restriction logically should allow for a more rapid recovery without depletion of the nutritional reserve and with minimal impairment of the normal role of the gut in the immune response.

Reduced abdominal wall pain from laparoscopic procedures compared with their conventional open alternative should result in a decreased narcotic requirement for the elderly [34,37,43,44]. Narcotic analgesic side effects are more problematic in elderly patients. Laparoscopic surgery has been shown in numerous studies across a spectrum of procedures to have lower postoperative analgesic requirements [22,40]. In the elderly population, this could reasonably be expected to result in less postoperative confusion and fewer falls [45]. Less narcotic suppression of pulmonary function should result in less postoperative pulmonary dysfunction and, therefore, reduce the incidence of postoperative atelectasis and pneumonia [33,46]. The reduced amount of abdominal wall pain is doubly important in the elderly because aging results in a much greater reliance on the abdominal muscles for respiration. Decreased abdominal discomfort should result in better pulmonary toilet and, again, a decreased incidence of postoperative atelectasis and pneumonia.

The improved cosmesis of laparoscopic surgical techniques is a benefit realized by young and old patients alike. Older patients are more prone to depression in the postoperative period. Avoiding significant changes in body image would be beneficial in reducing postoperative depression and the elderly patient's fear of becoming dependent.

Risks of Laparoscopic Surgery

An exhaustive discussion of all potential complications of laparoscopic surgery is beyond the scope of this chapter, so we focus on those that have special significance in geriatric patients. In all discussions of risks to geriatric patients, it must be kept in mind that their tolerance for technical mistakes and errors in general is lower than that for younger patients. The application of laparoscopic surgical techniques to an elderly patient without proper evaluation for his or her tolerance of the unique physiologic stresses imposed by the technique can be disastrous.

Risks associated with laparoscopic surgery include the creation of a pneumoperitoneum and the extreme positions required for exposure in many of the laparoscopic techniques. The negative effects of pneumoperitoneum and extreme body position are magnified in patients with cardiac or pulmonary dysfunction. These risks can be minimized by proper patient selection, patient preparation, and careful coordination with the anesthesiologist for optimal anesthetic technique.

Insufflation of the abdomen up to 15 mm Hg pressure with carbon dioxide, as is needed for most laparoscopic abdominal surgery, has several effects that can significantly alter a patient's cardiopulmonary function. The three immediate results of raising the intra-abdominal pressure to 15 mm Hg with carbon dioxide are an increase in $Paco_2$ due primarily to absorption of the carbon dioxide via the peritoneum, altered venous return to the heart, and venous stasis in the lower extremities due to venous hypertension.

The hemodynamic effects of a carbon dioxide pneumoperitoneum appear to be largely due to the effects of the absorbed gas with the resultant hypercarbia and acidosis. Studies on humans and animals using helium or nitrogen to create the pneumoperitoneum report only minimal hemodynamic changes at the pressures commonly used in laparoscopic surgery [47–49]. At this time, carbon dioxide is the preferred gas for laparoscopy due to its noncombustibility and rapid absorption from the peritoneal cavity after the procedure is completed. Unfortunately, the rapid development of hypercarbia and acidosis are the well-described and logical result of a carbon dioxide pneumoperitoneum [50]. The high Pco_2 in the peritoneal cavity relative to the Pco_2 in the bloodstream, coupled with the high solubility of carbon dioxide, results in the rapid establishment of a new elevated steady-state $Paco_2$. The net hemodynamic effect of this new hypercarbic state is determined by the physiologic summation of the direct effects on the vascular tree and myocardium and the indirect effects mediated by the sympathetic nervous system.

Induced hypercarbia alone, not associated with a pneumoperitoneum, has been shown to result in elevated systolic blood pressure and increased heart rate, cardiac output, mechanical cardiac activity, and cardiac oxygen demand [51]. This creates an unfavorable balance in myocardial oxygen consumption and supply. Direct application of these data from induced hypercarbia in patients undergoing carotid endarterectomy to laparoscopy patients, however, may not be entirely valid. Although these patients had increased cardiac output and decreased systemic vascular resistance, many human and animal studies of carbon dioxide pneumoperitoneum–induced hypercarbia have shown significant decreases in cardiac output and index and significant increases in systemic vascular resistance [52–55]. Reports on the effects of carbon dioxide pneumoperitoneum on these and other vital hemodynamic parameters vary greatly. Further study is needed to clearly define the hemodynamic effects of the carbon dioxide–induced pneumoperitoneum and then relate these findings to the elderly population.

In higher-risk patients, close monitoring of the intraoperative acidosis and cardiac depression is needed. End-tidal carbon dioxide monitoring may not be adequate or reliable in these patients [52]. This is due to decreased lung volumes and reduced pulmonary compliance. End-tidal carbon dioxide monitoring may be even less reliable in patients with chronic cardiopulmonary disease [56]. Therefore, high-risk patients, defined as patients with cardiopulmonary disease or American Society of Anesthesiologists class III or IV, should be considered for invasive monitoring and frequent blood gas determinations.

The second immediate effect of creating a carbon dioxide pneumoperitoneum is the alteration of splanchnic blood flow and flow through the inferior vena cava due to the increased intra-abdominal pressure. Increased intra-abdominal pressure may result in either increased or decreased venous return to the heart, depending on the patient's volume status, body position, and the level of intra-abdominal pressure achieved [57]. It is theorized that in hypervolemic patients, increased intra-abdominal pressure to levels commonly used for laparoscopic surgery results in increased extrinsic pressure on the capacitance vessels of the splanchnic circulation. This pump effect serves to increase venous return and may increase vascular resistance across the splanchnic bed. Increased venous return leads to increased mean pressure in the inferior vena cava, which serves to minimize the constriction of flow through the inferior vena cava caused by the elevated intra-abdominal pressure.

It is clear that hypovolemic patients experience a marked decrease in venous return immediately on establishing a pneumoperitoneum. This is theorized to occur because the unfilled capacitance vessels of the splanchnic circulation would have little volume to contribute to the pump effect. Therefore, the hydrostatic pressure within the inferior vena cava would not be augmented and the increased intra-abdominal pressure would lead to compression of the inferior vena cava. This extrinsic compression reduces venous return and ultimately, cardiac output.

The volume status of the patient clearly has bearing on the effects of a carbon dioxide pneumoperitoneum. Ho et al. [58] demonstrated the effects of a carbon dioxide pneumoperitoneum on pigs in different stages of hemorrhagic shock and volume resuscitation. On institution of the pneumoperitoneum, the hypovolemic animals not only had a decrease in stroke volume and cardiac index, they also had severe acidosis. Crystalloid resuscitation failed to prevent the development of the severe intraoperative acidosis. This has clear implications in the use of laparoscopy in the evaluation of abdominal trauma as well.

Positioning the patient in Trendelenburg's position augments venous return to the heart; positioning the patient in reverse Trendelenburg's position diminishes venous return. These effects are independent of intra-abdominal pressure within the pressure ranges routinely used for laparoscopic surgery [59].

The level of intra-abdominal pressure achieved can affect the degree of hypercarbia and hemodynamic change. Pressures <12 mm Hg do not appear to have any effect on pH or measurable hemodynamic parameters [60]. At some pressure >12 mm Hg—there is not agreement in the literature on a number—pH and hemodynamic function begin to be adversely affected. There may be altered solid organ perfusion and decreased renal function at relatively low intra-abdominal pressures.

Venous return from the lower extremities is impaired by increased mean venous pressure and extrinsic compression of the inferior vena cava as previously described. To demonstrate this, Millard et al. [61] measured peak systolic velocities in the common femoral vein of patients undergoing laparoscopic cholecystectomy. They demonstrated that a combination of pneumoperitoneum (13 to 15 mm Hg) and 30 degrees of reverse Trendelenburg's position caused a 42% decrease in peak systolic velocity. Similar findings were reported by Ido et al. [62]. This relative venous stasis could increase the risk for deep venous thrombosis (DVT). As elderly patients have a much higher risk of DVT, prophylaxis is essential. Sequential leg compression devices that are now routinely available are helpful devices. Millard et al. [61] showed that these were capable of returning peak systolic flow through the common femoral vein to the preoperative baseline level. Ido et al. [62] showed that graded elastic compression bandages were not effective if the intra-abdominal pressure exceeded 5 mm Hg. The use of minidose heparin is also advantageous.

Other poorly defined and poorly understood effects of a pneumoperitoneum may have significance in the elderly patient population. Regional blood flow to the liver, via the portal vein, to the intestines, through the superior mesenteric artery [60,63], and to the kidney [64] may be decreased via unclear mechanisms. Increased intracranial pressure [65,66] and hyperkalemia [67] have been noted in certain experimental models, and these too could have special significance in elderly patients.

General Recommendations for Laparoscopic Surgery

With some of the discussed benefits and risks in mind, certain general recommendations about undertaking laparoscopic surgery in the elderly can be made.

1. Preoperative pulmonary function testing is advised for patients with clinical evidence of respiratory impairment. Simple blood gas analysis is not enough because it has not been shown to correlate with the development of severe intraoperative acidosis.
2. Careful clinical cardiac examination is needed, with full cardiologic evaluation if the patient's history or clinical examination reveals an abnormality.

3. Preoperative preparation of the patient should include evaluation of the patient's home situation and current level of physical function, preparation of family members for their assistance in postoperative care, and a plan for any anticipated alterations in the patient's usual medications on discharge (e.g., liquids and elixirs in the place of pills if an esophageal procedure is planned).
4. Preoperatively, the surgeon and anesthesiologist should discuss the planned procedure, anticipated patient positioning, and types of invasive monitoring needed.
5. Plan to perform the operation on a day when other attending specialists will be available to monitor the patient's recovery. The use of a "geriatric team" has been supported in the literature [68].
6. DVT prophylaxis with lower-extremity sequential compression garments is strongly recommended, and minidose heparin should be considered.
7. If a special geriatric unit is available, plan to admit the patient there postoperatively rather than to a routine surgical unit.

Laparoscopic Procedures

Numerous laparoscopic procedures are now being performed around the world using widely varying techniques. Which of these procedures will ultimately be widely adopted has yet to be determined. However, there are several that hold great promise for the elderly and are mentioned here. For the details in surgical technique for each of these procedures, training courses by knowledgeable and experienced practitioners are available and the most current literature for newly identified risks and modifications of the procedure should be reviewed.

Biliary Tract

Since its introduction, laparoscopic cholecystectomy has become the standard of care for patients in many countries, including the United States [38,69–73]. It is the best characterized of the laparoscopic procedures and is a useful basis for comparison. It has been compared with open cholecystectomy in a multitude of studies, and its efficacy has been well established [74–76]. For those surgeons who have gained a significant experience with the technique, it is the preferred method for cholecystectomy in all situations. Previous contraindications for the choice of a laparoscopic approach such as obesity, acute cholecystitis [77,78], previous abdominal surgery [77], and hepatic cirrhosis [79] are no longer valid. Several studies evaluating laparoscopic cholecystectomy in older patient populations and in patients with high American Society of Anesthesiologists scores suggest that laparoscopic cholecystectomy is the preferred technique for these patients as well [80,81]. There may be a lower morbidity and mortality than reported for open cholecystectomy in these older and higher risk patients. Its application to elderly patients is reasonable, and the benefits of reduced postoperative morbidity are realized by the elderly population in the same manner as younger patients [82].

Laparoscopic common bile duct exploration is a useful technique in the hands of surgeons with advanced laparoscopic training [83]. Combined with intraoperative cholangiography, common duct stones may be extracted by several methods and, if necessary, a T-tube may be placed to allow further access to the duct [84]. In some cases, a papillotomy can be performed laparoscopically with the guidance of intraoperative upper GI endoscopy [85]. Elderly patients are generally suitable candidates for laparoscopic common bile duct exploration [86]; however, the benefits should be carefully weighed against the risks of prolonged intraoperative hypercarbia and acidosis. There is debate over the role of laparoscopic common duct exploration in patients of all ages in cases where endoscopic retrograde cholangiopancreatography is readily available. At this time, both procedures have merit, and decisions about how best to proceed in a patient with choledocholithiasis are influenced by local availability of services, preferences of individual surgeons and gastroenterologists, and individual patient considerations.

Other laparoscopic biliary tract procedures are being investigated that could have benefits for elderly patients. Patients with advanced pancreatic malignancies and biliary obstruction may be palliated by laparoscopic cholecystojejunostomy [87]. The number of patients undergoing this procedure is still small, but the reduced morbidity and shortened hospitalization afforded by this technique holds promise for these unfortunate patients.

Upper Gastrointestinal Tract

Laparoscopic Nissen fundoplication and several techniques for partial fundoplication are rapidly becoming standard operations for patients with severe gastroesophageal reflux disease. These procedures can be performed safely and rapidly with few side effects or complications in the vast majority of patients [88,89]. Hospitalization times are shorter than for the conventional open procedure [90,91], and clinical outcomes appear to be excellent [92–94]. Measurable physiologic parameters such as lower esophageal sphincter pressure and lower esophageal sphincter relaxation with deglutition are different after laparoscopic Nissen fundoplication when compared with the open technique. However, the clinical outcome after laparoscopic Nissen fundoplication is as good as or better than that seen in open fundoplications [95]. Many elderly patients suffer with free reflux of gastric contents into their esophaguses and mouths due to a patulous lower esophageal sphincter. This is made worse by an age-dependent decrease in salivary response to acid in the esophagus [96] and decreased amplitude and velocity of distal esophageal peristaltic waves [97]. Free gastroesophageal reflux into the oropharynx may result in aspiration and hospitalization. These elderly patients should be evaluated with upper GI endoscopy and esophageal motility and manometry studies, just as their younger counterparts would be. If an antireflux procedure is indicated, use of a partial fundoplication such as a Dor or Toupet procedure should be considered. A full 360-degree fundoplication, such as in a Nissen procedure, creates a significantly greater high-pressure zone at the gastroesophageal junction than does a partial fundoplication [98]. In elderly patients with weaker distal esophageal peristalsis, this theoretically could result in higher rates of postoperative dysphagia. In carefully selected patients we, as well as others, have achieved excellent results using either laparoscopic Nissen or partial fundoplication techniques.

Achalasia can now be treated laparoscopically. Extramucosal esophagomyotomy as initially described by Heller in 1913 [99] has proven to have excellent results. The majority of data comparing esophagomyotomy to forceful dilatation techniques has been from patients undergoing open surgical procedures. These studies have generally shown better, longer lasting results in the surgically treated patients [100–102]. Heller esophagomyotomy, with or without an antireflux procedure and performed entirely through a laparoscopic approach, has obvious advantages over more traditional approaches requiring a thoracotomy, or as performed more recently, thoracoscopically. We recently evaluated the results of our first 10 thoracoscopic and laparoscopic Heller esophagomyotomies [103]. Eight of 10 patients reported excellent results, one patient reported good results, and one patient reported fair results (continued mild dysphagia for some foods). Other groups are reporting similar results [104–106]. We are in the process of determining the need for simultaneous antireflux procedures on these patients. Some groups recommend routine fundoplication on all esophagomyotomy patients [105,107,108]; however, this may not be necessary [109–114] and certainly needs to be evaluated in the elderly population.

Spleen and Lymphatics

Laparoscopic splenectomy, with or without lymph node biopsies, for hematologic disorders or as part of staging for Hodgkin's lymphoma, has significant advantages over open splenectomy [115–117]. The shorter hospital stay and decreased postoperative morbidity are significant [115]. With current instrumentation and the increasing laparoscopic experience of the surgeons performing the procedure, clearly defined operative strategies are being developed [116,118] and operating times are decreasing. Removal of even very large spleens is now possible with current endoscopic pouches and intracorporeal morcellation techniques. Disruption of the gross structure of the specimen allows for better fixation of the tissues and excellent specimens for microscopy and staining.

The laparoscopic biopsy of lymphatic tissue, especially pelvic lymph nodes for the staging of prostate, bladder, and cervical cancer, is applicable to elderly patients [119–123]. If celiotomy can be avoided by determining lymphatic spread laparoscopically, not only will patients benefit from the lower morbidity, but there will be lowered costs by reducing the number of nontherapeutic celiotomies. The use of laparoscopic techniques for lymphatic biopsy in the staging of prostate cancer is a good example. Laparoscopic pelvic lymph node biopsy for the staging of prostatic cancer in most current studies has equivalent results when compared with open biopsy, and it is far more sensitive for nodal and regional metastasis than noninvasive imaging techniques [124–126]. When the biopsies are performed laparoscopically, they can be obtained separately from the planned therapeutic procedure. This allows for the added accuracy of permanent section pathology in the place of intraoperative frozen section analysis [125]. With this higher diagnostic accuracy, patients may be counseled more definitively about outcomes of planned operations and other possible therapies. If there are no nodal metastases, patients with prostatic malignancies may be offered transperineal prostatectomy, thus avoiding an abdominal procedure altogether [121]. These same benefits can be realized in the laparoscopic staging of cervical, bladder, pancreatic, and other intra-abdominal malignancies more common in elderly patients [122].

Colon and Rectum

Laparoscopic surgery of the colon and rectum is one of the greatest challenges for laparoscopic surgeons. Geriatric patients have the most to gain from advances in laparoscopic surgery of the colon and rectum because these diseases predominantly affect older patients. Great strides have been made; however, several serious issues are still to be resolved regarding laparoscopic surgery of the colon for malignant lesions. Problems with port site tumor implants [127] and questionable lymphatic dissections are being addressed. Although many groups have reported excellent results in the treatment of colon malignancies laparoscopically [128–131], at the present time, laparoscopic surgery of the colon and rectum for malignant disease is discouraged except as part of a research protocol.

Several benign conditions of the colon and rectum are currently being approached successfully via the laparoscope [128]. Rectal prolapse, ulcerative colitis, diverticulitis and diverticulosis, colostomy and Hartmann's pouch reversal, and appendicitis are all being treated successfully with laparoscopic surgical techniques.

Rectal prolapse is not uncommon in elderly patients, and there are several options for surgical correction. The primary open surgical techniques are the abdominal procedures (i.e., Wells and Ripstein–style proctopexy and sigmoid resection) and the perineal approaches (i.e., the Altemeier rectosigmoidectomy procedure, Delorme procedure, and Ivalon sponge technique popular in the United Kingdom). Laparoscopy has been applied to most of these techniques and generally been found to have good results [132–135]. Laparoscopic proctopexy alone, either by suture techniques or by securing the colon to pieces of prosthetic material anchored to the sacrum, has been shown to be effective and to decrease hospital stay, analgesic requirements, and time to enteral nutrition [136]. Whether performed as an open or laparoscopic procedure, some studies have indicated a greater degree of postoperative constipation in patients treated by proctopexy alone when compared with resectional techniques [137,138]. The best results seem to be achieved with a combination of sigmoid resection and proctopexy [139]. Baker et al. report their experience performing laparoscopically assisted anterior resection with and without proctopexy with results that compare favorably with the open procedure [140]. Open abdominal sigmoidectomy alone or in combination with proctopexy appears to be superior in long-term results when compared with the perineal approaches [141]. No direct comparisons have been made between the laparoscopic abdominal approaches and the perineal rectosigmoidectomies. Reports of laparoscopically assisted perineal rectosigmoidectomy have been made, and this appears to be another viable option with some advantages in both patient comfort and long-term results [130]. In severely ill patients, the perineal approaches may be best and have been carefully studied in high-risk situations in elderly patients [142,143].

Techniques for removal of part or all of the colon, either laparoscopically or with laparoscopic assistance for benign conditions such as ulcerative colitis, diverticular disease, and colonic inertia, have been developed. The techniques are similar to those used in open surgery. Laparoscopic removal of the colon has the advantages of earlier return to oral nutrition, decreased pain and analgesic requirements, earlier passage of flatus and return of bowel function, and earlier discharge from the hospital with earlier return to preoperative activity levels. The elimination of the large midline incision has great psychological benefits as well, stemming from the improved cosmetic appearance.

Colostomy takedown as well as anastomosis of the colon in patients with a Hartmann's pouch can be done laparoscopically.

Laparoscopic appendectomy can now be performed safely and rapidly [144]. Benefits of the laparoscopic approach include decreased incidence of wound infection, decreased length of hospitalization, reduced postoperative ileus, and reduced pain and nausea [145]. In cases in which the diagnosis is in question, diagnostic laparoscopy can be performed and the appendix can be removed laparoscopically [146]. In such cases, the use of a minimally invasive technique for diagnosis with a therapeutic option could result in a decrease in the usual delay in diagnosis and treatment of appendicitis in the elderly. However, if the diagnosis is clear preoperatively, the benefits are not as pronounced as those for laparoscopic cholecystectomy and fundoplication techniques. Its suitability for routine use in elderly patients, given their added risk of intraoperative complications related to carbon dioxide pneumoperitoneum, has not been established.

Hernia

Laparoscopic inguinal herniorrhaphy has been in use in various forms since the late 1980s. Just as open inguinal herniorrhaphy techniques have continued to evolve, so have the laparoscopic techniques. The two most commonly used laparoscopic herniorrhaphy techniques are the transabdominal preperitoneal repair (TAP procedure) and the totally extraperitoneal repair (TEP or EXTRA procedure). The TAP procedure allows for examination of the peritoneal cavity, a more familiar view of the anatomy, and a more straightforward approach to the operative site. The TEP procedure minimizes risk to the abdominal organs during the initial access, reduces the chance of creating intra-abdominal adhesions [147], and when mastered, may be quicker and easier to perform. Advocates of both procedures argue that there is a significant reduction in morbidity when compared with open procedures and that costs can be kept competitive with those incurred with open techniques [148–150]. Similar to laparoscopic appendectomy, laparoscopic inguinal herniorrhaphy may provide only a marginal decrease in postoperative morbidity in elderly patients. This benefit must be weighed carefully against the previously described risks of carbon dioxide pneumoperitoneum.

If laparoscopic inguinal herniorrhaphy is being considered for an elderly patient, the choice of TAP versus TEP is even less clear than in young patients. TEP herniorrhaphy appears to result in a higher level of hypercapnia than transabdominal procedures [151]. The effect of this apparent increased hypercapnia seen in pneumoperitoneum has yet to be defined. Until it is better understood, special consideration for performing a TAP instead of a TEP procedure should be made in geriatric patients.

Laparoscopic ventral herniorrhaphy is being developed as a potential option for the repair of large abdominal wall defects. This could be of great benefit to elderly patients because their abdominal wall fascia becomes attenuated with age. Ventral hernias can become particularly debilitating in elderly patients as they become increasingly dependent on abdominal wall muscles for respiration. A laparoscopic repair of large abdominal wall defects has the potential to repair the defect without the large soft tissue dissection generally required for a satisfactory open repair. Decreased opportunity for prosthetic graft infection should also result from placing the patch intra-abdominally and avoiding the large skin incision, soft-tissue defect, and typical postoperative seroma. There are few follow-up data available at this time, however, and this type of procedure should only be undertaken in a research setting.

Other Laparoscopic Procedures

Other laparoscopic procedures with special appeal for the elderly population are lysis of adhesions as treatment for intestinal obstruction, highly selective vagotomy for peptic ulcer disease [152], repair of perforated duodenal ulcer with suture techniques or Graham's patch [153], anterior lumbar diskectomy and fusion, bladder neck suspension (Burch's procedure) for urinary incontinence [154], nephrectomy [155–157], ureterolithotomy [158], placement of feeding tubes, GI bypass and biliary bypass as palliative procedures for inoperable malignancies, and staging for various gynecologic malignancies. As these procedures are developed and follow-up information is accrued, they may become the standard for surgical therapy.

Summary

The use of laparoscopic surgical techniques to perform common operations has been unquestionably established and proven to be beneficial in young healthy patients. Some of these procedures have been undertaken in elderly patients with good results. Others are just now being evaluated for safety and efficacy in the geriatric population.

In terms of overall care of the elderly patient, the potential benefits of laparoscopic surgery are many. Early return to preoperative activity levels and diet, decreased metabolic stress and immunosuppression, less pulmonary impairment and fewer analgesic requirements, and improved cosmetic outcome are the principal benefits currently identified. In terms of cost-benefit analyses, it appears that laparoscopic surgical techniques may be superior to open procedures in some stations and comparable in many. This type of cost analysis will most certainly be forthcoming in this era of managed care.

The risks of laparoscopic surgery in the elderly center around the cardiovascular stress placed on the patient by the carbon dioxide pneumoperitoneum. These risks are significant, and great care in patient selection, preoperative preparation, and perioperative monitoring must be taken. Geriatric patients have a much lower tolerance for technical errors and delays in treatment and careful consideration of these risks must be made when a laparoscopic technique is considered.

The long-term results of most advanced laparoscopic surgical procedures are not known yet. Durability of laparoscopic herniorrhaphies, longevity of laparoscopic fundoplications, and long-term cure rates for laparoscopic colon resections for cancer are unknown at this time. Careful patient tracking and ongoing outcomes analysis are vital to ensure that the long-term results are acceptable. The great benefits of laparoscopic surgery in the short-term and the reasonable expectation that these procedures will produce good long-term results are compelling reasons to promote these procedures now. However, patients being considered for laparoscopic surgical procedures must be carefully informed about the lack of long-term follow-up on these procedures and that more conventional open surgical options are available to them. Laparoscopic general surgery is a new and exciting field that holds great promise for the future of care in the elderly.

REFERENCES

1. Nath G, Ghorisch W, Kreitmair A, Kiefhaber P. Transmission of a powerful argon laser beam through a fiberoptic flexible gastroscope for operative gastroscopy. Endoscopy 1973;5:213–215.
2. Fleischer D, Kessler F. Endoscopic Nd:YAG laser therapy for carcinoma of the esophagus: a new form of palliative treatment. Gastroenterology 1983;85:600–603.
3. Fleischer D. Palliative Therapy of Esophageal Carcinoma. In Fleischer D, Jensen D, Bright-Asare P (eds), Therapeutic Laser Endoscopy in Gastrointestinal Disease. Boston: Martinus Nijhoff, 1983;117–129.
4. Pasricha PJ, Ravich WJ, Hendrix TR, et al. Intrasphincteric botulinum toxin for the treatment of achalasia. N Engl J Med 1995;322:774–778.
5. Savides TJ, Jensen DM. Endoscopic therapy for severe gastrointestinal bleeding. Adv Intern Med 1995;40:243–271.
6. Marks G. Guidelines for the use of flexible fiberoptic colonoscopy in the management of patients with colorectal neoplasia. Dis Colon Rectum 1979;22:302–305.
7. Warner ME, Warner MA, Leonard PF. Anesthesia for neodymium-YAG (Nd-YAG) laser resection of major airway obstructing tumors. Anesthesiology 1984;60:230–232.
8. Rontal M, Rontal E. Laser Treatment of Tracheal and Endobronchial Lesions. In Dent TL, Strodel WE, Turcotte JG (eds), Surgical Endoscopy. Chicago: Year Book, 1985;391–406.
9. Cuschieri A. Exploration of the Common Bile Duct. In Cuschieri A, Berci G (eds), Common Bile Duct Exploration. Boston: Martinus Nijhoff, 1984;81–84.
10. Berci G. Choledochoscopy. In Dent TL, Strodel WE, Turcotte JG (eds), Surgical Endoscopy. Chicago: Year Book, 1985;349–361.
11. Blocker WP Jr. Maintaining functional independence by mobilizing the aged. Geriatrics 1992;47:42, 48–50, 53.
12. Budny PG, Lavelle J, Regan PJ, Roberts AH. Pretibial injuries in the elderly: a prospective trial of early mobilisation versus bed rest following surgical treatment. Br J Plast Surg 1993;46:594–598.
13. Mahoney J, Sager M, Dunham NC, Johnson J. Risk of falls after hospital discharge. J Am Geriatr Soc 1994;42:269–274.
14. Bates DW, Pruess K, Souney P, Platt R. Serious falls in hospitalized patients: correlates and resource utilization. Am J Med 1995;99:137–143.
15. Callahan CM, Wolinsky FD. Hospitalization for major depression among older Americans. J Gerontol 1995;50:M196–M202.
16. Dunham NC, Sager MA. Functional status, symptoms of depression, and the outcomes of hospitalization in community-dwelling elderly patients. Arch Fam Med 1994;3:676–680.
17. Verbosky LA, Franco KN, Zrull JP. The relationship between depression and length of stay in the general hospital patient. J Clin Psychiatry 1993;54:177–181.
18. Friedman SM, Williamson JD, Lee BH, et al. Increased fall rates in nursing home residents after relocation to a new facility. J Am Geriatr Soc 1995;43:1237–1242.
19. Glaser F, Sannwald GA, Buhr HJ, et al. General stress response to conventional and laparoscopic cholecystectomy. Ann Surg 1995;221:372–380.
20. O'Dwyer PJ, McGregor JR, McDermott EW, et al. Patient recovery following cholecystectomy through a 6 cm or 15 cm transverse subcostal incision: a prospective randomized clinical trial. Postgrad Med J 1992;68:817–819.
21. Schauer PR, Sirinek KR. The laparoscopic approach reduces the endocrine response to elective cholecystectomy. Am Surg 1995;61:106–111.
22. Mealy K, Gallagher H, Barry M, et al. Physiological and metabolic responses to open and laparoscopic cholecystectomy. Br J Surg 1992;79:1061–1064.
23. Bolufer JM, Delgado F, Blanes F, et al. Injury in laparoscopic surgery. Surg Laparosc Endosc 1995;5:318–323.
24. Senagore AJ, Kilbride MJ, Luchtefeld MA, et al. Superior nitrogen balance after laparoscopic-assisted colectomy. Ann Surg 1995;221:171–175.
25. Busby J, Caranasos GJ. Immune function, autoimmunity, and selective immunoprophylaxis in the aged. Med Clin North Am 1985;69:465–474.
26. Delafuente JC. Immunosenescence. Clinical and pharmacologic considerations. Med Clin North Am 1985;69:475–486.
27. Redmond HP, Watson RW, Houghton T, et al. Immune function in patients undergoing open vs laparoscopic cholecystectomy. Arch Surg 1994;129:1243–1246.

28. Poulin EC, Mamazza J, Breton G, et al. Evaluation of pulmonary function in laparoscopic cholecystectomy. Surg Laparosc Endosc 1992;2:292–296.
29. Beecher HK. The measured effects of laparotomy on respiration. J Clin Invest 1993;12:63.
30. Latimer RG, Dickman M, Day WC, et al. Ventilatory patterns and cardiopulmonary complications after upper abdominal surgery determined by preoperative pulmonary spirometry and blood gas analysis. Am J Surg 1971;122:622–633.
31. Fowler RW. Ageing and lung function. Age Ageing 1985;14:209–215.
32. Hendolin H, Lahtinen J, Lansimies E, et al. The effect of thoracic epidural analgesia on respiratory function after cholecystectomy. Acta Anaesthesiol Scand 1987;31:645–651.
33. Da Costa ML, Qureshi MA, Brindley NM, et al. Normal inspiratory muscle strength is restored more rapidly after laparoscopic cholecystectomy. Ann R Coll Surg Engl 1995;77:252–255.
34. Farrow HC, Fletcher DR, Jones RM. The morbidity of surgical access: a study of open versus laparoscopic cholecystectomy. Aust N Z J Surg 1993;63:952–954.
35. Wittgen CM, Naunheim KS, Andrus CH, Kaminski DL. Preoperative pulmonary function evaluation for laparoscopic cholecystectomy. Arch Surg 1993;128:880–885.
36. Barnett RB, Clement GS, Drizin GS, et al. Pulmonary changes after laparoscopic cholecystectomy. Surg Laparosc Endosc 1992;2:125–127.
37. Ramos JM, Beart RW Jr, Goes R, et al. Role of laparoscopy in colorectal surgery. A prospective evaluation of 200 cases. Dis Colon Rectum 1995;38:494–501.
38. Eggleston JM, London SD, Glasheen WP, et al. A retrospective analysis of 6,387 cholecystectomies. Med Prog Technol 1995;21:85–90.
39. Tucker JG, Ambroze WL, Orangio GR, et al. Laparoscopically assisted bowel surgery. Surg Endosc 1995;9:297–300.
40. Hardy KJ, Miller H, Fletcher DR, et al. An evaluation of laparoscopic versus open cholecystectomy. Med J Aust 1994;160:58–62.
41. Moiniche S, Bulow S, Hesselfeldt P, et al. Convalescence and hospital stay after colonic surgery with balanced analgesia, early oral feeding, and enforced mobilisation. Eur J Surg 1995;161:283–288.
42. Bufo AJ, Feldman S, Daniels GA, Lieberman RC. Early postoperative feeding. Dis Colon Rectum 1994;37:1260–1265.
43. Wiesel S, Grillas R. Patient-controlled analgesia after laparoscopic and open cholecystectomy. Can J Anaesth 1995;42:37–40.
44. Stoker DL, Spiegelhalter DJ, Singh R, Wellwood JM. Laparoscopic versus open inguinal hernia repair: randomised prospective trial. Lancet 1994;343:1243–1245.
45. Gales BJ, Menard SM. Relationship between the administration of selected medications and falls in hospitalized elderly patients. Ann Pharmacother 1995;29:354–358.
46. Dauleh MI, Rahman S, Townell NH. Open versus laparoscopic cholecystectomy: a comparison of postoperative temperature. J R Coll Surg Edin 1995;40:116–118.
47. Ho HS, Saunders CJ, Gunther RA, Wolfe BM. Effector of hemodynamics during laparoscopy: CO_2 absorption or intra-abdominal pressure? J Surg Res 1995;59:497–503.
48. Bongard FS, Pianim NA, Leighton TA, et al. Helium insufflation for laparoscopic operation. Surg Gynecol Obstet 1993;177:140–146.
49. Leighton T, Pianim N, Liu SY, et al. Effectors of hypercarbia during experimental pneumoperitoneum. Am Surg 1992;58:717–721.
50. McDermott JP, Regan MC, Page R, et al. Cardiorespiratory effects of laparoscopy with and without gas insufflation. Arch Surg 1995;130:984–988.
51. Rasmussen JP, Dauchot PJ, DePalma RG, et al. Cardiac function and hypercarbia. Arch Surg 1978;113:1196–1200.
52. Wahba RW, Beique F, Kleiman SJ. Cardiopulmonary function and laparoscopic cholecystectomy. Can J Anaesth 1995;42:51–63.
53. Feig BW, Berger DH, Dougherty TB, et al. Phamacologic intervention can reestablish baseline hemodynamic parameters during laparoscopy. Surgery 1994;116:733–739.
54. Westerband A, Van De Water J, Amzallag M, et al. Cardiovascular changes during laparoscopic cholecystectomy. Surg Gynecol Obstet 1992;175:535–538.
55. Torrielli R, Cesarini M, Winnock S, et al. Modifications hemodynamiques durant la coelioscopie: étude menée par bioimpedance electrique thoracique. Can J Anaesth 1990;37:46–51.
56. Wittgen CM, Andrus CH, Fitzgerald SD, et al. Analysis of the hemodynamic and ventilatory effects of laparoscopic cholecystectomy. Arch Surg 1991;126:997–1000.
57. Ortega AE, Peters JH. Physiologic Alterations of Endosurgery. In Peters JH, Demeester TR (eds), Minimally Invasive Surgery of the Foregut. St. Louis: Quality Medical, 1994;23–37.
58. Ho HS, Saunders CJ, Corso FA, Wolfe BM. The effects of CO_2 pneumoperitoneum on hemodynamics in hemorrhaged animals. Surgery 1993;114:381–387.
59. Odegerg S, Ljungqvist O, Svenberg T, et al. Haemodynamic effects of pneumoperitoneum and the influence of posture during anaesthesia for laparoscopic surgery. Acta Anaesthesiol Scand 1994;38:276–283.
60. Ishizaki Y, Bandai Y, Shimomura K, et al. Safe intra-abdominal pressure of carbon dioxide pneumoperitoneum during laparoscopic surgery. Surgery 1993;114:549–554.
61. Millard JA, Hill BB, Cook PS, et al. Intermittent sequential pneumatic compression in prevention of venous stasis associated with pneumoperitoneum during laparoscopic cholecystectomy. Arch Surg 1993;128:914–918.
62. Ido K, Suzuki T, Taniguchi Y, et al. Femoral vein stasis during laparoscopic cholecystectomy: effects of graded elastic compression leg bandages in preventing thrombus formation. Gastrointest Endosc 1995;42:151–155.
63. Ishizaki Y, Bandai Y, Shimomura K, et al. Changes in splanchnic blood flow and cardiovascular effects following peritoneal insufflation of carbon dioxide. Surg Endosc 1993;7:420–423.
64. Chiu AW, Chang LS, Birkett DH, Babayan RK. The impact of pneumoperitoneum, pneumoretroperitoneum, and gasless laparoscopy on the systemic and renal hemodynamics. J Am Coll Surg 1995;181: 397–406.
65. Irgau I, Koyfman Y, Tikellis JI. Elective intraoperative intracranial pressure monitoring during laparoscopic cholecystectomy. Arch Surg 1995;130:1011–1013.
66. Josephs LG, Este-McDonald JR, Birkett DH, Hirsch EF. Diagnostic laparoscopy increases intracranial pressure. J Trauma 1994;36: 815–818.
67. Pearson MRB, Sander ML. Hyperkalaemia associated with prolonged insufflation of carbon dioxide into the peritoneal cavity. Br J Anaesth 1994;72:602–604.
68. White SJ, Powers JS, Knight FR, et al. Effectiveness of an inpatient geriatric service in a university hospital. J Tenn Med Assoc 1994; 87:425–428.
69. Vendenbergh HC, Wilson T, Adams SE, Inglis MJ. Laparoscopic cholecystectomy: its impact on national health economics. Med J Aust 1995;162:587–590.
70. Lucier MR, Lee K. Trends in laparoscopic cholecystectomy in Indiana. Indiana Med 1995;88:200–204.
71. Murphree S, Dakovic S, Mauchaza B, Raju V. Laparoscopic cholecystectomy in Zimbabwe: initial report. Cent Afr J Med. 1993;39: 85–88.
72. Soper NJ, Stockmann PT, Dunnegan DL, Ashley SW. Laparoscopic cholecystectomy. The new 'gold standard'? Arch Surg 1992;127:917–921.
73. Spaw AT, Reddick EJ, Olsen DO. Laparoscopic laser cholecystectomy: analysis of 500 procedures. Surg Laparosc Endosc 1991;1:2–7.
74. Dubois F, Berthelot G, Levard H. Coelioscopic cholecystectomy: experience with 2006 cases. World J Surg 1995;19:748–752.
75. Steiner CA, Bass EB, Talamini MA, et al. Surgical rates and operative mortality for open and laparoscopic cholecystectomy in Maryland. N Engl J Med 1994;330:403–408.
76. Kesteloot K, Penninckx F. The costs and effects of open versus laparoscopic cholecystectomies. Health Econ 1993;2:303–312.
77. Wongworawat MD, Aitken DR, Robles AE, Garberoglio C. The impact of prior intra-abdominal surgery on laparoscopic cholecystectomy. Am Surg 1994;60:763–766.
78. Cappuccino H, Cargill S, Nguyen T. Laparoscopic cholecystectomy: 563 cases at a community teaching hospital and a review of 12,201 cases in the literature. Surg Laparosc Endosc 1994;4:213–221.
79. D'Albuquerque LA, de Miranda MP, Genzini T, et al. Laparoscopic cholecystectomy in cirrhotic patients. Surg Laparosc Endosc 1995;5: 272–276.
80. Massie MT, Massie LB, Marrangoni AG, et al. Advantages of laparoscopic cholecystectomy in the elderly and in patients with high ASA classifications. J Laparoendosc Surg 1993;3:467–476.
81. Passone-Szerzyna N, Navez B, Cambier E, et al. Laparoscopic cholecystectomy in the elderly patient. Ann Chir 1995;49:291–295.
82. Saxe A, Lawson J, Phillips E. Laparoscopic cholecystectomy in patients aged 65 or older. J Laparoendosc Surg 1993;3:215–219.

83. Stoker ME. Common bile duct exploration in the era of laparoscopic surgery. Arch Surg 1995;130:265–268.
84. Rhodes M, Nathanson L, O'Rourke N, Fielding G. Laparoscopic exploration of the common bile duct: lessons learned from 129 consecutive cases. Br J Surg 1995;82:666–668.
85. Feretis C, Kalliakmanis B, Benakis P, Apostolidis N. Laparoscopic transcystic papillotomy under endoscopic control for bile duct stones. Endoscopy 1994;26:697–700.
86. Millat B, Fingerhut A, Deleuze A, et al. Prospective evaluation in 121 consecutive unselected patients undergoing laparoscopic treatment of choledocholithiasis. Br J Surg 1995;82:1266–1269.
87. Shimi S, Banting S, Cuschieri A. Laparoscopy in the management of pancreatic cancer: endoscopic cholecystojejunostomy for advanced disease. Br J Surg 1992;79:317–319.
88. Watson DI, Jamieson GG, Devitt PG, et al. Changing strategies in the performance of laparoscopic Nissen fundoplication as a result of experience with 230 operations. Surg Endosc 1995;9:961–966.
89. McAnena OJ, Willson PD, Evans DF, et al. Physiological and symptomatic outcome after laparoscopic gastric fundoplication. Br J Surg 1995;82:795–797.
90. Frantzides CT, Carlson MA. Laparoscopic versus conventional fundoplication. J Laparoendosc Surg 1995;5:137–143.
91. Laycock WS, Oddsdottir M, Franco A, et al. Laparoscopic Nissen fundoplication is less expensive than open Belsey Mark IV. Surg Endosc 1995;9:426–429.
92. Hinder RA, Filipi CJ, Wetscher G, et al. Laparoscopic Nissen fundoplication is an effective treatment for gastroesophageal reflux disease. Ann Surg 1994;220:472–483.
93. Jamieson GG, Watson DI, Britten-Jones R, et al. Laparoscopic Nissen fundoplication. Ann Surg 1994;220:137–145.
94. Bittner HB, Meyers WC, Brazer SR, Pappas TN. Laparoscopic Nissen fundoplication: operative results and short-term follow-up. Am J Surg 1994;167:193–200.
95. Anvari M, Allen C, Borm A. Laparoscopic Nissen fundoplication is a satisfactory alternative to long-term omeprazole therapy. Br J Surg 1995;82:938–942.
96. Dent J. Recent views on the pathogenesis of gastro-oesophageal reflux disease. Baillieres Clin Gastroenterol 1987;1:727–745.
97. Khan TA, Shragge BW, Crispin JS, Lind JF. Esophageal motility in the elderly. Dig Dis 1977;22:1049–1054.
98. Peters JH, Heimbucher J, Kauer WK, et al. Clinical and physiologic comparison of laparoscopic and open Nissen fundoplication. J Am Coll Surg 1995;180:385–393.
99. Heller E. Extramukose kardiaplastik beim chronischen kardiospasmus mit dilatation des oesophagus. Mitt Grensgeb Med Chir 1914; 27:141–149.
100. Rosato EF, Acker M, Curcillo PG, et al. Transabdominal esophagomyotomy and partial fundoplication for treatment of achalasia. Surg Gynecol Obstet 1991;173:137–141.
101. Ferguson MK. Achalasia: current evaluation and therapy. Ann Thorac Surg 1991;52:336–342.
102. Csendes A, Braghetto I, Burdiles P, Csendes P. Comparison of forceful dilatation and esophagomyotomy in patients with achalasia of the esophagus. Hepatogastroenterology 1991;38:502–505.
103. Holzman MD, Sharp KW, Ladipo JK, et al. Laparoscopic surgical treatment of achalasia. Am J Surg, 1997;173:308–311.
104. Swanstrom LL, Pennings J. Laparoscopic esophagomyotomy for achalasia. Surg Endosc 1995;9:286–292.
105. Ancona E, Anselmino M, Zaninotto G, et al. Esophageal achalasia: laparoscopic versus conventional open Heller-Dor operation. Am J Surg 1995;170:265–270.
106. Pellegrini C, Wetter LA, Patti M, et al. Thoracoscopic esophagomyotomy. Initial experience with a new approach for the treatment of achalasia. Ann Surg 1992;216:291–296.
107. Bonavina L, Nosadini A, Bardini R, et al. Primary treatment of esophageal achalasia. Long-term results of myotomy and/or fundoplication. Arch Surg 1992;127:222–226.
108. Jaakkola A, Ovaska J, Isolauri J. Esophagocardiomyotomy for achalasia. Long-term clinical and endoscopic evaluation of transabdominal vs. transthoracic approach. Eur J Surg 1991;157:407–410.
109. Ellis FH Jr, Watkins E Jr, Gibb SP, Heatley GJ. Ten to 20-year clinical results after short esophagomyotomy without an antireflux procedure (modified Heller operation) for esophageal achalasia. Eur J Cardiothorac Surg 1992;6:86–89.
110. Thomson D, Shoenut JP, Trenholm BJ, Teskey JM. Reflux patterns following limited myotomy without fundoplication for achalasia. Ann Thorac Surg 1987;43:550–553.
111. Murray GF, Battaglini JW, Keagy BA, et al. Selective application of fundoplication in achalasia. Ann Thorac Surg 1984;37:185–188.
112. Pai GP, Ellison RG, Rubin JW, Moore HV. Two decades of experience with modified Heller's myotomy for achalasia. Ann Thorac Surg 1984;38:201–206.
113. Ellis FH Jr, Crozier RE, Watkins E Jr. Operation for esophageal achalasia. Results of esophagomyotomy without an antireflux operation. J Thorac Cardiovasc Surg 1984;88:344–351.
114. Ellis FH Jr, Gibb SP, Crozier RE. Esophagomyotomy for achalasia of the esophagus. Ann Surg 1980;192:157–161.
115. Rhodes M, Rudd M, O'Rourke N, et al. Laparoscopic splenectomy and lymph node biopsy for hematologic disorders. Ann Surg 1995;222:43–46.
116. Cadiere GB, Verroken R, Himpens J, et al. Operative strategy in laparoscopic splenectomy. J Am Coll Surg 1994;179:668–672.
117. Phillips EH, Carroll BJ, Fallas MJ. Laparoscopic splenectomy. Surg Endosc 1994;8:931–933.
118. Lefor AT, Melvin WS, Bailey RW, Flowers JL. Laparoscopic splenectomy in the management of immune thrombocytopenia purpura. Surgery 1993;114:613–618.
119. Childers JM, Lang J, Surwit EA, Hatch KD. Laparoscopic surgical staging of ovarian cancer. Gynecol Oncol 1995;59:25–33.
120. Fowler JM, Carter JR, Carlson JW, et al. Lymph node yield from laparoscopic lymphadenectomy in cervical cancer: a comparative study. Gynecol Oncol 1993;51:187–192.
121. Levy DA, Resnick MI. Laparoscopic pelvic lymphadenectomy and radical perineal prostatectomy: a viable alternative to radical retropubic prostatectomy. J Urol 1994;151:905–908.
122. Kerbl K, Clayman RV, Petros JA, et al. Staging pelvic lymphadenectomy for prostate cancer: a comparison of laparoscopic and open techniques. J Urol 1993;150:396–398.
123. Matsuda T, Arai Y, Terachi T, et al. Laparoscopic pelvic lymphadenectomy in patients with localized prostate cancer. Hinyokika Kiyo-Acta Urologica Japonica 1992;38:419–424.
124. Haas GP, Shumaker BP, Haas PA, Toth C. The role of laparoscopy in the management of prostatic cancer. Orv Hetil 1995;136:2005–2007.
125. Rioja Sanz C, Blas Marin M, Minguez Peman JM, Rioja Sanz LA. Laparoscopic pelvic lymphadenectomy for prostatic cancer. Ann Urol 1995;29:73–80.
126. Parra RO, Andrus C, Boullier J. Staging laparoscopic pelvic lymph node dissection: comparison of results with open pelvic lymphadenectomy. J Urol 1992;147:875–878.
127. Cirocco WC, Schwartzman A, Golub RW. Abdominal wall recurrence after laparoscopic colectomy for colon cancer. Surgery 1994;116: 842–846.
128. Hoffman GC, Baker JW, Fitchett CW, Vansant JH. Laparoscopic-assisted colectomy. Initial experience. Ann Surg 1994;219:732–743.
129. Van Ye TM, Cattey RP, Henry LG. Laparoscopically assisted colon resections compare favorably with open technique. Surg Laparosc Endosc 1994;4:25–31.
130. Leach SD, Modlin IM, Goldstein L, Ballantyne GH. Laparoscopic local excision of a proximal rectal carcinoid. J Laparoendosc Surg 1994;4:65–70.
131. Gadaleta D, Fantini GA, Silane MF, Davis JM. Neutrophil leukotriene generation and pulmonary dysfunction after abdominal aortic aneurysm repair. Surgery 1994;116:847–852.
132. Reissman P, Weiss E, Teoh TA, et al. Laparoscopic-assisted perineal rectosigmoidectomy for rectal prolapse. Surg Laparosc Endosc 1995;5:217–218.
133. Senagore AJ, Luchtefeld MA, MacKeigan JM. Rectopexy. J Laparoendosc Surg 1993;3:339–343.
134. Kusminsky RE, Tiley EH, Boland JP. Laparoscopic Ripstein procedure. Surg Laparosc Endosc 1992;2:346–347.
135. Ballantyne GH. Laparoscopically assisted anterior resection for rectal prolapse. Surg Laparosc Endosc 1992;2:230–236.
136. Ratelle R, Vollant S, Peloquin AB, Gravel D. Abdominal rectopexy (Orr-Loygue) in rectal prolapse: celioscopic approach or conventional surgery. Ann Chir 1994;48:679–684.
137. Luukkonen P, Mikkonen U, Jarvinen H. Abdominal rectopexy with sigmoidectomy vs. rectopexy alone for rectal prolapse: a prospective, randomized study. Int J Colorectal Dis 1992;7:219–222.

138. McKee RF, Lauder JC, Poon FW, et al. A prospective randomized study of abdominal rectopexy with and without sigmoidectomy in rectal prolapse. Surg Gynecol Obstet 1992;174:145–148.
139. Huber FT, Stein H, Siewert JR. Functional results after treatment of rectal prolapse with rectopexy and sigmoid resection. World J Surg 1995;19:138–143.
140. Baker R, Senagore AJ, Luchtefeld MA. Laparoscopic-assisted vs. open resection. Rectopexy offers excellent results. Dis Colon Rectum 1995;38:199–201.
141. Deen KI, Grant E, Billingham C, Keighley MR. Abdominal resection rectopexy with pelvic floor repair versus perineal rectosigmoidectomy and pelvic floor repair for full-thickness rectal prolapse. Br J Surg 1994;81:302–304.
142. Ramanujam PS, Venkatesh KS, Fietz MJ. Perineal excision of rectal procidentia in elderly high-risk patients. A ten-year experience. Dis Colon Rectum 1994;37:1027–1030.
143. Johansen OB, Wexner SD, Nogueras JJ, Jagelman DG. Perineal rectosigmoidectomy in the elderly. Dis Colon Rectum 1993;36:767–772.
144. DesGroseilliers S, Fortin M, Lokanathan R, et al. Laparoscopic appendectomy versus open appendectomy: retrospective assessment of 200 patients. Can J Surg 1995;38:178–182.
145. Richards W, Watson D, Lynch G, et al. A review of the results of laparoscopic versus open appendectomy. Surg Gynecol Obstet 1993;177:473–480.
146. Cox MR, McCall JL, Padbury RT, et al. Laparoscopic surgery in women with a clinical diagnosis of acute appendicitis. Med J Aust 1995;162:130–132.
147. Eller R, Bukhari R, Poulos E, et al. Intraperitoneal adhesions in laparoscopic and standard open herniorrhaphy. An experimental study. Surg Endosc 1997;11:24–28.
148. Wilson MS, Deans GT, Brough WA. Prospective trial comparing Lichtenstein with laparoscopic tension-free mesh repair of inguinal hernia. Br J Surg 1995;82:274–277.
149. Payne JH Jr, Grininger LM, Izawa MT, et al. Laparoscopic or open inguinal herniorrhaphy? A randomized prospective trial. Arch Surg 1994;129:973–979.
150. Millikan KW, Kosik ML, Doolas A. A prospective comparison of transabdominal preperitoneal laparoscopic hernia repair versus traditional open hernia repair in a university setting. Surg Laparosc Endosc 1994;4:247–253.
151. Liem MS, Kallewaard JW, de Smet AM, van Vroonhoven TJ. Does hypercarbia develop faster during laparoscopic herniorrhaphy than during laparoscopic cholecystectomy? Assessment with continuous blood gas monitoring. Anesth Analg 1995;81:1243–1249.
152. Dallemagne B, Weerts JM, Jehaes C, et al. Laparoscopic highly selective vagotomy. Br J Surg 1994;81:554–556.
153. Lau WY, Leung KL, Zhu XL, et al. Laparoscopic repair of perforated peptic ulcer. Br J Surg 1995;82:814–816.
154. Frankel G, Kantipong M. Sixteen-month experience with video-assisted extraperitoneal laparoscopic bladder neck suspension. J Endourol 1995;9:259–264.
155. McDougall EM, Clayman RV, Elashry O. Laparoscopic nephroureterectomy for upper tract transitional cell cancer: the Washington University experience. J Urol 1995;154:975–979.
156. Parra RO, Perez MG, Boullier JA, Cummings JM. Comparison between standard flank versus laparoscopic nephrectomy for benign renal disease. J Urol 1995;153:1171–1173.
157. Eden CG, Haigh AC, Carter PG, Coptcoat MJ. Laparoscopic nephrectomy results in better postoperative pulmonary function. J Endourol 1994;8:419–22.
158. Harewood LM, Webb DR, Pope AJ. Laparoscopic ureterolithotomy: the results of an initial series, and an evaluation of its role in the management of ureteric calculi. Br J Urol 1994;74:170–176.

Surgical Care for the Elderly, 2nd ed., edited by
R. Benton Adkins, Jr., and H. William Scott, Jr.
Lippincott–Raven Publishers, Philadelphia © 1998.

CHAPTER 8

Medical Oncology

John D. Hainsworth

The treatment of some types of advanced inoperable cancer has improved greatly since the 1970s, due to the development of effective systemic chemotherapy. Some cancers (e.g., Hodgkin's disease, non-Hodgkin's lymphoma, testicular cancer, and ovarian cancer) are potentially curable with combination chemotherapy, while appropriate treatment of many other advanced neoplasms results in relief of symptoms and prolongation of survival.

During the 1970s, when rapid improvements occurred in the systemic treatment of cancer, elderly patients were usually not included in treatment trials. The most important reason for this was the assumption, based on limited data, that elderly patients could not tolerate the side effects produced by such treatments. In addition, many cancer types most sensitive to chemotherapy occur predominantly in children or young adults. Conversely, several cancer types that increase in incidence with advancing age (e.g., pancreas, lung, and prostate) were relatively insensitive to chemotherapy.

More recently, the systemic treatment of cancer in the elderly has received specific attention and has been the focus of many clinical trials. The side effects of most chemotherapeutic agents in elderly patients have not been as formidable as once feared, and improvements in supportive care (e.g., better antiemetics, antibiotics, colony-stimulating factors) have also improved patient tolerance of chemotherapy. Some elderly patients with Hodgkin's disease, aggressive non-Hodgkin's lymphoma, ovarian cancer, and small cell lung cancer have been cured with systemic combination chemotherapy originally proven effective in younger patients [1–4]. In a number of treatable malignancies, combination regimens have been designed specifically for elderly patients in an attempt to decrease toxicity while maintaining treatment efficacy. In some cancers (e.g., breast cancer), differences in the natural history in elderly versus younger patients has led to differences in treatment approach.

This chapter contains a brief documentation of the increased cancer incidence in the elderly, along with a summary of our current understanding of the molecular biological basis for this increased incidence. Specific problems involving the use of cytotoxic drugs and radiation therapy in the elderly are considered, followed by a discussion of several tumor types in which the tumor biology and therapy is distinctive in the elderly.

CANCER INCIDENCE AND MORTALITY IN THE ELDERLY

Cancer is one of the most serious and pervasive illnesses affecting persons 65 years of age and older. Approximately 20% of the U.S. population is 55 years of age or older, but more than 80% of invasive cancers occur in this age group. In addition, 60% of all cancer deaths occur after 65 years of age; the median age for all cancer deaths is 68 years [5]. Figure 8-1 illustrates the striking increase in cancer incidence with advancing age. The increase is particularly rapid after age 40 and continues to increase steadily thereafter. Further increases in cancer incidence are predicted in the future, paralleling the steadily increasing percentage of elderly people in the United States.

Although certain cancers occur only in children and young adults, these neoplasms are rare and account for only a small fraction of the total cancer incidence. In contradistinction, most of the common types of cancer occur rarely in children and young adults and increase in incidence in the elderly. The five cancer types associated with the highest mortality in the United States are shown in Table 8-1; in each of these cancer types, elderly patients account for a large majority of the patients affected [6].

In addition to the increased incidence of most cancers in the elderly, the associated mortality is also higher. The major factor accounting for this difference is the tendency of elderly patients to have a more advanced stage of disease at the time of diagnosis [7,8]. When the survival of patients with similar stages is compared, treatment outcomes in the elderly are similar to those in younger patients for most cancer types [5]. Compliance with recommended screening procedures for breast, prostate, cervix, and colon cancer is

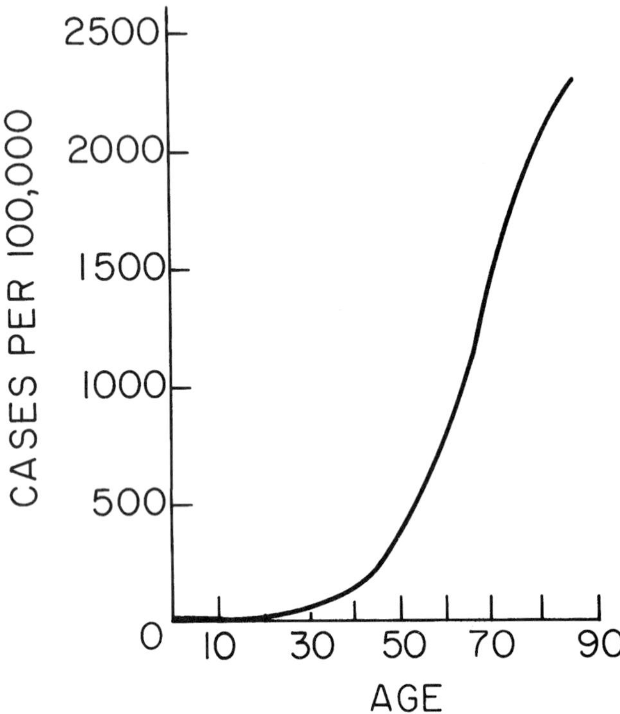

FIG. 8-1. Relationship of age and cancer incidence. (Data courtesy of Young JL, Percy CL, Asire AJ [eds]. Surveillance, epidemiology, and end results: incidence and mortality data, 1973–1977. Natl Cancer Inst Monogr 1981;57:1–1082.)

TABLE 8-1. *Mortality for the five leading cancer sites according to age, United States, 1991*

	Number of deaths by age group (%)		
Cancer type	<55	55–74	>75
Lung	14,418 (10)	86,044 (60)	43,296 (30)
Colon/rectum	4,777 (8)	25,005 (44)	27,413 (48)
Breast	9,849 (23)	19,900 (46)	13,834 (31)
Prostate	249 (1)	12,306 (37)	20,909 (62)
Pancreas	2,201 (9)	12,399 (49)	10,936 (42)

therefore of particular importance in the elderly, because of the higher incidence of these diseases and the proven effectiveness of treatment of early-stage cancer in this patient population. Various explanations for the later stage diagnosis in elderly patients include patient delay in seeking medical attention, increased difficulty in recognizing symptoms of cancer in the elderly, reluctance of the physician to refer the elderly cancer patient for treatment, and poor access by the elderly to the health care system.

PATHOGENESIS OF CANCER IN THE ELDERLY

From the mid-1980s through the mid-1990s, there has been a virtual explosion of knowledge concerning the molecular basis of carcinogenesis. Although a detailed discussion of the molecular basis of carcinogenesis is beyond the scope of this chapter, it is now firmly established that most cancers represent the endpoint of a multistep process of carcinogenesis that is manifest by sequential and progressive chromosomal abnormalities. A large number of oncogenes have been identified, which, when appropriately placed in the genome, can result in malignant transformation. Tumor suppressor genes have also been identified; inactivation of these genes also plays a role in malignant transformation [9,10]. Although molecular genetic changes within the individual cell are probably a result of random mutation, multiple genetic and environmental factors have been identified that increase the risk of these events occurring [11–13]. Vogelstein et al. proposed a genetic model of colorectal tumorigenesis, diagrammed in Figure 8-2. In this model, sequential and progressive genetic alterations are necessary before a carcinoma develops [14].

The large bulk of evidence therefore indicates that development of cancer in elderly patients is the culmination of a process that takes many years and requires multiple discrete intracellular changes to occur. According to this concept, age per se may not be associated with increased susceptibility to the process of carcinogenesis. However, others have noted subtle cytogenetic changes in the cells of older patients, in spite of the maintenance of a grossly stable diploid karyotype [15,16]. Age itself may therefore be an additional risk factor, with increased mutagenicity of aged cells increasing their susceptibility to malignant transformation.

Changes in immune function in elderly patients may also have a role in the development of some cancers. The concept of immune surveillance as a protection against the development of cancer was formerly popular [17]. According to this theory, one function of the normal immune system is to eliminate abnormal cells capable of giving rise to malignant tumors. The increased incidence of cancer in the elderly was explained by a decreased efficacy of the immune system in performing this function. Although some changes of the immune function are frequent in the elderly, little evidence exists to support this concept as a common explanation for the development of cancer [18,19].

USE OF CYTOTOXIC DRUGS IN THE ELDERLY

All drugs in current use for the systemic treatment of cancer, with the exception of a few hormonal agents, are cytotoxic agents. These drugs interfere with cell replication in a variety of ways including direct damage to DNA (alkylating agents), inhibition of synthesis of DNA and RNA precursors (antimetabolites), and interference with the mitotic mechanism (*Vinca* alkaloids, paclitaxel). Because cell replication in normal and neoplastic cells is similar, the therapeutic-to-toxic ratio of most antineoplastic agents is low, and side effects occur frequently with the use of these agents. Cancer patients with poor physical performance status at the time of

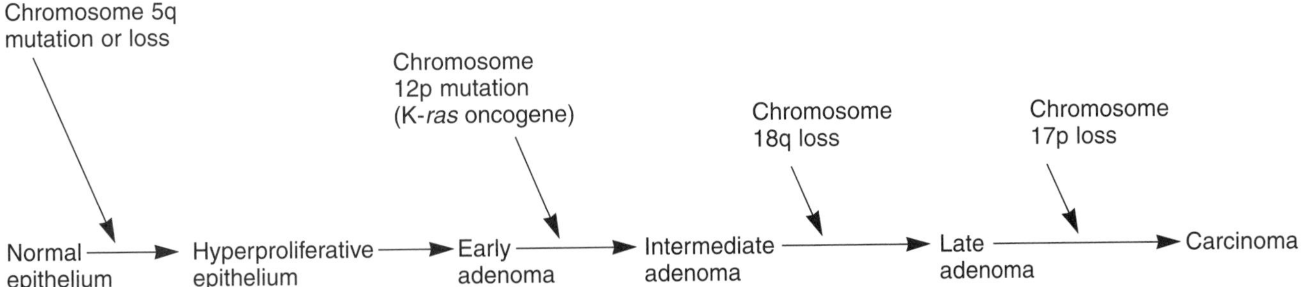

FIG. 8-2. Genetic model for colorectal tumorigenesis. Colorectal tumor arises through a series of genetic alterations involving oncogenes (*ras*) and tumor suppressor genes. Progression from early to late adenoma stages is characterized by increasing size, dysplasia, and villous content of the tumor. The accumulation of these events, rather than the order of their occurrence, is probably most important in carcinogenesis. (Adapted from Vogelstein B, Fearon ER, Hamilton SR, et al. Genetic alterations during colorectal tumor development. N Engl J Med 1988;319:525–530.)

TABLE 8-2. *Antineoplastic drugs associated with increased toxicity in the elderly*

Drug	Toxicity increased in elderly	Comment	Reference
Methotrexate	Myelosuppression	Decreased glomerular filtration rate causes delayed excretion	21, 22
Anthracyclines (doxorubicin, idarubicin); mitoxantrone	Congestive heart failure	Preexisting heart disease increases risk	25, 26
Bleomycin	Pulmonary fibrosis	Preexisting lung disease increases risk	28
Vinca alkaloids (vincristine, vinblastine); cisplatin; paclitaxel	Neurotoxicity	Preexisting neurologic dysfunction increases risk	29
Nitrosoureas	Myelosuppression	—	—
Glucocorticoids	Hyperglycemia	—	20

treatment experience more severe side effects when these agents are used.

Based on these observations, it was initially assumed that the use of antineoplastic agents in elderly patients would cause frequent and prohibitive side effects. Early clinical trials performed by cooperative groups routinely excluded patients over the age of 70 years and administered reduced doses of cytotoxic drugs if patients were between 60 and 70 years of age [20]. However, increased experience has indicated that age alone is not a good predictor of treatment-related toxicity, and patients are no longer excluded from clinical trials on this basis. However, specific chemotherapeutic agents and combinations remain problematic in the elderly; these are discussed in more detail.

Single Agents

Specific chemotherapy-related side effects more commonly experienced by elderly patients are outlined in Table 8-2. None of these side effects is peculiar to the elderly; rather, the incidence and severity increase with age.

Although many antineoplastic drugs cause myelosuppression, only methotrexate and the nitrosoureas have been particularly myelotoxic in the elderly [21]. Myelosuppression due to methotrexate is related to the dose administered and the duration of exposure; the decreased glomerular infiltration rate in most elderly patients delays excretion of methotrexate, increases duration of exposure, and therefore often results in increased myelosuppression [22]. Methotrexate can be used safely in elderly patients when the dose is modified based on the creatinine clearance [23]. The importance of adjusting dose based on creatinine clearance has also been recognized with other antineoplastic agents, including carboplatin [24]. The nitrosoureas can be associated with prolonged myelosuppression even in younger patients. This class of agents should be avoided in the elderly.

Cardiotoxicity associated with the use of the anthracyclines and related agents (e.g., doxorubicin, idarubicin, mitoxantrone) is a serious complication and is seen with increased frequency in the elderly [25,26]. The increased risk in elderly patients is probably related to preexisting compromise of cardiac function. Patients with significant congestive heart failure (i.e., ejection fraction <40%) are at high risk for early anthracycline-related cardiotoxicity. However, elderly patients with normal ejection fractions can safely receive doxorubicin and have a low incidence of clinically important cardiotoxicity at cumulative doses <450 mg/m^2. Alternate dosing schedules (e.g., low-dose weekly administration) have also proven less cardiotoxic [27].

Peripheral neuropathy is a toxicity associated with several antineoplastic agents including the *Vinca* alkaloids (vincristine, vinblastine), cisplatin, and paclitaxel. Peripheral neuropathy is related to the cumulative dose of these agents and is seen with greater frequency and severity in the elderly, particularly in those with preexisting neurologic deficits. The *Vinca* alkaloid–induced neurotoxicity can be particularly disabling in the elderly, and these drugs should therefore be used with great caution and promptly discontinued if significant peripheral neuropathy develops.

Bleomycin is associated with pulmonary fibrosis, which increases in frequency and severity when the cumulative dose exceeds 300 U [28]. Pulmonary fibrosis occurs with increased incidence in elderly patients and is probably related to preexisting chronic pulmonary disease. Because bleomycin-induced pulmonary fibrosis is irreversible, patients must be closely monitored with serial pulmonary function tests, particularly measurement of diffusing capacity. Patients of any age who have severe restrictive lung disease should not receive bleomycin therapy.

Combination Chemotherapy

The treatment of elderly patients with combination chemotherapy regimens has been approached with some trepidation, and only during the last decade has a substantial amount of data accumulated. In 1983, the Eastern Cooperative Oncology Group retrospectively reviewed the toxicity encountered by elderly versus younger patients participating in clinical trials [20]. Nineteen combination chemotherapy regimens used in studies involving eight different cancer types were retrospectively reviewed, and elderly patients (i.e., >70 years) were found to have identical rates of severe toxicity as their younger counterparts, with the exception of increased myelosuppression associated with methotrexate and methyl-lomustine. In addition, elderly patients had similar tumor response rates and survival rates when compared with the younger patients. It was recommended that physiologic functional parameters, such as measures of kidney, liver, and bone marrow function, or physical performance status be the basis of patient selection for chemotherapy, rather than age. Several more recent studies have confirmed these observations [29–31]. In a report from the Illinois Cancer Center, no differences were observed between elderly and younger patients participating in phase II trials when response rate, treatment-related toxicity, number of dose reductions, or number of treatment delays were compared [29].

Although these studies provide important data concerning the treatment of elderly patients, several factors must be considered before the data are generalized. Most of the types of cancer studied were incurable with chemotherapy, and the chemotherapy regimens used were of moderate intensity and administered with palliative intent. Only a minority of the patients enrolled in these cooperative group studies were older than 70 years, indicating a selection bias with inclusion of only unusually healthy elderly patients. It is doubtful that these results also apply to elderly patients with coexisting medical problems or poor performance status. Even though these data have resulted in a gradual change in the treatment offered to elderly patients with advanced malignancies, these patients remain under-represented in clinical trials. In 1990, only 29% of men and 26% of women enrolled in clinical trials were 65 years or older [32].

The treatment of elderly patients with the intensive combination chemotherapy regimens used for potentially curable neoplasms has been especially difficult. In these demanding regimens, drugs are administered in maximally tolerated doses, and the interval between doses is minimized. Specific problems with these intensive regimens when used in elderly patients include increased severity and duration of myelosuppression, declining physical performance status, severe muscular weakness, anorexia, and weight loss. These problems necessitate dose reductions and delays between doses, resulting in lower cure rates. Specific diseases in which these problems have been encountered include acute leukemia, Hodgkin's disease, non-Hodgkin's lymphoma, ovarian cancer, and adjuvant breast cancer treatment; several of these diseases are discussed more specifically in the remainder of this chapter.

In summary, the use of combination chemotherapy is feasible and beneficial in many elderly patients. Regimens of moderate intensity used to produce tumor remissions and prolongation of survival can be used with similar results and toxicity in patients of all ages. Certain chemotherapeutic agents must be used with caution in the elderly, particularly if specific organ dysfunction exists prior to treatment (Table 8-2). Although some elderly patients with Hodgkin's disease, non-Hodgkin's lymphoma, and acute leukemia can be cured with chemotherapy regimens, the intensive treatments required to cure these neoplasms are difficult to administer in the aged patient, and treatment results are still inferior in the elderly. Combinations designed specifically for elderly patients have recently been tested in non-Hodgkin's lymphoma and are discussed subsequently. Although increased toxicity is anticipated, elderly patients with reasonably good general health should be considered for curative chemotherapy for these diseases, because other curative modalities do not exist.

Radiation Therapy

Radiation therapy currently plays an integral role in the treatment of many cancers. Although most frequently used to provide palliation of local symptoms in patients with advanced cancer, radiation therapy may be used as the primary curative modality in several malignancies including testicular seminoma, early stage Hodgkin's disease, and some carcinomas of the head and neck, uterus, and cervix. Radiation therapy can produce distinctive acute and chronic tissue toxicity. Although radiation tolerance in elderly patients has not been specifically studied, it is generally accepted that the tolerance of normal tissues to irradiation is approximately 10% to 15% less in elderly patients.

Acute radiation effects are largely manifest in tissues with rapid rates of cell renewal such as bone marrow, skin, oropharyngeal mucosa, gastrointestinal tract, vaginal mucosa, and bladder mucosa. Acute radiation damage to these tissues depends not only on the radiation dose but also on the rate of administration. Short breaks between doses of radiation or decreases in the radiation fraction size can allow sufficient time for tissue repair and minimize acute toxicity. With modern radiotherapy equipment, acute toxicities can usually be minimized, particularly when a relatively low, palliative dose is being administered. In addition to direct tissue effects, elderly patients also experience increased constitutional symptoms such as fatigue, weakness, anorexia, and weight loss during radiation therapy.

The chronic side effects of radiotherapy are potentially more serious and are much more dependent on the total dose of radiation administered. Late effects include tissue necrosis, fibrosis, fistula formation, nonhealing ulceration, and damage to specific organs. Unfortunately, the effective tumoricidal radiation doses for some tumor types (e.g., head and neck cancers, cervical cancer, non–small cell lung cancer) are very close to the doses that produce major chronic tissue damage. Therefore, these problems are more likely to be encountered in patients receiving radiation therapy as definitive and potentially curative treatment for their cancer. In elderly patients, whose tissues are less tolerant of large doses of radiation, side effects are more frequent. In addition, preexisting impairment of specific organs can enhance their susceptibility to chronic radiation damage. A frequently encountered example of this problem is the difficulty in administering palliative doses of radiation therapy to elderly patients with non–small cell lung cancer in the face of significant preexisting pulmonary emphysema.

In spite of the mildly increased risk for chronic side effects, most elderly patients are able to receive radiation therapy without major problems. Tumor response to radiotherapy in the elderly seems to be identical to that in younger patients. The decision to use radiotherapy as either palliative or potentially curative treatment of cancer should not be made on the basis of age.

CANCERS WITH DISTINCTIVE CLINICAL FEATURES OR THERAPEUTIC CONSIDERATIONS IN THE ELDERLY

Breast Cancer

In recent years, recognition of a number of clinical and pathologic prognostic factors has helped explain the long-observed heterogeneity of patients with breast cancer. Age at the time of diagnosis is an important determinant of both tumor biology and prognosis; it is therefore not surprising that treatment recommendations for elderly women with breast cancer differ from those in younger women. This section highlights some of the differences in tumor biology and discusses recommended systemic therapy in elderly women with breast cancer.

TABLE 8-3. *Clinical profile of young versus elderly patients with breast cancer*

Clinical feature	Young	Elderly
Estrogen receptor	Negative	Positive
Histopathology	Poorly differentiated	Well differentiated
Growth rate	Fast	Slow
Metastatic sites	Viscera	Bone, soft tissue
Disease-free interval (mastectomy to recurrence)	Short	Long

Tumor Biology

The clinical profiles of young and old women with breast cancer are contrasted in Table 8-3. Considerable overlap exists; however, the differences in the parameters listed are substantial and help in part to explain the differences in response to therapy.

The measurement of cytosolic estrogen–receptor levels in breast cancer cells is of great value both prognostically and therapeutically. Estrogen receptors are present (>10 fmol/g of tumor tissue) in approximately 50% of patients with breast cancer; however, the incidence of estrogen receptor positivity increases steadily with age. Sixty percent of postmenopausal women have cancers that are positive for estrogen receptors; this figure increases to 70% to 80% in women over the age of 75 [33]. The estrogen receptor status of the tumor is the most powerful predictor of hormonal responsiveness; 60% of patients with tumors positive for estrogen receptors respond to hormonal therapy, whereas <10% of those with tumors negative for estrogen receptor respond [34]. Therefore, hormonal therapy is much more frequently an effective therapeutic option in elderly patients with metastatic breast cancer than it is in the younger patient.

The presence of estrogen receptors in breast cancer is also a favorable prognostic factor independent of therapy. Although the status of the axillary lymph nodes at the time of primary therapy remains the most important prognostic factor, patients with tumors positive for estrogen receptors have a lower recurrence rate than do those with tumors of similar stage that lack estrogen receptors. In patients with stage II estrogen receptor–positive breast cancer, the prognostic importance of the estrogen receptor status outweighs the importance of the axillary lymph node status. These patients have comparable or slightly better survival than do

TABLE 8-4. *Randomized trials comparing tamoxifen therapy with observation in patients with breast cancer*

Study [reference]	Tamoxifen dose (μg/day)	Duration of treatment (yrs)	Number of patients	Lymph nodes		Effect on survival	
				Positive	Negative	Disease-free	Overall
Copenhagen [90]	30	2	262	154	108	Increase	None
Christie [91]	20	1	961	349	297	Increase	Increase
NATO [92]	20	2	1,129	521	605	Increase	Increase
Scottish [93]	20	>5	1,312	456	751	Increase	Increase
ECOG [94]	20	2	170	168	0	Increase	None
Stockholm [95]	40	2 and 5	2,103	1,407	696	Increase	None
NSABP B-14 [44,45]	20	5	2,644	0	2,644	Increase	Increase
Toronto [96]	30	2	399	399	0	Increase	None
Caen/Royen [97]	40	3	179	179	0	Increase	None
Naples [98]	30	2	308	135	173	Increase	None
Cancer Research Campaign [99]	20	2	1,605	718	887	Increase	None

NATO = Nolvadex, Adjuvant Trial Organization; ECOG = Eastern Cooperative Oncology Group; NSABP = National Surgical Adjuvant Breast and Bowel Project.

patients with stage I estrogen receptor–negative tumors [35,36]. In addition, patients with tumors positive for estrogen receptors that do recur have a longer disease-free interval (i.e., time from mastectomy to recurrence) and longer survival with metastatic disease than do patients whose tumors are negative for estrogen receptors [34,37].

The other clinical and pathologic features listed in Table 8-3 are related to estrogen receptor status of the tumor as well as to patient age. Histologically well-differentiated tumors are much more likely to be positive for estrogen receptors [38]; these tumors also have a lower rate of proliferative activity [39]. Sites of recurrence are also related to estrogen receptor status. Recurrences in bone and soft tissue are more frequent in women with tumors positive for estrogen receptors, whereas visceral, particularly hepatic, involvement is seen more frequently in patients with tumors negative for estrogen receptors [40,41].

Two important prognostic factors are not age dependent. First, the stage at diagnosis is similar in young and elderly women in the United States. Second, the progesterone receptor status of the tumor, an independent prognostic variable, is unrelated to age [42,43]. Therefore, many elderly patients have adverse prognostic factors at the time of diagnosis and the cancer will recur despite optimal primary therapy.

Adjuvant Therapy

The administration of systemic therapy to breast cancer patients at risk for recurrence after primary surgical therapy has altered the natural history of breast cancer. Adjuvant therapy with either combination chemotherapy, hormonal therapy, or a combination of these treatments has been proven efficacious for most women following primary therapy. Based on the results of large randomized trials, treatment recommendations for premenopausal and postmenopausal women differ substantially.

Hormonal Therapy

Adjuvant therapy with tamoxifen is now firmly established as standard treatment for postmenopausal, estrogen receptor–positive patients following primary therapy. Results of large randomized studies comparing tamoxifen with observation alone are summarized in Table 8-4. Although the entry criteria differed somewhat in the various trials, all trials contained either exclusively or predominantly postmenopausal patients, most or all of whom had positive estrogen receptor status. Treatment with tamoxifen prolonged disease-free survival in all trials and also resulted in prolonged overall survival in several trials. Treatment benefits were observed in patients who had negative results for estrogen receptors as well as those who had positive results for estrogen receptors. The tamoxifen dose has varied in these studies, but there is no current evidence that doses >20 mg daily produce any additional benefit. Tamoxifen-related toxicity has been minimal. The optimal duration of therapy has not yet been established; however, results have generally been superior when tamoxifen is used for more than 2 years.

Most clinical trials have predominantly included patients with involved axillary lymph nodes (stage II), but recent data indicate that the magnitude of benefit is equivalent for patients with uninvolved axillary lymph nodes [44,45]. In studies of node-negative patients, most patients have had primary tumors >1 cm. Patients with node-negative breast cancer and primary tumors <1 cm have an extremely good prognosis, and therefore are unlikely to benefit from adjuvant therapy.

In summary, adjuvant tamoxifen therapy is now considered standard treatment for all postmenopausal patients, with the exception of patients whose lymph nodes test negative and who have very small (<1 cm) primary tumors. The magnitude of benefit is greater for patients with estrogen receptor–positive tumors. Long-term (5 years) treatment with tamoxifen is well tolerated, and may lead to decreased

TABLE 8-5. *Benefits of adjuvant therapy in premenopausal versus postmenopausal women*

	Age <50 years*		Age >50 years*	
Type of therapy compared	Recurrence (% + SD)	Death (% + SD)	Recurrence (% + SD)	Death (% + SD)
Combination chemotherapy vs. no treatment	37 ± 5	27 ± 6	22 ± 4	14 ± 5
Tamoxifen vs. no treatment	27 ± 7	NSD	30 ± 2	19 ± 3
Chemotherapy + tamoxifen vs. tamoxifen	NSD	NSD	26 ± 5	10 ± 7
Chemotherapy + tamoxifen vs. chemotherapy	7 ± 4	3 ± 5	28 ± 3	20 ± 4

*Data are expressed as a relative reduction in the annual odds of recurrence or death from any cause at 10 years.
NSD = not sufficient data.
Source: Data from Early Breast Cancer Trialists' Collaborative Group. Systemic treatment of early breast cancer by hormonal, cytotoxic, or immune therapy. 133 randomized trials involving 31,000 recurrences and 24,000 deaths among 75,000 women. Lancet 1992;339:1–15, 71–85.

cardiovascular events, decreased appearance of new primary breast cancer in the contralateral breast, and protection against the development of osteoporosis.

Combination Chemotherapy

The benefits of adjuvant combination chemotherapy have been more difficult to demonstrate in postmenopausal women than in premenopausal women. When examined individually, several trials that have demonstrated substantial benefits of chemotherapy in premenopausal women have failed to show statistically significant benefits in either disease-free survival or overall survival in elderly patients [46,47]. However, a recent meta-analysis of multiple published randomized trials including approximately 75,000 women revealed statistically significant reductions in the odds of recurrence or death from breast cancer in postmenopausal as well as premenopausal women receiving adjuvant chemotherapy [48]. From this analysis, summarized in Table 8-5, it is evident that the magnitude of benefit is less in postmenopausal than in premenopausal women, but that both groups derive a benefit from combination chemotherapy. Conversely, the benefit of hormonal therapy is greater in the postmenopausal women when compared with the premenopausal group. As with adjuvant hormonal therapy, the magnitude of benefit from adjuvant chemotherapy is similar in women whose nodes test positive and negative. Unfortunately, it is difficult to assess the benefits of chemotherapy in the very elderly (>70 years) group of women, because no trials have addressed this subgroup.

At present, adjuvant chemotherapy should be considered in postmenopausal women with estrogen receptor–negative breast cancer or in those with four or more lymph nodes that test positive if medical contraindications to such therapy do not exist. Adjuvant hormonal therapy should also be used in these women. Every effort should be made to use the same combination regimens at the same dose intensity as recommended for younger women. The benefit of adjuvant chemotherapy in women >70 years has not been adequately evaluated; at present, treatment in this group should be limited to patients who have excellent performance status and no major concurrent illnesses.

Metastatic Disease

The general guidelines for therapy of metastatic breast cancer in elderly women do not differ appreciably from those currently used in younger women. At present, metastatic breast cancer is considered to be an incurable disease, although appropriate treatment can palliate symptoms, provide meaningful remissions, and prolong survival in many patients. The goal of therapy for metastatic breast cancer is to provide patients with the best and longest remissions possible, while minimizing side effects of the palliative treatment.

In patients with hormonally responsive tumors, hormonal therapy usually provides longer remissions with less toxicity than does chemotherapy and should always be the first systemic treatment considered for estrogen receptor–positive breast cancer in postmenopausal women. A trial of hormonal therapy should also be considered in postmenopausal women with estrogen receptor–negative tumors who have other clinical features typical of estrogen receptor–positive tumors (e.g., well-differentiated histology, long interval from mastectomy to recurrence, and soft-tissue or bone metastases), because false-negative estrogen receptor determinations are well described [49]. The patient should receive a trial of hormonal therapy for at least 4 to 6 weeks; patients whose tumors respond favorably should then continue therapy as long as the response persists. Tamoxifen is usually the first drug used in hormonal therapy of breast cancer in postmenopausal women because of its ease of administration. Patients who relapse while on adjuvant tamoxifen or relapse after an initial response to tamoxifen for metastatic disease can achieve a second hormonal response with a different agent (e.g., progesterone, aminoglutethimide). The average duration of the first hormonal response is approximately 18 months; however, some patients have remissions that last several years.

Chemotherapy should be considered in patients whose tumors have become refractory to hormonal therapy or initially in patients who have visceral metastases and tumors that test negative for estrogen receptors. As in younger patients, chemotherapy with a combination of agents yields higher response rates and remissions of longer duration [50]. Approximately 60% of patients achieve a remission with initial chemotherapy; the average remission duration is 9 to 12 months. Problems with chemotherapy intolerance in elderly patients have been discussed earlier. In general, standard regimens for palliative treatment of breast cancer are of mild-to-moderate toxicity and can usually be tolerated by elderly patients. The recent development of chemotherapeutic agents with relatively favorable toxicity profiles, such as mitoxantrone and vinorelbine, has resulted in additional options for palliative therapy in breast cancer [51,52]. Pilot studies using combinations containing these new drugs have shown a high level of activity with considerably reduced toxicity, making these ideal regimens for use in elderly patients [53].

The patient with metastatic breast cancer, therefore, usually receives a series of treatments with various hormonal and chemotherapeutic agents and can have a series of remissions with sequential treatments. The use of combined chemotherapy and hormonal therapy or of more than one hormonal agent simultaneously does not increase remission duration or overall survival and should be avoided [54].

Hodgkin's Disease

The prognosis of Hodgkin's disease has been radically changed by the development of effective radiotherapy techniques and active combination chemotherapy. Optimal therapy now produces long-term, disease-free survival in at least 75% of patients, whereas this disease was formerly uniformly fatal. Important differences between young and elderly patients with respect to clinical features and treatment results have been appreciated as effective therapy has developed.

Hodgkin's disease is one of the few diseases that demonstrates a bimodal age incidence pattern, with the largest incidence peak occurring in young adults and a second small peak in the fifth and sixth decades of life. Several differences have been observed in the clinical and pathologic features of Hodgkin's disease in these two age groups. First, the histology differs, with young adults having a higher incidence of nodular sclerosing and lymphocyte-predominant subtypes, whereas elderly patients more often have tumors with mixed cellularity or lymphocyte-depleted histologic features [55]. Second, a higher percentage of elderly patients with Hodgkin's disease has advanced disease stage (III or IV) at the time of diagnosis. This difference in stage may be partially related to delay by older patients in seeking medical aid but is more probably related to the higher incidence of histologically unfavorable tumors in elderly patients [56]. Third, several epidemiologic features distinguish young and elderly persons developing Hodgkin's disease. Factors in the childhood environment associated with a higher incidence of Hodgkin's disease in the young age group include later age of exposure to common viruses, small sibship size, higher level of parental education, and living in single family dwellings [57]. None of these factors seems important in the elderly age group; in fact, the socioeconomic background of elderly patients with Hodgkin's disease was somewhat below average [57,58]. These differences have led to continued speculation that the etiology of Hodgkin's disease differs in the young and elderly age groups. Although the true etiology remains unknown, many investigators believe that Hodgkin's disease in young adults develops as a result of an abnormal response to certain viral exposures, whereas Hodgkin's disease in the elderly develops by a mechanism more similar to the development of other lymphomas in this age group [57,58].

Before the development of curative therapy for Hodgkin's disease, median survival in elderly patients was significantly worse than in younger patients [56]. This finding was not surprising because elderly patients tended to have higher stage disease and unfavorable histologic tumor types. However, age has remained an important prognostic factor in Hodgkin's disease even with the highly effective treatments currently available [1,59–63]. In a large Swedish study, the 5-year survival estimate was 28% in patients older than 50 years compared with 74% in younger patients [61]. In this study, marked differences persisted even in patients with early-stage disease (95% versus 55% actuarial 5-year survival) [64]. Other groups have reported more optimistic data for their elderly patients with early-stage Hodgkin's disease. Investigators at Stanford University reported an 86% 5-year survival in a small group of elderly patients with Hodgkin's disease who had pathologic stages I through IIIA and who were treated with definitive radiation therapy [1]. They stressed the importance of strict pathologic staging with laparotomy to determine optimal treatment in these patients. Patients with early-stage Hodgkin's disease who had only clinical staging also had a much lower survival (35%) with radiation therapy. Others have stressed the importance of using the same radiation therapy techniques in older patients as have proved effective in the treatment of early-stage Hodgkin's disease in younger patients. In one such comparison, actuarial 5-year disease-free survival rates were 61% in patients receiving radical radiation therapy versus only 6% receiving limited staging, limited field radiation, or both [65].

Results of treatment in elderly patients with advanced stage Hodgkin's disease (i.e., stages IIIB and IV) remain inferior to treatment results in younger patients. Difficulty in administering combination chemotherapy at optimal doses and schedules has been common. In one report, only eight of 18 elderly patients were able to receive 70% or more of the ideal calculated chemotherapy dose [1]. Recently, modified treatment approaches have included short courses of chemotherapy in combination with limited field radiation therapy and alternative chemotherapy regimens that are better tolerated in elderly patients [66,67]. It is likely that these approaches will improve the administration of optimal therapy to elderly patients and thereby improve cure rates. In spite of inferior treatment results, Hodgkin's disease nevertheless is a curable disease in some elderly patients. The approach to therapy in elderly patients should be the same as that recommended for younger patients, with careful initial staging followed by definitive radiation therapy or combination chemotherapy, dependent on the pathologic stage determined. Advances in supportive care, including cytokine therapy and improved antiemetics, will, it is hoped, enable elderly patients to tolerate the intensive combination chemotherapy required to cure Hodgkin's disease in a large percentage.

Non-Hodgkin's Lymphoma

Since the 1970s, substantial progress has been made in both the understanding and management of the non-Hodgkin's lymphomas. With improved pathologic techniques several types of non-Hodgkin's lymphoma have been recognized, each with a definable cell of origin and distinctive clinical behavior. Treatment for aggressive lymphomas has improved greatly; formerly, this group of lymphomas was uniformly fatal, with a median survival of 5 to 6 months. Current intensive combination chemotherapy allows 40% to 50% of patients to be cured [68].

The spectrum of non-Hodgkin's lymphoma in elderly patients differs from that in younger patients, because indolent (low-grade) lymphomas occur much more frequently in the elderly. Recognition and appropriate management of these lymphomas is important, because prolonged survival without treatment occurs in many patients [69]. The treatment of aggressive lymphomas in the elderly also poses special problems, because the intensive curative combination chemotherapy regimens are difficult to administer.

Indolent Non-Hodgkin's Lymphoma

Approximately 70% of lymphomas in patients >60 years of age are indolent or low grade. Histologically, most of these lymphomas retain nodular characteristics reminiscent of the nodules seen in normal lymph nodes. Immunologic typing reveals that most of these lymphomas are derived from B cells. Individual malignant cells are usually small and can either be cleaved cells derived from the follicular centers of the lymph nodes or have small round nuclei similar to the normal-appearing lymphocytes seen in chronic lymphocytic leukemia. Clinical presentation is variable, but most patients initially develop asymptomatic enlarging lymph nodes in multiple areas. Fluctuation in size of the lymph nodes is common, and spontaneous decrease in lymph node size is observed in 20% to 25% of patients. The majority of patients have asymptomatic bone marrow involvement with lymphoma at the time of diagnosis. Extranodal sites of involvement are uncommon early in the disease course but can become problematic in the later stages.

Although these lymphomas are sensitive to available chemotherapeutic agents and radiation therapy, these treatments are not curative in patients with indolent lymphomas. Even patients who achieve complete responses to therapy invariably relapse. In one series of patients with low-grade non-Hodgkin's lymphoma initially followed without treatment until symptoms occurred, the actuarial survival was 82% at 5 years and 73% at 10 years [70]. Because of the remarkable longevity of many patients, vigorous systemic therapy of indolent lymphomas is no longer used.

Indications for treatment in these patients include local symptoms due to bulky adenopathy, cytopenias due to bone marrow involvement, symptomatic extranodal involvement, or constitutional symptoms (e.g., fever, sweats, weight loss). Optimal treatment varies according to the clinical situation; local symptoms can often be effectively managed with a course of local radiation therapy, whereas systemic problems are usually managed with short courses of chemotherapy. Due to the indolent nature of many of these lymphomas, chemotherapy-induced partial remissions can provide prolonged palliation. Because achievement of complete remission is not an important goal, fewer drugs can be used at lower dosages. Therefore, effective management of these low-grade lymphomas is possible in elderly patients in whom local radiotherapy and moderate doses of chemotherapy are usually well tolerated. Because prolonged survival is the rule in these patients, careful follow-up and appropriate treatment of intercurrent problems are essential.

Aggressive Non-Hodgkin's Lymphoma

Most lymphomas in this group are large-cell lymphomas, formerly called *diffuse histiocytic lymphoma* in the Rappaport classification system. Almost all non-Hodgkin's lymphomas developing in young patients (<40 years of age) are aggressive lymphomas, compared with only 30% of all lymphomas in elderly patients. Although potentially curative treatments are available, even for patients with advanced stages, the effective treatment of aggressive lymphoma in the elderly has been difficult. Curative regimens for these lymphomas are among the most intensive regimens used in medical oncology and involve multiple cytotoxic agents given at frequent intervals [2,68]. These regimens have resulted in marked toxicity and increased treatment-related mortality when used in elderly patients [2,70,71]. Dose reductions and prolongations of the intervals between doses are often necessary due to increased myelosuppression [72,73].

Recent efforts have concentrated on the development of alternative combination chemotherapy regimens specifically tailored to elderly patients [71,74–78]. Most regimens have avoided specific drugs poorly tolerated by elderly patients (e.g., doxorubicin, vincristine) and have also limited the total duration of therapy. This approach has met with some success, and reported regimens are summarized in Table 8-6. Mortality has been generally low with these regimens, with high complete response rates and long-term, disease-free

TABLE 8-6. *Treatment results with combination chemotherapy regimens designed specifically for elderly patients with aggressive non-Hodgkin's lymphoma*

Investigator [reference]	Number of patients	Treatment regimen	Complete response rate (%)	Disease-free survival (%)
Heinz et al. [100]	34	CAOP (low dose)	62	27
Tirelli et al. [71]	25	ENPr	42	16
Solal-Celigny et al. [74]	34	CAP-T	56	24
Vose et al. [75]	112	CAP/BOP	61	34
McMaster et al. [76]	26	BECALM	50	27
O'Reilly et al. [77]	40	ACOP-B (low dose)	65	19
		VABE	63	34
Young et al. [78]	31	Chronic E/CNOP	64	56

C = cyclophosphamide; A = adriamycin; O = vincristine (Oncovin); P = prednisone; E = etoposide; N = mitoxantrone (Novantrone); Pr = prednimustine; T = teniposide; B = bleomycin; L = leucovorin; M = methotrexate; V = vinblastine.

survival in the 30% to 50% range. Active ongoing clinical research in this area is likely to further define optimal treatments for this population. These patients should therefore be treated with curative intent and given intensive supportive care to minimize side effects with therapy. Unlike breast cancer and Hodgkin's disease in the elderly, there is no suggestion that different tumor biology is responsible for the lower complete response rates; rather, inferior results are due to difficulties in administering effective treatment.

Acute Leukemia

The treatment of adult acute leukemia has improved since the 1970s, so that 70% to 80% of patients currently achieve complete remissions [79]. A variety of intensive regimens have been used to achieve 20% to 40% 5-year relapse-free survival [80–82]. In patients receiving optimal chemotherapy, age is the most important determinant of complete response rate and overall survival. Complete responses are currently achieved in >80% of young adults (16 to 40 years of age), in 65% of patients aged 40 to 60 years, and 30% to 55% of patients over the age of 60 [83].

The inferior treatment results in elderly patients stem from biological differences in the disease in elderly patients and from the difficulty in administering optimal therapy. Many elderly patients develop acute leukemia after a preleukemic prodrome, characterized by refractory cytopenias and a myelodysplastic bone marrow appearance. When acute leukemia arises in this setting, the leukemic cells carry specific chromosomal abnormalities associated with a lower complete remission rate and shorter survival [84]. Standard remission induction regimens are also difficult to administer to elderly patients because they produce approximately 4 weeks of chemotherapy-induced bone marrow aplasia. Serious infections and other treatment-related toxicity occur during this period with great frequency in elderly patients. Even after obtaining a complete remission, further intensive treatment is necessary to maximize remission duration. Two effective treatment approaches in this setting are allogeneic bone marrow transplantation and consolidation chemotherapy with high-dose cytarabine. Neither of these options is available to elderly patients, because of prohibitive toxicity [82,85,86].

Despite these difficulties, elderly patients without prohibitive coexistent medical problems deserve a trial of chemotherapy aimed at inducing complete remission. The achievement of complete remission remains the only treatment outcome that has any impact on survival. To date, attempts at lessening the intensity of chemotherapy have resulted only in a decrease in the complete response rate and are, therefore, a less effective therapy. As with other types of intensive therapy, improvements in supportive care techniques have decreased the risk of fatal complications related to myelosuppression.

Small Cell Lung Cancer

Combination chemotherapy is effective in prolonging survival in patients with small cell carcinoma of the lung. With optimal therapy, median survival is approximately 12 months compared with a median survival of 2 to 3 months in untreated patients. In this subset of patients with limited stage disease at diagnosis, combined modality therapy with chemotherapy and radiation to the chest results in a median survival of approximately 20 months, with 10% to 20% of patients disease-free at 3 years [4].

As with most other epithelial malignancies, the incidence of small cell lung cancer increases with age, and there is no evidence that the tumor biology is different in elderly patients. At the time of diagnosis, many elderly patients with small cell lung cancer also have poor performance status due to local and systemic tumor-related effects, as well as frequent coexistent chronic pulmonary disease. In these patients, the use of intensive combination chemotherapy regimens has been difficult. Again, regimens designed to minimize toxicity have been recently evaluated. The substitution of carboplatin for cisplatin in standard regimens results in decreased toxicity with equivalent efficacy [87]. The use of oral etoposide administered by chronic low-dose schedules has also provided an effective treatment alternative with minimal toxicity [88,89].

SUMMARY AND OVERVIEW

The field of medical oncology continues to undergo rapid change as new systemic treatments are developed. Since the mid-1980s, many problems peculiar to elderly patients have been recognized and addressed. Although this chapter focuses on differences that exist between young and elderly patients with cancer, it must be emphasized that *most* decisions in the treatment of the cancer patient should not be made on the basis of age. Surgical excision remains the only curative therapy for most types of cancer. All elderly patients with neoplasms amenable to surgical therapy should be considered for the same types of cancer operations offered to younger patients. Too often, elderly patients are thought to be poor candidates for radical cancer resections due to severe coexistent chronic medical problems. These patients receive lesser operations or nonsurgical palliative treatments and often die subsequently of metastatic cancer while the severe medical problems remain stable. Surgical therapy for most types of cancer is discussed elsewhere in this text.

The adult cancers for which potentially curative chemotherapy exists have been discussed separately in this chapter. In general, results of treatment of these neoplasms have been inferior in elderly patients. In some cancer types, differences in tumor biology play a role. However, the difficulties in administering intensive combination chemotherapy regimens to elderly patients, as well as bias against treating these patients intensively, are the major causes of treatment failure. All elderly patients with a reasonable performance status should receive a trial of therapy with the same potentially curative regimens used in younger patients. The proper dose and scheduling of drugs are crucial when administering these regimens, and the potential for cure is lost when doses are routinely decreased.

The majority of patients receiving chemotherapy have incurable neoplasms and are being treated to prolong survival or palliate symptoms. Chemotherapy regimens used in these situations are much less intensive than are those used in the treatment of potentially curable tumors. Elderly patients tolerate most palliative chemotherapy regimens as well as do younger patients, as long as their performance status is reasonably good. Recently, alternative regimens in selected malignancies have been developed for elderly and unfit patients, as discussed in this chapter.

Further advances in the field of medical oncology await the development of more effective and less toxic drugs. Elderly patients are now routinely included in trials of new therapeutic regimens; therefore, further improvements in our understanding of age-related differences in cancer biology and treatment are likely in the future.

REFERENCES

1. Austin-Seymour MM, Hoppe RT, Cox RS, et al. Hodgkin's disease in patients over sixty years old. Ann Intern Med 1984;100:13–18.
2. Klimo P, Connors JM. MACOP-B chemotherapy for the treatment of diffuse large-cell lymphoma. Ann Intern Med 1985;102:596–602.
3. Hainsworth JD, Burnett LS, Jones HW, et al. Advanced ovarian cancer: long-term results of treatment with intensive cisplatin-based chemotherapy of brief duration. Ann Intern Med 1988;108:165–170.
4. Johnson BE, lhde DC, Bunn PA, et al. Patients with small-cell lung cancer treated with combination chemotherapy with or without irradiation. Data on potential cures, chronic toxicities, and late relapses after a five to eleven year follow-up. Ann Intern Med 1985;103:430–438.
5. Young JL Jr, Percy CL, Asire AJ (eds). Surveillance, epidemiology, and end results: incidence and mortality data, 1973–77. Natl Cancer Inst Monogr 1981;57:1–1082.
6. Public Health Service. National Cancer for Health Statistics: Vital Statistics of the United States, 1991. Washington, DC: Public Health Service, 1994.
7. Holmes FF, Hearne E. Cancer stage-to-age relationship: implications for cancer screening in the elderly. J Am Geriatr Soc 1981;29:55–57.
8. Warnecke RB. The Elderly as a Target Group for Prevention and Early Detection of Cancer. In Yancik R, Yates JW (eds), Cancer in the Elderly: Approaches to Early Detection and Treatment. New York: Springer, 1989;3–14.
9. Fung Y-K T, Murphree AL, T'Ang A, et al. Structural evidence for the authenticity of the human retinoblastoma gene. Science 1987; 236:1657–1660.
10. Nigro JM, Baker SJ, Preisinger AC, et al. Mutations in the p53 gene occur in diverse tumor types. Nature 1989;342:705–706.
11. Mulkin D, Li FP, Strong LC, et al. Germline p53 mutations in a familial syndrome of breast cancer, sarcomas, and other neoplasms. Science 1990;250:1233–1236.
12. Bunney GE. Interactions of genes, environment and life-style in lung cancer development. J Natl Cancer Inst 1990;82:1236–1241.
13. Peto J, Seidman H, Selikoff IJ. Mesothelioma mortality in asbestos workers: implications for models of carcinogenesis and risk assessment. Br J Cancer 1982;45:124–135.
14. Vogelstein B, Fearon ER, Hamilton SR, et al. Genetic alterations during colorectal-tumor development. N Engl J Med 1988;319:525–532.
15. Shmookler Reis RJ, Goldstein S. Loss of reiterated DNA sequences during serial passage of human diploid fibroblasts. Cell 1980;21:739–749.
16. Lipschitz DA, Goldstein S, Reis R, et al. Cancer in the elderly: basic science and clinical aspects. Ann Intern Med 1985;102:218–228.
17. Burnet FM. Immunological Surveillance. Oxford: Pergamon, 1970.
18. Makinodan T, Adler WH. Effect of aging on the differentiation and proliferation potential of cells of the immune system. Fed Proc 1975;34:153–158.
19. Price GB, Makinodan T. Immunologic deficiencies in senescence: 1. Characterization of intrinsic deficiencies. J Immunol 1972;108:403–412.
20. Begg CB, Carbone PP. Clinical trials and drug toxicity in the elderly. The experience of the Eastern Cooperative Oncology Group. Cancer 1983;52:1986–1992.
21. Kristensen L, Wesimann K, Hutlers L. Renal function and the rate of disappearance of methotrexate from the serum. Eur J Clin Pharmacol 1975;8:439–444.
22. Hansen HH, Selawry OS, Holland JF, McCall CB. The variability of individual tolerance to methotrexate in cancer patients. Br J Cancer 1971;25:298–305.
23. Gelman RS, Taylor SG. Cyclophosphamide, methotrexate, and 5-fluorouracil chemotherapy in women more than 65 years old with advanced breast cancer: the elimination of age trends in toxicity by using doses based on creatinine clearance. J Clin Oncol 1984;2:1404–1413.
24. Calvert AH, Newekk DR, Gumbrell LA, et al. Carboplatin dosage: prospective evaluation of a simple formula based on renal function. J Clin Oncol 1989;7:1748–1756.
25. Praga C, Beretta G, Vigo PL, et al. Adriamycin cardiotoxicity: a survey of 1273 patients. Cancer Treat Rep 1979;63:827–837.
26. Von Hoff DD, Layard MW, Basa P, et al. Risk factors for doxorubicin-induced congestive heart failure. Ann Intern Med 1979;91:710–717.
27. Torti FM, Bristow MR, Howes AE, et al. Reduced cardiotoxicity of doxorubicin delivered on a weekly schedule: assessment by endomyocardial biopsy. Ann Intern Med 1983;99:745–749.
28. Haas CD, Coltman CA, Gottleib AJ, et al. Phase II evaluation of bleomycin: a Southwest Oncology Group Study. Cancer 1976;38:8–12.
29. Giovanazzi-Bannon S, Rademaker A, Lai G, Benson AB. Treatment tolerance of elderly cancer patients entered into phase II clinical trials: an Illinois Cancer Center Study. J Clin Oncol 1994;12:2447–2452.
30. Christman K, Muss HR, Case LD, et al. The relationship of age to treatment response in women with advanced breast cancer: the Pied-

mont Oncology Association experience [abstract]. Proc Am Soc Clin Oncol 1991;10:85.
31. Bicher A, Sarosy G, Kohn E, et al. Age does not influence Taxol dose intensity in recurrent carcinoma of the ovary. Cancer 1993;71:594–600.
32. Trimble EL, Carter CL, Cain D, et al. Representation of older patients in cancer treatment trials. Cancer 1994;74:2208–2214.
33. Kiang DT, Kennedy BJ. Factors affecting estrogen receptors in breast cancer. Cancer 1977;40:1571–1576.
34. Samaan NA, Buzdar AU, Aldinger KA, et al. Estrogen receptor: a prognostic factor in breast cancer. Cancer 1981;47:554–560.
35. Hahnel R, Woodings T, Vivian AB. Prognostic value of estrogen receptors in preliminary breast cancer. Cancer 1979;44:671–675.
36. Cooke T, George D, Shields R. Estrogen receptors and prognosis in early breast cancer. Lancet 1979;1:995–997.
37. Falkson G, Gelman RS, Pretorius FJ. Age as a prognostic factor in recurrent breast cancer. J Clin Oncol 1986;4:663–671.
38. Fisher ER, Redmond CK, Liu H, et al. Correlation of estrogen receptor and pathologic characteristics of invasive breast cancer. Cancer 1980;45:349–353.
39. Silvestrini R, Daidone MG, DiFronzo G. Relationship between proliferative activity and estrogen receptors in breast cancer. Cancer 1979;44:665–670.
40. Sherry MM, Greco FA, Johnson DH, Hainsworth JD. Metastatic breast cancer confined to the skeletal system: an indolent disease. Am J Med 1986;81:381–387.
41. Rosen PP, Menendez-Botet CJ, Urban JA, et al. Estrogen receptor protein (ERP) in multiple tumor specimens from individual patients with breast cancer. Cancer 1977;39:2194–2200.
42. Clark GM, McGuire WL, Hubay CA, et al. Progesterone receptors as a prognostic factor in stage II breast cancer. N Engl J Med 1993; 309:1343–1347.
43. Fisher B, Wickerham DL, Brown A, Redmond CK. Breast cancer estrogen and progesterone receptor values: their distribution, degree of concordance, and relation to number of positive axillary nodes. J Clin Oncol 1983;1:349–358.
44. Fisher B, Costantino J, Redmond C, et al. A randomized clinical trial evaluating tamoxifen in the treatment of patients with node-negative breast cancer who have estrogen receptor-positive tumors. N Engl J Med 1989;320:479–484.
45. Fisher B, Costantino J, Wickerham L, et al. Adjuvant therapy for node negative breast cancer: an update of NSABP findings [abstract]. Proc Am Soc Clin Oncol 1993;12:79.
46. Fisher B, Redmond C, Fisher ER. The contribution of recent NSABP clinical trials of primary breast cancer therapy to an understanding of tumor biology. Cancer 1980;46:1009–1025.
47. Bonadonna G, Rossi A, Tancini G, Valugussa P. Adjuvant chemotherapy in breast cancer [letter]. Lancet 1983;1:1157.
48. Early Breast Cancer Trialists' Collaborative Group. Systemic treatment of early breast cancer by hormonal, cytotoxic, or immune therapy. 133 randomized trials involving 31,000 recurrences and 24,000 deaths among 75,000 women. Lancet 1992;339:1–15, 71–85.
49. Hawkins RA, Hill A, Freedman B, et al. Reproducibility of measurements of oestrogen receptor concentration in breast cancer. Br J Cancer 1977;36:355–361.
50. Canellos GP, Pocock SJ, Taylor SG, et al. Combination chemotherapy for metastatic breast carcinoma: prospective comparison of multiple drug therapy with L-phenylalanine mustard. Cancer 1976;38:1882–1886.
51. Hainsworth JD. The use of mitoxantrone in the treatment of breast cancer. Semin Oncol 1995;22(Suppl 1):17–21.
52. Fumoleau P, Delgado FM, Delozier T, et al. Phase II trial of weekly intravenous vinorelbine in first-line advanced breast cancer chemotherapy. J Clin Oncol 1993;1:1245–1252.
53. Hainsworth JD, Andrews MB, Johnson DH, Greco FA. Mitoxantrone, 5-fluorouracil, and high-dose leucovorin: an effective, well tolerated regimen for metastatic breast cancer. J Clin Oncol 1991;9:1731–1736.
54. Australian and New Zealand Breast Cancer Trials Group. A randomized trial in postmenopausal patients with advanced breast cancer comparing endocrine and cytotoxic therapy given sequentially or in combination. J Clin Oncol 1986;4:186–193.
55. Hanson TAS. Histological classification and survival in Hodgkin's disease. Cancer 1964;17:1595–1603.
56. Tubiana M, Attie E, Flamant R. Prognostic factors in 454 cases of Hodgkin's disease. Cancer Res 1971;31:1801–1810.
57. MacMahon B. Epidemiology of Hodgkin's disease. Cancer Res 1966;26:1189–1200.
58. Gutensohn NM. Social class and age at diagnosis of Hodgkin's disease: new epidemiologic evidence for the "two-disease hypothesis." Cancer Treat Rep 1982;66:689–695.
59. Kaplan HS. Survival and relapse rates in Hodgkin's disease: Stanford experience, 1961–71. Natl Cancer Inst Monogr 1973;36:486–496.
60. Bjorkholm M, Holm G, Mellstedt H, et al. Prognostic factors in Hodgkin's disease. I. Analysis of histopathology, stage distribution, and results of therapy. Scand J Haematol 1977;19:487–495.
61. Wedelin C, Bjorkholm M, Biberfeld P, et al. Prognostic factors in Hodgkin's disease with special reference to age. Cancer 1984;53: 1202–1208.
62. Eghbali H, Hoerni-Simon G, Mascarel I. Hodgkin's disease in the elderly: a series of 30 patients aged older than 70 years. Cancer 1984;53:2191-2193.
63. Guinee VF, Giacco GG, Durand M, et al. The prognosis of Hodgkin's disease in older adults. J Clin Oncol 1991;9:947–953.
64. Collaborative Study. Survival and complications of radiotherapy following involved and extended field therapy of Hodgkin's disease stages I and II. Cancer 1976;38:288–305.
65. Zietman AL, Linggood RM, Brookes AR, et al. Radiation therapy in the management of early stage Hodgkin's disease presenting in later life. Cancer 1991;68:1869–1873.
66. Henkelmann GC, Hagemeister FB, Fuller LM. Two cycles of MOPP and radiotherapy for stage IIIA and stage IIIB Hodgkin's disease. J Clin Oncol 1988;6:1293–1302.
67. Horning SJ, Hoppe RT, Hancock SL, Rosenberg SA. Vinblastine, bleomycin, and methotrexate: an effective adjuvant in favorable Hodgkin's disease. J Clin Oncol 1988;6:1822–1831.
68. Fisher RI, Gaynor ER, Dahlberg S, et al. Comparison of a standard regimen (CHOP) with three intensive chemotherapy regimens for advanced non-Hodgkin's lymphoma. N Engl J Med 1993;328:1002–1006.
69. Horning SJ, Rosenberg SA. The natural history of initially untreated low-grade non-Hodgkin's lymphomas. N Engl J Med 1984;311: 1471–1481.
70. Armitage JD, Potter JF. Aggressive chemotherapy for diffuse histiocytic lymphoma in the elderly: increased complications with advanced age. J Am Geriatr Soc 1984;32:269–273.
71. Tirelli U, Zagonel V, Serraino P, et al. Non-Hodgkin's lymphoma in 137 patients aged 70 years or older: a retrospective European Organization for Research and Treatment of Cancer Lymphoma Group study. J Clin Oncol 1988;6:1708–1713.
72. Miller TP, Jones SE. Initial chemotherapy for clinically localized lymphomas of unfavorable histology. Blood 1983;62:413–418.
73. Vitolo U, Bertini M, Tarella C, et al. MACOP-B treatment for advanced stage diffuse large cell lymphoma: a multicenter Italian study. Eur J Cancer Clin Oncol 1989;25:1441–1449.
74. Solal-Celigny P, Chastang C, Herrera A, et al. Age as the main prognostic factor in adult aggressive non-Hodgkin's lymphoma. Am J Med 1987;83:1075–1079.
75. Vose JM, Armitage JD, Weisenburger DD, et al. The importance of age in survival of patients treated with chemotherapy for aggressive non-Hodgkin's lymphoma. J Clin Oncol 1988;6:1838–1844.
76. McMaster ML, Johnson DH, Greer JP, et al. A brief-duration combination chemotherapy for elderly patients with poor-prognosis non-Hodgkin's lymphoma. Cancer 1991;67:1487–1492.
77. O'Reilly SE, Klimo P, Connors JM. Low-dose ACOP-B and VABE: weekly chemotherapy for elderly patients with advanced-stage diffuse large cell lymphoma. J Clin Oncol 1991;9:741–747.
78. Young WA, Greco FA, Greer JP, Hainsworth JD. Aggressive non-Hodgkin's lymphoma in the elderly: an effective, well-tolerated treatment regimen containing extended-schedule etoposide. J Natl Cancer Inst 1994;86:1346–1347.
79. Gale RP, Foon KA, Cline MJ, Zighelboim J. Intensive chemotherapy for acute myelogenous leukemia. Ann Intern Med 1981;94: 753–757.
80. Peterson BA, Bloomfield CD. Long term disease-free survival in acute nonlymphocytic leukemia. Blood 1981;57:1144–1147.
81. Mayer RJ, Davis RB, Schiffer CA, et al. Intensive postremission chemotherapy in adults with acute myeloid leukemia. N Engl J Med 1994;331:896–903.
82. Zittoun RA, Mandelli F, Willemze R, et al. Autologous or allogeneic

bone marrow transplantation compared with intensive chemotherapy in acute myelogenous leukemia. N Engl J Med 1995;332:217–223.
83. Wiernik PH, Glidewell OJ, Hoagland HC, et al. A comparative trial of daunorubicin, cytosine arabinoside, and thioguanine, and a combination of the three agents for the treatment of acute myelocytic leukemia. Med Pediatr Oncol 1979;6:261–277.
84. Gajewski JL, Ho WG, Nimer SD, et al. Efficacy of intensive chemotherapy for acute myelogenous leukemia associated with a preleukemic syndrome. J Clin Oncol 1989;7:1637–1645.
85. Klingemann HG, Storb R, Fefer A, et al. Bone marrow transplantation in patients aged 45 years and older. Blood 1986;67:770–776.
86. Peterson BA, Bloomfield CD. Treatment of acute nonlymphocytic leukemia in elderly patients: a prospective study of intensive chemotherapy. Cancer 1977;40:647–652.
87. Gatzemeier V, Hossfeld DK, et al. Combination chemotherapy with carboplatin, etoposide and vincristine in first-line treatment in small cell lung cancer. J Clin Oncol 1992;10:818–823.
88. Clark PI, Cottier B. The activity of 10-, 14-, and 21-day schedules of single agent etoposide in previously untreated patients with extensive small-cell lung cancer. Semin Oncol 1992;19(Suppl 14):36–39.
89. Carney DN, Grogan L, Smit EF, et al. Single-agent oral etoposide for elderly small cell lung cancer patients. Semin Oncol 1991;17(Suppl 2):49–53.
90. Palshof T, Carstenson B, Morridshen HT, et al. Adjuvant endocrine therapy in pre- and postmenopausal women with operable breast cancer. Rev Endocrin Rel Cancer 1985;17(Suppl):43–50.
91. Ribeiro G, Swindell R. The Christie Hospital adjuvant tamoxifen trial—status at 10 years. Br J Cancer 1988;57:601–603.
92. Nolvadex Adjuvant Trial Organization. Controlled trial of tamoxifen as a single adjuvant agent in management of early breast cancer. Analysis at eight years by the Nolvadex Adjuvant Trial Organization. Br J Cancer 1988;57:608–611.
93. Breast Cancer Trials Committee, Scottish Cancer Trials Office. Adjuvant tamoxifen in the management of operable breast cancer: the Scottish Trial. Lancet 1987;2:171–175.
94. Cummings FJ, Gray R, Tormey DC, et al. Adjuvant tamoxifen versus placebo in elderly women with node-positive breast cancer: long-term followup and causes of death. J Clin Oncol 1993;11:29–35.
95. Rotqvist LE, Cedermark B, Glas U, et al. The Stockholm trial on adjuvant tamoxifen in early breast cancer: correlation between estrogen receptor level and treatment effect. Breast Cancer Res Treat 1987;10:255–266.
96. Pritchard K, Meakin JW, Boyd NF, et al. Adjuvant Tamoxifen in Postmenopausal Women with Axillary Node Positive Breast Cancer: An Update. In Salmon SE (ed), Adjuvant Therapy of Cancer V. Orlando, FL: Grune & Stratton, 1987;391–400.
97. DeLozier T, Julien J-P, Juret P, et al. Adjuvant tamoxifen in postmenopausal breast cancer: preliminary results of a randomized trial. Breast Cancer Res Treat 1987;7:105–110.
98. Bianco AR, DePlacido S, Gallo C, et al. Adjuvant therapy with tamoxifen in operable breast cancer: 10 year results of the Naples (GUN) study. Lancet 1988;2:1095–1099.
99. CRC Adjuvant Breast Trial Working Party. Cyclophosphamide and tamoxifen as adjuvant therapies in the management of breast cancer. Br J Cancer 1988;57:604–607.
100. Heinz R, Pawlicki M, Losonczy H, et al. Initial chemotherapy with an age-adjusted CHOP schedule in non-Hodgkin's lymphomas with an unfavorable prognosis. Haematologica 1986;71:473–479.

Surgical Care for the Elderly, 2nd ed., edited by
R. Benton Adkins, Jr., and H. William Scott, Jr.
Lippincott–Raven Publishers, Philadelphia © 1998.

CHAPTER 9

Nutrition and Aging

Richard Goldstein

The physician charged with caring for the elderly patient has the additional challenge of accounting for the physiologic changes that have occurred as part of the aging process. Some of these characteristic processes occur even in the well-nourished individual. However, in elderly patients, malnutrition occurs with alarming frequency. Malnutrition superimposed on the aging process appears to increase the risk of significant morbidity and mortality. Unresolved issues remain as to whether elderly patients with malnutrition can be identified preoperatively and whether preoperative interventions can then subsequently alter outcome. However, if preoperative interventions are failing to alter outcome, additional strategies may still be needed to improve the nutritional state of the geriatric patient. This chapter reviews the changes in metabolism and body composition that accompany aging, data on the nutritional state of the elderly population, assessments of the nutrient needs of elderly subjects, algorithms to determine nutritional status, and the relationship between malnutrition, morbidity, and mortality. Finally, this chapter reviews the data regarding nutritional intervention and outcome in elderly patients as well as possible future directions to improve the nutritional status of elderly patients.

CHANGES IN METABOLISM AND BODY COMPOSITION WITH AGING

A natural sequence of processes occurs with aging. They do not begin at one particular chronologic age, but manifest themselves as part of a continuum, often beginning in the third to fourth decade of life.

Overall, elderly patients take in fewer calories than younger patients [1]. This appears to take place in conjunction with a decline in the basal metabolic rate [2]. In the studies by Keys et al. [2], patients initially had their basal metabolic rates assessed at an average age of 49.8 years and then were followed for up to 25 years. These results were also compared with a population of young adults (average age, 21.9 years) followed for up to 19 years. The overall basal metabolic rate was 9.79% lower in the elderly compared with that of young patients. This equates to a decrease in the basal metabolic rate of 3.5% to 4% per decade. Similar findings have been reported by McGandy et al. [1]. However, if one views the basal metabolic rate in terms of fat-free mass [2], then the basal metabolic rate per kilogram of fat-free mass does decrease over time but to a lesser extent. Thus adjusted, this decrease is only 1% to 2% per decade of age. This reflects the fact that the percentage of fat as a component of body composition increases with age [2].

More significant than the decline in the overall basal metabolic rate is the change in overall body composition that accompanies aging. Cohn et al. [3] used measurements of total body potassium to determine the mass of muscle and nonmuscle lean tissue in normal male and female patients 20 to 80 years of age. The findings demonstrated that the skeletal muscle mass decreased 45% with age, whereas the nonmuscle lean mass did not change. Overall, lean body cell mass decreased 23% from the third decade to the eighth decade. Thus, muscle appears especially vulnerable to the normal aging process. This finding of decreased lean body mass with age has been supported by the findings of other investigators [4,5]. These studies have demonstrated a decrease in lean body mass with age and an increase in total body fat with age. The increase in total body fat with age has been extensively reviewed by Keys and Brozek [6].

One question that has yet to be definitively answered is whether this decrease in muscle mass is a mandatory manifestation of aging. The study by Evans and Campbell [7] specifically targeted the problem of sarcopenia or age-related loss in skeletal muscle mass. High-intensity resistance training was undertaken by a group of elderly men over a 12-week period. Within this group of patients, there was a significant increase in muscle strength. This correlated with an increase in the cross-sectional area of muscle as determined by computed tomographic scanning. Muscle biopsies demonstrated increases in type I and II fiber areas. This was accompanied by a 41% increase in the daily excretion of urinary 3-methylhistidine. 3-Methylhistidine is an amino acid produced during the synthesis of actin and myosin. During intracellular breakdown of actin and myosin, 3-methylhistidine is released and excreted in the urine. The urinary output of this methylated amino acid provides a reliable index of the rate of myofibrillar protein breakdown in the musculature of human patients [8]. An increase in this excretion rate, therefore, suggests an overall increase in total muscle mass. When an exercise program was applied to a group of frail, institutionalized elderly men and women, significant increases in strength and muscle area were observed [9]. This was particularly impressive in light of another study that showed that a substantial percentage of free-living elderly over age 75 could not lift 4.5 kg with their arms [10]. An extensive review [11] further examined the studies suggesting that resistance exercise can preserve both morphology and function in muscle. The structural changes attributable to aging include a decrease in total muscle mass, a decrease in the number and size of fast twitch fibers, loss of motor units, and neuropathic changes. All of these studies underscore the importance of preservation of muscle mass and suggest that programs could be designed that would help to preserve this mass. It remains unclear whether changes in body composition that accompany aging are entirely obligatory or whether cultural and societal patterns may influence body composition over several decades. The question could be raised as to whether changes in body composition merely follow changes in daily activities including exercise or whether intrinsic processes associated with aging are the dominant factor in changing body composition.

NUTRITIONAL STATE OF THE ELDERLY

In addition to changes in body composition associated with aging, there is a high incidence of nutritional abnormalities in the elderly. Zheng and Rosenberg [12] reviewed several studies in the literature, but also reported on a large group of elderly patients in the United States. Although the elderly patients had a slight decrease in total energy intake, of even more concern was that >40% of patients over 70 years of age took in less than two-thirds of the recommended daily allowance (RDA) of vitamin D, folic acid, vitamin B_6, and zinc. In another study of free-living middle-income elderly patients, approximately 13% of men and women took in less than the RDA of protein [13]. However, a substantial percentage of patients took in <50% of the RDA of vitamins and minerals including vitamins B_6, B_{12}, D, and E; folic acid; and zinc. To compensate for the deficiencies in dietary intake, most of the elderly patients in this study took supplementary vitamins and minerals such that only the intake of calcium and phosphorus lagged behind 1980 RDA. The concern remains that the total dietary intake in this population was only adequate as a result of vitamin and mineral supplements. A more economically disadvantaged population might find it more difficult to meet their nutritional requirements due to an inability to purchase the supplements.

Although the intake of vitamins and minerals has been shown to be particularly at risk in samplings of the healthy geriatric population, the intake of protein has been shown to be generally adequate in the healthy elderly population [13]. This finding was echoed in a study of apparently healthy elderly individuals in whom the intake of many nutrients was low whereas the intake of protein was generally thought to be adequate at 1.24 g of protein per kilogram of body weight [14]. Interestingly, although total caloric intake decreases with age, protein as a percentage of total caloric intake actually remains relatively constant [1].

Yet, further examination of protein intake in elderly patients raises other issues. There is a decrease in body cell mass with aging that correlates with decreased urinary creatinine excretion [5]. Measured body cell mass reflects metabolically active tissue including skeletal muscle. The decrease in body cell mass likely reflects a decrease in skeletal muscle mass with aging. A decrease in the absolute rate of whole-body protein breakdown in elderly patients was determined by using radiolabeled tracers. However, when the whole-body protein breakdown rate was expressed in terms of body cell mass, there was no change when compared with values obtained in young adults. Muscle protein breakdown was estimated by measuring 3-methylhistidine excretion. When expressed per unit of body weight, 3-methylhistidine excretion was decreased in the elderly. Furthermore, when muscle protein breakdown was expressed as a percentage of whole-body protein, values were significantly less in the elderly compared with young adults. Thus, muscle accounted for less of the whole-body protein breakdown in adults. This would suggest that there is less protein turnover in the skeletal muscle pool and, by inference, more turnover in the visceral pool. In another study, whole-body nitrogen flux was lower in elderly women compared with young women and tended to be lower in elderly men compared with young men [15]. Using sophisticated metabolic methodology to assess whole-body protein synthesis and breakdown, the data again suggested an increased reliance on visceral organs for whole-body protein flux compared with skeletal muscle. It can be argued that it is physiologically important for protein flux to remain at youthful levels. This turnover rate keeps free amino acids available to be used for new protein formation and gluconeogenesis as the situation demands. In younger patients, there is a greater reliance on skeletal muscle to contribute to this pool, whereas in the elderly, visceral organs such as the liver and intestine may be more at risk.

There are several other metabolic parameters that appear to change with age and that potentially place the aging subject at risk. Several studies have documented a decrease in total body water with age [16,17]. This decrease is fairly rapid over age 60 after beginning in middle age. Although the average water density of fat-free mass remains relatively constant with aging, the decrease in total body water with age likely reflects the decrease in lean body mass [17]. Because muscle has a greater amount of water per tissue mass than fat, the decrease in lean body mass translates into less total body water. Potentially, this decrease in total body water means that there is less fluid available for fluid shifts during stress. This may be the underlying reason that the elderly are more prone as a group to dehydration and electrolyte abnormalities [18] than younger patients. Superimposed on this decrease in total body water, there is a reduced sense of thirst in the elderly [18]. Thus, the elderly do not voluntarily rehydrate as well as younger patients. The mechanism for this is as yet unclear.

There is also a well-documented increase in insulin resistance that occurs with aging [19–21]. The result is that insulin, at a given concentration in the plasma, is not as effective in bringing about its metabolic effects. In addition to its function in regulating glycemia, insulin is an anabolic hormone and stimulates protein synthesis [22–26]. Thus, the increased insulin resistance that occurs with aging may impair the ability of elderly patients to effectively use metabolic substrates.

In looking more specifically at populations traditionally thought of as representing patients with greater surgical risk, several studies have examined the nutritional status of nursing home patients. In one study the incidence of malnutrition was 43%, with 16% of those characterized as severely malnourished [27]. Within the entire nursing home population sampled, 32% had a serum albumin of <3.5 g/dl and 19% were anergic to skin tests. Malnutrition is often categorized as either marasmus or kwashiorkor. Marasmus is defined in most studies as moderate-to-severe depletion of one or more somatic protein parameters. Kwashiorkor is generally defined as depletion of one or more visceral protein parameters. Both of these sets of parameters are discussed later in this chapter. In this group of nursing home patients, 48% of those determined to be malnourished had marasmus, 35% had both marasmus and kwashiorkor, whereas only 2% had kwashiorkor. The implication of this finding is that many of these patients had long-standing nutritional deficiencies. The data from this study of patients in the United States conflict with several Dutch studies [28,29] that examined the dietary intake in a large number of healthy independently living seniors. Although the elderly took in less energy and fewer nutrients, the overall intake of vitamins, minerals, and water was quite adequate. However, this was a fairly select group in that the patients had no chronic illnesses, had no recent hospitalizations, and 50% participated in regular exercise. Yet, the implication from virtually all of the previously mentioned studies is that adequate dietary intake can be achieved in significant segments of the elderly population. The issue may in part be the provision of adequate resources for this population.

Specifically looking at patients admitted to the hospital, several studies have documented surpassingly high rates of malnutrition in the elderly. One study looked at the nutritional status of 152 consecutive men admitted to a Veterans Administration (VA) hospital [30]; 59 of these patients were >65 years of age. According to their defined criteria, 41% of the overall group was malnourished. Focusing just on the elderly, 61% were malnourished. In an extensive study of 324 elderly patients admitted to a medical service [31], the overall presence of malnutrition was 30% in the men and 41% in the women. The presence of severe malnutrition was 16% in the men and 21% in the women. Of even more concern was the fact that nutritional parameters declined even further during the first 15 days of the admission, suggesting a tendency for the nutritional state of the patient to further deteriorate in the hospital.

Thus, in addition to occult or overt malnutrition that affects a significant percentage of elderly patients admitted to a hospital for elective and emergent surgery, the underlying assumption should be that these patients have a greater likelihood of dehydration than younger patients. This may increase the likelihood of perioperative hypotension and postoperative renal failure.

ENERGY ASSESSMENT IN THE ELDERLY

It is often necessary to determine the nutritional needs of elderly patients. In specifically assessing the nonprotein needs of humans, one of the most commonly known and used formulas is the Harris-Benedict formula [32,33]:

$$\text{Men: BEE (kcal/day)} = 66 + 13.7(W) + 5(H) - 6.8(A)$$

$$\text{Women: BEE (kcal/day)} = 655 + 9.6(W) + 1.7(H) - 4.7(A)$$

where BEE is basal energy expenditure, H is height in centimeters, W is weight in kilograms, and A is age in years. Remembering that the value derived is a *basal* value, it is common to then modify the BEE with a stress or activity factor [34,35].

The practical gold standard for estimating energy expenditure remains indirect calorimetry. Using this methodology, the oxygen consumption and carbon dioxide production are measured over a given period of time. A comprehensive review of indirect calorimetry was written by Ferrannini [36]. However, it is important to realize that the value derived is resting energy expenditure (REE). It is generally assessed while a subject is resting quietly for a period of 20 to 40 minutes [37]. Like the Harris-Benedict equation, various stress or activity factors [38–40] are then used to modify the value to arrive at the total metabolic energy expenditure. Therefore, the value derived is an estimate of the subject's true 24-hour energy expenditure.

Investigators at the University of Pennsylvania compared the REE determined using indirect calorimetry with 191 different published guidelines for nonprotein caloric requirements [41]. Assuming that the REE is the best estimation of the true energy needs of the patients [37], the concern was that only 48% of measured REE was within 90% to 110% of the requirements predicted by the Harris-

Benedict equation. In general, the formulas grossly overestimated the caloric needs of the patients. This overestimation would have led to significant overfeeding of the patients. The conclusion regarding overfeeding was made in the setting of fairly generous activity factors. In this study [41], patients received 25 to 35 nonprotein kcal/kg of body weight per 24 hours. In the patients determined to be relatively well nourished, 130% of their REE (REE × 1.3) was supplied. In the patients determined to be in need of fat repletion (current weight <95% of ideal body weight), 150% of their REE was supplied.

Further complicating the issue of caloric replacement is a recent finding suggesting that the caloric requirements necessary to repair a malnourished state may increase significantly with age [42]. In fact, if the goal is to maintain a steady body cell mass, which is considered the metabolically active pool, then caloric intake requirements may increase from 35 to 45 kcal/kg/day as the age of the subject increases from 60 to 80 years.

While the last study presented interesting data and future studies will almost certainly address caloric needs in the elderly, the delivery of approximately 30 to 35 kcal/kg of body weight per day is a reasonable initial target for adequately nourished patients. Within that delivery, carbohydrates should account for approximately 55% to 60% of the total caloric intake [43], with fat accounting for 30% to 40% of caloric intake. The elderly may be particularly in need of increased calories to combat malnutrition [42]. However, sudden overfeeding can bring about refeeding syndrome. The refeeding syndrome is extensively reviewed by Solomon and Kirby [44]. This syndrome is manifested by severe hypophosphatemia with potentially severe cardiac, neuromuscular, and hematologic dysfunction. The general mechanism appears to be initiated by total body depletion of phosphorus during starvation. With carbohydrate repletion and subsequent insulin release, there is movement of phosphorus from the extracellular space to the intracellular space, causing severe extracellular hypophosphatemia. This decrease in the extracellular phosphate pool may lead to depletion of phosphorylated compounds such as adenosine triphosphate in certain cells. Therefore, in the setting of long-standing severe malnutrition, nutritional intervention must be accompanied by close monitoring of electrolytes including phosphorus, magnesium, and potassium, as well as monitoring of the plasma glucose. Attention must also be paid to fluid overload and to watch for arrhythmias.

The protein requirements of elderly patients have been examined in several studies, but the results have not been in complete agreement. The most common approach has been to administer fixed amounts of protein to elderly patients for periods of 7 to 30 days and then to measure the patient's nitrogen balance. A positive nitrogen balance would suggest that adequate protein is being supplied in the diet and that the subject is anabolic. Thus, when assessing protein requirements as opposed to caloric requirements, there would appear to be simpler measurable endpoints that can be used to assess the general adequacy to protein supplementation. Such a graded intake approach was used to determine that in a group of elderly patients, protein intakes of 0.85 and 0.83 g/kg/day were appropriate for elderly men and women, respectively [45]. However, in another study, a diet providing 0.8 g/kg/day with an average energy intake of 32 and 29 kcal/kg/day for men and women, respectively, was provided [46]. In this study, approximately 50% of the patients were not in positive nitrogen balance after 30 days. Thus, the concern raised was that 0.8 g/kg/day may not be adequate. This same finding was echoed by two other studies [47,48]. In one of these studies [47], protein diets in elderly patients of 0.34 and 0.5 g/kg/day clearly left the patients in a negative nitrogen balance, whereas at 0.7 g/kg/day, one-third of patients still remained in negative nitrogen balance. In the other study, diets of various protein loads (0.4, 0.8, and 1.6 g/kg/day) were fed to young and elderly patients [48]. Nonprotein caloric intake was maintained at 40 kcal/kg/day. At a protein intake of 0.4 g/kg/day, all patients in both groups were in negative nitrogen balance. At 0.8 g/kg/day, five of eight of the elderly and six of nine young patients were in negative nitrogen balance. On the highest protein diet (1.6 g/kg/day) all patients were in positive nitrogen balance.

In another study of seven chronically ill elderly patients studied over 6 months, it was concluded that the best estimate of protein required to maintain nitrogen equilibrium was 0.8 g/kg/day. However, this estimate was based on regression analysis where the patient's mean protein intake ranged from 1.0 to 1.9 g of protein per kg. When a slightly different estimate of nonurinary nitrogen loss was introduced into the equations, the estimate of daily protein needs increased to 1.2 g/kg/day. Thus, although the current recommended dietary intake for the elderly (RDA) is 0.8 g/kg/day [32], there is considerable evidence that at 0.8 g/kg/day, there is a significant chance that the elderly subject will not be in an anabolic state. Therefore, it is probably reasonable to suggest that a protein intake closer to 1.0 to 1.25 g/kg/day [49] is necessary and reasonable for maintenance of an anabolic state in the elderly under nonstressed conditions.

However, many of the elderly who present for surgical care are significantly stressed. Under these conditions, protein requirements can increase significantly. Clark et al. have estimated that surgery alone increases baseline protein requirements by 30% [50,51]. Trauma and sepsis can double daily urinary nitrogen excretion, whereas a major burn injury can increase daily urinary nitrogen excretion fourfold [52]. In stressed patients, weekly determination of 24-hour urinary urea nitrogen excretion remains one of the most reasonable methods of following protein supplementation [52].

Thus, the current data would suggest that maintenance of normal protein needs in a healthy individual can likely be met by supplying approximately 0.8 to 1.2 g/kg/day of protein [53]. However, in the stressed or malnourished state, these needs increase to approximately 1.5 g/kg/day.

VITAMIN REQUIREMENTS IN THE ELDERLY

The RDA of vitamins and minerals for adults >51 years of age are reviewed in Table 9-1 [32]. It is important to realize that these recommendations encompass a wide age range. Thus, the issue of whether vitamin requirements are different in the age group of those >70 years of age compared with those between age 51 and 70 years is not yet known but is controversial. This is because there is evidence that requirements for certain vitamins may change with advanced age [54]. In particular, requirements for vitamins D, B_{12}, and B_6 may increase with age, whereas requirements for vitamin A and folic acid may decrease with age.

Vitamin A appears to be important for certain aspects of the immunologic response to infection [55]. It also appears to play a role in wound healing and cell growth [56]. There is evidence that elderly patients may not be able to clear retinyl esters, produced as a product of vitamin A metabolism, through the liver as efficiently as younger patients. Thus, elderly patients may be particularly susceptible to vitamin A toxicity [57]. However, although it appears that vitamin A requirements in the elderly should be lowered, specific target levels have not been identified [55,58].

As noted earlier in this chapter, surveys of elderly patients have demonstrated that significant percentages of the population have suboptimal vitamin D intake [13]. In addition to poor dietary intake of vitamin D, a decrease in the active form of vitamin D may coexist due to a decreased ability of senile skin to synthesize vitamin D combined with poor sun exposure [57]. Vitamin D supplementation has been shown to be an effective and practical method to achieve vitamin D prophylaxis in elderly patients [59,60].

The elderly are also prone to have decreased vitamin B_{12} levels [57]. Vitamin B_{12} is perhaps best known for its association with pernicious anemia [56]. Vitamin B_{12} is essential for DNA synthesis as well as for several aspects of fat and carbohydrate metabolism [56]. Several studies have documented a high incidence of B_{12} deficiency as a cause of anemia in elderly patients [61,62]. This may be further complicated by malabsorption, a condition that affects a significant number of elderly men and women [63]. In one study, many elderly patients with malabsorption also had vitamin B_{12} deficiency [64]. Parenteral vitamin B_{12} therapy corrected the malabsorption. This suggests that intestinal epithelial cells depleted of B_{12} may have impaired enterocyte function, leading to further malabsorption.

As the previously mentioned studies suggested, it is important to realize that although requirements for vitamins may change with age, malabsorption further exacerbates nutritional deficiencies. In fact, malabsorption from the gastrointestinal tract is more prevalent in the elderly [63]. This incidence of unsuspected malabsorption in the elderly has

TABLE 9-1. *Recommended daily dietary allowances for adults over 51 years of age*

	Men	Women
Protein (g/kg)	0.8	0.8
Vitamin A (μg RE)	1,000	800
Vitamin D (IU)	400	400
Vitamin E (mg)	10	8
Vitamin C (mg)	60	62
Thiamine (mg)	1.2	1.0
Riboflavin (mg)	1.4	1.2
Niacin (mg)	16	13
Vitamin B_6 (mg)	2.2	2.0
Folic acid (μg)	400	400
Vitamin B_{12} (μg)	3.0	3.0
Calcium (mg)	800	800
Phosphorus (mg)	800	800
Magnesium (mg)	350	300
Iron (mg)	10	10
Zinc (mg)	15	15
Chromium (μg)	50–200	50–200
Selenium (μg)	50–200	50–200
Iodine (μg)	150	150
Water	30 ml/kg/day	30 ml/kg/day
Energy 51–75 yrs	2,400 kcal	1,800 kcal
Energy >75 yrs	2,050 kcal	1,600 kcal

Source: Adapted from Nelson R, Franzi L. Nutrition and aging. Med Clin North Am 1989;73:1531–1550.

been estimated at 5% to 12%. In patients with suspected malabsorption, the incidence of documented malabsorption was 50% [65]. Folic acid is another vitamin whose requirements may decrease with age [55]. Folates are extremely important, as they are involved in many metabolic pathways and are needed for DNA synthesis [56]. Despite evidence that the nutritional requirement for folic acid decreases with age, many elderly patients are identified with folic acid deficiency [63,66]. In addition to poor dietary intake, malabsorption can result in impaired folic acid intake despite decreased whole-body folic acid needs [63,66].

Malnutrition remains a major problem in the geriatric population. In addition to protein-calorie malnutrition, the elderly are at risk for vitamin deficiencies. Although there is evidence that the daily requirements of certain vitamins may change with age, the most common problem facing physicians taking care of the elderly relative to vitamins are vitamin deficiencies. The causes can include both decreased dietary intake and malabsorption. In particular, in those elderly patients either admitted to the hospital or institutionalized, the incidence of malnutrition is disturbingly high. As is discussed later in this chapter, there is a correlation between significant malnutrition and poor outcome in the hospital.

ALGORITHMS TO DETERMINE NUTRITIONAL STATUS

One of the issues in the field of nutrition has been whether those patients who are malnourished can be prospectively identified and whether patients with nutritional deficiencies can be objectively categorized. The goal is to identify those patients at greatest risk for subsequent morbidity and mortality based on their malnourished state. One component of such a nutritional assessment is to use measurements of the physical body. These measurements are known as anthropometric data, and the anthropometric norms are affected by age [67]. In addition to height and weight, anthropometric data also encompass such parameters as percent of ideal body weight, mid-arm circumference, mid-arm muscle area, and triceps skinfold measurements [32,68]. Some formulas also take into account the fact that the physique of patients changes with age. With age, there is a progressive decrease in height. In some patients, obtaining a true height can prove difficult. Formulas that address these changes allow a determination of height based on knee height, age, and sex [69].

$$\text{Stature for men} = 64.19 - (0.04 \times \text{age}) + (2.02 \times \text{knee height})$$

$$\text{Stature for women} = 84.88 - (0.24 \times \text{age}) + (1.83 \times \text{knee height})$$

One of the most comprehensive nutritional and metabolic assessments using anthropometric as well as biochemical data was that proposed by Blackburn et al. [70]. To complete the profile, an extensive database was obtained on each patient. A representative sample of nutritional and metabolic parameters used to determine the nutritional profile on a hospitalized patient is presented here. The complete list of parameters is reported by Blackburn et al. [70].

- Height in centimeters
- Weight in kilograms
- Basal energy expenditure in kilocalories per day
- Actual weight as a percentage of ideal weight
- Actual triceps skinfold thickness as a percent of the norm
- Actual mid-upper arm muscle circumference as a percent of the norm
- Creatinine/height index
- Serum albumin level
- Serum transferrin level or total iron-binding capacity
- Total lymphocyte count
- Skin testing for anergy
- Nitrogen balance
- Apparent net protein use
- Weight change as a percent of usual weight
- Body surface area in square meters
- Caloric intake as a multiple of BEE

Using these parameters, various nutritional parameters were derived. An estimation of the arm muscle circumference was derived from the arm circumference and the triceps skinfold [70]. The creatinine height index was determined by comparing the actual daily urinary creatinine excretion with an ideal value based on height and sex. The major markers of visceral protein status included the serum albumin, serum transferrin, immune function including total lymphocyte count, and the response to skin testing. The skin tests consisted of streptokinase-streptodornase, mumps, and *Candida* antigens. The BEE was based on the Harris-Benedict equation. Using this extensive database, a nutritional profile was then generated by the computer. The two major categories for malnutrition were marasmus and kwashiorkor. As discussed elsewhere in this chapter, marasmus is a variant of protein-calorie malnutrition characterized by the depression of anthropometric measurements. A kwashiorkor-like syndrome is characterized by a depletion of visceral protein stores. Patients can also exhibit characteristics of both syndromes [70]. Using these criteria, patients were grouped within these two categories as depicted in Table 9-2. The significance of this assessment was the establishment of parameters that allowed objective criteria used to define patients. Such criteria are essential for monitoring the response to nutritional therapy.

TABLE 9-2. *Classification of malnutrition based on parameters used to assess the severity and type of malnutrition*

Marasmus	% Ideal weight	Creatinine height index (%)	Skin test (mm)
Moderate	60–80	60–80	—
Severe	<60	<60	<5

Kwashiorkor-like	Serum albumin	Serum transferrin	Total lymphocyte count	Skin test (mm)
Moderate	2.1–3.0	100–150	800–1,200	<5
Severe	<2.1	<100	<800	<5

Source: Adapted from Blackburn GL, Bistrian BR, Maini BS, et al. Nutritional and metabolic assessment of the hospitalized patient. JPEN J Parenter Enteral Nutr 1977;1:11–22.

However, this level of monitoring is quite intense and cannot easily be performed in most physician or hospital practices. A study was performed that compared clinical judgment with the objective measurements [71]. The objective criteria were the same used by Blackburn et al. [70]. Clinical judgment was made after a careful history was taken and a physical examination was performed. The history and physical examination placed emphasis on manifestations and signs of malnutrition. The authors concluded that there was very good correlation between clinical judgment and objective measurements of malnutrition. In the group of patients clinically judged to be malnourished, subsequent rates of infection and length of hospital stay were markedly elevated. These authors subsequently named this the Subjective Global Assessment [72] and listed the specific items to be included in the history and physical assessment that could help identify those patients at greatest risk for malnutrition. The items evaluated in the patient history included weight loss, change in dietary intake, gastrointestinal symptoms, functional capacity, and the metabolic demands of the patient's underlying disease state. There were four features of the physical examination that were rated on a four-point scale from normal (0) to severe (3+). These features included loss of subcutaneous fat in the triceps region and the midaxillary line at the level of the lower ribs, muscle wasting in the quadriceps and deltoids, the presence of edema in both the ankles and the sacral region, and the presence of ascites. Based on this evaluation, the clinician then can assign one of three nutritional categories to the subject: well nourished, moderately malnourished, or severely malnourished.

Another approach is to focus on only a few objective laboratory tests that are usually routinely obtained as part of a hospital admission. This evaluation is known as the *instant nutritional assessment* [73]. The laboratory tests include the complete blood count with differential and what is commonly known as the SMA-12. From these, the total lymphocyte count and the serum albumin level are obtained. In those patients with an abnormal serum albumin (<3.5 g/dl), there was a fourfold increase in hospital complications and a sixfold increase in death. In those patients with an abnormal total lymphocyte count (<1,500/mm^2), there was no statistical increase in complications but a fourfold increase in the probability of hospital mortality. When both of these were abnormal, there was a fourfold increase in the probability of complications and a 20-fold increase in death. When Blackburn and Harvey used the serum albumin level as the primary objective indicator of outcome in patients at risk for malnutrition, they determined that a serum albumin level of 3.1 to 3.2 g/dl was the 50% point for probability of anergy, sepsis, and death [35]. An initial serum albumin level of <2.2 g/dl was associated with >75% risk of having concurrent anergy, sepsis, and subsequent death [74].

Another nutritional assessment, the prognostic nutritional index (PNI), was developed by Buzby et al. [75]. A computer-based stepwise regression procedure was used to select the most important predictive variables relating the risk of operative morbidity, mortality, or both to nutritional status. The PNI (percent) was defined as:

$$\text{PNI}(\%) = 158 - 16.6(\text{ALB}) - 0.78(\text{TSF}) - 0.20(\text{TFN}) - 5.8(\text{DH})$$

where PNI is the risk of a complication occurring in an individual patient, ALB is serum albumin level (g/100 ml), TSF is triceps skinfold (mm), TFN is serum transferrin level (mg/dl), and DH is cutaneous delayed hypersensitivity reactivity to any of the three antigens: streptokinase-streptodornase, mumps, and *Candida* antigens. One hundred patients were then classified as high risk (PNI ≥50), intermediate risk (40 ≤ PNI ≤ 49), or low risk (PNI <40). A highly significant increase in the actual incidence of death, complications, and sepsis was noted as PNI increased.

More recently, Buzby et al. [76,77] have described the nutritional risk index calculated according to the following formula:

$$\text{Nutritional risk index} = 1.519 \times \text{ALB (g/liter)} + 0.417 \times \text{(current weight per usual weight)} \times 100$$

A score ≤100 is suggestive of malnutrition. This formula was used in the Veterans Affairs Parenteral Nutrition Cooperative Study and is discussed later in this chapter [77].

MALNUTRITION, MORBIDITY, AND MORTALITY

As discussed earlier, the incidence of both occult and overt malnutrition in the elderly can be surprisingly high. As discussed briefly in the previous section, there is a relationship between malnutrition and outcome parameters including mortality. In a study of geriatric patients admitted to a VA hospital [30], hospital mortality was 28% in the group of malnourished geriatric patients versus only 4% in the nonmalnourished group. In a study of geriatric nursing home patients [27], 19% were anergic to skin testing. Prospectively over the next 6 months, anergic patients had a mortality of 48%, whereas those in the immunocompetent group had a mortality of 12.5%. In another study of elderly patients admitted to the geriatric unit of a VA hospital, the top three predictors of subsequent complications were the serum albumin level, an index of function known as the Katz Index of Activities of Daily Living, and the total amount of weight lost over the past year [78]. The Katz Index measures functional independence in six categories including bathing, dressing, toileting, transferring, continence, and feeding. Another study looked specifically at the predictive value of a low serum albumin level [79]. This study first identified 509 VA patients with a serum albumin level of ≤3.4 g/dl. The mean age of this group was 59.4 years. The overall 30-day mortality from all causes in these patients was 24.6%. The results also demonstrated that mortality was linearly inversely related to the serum albumin level. The highest mortality was present in those patients with a serum albumin level of ≤2.0 g/dl. In this group, the all-cause 30-day mortality was 62%.

Several studies have focused on the relationship between malnutrition and morbidity rather than mortality. One study focused on elderly nursing home patients with pressure sores [80]. In this study of 232 patients with an average age of 73 years, the overall incidence of malnutrition was 59%. These were grouped into mild, moderate, and severe malnutrition categories according to referenced methods. Seventeen of the 232 patients had pressure sores. Of these patients with pressure sores, 100% were anergic to skin testing and 71% had primarily kwashiorkor as the predominant manifestation of their malnutrition. All of these patients also had a serum albumin level of 2.6 g/dl or less. In reporting those patients who were malnourished but without pressure sores, the incidence of anergy was only 25%, and the average serum albumin level was 3.3 g/dl. Finally, in those patients who were well nourished, no patients had pressure sores. Thus, in this study, parameters suggesting severe malnutrition correlated with patients who had developed the morbid complication of pressure sores.

A Swedish study examined whether nutritional parameters were predictive for subsequent morbidity [81]. The overall rate of hospital complications was 48% in those patients with abnormal nutritional parameters while it was 23% in those with normal nutritional parameters. Correlating with the increased rate of complications, the length of hospital stay was doubled in those patients with malnutrition. The serum albumin level again emerged as one of the most predictive parameters, although the serum prealbumin level was strongly predictive for subsequent complications.

A good review of the link between nutritional status and clinical outcome was published by Dempsey et al. [82]. One of the points the authors make is that the more parameters measured in a study, the higher the probability that one or more of the nutritional parameters will be abnormal. Thus, the incidence of malnutrition in any given subject pool can vary markedly based on what parameters are being assessed. These authors developed the PNI discussed previously [75]. Using their predictive parameters, those patients with a PNI value of >40 had a very high probability of subsequent morbidity.

Thus, numerous studies have established a clear link between malnutrition and subsequent risk for major morbidity and death. This relationship holds in the adult population as a whole as well as in elderly patients. The next question is whether nutritional intervention can decrease the rate of complications and death in the general population and, specifically, whether nutritional intervention can alter outcome in the geriatric population.

NUTRITIONAL INTERVENTION

In many cases, surgical care of the elderly must be provided on an emergent or urgent basis. Thus, for the geriatric malnourished patient with a hip fracture, there is little time to "beef up" that patient. While the elderly subject presenting with a gastric carcinoma may be able to receive nutritional support for several weeks prior to operative resection, it would be less likely that a period of over 1 month without either operative or chemotherapeutic intervention could be contemplated. From the discussion earlier in the chapter, most patients with significant malnutrition can be identified preoperatively. The question then becomes what type of nutritional intervention and for what period of time is clinically effective and, perhaps, cost-effective.

In most cases, nutritional intervention needs to be in the form of enteral tube feeding or total parenteral nutrition (TPN). The intact gut should be used whenever possible [83], and there are studies that document the relative safety of enteral feedings [84,85]. Although catheter sepsis can be a significant problem for patients supported with TPN [86], there are a few reports of significant complication rates, primarily aspiration pneumonia, in patients enterally fed via a nasogastric tube [87]. Even after placement of a gastrostomy tube, aspiration pneumonia can still be a significant problem [87]. There is also evidence that during intravenous alimentation, forearm metabolism bears many similarities to that which occurs after a mixed meal in normal patients [88]. This finding is reflected in another study in which whole-body substrate oxidation rates were similar regardless of whether nutrition was administered enterally or parenterally [89]. Probably most importantly, however, there are no data to substantiate claims that outcome is improved with enteral versus parenteral feeding [90]. Thus, although an enteral route is the generally preferred route of nutritional support, individual patient circumstances often dictate the mode of nutritional supplementation, and in some cases parenteral administration will be the only available route to provide substrates. Despite the reported safety of enteral feeding, most outcome studies have focused on TPN and its effect on subsequent morbidity and mortality. However, to date, there have been few studies that have specifically focused on nutritional support and outcome in elderly patients.

NUTRITIONAL SUPPORT, MORTALITY, AND MORBIDITY

First, focusing on TPN in the adult surgical patient, Mullen et al. [91] applied the PNI retrospectively to stratify patients who either received or did not receive preoperative TPN before a surgical procedure. Approximately 45% of the patients in each group had a PNI ≥50 and thus were considered severely malnourished. The rate of major complications was 18% in the group that received at least 7 days of preoperative TPN, whereas the rate of major complications was significantly increased at 38.9% in the group that did not receive preoperative TPN. In the group that received preoperative TPN, the mortality was 4%, and in the group that did not receive preoperative TPN the mortality was 29.4%. When outcome was compared for patients who received preoperative TPN relative to those who received no preoperative TPN, there was a significant difference only for those patients identified as high risk (PNI ≥50). However, most of the patients who did not receive TPN preoperatively did receive TPN postoperatively. Thus, some nutritional support was provided to most patients in the immediate perioperative period. One could argue that greater differences may have been detected between the two groups in terms of morbidity and mortality if postoperative TPN was not administered in the group that did not receive preoperative TPN.

Fairly similar conclusions were reached by the well-publicized Veterans Affairs Study [77]. In this study, patients admitted before nonemergency laparotomy or thoracotomy underwent nutritional screening. A component of the nutritional screening included the nutrition risk index described earlier in this chapter. Patients who appeared to meet the criteria for malnourishment were then randomized to either receive preoperative TPN or no TPN. The patients receiving TPN underwent surgery after receiving what was defined as adequate TPN for at least 7 days. These patients also received TPN for at least 3 days postoperatively. Of 3,259 potentially eligible patients, 782 patients were eligible for the study; 459 of those were entered. Although this was not a study of geriatric patients per se, the mean age of this study group was 63 years.

Overall, the rates of major complications during the first 30 days after surgery in the groups were similar, as was the rate of mortality. In fact, there were more infectious complications in the TPN group compared with the control group. However, when the patients were subdivided by degree of malnutrition, a different picture emerged. In the severely malnourished group, infectious complications were no higher in the TPN group compared with the control group. More importantly, the incidence of noninfectious complications was decreased in the TPN group (5% vs. 43%). Thus, these two studies [77,91] suggest that nutritional support can positively alter outcome and hospital course in surgical patients. However, patients most likely to benefit are the severely malnourished patients when nutritional support is instituted at least 7 days prior to their operative procedure. The converse conclusion would be that TPN should not be used in nonseverely malnourished patients [92]. Further information on clinical trials of TPN is summarized in three recent reviews on this subject [90,93,94]. Another issue is whether the elderly are more subject to complications when nutrition is withheld. In one study suggesting that underfeeding places patients at risk for pulmonary complications, normal patients were infused with just enough of an amino acid solution to prevent a negative nitrogen balance [95]. One group received only this amino acid solution with no nonprotein calories, whereas the control group received 550 kcal per day of additional nonprotein calories. In the group receiving only amino acids, there was noted a severe depression in hypoxic drive. In the group receiving nonprotein calories in addition to amino acids, hypoxic drive was preserved. Thus, when the study is designed to look at the impact of withholding nutritional support, at least this one report would suggest there is a negative impact. The perhaps more practical issue of how long nonseverely malnourished patients can go without adequate nutritional support has not been addressed to any significant extent [90].

Although the previously referenced studies on the efficacy of TPN dealt with general surgical populations with mean ages of approximately 63 years, there have been a few studies that have specifically addressed nutritional support and outcome in the geriatric population. Two studies have addressed dietary supplementation in elderly patients who had sustained femur fractures [96,97]. The first study focused on a severely malnourished group of elderly patients with femur fractures, and showed that nightly enteral nutritional supplementation significantly decreased mortality, rehabilitation time, and length of hospital stay [96]. These improvements appeared to correlate with faster recovery of the prealbumin level, as well as positive changes in anthropometrics. Similar improvements in terms of hospital length of stay, rehabilitation progress, and the complication rates were also detected in the second study [97]. Another study assessed protein breakdown and amino acid (leucine) incorporation into protein in elderly patients who had sustained hip fractures [98]. In this study, measurable increases in protein synthesis were detected in elderly patients supplemented with TPN. Although the study lacked a true control group, the results suggest that protein synthesis can be augmented in the elderly through nutritional supplementation.

FUTURE DIRECTIONS

Significant mortality and morbidity are still observed in elderly patients even in the setting of adequate nutritional supplementation. It has also been difficult to prove that nutritional support in the perioperative period is efficacious in well-nourished to moderately malnourished patients. One can take the pessimistic view and conclude that nutritional support should rarely be instituted because it can be an expensive and potentially cost-ineffective treatment modality. The other point of view is that malnutrition, or lack of acute nutrition, is only one of many factors that affect the elderly patient. Perhaps other formulations of nutritional support or additional pharmacologic intervention are needed and will prove to be beneficial.

Growth Hormone and Insulin-Growth Factor 1

Carter [99] provided an excellent review in which several potential lines of research that may eventually have significant payoffs for elderly patients were presented. One of these lines has focused on growth hormone (GH) and insulin-growth factor 1 (IGF-1) supplementation. Interest in its use in the elderly has been prompted in part by the observation that GH secretion decreases with age [100] and that GH and IGF-1 levels decrease with age [101]. Fairly extensive reviews of the physiology [102] and clinical uses of GH and IGF-1 [103] have been published. GH is released from the anterior pituitary gland in response to a wide variety of hormones including stimulation from the hypothalamic hormone, GH-releasing hormone. GH release is inhibited by another hypothalamic hormone, somatostatin. GH secretion results in the secretion of IGF-1 from the liver [103]. IGF-1 then feeds back to suppress the secretion of GH and insulin. GH is essential for postnatal growth and for normal carbohydrate, lipid, and mineral metabolism. GH also increases the transport of amino acids into muscle cells and increases protein synthesis. However, because GH results in increased IGF-1 levels, it is often difficult to sort out direct effects of GH versus those caused by IGF-1.

One of the most active laboratories investigating the potential benefits of GH has been that of Wilmore [104–108]. When patients receiving hypocaloric feedings were supplemented with GH, overall nitrogen balance was improved [106]. There was also a detectable increase in protein synthesis. When GH was administered to patients after elective gastrointestinal surgery, nitrogen loss was significantly attenuated compared with those patients not receiving GH [105].

This study also demonstrated increased protein synthesis, increased amino acid uptake across the forearm, and maintenance of muscle strength in those patients receiving GH. Recombinant human GH has been administered in a multicenter study of patients receiving TPN [104]. In those patients receiving GH in addition to TPN, there was a significant improvement in the cumulative nitrogen balance during the study period. Overall, the GH therapy in this study was well tolerated by the study patients.

There have also been several recent studies that have specifically investigated the use of GH in elderly patients. In one study, elderly men were placed on a 14-week exercise program [101]. During this initial weight training period, muscle strength increased 24% to 62%, after which the men were randomized to receive either GH or placebo for an additional 10 weeks while the exercise program continued. Although the patients who received GH experienced an increase in lean body mass and a decrease in body fat, there was no further increase in muscle strength after the initial weight training period. In another study, synthetic GH was administered to elderly men for 6 months [109]. Compared with a similar group of elderly men receiving no GH, the study group experienced increased lean body mass, decreased adipose tissue mass, and increased lumbar vertebral bone density. Other studies have also demonstrated positive effects on body composition when GH was administered to elderly men [110,111]. In a study of elderly women, GH or placebo was administered over a 6-month period [112]. Surprisingly, in this study GH had little effect on body composition, neither increasing lean body mass nor decreasing body fat. Markers of bone turnover were increased in those patients receiving GH, although there was no clear increase in bone mineral density. Of further concern was the fact that 58% of those patients initially receiving GH experienced unacceptable fluid retention and edema, and some patients developed carpal tunnel syndrome. Similar complications, though not necessarily at the same rate, have been previously reported by other investigators [111]. The failure to detect positive changes in lean body mass is somewhat at odds with a short-term study that incorporated elderly women receiving GH [113] and is certainly at odds with the studies described earlier where GH was administered to elderly men. Further studies of GH in elderly men and women are certainly warranted.

In all of the studies in which GH was administered, serum IGF-1 levels rose in response to the increased GH levels. The question therefore arises as to whether administering IGF-1 rather than GH may have beneficial effects, possibly without the detrimental effects. Now that recombinant IGF-1 has been made available for clinical studies, data of its effects on protein metabolism are beginning to be available. In a study of burn patients, IGF-1 decreased protein oxidation and protein breakdown rates while improving nitrogen balance [114]. In another study of human volunteers fed a hypocaloric diet, infusions of GH or IGF-1 appeared to have similar effects on improving nitrogen balance [115]. Regarding side effects, IGF-1 tended to cause hypoglycemia, whereas GH infusion tended to cause hyperglycemia. An intriguing recent study has suggested that IGF-1 administration can combat glucocorticoid-induced nitrogen wasting in animals [116]. However, a similar finding has been reported when GH was administered to human patients [117]. The combination of GH and IGF-1 has also been tried in human patients [118]. Surprisingly, this combination resulted in greater nitrogen retention than when only IGF-1 was administered. This suggests that GH may exert positive effects on protein metabolism that are not solely mediated by IGF-1.

Clearly, some of the data involving both GH and IGF-1 are encouraging. Many of the studies are short term or fairly small. Additional studies are needed to further elucidate whether either of these modalities is efficacious in the elderly as well as whether certain subsets of this population are most likely to benefit from this pharmacologic intervention.

Anabolic Steroids

Several studies have documented that the serum level of the androgen testosterone is decreased in both healthy elderly men as well as institutionalized elderly men [119–122]. Some studies have correlated decreasing testosterone levels with decreasing bone mineral density [120], whereas others did not find such a correlation [121].

A few studies have administered testosterone to elderly men with mixed results. In a small study, testosterone treatment resulted in elevated testosterone levels and a slight increase in right hand muscle strength [123]. In another small study, testosterone administration to elderly men resulted in a modest increase in fat-free mass while muscle strength and bone density showed minimal, if any, improvement [124]. Another study also detected an increase in lean body mass after 3 months of testosterone supplementation [125]. However, the serum prostate-specific antigen level rose slightly in response to testosterone treatment. This finding raises the concern that testosterone supplementation could stimulate the growth of clinically undetected prostate cancer in elderly men and could ultimately limit its use.

Another anabolic steroid, oxandrolone, has been used in several studies investigating nutrition in cirrhotic patients, but not specifically in elderly patients [126,127]. The cirrhotic patient is, however, frequently malnourished [126]. These studies demonstrated improved survival when oxandrolone was combined with nutritional support in those patients with moderate malnutrition [126], and treatment with the anabolic corticosteroid resulted in an increased prealbumin level, suggesting improved protein synthesis [127]. To date, there have been no major studies reporting the use of this agent in elderly patients. This very likely will be an area of future investigation.

Amino Acid and Fat Mixtures

Research in the next decade will also focus on potential changes in the amino acid and lipid formulations provided to patients. Current parenteral lipid replacement consists of esterified fatty acids composed of long chain fatty acids. Structured lipids incorporate medium chain fatty acids as well as long chain fatty acids in the triglyceride moiety. There are theoretical reasons why medium chain fatty acids may be more efficiently oxidized by the body than long chain fatty acids [128]. Increased oxidation of fatty acids may have a protein sparing effect and improve protein metabolism [129]. Some future studies will likely focus on whether the type of lipid supplementation alters hospital morbidity and mortality. In addition, there is also data that lipids, particularly long chain fatty acids, may exert negative effects on the immune system [130,131]. Thus, protocols that decrease the percentage of nonprotein calories supplied as lipids or protocols that alter the type of lipids supplied may be particularly indicated for those elderly patients with sepsis.

When nutrition is supplemented parenterally, the amino acid glutamine has not been administered routinely. Glutamine appears to be important as a fuel for the small intestine and may help to maintain gut barrier function [132,133]. There are now some data to suggest that parenterally administered glutamine may improve nitrogen balance and decrease the infection rate of patients [134–136]. However, the stability of glutamine in solution has been the subject of debate. Therefore, there is also interest in supplying glutamine as a dipeptide such as alycylglutamine or alanylglutamine [137], which appears to be quite stable in solution. Most certainly, there will be further studies investigating the role of glutamine in nutritional support.

CONCLUSIONS

Elderly patients will continue to represent an increasing percentage of the population. They will also be the recipients of an increasing amount of surgical care. However, what appears to be a natural process of aging brings about changes in body composition that likely adversely affect elderly patients, namely, a loss of lean body mass and, perhaps, a consequential loss in muscle strength. Superimposed on the physiologic changes that occur with aging is the fact that poor nutrition and frank malnutrition are surprisingly common in this population. Studies have universally demonstrated significantly higher morbidity and mortality when elderly patients present for surgical care in a malnourished state.

There is, however, considerable debate as to the best method to assess the nutritional status of individuals as well as whether nutritional intervention can alter the outcome of those patients deemed to be malnourished. There are data to suggest that preoperative as well as perioperative nutritional support can significantly alter morbidity and mortality in elderly patients. This appears particularly true in those patients who are severely malnourished.

The difficulty in demonstrating the efficacy of nutritional support may be due in large part to the fact that the nutritional state may not be the only variable that is significantly altered in elderly patients. There are many other changes in physiology that accompany aging, many of which are reviewed elsewhere in this book. There is now encouraging preliminary evidence that altering this physiology through pharmacology may play an additional role in combating the deleterious effects of malnutrition.

The most effective modality in preventing the increased morbidity and mortality brought about by malnutrition in the elderly may be increased efforts to recognize malnutrition and take preventative measures. Efforts should likely be directed at both preventing malnutrition in the elderly and at designing regimens aimed at helping the elderly to maintain a greater degree of muscle mass and strength.

REFERENCES

1. McGandy RB, Barrows CH Jr, Spanias A, et al. Nutrient intakes and energy expenditure in men of different ages. J Gerontol 1966;21: 581–587.
2. Keys A, Taylor HL, Grande F. Basal metabolism and age of adult man. Metabolism 1973;22:579–587.
3. Cohn S, Vartsky D, Yasumura S, et al. Compartmental body composition based on total-body nitrogen, potassium, and calcium. Am J Phys Endocrinol Metab 1980;239:E524–E530.
4. Forbes RM, Reina JC. Adult lean body mass declines with age: some longitudinal observations. Metabolism 1970;19:653–663.
5. Uauy R, Winterer J, Bilmazes C, et al. The changing pattern of whole body protein metabolism in aging humans. J Gerontol 1978;33:663–671.
6. Keys A, Brozek J. Body fat in adult man. Physiol Rev 1953;33:245–325.
7. Evans W, Campbell W. Sarcopenia and age-related changes in body composition and functional capacity. J Nutr 1993;123:465–468.
8. Martin DW Jr, Mayes PA, Rodwell VW, Granner DK. Harper's Review of Biochemistry (20th ed). Los Altos, CA: Lange Medical, 1985.
9. Fiatarone M, Marks E, Ryan N, et al. High-intensity strength training in nonagenarians. JAMA 1990;263:3029–3034.
10. Jette A, Branch L. Impairment and disability in the aged. J Chron Dis 1985;38:59–65.
11. Fiatarone M, Evans W. The etiology and reversibility of muscle dysfunction in the aged. J Gerontol 1993;48:77–83.
12. Zheng J, Rosenberg I. What is the nutritional status of the elderly? Geriatrics 1989;44:57–64.
13. Garry PJ, Goodwin JS, Hunt WC, et al. Nutritional status in a healthy elderly population: dietary and supplemental intakes. Am J Clin Nutr 1982;36:319–331.
14. Davidson CS, Livermore J, Anderson P, Kaufman S. The nutrition of a group of apparently healthy aging persons. Am J Clin Nutr 1962;10: 181–199.
15. Winterer J, Steffee W, Davy W, et al. Whole body protein turnover in aging man. Exp Gerontol 1976;11:79–87.
16. Reiff T. Water loss in aging and its clinical significance. Geriatrics 1987;42:53–62.
17. Schoeller D. Changes in total body water with age. Am J Clin Nutr 1989;50:1176–1181.
18. Phillips PA, Rolls BJ, Leddingham JGG, et al. Reduced thirst after water deprivation in healthy elderly men. N Engl J Med 1984;311: 753–759.
19. Miller J, Pratley R, Goldberg A, et al. Strength training increases insulin action in healthy 50- to 65-yr-old men. J Appl Physiol 1994;77:1122–1127.
20. Gumbiner B, Thorburn A, Ditzler T, et al. Role of impaired intracellular glucose metabolism in the insulin resistance of aging. Metabolism 1992;41:1115–1121.
21. Frank S, Roland D, Sturis J, et al. Effects of aging on glucose regulation during wakefulness and sleep. Am J Phys Endocrinol Metab 1995;269:E1006–E1016.
22. Miller DS. Stimulation of RNA and protein synthesis by intracellular insulin. Science 1988;240:506–508.

23. Jefferson LAS. Role of insulin in the regulation of protein synthesis. Diabetes 1980;29:487–496.
24. Fukagawa NK, Minaker KL, Rowe JW, et al. Insulin-mediated reduction of whole body protein breakdown. J Clin Invest 1985;12:2306–2311.
25. Gelfand RA, Barrett EJ. Effect of physiologic hyperinsulinemia on skeletal muscle protein synthesis and breakdown in man. J Clin Invest 1987;80:1–6.
26. Biolo G, Fleming RYD, Wolfe RR. Physiologic hyperinsulinemia stimulates protein synthesis and enhances transport of selected amino acids in human skeletal muscle. J Clin Invest 1995;95:811–819.
27. Shaver HJ, Loper JA, Lutes RA. Nutritional status of nursing home patients. JPEN J Parenter Enteral Nutr 1980;4:367–370.
28. Lowik M, Westenbrink S, Hulshof K, et al. Nutrition and aging: dietary intake of "apparently healthy" elderly (Dutch nutrition surveillance system). J Am Coll Nutr 1989;8:347–356.
29. Lowik M, Schrijver J, Odink J, et al. Nutrition and aging: nutritional status of "apparently healthy" elderly (Dutch surveillance system). J Am Coll Nutr 1990;9:18–27.
30. Bienia R, Ratcliff S, Barbour G, Kummer M. Malnutrition in the hospitalized geriatric patient. J Am Geriatr Soc 1992;30:433–436.
31. Constans T, Bacq Y, Brechot J, et al. Protein-energy malnutrition in elderly medical patients. J Am Geriatr Soc 1992;40:263–268.
32. Nelson R, Franzi L. Nutrition and aging. Med Clin North Am 1989; 73:1531–1550.
33. Van Way C. Variability of the Harris-Benedict equation in recently published textbooks. JPEN J Parenter Enteral Nutr 1992;16:566–568.
34. Long C, Schaffel N, Geiger J. Metabolic response to injury and illness: estimation of energy and protein needs from indirect calorimetry and nitrogen balance. JPEN J Parenter Enteral Nutr 1979;3: 455–456.
35. Blackburn GL, Harvey KB. Nutritional assessment as a routine in clinical medicine. Nutr Assess 1982;71:46–63.
36. Ferrannini E. The theoretical bases of indirect calorimetry: a review. Metabolism 1988;37:287–301.
37. McClave S, Snider H. Use of Indirect Calorimetry in Clinical Nutrition. In Schneider P, Bell S (eds), Selected Reviews in Nutrition Support. Silver Spring, MD: Aspen, 1993;1–15.
38. Weissman C, Kemper M, Askanazi J, et al. Resting metabolic rate of the critically ill patient: measured versus predicted. Anesthesiology 1986;64:673–679.
39. Weissman C, Kemper M, Damask M. Effect of routine intensive care interactions on metabolic rate. Chest 1984;86:815–816.
40. Mann S, Westenkow D, Houtchens B. Measured and predicted caloric expenditure in the acutely ill. Crit Care Med 1985;13:173–177.
41. Foster GD, Knox LS, Dempsey DT, Mullen JL. Caloric requirements in total parenteral nutrition. J Am Coll Nutr 1987;6:231–253.
42. Shizgal H, Martin M, Gimmon Z. The effect of age on the caloric requirement of malnourished individuals. Am J Clin Nutr 1992;55:783–789.
43. Chernoff R. Effects of age on nutrient requirements. Clin Geriatr Med 1995;11:641–651.
44. Solomon S, Kirby D. The refeeding syndrome. JPEN J Parenter Enteral Nutr 1990;14:52–59.
45. Uauy R, Scrimshaw NS, Young VR. Human protein requirements: nitrogen balance response to graded levels of egg protein in elderly men and women. Am J Clin Nutr 1978;31:779–785.
46. Gersovitz M, Motil K, Munro HN, et al. Human protein requirements: assessment of the adequacy of the current recommended dietary allowance for dietary protein in elderly men and women. Am J Clin Nutr 1982;35:6–14.
47. Kountz W, Hofstatter L, Ackermann P. Nitrogen balance studies in four elderly men. J Gerontol 1951;6:20–33.
48. Cheng A, Gomez A, Bergan J, et al. Comparative nitrogen balance study between young and aged adults using three levels of protein intake from a combination wheat-soy-milk mixture. Am J Clin Nutr 1978;31:12–22.
49. Campbell W, Crim M, Dallal G, et al. Increased protein requirements in elderly people: new data and retrospective measurements. Am J Clin Nutr 1994;60:501–509.
50. Clark NG, Rappaport JI, DiScala C, et al. Nutritional support of the chronically ill elderly female at risk for elective or urgent surgery. J Am Coll Nutr 1988;7:17–26.
51. Vente JP, Soeters PB, von Meyenfeldt MF, et al. Prospective randomized double-blind trial of branched chain amino acid enriched versus standard parenteral nutrition solutions in traumatized and septic patients. World J Surg 1991;15:128–133.
52. Long CL, Schaffel N, Geiger JW, et al. Metabolic response to injury and illness: estimation of energy and protein needs from indirect calorimetry and nitrogen balance. JPEN J Parenter Enteral Nutr 1979;3:452–456.
53. Protho J. Protein and Amino Acid Requirements of the Elderly. In Murphy C, Cain W, Hegsted DM (eds), Nutrition and the Chemical Senses in Aging: Recent Advances and Current Research Needs. New York: New York Academy of Sciences, 1989;143–156.
54. Chernoff R. Physiologic Aging and Nutritional Status. In Schneider P, Bell S (eds), Selected Reviews in Nutrition Support. Silver Spring, MD: Aspen, 1993;103–108.
55. Stephensen C, Blount S, Schoeb T, Park J. Vitamin deficiency impairs some aspects of the host response to influenza A virus infection in BALB/c mice. J Nutr 1993;123:823–833.
56. Demetriou A, Jones L. Vitamins. In Rombeau J, Caldwell M (eds), Clinical Nutrition: Parenteral Nutrition. Philadelphia: Saunders, 1993;184–202.
57. Mason J, Russell R. Parenteral Nutrition in the Elderly. In Rombeau J, Caldwell M (eds), Clinical Nutrition: Parenteral Nutrition. Philadelphia: Saunders, 1993;737–747.
58. Krasinski S, Russell R, Otradovec C, et al. Relationship of vitamin A and vitamin E intake to fasting plasma retinol, retinol-binding protein, retinyl esters, carotene, alpha-tocopherol, and cholesterol among elderly people and young adults: increased plasma retinyl esters among vitamin A–supplement users. Am J Clin Nutr 1989;49:112–120.
59. Davies M, Mawer E, Mann J, et al. Vitamin D prophylaxis in the elderly: a simple effective method suitable for large populations. Age Ageing 1985;14:349–354.
60. Norman RW. Vitamin D supplementation in the elderly. Lancet 1987;306–307.
61. Craig GM, Elliot C, Hughes KR. Masked vitamin B12 and folate deficiency in the elderly. Br J Nutr 1985;54:613–619.
62. Elsborg L, Lund V, Bastrup-Madsen P. Serum vitamin B12 levels in the aged. Acta Medica Scandia 1976;200:309–314.
63. Baker H, Jaslow SP, Frank O. Severe impairment of dietary folate utilization in the elderly. J Am Geriatr Soc 1978;26:218–221.
64. Montgomery BB, Haboubi HE, Mixe H, et al. Causes of malabsorption in the elderly. Age Ageing 1986;15:235–240.
65. Montgomery RD, Haeney MR, Ross IN, et al. The ageing gut: a study of intestinal absorption in relation to nutrition in the elderly. Q J Med 1978;186:197–211.
66. Marcus DL, Freedman ML. Folic acid deficiency in the elderly: geriatric bioscience. J Am Geriatr Soc 1985;33:552–558.
67. Burr ML, Phillips KM. Anthropometric norms in the elderly. Br J Nutr 1984;51:165–169.
68. Heymsfield S, McManus C, Smith J. Anthropometric measurement of muscle mass: revised equations for calculating bone-free arm muscle area. Am J Clin Nutr 1982;36:685.
69. Chumlea W, Roche A, Mukherjee D. Nutritional Assessment of the Elderly Through Anthropometry. Columbus, OH: Ross Laboratories, 1984;10.
70. Blackburn GL, Bistrian BR, Maini BS, et al. Nutritional and metabolic assessment of the hospitalized patient. JPEN J Parenter Enteral Nutr 1977;1:11–22.
71. Baker JP, Detsky AS, Wesson DE, et al. Nutritional assessment: a comparison of clinical judgment and objective measurements. N Engl J Med 1982;306:969–972.
72. Detsky A, McLaughlin J, Baker J, et al. What is subjective global assessment of nutritional status? JPEN J Parenter Enteral Nutr 1987;11:8–13.
73. Seltzer MH, Bastidas JA, Cooper DM, et al. Instant nutritional assessment. JPEN J Parenter Enteral Nutr 1979;3:157–159.
74. Harvey K, Moldawer L, Bistrian B, Blackburn G. Biological measures for the formulation of a hospital prognostic index. Am J Clin Nutr 1981;34:2013–2022.
75. Buzby G, Mullen J, Matthews D, et al. Prognostic nutritional index in gastrointestinal surgery. Am J Surg 1980;139:160–167.
76. Buzby G, Williford W, Peterson O, et al. A randomized clinical trial of total parenteral nutrition in malnourished surgical patients: the rationale and impact of previous clinical trials and pilot study on protocol design. Am J Clin Nutr 1988;47:357–365.
77. The Veterans Affairs TPN Cooperative Study Group. Perioperative total parenteral nutrition in surgical patients. N Engl J Med 1991; 325:525–532.

78. Sullivan DH, Patch GA, Walls RC, Lipschitz DA. Impact of nutrition status on morbidity and mortality in a select population of geriatric rehabilitation patients. Am J Clin Nutr 1990;51:749–758.
79. Reinhardt GF, Myscofski JW, Wilkens DB, et al. Incidence and mortality of hypoalbuminemic patients in hospitalized veterans. JPEN J Parenter Enteral Nutr 1980;4:357–359.
80. Devin GD, Kaminski MV. Correlation of pressure sores and nutritional status. J Am Geriatr Soc 1986;34:435–440.
81. Warnold I, Lundholm K. Clinical significance of preoperative nutritional status in 215 noncancer patients. Ann Surg 1984;199:299–305.
82. Dempsey D, Mullen J, Buzby G. The link between nutritional status and clinical outcome: can nutritional intervention modify it? Am J Clin Nutr 1988;47:352–356.
83. Daly JM, Lieberman MD, Goldfine J, et al. Enteral nutrition with supplemental arginine, RNA, and omega-3 fatty acids in patients after operation: immunologic, metabolic, and clinical outcome. Surgery 1992;112:56–67.
84. Souba W. Enteral nutrition after surgery. BMJ 1996;312:869–871.
85. Kudsk K. Clinical applications of enteral nutrition. Select Rev Nutr Support 1995;2:13–19.
86. Cahill S, Benotti P. Catheter infection control in parenteral nutrition. Select Rev Nutr Support 1993;61:43–45.
87. Ciocon JO, Silverstone FA, Graver LM, Foley CJ. Tube feedings in elderly patients. Arch Intern Med 1988;148:429–433.
88. Khan K, Baker BA, Elia M. Nutrient utilisation in muscle and in the whole body of patients receiving total parenteral nutrition. Clin Nutr 1992;11:345–351.
89. Vernet O, Christin L, Schutz Y, et al. Enteral versus parenteral nutrition: comparison of energy metabolism in healthy subjects. Am J Physiol 1986;250:E47–E54.
90. Campos A, Meguid M. A critical appraisal of the usefulness of perioperative nutritional support. Am J Clin Nutr 1992;55:117–130.
91. Mullen J, Buzby G, Matthews D, et al. Reduction of operative morbidity and mortality by combined preoperative and postoperative nutritional support. Ann Surg 1980;192:604–613.
92. Williford W, Krol W, Buzby G. Comparison of eligible randomized patients with two groups of ineligible patients: can the results of the VA total parenteral nutrition clinical trial be generalized? J Clin Epidemiol 1993;46:1025–1034.
93. Buzby G. Overview of randomized clinical trials of total parenteral nutrition for malnourished surgical patients. World J Surg 1993;17:173–177.
94. Sullivan D. The role of nutrition in increased morbidity and mortality. Clin Geriatr Med 1995;11:661–674.
95. Baier H, Somani P. Ventilatory drive in normal man during semistarvation. Chest 1984;85:222–225.
96. Bastow M, Rawlings J, Allison S. Benefits of supplementary tube feeding after fractured neck of femur: a randomised controlled trial. BMJ 1983;287:1589–1592.
97. Delmi M, Rapin C, Benoga J, et al. Dietary supplementation in elderly patients with fractured neck of the femur. Lancet 1990;335:1013–1016.
98. Nelson KM, Richards EW, Long CL, et al. Protein and energy balance following femoral neck fracture in geriatric patients. Metabolism 1995;44:59–66.
99. Carter W. Effect of anabolic hormones and insulin-like growth factor-I on muscle mass and strength in elderly persons. Clin Geriatr Med 1995;11:735–748.
100. Iranmanesh A, Lizarralde G, Veldhuis J. Age and relative adiposity are specific negative determinants of the frequency and amplitude of growth hormone (GH) secretory bursts and the half-life endogenous GH in healthy men. J Clin Endocrinol Metab 1991;73:1081–1088.
101. Taafe D, Pruitt L, Reim J, et al. Effect of recombinant human growth hormone on the muscle strength response to resistance exercise in elderly men. J Clin Endocrinol Metab 1994;79:1361–1366.
102. Williams RH. Williams Textbook of Endocrinology (8th ed). Philadelphia: Saunders, 1992.
103. Bondy C. Clinical uses of insulin-like growth factor I. Ann Intern Med 1994;120:593–601.
104. Ziegler TR, Rombeau JL, Young LS, et al. Recombinant human growth hormone enhances the metabolic efficacy of parenteral nutrition: a double-blind, randomized controlled study. J Clin Endocrinol Metab 1992;74:865–873.
105. Jiang Z, He G, Zhang S, et al. Low dose growth hormone and hypocaloric nutrition attenuate the protein-catabolic response after major operation. Ann Surg 1989;210:513–524.
106. Manson JM, Smith RJ, Wilmore DW. Growth hormone stimulates protein synthesis during hypocaloric parenteral nutrition. Ann Surg 1988;208:136–142.
107. Byrne T, Morrissey T, Gatzen C, et al. Anabolic therapy with growth hormone accelerates protein gain in surgical patients requiring nutritional rehabilitation. Ann Surg 1993;218:400–418.
108. Ziegler TR, Barbieri RL, Young LS, et al. Effects of growth hormone administration on dehydroepiandrosterone sulphate, androstenedione, testosterone and cortisol metabolism during nutritional repletion. Clin Endocrinol 1991;34:281–287.
109. Rudman D, Feller A, Nagraj H, et al. Effects of human growth hormone in men over 60 years old. N Engl J Med 1990;323:1–6.
110. Borst S, Millard W, Lowenthal D. Growth hormone, exercise, and aging: the future of therapy for the frail elderly. J Am Geriatr Soc 1994;42:528–535.
111. Rudman D, Feller A, Cohn L, et al. Effects of human growth hormone on body composition in elderly men. Horm Res 1991;36(Suppl):73–81.
112. Holloway L, Butterfield G, Hintz R, et al. Effects of recombinant human growth hormone on metabolic indices, body composition, and bone turnover in healthy elderly women. J Clin Endocrinol Metab 1994;79:470–479.
113. Previs S, Fernandez C, Yang D, et al. Limitations of the mass isotopomer distribution analysis of glucose to study gluconeogenesis. J Biol Chem 1995;270:19806–19815.
114. Cioffi W, Gore D, Rue L, et al. Insulin-like growth factor-I lowers protein oxidation in patients with thermal injury. Ann Surg 1994;220:310–319.
115. Clemmons D, Smith-Banks A, Underwood L. Reversal of diet-induced catabolism by infusion of recombinant insulin-like growth factor-I in humans. J Clin Endocrinal Metab 1992;75:234–238.
116. Yang H, Grahn M, Schalch D, Ney D. Anabolic effect of IGF-I coinfused with total parenteral nutrition in dexamethasone-treated rats. Am J Phys Endocrinol Metab 1994;266:E690–E698.
117. Horber F, Haymond M. Human growth prevents the protein catabolic side effects of prednisone in humans. J Clin Invest 1990;86:265–272.
118. Kupfer S, Underwood L, Baxter R, Clemmons D. Enhancement of the anabolic effects of growth hormone and insulin-like growth factor I by the use of both agents simultaneously. J Clin Invest 1993;91:391–396.
119. Abbasi A, Drinka P, Mattson D, Rudman D. Low circulating levels of insulin-like growth factors and testosterone in chronically institutionalized elderly men. J Am Geriatr Soc 1993;41:975–982.
120. Rudman D, Drinka P, Wilson C, et al. Relations of endogenous anabolic hormones and physical activity to bone mineral density and lean body mass in elderly men. Clin Endocrinol 1994;40:653–661.
121. Rudman D, Mattson D, Nagraj H, et al. Plasma testosterone in nursing home men. J Clin Epidemiol 1988;41:231–236.
122. Gray A, Feldman H, McKinlay J, Longcope C. Age, disease, and changing sex hormone levels in middle aged men: results of the Massachusetts Male Aging Study. J Clin Endocrinol Metab 1991;73:1016–1025.
123. Morley J, Perry M, Kaiser F, et al. Effects of testosterone replacement therapy in old hypogonadal males: a preliminary study. J Am Geriatr Soc 1993;41:149–152.
124. Young N, Baker H, Liu G, Seeman E. Body composition and muscle strength in healthy men receiving testosterone enanthate for contraception. J Clin Endocrinol Metab 1993;77:1028–1032.
125. Tenover J. Effects of testosterone supplementation in the aging male. J Clin Endocrinol Metab 1992;75:1092–1098.
126. Mendenhall CL, Moritz TE, Roselle GA, et al. A study of oral nutritional support with oxandrolone in malnourished patients with alcoholic hepatitis: results of a Department of Veterans Affairs cooperative study. Hepatology 1993;17:564–576.
127. Bonkovsky HL, Singh RH, Jafri IH, et al. A randomized, controlled trial of treatment of alcoholic hepatitis with parenteral nutrition and oxandrolone. II. Short-term effects on nitrogen metabolism, metabolic balance, and nutrition. Am J Gastroenterol 1991;86:9: 1209–1218.
128. Sandstrom R, Hyltander A, Korner U, Lundholm K. Structured triglycerides were well tolerated and induced increased whole body

fat oxidation compared with long-chain triglycerides in postoperative patients. JPEN J Parenter Enteral Nutr 1995;19:381–386.
129. Mendez B, Ling PR, Istfan NW, et al. Effects of different lipid sources in total parenteral nutrition on whole body protein kinetics and tumor growth. JPEN J Parenter Enteral Nutr 1992;16:545–551.
130. Goldstein RE, Flakoll PJ. Effects of dietary components on cellular elements and metabolism. Curr Opin Gastroenterol 1994;10:193–198.
131. Bower R. Nutrition and immune function. Select Rev Nutr Support 1993;5:16–22.
132. van der Hulst R, van Kreel B, von Meyenfeldt M, et al. Glutamine and the preservation of gut integrity. Lancet 1993;341:1363–1365.
133. Souba W. Drug therapy: nutritional support. N Engl J Med 1997;336: 41–48.
134. Stehle P, Zander J, Mertes N, et al. Effect of parenteral glutamine peptide supplements on muscle glutamine loss and nitrogen balance after major surgery. Lancet 1989;1:231–233.
135. Ziegler T, Young L, Benfell K, et al. Clinical and metabolic efficacy of glutamine-supplemented parenteral nutrition after bone marrow transplantation: a randomized, double-blind, controlled study. Ann Intern Med 1992;116:821–828.
136. Byrne T, Persinger R, Young L, et al. A new treatment for patients with short-bowel syndrome: growth hormone, glutamine, and a modified diet. Ann Surg 1995;222:243–255.
137. Abumrad NN, Morse EL, Lochs H, et al. Possible sources of glutamine for parenteral nutrition: impact on glutamine metabolism. Am J Physiol 1989;20:E228–E234.

Surgical Care for the Elderly, 2nd ed., edited by
R. Benton Adkins, Jr., and H. William Scott, Jr.
Lippincott–Raven Publishers, Philadelphia © 1998.

CHAPTER 10

Neuropsychiatric Aspects of Surgery

Richard A. Margolin and Joseph A. Kwentus

Surgical treatment may have a profound influence on the mental well-being of the elderly patient. Normal elderly patients encounter the same stresses of surgical procedures that younger patients experience. Older patients, however, often do not have the same mental capacity that younger patients have. Therefore, seniors may need special attention before and after surgery. Before surgery, the surgeon must be aware that elderly patients process information more slowly than younger people. They may need more careful explanations to understand and prepare for the procedure. After surgery, certain complications, such as delirium, occur more commonly in the elderly patient. Psychiatric symptoms, such as confusion or depression, can be the first sign of physical complications. These symptoms can interfere with management and delay recovery [1]. In addition, elderly patients may have extra needs for home health nursing postoperatively. Elderly patients who have psychiatric disease or dementia pose special additional problems for the surgeon. The surgeon who understands the ways in which psychiatric symptoms and psychiatric illness can interfere with recovery will be able to deal with these issues in a way that ensures a more favorable outcome.

Psychiatric illness is fairly common among the elderly [2]. Psychopathology and physical illnesses often go hand in hand in this population [3]. Therefore, when surgeons work with old people they will inevitably encounter psychiatric problems. In the elderly, psychiatric symptoms can reflect organic brain disease as easily as a functional psychiatric disorder. A review of normal aging provides a basis for understanding the causes for psychiatric symptoms in the older surgical patient. The psychiatric symptoms and illnesses that are especially important in the management of surgical patients are stressed in the context of the process of normal aging.

NORMAL AGING PROCESS

Normal aging involves change in both the mind and the brain. Unfortunately, a full developmental conception of the psychology of aging has yet to be developed. The same is true of the age-associated anatomic and physiologic changes in the brain. Despite lapses in our knowledge, an understanding of normal aging still provides the framework for exploring the psychiatric diseases in later life.

The maintenance of good mental health in the senescent years clearly requires intact neurologic function. There is a complex and poorly understood interplay between microanatomic and physiologic changes of the brain, on the one hand, and the psychological variable in behavior, on the other. In healthy people, personality, cognition, and affective style continue to grow well into later life. Most elderly people in the United States possess good general physical and mental health. In many other elderly people, however, the impact of acute or chronic disease significantly affects the psychological capacity to handle new situations.

Although mental capacity may be more limited, the older person may also face considerable psychological stress. Many elderly people are forced to face significant losses, including the death of a spouse or another important relative. Financial considerations are also important and add to poor health, isolation, and other social burdens. When stress overtaxes the older person's ability to solve life's problems, psychiatric disease often ensues.

Stereotypes, mostly of a negative sort, have long characterized society's perception of the elderly. Butler and Lewis referred to these negative views generally as *ageism* [4]. Recent research has debunked many myths about the limitations of the elderly. An important finding is that variability is increased in the aged in many physiologic and psychological processes [5]. Therefore, stereotypes and ageism are dangerous and often unfounded.

NORMAL PSYCHOLOGY OF AGING

The psychology of aging is best approached from a developmental perspective—that is, one that views senescence as representing a further stage of adult individualization. There are several theories regarding psychological development.

However, it is generally agreed that adult psychological function comprises at least the basic components of cognition and related skills, such as memory and learning, mood, and affect. These building blocks are organized into the comprehensive and stable attributes of intelligence, personality, and behavior. Although it is possible to consider the psychology of aging from a biological standpoint that stresses brain-behavior relationships, a psychosocial standpoint, stressing the relationship between an individual and the community, is equally important. Both perspectives are revealing for the geriatric surgeon. The field of geriatric psychology has grown rapidly; our review is selective and targeted at those aspects of the field likely to be important to the surgeon.

Cognition

Cognition actually means knowing, particularly with regard to the outside world. It is a generic term, encompassing a set of discrete mental processes. Cognitive skills include perceiving, recognizing, reasoning, and judging. Memory and learning are closely related mental capabilities. Intact consciousness and attention are also obvious prerequisites for successful cognition. Normal aging is associated with a mild detriment in cognitive abilities.

Changes in cognitive performance related to age differ greatly among seniors. Information processing shows the most pronounced changes. Verbal speed and working memory account for much of the age-related performance decrements [6,7]. Older people who have highly developed abilities, such as verbal intellect, can probably mask some age-related memory defects [8]. After age 70, brain functions and capabilities decline more rapidly. Cognitive decline related to aging produces impaired memory, diminished apprehension of complex ideas, mental rigidity, cautious responses, and behavioral slowing [9,10]. Slowing of responses is the most consistent cognitive change in elderly people [11]. Therefore, the time required for providing professional services to older people is greater than that required for younger people.

Physicians who take sufficient time to test the mental status in older individuals are more likely to obtain accurate results than physicians who rush through the examination. If given enough time, normal seniors can be expected to do the following tasks accurately: (1) repeat up to random digits forward, (2) solve untimed serial arithmetic problems, (3) solve simple vigilance tests, (4) display basic orientation, and (5) recall immediate memories [12]. Unfamiliar stimuli, complex tasks, and time limitations cause trouble for the normal elderly. Seniors who are forced to reorganize material have more trouble. Thus, seniors have some difficulty presenting digits backward.

Many tasks of modern life, such as driving a car, may require speed as well as dexterity. Response impairments interfere with the performance of such tasks by the elderly. Not all cognitive tasks of daily life require response speed, however. Reading and gardening are examples of activities that the elderly may find enjoyable and at which they may excel, but for which time is not a critical factor.

Memory and Learning

The study of memory is a great challenge because the systems that underlie memory function are complex and not well understood. Patients are diagnosed with an amnestic disorder when they are unable to learn new information or recall previously learned facts or events. To diagnose an amnestic disorder, a coexisting dementia delirium must be absent. The *Diagnostic and Statistical Manual of Mental Disorders*, 4th edition (DSM-IV), classifies amnestic disorders according to etiology [13]. The amnestic disorder may thus be due to a general medical condition or induced by a particular substance. Amnestic disorders due to a general medical condition must be the direct consequence of the medical illness. The physician also reports the responsible medical condition as part of the axis I diagnosis. Amnestic disorders that are mild are difficult to categorize and may be difficult to distinguish from a mild generalized cognitive impairment.

A great deal of controversy exists about the nature and measurement of memory. Clinically, we usually divide memory into long-term and short-term components. Short-term memory consists of registration and immediate memory. Registration holds information briefly for approximately 1 or 2 seconds. Immediate memory, or working memory, is retained for 30 seconds to a few minutes. Immediate memory retains information in reverberating neural circuits. If it is not converted to long-term storage, it is lost. Memories are ultimately stored in long-term memory through a process called *consolidation*. These memories are organized in the brain according to meaning. Long-term memory is a biochemical process that depends on the protein synthesis and development of dendritic connections.

Patients who have difficulty with short-term memory generally have anterograde amnesia. Patients with anterograde amnesia are unable to learn new material. Patients who have difficulty recalling information stored before the onset of an illness or injury have retrograde amnesia. These patients have impairment in long-term memory. The retention of material in long-term storage depends on the part of the cerebral cortex related to the specific sensory modality retained in long-term memory. Thus, if the occipital cortex and the occipital parietal cortex are involved in an injury, visual memories may be significantly impaired.

Memory can be classified according to many different paradigms. One common system divides memory into implicit and explicit types. Explicit memory is sometimes called *declarative memory*. Explicit measures of human memory reflect conscious recollection of the past. Recall and recognition are explicit memory functions. We can state or declare these memories. Declarative memory is concerned with the accumulation of facts. Declarative memory is used to remember the facts read in this chapter. However, declarative memory contains facts not only about verbal material but about all sensory modalities. Declarative facts can be about size, color, or shape. Declarative memory is ultimately about relationships. An example of declarative memory would be the recollection that a certain bird has blue feathers and stands 4 in. tall. Declarative memory combines information about the bird with its attributes. Declarative memories are consciously known and are therefore explicit. Declarative facts can be stated. Lesions in the medial temporal lobes, midline diencephalon, or basal forebrain can cause difficulty with declarative memory. This is because relationships between sensory modalities are processed through the hippocampal diencephalic system.

We can further subdivide declarative memory into episodic memory and semantic memory. Episodic memory contains information about events. Semantic memory is a deeper form of memory. Semantic memory refers to memory for knowledge about language structure or about the significance of events in the world around us. Semantic memory has meaning. Patients with the classic amnestic syndromes have well-defined problems with episodic memory. On the other hand, patients who suffer from Alzheimer's disease have significant deficiencies in semantic memory.

The nondeclarative memory category is sometimes called *implicit memory*. Implicit memory is not usually tested in depth at the bedside because it requires more sophisticated neuropsychological testing. Implicit memory does not require conscious recollection of recent experiences for execution of tasks. Procedural learning is an example of the implicit memory system. Apraxias provide examples of deficits in implicit memory. Amnestic patients can learn certain skills or acquire problem-solving abilities. This learning occurs although the amnestic patient is unable to recall that he or she has learned the behavior. The basal ganglia, cerebellum, and frontal lobes have been linked to procedural learning. Procedural learning functions independently of the hippocampal diencephalic system. Procedural learning is more severely affected in subcortical dementias such as Huntington's chorea and Parkinson's disease. Another example of implicit learning is classical or operant conditioning. Amnestic patients are also able to learn through classical conditioning techniques. Again, they are not able to recollect the experience of learning when questioned later.

Recently, neural network theories of memory have been developed. These systems are based on mathematical and logical descriptions of network architectures that computer programs can apply within certain limitations. In these models, dissociable systems that accomplish different forms of learning work together to form memories. Different memory modalities are mediated by distinct neural networks. Evidence for this comes from the fact that damage to specific areas of association cortex affects individual sensory memory modalities. Currently, research in functional brain imaging is being combined with these theories to provide a new source of information about how memory systems function.

From a practical standpoint, amnestic disorders continue to be understood through well-known anatomic pathways. These structures include the medial temporal lobes, mamillary bodies, fornix, medial dorsal nucleus of the thalamus, and frontal lobes [14–17]. Damage to these pathways by neurologic insults or toxins causes clinical memory problems. Injuries and toxic exposures can produce either reversible or irreversible amnestic conditions. In patients with amnestic syndromes, neuropsychological testing reveals normal perception, language, motor functions, and preserved intellectual skills. Explicit memory disorders are well recognized clinically.

Memory loss in nondemented seniors is a common complaint. Many of these patients become terrified that they have Alzheimer's disease and seek medical help. Physicians have difficulty distinguishing normal age-associated memory loss, benign forgetfulness, and early Alzheimer's disease. Benign senile forgetfulness has effects on memory that are greater than expected [18]. Elderly persons who have benign forgetfulness forget unimportant details. This contrasts with patients with Alzheimer's disease who forget events randomly. In addition, seniors who suffer from benign senile forgetfulness have trouble remembering recent information. Typically, patients with Alzheimer's disease have difficulty with recent *and* remote memory. For DSM-IV purposes, benign senile forgetfulness usually qualifies as a mild cognitive impairment. The most important aspect in the treatment of these patients is reassurance, but cognitive retraining can also sometimes be helpful. Nonetheless, physicians must be vigilant because some of these patients later develop more serious disorders.

Memory is a complex process. There is age-related decline in memory, as documented by formal laboratory experiments [19]. Visual and verbal memories demonstrate different patterns of change with aging; verbal and especially numeric retention is relatively well preserved [20]. Predictably, the elderly perform most poorly on memory tasks that are time constrained; their deficit is less apparent when response is not limited.

Mood and Affect

Mood refers to a feeling state that is stable over a reasonable period of time. Affect reflects feeling states that may change in response to external or internal stimuli. Elderly people have as wide a variation in temperament as their younger counterparts. Stereotypes of elderly as cantankerous, crotchety, irritable, or stubborn are inaccurate. When older people retain the ability to show a wide range of moods and affects, they are likely to demonstrate capacity in other aspects of psychological function.

Elderly people who demonstrate an altered mood that persists for days or weeks are likely to suffer from an affective disorder. Such mood changes should not be taken as part of normal aging. Affective lability refers to frequent swings in mood. Frequent mood swings are not a part of normal aging and often represent a psychiatric disorder.

Intelligence

The aging process has a detrimental effect on some intellectual processes; however, not all intellectual abilities are affected in the same degree. Verbal skills such as vocabulary decline little with aging. However, perceptual-integrative intelligence does decline progressively with age. This type of intelligence is measured by performance on tests like block design (object assembly) [21]. Executive functions, such as mental flexibility, attention, and drive, may also decline with aging.

Personality

Aging is characterized by a progressive loss of coordinated functions with a loss of psychological flexibility. There is a gradual decrease in adaptability to the environment. Nonetheless, normal aging is associated with a preservation of long-standing personality traits. Sometimes, personality traits become accentuated. This may have either a positive or negative impact on the ability of older people to function in their environment. Premorbid personality can contribute to social isolation if the personality traits are pronounced. This is particularly true of alcoholics. One of the factors associated with aging is loss of control. For the most part, senior citizens tend to have a healthy overall sense of control. However, they are more likely to handle their concerns by acceptance. As a result, they are also more willing to perceive control as coming from others, including God or a higher power [22]. Acceptance helps the individual to cope with failure and helps channel motivational resources toward obtainable goals throughout life.

Paradoxically, older people who accept the things they cannot change are more likely to engage in behaviors directed to change the world to fit their own needs and desires. Different perceptions of control are associated with significant differences in health practices and health status. The physician is in a unique position to help educate the older patient about the health concerns he or she can affect by corrective action and those that the patient must accept. The personality of the individual affects his or her ability to process the information in a constructive way.

In general, those who have been optimistic throughout their lives will remain so and will deal with aging better than those who have been pessimistic. Optimism and pessimism affect the attitudes that older people bring to surgery. More pessimistic people may feel that life has passed them by or that they have lived long enough. The will to live is certainly not directly related to chronologic age. Pessimistic views about the future do not necessarily equate with depression.

Behavior

Changes in mental function translate into behavioral differences between the elderly and their younger counterparts. Some evidence suggests that older individuals are more cautious. In psychological tests, for example, the elderly are more likely to avoid responding, whereas the young more readily guess, even if they guess incorrectly. These stylistic differences have practical ramifications for surgeons. The elderly are less willing to accept risks.

Stress and Coping

The effect of aging on the ability to cope with life's problems is unclear. On the one hand, the elderly are buffeted by increasingly stressful circumstances (i.e., loss of independence, health, and social standing). At the same time, older people have fewer and fewer resources to deal effectively with these stresses. The elderly are, by definition, survivors, who must have at least a minimally adequate repertoire of skills to have been able to attain advanced age. Love is a human need that is especially important for the elderly. In times of stress it is important that older people have those around them who care the most. It is equally important that physicians project an attitude of caring.

Activity Level

Physical and mental activities are reduced in most old people. The reasons for this are both anatomic and psychological. People who complain of fatigue may have underlying disorders such as anemia or heart failure. Excessive use of sedative drugs also leads to lower levels of activity.

If a person has a negative outlook, there can be a big difference between his or her actual physical capabilities and the perception of capabilities. Reduced physical and mental activity may be caused by depression or boredom. Conversely, inactivity can cause mood disturbances by increasing isolation. It is important for physicians to encourage elderly patients to engage in some form of exercise. Exercise has unique beneficial effects on musculoskeletal disorders and mood state. Perhaps most importantly, it improves the quality of life, helping to maintain physical abilities and thus independence into extreme old age [23]. Forty years of population studies have shown that physical activity can protect against coronary heart disease in men of middle and early old age [24]. Exercise helps reduce the risk of osteoporosis. Endurance training in later life is associated with a lesser age-related decline in certain immune system functions [25]. High-intensity resistance exercise training is an effective means of counteracting muscle weakness and physical frailty in very elderly people. In contrast, multinutrient supplementation without concomitant exercise does not reduce muscle weakness or physical frailty [26].

Social and Economic Factors

The well-recognized increase in longevity in recent decades has been paralleled by not so well-appreciated changes in social structure. Thirty years ago most elderly lived as part of an extended family; today this is less likely to be the case. Changes in family structure, especially divorce, coupled with the remarkable physical mobility in American society, mean that more elderly are entirely alone and others have relatives living only at a great distance. Such social isolation can readily affect their attitudes toward illness and health care.

Economic considerations cannot be ignored by the elderly. The percentage of elderly living in poverty has recently declined. However, most old people in the United States still live on fixed incomes. Most elderly patients rely on Medicare for reimbursement of medical costs. Despite this fact, the percentage of costs reimbursed by Medicare has decreased in recent years. Policy developments occurring as a result of the federal budget deficit threaten to increase the elderly population's costs for medical and surgical therapy and to decrease their access to these services.

Concurrent Medical Illness and Psychological Function in the Aged

The presence of concomitant chronic medical illness is important in surgical decision making. It has been estimated that 75% of surgical patients over the age of 70 have one or more associated diseases [27]. The presence of these diseases often adversely affects the response to surgical care. Whereas there are surely many reasons for this adverse effect, the impact of chronic illness on the psyche may be one of the mechanisms involved. For example, chronic cardiac, pulmonary, or renal disease, as well as poor nutritional status, have been correlated with relatively impaired cognition in elderly populations. Recovery from illness and operation includes both subjective and objective aspects. The elderly take longer to recover fully. Again, psychological factors may mediate this finding.

For many frail old people, the simplest and most basic capabilities may be extremely important, both for maintaining self-esteem and for preservation of a minimally adequate quality of life. Intact mental functioning and the ability to move are perhaps the most basic attributes necessary for a meaningful existence [28].

In summary, the mental health of the elderly is influenced by at least four kinds of factors: psychological, social, economic, and physical. When one or more of these factors become seriously disturbed, psychopathology is likely to ensue.

NORMAL AGING CHANGES IN STRUCTURAL AND PHYSIOLOGIC ATTRIBUTES OF THE BRAIN

Anatomic and physiologic changes of the brain associated with aging are important to geriatric surgery because the brain is the substrate for higher mental processes. The past several decades have witnessed dramatic advances in our ability to determine parameters of human cerebral structure and function. Certain morphologic changes are now well documented in the aging human brain, both at the macroscopic and microscopic levels.

As a person ages, the brain becomes more vulnerable to a variety of insults. The weight and volume of the brain attain their maximum in the early teens, but the brain loses both weight and volume as it ages. Gradual shrinkage of the brain has begun by the time that most people reach their 60s. By the tenth decade, the ratio of the brain to the skull cavity has decreased from 93% to 80% [29]. When the cortical neurons decrease in number, the cortical ribbon also begins to thin [30]. The number of large neurons decreases, while the number of small neurons increases [31].

Normal aging affects the frontal and temporal lobes more than the parietal lobe. The limbic system, substantia nigra, and locus ceruleus all experience a sizable loss of neurons. In spite of the loss of neurons, the aged brain continues to undergo dynamic remodeling. In normal old people, dendrites in hippocampal regions continue to show plasticity. It is when dendritic arborization fails that mental powers also decline [32].

The relationship between the morphologic changes that occur as the brain ages and cognitive function remains unclear. The volume of the cerebral ventricles increases with age, but the range of ventricular size is greater in old age than in youth. Increases in the size of ventricles, sulci, and subarachnoid spaces are observed easily with modern imaging techniques [33].

On a microscopic level, lipofuscin granules collect in neurons [34]. Fibrous astrocytes increase in size and number. The hippocampus shows granulovacuolar changes. Normal elderly brains have senile plaques and neurofibrillary tangles. The number of plaques and tangles in the brains of normal elders overlaps with the numbers of these structures observed in patients with Alzheimer's disease [35]. Small infarcts are found in the brains of many normal old people.

Age-related biochemical changes also occur in the brain. Postmortem neurochemical studies have shown age-related reductions in most neurotransmitter levels and in levels of their synthetic enzymes [36]; an important exception is monoamine oxidase, which increases with age.

These structural and chemical changes are compensated for by the physiologic reserve capacity of the brain. Such mechanisms as redundant neural circuitry work to preserve the functional integrity of the brain. It is evident that the brain's reserve properties are substantial and that the higher mental functions are frequently preserved despite age-associated structural disruption of neuronal architecture. Only when damage is severe or focal does mental aberration result.

Newer imaging modalities, especially positron emission tomography, have shown age-related differences in a number of physiologic processes such as cerebral blood flow (CBF), glucose and oxygen metabolism, and neurotransmitter function. Several groups have documented modestly declining CBF with advancing age [37,38]. It is known that CBF and neuropsychological function are significantly correlated [39,40].

Not all neurophysiologic processes deteriorate with age, however. Recent research suggests that healthy elderly persons have no significant decrements in the basal level of cerebral glucose metabolism [41]. This is important because under ordinary circumstances glucose is the sole fuel for oxidative metabolism in the brain. Thus, the ability of the brain to support higher mental processes should not be considered intrinsically impaired by the aging process. More typical elderly persons, such as those with chronic disease, do show age-dependent decrements in the cerebral metabolic rate of glucose (CMR_{glu}) [42]. CMR_{glu} has likewise been shown to be significantly correlated with neuropsychological function [43].

Acetylcholine has been the subject of study because of its role in memory. Older people experience a decrease in the synthesizing enzyme for acetylcholine, choline acetyl transferase. Uptake of circulating choline into the brain decreases with age [44]. Deficits of acetylcholine in the hippocampus may account for the age-related decline in short-term memory. In Alzheimer's disease, damage to the ascending cholinergic system plays an important role in the loss of memory and other cognitive deficits [45].

Decrease in catecholamines is more closely linked to affective changes than to cognitive changes in elderly people. An age-related loss of noradrenergic cell bodies from the locus ceruleus occurs, but concentrations of noradrenaline appear to remain normal in target areas. On the other hand, monoamine oxidase increases [46] while tyrosine hydroxylase decreases [47]. Research also suggests reduced serotonergic innervation in the neocortex.

Loss of dopaminergic innervation of the neostriatum is a prominent age-related change that corresponds with the age-related loss of dopaminergic cell bodies from the substantia nigra [48]. Age-related decrease in basal ganglia dopamine makes seniors more sensitive to neuroleptic side effects [49]. Dopaminergic innervation of the neocortex and the neostriatum are not affected.

Studies of the brains of old people display a decrease in beta-adrenergic, serotonin, cholinergic, and dopamine receptors [50–53]. A decrease in beta-receptor density results in reduced cyclic adenosine monophosphate and decreased adaptability to the external environment [54]. Brain receptors sensitive to hormones such as glucocorticoids, estrogens, and androgens diminish. On the other hand, old people have an increase in benzodiazepine–gamma aminobutyric acid receptor inhibitory activity and sensitivity to benzodiazepines.

SENILE SENSORY AND PERCEPTUAL CHANGES

Vision Loss (Presbyopia) and Hearing Loss (Presbycusis)

Age-associated impairments in sensory modalities are quite frequent; visual and auditory deficits are the most significant. Most elderly persons demonstrate presbyopia, the lengthening of the minimal focal point for accurate vision. The effect of this condition is to interfere with visual acuity for close objects, such as written text. Other common ophthalmologic and neuro-ophthalmologic disorders in the elderly include cataracts, glaucoma, and diabetic and other retinopathies. Stroke can affect vision by involvement of the visual cortex. Visual deficits are readily linked to behavioral changes by promoting isolation and insecurity. Partial or complete treatment exists for many senile visual disorders and aggressive management is indicated.

Presbycusis is also common in older people. Acuity for high-frequency sounds is reduced. Generally, perception of spoken words is more impaired than perception of less-organized sounds. The old person usually has more difficulty with speech discrimination in group conversations than in individual discourse. Most senile hearing loss is of the sensory neural type, and men are more frequently affected than women [55]. Hearing problems can lead to social withdrawal and have a tendency to accentuate paranoid disorders. Some older people use their hearing aids selectively and turn off the hearing aid when the conversation is not to their liking.

Pain Sensitivity

There is little age-related difference in pain sensitivity. Although there may be some minimal increase in threshold to some stimuli, pain is a subjective experience and older individuals seem to experience it as intensely as younger people. Myths about changes in pain perception thresholds combined with age-related changes in the body's response to physiologic stress can lead to misdiagnosis of certain conditions, with subsequent adverse outcomes. The pain associated with appendicitis presents in a similar fashion regardless of the patient's age [56]. This is not always recognized in clinical situations, and late diagnosis can result. In addition, older people do not develop fever as readily as younger people [57]. The peripheral white cell count changes associated with acute processes are not as dramatic. Pain complaints might dissipate as the patient's mental status changes in response to the stress, a phenomenon that occurs somewhat frequently.

Fortunately, there have been studies on the effects of age on analgesic pharmacotherapy. The elderly are more sensitive to the effects of narcotics [58]. In the case of morphine, elderly patients may respond as if given several times the dose given to young adults. In addition, clearance of morphine from the plasma is only half that seen in younger patients. As a result, older patients are more prone to morphine intoxication. This further complicates the management of these patients, because a change in mental status could be the result of worsening of the underlying condition or of opiate intoxication. Narcotic analgesics must be carefully titrated in older patients. Doses should be increased gradually. A regular dosing schedule is advantageous because it produces a sustained level of analgesia, thus precluding anticipatory anxiety and behavior reinforcement of drug use [59]. The total dose of narcotic can be reduced by using synergistic compounds such as a nonsteroidal anti-inflammatory drug (NSAID), hydroxyzine, or less commonly, a tricyclic antidepressant.

The clinician who chooses non-narcotic analgesics must remember that the safety margin between therapeutic and toxic levels is reduced in the elderly. NSAIDs are bound to serum proteins and can displace other drugs from protein-binding sites. Elderly patients can be more prone to toxic reactions because of low serum albumin levels. They are also at risk because concurrent antihypertensive, anticoagulant, and other drug therapies can have significant interactions with NSAIDs. These drugs can also cause confusion in predisposed elderly individuals.

Sleep Changes in Aging

Adequate sleep is required for good physical and psychological health. Sleep disturbance is common and its prevalence increases with advancing age. Changes in sleep-wake patterns are among the hallmarks of biological aging. Physiologically, sleep in elderly adults differs from that in younger adults, both in terms of quantity and quality. Rapid eye movement (REM) sleep latency is slightly prolonged, and there is a slight decrease in the total amount of REM sleep. This is consistent with the changes that occur throughout the life cycle. REM sleep is more prominent in children and becomes progressively less prominent in late life. In addition, elderly people have increased sleep fragmentation, with more frequent arousals than young people. They also have substantially less deep sleep.

The elderly often complain about sleep problems. Sleep disturbance in old age may be associated with many physical and psychological conditions. The evaluation of a patient with a sleep disorder requires full medical psychiatric and social histories, mental state and physical examinations, and appropriate investigations. If present, an underlying condition should be treated [60]. The patient with excessive daytime sleepiness is at highest risk. Sleep apnea is the most common sleep disorder in older people. It can present with psychiatric symptoms, particularly depression.

Many elderly people have unrealistic expectations that they will sleep for as long and as soundly as when they were younger. Some of these patients respond to simple reassurance and counseling. Chronic administration of hypnotic drugs is counterproductive in the aged patient and produces daytime sedation and memory disturbance. In addition, hypnotic drugs can cause falls because these medications tend to impair the balance of older people. Whenever hypnotics are used, it is important to keep in mind that many of these drugs have prolonged half-lives in elderly people and may accumulate over time. A relationship between excess mortality and use of sleep medication has been described. Among elderly people, however, this relationship does not derive from the pharmacologic characteristics of prescription hypnotics. Rather, it appears that reported self-medication to promote sleep, using a variety of nonsedative products, provides an epidemiologic marker for a group within which levels of morbidity and mortality are particularly high [61]. At any age, hypnotic drug use can give rise to three major problems: (1) unwanted effects on daytime cognition; (2) rebound effects associated with drug withdrawal; and (3) dependency associated with long-term drug use. Age-related changes in pharmacodynamic and pharmacokinetic processes amplify the behavioral effect of many hypnotics [62]. Ideally, a hypnotic should be prescribed for a limited period and then in the smallest effective dose. Impaired melatonin secretion has been reported in sleep disorders of old age. Melatonin replacement therapy can be effective for sleep initiation and maintenance in elderly insomniacs [63].

PATHOLOGIC BRAIN AGING

It is difficult to delineate a clear division between changes in brain structure related to normal aging and pathologic changes. The differences encountered are usually quantitative and statistical, not qualitative or absolute. With regard to structure, clearly more cell loss and atrophy are present in dementia, for example, than in normal aging. Efforts to translate this fact into a reliable clinical tool has not been successful. Cell loss and degeneration are clearly linked to age-related brain disease in at least one case, namely that of the decreased volume of the nigrostriatal tract associated with Parkinson's disease.

Physiologically, substantially supernormal declines in CBF and CMR_{glu} have been shown in dementia. Imaging of these processes has become a useful clinical tool. Positron emission tomography and single photon emission computed tomography scans tend to show decreased temporal parietal activity in patients with Alzheimer's disease.

Functional Status

A useful term that incorporates both psychological and neurologic components of age-related change is that of *functional status*. This term refers to the overall capacity of an elderly individual to act in the world as an independent agent. Both psychological and neurologic aspects of functional status are relevant in the setting of geriatric surgery.

An important distinction is that of the old versus the very old, although no exact chronologic age boundary had biological significance. The important point to understand is that the very old may be physiologically different from the young old, who are more like middle-aged persons. The age of 85 years is generally used to distinguish the very old group.

GERIATRIC PSYCHOLOGY AND SURGICAL THERAPY

Specific Normal Psychiatric Responses to Surgical Trauma

An operation is a major traumatic occurrence for anyone. Regardless of the circumstances, certain strong emotions are a natural part of the surgical experience for the elderly. Anxiety and fear in moderate degrees, as well as feelings of isolation, are certainly common and need not be considered intrinsically pathologic. There are many reasons for fear and anxiety in the elderly surgical patient. Many older persons have known someone who has died during an operation. Some may be more afraid of dying during anesthesia than the operation itself [64]. The distinction between fear and anxiety is subtle. Fear is defined as an unpleasant, often strong emotion caused by awareness of danger; anxiety adds an element of anticipatory apprehension. Although fear closely corresponds to a real danger, anxiety is often chronic and apart from the reality of a present danger. Anxiety is also associated with other mental processes, such as worry and rumination. Depressed mood and denial of illness are frequently observed psychopathologic symptoms.

The boundary between the presence of such symptoms as normal reactions to a stressful experience and as features of more serious psychiatric illness may be subtle. The essential distinction is whether or not the symptoms interfere with normal functioning for an individual. Thus, to feel anxious when facing a surgical procedure is normal for many elderly patients. However, additional behavioral aberrations, such as anorexia or persistent insomnia, may indicate the presence of a psychiatric disorder.

What is the incidence of psychopathology among the elderly in the surgical setting? Estimates have varied. In a study of surgical patients of all ages, Titchener and colleagues found a 15% incidence of postoperative psychosis [65]. Furthermore, Heller and associates found a 33% incidence of organic brain syndrome after open heart procedures [66]. There is reason to believe that the elderly are a high-risk group for the development of preoperative psychopathology. Millar evaluated 100 consecutive elective general surgical cases in patients over age 65 [1]. He correlated a preoperative standardized psychiatric interview with postoperative nursing notes and repetition of the standardized interview. Thirteen of his patients showed preoperative psychiatric disturbance, and 212 demonstrated abnormalities postoperatively. Advanced age (>80 years), a major surgical procedure, and polypharmacy were all significantly associated with increased psychiatric morbidity.

Psychological and Psychiatric Components of the Preoperative Evaluation

Psychiatric aspects of the preoperative evaluation should include a history and mental status examination. The patient's family often needs to be contacted. Although necessarily brief, there is much evidence to suggest that this part of the evaluation is essential and of practical value to the surgeon. In addition, some data for psychiatric assessment can be obtained during other parts of the patient's evaluation through careful listening.

There are various parts to a preoperative psychiatric history. The process begins with identification of past or present psychiatric disease and clarification of whether it has any direct bearing on the current surgical problem. For example, surgical repair of wounds resulting from a self-inflicted injury sustained in a suicide attempt would be a setting in which inquiry about mental and emotional symptoms would be obviously germane. Depression, anxiety, and psychosis may be easily explored. A past history of major psychiatric disease is important to elicit because of its possible impact on the patient's behavior in the current setting. The stress of an operation can reactivate dormant psychiatric illness.

A behavioral history is important in the elderly. Alcohol or drug abuse is not rare in the aged. The unexpected development of a postoperative withdrawal state can have serious associated morbidity. A complete medication history is crucial for preventing adverse behavioral reactions to medication. The elderly frequently consume both prescribed and over-the-counter medications. They also use psychotropic medications at a higher rate than the young.

Indications for including the family in the psychiatric assessment are more frequent for an elderly patient than for a younger one. This is so because a family member may have valuable historic data to offer that the patient has forgotten or neglected to mention [67]. The family can also provide information about the patient's overall situation, including the social situation to which the patient is returning.

The mental status examination need not be a forbidding procedure for the surgeon. Key components to be assessed are orientation; mood and affect; cognitive skills, such as the ability to reason; memory (especially short-term memory); and the presence of symptoms of psychosis, such as hallucinations and delusion.

As an adjunct to the mental status examination, brief quantitative cognitive function rating scales might be used. These measures have the advantage of reproducibility. An excellent example of such scales is the mini-mental state examination, developed by Folstein and colleagues [68]. It can be administered in approximately 5 minutes and has been validated by application to a large and diverse patient population.

Although the surgeon's mental status examination is necessarily brief, the assessment of preoperative cognitive function provides a baseline for comparison in the event of complications. The preoperative assessment should be comprehensive and also include consideration of emotional well-being and sensory function. There are certain qualitative factors that must be included. One is the evaluation of the contribution of a surgical procedure not only to the extension of life but also to its qualitative improvement. The surgeon should reflect on the comparative risk of an operation versus conservative treatment. In the older patient, the patient's psychological limitations require careful consideration. The timing and the magnitude of the procedure may need to be modified by factors associated with mental or emotional illness [69].

Others involved in preoperative assessment can complement the surgeon's evaluation. The anesthesiologist is especially important in this regard, both as a backup for the completeness of data gathering and as another source of reassurance when discussing specific anesthesia-related issues with the patient. The patient's own wishes and opinions are germane and should be sought preoperatively. The medical ethicist can play a valuable role in assisting the surgeon in difficult cases.

Surgical Style and the Surgeon's Attitude Toward the Elderly

Certain intangible aspects of the doctor-patient relationship are especially important in geriatric surgery. These include the style of communication, sensitivity to the values and wishes of the patient, and the creation of a real rapport. Beard, for example, has stressed the importance of unhurried and proper communication with an elderly patient [70]. Communication is a two-way street. The surgeon must be a sincere, active listener to the patient's concerns, as well as a provider of facts and opinions for the elderly patient's consideration. The surgeon's explanations of the reasons for the surgical procedure, the process itself, associated risks, some preliminary aspects of postoperative recovery, and the likely outcome must be presented in a straightforward way and in common sense, layperson's language. Specific unfamiliar procedures that the patient is likely to encounter should be explained in advance. These might include cardiac catheterization, endotracheal intubation, artificial ventilation, central line placement, and so forth. Advance explanations can diminish anticipatory anxiety and surprise. In view of the frequent coexistence of cognitive impairment, sensory loss, and cautious behavior among the elderly, the value of patience and attention on the surgeon's part is obvious.

Similarly, communication with the family is crucial. The older patient may rely on family members to help with the final decision. The surgeon's instructions can also be reinforced by the family when the instructions are not assimilated by the elderly patient because of poor memory or lack of attention. Admittedly, communication with an elderly surgical patient and the family is not always possible and is seldom easy. Surgical emergencies are more common in the elderly and under many of these circumstances no family or friend may be readily available [70]. An individual's dignity and self-esteem are closely connected to decision making. A surgeon will maximize his or her effectiveness if the patient is involved in the act of decision making as much as possible. Rapport between the surgeon and the elderly patient enhances the chances for a favorable surgical outcome. This relationship is the best safeguard for the surgeon in the event of an unfavorable outcome.

A final point on this issue is the advisability of involving the patient's internist or other primary care physician during all phases of the surgical process. Such consultation is reasonable with compromised patients of any age, but there are specific reasons for it in the geriatric surgical situation. The patient will presumably have ready rapport with his or her own family physician. Elderly patients may more easily trust and have confidence in the surgeon if they know that their own physician is involved. The primary care physician who knows the patient well can also alert the surgeon to the patient's idiosyncrasies.

TABLE 10-1. *Common psychiatric disorders in the elderly surgical patient*

Organic mental syndromes
Delirium
Dementia
Affective disorders
Unipolar depression
Bipolar affective disorder (manic-depressive illness)
Psychosis (including schizophrenia and psychosis secondary to depression, mania, or organic brain disease)
Adjustment disorder
With depressed mood
With anxiety

PSYCHIATRIC DISEASES IN THE ELDERLY IN THE SURGICAL SETTING

The surgeon may face psychopathology in the elderly age groups from patients with known psychiatric disease and also in the previously mentally healthy individual. Furthermore, psychopathology may present due to anxiety incurred preoperatively, in the hectic perioperative period, or during a prolonged postoperative course. The presence of a known psychiatric condition in an elderly patient is not in itself a contraindication to an operation; however, the involvement of a psychiatrist may be desirable. All the commonly occurring psychiatric disorders of adult life occur in the elderly. Moreover, certain conditions are especially frequent in this phase of life. Table 10-1 summarizes the psychiatric illness that the geriatric surgeon is likely to encounter.

Delirium

Definition and Presentation

The phenomenon of delirium suggests the acute failure of the brain as a bodily organ. In the DSM-IV, the essential feature of this brain failure is an alteration in attention associated with disturbed consciousness and cognition [13]. Delirium is a common occurrence in medical and surgical patients. Terms like *encephalopathy* or *acute confusional state* are synonyms for *delirium* in the DSM-IV.

One of the most disconcerting clinical characteristics of delirium is the fluctuating course. Symptoms are ever changing, and the patient's mental status varies considerably from time to time. Cognitive deficits develop quickly and disappear just as quickly. Patients may be apathetic at one moment, and a short time later they may be restless, anxious, or irritable. Other patients become agitated and begin hallucinating without any apparent change in the underlying medical condition. Waxing and waning of symptoms and perceptual disturbances may reflect the fact that the nondominant cortex is involved. Delirium has been divided into hypoactive and hyperactive subtypes based on psychomotor activity [71], but almost no research data are available to support this division [72].

Sleep disturbance and decreased consciousness are quite common. Delirium may first present as sundown syndrome with daytime drowsiness and nighttime insomnia with confusion. However, as the patient becomes more ill, disorientation and inattention become more consistent. Nonetheless, the level of consciousness does not always follow the course of the underlying illness. When sleep is disturbed and affect is labile, delirium usually lasts longer. This cluster of delirious symptoms points to involvement of brain stem ascending pathways [74]. Symptoms usually resolve quickly when the underlying problem is treated but can last as long as a month after the medical illness has been treated.

Etiology

A variety of conditions lead to delirium. We can organize these causes into four major groups: (1) systemic disease secondarily affecting the brain, (2) primary intracranial disease, (3) exogenous toxic agents, and (4) withdrawal from substances of abuse. The DSM-IV classifies delirium according to the presumed etiology [13]. If delirium is due to a systemic medical condition or primary intracranial disease, then the medical cause is listed in the axis I diagnosis. Substance-induced delirium and substance withdrawal delirium are classified separately. Substance-induced delirium includes delirium caused by toxins and by drugs of abuse. If the etiology cannot be determined, then the delirium is classified as "Not otherwise specified." In most clinical situations, delirium is caused by multiple factors. Thus, the DSM-IV system improves on the DSM-III system because it includes delirium due to multiple etiologies. The list of factors that can produce delirium in the surgical setting is long (Table 10-2).

TABLE 10-2. *Common causes of postoperative confusion in the elderly*

Environmental
Intensive care unit
Intubation
Restraints
Isolation
Traction devices
Sensory deprivation
Decreased auditory acuity
Decreased visual acuity
Bandages and dressings
Drug reactions
Anticholinergic agents and anticholinergic side effects of other drugs
Metabolic
Hypoxia
Acid-based disturbances
Hyponatremia
Hyperosmolar coma
Acute renal failure
Fever
Dehydration
Infection
Sepsis
Pneumonia
Urinary tract infection
Wound infection
Meningitis
Anesthetic agents
Narcotics
Hypnotics
Antiemetics
Tranquilizers
Vascular
Myocardial infarction
Stroke, especially embolic
Pulmonary embolism
Hemorrhage
Shock
Heart failure
Miscellaneous
Trauma
Unrelieved pain
Anxiety

Incidence and Significance

Delirium is highly prevalent in hospitalized patients. The prevalence of delirium in general hospital patients is 10% to 30% [74]. Up to 50% of surgical patients become delirious in the postoperative period [75]. Delirium accompanies the terminal stages of many illnesses. It occurs in 25% to 40% of patients with cancer and in up to 85% of patients with advanced cancer [76]. Close to 80% of terminal patients become delirious before they die [77].

Age is the most widely identified risk factor for delirium. Patients with dementia are at even higher risk for delirium. Forty-one percent of dementia patients have delirium on admission to the hospital. Twenty-five percent of patients admitted with delirium will ultimately be diagnosed with coexisting dementia [78]. The incidence of delirium in nursing homes is also quite high. In seniors, delirium onset is more insidious than in young people, so there is an even higher probability that delirium will be overlooked in nursing homes. Illnesses that cause delirium can be life-threatening. The staff must be able to recognize delirium at an early stage so that they can identify and treat the primary medical conditions promptly. Some conditions that may lead to a rapid death if left untreated include hypoxia, hypoperfusion of the brain, hypoglycemia, hypertensive encephalopathy, intracranial hemorrhage, central nervous system infection, and toxins. Even when delirium is promptly recognized and treated it remains a marker for future cognitive decline. Many elderly patients who become delirious do not fully recover.

Treatment

The correct treatment of delirium entails a search for the underlying causes and an attempt to treat the acute symptoms. Close nursing supervision to protect the patient is essential for efficient evaluation and treatment of delirious seniors. Staff should remove all dangerous objects. Brief visits from a familiar person and a supportive environment with television, radio, calendar, and proper lighting help orient the patient. The physician should stop unnecessary drugs and monitor electrolyte balance, hydration, and nutrition.

Although the evaluation of delirium involves the analysis of straightforward data, physicians often miss the diagnosis [79]. The physician must be careful to obtain a careful history, perform a relevant physical examination, conduct a mental status examination, and review the patient's medication. Physicians who do not do a careful physical examination may overlook asterixis, tremors, psychomotor retardation, and other motor manifestations of delirium. An organized mental status, however, is the cornerstone of the assessment. The clinician who makes assumptions about the patient's cognitive status will make mistakes. This is particularly true in apathetic patients. Sometimes, clinicians who are otherwise quite capable do a careless mental status examination and are thus unaware of the patient's confusion. After the physician has assessed the mental status, a careful review of laboratory data and medications will yield important information about the cause.

Drugs that have anticholinergic properties commonly contribute to delirium. In patients in medical wards, symptoms of delirium occur when serum anticholinergic activity is elevated [80]. Total serum anticholinergic activity also helps predict which patients will be likely to be confused in intensive care units [81]. Symptoms of anticholinergic delirium include agitation, mydriasis, dry skin, and memory impairment.

Physicians must be cautious when prescribing psychotropic drugs for seniors because one of the most common causes of delirium is medicine. Common agents, such as digoxin, may induce cognitive dysfunction in older people even when digoxin serum concentrations are therapeutic. In the intensive care unit, antiarrhythmics such as lidocaine or mexiletine may cause confusion. Among the narcotics, meperidine (Demerol) is particularly likely to cause confusion and hallucinations. Benzodiazepines, narcotics, and antihistamines are also frequent contributors to delirium. The list of other drugs that may induce confusion is too extensive to warrant discussion.

Misuse of psychotropic drugs causes as many as 20% of psychogeriatric admissions [82]. Odds of an adverse cognitive response increase as the number of drugs increases. Adverse drug reactions are a source of excess morbidity in elderly patients. A high index of suspicion, drug-free trials, and careful monitoring of drug therapy reduce this problem [83].

Occasionally a specific antidote is available for drug-induced delirium. Reversal of anticholinergic delirium occurs with physostigmine or with neuroleptics [84]. Narcotic-induced delirium can be reversed with naloxone (Narcan). Flumazenil is an imidazobenzodiazepine that antagonizes the effects of benzodiazepine agonists by competitive interaction at the cerebral. Narcan and flumazenil have short half-lives and may have to be readministered.

When delirious patients become agitated, they may resist treatment, threaten staff, or place themselves in danger. Of equal importance is the fact that these patients have increased circulating catecholamines that cause an increase in heart rate, blood pressure, and ventilation.

Hospital personnel must protect patient rights and apply the least restrictive intervention when dealing with an agitated patient. The use of mechanical restraints increases morbidity, especially if the restraints are applied longer than 4 days [85]. Use of a sitter, although expensive, can sometimes prevent the use of physical restraint. Specially designed beds can also reduce the need for restraints.

Chemical sedation is usually more effective and less dangerous than physical restraint when other methods fail to control agitated patients. According to the practice parameters of the Society of Critical Care Medicine, haloperidol is the preferred agent for the treatment of delirium in the critically ill adult [86]. Haloperidol and other high-potency neuroleptics are less likely to produce adverse reactions than low-potency agents.

In emergencies, haloperidol should be administered intravenously to achieve a painless, more rapid, and more reliable onset of action [87]. The onset of action is approximately 11 minutes. The dose regimen can therefore be adjusted every 30 minutes until the patient is under control. For mildly agitated patients 1 to 2 mg may suffice. In severely agitated patients, 4 mg may be started. Every 30 minutes the dose is doubled until the patient is contained. Approximately 80% of patients respond to <20 mg of intravenous haloperidol per day. Although safe, significant QTc prolongation and torsade de pointes are possible complications of high-dose intravenous haloperidol therapy [88]. Hypotension may also occur rarely. The prevalence of acute dystonic reactions occurs in <1% of cases.

Patients admitted to the intensive care unit are often anxious and in pain, conditions that make delirium worse. Anxiety and delirium often exist together and may be difficult to distinguish from one another. The interplay between confusion and anxiety may cause patients to become agitated when obliged to engage in stressful activities such as weaning from mechanical ventilation [89]. Benzodiazepines can help calm patients who face these situations.

If benzodiazepines are given intravenously they can cause respiratory depression or hypotension. However, these drugs can be easily titrated when monitoring is appropriate [90]. As a result, this class of drugs is effective in the treatment of many delirious patients [91]. Neuroleptic agents such as haloperidol may act synergistically with benzodiazepines, resulting in control of agitation without significantly depressing the patient's level of consciousness or respiratory drive. Once sedation has been achieved, control usually can be maintained by intermittently administering a neuroleptic agent in combination with a continuous intravenous infusion of a benzodiazepine.

It is important for the physician to be aware of the side effects of benzodiazepines. Even when these medications are used for sleep, they may cause a drop in the mini-mental score [92]. The pharmacokinetics of some benzodiazepines are modified in seniors by impaired hepatic conjugation. Lorazepam and oxazepam do not require hepatic conjugation and are therefore preferred. Midazolam has been used as an intravenous infusion in intensive care units because of its margin of safety and short half-life [93].

Dementia

Definition and Presentation

Dementia is characterized by a loss of intellectual ability of sufficient severity to interfere with social or occupational functioning [13]. By definition, it presumes prior normal development of such ability. It presents along a continuum from mild deficits in specific cognitive capacity through global impairment of higher mental functions, to loss of control of even basic human bodily functions (e.g., bowel and bladder control and personal hygiene). In contrast to delirium, dementia is not an acute or subacute process, but rather a chronic one. Thus, it should always be identifiable preoperatively.

The demented patient can display inappropriate behaviors or behaviors dangerous to himself or herself or to the care-giving staff. These activities can include cursing, kicking, scratching, spitting, and attempting to loosen or remove restraints, arise from a bed over or through the side rails, or remove intravenous or other catheters. Urinary and fecal incontinence are especially challenging behaviors to manage. Elderly demented patients can easily become dehydrated or malnourished because of poor fluid and food intake. Although cognitive skills and memory are the most regularly affected mental functions, demented patients are often emotionally disturbed. A so-called catastrophic reaction has been identified in dementia. A stress that would be considered relatively minor by the nondemented person instead provokes severe behavioral decompensation. Typical stresses capable of producing a catastrophic reaction include hospitalization, physical restraint, and separation from the family. Agitation paranoia and wandering are regularly encountered in advanced dementia. It should also be noted that dementia and delirium are not mutually exclusive.

Etiology

Dementia syndromes share many common symptoms, but have varied etiology. The DSM-IV lists the dementias according to presumed etiology [13]. There are several subtypes: dementia of the Alzheimer's type, vascular dementia, dementia due to human immunodeficiency virus (HIV), dementia due to head trauma, dementia due to Parkinson's disease, dementia due to Huntington's disease, dementia due to Pick's disease, dementia due to Creutzfeldt-Jakob disease, dementia due to other general medical conditions, substance-induced persisting dementia, and dementia due to multiple etiologies. In the elderly, Alzheimer's disease and vascular dementia are the most prevalent forms.

Incidence and Significance

The incidence and prevalence of dementia increase steadily with advancing age. Although <7% of all people over age 65 are afflicted, as many as 20% of persons aged 85 and older may have significant dementia.

Operating on an elderly patient with dementia may be one of the most challenging tasks a surgeon can face. Issues that must be considered include those of a medicolegal nature (e.g., informed consent and competency) and postoperative management techniques. Although methodologically sound studies are lacking, it is widely believed that demented patients tolerate surgical procedures less well than nondemented patients of comparable age.

Treatment

Although there is currently no successful treatment for Alzheimer's disease, some other conditions that can cause dementia are remediable [94]. Regardless of etiology, the symptoms of dementia that can interfere with surgical therapy are relatively treatable acutely. Quite low doses of antipsychotic agents, such as haloperidol, can usually contain agitation. Tardive dyskinesia is a significant risk in the elderly. A clearly positive clinical response is the exception rather than the rule in elderly patients who have dementia. As a result, many other drugs have been used to treat agitated demented patients.

Short-acting benzodiazepines also control agitation and on occasion may provide short-term therapy of agitation in severely demented patients [95]. Benzodiazepines may be used in conjunction with antipsychotics. Benzodiazepines are often used to help agitated patients sleep. Benzodiazepines are effective only for a minority of patients, and side effects frequently make patients worse [96]. Even when used only at night, these drugs have an adverse effect on cognition and are a common cause of incoordination and falls in older hospitalized patients.

Trazodone [97], doxepin [98], carbamazepine [99,100], valproate [101], and buspirone [102] may reduce agitation in dementia patients. There are no placebo-controlled studies, but the use of these drugs is appropriate in patients who have failed conventional treatment. Choice of the drug can be based on the predominant target symptom. Carbamazepine or valproate may be best for patients with manic symptoms, buspirone for patients with anxiety, and antidepressants for patients who appear lonely or depressed. The use of these medications for control of behavior in dementia patients is best reserved for the psychiatric consultant.

Psychosis

Psychosis is an acute or chronic mental state of faulty relation to reality. A psychotic person may have false perceptions and beliefs about himself or herself and the world that he or she holds despite contradictory evidence. Psychotic symptoms in the elderly include hallucinations and delusions, particularly of the paranoid type. It is important to recognize that psychotic symptoms appearing de novo postoperatively may actually reflect the existence of delirium, and a thorough search for organic causes must be undertaken before presuming these symptoms to be functional in nature.

Etiology

Preoperatively diagnosed psychosis may reflect a long-standing psychiatric disorder, such as schizophrenia. Psychosis can also be seen in major depression or mania. Postoperative psychosis is an entity long known to surgeons. Whether it reflects a distinct diagnostic entity, however, is controversial.

Incidence and Significance

Because schizophrenia has an approximately 0.8% prevalence worldwide and afflicted patients in industrialized societies are living longer, it is not rare to encounter such patients in late life. The new-onset psychosis in late life is also a recognized clinical entity [103]. The significance of psychosis for the geriatric surgeon is primarily the need for diligent attention to the patient's behavior. Psychotic patients frequently behave unpredictably and may be uncooperative or noncompliant with instructions.

Treatment

The management of psychosis includes both pharmacologic and supportive components. Antipsychotic drugs are often necessary, but the lowest doses possible should be used to prevent side effects to which the elderly are more susceptible. Useful supportive measures are substantially the same as those listed for dementia.

Depression

Definition and Presentation

Depression is a vague term, referring both to a symptom and to specific clinical disorders. Feelings of loneliness, isolation, and sadness, as well as loss of energy, appetite, and interest in formerly enjoyable activities, are typical symptoms. Other symptoms include feelings of guilt or worthlessness; impaired ability to concentrate; recurrent unpleasant thoughts, especially of suicide; and reduction in sexual interest. Signs of depression include weight loss, sleep disturbance, and psychomotor agitation or retardation. A major depressive episode is diagnosable given the presence of one or more such signs and symptoms to a significant degree over a period >2 weeks. Chronic depressed mood in the absence of severe functional impairment suggests a related diagnosis, dysthymic disorder. Exaggerated grief and bereavement reactions are also encountered in the elderly. Depression may be manifested preoperatively or it may arise postoperatively.

Etiology

The etiology of geriatric depression is certainly multifactorial, with biochemical, psychodynamic, interpersonal, sociologic, existential, and genetic factors contributing to different degrees. Depression in the elderly is much more likely to be due to a general medical condition. The history and physical examination can suggest specific causes of mood disorders in the elderly. Endocrine disease, neurologic diseases, and even HIV infection can cause depressive illness in the older patient. Depression also occurs frequently in the early stages of dementia, particularly in vascular dementia and Alzheimer's disease. Parkinson's disease and stroke are also frequent contributors to depressive syndromes. Many medications are known to produce depressive symptoms in the elderly, but the antihypertensives should be mentioned in particular because of the frequency of this side effect and the frequency of their use in the elderly.

Incidence and Significance

Epidemiology studies have shown a considerable prevalence of depression among the aged and have in fact identified it as the most common geropsychiatric disorder. Blazer and Williams [104] found an almost 15% rate of dysphoric symptoms in one representative group of elderly, but only 4% of the individuals they studied met criteria for diagnosis of a major depressive episode. Cheah and Beard [105] noted a much higher prevalence of depression—31% in hospitalized patients on a medical unit.

Although it varies considerably in severity, the surgeon should consider the presence of depression as serious. Shuckitt and associates found a 60% 3-year mortality in a depressed geriatric group, but only a 32% mortality in a nondepressed group [106]. The presence of depression during preoperative evaluation may interfere with patient participation in rational decision making concerning an operation. Depression developing postoperatively can interfere with compliance with recuperative instructions, including medication use. Anorexia and resulting weight loss can induce a catabolic state that can impair wound healing. A major aspect of the significance of depression is its association with suicide. A number of studies in Europe and North America have shown a progressively increasing incidence of suicide with advancing age, at least in men. Although sometimes suicide occurs in nondepressed psychotic patients, it usually results from severe depression.

Treatment

Transitory depressive symptoms do not necessarily warrant treatment: Significant depression, however, should be treated with a combination of psychotherapy and antidepressant drugs. The newer antidepressants including the selective serotonin reuptake inhibitors are safe in older people. Sertraline has the advantage of not affecting the metabolism of other drugs as much as fluoxetine or paroxetine while having a relatively short half-life. Bupropion is preferred when there is a history of bipolar depression. The standard tricyclics are usually reserved for more severe depressions because their side effects are problematic in the older population. Even within this group, drugs such as amitriptyline have significant anticholinergic activity and should probably be avoided. Electroconvulsive therapy is thought to be particularly helpful in refractory geriatric depression and may also be used when antidepressant medication is contraindicated. Psychiatry consultation is useful in moderate or severe depression; sometimes delaying an operation to allow pharmacologic and psychotherapeutic treatment to take effect may be desirable.

Bipolar Disorder

Bipolar affective disorder (manic-depressive disorder) is also commonly encountered in the elderly. Mania is treated acutely with antipsychotic drugs and lithium salts. Patients are then maintained on lithium. More recently, sodium valproate has been approved for use in mania. This medication is safe in most geriatric patients, but it does have significant drug-drug interactions, particularly with anticoagulants. Sometimes lithium and valproate are used in combination for more intractable cases. Because mania interferes with the patient's ability to comply with treatment, it is advisable to control mania preoperatively if possible.

Anxiety Disorders

Some anxiety is expected in the surgical setting. In fact, its absence would be surprising. However, anxiety that interferes with rational behavior should be treated. The benzodiazepines are the preferred agents for anxiety, and scheduled dosages are recommended. Fears of inducing drug dependence by prescription of these agents are usually unwarranted in geriatric surgery. Lorazepam and oxazepam are preferred in geriatric patients because they are better metabolized. Long-acting benzodiazepines may accumulate and cause memory problems. Benzodiazepines are more likely to cause an increase in falls in the geriatric population because balance is already compromised in many old people.

Miscellaneous Conditions

Many other psychiatric conditions may of course be encountered by the geriatric surgeon. Medical progress has enabled individuals with developmental disabilities, such as Down syndrome, to survive into advanced age. Elderly patients with personality disorders, alcohol and substance abuse, and Munchausen syndrome may also be seen.

Psychopathology and Specific Surgical Procedures

Although no psychiatric syndromes occur exclusively in relation to specific surgical procedures, it is true that certain problems may more likely be encountered after certain operations. One of the most intriguing such associations is the development of cognitive deficits, affective disturbance, or personality changes after cardiac procedures and carotid endarterectomy [107]. Microemboli and hypoxia have been postulated as causes. Emotional incontinence and emotional lability are two important mood disturbances that may typically be seen after such events. Emotional incontinence describes a syndrome in which there is a sudden expression of emotion that is rapid in onset and that is not subjectively experienced by the patient. It is common when there has been damage to frontal lobe systems.

Colostomy, amputation of an extremity, and oral, esophageal, or laryngeal procedures that result in speech or swallowing impairment all are difficult operations for the elderly physically and psychologically. Procedures resulting in cosmetic deformity may produce depression. This is particularly true with mastectomy, even for women well past menopause.

SPECIAL TOPICS

Impact of Anesthesia

Although specifically covered in another chapter, the effect of anesthesia on mental function in the elderly is worth a brief comment here. Conflicting reports about the impact of different types of anesthesia have appeared in the literature. Some authors have suggested that general anesthesia has an adverse effect on postoperative mental function when compared with local or regional techniques [108,109]. Others have not confirmed this effect in elective procedures [110,111]. Bigler and colleagues, in a study of emergency hip repair in the elderly, found no difference in postoperative mental function between general and epidural anesthesia [112]. Some confusion in the literature undoubtedly results from lumping early and late differences in postoperative mentation together, because most studies found some early differences. Those differences, even if transient, could negatively affect the course of recovery by interfering with compliance and increasing the risk of complications.

Pharmacologic Considerations

The importance of pharmacologic factors in geriatric surgery cannot be overemphasized. The elderly use many drugs in general, both those prescribed by physicians and those purchased over the counter. One group of researchers found that 78% of an elderly cohort were taking at least one prescribed drug, and another study revealed that 7% of an elderly population were consuming 12 or more drugs simultaneously [113]. The elderly are also among the most frequent users of psychotropic drugs [114].

Complications of drug use in the elderly are both frequent and serious. Hurwitz and Wade found a drug complication rate of 15% in a group of elderly inpatients versus a rate of only 6% in a younger group [115]. Drugs are even important in the etiology of surgical problems themselves. Drugs play a large role in hip fractures and in bowel obstruction.

In the surgical setting, many classes of psychoactive drugs are used. Preoperative preparation includes anticholinergics, sedatives, and narcotics. The preoperative period involves anesthetics, and the postoperative period sees further use of sedatives, hypnotics, narcotics, and tranquilizers.

Both pharmacokinetic and pharmacodynamic factors are important in geriatric pharmacology in the surgical setting. Pharmacokinetics refers to the disposition of administered drugs, including such processes as absorption, distribution, metabolism, and excretion, whereas pharmacodynamics refers to the responsiveness of the body to drug action. Our discussion is confined to the psychopharmacologic domain and factors likely to be significant in the surgical setting.

Absorption and First-Pass Effect

Although no age-related changes in absorption of psychotropic medications have been convincingly demonstrated, a number of orally administered drugs are affected by first-pass hepatic enzymatic activity. These include some commonly used antidepressants (desipramine and nortriptyline) and narcotic analgesics (meperidine, morphine, and propoxyphene) [116]. Decrements in hepatic function can at least theoretically lead to increased blood levels of these agents.

Distribution

Most psychotropic drugs are quite lipid soluble. The age-associated decreases in lean body mass and water are coupled with a trend to increased lipid stores. Thus, fat-soluble drugs have a larger volume of distribution, a fact linked to their tendency to accumulate in the body during steady-state dosing periods. An important exception to the lipid solubility of psychotropics is that of lithium; as an ion it is water soluble.

Metabolism

Specific differences in pathways of drug metabolism associated with aging are not clearly evident; however, the rate of metabolism of many drugs is diminished by age. Many psychotropics are metabolized by liver to other active compounds. When possible, drugs that are metabolized only to inactive compounds are therefore preferable.

Excretion

Most psychotropics are excreted by the liver; exceptions are lithium and oxazepam, which are renally cleared. Because creatinine clearance decreases with age, a smaller margin of error exists before toxicity ensues. The final common pathway of these various pharmacokinetic processes is the blood level of drugs and their active metabolites. A secondary factor is their level of protein binding, because it is the unbound drug that is active. Blood levels are often higher in the elderly after a given dosing schedule. Thus it is important in many cases to measure blood levels. Diazepam, for example, has a fourfold increased half-life in the aged.

Adverse Reactions

Some specific frequently encountered adverse reactions to psychotropic agents merit attention. Long-acting benzodiazepines, such as diazepam and chlordiazepoxide, when given as anxiolytics or hypnotics, can produce daytime sedation. A number of antihypertensive agents have been linked to depression. The most notorious is reserpine, which is fortunately little used today. However, alpha-methyldopa and the beta-adrenergic receptor blocking agent propranolol have also demonstrated this property. The beta-blocking agent atenolol can be substituted for propranolol in many cases. Cimetidine has been linked to delirium in the elderly; the newer agents may not share this property. The cardiotoxicity of the tricyclic antidepressants in overdose is well appreciated. Their most important cardiac effects when given in therapeutic concentrations are prolongation of the PR and QRS intervals. Although use of these drugs in the elderly requires careful monitoring, it is usually possible to administer them. In particular, they can generally be used in patients with preexisting cardiovascular disease. Important exceptions are patients in the first several months following myocardial infarction and patients with bundle branch blocks. The introduction of newer antidepressants such as the selective serotonin reuptake inhibitors and bupropion allows for greater flexibility in the management of geriatric depression. These drugs do not have significant cardiac side effects.

A potentially serious adverse reaction to tricyclic antidepressants and antipsychotic agents is the anticholinergic syndrome, which is much more common in the elderly. Tricyclic antidepressants and low-potency neuroleptics can also produce orthostatic hypotension. Orthostatic hypotension predisposes the patient to falls. The safest course is the careful monitoring of orthostatic blood pressures and pulse when introducing these agents. With the new drugs, however, the use of these agents has become relatively uncommon in older patients.

Drug Interactions

Some specific drug interactions merit attention: Alcohol increases benzodiazepine levels and potentiates the effects of these drugs. Cimetidine increases diazepam levels. Tricyclic antidepressants antagonize the effect of guanethidine, alpha-methyldopa, and clonidine. Certain psychotropic drugs such as tricyclic antidepressants interact significantly with anesthetics. The anticholinergic effects of tricyclic antidepressants may add to that of preoperative anticholinergic agents, producing tachycardia and anticholinergic delirium.

Several important interactions are associated with the monamine oxidase inhibitors. They are known to potentiate the central nervous system depression of anesthetics, barbiturates, and narcotics, as well as the action of vasopressors. Fatalities have occurred when they are combined with meperidine, although the mechanism is unclear. Duncalf and Kepes recommend that monamine oxidase inhibitors be discontinued at least a week before surgery [64]. Valproic acid prolongs the half-life of many common medications, particularly anticoagulants. A final important interaction is that of lithium with muscle relaxants and succinylcholine; this combination should be used with great care.

Indications for Psychiatric Consultation

It is useful to consider the role of the psychiatrist in geriatric surgery. Certain situations that a surgeon may face naturally suggest psychiatric consultation. These include the prospect of operating on a patient with known psychiatric disease who has symptomatic psychopathology or who uses more than the simplest regimen of psychotropic drugs. The unexpected development of significant mental or emotional symptoms in a surgical patient may also be an occasion for consultation, as for example in many medicolegal problems, such as the determination of competence to consent to or refuse proposed treatment. Finally, the question of surgical consideration in the terminally or chronically ill patient may be an indication for using psychiatric expertise. Research indicates that psychiatric consultation in elderly inpatients is an underused service relative to the incidence of significant psychopathology [117]. Yet the value of such consultation, when indicated, is substantial.

Medicolegal Considerations: Competence and Informed Consent

A number of psychiatric diagnoses, either intrinsically or in severe form, call into question a patient's competence to participate in surgical decision making. Competence is actually a legal term, and as such it must ultimately be determined by a court of appropriate jurisdiction. In practice, however, psychiatric evaluation, including a formal mental status examination, plays a key role in determining competence.

A particularly thorny area in geriatric surgery is that of informed consent. Cognitive, affective, and behavioral changes in the elderly may interfere with a patient's capacity to reason. The depressed or paranoid patient may refuse an operation when it is life-saving. The demented patient may be unable to comprehend the nature of the surgical intervention proposed [118]. In such cases, a psychiatric evaluation is indicated to assist in determining the patient's competence to give informed consent. Family support at such times, if available, helps substantially to promote the chance of a favorable outcome. Legal steps are available to the care-giving team in cases in which a patient is not able to act independently or intends actions contrary to his or her best interest. Yet a patient's will should be respected if competence is determined to exist, even if the patient's intent is at odds with the surgeon's opinion [119].

Philosophy and Medical Ethics in Geriatric Surgery

Philosophical and ethical issues and questions of values often arise in geriatrics. The prospects of a surgical procedure, which has the quality of drama, is thus frequently the stage on which conflicts in these areas are played out. It therefore behooves the geriatric surgeon to consider philosophical and ethical issues. In doing so, twin perils greet the surgeon. On the one hand, ageism has long engendered a defeatist attitude in which valuable procedures were denied the elderly because of mistaken beliefs about their frailty. On the other hand, the rapid technological advances of recent decades have sometimes led to overly aggressive surgical approaches to medical problems. This has led to a situation of surgically cured but still chronically ill and disabled individuals.

Surgical procedures in the elderly should be oriented toward preservation of functional integrity. An operation should be considered not only for what it might achieve but also in light of what harm complications might cause. There is less margin for error in the elderly. Knowledge of geriatric physiology and broad experience will guide the thoughtful surgeon to an appreciation of the indications for aggressive or limited operations, or no surgical procedure at all. In very difficult cases, a referral to the hospital ethicist may help clarify issues.

CONCLUSION

Various neuropsychiatric aspects of surgical care in the elderly have been reviewed. Consideration of the normal aging process, both psychological and neuropsychological, is the foundation for understanding the reaction of normal elderly individuals subject to surgical treatment. Certain common pathologic reactions occur frequently; delirium is especially important. The surgeon faces special challenges when operating on patients with known psychiatric diseases, such as dementia, psychosis, and depression, as well as those of extremely advanced age with multiple system dysfunction. Psychopharmacologic expertise is essential because of its implications for patient management and recovery. Other topics such as legal competence, informed consent, and ethics are also important concerns for the geriatric surgeon.

REFERENCES

1. Millar HR. Psychiatric morbidity in elderly surgical patients. Br J Psychiatry 1981;138:17–20.
2. Blazer D. Psychiatric Disorders. In Rossman I (ed), Clinical Geriatrics (3rd ed). Philadelphia: Lippincott, 1986;593–605.
3. Knights EB, Folstein MF. Unsuspected emotional and cognitive disturbance in medical patients. Ann Intern Med 1977;87:723–724.
4. Butler RN, Lewis MI. Aging and Mental Health (2nd ed). St. Louis: Mosby, 1977.
5. Rowe JW. Physiological changes of aging and their clinical impact. Psychosomatics 1984;25:6–11.
6. Stine EL, Wingfield A. Process and strategy in memory of speech among younger and older adults. Psychol Aging 1987;2:272–279.
7. Hartlely JT. Individual Differences in Memory for Written Discourse. In Light LL, Burke DM (eds), Language, Memory, and Aging. New York: Cambridge University Press, 1977;36–57.
8. Meyer BJF. Reading Comprehension and Aging. In Schaie KW (ed), Annual Review of Gerontology and Geriatrics (Vol. 7). New York: Springer, 1987;93–116.
9. Botwinick J. Aging and Behavior (2nd ed). New York: Springer, 1978;185–205.
10. Kermis MD. The Psychology of Human Aging: Theory, Research, and Practice. Boston: Allyn and Bacon, 1985;190–212.
11. Salthouse TA. Speed of Behavior and Its Implications for Cognition. In Birren JE, Schaie W (eds), Handbook of the Psychology of Aging. New York: van Nostrand, 1985;400–426.
12. Craik FIM. Age Differences in Human Memory. In Birren JE, Schaie W (eds), Handbook of the Psychology of Aging. New York: van Nostrand Reinhold, 1977;384–421.
13. American Psychiatric Association. Diagnostic and Statistical Manual of Mental Disorders (4th ed). Washington, DC: American Psychiatric Association, 1994.
14. Damasio A. The anatomical basis of memory disorders. Semin Neurol 1984;4:223–225.
15. Butters N, Cermak LS. Alcoholic Korsakoff's Syndrome. New York: Academic Press, 1980.
16. Squire LR. Two forms of human amnesia: an analysis of forgetting. J Neurol Sci 1981;6:635–640.
17. Milner B. Visually-guided maze learning in man: effect of bilateral hippocampal, bilateral frontal, and unilateral cerebral lesions. Neuropsychologica 1965;3:317–338.
18. Kral BA. Forgetfulness: benign and malignant. Can Med Assoc J 1962;86:257–260.
19. Poon L. Differences in Human Memory with Aging: Nature, Causes, and Clinical Implications. In Birren JE, Schaie KW (eds), Handbook of the Psychology of Aging (2nd ed). New York: van Nostrand, 1985.
20. Arenberg D. Changes with Age in Problem Solving. In Craik FIM, Trehub S (eds), Aging and Cognitive Processes. New York: Plenum, 1982;221–235.
21. Storandt M. Psychological Aspects of Aging. In Rossman I (ed), Clinical Geriatrics (3rd ed). Philadelphia: Lippincott, 1986;606–617.
22. Shapiro DH Jr, Sandman CA, Grossman M, Grossman B. Aging and sense of control. Psychol Rep 1995;77:616–618.
23. Shephard RJ. Physical activity and reduction of health risks: how far are the benefits independent of fat loss? J Sports Med Phys Fitness 1994;34:91–98.
24. Morris JN. Exercise in the prevention of coronary heart disease: today's best buy in public health. Med Sci Sports Exerc 1994;26:807–814.
25. Shinkai S, Kohno H, Kimura K, et al. Physical activity and immune senescence in men. Sports Exerc 1995;27:1516–1526.
26. Fiatarone MA, O'Neill EF, Ryan ND, et al. Exercise training and nutritional supplementation for physical frailty in very elderly people [see comments]. N Engl J Med 1994;330:1769–1775.
27. Weiss MF, Lesnick GJ. Surgery in the elderly: attitudes and facts. Mt Sinai J Med 1980;47:208–214.
28. Haavisto MV, Heikinheimno RJ, Mattila KH, Rajala SA. Living conditions and health of a population aged 85 years or over: a five year follow-up study. Age Ageing 1985;14:202–208.
29. Davis PJM, Wright EA. A new method for measuring cranial cavity volume and its application to the assessment of cerebral atrophy at autopsy. Neuropathol Appl Neurobiol 1977;3:341–358.
30. Coleman PD, Flood DG. Neuron numbers and dendritic extent in normal aging and Alzheimer's disease. Neurobiol Aging 1987;8:521–545.
31. Terry RD, DeTeresa R, Hansen LA. Neocortical cell counts in normal human adult aging. Ann Neurol 1987;21:530–539.
32. Flood DG, Coleman PD. Hippocampal plasticity in normal aging and decreased plasticity in Alzheimer's disease. Prog Brain Res 1990;83: 435–443.
33. Wippold FJ II, Gado MH, Morris JC, et al. Senile dementia and healthy aging: a longitudinal CT study. Radiology 1991;179:215–219.
34. Wisniewski HM, Wen GY. Lipopigment in the aging brain. Am J Med Genet Suppl 1977;5:183–916.
35. Tomlinson BE. Morphological Brain Changes in Non-Demented Old People. In van Praag HM, Kalverboer AF (eds), Ageing of the Central Nervous System. Biological and Psychological Aspects. Bohn: Haarlem, 1972;38–57.
36. Waller SB, London ED. Noninvasive Diagnostic Techniques to Study Age-Related Cerebral Disorders. In Bergener M (ed), Psychogeriatrics: An International Handbook, New York: Springer, 1987.
37 Naritomi H, Meyer JS, Sakai F, et al. Effects of advancing age on regional cerebral blood flow. Studies in normal subjects and subjects with risk factor for atherothrombotic stroke. Arch Neurol 1979;36:410–416.
38. Obrist WD. Noninvasive Studies of Cerebral Blood Flow in Aging and Dementia. In Katzman R, Terry RD, Bick KL (eds), Aging (Vol. 7). New York: Raven, 1978;213.
39. Ingvar DH. Patterns of Brain Activity by Measurements of Regional Cerebral Blood Flow. In Ingvar DH, Lassen NA (eds), Brain Work: The Coupling of Function, Metabolism, and Blood Flow in the Brain. New York: Academic, 1975;397.
40. MacInnes WD, Golden CJ, Gillen RW, et al. Aging, regional cerebral blood flow, and neuropsychological functioning. J Am Geriatr Soc 1984;32:712–718.
41. Duara R, Margolin RA, Robertson-Tchabo EA, et al. Cerebral glucose utilization, as measured with positron emission tomography in 21 resting healthy men between the ages of 21 and 83 years. Brain 1983;106:761–765.
42. Kuhl DE, Metter EG, Riege WH, Phelps ME. Effects of human aging on patterns of local cerebral glucose utilization determined by the F-18 fluoro-deoxyglucose method. J Cereb Bood Flow Metab 1982;2:163–171.
43. Reige WH, Metter EJ, Kuhl DE, Phelps ME. Brain glucose metabolism and memory functions: age decreases in factor scores. J Gerontol 1985;40:459–467.
44. Cohen BM, Renshaw PF, Stoll AL, et al. Decreased brain choline uptake in older adults. An in vivo proton magnetic resonance spectroscopy study. JAMA 1995;274:902–907.
45. Bartus RT, Dean RL, Beer P, Lippa AS. The cholinergic hypothesis of geriatric memory dysfunction. Science 1982;217:408–412.
46. Robinson D, Davis J, Nies A, et al. Relation of sex and aging to monoamine oxidase activity on human brain plasma and platelets. Arch Gen Psychiatry 1971;24:536–539.
47. McGeer PL, McGeer EG. Aging and Neurotransmitter Systems. In Finch CE, Potter DE, Kenny AD (eds), Parkinson's Disease-II Aging and Neuroendocrine Relationship. New York: Plenum, 1978;1–57.

48. Palmer AM, DeKosky ST. Monoamine neurons in aging and Alzheimer's disease. J Neural Transm Gen Sect 1993;91:135–159.
49. Carlsson A. Neurotransmitter changes in the aging brain. Dan Med Bull 1985;32(Suppl 1):40–43.
50. Roth GS. Steroid and Dopaminergic Receptors in the Aged Brain. In Enna SJ, Samorajski T, Beer B (eds), Aging (Vol. 17). New York: Raven, 1981;163–169.
51. Severson J. Neurotransmitter receptors and aging. J Am Geriatr Soc 1984;32:24–27.
52. Iyo M, Yamasaki T. The detection of age-related decrease of dopamine D1, D2 and serotonin 5-HT2 receptors in living human brain. Prog Neuropsychopharmacol Biol Psychiatry 1993;17:415–421.
53. Blin J, Baron JC, Dubois B, et al. Loss of brain 5-HT2 receptors in Alzheimer's disease. In vivo assessment with positron emission tomography and [18F] setoperone. Brain 1993;116(Pt 3):497–510.
54. Swift CG. Pharmacodynamics: changes in homeostatic mechanisms, receptor and target organ sensitivity in the elderly. Br Med Bull 1990;46:36–52.
55. Agate J. Common Symptoms and Complaints. In Rossman I (ed), Clinical Geriatrics (3rd ed). Philadelphia: Lippincott, 1986;38–149.
56. Albano WA, Zielinski CM, Organ CH. Is appendicitis in the aged really different? Geriatrics 1975;30:81–88.
57. Gleckman R, Hibert D. Afebrile bacteremia. A phenomenon in geriatric patients. JAMA 1982;248:1478–1481.
58. Kaiko RF, Wallenstien SC, Rogers AG. Narcotics in the elderly. Med Clin North Am 1982;66:1079–1089.
59. Harkis SW, Kwentus J, Price D. Pain and Suffering in the Elderly. In Bonica J (ed), The Management of Pain. Philadelphia: Lea & Febiger, 1990;552–559.
60. Mullan E, Katona C, Bellew M. Patterns of sleep disorders and sedative hypnotic use in seniors. Drugs Aging 1994;5:49–58.
61. Rumble R, Morgan K. Hypnotics, sleep, and mortality in elderly people. J Am Geriatr Soc 1992;40:787–791.
62. Morgan K. Hypnotics in the elderly. What cause for concern? Drugs 1990;40:688–696.
63. Haimov I, Lavie P, Laudon M, et al. Melatonin replacement therapy of elderly insomniacs. Sleep 1995;18:598–603.
64. Duncalf D, Kepes ER. Geriatric Anesthesia. In Rossman I (ed), Clinical Geriatrics (3rd ed). Philadelphia: Lippincott, 1986;494–510.
65. Titchener JL, Zwerling I, Gottschalk L, et al. Psychosis in surgical patients. Surg Gynecol Obstet 1956;102:59–65.
66. Heller SS, Frank KA, Malm JR, et al. Psychiatric complication of open-heart surgery: a re-examination. N Engl J Med 1970;283:1015–1020.
67. Djokovic JL. Preoperative assessment of the elderly. Wis Med J 1983;82:20–22.
68. Folstein MF, Folstein SE, McHugh PR. "Mini-mental state." A practical method for grading the cognitive state of patients for the clinician. J Psychiatr Res 1975;12:189–198.
69. Morrissey K, Schein CH. Surgical Problems in the Aged. In Rossman I (ed), Clinical Geriatrics (3rd ed). Philadelphia: Lippincott, 1986; 472–493.
70. Beard BH. Management of Psychiatric Problems. In Greenfield LHJ (ed), Major Problems in Clinical Surgery (3rd ed). Philadelphia: Saunders, 1975;124–138.
71. Lipowski ZJ. Transient cognitive disorders (delirium, acute confusional states) in the elderly. Am J Psychiatry 1983;140:1426–1436.
72. Trzepacz PT. The neuropathogenesis of delirium: a need to focus our research. Psychosomatics 1994;35:374–379.
73. Trzepacz PT, Dew MA. Further analyses of the delirium rating scale. Gen Hosp Psychiatry 1995;17:75–79.
74. Lipowski AJ. Delirium (acute confusional states). JAMA 1987;258: 1789–1792.
75. Tune LE. Post-operative delirium. Int Psychogeriatr 1991;3:325–352.
76. Weinrich S, Sarna L. Delirium in the older person with cancer. Cancer 1994;74(Suppl 7):2079–2091.
77. Massie MJ, Holland J, Glass E. Delirium in terminally ill cancer patients. Am J Psychiatry 1983;140:1048–1050.
78. Erkinjuntii T, Wikstrom J, Palo J, et al. Dementia among medical inpatients. Arch Intern Med 1986;146:1923–1926.
79. Inouye SK. The dilemma of delirium: clinical and research controversies regarding diagnosis and evaluation of delirium in hospitalized elderly medical patients. Am J Med 1994;97:278–288.
80. Mach JR Jr, Dysken MW, Kuskowski M, et al. Serum anticholinergic activity in hospitalized older persons with delirium: a preliminary study [see comments]. J Am Geriatr Soc 1995;43:491–495.
81. Golinger RC, Peet T, Tune LE. Association of elevated plasma anticholinergic activity with delirium in surgical patients. Am J Psychiatry 1987;144:1218–1220.
82. Learoyd BM. Psychotropic drugs and the elderly patient. Med J Aust 1972;1:1131–1133.
83. Larson EB, Kukull WA, Buchner D, Reifler BV. Adverse drug reactions associated with global cognitive impairment in elderly persons. Ann Intern Med 1987;107:169–173.
84. Granacher RP, Baldessarini RJ, Messner E. Physostigmine treatment of delirium induced by anticholinergics. Am Fam Physician 1976;13:99–103.
85. Lofgren RP, MacPherson DS, Granieri R, et al. Mechanical restraints on the medical wards: are protective devices safe? Am J Public Health 1989;79:735–738.
86. Shapiro BA, Warren J, Egol AB, et al. Practice parameters for intravenous analgesia and sedation for adult patients in the intensive care unit: an executive summary. Society of Critical Care Medicine [see comments]. Crit Care Med 1995;23:1596–1600.
87. Frye MA, Coudreaut MF, Hakeman SM, et al. Continuous droperidol infusion for management of agitated delirium in an intensive care unit. Psychosomatics 1995;36:301–305.
88. Di Salvo TG, O'Gara PT. Torsade de pointes caused by high-dose intravenous haloperidol in cardiac patients. Clin Cardiol 1995;18:285–290.
89. McCartney JR, Boland RJ. Anxiety and delirium in the intensive care unit. Crit Care Clin 1994;10:673–680.
90. Levine RL. Pharmacology of intravenous sedatives and opioids in critically ill patients. Crit Care Clin 1994;10:709–731.
91. Ayd FJ. Intravenous haloperidol-lorazepam therapy for delirium. Drug Ther Newsletter 1984;19:33–35.
92. Foy A, O'Connell D, Henry D, et al. Benzodiazepine use as a case of cognitive impairment in elderly hospital inpatients. J Gerontol A Biol Sci Med Sci 1995;50:M99–M106.
93. Feldmeier C, Kapp W. Comparative clinical studies with midazolam, oxazepam and placebo. Br J Clin Pharmacol 1983;1:S151–S155.
94. Wells CE. The Differential Diagnosis of Psychiatric Disorders in the Elderly. In Cole JO, Barrett JE (eds), Psychopathology in the Aged. New York: Raven, 1980;19–31.
95. Coccaro EF, Kramer E, Zemishlany Z, et al. Pharmacologic treatment of noncognitive behavioral disturbances in elderly demented patients. Am J Psychiatry 1990;147:1640–1645.
96. Risse SC, Barnes R. Pharmacologic treatment of agitation associated with dementia. J Am Geriatr Soc 1986;34:368–376.
97. Lebert F, Pasquier F, Petit H. Behavioral effects of trazodone in Alzheimer's disease. J Clin Psychiatry 1994;55:536–538.
98. Friedman R, Gryfe CI, Tal DT, Freedman M. The noisy elderly patient: prevalence, assessment, and response to the antidepressant doxepin. J Geriatr Psychiatry Neurol 1992;5:187–191.
99. Gleason RP, Schneider LS. Carbamazepine treatment of agitation in Alzheimer's outpatients refractory to neuroleptics [see comments]. J Clin Psychiatry 1990;51:115–118.
100. Essa M. Carbamazepine in dementia. J Clin Psychopharmacol 1986; 6:234–236.
101. Mellow AM, Solano-Lopez C, Davis S. Sodium valproate in the treatment of behavioral disturbance in dementia. J Geriatr Psychiatry Neurol 1993;6:205–209.
102. Holzer JC, Gitelman DR, Price BH. Efficacy of buspirone in the treatment of dementia with aggression [letter]. Am J Psychiatry 1995;152:812.
103. Roth M. The natural history of mental disorder in old age. J Ment Sci 1955;101:281–301.
104. Blazer D, Williams CD. Epidemiology of dysphoria and depression in an elderly population. Am J Psychiatry 1980;137:439–444.
105. Cheah KC, Beard OW. Psychiatric findings in the population of a geriatric evaluation unit: implications. J Am Geriatr Soc 1980;28: 153–156.
106. Shuckitt MA, Miller PL, Berman J. The three year course of psychiatric problems in a geriatric population. J Clin Psychiatry 1980;41: 27–32.
107. Folks DG, Franceshini J, Sokol RS, et al. Coronary artery bypass surgery in older patients: psychiatric morbidity. South Med J 1986;79: 303–306.
108. Blundell E. A psychological study of the effect of surgery on eighty-six elderly patients. Br J Soc Clin Psychol 1967;6:297–303.

109. Hole A, Terjesen T, Breivik L. Epidural versus general anesthesia for total hip arthroplasty in elderly patients. Acta Anesthesiol Scand 1982;26:291–296.
110. Karhunen U, John G. A comparison of memory function following local and general anaesthesia for extraction of senile cataract. Acta Anaesthesiol Scand 1982;26:291–296.
111. Riis J, Lomholt B, Haxholdt O, et al. Immediate and long-term mental recovery from general versus epidural anesthesia in elderly patients. Acta Anaesthesiol Scand 1983;27:44–49.
112. Bigler D, Adelhoj B, Petring OU, et al. Mental function and morbidity after acute hip surgery during spinal and general anaesthesia. Anaesthesia 1985;40:672–676.
113. Skoll SL, August RJ, Johnson G. Drug prescribing for the elderly in Saskatchewan during 1976. Can Med Assoc J 1979;121:1074–1081.
114. Richelson E. Psychotropics and the elderly: interaction to watch for. Geriatrics 1984;39:30–42.
115. Hurwitz N, Wade OL. Intensive hospital monitoring of adverse reactions to drugs. Br Med J 1969;1:531–536.
116. Carruthers SG. Principles of Drug Treatment in the Aged. In Rossman I (ed), Clinical Geriatrics (3rd ed). Philadelphia: Lippincott, 1986; 114–124.
117. Rabins P, Lucas MJ, Teitelbaum M, et al. Utilization of psychiatric consultation for elderly patients. J Am Geriatr Soc 1983;31:581–585.
118. Hamerman D, Dubler NN, Kennedy GJ, Masdeu J. Decision making in response to an elderly woman with dementia who refused surgical repair of her fractured hip. J Am Geriatr Soc 1986;34:234–239.
119. Abernathy V. Compassion, control, and decision about competency. Am J Psychiatry 1984;141:53–60.

Surgical Care for the Elderly, 2nd ed., edited by
R. Benton Adkins, Jr., and H. William Scott, Jr.
Lippincott–Raven Publishers, Philadelphia © 1998.

CHAPTER 11

Surgical Nursing

Sarah J. White

Increasing numbers of individuals are living well past retirement age. Many seniors are remaining healthy and active into their 80s and beyond. In fact, the fastest growing segment of the population in the United States is the >85 age group, increasing at an average rate of approximately 4% per year [1,2]. Surgical procedures that might once have been contraindicated based on chronologic age are now considered in light of a person's general health and functional status, the risks and benefits of the procedure, and the expected outcome in terms of quality of life. Age alone is not a deterrent to a major surgical procedure. As research into aging provides more information about the unique nature of this population, nursing is challenged to adapt its approaches to perioperative care to meet the needs of elderly patients.

SPECIALIZED CARE NEEDS

Physiologic Changes

Aging is a complex process of physiologic, psychological, developmental, and social changes that occurs at varying rates in different individuals. Different organ systems can age at different rates within the same individual. Superimposed on the aging process are the effects of life-style choices, chronic diseases, and acute illnesses. The nurse must recognize normal aging changes and secondary effects of illness to develop and implement a comprehensive plan of care for the older surgical patient. Table 11-1 summarizes some of the specific changes associated with aging, along with suggested adaptations in nursing care.

Changes occur in every body system with aging. Changes in vision and hearing decrease acuity and affect how we interview and educate patients. Integumentary changes predispose the patient to slower wound healing and the development of pressure ulcers. Cardiopulmonary alterations limit reserve in those systems and increase the risk of complications perioperatively. Nutritional status is a multifactorial phenomenon often negatively affected by poor dentition and changes in the gastrointestinal tract. Medication metabolism and excretion are affected by changes in hepatic enzyme activity, decreased creatinine clearance secondary to renal changes, and reduction in the percentage of lean body mass associated with aging. Changes in the neurologic and musculoskeletal systems increase the risk of falls and fractures in the elderly.

With aging there is a general loss of reserve functional capacity in all organ systems. This loss of reserve is well tolerated by the healthy older individual. Chronic diseases such as chronic obstructive pulmonary disease, coronary artery disease, and osteoarthritis further limit functional reserve. During any type of physiologic stress, even the healthy older patient may not be able to respond as promptly and appropriately as a younger patient. Stress may occur in the form of fever, surgery, dehydration, or infection. This loss of functional reserve accounts for many of the atypical presentations of illness in the older patient. For example, the older patient who develops a urinary tract infection postoperatively may exhibit only a subtle change in mental status rather than the classic symptoms of fever, chills, and dysuria. Nurses must develop a high degree of suspicion in assessing and interpreting information with older patients.

Care needs in older patients are also influenced by chronic diseases that become more prevalent as we age. Over 85% of those over age 65 have at least one significant chronic health problem, with many having multiple chronic diseases. Cardiovascular disease remains the number one cause of death in the elderly population. Other common chronic illnesses that may affect the decision to undergo surgery and the postoperative recovery include osteoarthritis, chronic obstructive pulmonary disease, chronic renal insufficiency, hypertension, and diabetes mellitus [3]. Although these diseases do not necessarily prevent an individual from benefiting from a surgical procedure, they must be well managed and monitored perioperatively. Careful explanation to the patient and family of the risks and benefits of the surgical procedure is warranted. The nurse may find himself or herself in the role of patient advocate during this process, providing additional information, support, and education as appropriate.

TABLE 11-1. *Common aging changes and care adaptations*

Changes	Adaptations
Sensory	
Decreased pupil size	Provide direct, adequate lighting
Narrowing of visual fields	Avoid monochromatic color schemes
Yellowing, opacity, rigidity of lens	Provide educational materials in large print
Presbyopia (farsightedness)	Address safety concerns in the environment
High-frequency hearing loss	Correct use of glasses and hearing aids
Tone discrimination loss	Lower the pitch of your voice
Increased production of cerumen	Face the patient at eye level
Decreased elasticity of tympanic membrane	Check for and remove cerumen impaction
Integumentary	
Epidermis thins and atrophies	Assess risk of pressure ulcers
Increased vascular fragility	Use appropriate pressure reduction devices
Loss of subcutaneous fat	Avoid the use of tape on fragile skin
Decreased perception to touch, pain, etc.	Avoid frequent bathing; use emollients
Slower wound healing	Maximize nutrition to promote wound healing
Cardiovascular	
Decreased stroke volume and cardiac output	Frequent small meals
Decreased ability to increase heart rate in response to stress	Avoid extremes and sudden changes in temperatures
Increased amount of collagen and fat	Provide frequent rest periods
Thickening and rigidity of heart valves	Be aware of effect of fever, stress on limited cardiac reserve
Respiratory	
Decreased elasticity and number of alveoli	Schedule rest periods with activities
Decreased vital capacity	Careful assessment of respiratory status
Decreased mobility of bony thorax	Aggressive pulmonary toilet postoperatively
Weakening of respiratory muscles	Monitoring of pulse oximetry
Decreased ciliary action	—
Gastrointestinal	
Poor dentition	Careful assessment of nutritional status
Decreased taste sensation and appetite	Minimize dietary restrictions
Decreased emptying time	Encourage upright position for meals
Decreased gastric acid and hepatic enzymes	Appropriate texture and consistency of meals
Increased incidence of malnutrition	Consider need for bowel regimen
Genitourinary	
Decreased blood flow to kidneys	Encourage adequate fluid intake
Decreased number of nephrons	Investigate incontinence for cause
Decreased creatinine clearance	Monitor for atypical presentation of fluid and electrolyte imbalances
Bladder capacity decreased from 500 to 250 ml	Monitor medications closely, especially those cleared through the kidneys
Decreased bladder tone and elasticity	Avoid diapers
Musculoskeletal	
Decreased muscle strength and symmetrical muscle wasting	Avoid bedrest, promote early mobilization and involvement of physical therapy
Demineralization of bones with loss of height (2 in. between 20 and 70 years)	Initiate fall prevention strategies when appropriate
Decreased flexibility and mobility	Proper fitting and use of assistive devices
Increased risk for falls	Proper fitting and use of shoes; proper nail care
Changes in gait	Modify the environment for safety
Neurologic	
Decreased number of neurons	Assess baseline cognitive function
Decreased size and weight of brain, but dementia is not normal aging	Teach in multiple, short sessions
Change in sleep patterns	Adjust care to avoid disturbing sleep
Slower response to stimuli	Use schedules and memory aids as needed
Decreased sensation	Change positions frequently

Functional Status

As an individual ages, functional disability often increases. These functional losses may consist of visual or hearing deficits, incontinence, difficulty with mobility and transfers, cognitive impairment, or limitations with activities of daily living (ADLs). ADLs consist of basic day-to-day tasks such as bathing, dressing, feeding, toileting, and ambulating. Approximately one-half of all older individuals have at least one personal-care activity limitation. Those living in long-term care facilities generally have three or more functional limitations [4]. Functional ability is strongly correlated with numerous outcome measures including hospital length of stay, severity of disease process, mortality, morbidity, and physiologic reserve. Measurement of function is also an important indicator of overall progress during treatment [5]. Understanding the patient's baseline functional status and the degree of functional deficits is an important component of the decision-making process and will help the nurse plan for care during the perioperative period. For example, an 85-year-old man who is nonambulatory as a result of a stroke falls out of bed and fractures his hip. With this patient's limited baseline functional status, a decision may be made not to surgically intervene to repair the hip fracture. On the other hand, an 85-year-old woman who lived alone but walked with a walker was hospitalized for acute cholecystitis. Surgery followed by aggressive mobilization and nutrition may be warranted to restore her to her pre-illness function and to independent living.

Developmental Issues

Social, psychological, and economic concerns related to aging affect decision making before surgery, postoperative care, and planning for discharge. Assessing and meeting identified needs in these arenas is a primary nursing role. Developmental tasks to be considered for the younger old, up to age 75, include preparing for the retirement role, adjusting to a fixed income, establishing living arrangements appropriate to one's health, adjusting to new relationships with spouse and offspring, developing leisure time activities, adjusting to slower physical and intellectual responses in ADLs, dealing with one's own mortality, and dealing with the losses inherent in aging. The vulnerable old, over age 75, have the additional tasks of combining new dependency needs with the continuing need for independence, adapting to living alone without becoming socially isolated, adjusting to possible institutional living, adjusting to decreased physical and emotional reserve, and accepting one's own approaching death [6].

These developmental tasks can be used in a practical approach as the nurse assists the older patient in preparing for surgical treatment and going home after surgery. Key questions to ask before surgery include the following: Where does the patient live and with whom, what social supports exist, what is the home environment like, what financial concerns exist, what home care needs may exist and what is covered by insurance, what concerns and goals do the patient and family express, and does the patient have advance directives that have been communicated to all care providers?

RESTORATIVE CARE

Principles and Goals of Restorative Care

Restorative care is a model of care that incorporates the biological, psychological, and social aspects of the individual patient and builds a plan of care based on the patient's strengths. The goals of care are patient oriented rather than problem oriented. The problem-oriented model of care focuses on disease and uses the traditional biomedical approach whereas the restorative or functional approach allows for the incorporation of the principles of the biopsychosocial model into clinical practice. At any point in time, functional status can be conceptualized as an individual's overall level of functioning and depicted as the composition of various biological, psychological, and social capabilities. The biological component includes the combined level of functioning of specific organs and organ systems. The psychological component consists of cognitive and perceptual capabilities as well as personality traits. The social component can be viewed as a support network that includes people, places, programs, policies, attitudes, and economic resources [7,8].

The restorative model, therefore, views the individual holistically. It uses functional assessment to identify a patient's strengths and weaknesses regardless of the medical diagnosis or surgical procedure. The plan of care is based on this assessment and is designed to restore, promote, maintain, or improve function. Nursing care helps the older adult maintain or return to a desired lifestyle.

This model is based on several premises. First, remaining functionally independent is a common goal of all adults. Second, most people use functional ability to define their health status, rather than or in spite of, specific pathology. Third, the language used in discussing functional assessment is easily understood and promotes improved communication among the patient, family, and all health team members [8].

Preoperative Assessment

A preoperative nursing assessment using the restorative model, therefore, focuses on selected parameters in a variety of functional domains. The information obtained forms the basis for an individualized plan of care. The American Nursing Association Standards for Gerontological Nursing Practice provide guidelines for a comprehensive history and

TABLE 11-2. *Activities of daily living: Katz Index*

Activity	Independent	With assistance*	Dependent
Bathing	Receives no assistance	Receives assistance with one part of body	Receives assistance with more than one part of body
Dressing	Gets clothes and gets dressed with no assistance	Gets clothes and gets dressed except for tying shoes	Receives assistance in getting clothes or in dressing
Toileting	Receives no assistance	Receives assistance in getting to toilet, cleaning self, or in arranging clothes	Does not go to room termed *toilet*
Transfer	Moves in and out of bed without assistance	Moves in or out of bed or chair with assistance	Does not get out of bed
Continence	Controls elimination completely by self	Has occasional accidents	Catheter is used or is incontinent
Feeding	Feeds self without assistance	Receives assistance in cutting meat or buttering bread	Receives assistance in feeding or is fed enterally

**Assistance* means supervision, direction, or personal assistance.

Sources: Adapted from Katz S, Downs TD, Cash HR, et al. Progress in development of the index of ADL. Gerontologist 1970;10:20–30; and Katz S. Assessing self-maintenance: activities of daily living, mobility, and instrumental activities of daily living. J Am Geriatr Soc 1983;31:721–727.

assessment. These standards stress the individualization of the nursing process for older patients [9].

The general history and physical assessment obtained by the nurse should complement the medical history. Most health care facilities use a standardized history and physical examination form to gather pertinent information. These may be organized by a traditional medical history format, by body systems, in a head-to-toe format, by selected domains of care, or some combination of these formats. Adapting interview and assessment techniques to the needs of the older patient is often necessary. Older patients frequently have lengthy and complicated health histories. They may have limited endurance related to age and health problems that prohibit them from participating fully in a prolonged interview session. Focusing the history and physical examination on targeted information based on the admission diagnosis, the patient's stated concerns, and the planned surgical procedure may be the most effective use of time and energy.

There are fundamental differences in adapting a medical history to older patients. The history of the present illness, rather than focusing on symptoms, is more appropriately focused on changes in function. Because many aging problems are multifactorial, the history may need to be expanded to include additional pertinent information. For example, the 85-year-old man who fell and fractured his hip may have done so as a result of a combination of such factors as medication use, arthritis, use of a cane, impaired vision, and environmental hazards in his home. Failing to address these contributing elements limits the ability of the nurse to comprehensively plan for the care of this patient.

A functional assessment is the core of geriatric care. Again, a standardized format will assist in obtaining information in a systematic and comprehensive manner. This assessment is best obtained from actual observation of the patient performing selected activities, but may at times be based on self- or family reporting. There are many simple tools available for ADL assessment that can be completed quickly and easily by the nurse. The Katz Index of ADL, the Barthel Index, and the PULSES profile all combine various aspects of function into a simple format [10,11]. These tools assess the patient's level of independence in the basic activities of bathing, dressing, toileting, transferring, feeding, and continence. PULSES adds the general physical condition, other mobility and sensory components, and social supports. Table 11-2 provides the Katz Index of ADL as an example of a simple screening tool.

Instrumental ADLs are higher level functions needed to live independently. Instrumental ADLs include using the telephone, shopping, preparing meals, doing housework, taking medications, handling money, and getting to places outside of walking distance [12]. Figure 11-1 provides a simple scale for screening for difficulties in performing these tasks. A more detailed evaluation may be provided by an occupational therapist. One tool that can be used is the Kohlman Evaluation of Living Skills. This takes approximately 20 to 30 minutes to administer and includes assessments of self-care, safety, money management, use of the telephone, and means of transportation. This tool uses photographs to assess the patient's ability to recognize dangerous household situations. It tests for knowledge of emergency numbers and appropriate action in the event of sickness or accidents. The patient is evaluated on money management using a check, checkbook, a copy of an actual bill, and actual money in making change [13]. If the patient is found to have difficulty with these tasks, the discharge plan should identify other mechanisms for providing these services safely. Family members are often able to assist but may be required to provide more supervision and assistance than was required before the surgery.

Baseline cognitive function should be included in a general functional assessment. The incidence of postoperative delirium is 10% to 15% in elderly patients undergoing any surgical procedure and up to 50% of older individuals undergoing total hip replacement [14]. Distinguishing subtle

Activity	Independent	Needs assistance	Unable to do
Use telephone			
Travel			
Shop for groceries			
Prepare meals			
Do housework			
Make home repairs			
Do laundry			
Take medicines			
Manage finances			

FIG. 11-1. Checklist for instrumental activities of daily living. (Modified from Lawton MD, Brody EM. Assessment of older people: self maintaining and instrumental activities of daily living. Gerontologist 1969;9:179–185.)

changes in cognition from the baseline measurement is an important clue to possible medication reactions, early postoperative infections, or other complications. Clues that may alert the nurse to the need for a more standardized evaluation include difficulty with word finding, inaccurate or incomplete responses to history questions, poor attention span, recent memory deficits, and spatial deficits. Concern about cognitive functioning should be followed up with a more systematic screening such as a mini-mental state examination or the modified mini-mental state examination [15,16]. The mini-mental state examination is provided in Fig. 11-2. Referral for a thorough dementia workup may be indicated.

General observations can yield pertinent information about mental health. Grooming and appropriate dress, posture, facial expression, and nonverbal body language during the assessment process are indicators of mood and cognitive functioning. Specific questions regarding mood and previous coping behaviors can be included in the interview. Depression is a frequently undiagnosed illness in the elderly and one that greatly affects motivation for participation in recovery [17]. The geriatric depression scale is an easily administered tool that can be used to further assess the presence of depression in older patients [18].

An assessment of current nutritional status is essential. Twenty percent to 60% of older patients in hospitals and nursing homes have been noted to suffer from inadequate nutrition, protein calorie malnutrition, or both [19]. This is reflected in a serum albumin of <3.5 g/dl. Low admission serum albumin level and weight loss in the year prior to the hospitalization have been found to be highly predictive of complications during hospitalization [20]. The following list details some of the contributing causes to malnutrition that should be included in an evaluation of nutritional status in the elderly:

- Eating habits
- Dentition
- Economics
- Mobility
- Housing/isolation
- Sensory: vision, taste, and smell
- Transportation
- Constipation
- Information and education
- Health problems
- Motivation
- Medications
- Confusion
- Depression

A review of the patient's medication regimen is a key component of a preoperative assessment. The >65 population uses 25% to 31% of prescription drugs and an even higher percentage of over-the-counter drugs. They have a higher incidence of adverse reactions and drug-drug interactions than younger patients [21,22]. Doses acceptable for younger patients can be excessive and even toxic in older individuals. Medications are often adjusted, added, or deleted during hospitalization. Understanding the indications and potential adverse reactions for each medication enhances the preoperative nursing assessment.

A thorough evaluation of the patient's home and social supports will help in anticipating discharge needs and planning for posthospital care. It is important to know where the patient lives and with whom. Only 5% of those >65 live in long-term care facilities, although about one in four older adults will spend some time in a nursing home during the last years of his or her life [23]. The majority live independently,

Patient: ____________ **Examiner:** ____________ **Date:** ____________

Maximum score	Score	
		Orientation
5	( )	What is the (year) (season) (date) (day) (month)?
5	( )	Where are we (state) (country) (town) (hospital) (floor)?
3	( )	Registration Name three objects: 1 second to say each. Then ask the patient all three after you have said them. Give 1 point for each correct answer. Then repeat them until he/she learns all three. Count trials and record. Trials:
5	( )	Attention and calculation Serial 7s. One point for each correct answer. Stop after five answers. Alternatively, spell "world" backward.
3	( )	Recall Ask for the three objects repeated above. Give 1 point for each correct answer.
2	( )	Language Name a pencil and watch.
1	( )	Repeat the following: "No ifs, ands, or buts."
3	( )	Follow a three-stage command: "Take a paper in your hand, fold it in half, and put it on the floor."
1	( )	Read and obey the following: CLOSE YOUR EYES.
1	( )	Write a sentence.
1	( )	Copy design.
		Total score

ASSESS level of consciousness along a continuum: Alert Drowsy Stupor Coma

FIG. 11-2. Mini-mental state examination. (Reprinted with permission from Folstein ME, Folstein SE. Mini-mental state: a practical method for grading the cognitive state of patients for the clinician. J Psychiatr Res 1975;12:189–198. Elsevier Science Ltd, Oxford, England.)

alone or with family, in assisted living arrangements, or in boarding home situations. Each living situation presents specific limitations and challenges in providing needed post-hospital care. With shorter hospital stays, much of the postoperative recovery may need to occur outside of the hospital. Many patients will need ongoing wound care, intravenous therapy, rehabilitative therapy, or other complex care following surgery. Identifying those needs early and working with the patient and family to determine where these needs can best be met is important for the efficient use of health care resources and optimal outcomes for the patient.

The following list summarizes the major components of a comprehensive preoperative assessment. Data may be obtained from the patient directly, from the family or other social supports, from previous hospital records, or from other health care providers, such as home health nurses who have cared for the patient.

- Patient history
- Physical assessment
- Functional assessment: ADLs, instrumental ADLs
- Nutritional status
- Medications
- Mental status
- Mood
- Home environment
- Social supports
- Finances and insurance
- Use of assistive devices

Interdisciplinary Approach

The multiple needs of the elderly surgical patient cross many different disciplines and can best be met through an interdisciplinary geriatric evaluation team. A geriatric team is usually made up of representatives from medicine, nursing, social work, nutrition services, rehabilitative services, and pharmacy. Medical ethics, chaplain services, and clinical psychology may be available or serve on an as-needed basis. The team offers expertise in aging issues along with a coordinated approach.

Although the coordinated geriatric team may be the ideal approach, not every hospital has such a resource. Nursing must then play an integral role in advocating for the input of other disciplines to meet the needs of the elderly surgical patient.

The registered dietitian offers an in-depth assessment of the patient's current nutritional and hydration status and the possible causes of malnutrition or dehydration. He or she obtains information on dietary habits and preferences, access to groceries, difficulties with meal preparation, and difficulties with dentition or swallowing. The dietitian will calculate ideal body weight, calorie needs, and protein needs, taking into account the need for additional calories and protein for wound healing. The dietitian makes recommendations about the appropriate diet order, nutritional supplements, or more aggressive nutritional support such as enteral feedings or total parenteral nutrition.

The social worker should be consulted early in the hospitalization in the case of complex psychosocial concerns or potential posthospital needs. The social worker completes a psychosocial assessment focusing on the patient and family and their perception of needs. The social worker evaluates the home, social supports, and financial situation and educates the patient on available community resources for home care. If nursing home care or a stay in a rehabilitation facility is expected after hospitalization, the social worker provides the patient and family with in-depth information on admission criteria, reimbursement mechanisms, and facilities that meet the patient's needs and resources. The social worker also is trained to provide counseling and support to families during crises.

Physical and occupational therapists promote early mobilization and prevention of functional decline during the hospitalization. The therapists focus on maintaining and improving function, assessing the need for assistive devices to promote independence, evaluating skills needed to return home, and addressing home safety issues. A preoperative assessment should be recommended in the elderly patient who has functional limitations going into a surgical procedure.

Reviewing the medication regimen periodically throughout the hospitalization can best be done by the clinical pharmacist. The clinical pharmacist considers each medication and reviews the dose, frequency, schedule, form, reason the medication was prescribed, potential interactions with other drugs, possible adverse reactions, and the cost to the patient. The clinical pharmacist follows pertinent laboratory data such as the patient's creatinine clearance or specific drug levels and makes recommendations on appropriate drug therapy. The pharmacist is extremely helpful in simplifying the medication regimen and offering suggestions to ensure patient compliance.

The clinical psychologist may be needed to further assess cognitive functioning or address the question of depression in an older patient. Complex ethical decisions may require input from the medical ethicist or chaplain. Counseling and support through the chaplain's office is often needed in the event of a diagnosis of a condition such as cancer, an unexpected death, or during terminal supportive care in the hospital.

Coordinating needed services requires a facilitative approach and is a role often filled by the nurse. In the absence of a geriatric team, the nurse can mobilize a variety of resources within the hospital to assist with meeting the complex and varied needs of the older surgical patient.

PREOPERATIVE TEACHING

Preparation of a patient for a surgical procedure includes preoperative teaching. An essential first step in developing a teaching plan is assessing the patient's current knowledge and learning needs, educational level, and ability to read, any changes in sensory or cognitive function that may affect learning, the patient's preferred learning style, any sociocultural values, religious beliefs, or economic constraints that may affect teaching, any family member or other caregiver who needs to be included in the teaching, and the patient's motivation and interest in learning [24].

The patient anticipating a surgical procedure should understand what the surgery entails, along with the potential risks and benefits of that surgery. The patient should be taught what to expect before, during, and after the operative procedure including any preoperative preparations such as laboratory tests, scrubs, medications, and restrictions on oral intake. Anticipated postoperative care may include dressings and drainage tubes that will be in place; presence of a Foley catheter, oxygen, or an intravenous line; where the patient will go initially following surgery and how long before he or she will return to the floor; any expected stay in an intensive care unit and what policies exist that affect family visitation; and specific measures that will be used to manage his or her care and prevent postoperative complications. Special instructions in coughing and deep breathing, early mobilization, and the importance of adequate pain management should be taught.

Preoperative teaching should ideally begin in the outpatient setting and be reviewed and expanded in the hospital. With increasing emphasis on shortening the length of the hospital stay, many patients are now being admitted to the hospital on the morning of surgery. Additionally, teaching is more effective in older patients in shorter sessions and in an environment of minimal stress [25]. Nurses' involvement in teaching may, therefore, be primarily in a clinic, home, or office setting. There may only be time for the nurse in the hospital to review what the patient knows and reinforce selected concepts. Because of these time constraints, a greater emphasis should be placed on using teaching tools that can be customized for patients. These tools promote gradual learning through a more consistent approach, regardless of the teacher.

Older adults often require adaptations of teaching methodology due to sensory deficits and limited endurance. How we teach becomes increasingly important. Using a variety of materials and strategies to compensate for deficits is recommended. Large-print materials with bold, dark type against a white or yellow background is most easily visualized by the elderly who often have a decreased ability to discriminate between colors, decreased visual acuity, and decreased light reaching the retina via the smaller pupil. Teaching materials should generally be written at a fifth grade level in nonmedical terminology for ease of comprehension by all patients. Audio and video presentations and charts can be effectively used to supplement teaching. Patient education handouts, booklets, or instruction sheets that can be taken home for further review are useful tools and help reinforce teaching.

Careful attention should be paid to the learning environment. A quiet, well-lit space with limited extraneous noise and minimal interruptions is more conducive to learning. Soft white light focused directly on teaching materials helps decrease glare and improve visualization. A comfortable chair and concern about comfort measures such as pain, toileting needs, thirst, hunger, room temperature, and frequent breaks enhance learning in the older individual as well [26].

Evaluation of the success of patient education in terms of patient understanding and retention of the content is essential. Simple, measurable behavioral objectives aid in this evaluation. Sample behavioral objectives include the following: (1) the patient will demonstrate correct use of incentive spirometry; (2) the patient will describe the purpose of the surgery; and (3) the patient will demonstrate the correct use of a walker or crutches.

POSTOPERATIVE CARE

Assessment

Immediately following surgery, the nurse should focus on a systematic assessment of the patient's respiratory status, cardiac status, fluid and electrolyte status, the surgical wound, and the level of pain. Ensuring adequate ventilation and aeration through an evaluation of respiratory rate and effort, auscultation and interpretation of breath sounds, and monitoring of oxygen saturations through pulse oximetry is important. The nurse must initiate measures to prevent pulmonary complications and promote good air exchange as soon as possible. Respiratory complications that are common in the older patient include atelectasis, pulmonary emboli, and pneumonia. Preventive measures consist of frequent turning and repositioning, early mobilization, reminders to cough and breathe deeply, and assisting the patient with the use of incentive spirometers. Any alterations in respiratory function or signs of infection should be reported promptly.

Patients over age 80 have a higher incidence of postoperative cardiovascular complications than younger patients. Changes in the aging heart contribute to myocardial irritability, valvular and myocardial disease, and the incidence of arrhythmias. Preexisting cardiovascular diseases such as hypertension or coronary artery disease along with the stress of surgery add to the risk of cardiac complications [27]. Monitoring should include close assessment of vital signs, breath sounds, and heart sounds. Central monitoring via a central venous pressure catheter is often indicated. The nurse should carefully monitor fluid status through intake and output, as well as reviewing pertinent laboratory data. The nurse should also be alert to any subtle change in mental status that may represent an atypical presentation of cardiac problems such as ischemia and arrhythmias.

Changes in the kidneys predispose older patients to a higher sensitivity to fluid and electrolyte disturbances. Careful monitoring of intravenous and oral intake, urine output, amount of drainage from wounds or drainage tubes, fluid losses through diarrhea or emesis, and estimates of insensible water losses through sweating or rapid respirations is essential during the initial postoperative period. Assessment of laboratory electrolyte values, vital signs, daily weights, and skin turgor adds to the overall assessment of fluid and electrolyte status. Fluid balance may be fragile in an older individual with impaired cardiac and renal functions. More gentle hydration at lower rates is generally indicated. The need for accurate urine output information should be balanced with the risk of infection with indwelling Foley catheters. Every effort should be made to remove Foley catheters within the first 24 to 48 hours following surgery. Thirty-five percent to 40% of all nosocomial infections are catheter-associated urinary tract infections, with one half of catheterized patients developing bacteriuria within the first 24 hours of having a catheter [28]. If the patient is stable, estimates of urine output along with weights should provide adequate information. Scheduled toileting for the incontinent patient often minimizes incontinent episodes and allows for continued monitoring of output. Scheduled toileting consists of offering the patient a bedside commode or urinal at scheduled frequencies throughout the day. Scheduled toileting in long-term care settings has been found to reduce the number of incontinent episodes by as much as 26%. Those who benefited most were those with normal bladder capacity and more intact cognitive functioning [29].

Postoperative delirium occurs in 10% to 15% of older patients and 30% to 50% of hip fracture patients [30]. Delirium can be defined as an acute alteration in mental status that develops over a short period of time and always includes attention span deficits. The most common causes of delirium are fluid-electrolyte abnormalities, infection, medications, metabolic disturbances, and environmental disturbances [31]. Delirium is often poorly understood and overlooked by nurses and underdiagnosed by physicians [32]. Acute changes in mental status are often the first indication in older patients of a change in physical status and should always be evaluated for potentially reversible causes.

Wound and Skin Care

Assessment of the surgical site is an immediate consideration postoperatively. The type of incision, placement of drains, location and type of dressing, as well as the amount and character of drainage should be evaluated immediately postoperatively and at frequent intervals during the immediate postoperative period. Ongoing wound management with appropriate dressing changes and assessment of the incision for signs of infection are equally important. A decreased epi-

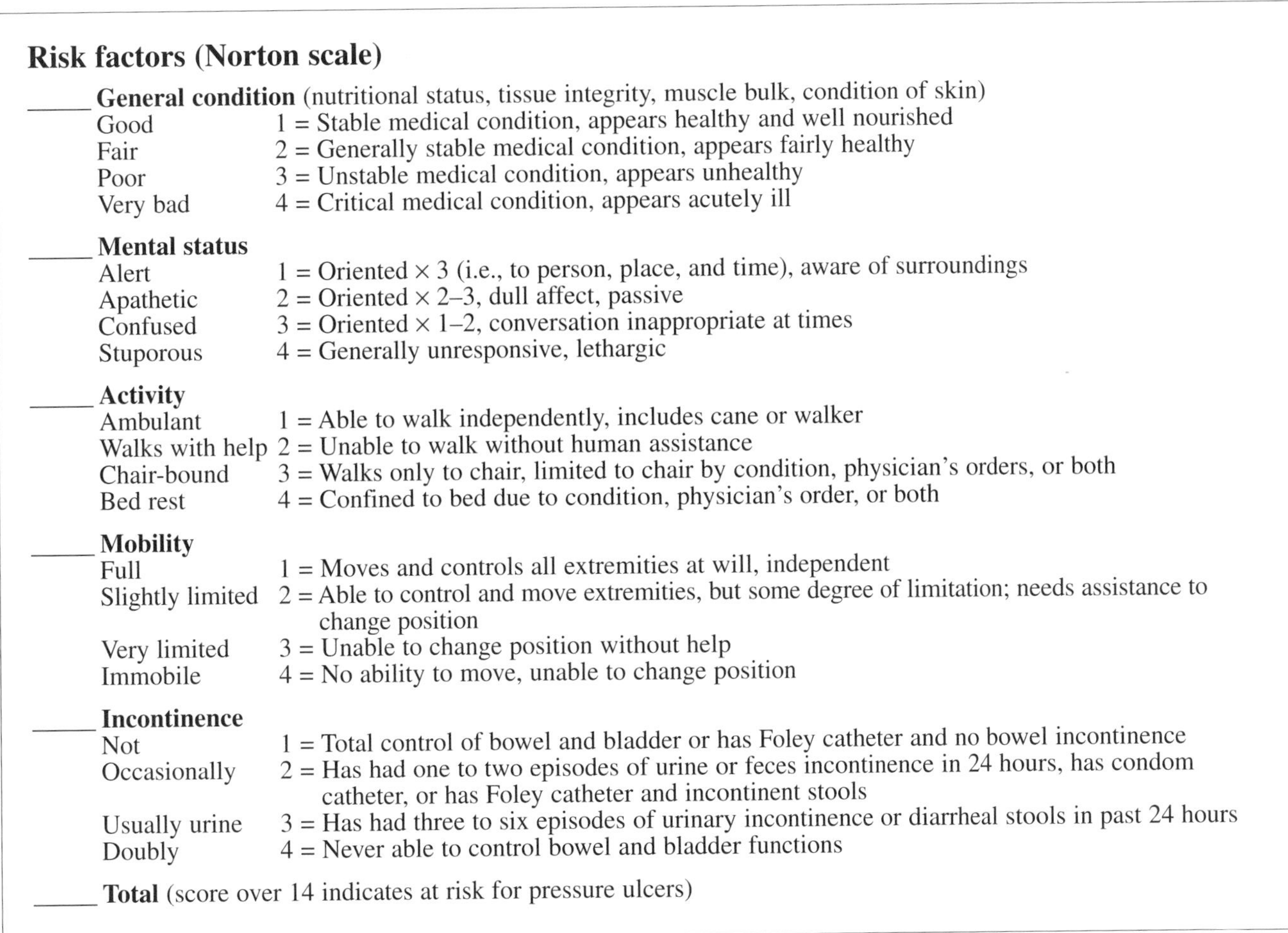

Risk factors (Norton scale)

_____ **General condition** (nutritional status, tissue integrity, muscle bulk, condition of skin)

Good	1 = Stable medical condition, appears healthy and well nourished
Fair	2 = Generally stable medical condition, appears fairly healthy
Poor	3 = Unstable medical condition, appears unhealthy
Very bad	4 = Critical medical condition, appears acutely ill

_____ **Mental status**

Alert	1 = Oriented × 3 (i.e., to person, place, and time), aware of surroundings
Apathetic	2 = Oriented × 2–3, dull affect, passive
Confused	3 = Oriented × 1–2, conversation inappropriate at times
Stuporous	4 = Generally unresponsive, lethargic

_____ **Activity**

Ambulant	1 = Able to walk independently, includes cane or walker
Walks with help	2 = Unable to walk without human assistance
Chair-bound	3 = Walks only to chair, limited to chair by condition, physician's orders, or both
Bed rest	4 = Confined to bed due to condition, physician's order, or both

_____ **Mobility**

Full	1 = Moves and controls all extremities at will, independent
Slightly limited	2 = Able to control and move extremities, but some degree of limitation; needs assistance to change position
Very limited	3 = Unable to change position without help
Immobile	4 = No ability to move, unable to change position

_____ **Incontinence**

Not	1 = Total control of bowel and bladder or has Foley catheter and no bowel incontinence
Occasionally	2 = Has had one to two episodes of urine or feces incontinence in 24 hours, has condom catheter, or has Foley catheter and incontinent stools
Usually urine	3 = Has had three to six episodes of urinary incontinence or diarrheal stools in past 24 hours
Doubly	4 = Never able to control bowel and bladder functions

_____ **Total** (score over 14 indicates at risk for pressure ulcers)

FIG. 11-3. Assessment of risk for pressure ulcers. (From Norton D, McLaren R, Exton-Smith AN. An investigation of geriatric nursing problems in the hospital. London: National Corporation for the Care of Old People, 1962.)

dermal turnover rate of approximately 50% between the third and seventh decades, reduced vascularity of the dermis, and changes in the histology of aging skin result in a tendency for decreased wound healing and increased risk of skin breakdown [33]. Frequent systematic assessment of the wound and high-pressure areas such as the sacrum, heels, shoulders, and hips is imperative.

The incidence of pressure ulcers in hospitals ranges from 2.7% to 29.5%. Elderly patients admitted for femoral fractures have been noted to have an incidence of pressure ulcers as high as 66% [34–36]. A number of simple assessment tools exist. The Norton scale provides a simple instrument for assessment of risk for pressure ulcers and is provided in Fig. 11-3 [37,38]. This tool summarizes the patient's physical condition, mental condition, activity level, mobility level, and degree of incontinence to provide a score that correlates with risk of pressure ulcers. The assessment should be documented and repeated at appropriate intervals. Pressure ulcers should be carefully assessed and the following parameters documented: location, size, stage, presence of undermining, color, odor, and drainage. Staging is a system of grading the degree of tissue damage present. The National Pressure Ulcer Advisory Panel recommendations for staging pressure ulcers are noted in Table 11-3, along with basic treatment modalities [39].

Early and aggressive interventions to prevent or manage pressure ulcers should be initiated. These measures include minimizing skin exposure to moisture due to incontinence, perspiration, or wound drainage; reduction of friction and shear forces through proper positioning, transferring, and turning techniques; appropriate use of lubricating and protective creams; appropriate use of protective dressings and pressure-reduction devices such as mattresses and chair cushions; and careful attention to increasing mobility and improving nutrition [40]. If a pressure ulcer develops, aggressive management with a consistent plan of care will help prevent further deterioration and promote healing. Referral to a wound management team or enterostomal therapist, if available, may be warranted, particularly if worsening or no improvement is noted.

Pain Management

Adequate pain management enhances patient compliance in turning, transferring from the bed, and participating in pulmonary toileting activities, dressing changes, and other

TABLE 11-3. *Staging and treatment of pressure ulcers*

Staging	
Stage I	Nonblanchable erythema of intact skin
Stage II	Partial thickness skin loss involving epidermis, dermis, or both
Stage III	Full-thickness skin loss involving damage to or necrosis of subcutaneous tissue that may extend down to, but not through, underlying fascia
Stage IV	Full-thickness skin loss with extensive destruction, tissue necrosis, or damage to muscle, bone, or supporting structures
Treatment	
Modify risk factors when possible (nutrition, mobility, continence)	
Reduce surface pressure (mattresses, chair cushions, positioning)	
Treat topically (cleansing, drying, protecting skin)	
Apply topical dressing (stages I and II)	
Debride, dress, or pack wound (stages III and IV)	

Source: Agency for Health Care Policy and Research, Public Health Service. Treatment of Pressure Ulcers. Clinical Practice Guideline, Number 15. AHCPR Pub. No. 95-0652. Rockville, MD: U.S. Department of Health and Human Services, December 1994.

aspects of care. An initial assessment of level of comfort postoperatively may rely on nonverbal cues such as restlessness, guarding, protective posturing, and facial grimacing. As a patient's level of consciousness returns, the patient should be questioned about his or her level of comfort, frequently assessed for nonverbal manifestations of pain, and offered medication at appropriate intervals. Accurate pain assessment is critical in identifying appropriate interventions and evaluating the effectiveness of those interventions. A number of pain scales are available to aid in more objective assessment of pain. The most commonly used scales are numeric (1 to 10, with 1 meaning no pain and 10 the worst pain possible), descriptive, or based on facial expressions [41].

Elderly patients may be reluctant to report pain for a number of reasons. They may believe that pain is to be expected and is something they must live with. Some patients may fear presumed consequences of reporting pain: prolonged hospitalization, institutionalization, or additional diagnostic procedures. Others may fail to acknowledge pain to avoid confronting the possibility of a life-threatening condition or to avoid potentially addicting pain medication. Some elderly patients may exhibit a stoic demeanor, believing it is not acceptable to acknowledge pain [42].

Appropriate pain management in the elderly is further complicated by the nurse's own beliefs and knowledge about pain. Research suggests that nurses often underestimate the degree of pain and do not appropriately use narcotics to achieve effective pain management. Inadequate control of pain by health professionals has been attributed to their fears of addiction and respiratory depression, attitudes regarding the degree of pain the patient is really experiencing and what constitutes adequate pain relief, and misunderstandings about physiologic and psychological components of pain [43,44].

Early Mobilization

As the patient progresses and stabilizes during the immediate postoperative period, nursing interventions should focus on promoting recovery and preventing complications. Early mobilization is a key intervention. The hazards of immobility are well documented. Muscle strength has been found to decrease by a rate of 5% per day with inactivity, and in older patients, there is a tendency for limitation of range of motion and contractures. Bed rest contributes to postural hypotension and syncope, reduced ventilatory effort and aerobic capacity, accelerated loss of calcium from the bones, and an increased incidence of urinary incontinence and pressure ulcers [45]. Bed rest combined with a reduced functional reserve in the elderly and the stress of a surgical procedure can predispose the older patient to more iatrogenic complications, a prolonged recovery period, and an inability to return to their presurgical level of function and living arrangements. Getting a patient out of bed as soon as possible postoperatively goes a long way toward preventing these problems.

Safety Issues

Falls in the elderly are generally caused by many factors. Host factors include pain, medications, underlying medical conditions, and impaired vision and hearing. Environmental factors contributing to an increased risk of falling in the hospital include bed rails; high beds; low lighting; ill-fitting shoes or slippers; low chairs that are difficult to get out of; assistive devices such as walkers; tethers such as intravenous lines, feeding tubes, and oxygen tubes; pulse oximeters; telemetry devices; and "elder-unfriendly" hospital rooms, corridors, and bathrooms. The third set of factors has to do with the activity the patient was engaged in at the time of the fall. Often this activity is not a hazardous activity in and of itself. Typical activities during which a fall may occur include moving from the chair to the bed or the bed to the chair unaided or moving to the bathroom to prevent an incontinent episode.

The key to falls in the elderly is prevention. A falls prevention program designed to identify those at risk for falling, the degree of risk, and specific nursing interventions to prevent falls is a recognized strategy in a variety of settings. Preoperatively, this tool can alert nurses to patients who may be at risk for falling after surgery when they are weaker, possibly sedated, in pain, or disoriented. The goal in any fall prevention program is to minimize the risk of falling without compromising mobility or functional independence. Table 11-4 lists suggested fall prevention strategies [46].

One mechanism often used to prevent falls is physical restraints. This has been a common practice in the acute setting to protect the patient from harm, to prevent disruption of therapy, to prevent wandering, or to manage behavioral problems. The prevalence of restraint use in the older hospitalized population has been found to increase with increasing age to an estimated 22%, or one in five, for those 75 years or older [47]. Physical restraints are more likely to be used in a patient with at least one of the following characteristics: severe acute illness, cognitive impairment, physical impairment, psychiatric condition, recent surgical procedure, or medical devices that restrict mobility (i.e., intravenous lines and feeding tubes).

Recent research, however, indicates that individuals continue to fall and sustain injuries even with the use of physical restraints and that injuries from falls are actually greater with the presence of physical restraints. Other complications associated with the use of physical restraints include bowel and bladder incontinence, pressure ulcers, contractures, nerve damage, complications from immobility, and increased confusion. The Omnibus Reconciliation Act of 1987 and the most recent guidelines from the Joint Commission on Accreditation of Hospitals support these data by restricting the use of physical restraints [48]. As a component of the Hartford Foundation's Nurses Improving Care of the Hospitalized Elderly Project, a standard of practice for the use of physical restraints in the acute care setting was developed by a panel of nurse experts. The standard essentially states that physical restraints will be applied only after exhausting all reasonable alternatives and then for a specific reason. When a restraint is necessary, the nurse should choose the least restrictive device, reassess the need and the patient's response to restraints every 1 to 2 hours, remove the restraints every 2 hours, and renew the restraint order every 24 hours. The standard goes on to offer alternative approaches to care such as modified chairs, adaptive cushions, removal of wheels from beds to position the bed closer to the floor, use of gauze wrappings to disguise intravenous lines, use of abdominal binders to disguise gastrostomy tubes, and a calm, consistent approach to the confused patient [47].

Rehabilitation Focus

Identification and agreement of treatment goals, both short and long term, should occur before admission for the surgical procedure. The patient and family should be informed of the expected length of stay, the expected hospital course, and their role in meeting those goals. Acute care goals will be limited and may include adequate pain management, tolerating oral feedings, nearing target goal of enteral feedings, or transferring from bed to chair with minimum assistance. The specific goals for a patient will, of course, depend on the type of procedure, the patient's underlying medical condition, the patient's level of independence and function before surgery, and the patient's discharge plan. For example, a patient going home alone must be at a higher level of function than the patient going to a skilled nursing facility for a 2- to 3-week recovery period.

TABLE 11-4. *Fall prevention strategies*

Assess risk factors
Patient factors: confusion, visual and hearing deficits, medications, functional deficits, pain, lack of proper footwear, orthostasis, thirst, hunger, gait disturbances, and improper use of assistive devices (cane or walker)
Environmental factors: lighting, use of side rails, accessibility of bathroom, food or water, and flooring
Activity factors: toileting, transferring, and ambulating activities
Correct visual and hearing deficits
Provide assistance with toileting
Meet basic needs: food, water, toileting, comfort
Promote mobility: gait training, appropriate adaptive equipment
Promote optimal nutrition
Reduce tethers: intravenous lines, catheters, oxygen
Assess medication regimen
Provide "senior-friendly" environment: adequate lighting, appropriate colors, avoidance of glare, appropriate seating for ease and safety of transfers, elimination of clutter
Provide safe, well-fitting footwear
Avoid use of restraints

Daily goals should address pain control, progressive mobilization, nutritional status, bowel and bladder function, fluid status, wound and skin integrity, and absence of signs of complications. Communicating these goals to all care providers, the family, and the patient will aid in ensuring a consistent approach to care. Posting daily goals and a daily schedule in the room is a good way to communicate this approach.

Restorative techniques help patients reach the identified goals. All care providers must be attuned to the goals and these strategies. These techniques are often simple. For example, avoiding the use of the bedpan and having the patient get up to the bedside commode or bathroom affords the patient a more normal toileting routine, as well as provides frequent exercise and mobility to lessen functional decline. Encouraging the patient to do whatever the patient can for himself or herself and advancing those skills daily promotes independence rather than teaching the patient dependency.

Enlisting the aid of other health team members enhances the restorative approach. Occupational therapy offers a thorough evaluation of the patient's functional status and recommends adaptive equipment as needed to restore independence. Physical therapy can recommend bed and chair exercises, teach range of motion exercises, assess the need for assistive devices, and teach the family correct body mechanics and transfer techniques for the patient. A registered dietitian provides in-depth screening related to nutritional issues and recommends appropriate supplements and diet modifications geared toward promoting improved nutritional status as well as better wound healing. The dietitian's input into food preferences and scheduling can also enhance oral intake and improved nutrition.

The nurse caring for the postoperative patient participates in coordinating this team approach. This coordination may mean that the nurse talks to the therapists and negotiates an

TABLE 11-5. *Potential home care needs*

Equipment
- Hospital bed
- Pressure-reduction device for bed and chair
- Bedside commode
- Wheelchair, walker, cane
- Lifts
- Dressing supplies
- Supplies for enteral feeding, etc.
- Oxygen

Assessment
- Skilled assessment of medical status, wounds and incisions, tolerance to therapy, acute problems
- Home safety

Basic needs
- Meals on Wheels
- Transportation
- Assistance with physical care: bathing, preparing meals, lifting, transferring, toileting
- Transportation for follow-up treatments
- Obtaining medications, adapting medication schedule, use of devices to promote compliance

Specialized needs
- Venipuncture for laboratory monitoring
- Specialized diet or enteral feeding supplies
- Total parenteral nutrition, intravenous fluids and antibiotics, pain management
- Administration of medications
- Wound care and dressing changes
- Physical therapy, occupational therapy, speech therapy
- Social work evaluation for finances, benefits, community resources
- Hospice

Safety
- Modifications of the home environment: ramps, wide doorways, handrails, bathroom safety devices
- Use of assistive devices

Education
- Patient/family/care-giver education
- Care-giver support and counseling

appropriate schedule so that the patient is medicated for pain before active therapy and has built-in rest periods to avoid becoming overly fatigued. The nurse may need to advocate for a rest period before meals in an effort to improve oral intake or coordinate all therapies in the morning when the patient is at his or her strongest. The nurse must have a good understanding of the overall goals, the patient's needs, the patient's limitations, and the role of all team members.

Throughout the hospital stay, the nurse should be aware of the patient's potential for benefiting from more intensive rehabilitation. For example, a patient who has just undergone a total hip replacement may certainly benefit from a short stay in an inpatient rehabilitation unit or a skilled nursing facility for additional physical therapy. The patient who was previously living independently but is now debilitated with decreased endurance may also benefit from such intensive occupational and physical therapy with the goal of returning to independent living. The nurse should have a general understanding of the criteria for admission to such units under Medicare. A patient must have the potential of improving with therapy, must need at least two therapies (occupational therapy, physical therapy, and speech therapy), and must be able to participate in a minimum of 3 hours of therapy per day. Older patients often require a customized therapy program until their endurance improves. The 3 hours of therapy can be broken down into shorter, less intensive time periods. Working with the physician, patient and family, therapists, and social services to document need, current status, and progress with therapy is a key role for nursing.

DISCHARGE PLAN

Planning for discharge should begin before admission for a surgical procedure. The patient and family should be informed of the anticipated length of stay and the expected posthospital needs. Early involvement of social services with patients whose level of care may change with this surgery and hospitalization is important. This includes the patient who may not be able to return to living independently immediately after the hospitalization, as well as the patient who resides in a long-term care facility but whose level of care may change from an intermediate level (e.g., intermediate care facility) to a skilled level (e.g., skilled nursing facility) and who may, therefore, need to change facilities. Many factors influence the decision for nursing home care rather than home care. The most commonly identified are presented in the following list.

- Incontinence of urine and stool
- Enteral feeding
- Immobility
- Severe disorientation or dementia
- Behaviors that are difficult to manage (i.e., alteration in sleep-wake cycle, wandering, yelling, aggressive or violent behavior)
- Complex medical therapy or dressing changes
- Unavailability of family care-giver

The social worker can provide the patient and family with information about available facilities and programs, criteria for admission, and reimbursement for needed services.

Identification of home needs should also occur early in the hospital stay. Table 11-5 lists potential home care needs. Medicare typically provides these services with documented needs and with certain limitations. In the managed care environment, however, these services may require prior approval from secondary insurance providers. Nursing and social services must work together to provide the patient with accurate information about what home care and equipment is available, what is reimbursable, and what out-of-pocket expenses the patient can expect. Table 11-6 provides basic criteria the patient must meet for selected durable medical equipment.

CONCLUSION

Nursing care of the elderly surgical patient encompasses a wide array of specialized knowledge and skills. An understanding of the unique care needs of this population based on up-to-date, comprehensive data that include the physiologic changes of aging, the effects of chronic illnesses, and the impact of functional, developmental, and psychosocial issues provides the foundation for care. Incorporating a restorative approach throughout the hospitalization is vital to maximizing outcomes. Nursing care should be focused on maintaining or improving functional status, preventing complications such as pressure ulcers and falls, and recognizing atypical changes in status that might indicate an underlying infection or fluid and electrolyte imbalance.

Coordination of patient education and discharge planning with the team of care providers is a nursing responsibility. As we enter an era of health care in which length of stay, appropriate resource use, and cost-effective care play an even greater role, nurses must understand and work to meet these goals as they ensure high-quality care for older surgical patients.

TABLE 11-6. *Durable medical equipment requirements*

Equipment	Requirements
Enteral feeding	20–35 cal/kg/day
Home oxygen	Po_2 <55 (59 with heart failure) or O_2 saturation <88 (90 with heart failure)
Pressure-reduction mattress	Varies with product, usually requires presence of stage III or IV pressure ulcers
Hospital bed	Change of position required for medical condition
Specialized wheelchair	Unique need such as amputation, with preservation of self-care ability

REFERENCES

1. U.S. Senate Special Committee on Aging, American Association of Retired Persons, Federal Council on the Aging, U.S. Administration on Aging. Aging America, Trends and Projections. Pub No. 91-28001. Washington, DC: U.S. Department of Health and Human Services, 1991.
2. Coroni-Huntley J, Brock DB, Ostfeld AM, et al. Established Populations for Epidemiologic Studies of the Elderly: Resource Data Book. Pub No. NIH 86-2443. Washington, DC: U.S. Department of Health and Human Services, 1986.
3. U.S. Department of Commerce. Statistical Abstract of the U.S. (110th ed). Washington, DC: Bureau of the Census, 1990.
4. U.S. Department of Health and Human Services. Vital and Health Statistics. Series 13, No. 104. Hyattsville, MD: National Center for Health Statistics, 1990.
5. Narain P, Robenstein LZ, Weiland GD, et al. Predictors of immediate and six month outcomes in hospitalized elderly patients: the importance of functional status. J Am Geriatr Soc 1988;36:775–783.
6. Peterson BH. Counseling for growth in mid-life. Aust J Sex Marriage Family 1983;4:85–93.
7. Becker PM, Cohen HJ. The functional approach to the care of the elderly: a conceptual framework. J Am Geriatr Soc 1984;32:923–929.
8. Panicucci CL. Functional assessment of the older adult in the acute care setting. Nurs Clin North Am 1983;18:355–363.
9. American Nurses Association. Standards and Scope of Gerontological Nursing. Kansas City, KS: American Nurses Association, 1987.
10. Katz S, Ford AB, Moskowitz RS, et al. Studies of illness in the aged. The index of ADL: a standardized measure of biological and psychosocial function. JAMA 1963;185:94–98.
11. Granger CV, Albrecht GL, Hamilton BB. Outcome of comprehensive medical rehabilitation: measures of PULSES profile and the Barthel index. Arch Phys Med Rehab 1979;60:145–154.
12. Lawton HP, Brody EM. Assessment of older people: self-maintaining and instrumental activities of daily living. Gerontologist 1969;9: 179–186.
13. American Occupational Therapy Association. Kohlman Evaluation of Living Skills (KELS). Rockville, MD: American Occupational Therapy Association, 1992.
14. Gustafson Y, Berggren D, Brannstrom B, et al. Acute confusional states in elderly patients treated for femoral neck fractures. J Am Geriatr Soc 1988;36:525–530.
15. Folstein ME, Folstein SE. Mini-mental state: a practical method for grading the cognitive state of patients for the clinician. J Psychiatr Res 1975;12:189–198.
16. Teng EL, Chui HC. The modified mini-mental state (3MS) examination. J Clin Psychiatry 1987;48:314–318.
17. Buckwalter KC. How to unmask depression. Geriatr Nurs 1990;11: 179–181.
18. Yesavage JA, Brink TL, Rose TL, et al. Development and validation of a geriatric depression screening scale: a preliminary report. J Psychiatr Res 1983;17:37–49.
19. Sullivan DH, Walls RC. Impact of nutritional status on morbidity in a population of geriatric rehabilitation patients. J Am Geriatr Soc 1994;42:471–477.
20. Remig VM, Shumaker NS, St. Jeor S. Weight as a clinical indicator: elderly. Top Clin Nutr 1992;8:16–25.
21. Santo-Novak D, Edwards RM. Rx: take caution with drugs for elders. Geriatr Nurs 1989;10:72–75.
22. Eliopoulos C. Safe Drug Use in the Elderly. In Eliopoulous C (ed), Caring for the Elderly in Diverse Care Situations. Philadelphia: Lippincott, 1990.
23. Matteson MA, McConnell ES. Gerontological Nursing: Concepts and Practice. Philadelphia: Saunders, 1988.
24. Dellasega C, Clark D, McCreary D, et al. Nursing process: teaching elderly clients. J Gerontol Nurs 1994;20:31–38.
25. Kick E. Patient teaching for elders. Nurs Clin North Am 1989;24: 681–686.
26. Weinrich SP, Boyd M, Nussbaum J. Continuing education: adapting strategies to teach the elderly. J Gerontol Nurs 1989;15:17–21.
27. Saleh KL. The elderly patient in the post anesthesia care unit. Nurs Clin North Am 1993;28:507–518.
28. Bush LM, Kaye D. Epidemiology and Pathogenesis of Infectious Diseases. In Abrams WB, Berkow R (eds), The Merck Manual of Geriatrics. Rahway, NJ: Merck Sharpe and Dohme Research Laboratories, 1990.
29. Wells T. Conquering incontinence. Geriatr Nurs 1990;11:133–135.
30. Seymour DG, Vaz FG. A prospective study of elderly surgical patients: post operative complications. Age Ageing 1989;18:316–325.
31. Schor J, Levkoff SE, Lipsitz, et al. Risk factors for delirium in hospitalized elderly. JAMA 1992;267:827–831.
32. Gustafson Y, Brannstrom B, Norberg A, et al. Underdiagnosis and poor documentation of acute confusional states in elderly hip fracture patients. J Am Geriatr Soc 1991;39:760–765.
33. Kaminer MS, Gilchrest BA. Aging of the Skin. Principles of Geriatric Medicine and Gerontology. New York: McGraw-Hill, 1994;411–429.
34. Clarke M, Kadhom HM. The nursing prevention of pressure sores in hospital and community patients. J Adv Nurs 1988;13:365–373.
35. Meehan M. Multisite pressure ulcer prevalence survey. Decubitus 1990;3:14–17.
36. Versluysen M. Pressure sores in elderly patients. The epidemiology related to hip operations. J Bone Joint Surg 1985;67:10–13.
37. Goodridge DM. Pressure ulcer risk assessment tools: what's new for gerontological nurses. J Gerontol Nurs 1993;19:23–27.
38. Norton D, McLaren R, Exton-Smith AN. An Investigation of Geriatric Nursing Problems in the Hospital. London: National Corporation for the Care of Old People, 1962.

39. Agency for Health Care Policy and Research, Public Health Service. Treatment of Pressure Ulcers. Clinical Practice Guideline, Number 15. AHCPR Pub No. 95-0652. Rockville, MD: U.S. Department of Health and Human Services, December 1994.
40. Agency for Health Care Policy and Research, Public Health Service. Pressure Ulcers in Adults: Prediction and Prevention. Clinical Practice Guideline, Number 3. AHCPR Pub No. 92-0047. Rockville, MD: U.S. Department of Health and Human Services, May 1992.
41. Agency for Health Care Policy and Research, Public Health Service. Acute Pain Management in Adults: Operative Procedures. AHCPR Pub No. 92-0019. Rockville, MD: U.S. Department of Health and Human Services, February 1992.
42. Herr KA, Mobily PR. Complexities of pain assessment in the elderly: clinical considerations. J Gerontol Nurs 1991;17:12–18.
43. Brockopp DY, Warden S, Colclough MD, Brockopp GW. Nursing knowledge: acute postoperative pain management in the elderly. J Gerontol Nurs 1993;19:31–37.
44. McCaffery M, Beebe A. Pain: Clinical Manual for Nursing Practice. St. Louis: Mosby, 1989.
45. Creditor MC. Hazards of hospitalization in the elderly. Ann Intern Med 1993;118:219–223.
46. Hendrich AL. An effective unit-based fall prevention plan. J Nurs Qual Assur 1988;3:28–36.
47. Mion LC, Strumpf N. Use of physical restraints in the hospital setting: implications for the nurse. Geriatr Nurs 1994;15:127–132.
48. The Joint Commission Comprehensive Accreditation Manual for Hospitals. Volume 1: Standards. Oakbrook Terrace, IL: Joint Commission for the Accreditation of Hospitals, 1997.

Surgical Care for the Elderly, 2nd ed., edited by
R. Benton Adkins, Jr., and H. William Scott, Jr.
Lippincott–Raven Publishers, Philadelphia © 1998.

CHAPTER 12

Extended Care and Rehabilitation

Horace E. Watson and Thomas E. Groomes

Rehabilitation is a term used in such a wide variety of contexts that one must specifically indicate what is meant when using the word. The terminology *geriatric rehabilitation* should connote a process by which an elderly person achieves maximum function. As the population of older people throughout the world grows progressively larger, there is an increasing need for extended care and rehabilitation. Extended care involves the provision for the basic needs of the recipients, including a home, clothing, food, transportation, and a loving, caring environment. Rehabilitation involves the physical, mental, emotional, and spiritual restoration of individuals to a maximum level of function.

EXTENDED CARE DELIVERY SYSTEMS NOW AVAILABLE TO THE ELDERLY

When treating elderly patients who have diseases or injuries, it is useful to think about the extended health care needs of these patients during rehabilitation. However, frequently these elderly patients must make long-term and even lifetime adjustments in their living circumstances as a consequence of disabling disease or injury. Ideally, loving and caring family members are willing to make necessary adjustments in their lives to provide for their loved ones. Realistically, however, many elderly persons must make arrangements for their extended care without any help from family members.

Extended care facilities generally fall into two categories: skilled care and unskilled care. Elderly patients discharged from acute care hospital settings may be considered for skilled or unskilled nursing home care in an extended care facility. To qualify for skilled care, one must require the services of nurses for such skilled procedures as administration of intravenous fluids, open wound dressing changes, catheterization, or total parenteral nutrition. A patient with good rehabilitation potential may qualify for skilled care because of documented progressive improvement with ongoing physical, occupational, or speech therapy. Medicare offers limited financial coverage for skilled nursing and home health care but will not pay for custodial, personal, or homemaking services. Medicaid is the primary payer of indigent nonskilled long-term care in this country [1]. Various types of daycare programs have been established in an effort to meet the needs of the noninstitutionalized elderly.

PROBLEMS THAT CONFRONT THE ELDERLY

In general, as we grow older, we have increasing health care needs. Vision and hearing become less acute and the sense of taste and smell are diminished [2,3]. Muscle strength is reduced, and joint range of motion is frequently diminished [2,3]. Balance may become impaired, increasing the likelihood of falling [2–4]. The ability to carry out the activities of daily living (ADLs) may become progressively impaired. Bone mass and thereby skeletal strength diminishes with increasing age [2,3]. All of these anatomic and physiologic effects of aging contribute to increased health care needs and the need for the provision of long-term care. Many elderly people do not have the financial means to pay for these health care services.

REHABILITATION OF THE ELDERLY FROM SPINAL CORD INJURY

Spinal cord injury is devastating at any age. Certainly it occurs much more frequently in young adults than in the elderly. It is a sudden, life-changing injury that affects not only physical functions but also visceral functions, sensations, family relationships, socioeconomic considerations, and career options. When it does occur to an elderly person, that individual needs to muster all the motivation and physical stamina possible to cope with the effects of the injury. A predisposing condition frequently present in the elderly, degenerative joint disease of the spine, may result in spinal cord injury associated with minimal trauma. Spinal cord injury may be classified as complete or incomplete depending on the early clinical manifestations of the injury. If at the end of spinal shock there has been no return of function below the level of the spinal cord injury, the injury is considered complete (Frankel A) and the prognosis for recovery is practically nil. If at the end of spinal shock there has been some evidence of return of function below the level of the spinal cord injury, either motor or sensory, the injury is considered incomplete. In these cases, the prognosis is extremely variable between minimal return of sensation (Frankel B), minimal return of motor function (Frankel C), useful return of motor function (Frankel D), and full return of motor and sensory function (Frankel E) [5].

A form of incomplete spinal cord injury frequently encountered in the elderly is the central cervical spinal cord syndrome. This injury may occur as the result of a fall or other type of blow to the head, usually with hyperextension of the neck. With preexisting hypertrophic changes and resultant cervical spinal stenosis, the spinal cord may be acutely injured, with hemorrhage, edema, and necrosis of neural elements beginning in the center of the cord and progressing outward. The ascending and descending tracts are so arranged in the cord that the central cord damage is much more pronounced to the medially arranged fibers to the upper extremities than to the more peripherally arranged fibers to the lower extremities. Therefore, these patients generally experience rapid improvement in lower extremity function after spinal shock ends, but may experience delayed improvement in the upper extremity function [6]. The other frequently encountered forms of incomplete spinal cord injury include anterior spinal cord syndrome and the Brown-Séquard's hemisection type of spinal cord injury. In general, the Brown-Séquard's type has the best prognosis for long-term improvement, whereas the anterior spinal syndrome has the poorest prognosis for long-term improvement [6].

REHABILITATION FROM A FRACTURED HIP

Hip fractures may occur at any age, but are much more frequently encountered in the elderly. There are numerous reasons for this including balance problems, muscular weakness, osteopenia, defective vision, and cognitive deficits. Because most fractured hips result from falls, older people with balance problems, musculoskeletal weakness, or cognitive or visual deficit should use an assistive device in an effort to prevent falls.

There are basically three types of hip fractures: (1) femoral neck, (2) intertrochanteric, and (3) subtrochanteric. Any of these fractures may be undisplaced, impacted, or displaced. A femoral neck fracture is intracapsular and may be located anywhere in the femoral neck from the subcapital to the base of the neck. A displaced fracture is more susceptible to complications including avascular necrosis of the femoral head, delayed union or nonunion, hardware failure, and deformity [7]. Frequently, displaced femoral neck fractures in the elderly are treated with prosthetic implant replacement of the femoral head, either unipolar or bipolar. Undisplaced, impacted, or incomplete femoral neck fractures are generally treated by internal fixation with lag screws or pins.

Intertrochanteric fractures are generally treated with dynamic hip screw fixation, using a plate that is affixed to the proximal shaft of the femur with several cortical screws [7]. Subtrochanteric hip fractures are generally best treated with an intramedullary nail, which allows early weight bearing as tolerated [7]. Rehabilitation of the elderly from hip fracture is greatly facilitated by early full-weight bearing. However, the nature of the fracture and the type of fixation used frequently require a period of several weeks of essentially no weight bearing for healing to progress sufficiently to allow weight bearing. It is during this time that physical and occupational therapy in a subacute intensive rehabilitation program should allow these patients to gain confidence, strength, endurance, flexibility, and mobility, as well as to progressively resume ADLs. On the achievement of inpatient rehabilitation goals, either outpatient or home health rehabilitation therapy is usually indicated for a few weeks or until the patient is able to continue with a home program.

Most patients with a hemiarthroplasty are allowed to bear weight as tolerated almost immediately postoperatively. However, these patients also need specific physical and occupational therapy in a subacute or intensive rehabilitation program with emphasis on safe positioning of the extremity in an effort to prevent dislocation of the implant. As safety awareness, strength, and endurance improve, these patients may be progressively advanced in the use of assistive devices from a walker to a cane.

REHABILITATION FROM TOTAL JOINT REPLACEMENT ARTHROPLASTY

Total joint replacement arthroplasty has been done extensively in the United States for approximately 25 years. Many patients with disabling osteoarthritis or rheumatoid arthritis of the hip or knee joint have greatly benefited from these operations. In general, surgical techniques and implant technology have progressively improved over the years. Controversy continues regarding the merits of cemented versus uncemented implants [7]. These operations have particularly benefited elderly patients because their limited activity allows the implants to last longer. It has been generally believed that a total hip or total knee replacement implant will last approximately 15 years. However, with improved technology and surgical techniques, these implants will likely last longer. The usual postoperative protocol allows for weight bearing as tolerated for cemented implants, but essentially no weight bearing for 6 weeks for press fit implants to allow for early bone ingrowth to help stabilize the implant [7].

Total shoulder and total elbow joint replacements are also done, but much less frequently than hips and knees. Total ankle joint replacement arthroplasty, once considered a good operation for specific indications is hardly ever done now because of a high percentage of implant failures.

REHABILITATION FROM MULTIPLE FRACTURES

Multiple trauma occurs all too frequently in our highly mechanized society. When elderly persons sustain multiple injuries in a motor vehicle accident or from another cause, rehabilitation may be much more difficult than for younger healthy individuals. An older person may have early failure in a number of organ systems or bodily functions that do not present major problems until the stresses of multiple injuries are superimposed. Borderline diabetes mellitus, early congestive heart failure, early hepatic or renal failure, or early emphysema may become a major clinical problem for a patient with multiple trauma. In general, the best course of management for multiple trauma in an elderly individual is early surgical repair of the injury. Certainly, early surgical intervention when indicated for traumatic brain injuries or for traumatic intrapelvic injuries should reduce the incidence of complications inherent with bed rest and immobility. It is well recognized that early surgical stabilization of multiple fractures should reduce the incidence of pneumonia, deep vein thrombosis, and pulmonary embolism [8,9]. It also reduces the incidence of neurovascular injuries from displaced fractures, osteomyelitis, malunion, delayed union, and nonunion of fractures [8,9]. With early surgical stabilization of fractures, patients may be mobilized much more effectively in an intensive inpatient rehabilitation setting. Physical therapy designed to facilitate mobility skills, transfers, wheelchair mobility, assisted ambulation, strengthening, flexibility, and endurance training should be started as early as is feasible. Occupational therapy, with emphasis on ADLs such as dressing, bathing, grooming, and self-feeding, along with upper extremity functional tasks, strengthening, and endurance training should also be started early. Recreation therapy, designed to help the patient reenter the community in a productive and fulfilling manner, is also an important rehabilitation component.

REHABILITATION OF THE ELDERLY AMPUTEE

Amputation surgery necessitated by severe trauma to the limbs is much more frequently encountered in younger age groups, but does occur in the elderly population. Amputation surgery for dysvascular limbs is much more common in the older age groups. Because of increased longevity, patients with ischemic lower extremities, diabetic peripheral neuropathy, and patients with end-stage renal disease account for progressively increasing numbers of lower extremity amputees [10]. The consideration for amputation surgery involves an interdisciplinary approach including the primary care physician, orthopedic surgeon (or other amputation surgeon), vascular surgeon, prosthetist, and physical therapist. Knowing as much as possible about the patient will help in the decision making regarding prosthetic rehabilitation potential and in the selection of the level for amputation. In general, the level of amputation should be the longest level that will allow for reasonably healthy soft tissues to be approximated [10]. It has been established that longer residual limbs provide more proprioceptive feedback and improved self-esteem and require less energy consumption than do shorter residual limbs [11]. Partial foot amputations are preferable to amputations at a higher level if sufficient healing potential is present. Syme's amputation (i.e., disarticulation at the ankle joint with preservation of the heel pad) is preferable to any transtibial level of amputation [10]. Even a short transtibial level, if it preserves the attachment of the patellar tendon, is preferable to any higher level of amputation. A knee disarticulation amputation is preferable to a higher level and should be considered for any patient who is not a rehabilitation candidate for ambulation at a transtibial level. This level provides for a good sitting surface in a wheelchair and eliminates the problem of knee flexion contracture, delayed healing, and continued ischemia in a transtibial level. If transfemoral amputation is necessary, the long transfemoral residual limb is preferable and provides for good cosmesis if at a level of 2 in. above the joint line. Hip disarticulation amputation and hemipelvectomy are usually reserved for malignant disease or severe trauma that does not allow for salvage at a longer level. The elderly patient who becomes an amputee generally benefits from an intensive inpatient program beginning within a few days of surgery. For lower-extremity amputations, the patient needs to strengthen the remaining limbs and trunk to facilitate balance, ADLs, and assisted ambulation as part of the preprosthetic training program. The use of rigid plaster or fiberglass dressing for transtibial or longer levels helps to provide protection and total contact, reduce swelling, and maintain knee extension to prevent flexion contractures [12]. Early prosthetic fitting with a temporary prosthesis facilitates rehabilitation efforts and hastens the shaping and shrinking of the residual limb necessary for fabrication of the definitive prosthesis. With dysvascular amputees, it is advisable to await soft-tissue healing before suture removal. At that point, the patient is ready for application of a stump shrinker, followed soon by the temporary (preparatory) prosthesis [12]. When inpatient rehabilitation goals have been accomplished, the patient may then benefit from home health or outpatient physical and occupational therapy. With ongoing follow-up, the patient will probably be ready for the definitive prosthesis in 4 to 6 months. By that time, shaping and shrinking of the residual limb usually necessitates the fabrication of a definitive socket. In recent years technological advances in the space industry have provided improved, stronger, and lighter weight materials that have been used in prosthetics [13]. Dynamic elastic response feet that are lightweight, strong, and flexible offer energy-storing capability that provides the amputee with improved prosthetic gait and less energy expenditure [14]. Examples of such prosthetic feet include the Flex-foot (Aliso Viejo, CA), the Seattle light foot (Seattle Limb Systems, Poulsbo, WA), and the Carbon Copy II Foot (Ohio Willow Wood Co., Mt. Sterling, OH). Knee components that provide safer, smoother, and more energy-efficient gait include the Total Knee (seven bar linkage with hydraulic action, available from Century XXII Innovations, Inc.) and the weight-activated, stance-control knee [15]. Lightweight materials that provide much improved strength in the fabrication of prostheses include carbon fiber and titanium. Silicone suction sockets and silicone socket liners have provided improved suspension and fewer shear forces at the limb-socket interface. Upper-extremity amputees also benefit from intensive rehabilitation efforts to improve overall strength, coordination, and use of the prosthesis in ADLs. Prosthetic upper-extremity training needs to be instituted as early as possible following amputation surgery so that the patient will not become one-handed. In general, the occupational therapist will need to work intensively with upper-extremity amputees in an effort to help patients adapt to and become proficient with the use of the prosthetic arm.

REHABILITATION OF THE ELDERLY FROM MULTIPLE TRAUMA

Multiple trauma may include any and all combinations of trauma to various parts of the anatomy, including traumatic brain injury; spine injury; and intrathoracic, intra-abdominal, intrapelvic, and long bone fractures. It is especially important to diagnose each and every injury as early as possible in the elderly patient so that early appropriate management will result in stabilization of the injury. Intracranial injuries such as subdural or epidural hematoma may require surgical intervention promptly. Intrathoracic injuries requiring such measures as chest tube insertion for hemopneumothorax require early detection and intervention. Intra-abdominal trauma may be detected by diagnostic peritoneal lavage, computed tomographic imaging, or both. Early surgical management of intra-abdominal and intrapelvic injuries will greatly enhance the possibility of recovery. In the case of multiple fractures, early surgical stabilization will greatly facilitate early rehabilitation efforts. It is important to mobilize older patients as early as possible following multiple trauma in an effort to prevent such complications as deep vein thrombosis and pulmonary embolism. Chest tubes, intravenous catheters, and indwelling urethral catheters should be removed as early as possible.

GERIATRIC REHABILITATION

The focus of rehabilitation services is to improve the physical and psychosocial functioning in individuals affected by chronic disease and disability. Between 1989 and 2030 the U.S. population over the age of 65 is expected to more than double such that by the year 2030, over 20% of the population will be 65 years old or older. In addition, the subgroup of persons 85 years or older is predicted to triple in number over the same period [16]. Due to the increased prevalence of chronic diseases in persons >65 years old, there is an increased prevalence of impairments leading to disabilities in this age group. Approximately 13% of persons age 65 and older who live in the community report limitations in walking or in basic ADLs (e.g., bathing, dressing, toileting, feeding). In addition, approximately 5% of persons in the United States aged 65 and older reside in a nursing home, with 85% of those persons requiring assistance with at least one ADL [16]. The goal of rehabilitative services is predominately functional improvement as opposed to cure of a specific disease. The ability to function independently in ADLs is one measure of a person's health status or quality of life. Geriatric rehabilitation may be divided into three main components: development of a proper exercise program for the well elderly, assessment and treatment of minor musculoskeletal complaints before development of a disability, and development of a program to restore a person impaired from injury or disease to the pre-illness environment and level of functioning [17]. This chapter focuses on the latter component.

TRAUMATIC BRAIN INJURY

The age distribution for traumatic brain injury is bimodal, with the elderly over age 70 having the second highest incidence of any age group [18]. Possible reasons for the higher incidence in this age group include the increased occurrence of falls and the increased susceptibility to assaults. Motor vehicle accidents and pedestrian accidents are the second most common cause of traumatic brain injury in the elderly. Impaired vision, hearing, and reaction time may all contribute to the occurrence of this form of injury [19].

Due to the lower velocity of impact typically seen in the elderly (from falls or lower speed motor vehicle accidents), there is less occurrence of diffuse axonal injury as the main pathology [3]. Focal injuries are more prevalent, with intracranial hemorrhages up to four times more likely in the elderly than in those injured <45 years of age [20,21].

Mortality and morbidity from traumatic brain injury are both increased in the elderly [19,21]. Mortality from traumatic brain injury greatly increases over the age of 75, and age is in fact as good a predictor of mortality as pupillary reactivity or Glasgow Coma Score [19]. Mortality is often secondary to complications including adult respiratory distress syndrome, pneumonia, cardiac failure, or pulmonary embolism.

Before rehabilitative services are initiated, a pertinent history should be obtained including the patient's preinjury level of functioning, endurance, impairments, and social and family support. An estimation of cardiac and pulmonary functioning from previous medical history and deconditioning from the acute injury event is helpful in guiding therapists to the appropriate level of activity that the patient may be able to tolerate. Treatment for agitation should focus on establishing a proper sleep-wake cycle, providing adequate pain relief, and removing medications (e.g., anticholinergics, benzodiazepines, and major tranquilizers) that may increase confusion. Therapies should be provided in a quiet, undistracting environment that is consistent and structured. The patient, family, and treatment staff should set appropriate goals, not only for basic self-care skills but for recreational and vocational issues. Social and behavioral deficits from traumatic brain injury are often more stressful to family members than are cognitive deficits. Although in general, overall recovery from traumatic brain injury in the elderly is less than that seen in the younger population, the elderly have been shown to make significant functional progress with rehabilitative services [19].

STROKE

Cerebrovascular accident (CVA) is the third most common cause of death in the United States (after heart disease and cancer) and is second only to head trauma as the leading cause of neurologic disability [18]. The incidence of CVA increases steadily with age. Age, along with hypertension, cardiac disease, and diabetes, is a major risk factor for stroke [22].

The benefits of rehabilitation services following CVA remain controversial. It is unclear if rehabilitation has any effect on neurologic motor recovery or improvement in language skills [18,23]. Several studies, however, have supported the benefits of rehabilitation, including decreased use of medications, improved diagnosis of depression, improvement in functional status, and increased likelihood of returning to live in the community [18,24,25]. It is often easier to predict who will not benefit from rehabilitation services than to predict who will. Because learning is a required component for rehabilitation services, patients with severe global aphasia unable to follow simple verbal or gestural instructions are highly unlikely to benefit from rehabilitation services. Other predictors of poor outcome include bowel and bladder incontinence and severe visual-perceptual deficits [18].

There are several neurophysiologic facilitating techniques that may improve motor control. These techniques are based on the motor recovery patterns of CVA described by Twitchell [26] in the 1950s and based on the supposition that sensory input affects motor output and that voluntary movement is influenced by reflex activity. Brunnstrom's technique emphasizes specific stages of stroke recovery from flaccidity to hyperreflexivity to synergistic movement (gross movement patterns of an entire extremity as opposed to isolated movement across a single joint) to voluntary discrete movement. Brunnstrom emphasizes that synergistic patterns are part of a normal recovery and should be enhanced through cutaneous stimuli to achieve functional outcomes [27]. The Bobath technique discourages synergistic patterns, describing them as abnormal movement patterns. This technique emphasizes the importance of strengthening on specific task-related functional positions, with the majority of therapy performed in a sitting position (the most common position for the majority of ADL skills) [28]. Rood, whose theories are no longer widely practiced, emphasized the use of cutaneous sensory stimulation to attempt to modify tone and thereby influence voluntary muscle movement [29]. Kabat, Knott, and Voss helped develop the concept of proprioceptive neuromuscular facilitation, which makes use of diagonal mass movement patterns for both upper and lower extremities and emphasizes the concept that early motor movement is dominated by reflex activity [29]. The therapist provides manual contact and makes use of tonic reflexes to facilitate movement and theoretically to promote coordinated motor performance [30]. Other therapeutic procedures include biofeedback and functional electrical stimulation. Despite the extensive variety of facilitating techniques, no one technique has been proven to be more efficient or successful than another [31–33].

Due to time constraints and concern for health care costs, rehabilitation of stroke patients has shifted from the previously mentioned facilitatory techniques to a higher percentage of time spent on compensatory techniques (strengthening of weakened muscle groups or compensatory muscle groups to enable the patient to achieve specific functional goals).

Due to financial constraints with health care funding, length of stay for inpatient rehabilitative services has decreased significantly since 1980, with an increasing shift toward outpatient therapies, home care services, and skilled nursing facilities. It is important to realize that functional outcome does not always predict placement after discharge from acute rehabilitation. Disposition is heavily influenced by family and social support as well as financial constraints [18].

EFFECTS OF AGING AND RESPONSE TO EXERCISE

In planning a rehabilitation program for the geriatric population it is important to know what changes in organ systems are typically seen with aging. Cardiac output decreases at approximately 1% per year after the third decade in normal subjects otherwise free of cardiac disease. Theories for the cause of decreased cardiac output with aging include decreased inotropic response of cardiac muscle to catecholamines, an increase in myocardial stiffness possibly secondary to increased interstitial fibrosis, and increased afterload secondary to progressive stiffening of the thoracic aorta [34]. A linear decrease in vital capacity also is found after the third decade of life (approximately 20 to 25 ml per year). There is also a 20% to 30% decrease in maximum voluntary ventilation during adult life [34]. The changes in cardiac and pulmonary functioning result in an overall decreased maximum aerobic capacity [35]. The elderly are more greatly affected by the cardiovascular deconditioning associated with bed rest. Degenerative joint disease is present in 85% of persons over the age of 70. Characterized by degeneration of cartilage, subchondral bone thickening, and remodeling of bone with formation of subarticular bone cysts, degenerative joint disease has a predilection for weight-bearing joints and can greatly limit the activities of an elderly person. The decrease in muscle mass commonly seen with aging in combination with the skeletal changes mentioned previously can contribute to decreased locomotion [34].

The skin is also affected by aging. Thinning of the epidermis is noted, with flattening of the dermal-epidermal junction. Dermal collagen is stiffer and elastin has a higher degree of calcification leading to a loss of skin elasticity. This combined with a decrease in the number of dermal blood vessels leads to an increased susceptibility to decubitus ulcers from ischemia and immobility. Decreases in epidermal cell growth and division lead to slower wound healing in the elderly [34].

The role of exercise in the elderly is often to prevent age-related decline in health status and function or to restore lost function. Exercise can be classified as endurance training (i.e., focusing on aerobic capacity) or strength training (i.e., focusing on skeletal muscle strength). Intensity of endurance exercises is often monitored by heart rate or the person's perceived level of exertion. Moderate intensity (60% to 70% maximal heart rate) is generally recommended for the elderly. Moderate intensity exercises have been demonstrated to slow the loss of aerobic capacity seen with aging and have a higher chance of compliance and less risk of injury than high-intensity exercise. Although one can observe a more rapid increase of aerobic capacity with high-intensity exercise, there is little net difference observed over a 1-year period when compared with moderate intensity exercise [36]. Strength training is often a major component of a therapy program for the elderly. Biomechanical study results can be used to estimate the strength required for a functional task. In general, high-intensity strength training (70% to 80% of one repetition maximum weight) is well tolerated. Muscle strength can increase as much as 40% to 60% over a 6-week training period. For those who can only tolerate low- or medium-intensity exercise, a gain of only 5% to 20% should be expected, with an early plateau of gains. Muscle hypertrophy with exercise has been documented in individuals up to age 90. It is important to realize that there is a varied range of response to exercise in the elderly that is not related to age, sex, or initial level of fitness. In addition, the absolute gains of exercise late in life will not equal or exceed the loss of aerobic capacity from sedentary aging [36,37].

ATTITUDES OF AGEISM

Unfortunately, misconceptions and negative attitudes concerning health status in the elderly exist and can interfere with providing adequate and complete health care services. Health problems are frequently under-reported by the elderly, partly due to the misconception that a decline in health or functional status is a normal part of the aging process. This misconception can falsely lead to the conclusion that functional decline should be expected and not treated. Other factors that can contribute to under-reporting include fear of the underlying illness, cost and discomfort of treatment, and fear of institutionalization [38].

In the rehabilitation setting, progress can be limited by the "right of dependency" often associated with the elderly. Staff as well as the elderly patient often express the feeling that the elderly person has worked hard all his or her life and now deserves to be cared for as opposed to the patient taking a more active role in regaining independence. When this attitude is noted, it is best to provide staff education and have frank conversations between the patient and his or her family to decide on common goals and to help the patient realize the amount of independence required to return to community dwelling [39].

Too often, patients may be thought of as poorly motivated. It is not uncommon for the elderly patient to be physically exhausted from the acute hospitalization. In addition, emotional exhaustion can occur as the person attempts to adjust to the new level of impairment during a time when he or she is often separated from spouse or immediate family. Sleep disturbance and depression can compound the situation, contributing to an "apathy of fatigue." Social and psychosocial support should be readily available to the elderly to help counteract this apathy. Under present health funding systems, the patient must show a timely, progressive improvement to receive continued funding for health services. Therefore, one should actively address the previously mentioned attitudes to allow the elderly patient to receive full health care services [38,39].

REFERENCES

1. Bacon B, McKnight W. Extended Care and Rehabilitation for the Elderly. In Adkins RB, Scott HW (eds), Surgical Care for the Elderly. Baltimore: Williams & Wilkins, 1988;524–534.
2. Clark GS, Murray PK. Rehabilitation of the Geriatric Patient. In DeLisa JA (ed), Rehabilitation Medicine. Philadelphia: Lippincott, 1988;410–427.
3. Hong C, Tobis J. Physiatric Rehabilitation and Maintenance of the Geriatric Patient. In Kottke FJ, Lehmann JF (eds), Krusen's Handbook of Physical Medicine and Rehabilitation (4th ed). Philadelphia: Saunders, 1990;1209–1215.
4. Nardone A, Siliotto R, Grasso M, Schieppati M. Influence of aging on leg muscle reflex. Responses to stance perturbation. Arch Phys Med Rehab 1995;76:158–165.
5. Freed M. Traumatic and Congenital Lesion of the Spinal Cord. In Kottke FJ, Lehmann JF (eds), Krusen's Handbook of Physical Medicine and Rehabilitation (4th ed). Philadelphia: Saunders, 1990;717–744.
6. Yarkony G. Spinal Cord Injury Rehabilitation. In Lee BY, Ostrander, Cochran GVB, Shaw WH (eds), The Spinal Cord Injured Patient: Comprehensive Management. Philadelphia: Saunders, 1991;265–280.

7. Lowrey C, Coutts R. Rehabilitation of the Hip. In Nickel VL, Botte MJ (eds), Orthopaedic Rehabilitation (2nd ed). New York: Churchill Livingstone, 1992;779–789.
8. Mooney V, Becker S. Major Fractures. In Nickel VL, Botte MJ (eds), Orthopaedic Rehabilitation (2nd ed). New York: Churchill Livingstone, 1992;601–610.
9. Young M, O'Young B, McFarland E. Rehabilitation of the orthopaedic trauma patient: general principles. Phys Med Rehab State Art Rev 1995;9:185–199.
10. McCollum P, Walker M. Major Limb Amputation for End-Stage Peripheral Vascular Disease. In Bowker JH (ed), Atlas of Limb Prosthetics: Surgical, Prosthetic, and Rehabilitation Principles / American Association of Orthopaedic Surgeons (2nd ed). St. Louis: Mosby, 1992;25–36.
11. Waters RL. The Energy Expenditure of Amputee Gait. In Bowker JH (ed), Atlas of Limb Prosthetics: Surgical, Prosthetic, and Rehabilitation Principles / American Association of Orthopaedic Surgeons (2nd ed). St. Louis: Mosby, 1992;381–386.
12. Wekoff E. Preprosthetic management. Phys Med Rehab State Art Rev 1994;8:61–71.
13. Leonard J. Lower limb prosthetic sockets. Phys Med Rehab State Art Rev 1994;8:129–145.
14. Czernieckis J, Gitley A. Prosthetic feet. Phys Med Rehab State Art Rev 1994;8:109–127.
15. Michael J. Prosthetic knee mechanisms. Phys Med Rehab State Art Rev 1994;8:147–163.
16. U.S. Senate Special Committee on Aging, American Association of Retired Persons, Federal Council on the Aging, U.S. Administration on Aging. Aging America, Trends and Projections. Pub No. 91-28001. Washington, DC: U.S. Department of Health and Human Services, 1991.
17. Steinberg FU. Principles of geriatric rehabilitation. Arch Phys Med Rehab 1989;70:67–68.
18. Delisa JA (ed). Rehabilitation Medicine: Principles and Practice. Philadelphia: Lippincott, 1988.
19. Goodman H, Englander J. Traumatic Brain Injury in Elderly Individuals. Phys Med Rehab Clin North Am 1992;3:441–461.
20. Kalsbeek WB, McLaurin PL, Harris SH, et al. The National Head and Spinal Cord Injury Survey: major findings. J Neurosurg 1980;53:S19–S31.
21. Cifu DX, Means KM, Currie DM, et al. Geriatric rehabilitation, 2. Diagnosis and management of acquired disabling disorders. Arch Phys Med Rehab 1993;74:S406–S411.
22. National Institute of Neurological Disorders and Stroke. Stroke—1989. Washington, DC: U.S. Department of Health and Human Services, Public Health Service, National Institutes of Health,1989.
23. Dobbin BH. Focused stroke rehabilitation programs do not improve outcome. Arch Neurol 1989;46:701–703.
24. Applegate WB, Craney MJ, Miller ST, Elam JT. Impact of a geriatric assessment unit on subsequent health. Am J Public Health 1991;81:1302–1306.
25. Reding MJ, McDowell FH. Focused stroke rehabilitation programs improve outcome. Arch Neurol 1989;46:700–701.
26. Twitchell T. The restoration of motor function following hemiplegia in man. Brain 1951;74:443–480.
27. Sawner K, LaVigne J (eds). Brunnstrom's Movement Therapy in Hemiplegia: A Neurophysiological Approach (2nd ed). Philadelphia: Lippincott, 1992.
28. Bobath B. Adult Hemiplegia Evaluation and Treatment (3rd ed). Oxford: Heinemann, 1990.
29. Basmajian J (ed). Therapeutic Exercise (4th ed). Baltimore: Williams & Wilkins, 1984.
30. Voss DE, Ionta ME, Myers BJ. Proprioceptive Neuromuscular Facilitation (3rd ed). Philadelphia: Harper & Row, 1985.
31. Kraft GH, Fitts SS, Hammond MC. Techniques to improve function of the arm and hand in chronic hemiplegia. Arch Phys Med Rehab 1992;73:220–227.
32. Dickstein R, Hocherman S, Pillar T, et al. Stroke rehabilitation: three exercise therapy approaches. Phys Ther 1986;66:1233–1238.
33. Wagenaar RC, Meijer OG, van Wieringen PCW, et al. The functional recovery of stroke: a comparison between neuro-developmental treatment and the Brunnstrom method. Scand J Rehabil Med 1990;22:1–8.
34. Boss GR, Seegmiller JE. Age-related physiological changes and their clinical significance. West J Med 1981;135:433–440.
35. Bortf WM II. Disuse and aging. JAMA 1982;248:1203–1208.
36. Buchner D, Coleman E. Exercise Considerations in Older Adults: Intensity, Fall Prevention, and Safety. Phys Med Rehab Clin North Am 1994;5:357–377.
37. Pasner JD, Gorman K, Klein H, et al. Exercise capacity in the elderly. Am J Cardiol 1986;57:52C–58C.
38. Williams ME. Clinical implications of aging physiology. Am J Med 1984;76:1049–1054.
39. Hesse KA, Compion EW, Karamout N. Attitudinal stumbling blocks to geriatric rehabilitation. J Am Geriatr Soc 1984;32:747–750.

SECTION III

Surgical Conditions in the Elderly

Surgical Care for the Elderly, 2nd ed., edited by R. Benton Adkins, Jr., and H. William Scott, Jr. Lippincott–Raven Publishers, Philadelphia © 1998.

CHAPTER 13

Rhinolaryngologic Problems

D. Scott Fortune and James L. Netterville

Maladies of the nasal and laryngeal regions are a common health care demand in patients of all ages. The sequelae of aging exact a heavy toll on the nose and larynx, resulting in an increased incidence of rhinolaryngologic disease in elderly patients. Rhinolaryngologic disease in the elderly may be of degenerative, idiopathic, metabolic, infectious, inflammatory, neoplastic, traumatic, or toxic etiology. Many of these problems are amenable to surgical therapy. The goal of this chapter is to address common problems of the nose and larynx and their surgical therapy. Sinusitis, epistaxis, laryngeal cancer, functional disorders of the larynx, and cranial nerve deficits are discussed. Rather than provide a superficial overview of many uncommon diseases, we cover these common problems in sufficient detail to be useful to the reader.

SINUSITIS

A large proportion of medical care delivered to elderly patients relates to conditions of the upper aerodigestive tract [1]. Indeed, chronic sinusitis has been found to be one of the 10 most common chronic conditions among persons aged >65, along with such conditions as arthritis, hypertension, heart disease, hearing loss, orthopedic impairment, cataracts, diabetes, vision loss, and varicose veins [2]. To understand the pathophysiology and treatment of sinusitis, a fundamental knowledge of paranasal sinus and lateral nasal wall anatomy and physiology is required. A complete review of this subject is available elsewhere [3]; we provide a brief overview of sinus anatomy and function, followed by a discussion of surgical management of sinusitis.

Paranasal Sinus Anatomy and Physiology

There are four paired paranasal sinuses: the maxillary, ethmoid, frontal, and sphenoid sinuses. The maxillary and ethmoid sinuses are generally present at birth; the frontal and sphenoid sinuses generally begin development in the second or third year of life. Sinus development is normally complete by age 18.

Functionally, the sinuses are divided into two groups, anterior and posterior, depending on the region of their drainage. The anterior group drains into the middle meatus and comprises the maxillary, anterior ethmoid, and frontal sinuses. The posterior group drains into the superior meatus and is made up of the posterior ethmoid and sphenoid sinuses. Each sinus has its own unique ostium through which its secretions emanate. A meatus is an anatomic area located underneath the three conchal bones (turbinates) that line the lateral nasal wall. A meatus and the sinuses that drain into it form an anatomic unit known as the *ostiomeatal complex*. This concept is important because sinusitis is currently thought to be due in most cases to disease within the ostiomeatal complex [4].

The physiologic function of the paranasal sinuses is not precisely known. Various theories have been proposed including humidification and warming of ambient air, clearance of particulate debris, olfaction, and maintenance of proper head balance. It is clear, however, that the sinuses produce mucus, which aids in keeping the nasal cavity moist. Mucus is secreted by the sinus epithelium, which is a pseudostratified columnar type with goblet cells and cilia typical of respiratory epithelium elsewhere in the upper aerodigestive tract. The mucus is swept along toward the sinus ostium by the motion of the cilia. From this brief overview of sinus anatomy and function, it should be clear that disturbances in mucous production, mucous composition, ciliary function, sinus ostium patency, or ostiomeatal complex anatomy may be involved individually or collectively in the pathophysiology of sinusitis [3,4].

Pathologically, sinusitis may be considered as acute, subacute, or chronic. For purposes of this discussion, we address acute and chronic sinusitis. In general, acute sinusitis may be medically managed, whereas chronic sinusitis more often requires surgical management.

TABLE 13-1. *Treatment of acute sinusitis*

Medical
- Antibiotics
- Saline irrigation
- Humidification
- Decongestants: topical, systemic
- Corticosteroids: topical, systemic (selected cases)
- Dependent drainage: elevate head of bed 30 to 45 degrees
- Mucolytics: guaifenesin

Surgical
- Indications
  - Orbital and periorbital cellulitis
  - Orbital abscess
  - Intracranial or extracranial abscess
  - Maxillary sinus empyema
- Procedures
  - Incision and drainage of abscess
  - Frontal sinus trephination
  - External ethmoidectomy
  - Maxillary sinus paracentesis

Acute Sinusitis

Acute sinusitis is most often a sequela of viral upper respiratory tract infection (URI) that lasts from 1 day to 4 weeks. URI results in mucosal inflammation and edema, which leads to obstruction of the sinus ostium. Mucosal hypoxia ensues, resulting in ciliary dysfunction and thick, retained secretions. Bacteria already present in the sinus or those inoculated by sneezing, nose blowing, or sniffling overgrow and invade the sinus, resulting in clinical infection [4].

URIs are underdiagnosed and often inappropriately treated in the elderly, which may predispose them to an increased incidence of acute sinusitis. Appropriate management may also be delayed by self-treatment with ineffective, over-the-counter remedies [1]. Systemic predisposing factors are often present in elderly patients including age-related immune deficiency [5], long-term corticosteroid therapy (for arthritis or reactive airways disease), poorly controlled diabetes, malnutrition, immunoglobulin deficiency (e.g., multiple myeloma), nasal or facial fractures, allergic rhinitis, atrophic rhinitis (ozena), dehydration (causing thick, inspissated secretions), poor dentition (with dental abscess), frequent use of topical nasal sprays (rhinitis medicamentosa), immotile cilia syndromes (e.g., Kartagener's syndrome), previous sinus surgery (synechiae), and nasal intubation (in nosocomial sinusitis). Although quite curable, early and aggressive treatment of acute sinusitis is indicated to prevent life-threatening complications.

Patients with acute sinusitis present with headache, purulent rhinorrhea, recent URI, and constitutional symptoms. Pain from the paranasal sinuses may be referred to the following areas: teeth, malar area, or retro-orbital area for maxillary sinus; periorbital, retro-orbital, paranasal, or frontal area for ethmoid sinuses; forehead or paranasal area in frontal sinusitis; and retro-orbital or vertex area for sphenoid sinusitis. Other possible symptoms include epistaxis, facial pain and tenderness, dental pain, eye pain, vertigo, disturbed sleep, cough, wheezing, hemoptysis, gastroesophageal reflux, nasal crusting, halitosis, and mouth breathing [1]. Fever and leukocytosis are atypical features and should alert the clinician to the possibility of complications [6]. Physical examination with both anterior rhinoscopy (speculum examination) and nasal endoscopy (rigid or flexible) usually reveals edematous, erythematous mucosa with purulent secretions emanating from the ostia of the affected sinuses. Palpation tenderness may also be present over the malar, periorbital, frontal, or superior alveolar regions. In patients with dental apical abscess, pain may be elicited by tapping the offending tooth with a dental mirror. Physical examination findings can be confirmed and correlated with computed tomographic (CT) imaging of the paranasal sinuses. In addition to the traditional axial and coronal views, many centers have developed a protocol for "screening sinus" CT scans; screening views give adequate views of the paranasal sinuses at less cost and radiation exposure to the patient [4]. CT scans are not a necessary step in the diagnosis and treatment of sinusitis; however, they are quite useful in cases in which the diagnosis is in question and are essential in cases in which surgery is to be performed or complications are suspected.

As alluded to previously, medical management is the mainstay of therapy for acute sinusitis (Table 13-1). Antibiotics, saline irrigation, humidification, topical and systemic decongestants, topical and systemic corticosteroids (in selected cases), dependent drainage, and mucolytics are the elements of the medical armamentarium. The bacteriology of community-acquired sinusitis is predictable and typically includes pneumococcus, *Streptococcus pyogenes*, *Staphylococcus aureus*, *Haemophilus influenzae*, and *Branhamella catarrhalis;* less commonly, anaerobic species are involved, in which case a dental origin should be suspected. Nosocomial pathogens tend to be aerobic gram-negative bacilli or mixed aerobic and anaerobic infections. Antibiotics, therefore, should be chosen empirically for the clinical setting (i.e., community-acquired versus nosocomial sinusitis), and then appropriately adjusted following culture and sensitivity results. Cultures obtained directly from the affected sinus or from the affected sinus ostium more accurately reflect the offending flora than random cultures of the nasal cavity and nasopharynx [4]. The duration of antibiotic therapy should last a minimum of 10 to 14 days and for 7 days after symptoms subside to prevent relapse. This recommendation is based on the fact that antibiotic penetration into infected sinuses may be decreased. Topical and systemic decongestants help relieve mucosal edema; however, topical agents should be limited to 4 to 5 days' duration to prevent rhinitis medicamentosa. Elevation of the head of the patient's bed 30 to 45 degrees encourages dependent drainage. Rarely, mucolytics (e.g., guaifenesin) are helpful in patients with exceptionally tenacious mucus. Successful management also necessitates control of predisposing factors. Diabetes should be tightly controlled; malnutrition and dehydration should be reversed; and poor dentition should be addressed.

Perhaps two of the most common scenarios in which surgeons encounter sinusitis are in nasally intubated patients (nasogastric tubes, endotracheal tubes, feeding tubes, etc.) and post-traumatic patients with nasal or facial fractures and hemorrhagic sinus effusions. For nasally intubated patients, decannulation, saline irrigations, dependent drainage, and occasionally topical decongestants are sufficient to relieve sinus ostial blockage. Post-traumatic patients usually respond well to saline irrigations, humidification, dependent drainage, and topical decongestants for 48 hours. For nasally intubated and post-traumatic patients, antibiotic therapy is not indicated, unless there is purulent rhinorrhea, and may lead to adverse sequelae, such as antibiotic resistance or antibiotic-associated colitis [1,4,6]. Otolaryngologic consultation is recommended for patients who do not respond to these first-line measures.

Surgical therapy is infrequently necessary for patients with acute sinusitis. When necessary, it is usually in the setting of a patient with impending complications, or cases that are refractory to maximal medical therapy. Due to the proximity of the paranasal sinuses to orbital and intracranial structures, there is a potential for significant morbidity and mortality. The lamina papyracea and cribriform plate are two thin shelves of bone separating the sinuses from the orbit and cranial vault, respectively. Fulminant infections in elderly patients often with coexisting osteopenia can erode these tenuous, already paper-thin laminae of bone, with resultant extension of infection. Possible complications include inflammatory edema; orbital and periorbital cellulitis; orbital abscess; cavernous sinus thrombosis; and epidural, subdural, subperiosteal, or intracranial abscess. Pott's puffy tumor, originally described by Sir Percival Pott in 1760, results from progressive frontal sinusitis with frontal osteomyelitis and erosion of the anterior table of the frontal bone. Cellulitis may be initially managed conservatively with CT scanning to rule out abscess, antibiotics, and hourly visual acuity checks. Surgery is indicated when visual acuity worsens, vision is lost, symptoms progress over 24 hours, symptoms do not respond after 48 to 72 hours of aggressive therapy, or when imaging reveals abscess formation. Surgical therapy includes drainage of the abscess, external ethmoidectomy via a medial canthal incision [7], and possibly frontal sinus trephination, depending on CT scan findings. Early consultation with an otolaryngologist, ophthalmologist, or neurosurgeon is mandatory.

Cases of acute sinusitis that are refractory to medical therapy or in which there is total (empyema) or near-total opacification of the maxillary sinus may be amenable to paracentesis (so-called sinus tap). This can be accomplished via either a transnasal or sublabial transmaxillary needle puncture with a 16-gauge needle under topical and local anesthesia. Paracentesis is both diagnostic and therapeutic: Material is obtained for culture and empyema is drained. A critical step in this procedure is to ascertain placement of the needle within the maxillary sinus before any irrigation. Placement is confirmed by return of air or purulent material. Irrigation prior to this step may result in air embolism or dissemination of infection into soft tissues. Otolaryngologists use both methods depending on the clinical circumstances, but in general the sublabial approach is preferred because it affords a direct route into the sinus. The aspirate should be sent for bacterial, fungal, acid-fast bacilli, and anaerobic culture and sensitivity. In cases of unexplained, isolated maxillary sinus opacification, malignancy should be considered; the sinus irrigant may also be sent for cytology [4,6].

In summary, acute sinusitis is most often medically managed. Surgery is reserved for refractory cases or impending complications. In these instances, surgical procedures may be both diagnostic and therapeutic. Early aggressive management of acute sinusitis in elderly patients may prevent complications.

Chronic Sinusitis

In contrast to acute sinusitis, chronic sinusitis most often requires surgical therapy. Chronic sinusitis is defined as persistent sinus inflammation lasting >3 months. Subacute sinusitis is defined as persistent sinus inflammation lasting 4 weeks to 3 months; pathologic changes in this condition are medically reversible with treatment similar to that appropriate for acute sinusitis and therefore are not discussed further. When sinus inflammation reaches the chronic stage, the process is irreversible with medical management alone. Successful management in these cases likely requires a combination of surgical intervention and medical therapy. Elderly patients may be at increased risk for chronic sinusitis due to delays in seeking treatment for early symptoms, acquired distortions in normal nasal anatomy, nasal polyposis associated with the use of aspirin and nonsteroidal anti-inflammatory drugs (NSAIDs), or multiple bouts of acute sinusitis with inadequate treatment [1,2].

Patients with chronic sinusitis present with complaints of persistent mucopurulent rhinorrhea and nasal obstruction that may be bilateral or unilateral. In contrast to acute and subacute sinusitis, pain (i.e., headache, facial pain) is not a feature of chronic sinusitis, except in cases of chronic sinusitis complicated by the superimposition of acute infection [1,6]. Physical examination findings are variable and may include mucosal edema and erythema, nasal polyps, purulent rhinitis, facial or periorbital edema, posterior pharyngeal drainage, intranasal synechiae, septal deformity, paradoxically curved middle turbinates, or other abnormal anatomy. Intranasal examination has been greatly enhanced by the development of flexible and rigid endoscopes. These instruments improve visualization of obscure abnormalities, allow videographic and photographic documentation of pathology, and facilitate teaching of house staff, students, and nurses [1].

CT and magnetic resonance imaging (MRI) of the paranasal sinuses aid in the diagnosis of chronic sinusitis. CT is the modality of choice for evaluation of intranasal anatomy, bony detail, trauma, and the ostiomeatal complex. MRI is the modality of choice for evaluation of neoplastic disease and complicated inflammatory disease [8]. Anatomic variations

TABLE 13-2. *Treatment of chronic sinusitis*

Maximal medical therapy
Radiography
Computed tomographic scan
Magnetic resonance imaging
Sinus plain films
Surgery
Functional endoscopic sinus surgery
Caldwell-Luc operation
Intranasal and external ethmoidectomy
Frontal sinus obliteration
Postoperative
Medical management
Flexible and rigid sinus endoscopy
Frequent debridement of crusting, synechiae, etc.

TABLE 13-3. *Complications of endoscopic sinus surgery*

Minor
Synechiae
Orbital emphysema
Dental pain or hypesthesia
Asthma exacerbation
Epiphora
Hyposmia or anosmia
Major
Cerebrospinal fluid leak
Carotid artery injury
Blindness
Orbital hematoma
Meningitis
Diplopia
Intracranial hemorrhage
Death

Source: Lanza DC, Kennedy DW. Endoscopic Sinus Surgery. In Bailey BJ (ed), Head and Neck Surgery—Otolaryngology (Vol I). Philadelphia: Lippincott, 1993.

that can be identified with CT include concha bullosa cells (aerated middle turbinate), septal deflections and spurs, paradoxically curved middle turbinates, pneumatization of the uncinate process, agger nasi cells (ethmoid cells anterior to the frontal sinus ostium), prominent bulla ethmoidalis, Haller cells (pneumatized orbital floor), Onodi cells (sphenoid bone pneumatized by ethmoid cell), exposed optic nerve in the sphenoid sinus, bony defects of the parasphenoid carotid canal, and aplasia of the maxillary sinus. Radiographic imaging is thus an important part of the workup of chronic sinusitis because it helps define the extent of sinus disease and allows preoperative identification of potential surgical hazards [8].

Patients with chronic sinusitis who have failed a trial of maximal medical therapy are considered for surgical therapy. Preoperative screening of these patients is similar to that for other patients being considered for general anesthesia: Sinus surgery may also be performed under local and topical anesthesia in the otolaryngologist's office for those patients unsuitable for general anesthesia or those who require minor procedures. In general, patients with chronic sinusitis are ambulatory; rarely, a surgeon will be confronted with an inpatient case of chronic sinusitis that is exacerbated by trauma, nasal intubation, or acute infection. Surgery, depending on the extent, may be performed on an outpatient basis—that is, same-day surgery—or may require a postoperative hospital stay lasting from 23 hours to several days. It should be noted that surgery for chronic sinusitis is elective, unless complications have developed. The management of chronic sinusitis is summarized in Table 13-2.

The goal of surgery in chronic sinusitis is to provide adequate drainage of the affected sinus(es), allowing reaeration of the sinus, return of normal sinus function, and re-establishment of mucociliary flow [9]. Traditional approaches to sinus surgery were intranasal or extranasal and mainly addressed disease of the maxillary and ethmoid sinuses. These procedures included inferior meatus (maxillary) antrostomy, intranasal ethmoidectomy, external ethmoidectomy, transantral ethmoidectomy, and the Caldwell-Luc operation. These procedures were formerly the gold standard against which other sinus operations were measured [10]. Following the advent of nasal endoscopes, these procedures have become less common, having been largely supplanted by endoscopic sinus surgery. In particular, the inferior meatus antrostomy has been shown to be inferior to intranasal endoscopic middle meatus antrostomy except in cases where there is no hope of restoring normal mucociliary clearance, as in immotile cilia syndrome; for these patients gravity-dependent inferior meatus antrostomies are required [9].

Endoscopic sinus surgery was introduced into the United States in 1984 by Kennedy [9]. It has since continued to gain popularity [9] because it is less traumatic and well tolerated, even in elderly patients [1]. Reversal of maxillary, ethmoid, sphenoid, and frontal sinus disease is possible via an endoscopic approach. The indications for this approach are similar to those for other forms of sinus surgery. However, extensive training and experience in these techniques are required to perform the surgery safely [1], and thus this technique may not be offered by every otolaryngologist. Endoscopic sinus surgery is contraindicated in instances where the patient or physician are not committed to meticulous and frequent postoperative debridement [9] and medical management of disease [1].

Complications from endoscopic sinus surgery are infrequent but can be disastrous. Major negative outcomes include death, intracranial bleeding, direct brain injury, blindness or partial vision loss, diplopia, meningitis, massive epistaxis, orbital hematoma, cerebrospinal fluid leak, and carotid artery and optic nerve injury. Minor complications include intranasal synechiae, orbital emphysema, tooth pain, supraorbital or infraorbital hypesthesia, asthma exacerbation, epiphora secondary to nasolacrimal duct injury, and other complications [7,9,11]. Table 13-3 summarizes the complications of endoscopic sinus surgery. Synechiae are a particularly bothersome and common postoperative complication. Frontal recess stenosis after endoscopic surgery occurs in approximately 12% of patients. Refractory frontal sinus symptoms and their treatment are somewhat controversial. Techniques for treatment of frontal recess stenosis include frontal sinus trephination or frontal sinus obliteration, with osteoplastic flap and abdominal fat graft [12]. For sphenoid sinus restenosis the approach may be endoscopic, intranasal transseptal, sublabial transseptal, or transpalatal.

In summary, surgery for chronic sinusitis is indicated for patients who fail an adequate trial of maximal medical therapy. Standard intranasal or endoscopic surgery may be necessary. The overall rate of complications is low; however, complications can be devastating and are best avoided by an extensive, practical knowledge of intranasal and paranasal anatomy. Meticulous postoperative care is required to achieve satisfactory results.

EPISTAXIS

Few disorders treated by otolaryngologists provoke as much anxiety in patients and physicians as epistaxis. Often by the time the patient seeks medical care for the problem, it has become a medical emergency [13] requiring prompt control to prevent sequelae such as exsanguination, shock, myocardial infarction, aspiration, syncope, or even death. Although rarely life-threatening [14], epistaxis may result in significant blood loss with secondary hypoxia that may not be well tolerated in elderly patients with comorbid factors such as coronary artery disease, hypertension, or chronic obstructive lung disease. Epistaxis occurs at least once in an estimated 7% to 14% of the U.S. population [14]. However, the incidence in elderly patients is increased because aging leads to nasal mucosal atrophy. The result is an increased tendency toward desiccation and ulceration [15]. Atrophic mucosa predisposes the elderly patient to bleeding from other etiologies (discussed in the following section). Epistaxis is most common during the cold months; likewise the incidence in patients living in the northeast United States is higher than in other areas [14,15]. Most cases of epistaxis are handled by the patient with time-honored remedies such as ice packs and digital pressure. Those patients who present to a physician require rapid treatment and a search for primary causes such as neoplasm.

Etiology of Epistaxis

For classification purposes as well as clinical purposes, the etiology of epistaxis can be broken down into two categories: local and systemic factors (Table 13-4). Local factors include trauma, inflammatory reactions, anatomic or structural deformities, foreign bodies, toxic or chemical irritants, low-humidity environments, surgery, and intranasal tumors [14]. Trauma is the most common cause of nasal hemorrhage whether from nose picking or blunt trauma. Nasal and midface fractures are also frequent causes [14,16]. In wintertime indoor heating units decrease the humidity in ambient air, resulting in crusting and desiccation of the nasal mucosa. This accounts for the increased incidence of epistaxis in cold months and in the Northeast. Occasionally, intranasal or nasopharyngeal tumors present with epistaxis. A thorough physical examination will aid in making the diagnosis.

TABLE 13-4. *Exacerbating factors in epistaxis*

Local factors
Trauma
Inflammatory reactions
Anatomic and structural deformity
Foreign body
Local toxins
Low humidity
Intranasal tumors
Surgery
Systemic factors
Vascular malformations
Hypertension
Atherosclerosis
Blood dyscrasias
Drugs
Alcoholism
Systemic toxins

Systemic factors involved in epistaxis include vascular malformations, hypertension, atherosclerosis, blood dyscrasias, drugs, ethanol, and systemic toxic agents such as phosphorous, mercury, and chromium [13–16]. Hereditary hemorrhagic telangiectasia (HHT; Osler-Weber-Rendu disease) is by far the most common vascular malformation leading to epistaxis. It is an autosomal dominant disease and is characterized by a lack of contractile elements in vessel walls. HHT is often more problematic in elderly patients than in younger ones due to the mucosal atrophy present in this age group, which leaves the disordered blood vessels relatively exposed. It is teleologically impossible to know whether hypertension initiates or merely exacerbates epistaxis; what is known is that epistaxis is much more difficult to control in the hypertensive patient. Arteriosclerosis leads to friable vessels within the nose, usually located posterior to the inferior aspect of the middle turbinate [17]. Clearly, hypertension and arteriosclerosis are more common in elderly patients. Blood dyscrasias that contribute to epistaxis include leukemia, von Willebrand's disease, hemophilia, multiple myeloma, idiopathic and thrombotic thrombocytopenic purpura, and chronic renal failure. These entities vary in their ability to lead to nasal hemorrhage and usually involve dysfunction of platelets or clotting factors or thrombocytopenia. Common medications predisposing to epistaxis include aspirin, warfarin (Coumadin), and NSAIDs. Aspirin and NSAIDs are frequently used medications in elderly patients with atherosclerosis or arthritis. Heavy consumption of ethanol may lead to nose bleeds due to hepatic synthetic dysfunction or thrombocytopenia [14].

As previously mentioned, both local and systemic factors combine with atrophic nasal mucosa in elderly patients to increase the incidence of epistaxis. Knowledge of these factors is important because successful management depends

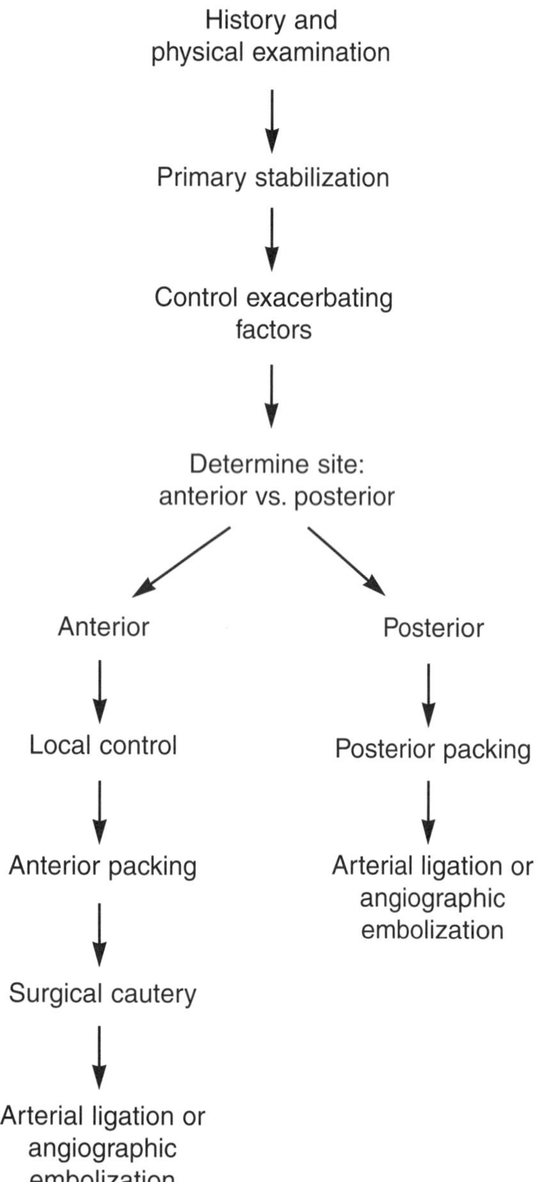

FIG. 13-1. Management of epistaxis.

on control of predisposing factors. These factors should be diligently sought when the physician is taking the history.

Anatomy

To treat epistaxis appropriately, the anatomy of the entire nose, as well as its vascular supply, must be well understood. The nasal mucosa derives its rich blood supply from both the internal and external carotid arteries. The two major sources of blood supply are the internal maxillary artery and the facial artery, which are branches of the external carotid artery. The internal maxillary artery ascends on the posterior wall of the maxillary sinus and branches into the sphenopalatine artery, the descending palatal arteries, and the infraorbital artery. The sphenopalatine artery passes through the sphenopalatine foramen to enter the nasal cavity at the posterior aspect of the middle turbinate. The artery then branches, sending a lateral branch to supply the middle and inferior turbinates and the medial wall of the ethmoid and maxillary sinuses. The second branch, the posterior septal artery, crosses over the posterior roof of the posterior choanae and supplies the nasal septum. It anastomoses distally in the anterior septum with the incisive artery—the distal branch of the greater palatine artery—to form the rich vascular supply to the anterior septum. The facial artery adds a portion of the blood supply to the anterior septum also via the septal branch of the superior labial artery. Blood supply from the internal carotid is contributed through two branches of the ophthalmic artery, the anterior and posterior ethmoidal arteries. Both of these vessels pass through the medial wall of the orbit into the superior aspect of the ethmoid sinuses. They continue along the cribriform plate to supply the superior aspect of the lateral nasal wall, including the superior turbinate [17]. From this description of the intranasal blood supply, it should be clear that two highly vascularized regions of nasal mucosa are the most common sites of intranasal hemorrhage. The most common site of all cases of intranasal bleeding in all age groups is Kiesselbach's plexus in the region of the anterior septum. The portion of the anterior septum that represents the confluence of three major arterial branches is known as *Kiesselbach's area* and is also occasionally referred to as *Little's area.* In addition to being the most common site overall for nasal bleeding, this region is the most common site of an anterior bleed. Posterior bleeding is more common in elderly patients than in other groups. The second most common area for epistaxis to occur, therefore, lies posterior in the nasal cavity where the sphenopalatine artery divides within the mucosa, just posterior to the middle turbinate [17]. Familiarity with the nasal vascular anatomy is imperative because anterior and posterior epistaxis are treated differently.

Management of Epistaxis

The management of epistaxis can be broken down into three main steps: (1) initial evaluation; (2) outpatient management, including medical management and anterior nasal packing; and (3) inpatient management, including posterior nasal packing and surgical ligation or catheter embolization of feeding arteries. A key distinction, which should be made early in the evaluation of a patient with epistaxis, is whether the bleed is anterior or posterior. This distinction largely determines management of the individual patient. A simplified treatment algorithm is presented in Fig. 13-1.

The initial step in management of a patient with epistaxis is to calm the patient and family, allay their fears, and develop rapport with them. The patient and family should be assured that you can control the problem. Next, the degree of urgency should be assessed by reviewing the vital signs and hematocrit or hemoglobin concentration (if available at the time of the initial evaluation). The physician then obtains a thorough history of the current episode. Factors that should be sought include previous history of epistaxis; history of sinus disease; predisposing factors such as HHT, blood dyscrasias, aspirin or NSAID use, ethanol use, nasal trauma or surgery; history of hypertension, atherosclerosis, or coronary artery disease; the duration of the current episode and the patient's estimation of the actual amount of blood loss; other symptoms such as dizziness, syncope, chest pain, dyspnea, and so forth; and past medical history including allergies and medication use. In evaluating patients with epistaxis, it is important to remember the assessment and protection of the airway. It is also important to establish intravenous access early in the course of evaluation for rapid institution of intravenous fluid replacement, which is usually necessary for patients who bleed long enough to present to a physician, as well as for administration of antihypertensive or sedating medications.

In severe episodes of epistaxis with massive hemorrhage, unstable vital signs, and shock, one may institute rapid pressure on the bleeding site by placing Foley catheters into both nares with the balloons positioned in the nasopharynx. The balloons are then filled with 10 to 15 ml of saline and pulled forward snugly against the posterior choanae. Tight anterior packing is then placed bilaterally and left in place until the situation has stabilized. This is a rare instance because epistaxis is usually limited by the patient's hemodynamic stability; that is, intranasal bleeding is often markedly decreased when the patient becomes hypotensive. Controlling epistaxis with Foley catheters is a rare occurrence and is most often seen in the setting of a polytrauma patient with severe facial injuries who is hemodynamically unstable, or in those patients with life-threatening nasal exsanguination from a cause other than trauma. This manner of controlling bleeding is quite effective in emergency situations and allows one to exert an extreme amount of pressure on the nasopharyngeal and intranasal tissues. For this reason, these packs should not be used for chronic control of epistaxis or in nonemergent bleeds. These packs have been known to cause septal and turbinate necrosis within 48 hours. Most emergency departments have commercially manufactured double-balloon catheters (with intranasal and pharyngeal balloons) in stock that may be more expedient than a Foley catheter and anterior pack in the emergency situation.

In moderately severe epistaxis, the history and initial stabilizing steps should take place concurrently. Elderly patients with epistaxis should be treated expediently because the rate of complication increases with the amount of time required to control bleeding [14]. At our institution, this is accomplished by having the nursing staff establish intravenous lines and administer antihypertensive drugs while the physician takes the history and begins the physical examination. Blood pressure should always be addressed first. Blood pressures >140/80 may exacerbate bleeding. Blood pressure can be safely and rapidly controlled with sublingual nifedipine in those patients without calcium channel blocker allergies.

After initial stabilization, the physician should progress to physical examination of the nose and nasopharynx to determine the actual site of bleeding. A brilliant light source is an absolute prerequisite; the beam of light should be parallel to the vision of the examiner. Using a Frazier suction and a nasal speculum, both sides of the nasal cavity are systematically examined in an effort to identify the site of hemorrhage. If this inspection does not reveal the site, then nasal pledgets soaked in a topical solution that causes both vasoconstriction and anesthesia of the nasal mucosa are placed in each nostril. The most common solution used for this purpose is 4% cocaine. To prevent a catastrophic disaster from cocaine overdose, the dose should be limited to 200 mg (i.e., 5 ml of 4% solution). The pledgets are then removed and the nose is reexamined. If the bleeding is anterior then electrical or topical cautery with silver nitrate may be performed. This is done accurately by cauterizing the bleeding point as well as a rosette pattern around it for a distance of 3 mm. The most common cause of failure using cautery is the inappropriate use of silver nitrate [14,17]. The chemical should be applied to the area for 20 seconds; application for 5 to 10 seconds inevitably results in rebleeding within minutes. The cauterized area is then covered with absorbable knitted fabric (Surgicel) or gelatin sponge (Gelfoam) impregnated with bacitracin ointment. These measures usually suffice for mild-to-moderate anterior bleeding. The patient is then managed on an ambulatory basis with saline nasal irrigations, instillation of antibiotic or petroleum ointment into the nasal vestibule at night, vasoconstricting nasal sprays (oxymetazoline or phenylephrine) on an as-needed basis for 72 hours, stool softeners, and limited activity with no heavy lifting, bending over, or straining.

If the bleeding is posterior—located posterior to the posterior aspect of the middle turbinate—a flexible or rigid nasal endoscope may be used to aid examination. Epistaxis is rarely bilateral, except in traumatic cases. However, blood passes behind the nasal septum into the unaffected side, giving the appearance of bilaterality. The history of the side of onset and the endoscopic examination often are helpful in localization [16]. If a discrete posterior lesion can be identified, it may be treated with posterior endoscopic cautery. This is accomplished using the standard nasal cautery armamentarium under endoscopic guidance with a 2.7- or 4-mm straight or angled nasal endoscope and a suction cautery apparatus [13]. The success rate with this technique approaches 90%. Complications, which are infrequent, include palatal numbness, synechiae, mucosal sloughing, and permanent serous otitis media if the eustachian tube orifice is cauterized.

If a discrete anterior or posterior bleeding site cannot be identified, then packing is the next step in management. If the bleeding is in the anterior nasal cavity, from between the nasal vestibule to the posterior aspect of middle turbinate, then an anterior pack is indicated. Pledgets are again placed in the nose while preparing the nasal pack. An anterior pack is usually formed from 0.5 × 72–in. plain or petroleum jelly gauze impregnated with antibiotic ointment with antistaphylococcal activity. The antibiotic ointment reduces crusting and prevents toxic shock syndrome, which has been reported in patients with nasal packing. During placement of the pack, both ends are carefully monitored to prevent it from prolapsing through the posterior choanae into the hypopharynx. The initial portion is placed into the superior nasal recess along the superior and middle turbinate to the posterior choana and then the remainder is layered from posterior to anterior until the cavity is tightly filled. Anterior packing is left in place for 3 to 5 days to allow formation of a mature clot. With only an anterior pack in place, the patient may be observed at home. During the period of observation with packing in place, oral antibiotics and decongestants should be prescribed to prevent paranasal sinusitis. Management after pack removal is similar to that following successful cautery [14,16,17].

Well-placed anterior packs can often control posterior bleeding. If anterior packing fails, however, posterior packing must be instituted. Posterior packing accomplishes two objectives: (1) It places pressure on the nasopharyngeal region and the posterior aspect of the turbinates, and (2) it forms a buttress for the anterior pack, allowing increased pack pressure in the posterior aspect of the nasal cavity. Various posterior packing techniques have been described. Foley catheters, gauze, or commercial pneumatic nasal catheters may be used [14]. A 16-French Foley catheter with a 30-ml balloon is passed through the site of major bleeding and into the nasopharynx. After 10 to 15 ml of saline is instilled into the balloon, the catheter is pulled anteriorly to snug the balloon against the posterior choana. Anterior packing as previously described is then placed around the catheter in the nasal cavity. A piece of plastic tubing, either the flared end of a Foley catheter or a cut endotracheal tube can be placed around the Foley and pushed up against the nasal packing before clamping the catheter tube against this supplemental ring. This allows countertension to be applied to the intranasal pack and not against the alar rim. This should prevent necrosis of the alar rim from the pressure over the period that the pack remains in place. The technique of posterior packing using gauze is described elsewhere [14]. Posterior nasal packing activates the nasopulmonary reflex, resulting in abnormalities of the cardiac and respiratory systems. These abnormalities range from altered respiration to hypoxia, syncope, dysrhythmias, myocardial infarction, cerebrovascular accident, and cardiac arrest. Elderly patients should be admitted to a monitored bed with continuous pulse oximetry and be provided with humidified oxygen (we use 40% by face tent). The combination of anterior and posterior packing is uncomfortable, and adequate analgesia must be provided. At our institution this usually consists of patient-controlled analgesia in the demand mode only without a basal rate. Prophylactic antibiotics, nasal decongestants (if the patient's blood pressure is controlled), and stool softeners are also provided. These packs remain in place for 3 to 5 days depending on the severity of the bleeding and whether exacerbating factors have been controlled.

For patients with blood dyscrasias, coagulopathy, or HHT, using a packing material that will eventually dissolve is helpful to prevent further intranasal trauma during packing removal. Agents such as oxidase cellulose, Gelfoam sponges coated with topical thrombin, or microfibrillar collagen (Avitene) all work well in this situation [14].

At the time of packing removal, whether anterior or anterior and posterior, if there is no further hemorrhage, management is similar to other outpatient measures described previously (i.e., saline irrigation, ointment application to the vestibule, stool softeners, limited activity, and topical vasoconstricting agents). If, however, bleeding resumes interventional management is indicated.

Options for interventional management of epistaxis in elderly patients include arterial ligation, angiographic embolization, laser coagulation, and septodermoplasty. When considering ligation or catheter embolization, the physician must ascertain whether the bleeding is anterior, posterior, or superior in location. Anterior bleeding indicates involvement of branches of the facial artery, posterior inferior bleeding indicates involvement of the internal maxillary system, and superior anterior bleeding indicates involvement of the ethmoid arteries. In recurrent epistaxis, early ligation or embolization of the feeding vessel is efficacious and prevents multiple repacking of the already traumatized mucosa [17]. Preoperative evaluation of these patients is similar to other surgical patients. However, one must keep in mind that comorbid conditions such as hypertension, coronary atherosclerosis, and others are more frequent in the elderly population. These conditions should be medically optimized, if possible, before operation.

The ethmoid arteries are usually the supplying vessels for superior nasal bleeding. The ethmoid arteries are surgically approached through an incision halfway between the nasion and the medial canthus (i.e., a Lynch incision). The periosteum is elevated off the medial canthal region and along the lamina papyracea until the anterior ethmoid artery is identified. This artery is usually 2 cm from the anterior lacrimal crest. It is coagulated with bipolar cautery and ligated with surgical ties or vascular clips. Careful ligation is necessary to prevent the proximal end of the artery from retracting into the orbital floor, causing a retro-orbital hematoma and possibly blindness. The posterior ethmoid artery is located 10 mm posterior to the anterior ethmoid artery and approximately 5 mm anterior to the optic nerve. Due to its proximity to this vital structure, it is rarely ligated. During this procedure it is necessary to monitor the degree of pressure placed on the globe and orbit to prevent ocular damage. Rarely, it is necessary to ligate both anterior ethmoid arteries when bleeding cannot be localized to one side [14,17].

If the hemorrhage can be localized to the posterior inferior aspect of the nasal cavity and it has failed to respond to posterior nasal packing, then internal maxillary artery ligation is the procedure of choice. With the patient under general anesthesia, an incision is made in the buccal mucosa identifying the anterior surface of the maxilla. After removing the anterior wall, the posterior wall of the maxillary sinus is removed under microscopic guidance, leaving the posterior periosteum intact. After careful incision of the posterior periosteum, the maxillary artery and its several branches, the infraorbital artery, and the sphenopalatine artery can be identified. These vessels are then ligated with vascular clips. Patients can often be discharged 24 hours after the procedure [13]. The procedural failure rate is 5% to 13% with inadequate clipping, development of collateral circulation, and inadequate identification of the arterial landmarks accounting for the majority of failures [14]. Alternatively, the internal maxillary artery can be approached intraorally. It is identified as it passes between the lateral and medial pterygoid muscles where it is ligated with surgical clips. Before the operation, a Waters' view of the maxillary sinus or other sinus imaging study may be obtained to rule out neoplasm or congenital absence of the sinus [13]. Infraorbital neuropraxia and anesthesia have been reported following this procedure, as well as sinusitis, oroantral fistula, and, rarely, blindness [13–14,16,17].

Routine ligation of the external carotid artery for prevention of posterior epistaxis has fallen into disfavor because the collateral blood flow that feeds into the artery distal to the point of ligation sustains a high rate of flow in the artery. This leads to a high failure rate with this procedure [17]. In cases of severe facial trauma, ligation of the external carotid artery and the anterior ethmoid artery—a major source of collateral flow—may be life-saving [14]. The external carotid artery is exposed via a standard incision along the anterior border of the sternocleidomastoid muscle. The ligation is performed distal to the superior thyroid artery.

Recently, laser coagulation of nasal vessels has been successfully used to control epistaxis. This technique is particularly useful for patients with HHT or other blood dyscrasia. Laser coagulation in these patients allows control of bleeding using a virtually no-touch technique, without the requirement for post-treatment nasal packing. The lasers best suited for this purpose are the potassium titanyl phosphate, argon, and neodymium:yttrium-aluminum-garnet lasers. This technique may be performed under local anesthesia with the patient awake or under general anesthesia. The surgeon must apply all proper safety precautions for laser-assisted procedures while using this technique [18].

Another useful technique for HHT patients is septodermoplasty. It has been shown to be effective in controlling the number of bleeding episodes in these patients. The anterior nasal septum, floor of the nose, and medial portion of the inferior turbinate are stripped of their mucosa. These areas are then resurfaced with a dermal graft harvested from the thigh. Cross-matched blood should be available for this operation because blood loss may be high [17].

Arteriographic embolization is an interventional alternative to surgery for refractory epistaxis. The advantages of angiography include obliteration of distal vessels, definition of bleeding sites, identification of collateral flow, performance under local anesthesia, and embolization of surgically inaccessible vessels. In addition, the procedure is a good alternative for poor surgical candidates and can be repeated with relative ease if bleeding recurs. A variety of embolization materials are currently in use including polyvinyl alcohol, Gelfoam, and coiled springs. Gelfoam has the disadvantage of being resorbable. The complications of this procedure are similar to other arteriographic procedures [14,17].

In summary, epistaxis is a common malady affecting up to 7% to 14% of the population. The incidence in elderly patients is increased due to nasal mucosal atrophy and other comorbid conditions. Although it is most often handled without the aid of a physician, it is a common problem dealt with by the otolaryngologist. When conservative control measures are ineffective, interventional management is indicated. Rarely, epistaxis can lead to complications such as hypoxia, myocardial infarction, exsanguination, and death if not dealt with swiftly. The key to successful management of epistaxis is to be prepared to deal with it before the patient presents; this cannot be overemphasized. The treating physician must have an algorithm for managing patients with epistaxis. Early otolaryngologic consultation is recommended.

FUNCTIONAL ANATOMY OF THE LARYNX

The larynx is divided into three anatomic subunits based on embryology, function, and lymphatic drainage. The supraglottic larynx extends from the tip of the epiglottis down to and including the superior half of the laryngeal ventricle, separating the true and false vocal cords. The glottic larynx includes the lower half of the ventricle, true vocal cords, mucosa covering the arytenoid vocal processes, anterior and posterior commissure, and mucosa that extends 10 mm below the free margin of the true vocal cord. Finally, the subglottis consists of the mucosa overlying the internal aspect of the cricoid cartilage.

The supraglottic region develops from the buccopharyngeal anlage. This area has a rich lymphatic drainage to both contralateral and ipsilateral lymph nodes. The glottic and subglottic regions originate from the laryngotracheal anlage. The true vocal cord, which has a sparse lymphatic network, drains through the ligament at the anterior commissure through the thyroid cartilage to the pretracheal Delphian lymph node. The subglottic region has a richer lymphatic supply than the glottis and drains to the ipsilateral paratracheal nodes with extension toward the mediastinal nodes. The pattern of lymphatic drainage for each subunit of the larynx has implications for treatment of laryngeal cancer.

The true vocal cord is composed of five layers: the epithelium; the superficial, middle, and deep layers of the lamina propria; and the vocalis muscle. Normally, these layers glide over one another during phonation, allowing a fluidlike motion of the epithelial layer that results in the pleasing quality of the human voice. Abnormalities of these layers such as nodules, cysts, polyps, or scar tissue prevent the normal motion of these layers, resulting in hoarseness.

The intrinsic musculature of the larynx includes the posterior and lateral cricoarytenoid, the transverse and oblique arytenoids, and the thyroarytenoids. These muscles, which are innervated by the recurrent laryngeal nerve, function conjointly in a complex fashion to control both adduction and abduction of the true vocal cords. The extrinsic laryngeal muscle is the cricothyroid, which is innervated by the external branch of the superior laryngeal nerve. It extends from the anterior inferior of the thyroid cartilage to the anterior surface of the cricoid cartilage. Contraction of this muscle tilts the laryngeal cartilage forward, producing increased tension of the true vocal cords. The internal branch of the superior laryngeal nerve passes through the thyrohyoid membrane to provide sensory innervation to the pyriform sinus and supraglottic larynx. Sensation to the endolarynx is provided by the recurrent laryngeal nerve. The superior and recurrent laryngeal nerves are connected via the endolaryngeal nerve of Galen [19].

Functional Disorders of the Larynx

The human larynx has three basic functions. The primary function is protective: The larynx acts as a sphincter, protecting the tracheobronchial tree from various insults. Another primary function is ventilation. The larynx may alter the pattern of airflow to and from the bronchi as in coughing. Secondarily, the larynx serves a phonatory role, providing the sound source for voicing [20]. Functional disorders of the larynx may affect one, several, or all of these laryngeal functions. Functional disorders of the larynx are most often degenerative in etiology, but may be secondary to neoplastic processes (e.g., vocal cord paralysis due to lung cancer), inflammatory conditions (e.g., rheumatoid arthritis with cricoarytenoid ankylosis), infectious conditions, or traumatic illnesses. There are numerous functional disorders of the human larynx. We concentrate on the more common problems evaluated by otolaryngologists, including aspiration, vocal cord paralysis, and cranial nerve disorders.

Aspiration

The airway and the alimentary tract are intimately associated in the upper aerodigestive tract. Consequently, the laryngeal sphincter must be competent to prevent life-threatening aspiration. Hypoxia, diffuse chemical pneumonitis, tracheobronchitis, bacterial pneumonia, and death are the possible sequelae of chronic aspiration. Aspiration in elderly patients is most often due to neurologic dysfunction. Brain stem cerebrovascular accidents are the most common cause, followed by posterior fossa tumors, head injury, bulbar palsy, muscular dystrophy, amyotrophic lateral sclerosis, and multiple sclerosis [21]. Other cases may be secondary to extirpative resections of the pharynx, hypopharynx, larynx, or skull base. Recently, several investigators have shown that age-related changes in pharyngeal and supraglottic sensation may also play a role in chronic aspiration [22]. Other more readily treatable causes of aspiration in elderly patients include Zenker's diverticulum, cricopharyngeal dysfunction, achalasia, and gastroesophageal reflux. Rare cases are due to cricoarytenoid joint dislocation [23] or cricoarytenoid joint ankylosis in patients with rheumatoid arthritis. Finally, neoplasms of the upper aerodigestive tract may cause aspiration.

Treatment of chronic aspiration must be individualized to each patient. Important considerations prior to therapy include the site of the lesion, the severity of aspiration, and the patient's mental status. Functional disability worsens as the vagus nerve lesion moves proximally. For example, base of skull lesions that affect both the superior and recurrent laryngeal nerves are more severe than recurrent laryngeal nerve dysfunction alone; likewise, central lesions after brain stem strokes produce far greater disability than vagal lesions [23].

In cases of unilateral vocal cord paralysis, elderly patients respond well to vocal fold medialization. Several techniques are available for this procedure. When return of function is possible, Gelfoam may be injected into the true vocal cord. This results in temporary medialization. Autologous fat harvested from the abdomen or periumbilical area may also be used to position the true vocal cord medially. If the fat is to be harvested from the abdomen, it should be taken from the periumbilical region or left lower quadrant to prevent mistaking the scar for an appendectomy scar. Unlike Gelfoam, this technique allows permanent medialization. Teflon, once the most commonly used substance for vocal cord medialization, has fallen out of favor due to the high incidence of granuloma formation and the difficulty in treating the granulomas [24]. Many patients with aspiration due to vocal cord paralysis can benefit from polymeric silicone substance (Silastic) medialization of the paralyzed cord. The technique is described elsewhere by Netterville et al. [25]. The procedure is performed under local anesthesia with flexible laryngoscopic guidance. A Silastic implant is positioned between the inner table of the thyroid cartilage and the true vocal cord, resulting in restored glottal competence. The contralateral cord is able to adduct to allow phonation and airway protection. Thus, this technique does not require insertion of instrumentation into the substance of the vocal fold [25] as do fat and Gelfoam injection. Should normal vocal fold function return, Silastic medialization is reversible. Netterville et al. reported a series of 116 phonosurgical procedures with excellent results and only one complication [26].

Tracheotomy is a poor long-term solution for aspiration. However, it can be used in emergent situations. Tracheotomy is often required for airway control and pulmonary toilet in ventilator-dependent elderly patients with aspiration pneumonia. The tube cuff will prevent some but not all secretions or food particles from entering the airway. Care must be taken when deflating the cuff because this could result in a large bolus of secretions or food entering the distal airway. Careful and frequent suctioning is necessary to prevent ongoing aspiration while the cuff is deflated. Periodic cuff deflation is necessary to prevent tracheal necrosis. Over time the pressure from the tracheotomy tube cuff results in tracheomalacia and inability to effectively seal the trachea from continuous insult. Tracheotomy tethers the larynx and trachea to the skin, preventing the normal physiologic protection mechanisms. Thus, tracheotomy should only be used as a bridge to a more permanent solution [23].

Several methods of laryngeal closure for treatment of chronic aspiration have been described. These include laryngeal suspension, glottic prosthesis, glottic and supraglottic closure, laryngeal diversion, laryngectomy, and cricoid resection [23]. The ideal treatment would provide reliable, durable protection from aspiration, be reversible, and have low morbidity and mortality. As will be shown, few of the aforementioned options meet all of these criteria.

Laryngeal suspension is most often used after cancer surgery or trauma to partially recreate the physiologic elevation of the larynx during deglutition. Several techniques have been described in which the thyroid lamina is sewn to the mandible or other anterior structure. This tilts and raises the larynx under the base of tongue. Laryngeal suspension is potentially reversible, which is its major advantage; morbidity is dependent on the extent of resection or associated injuries in the case of trauma.

Glottic prostheses can only be used in patients with a tracheotomy. They may be inserted endoscopically and are usually held in place with percutaneous sutures tied over Silastic buttons. Although easily reversible, there can be numerous problems with these stents such as local inflammation, discomfort, glottic scarring, inability to phonate, and leakage due to incomplete seal. One-way valve prostheses are now available that allow phonation [23].

Laryngeal closure can be performed to prevent aspiration, but it requires a permanent tracheotomy and does not allow phonation. Subsequently, it is reserved for elderly, debilitated patients with no ability to phonate. These techniques provide complete separation of the digestive and ventilatory passages, and some of them are reversible [23]. However, there is a high rate of wound dehiscence and recurrent aspiration [27]. Debilitated, elderly patients may be poor candidates for these procedures due to comorbid conditions. For a full description of these techniques, the reader is referred elsewhere [23].

Lindeman initially described laryngeal diversion for treatment of chronic aspiration in 1975 [28]. It is indicated for relief of severe aspiration secondary to combined pharyngeal and laryngeal dysfunction. The trachea is divided at the third or fourth interspace, and the distal trachea is used to create a tracheostoma. Two options are available for the proximal trachea: It can be anastomosed in an end-to-side fashion to the anterior cervical esophagus, or it can be sewn to the cervical skin. Both forms of this procedure work well for aspiration, but the neck diversion technique results in a cutaneous salivary fistula that complicates the care of an already debilitated patient. Another attractive feature of this procedure is its reversibility. Lindeman has reported successful reversal of this procedure. A disadvantage of this technique is that it does not allow phonation because a permanent tracheostoma is required [23].

Total laryngectomy is the most definitive procedure for control of aspiration. It is not reversible, eliminates phonation, and may have high morbidity and mortality in an elderly, debilitated patient. Blitzer et al. have performed a modified small field laryngectomy that preserves the strap muscles, postcricoid mucosa, and arytenoid mucosa [23]. Although it efficiently controls aspiration, some of the previously mentioned techniques may be accomplished in a more efficient manner with equal success and less morbidity. Total laryngectomy may be used as a salvage therapy for patients who fail other forms of therapy for chronic aspiration.

Other techniques for control of aspiration in the elderly that have not been mentioned include cricoid resection, feeding gastrostomy and jejunostomy, fundoplication, and cricopharyngeal myotomy. Cricoid resection is most often used after head and neck cancer resections for patients who develop intractable aspiration [23]. Gastrostomy, jejunostomy, fundoplication, and cricopharyngeal myotomy are covered elsewhere and are not discussed further here. Ancillary services such as speech therapy are extremely important in the treatment of chronic aspiration. Use of these services is strongly encouraged.

Vocal Cord Paralysis

Vocal cord paralysis, like aspiration, is a functional disorder of the human larynx. It is often associated with chronic aspiration, and on occasion a single treatment may be used for both disorders. Vocal cord paralysis may be bilateral or unilateral, although unilateral paralysis is more common. The most common cause of vocal cord paralysis is surgical trauma, specifically injury of the recurrent laryngeal nerve, which may occur in the chest, neck, or skull base. Other common causes of vocal cord paralysis in the elderly include cerebrovascular accident and other neurologic disorders such as poliomyelitis; neoplasms of the thyroid, esophagus, larynx, lung, mediastinum, or brain; inflammatory diseases; and trauma. Idiopathic vocal cord paralysis is also common. The most common cause of bilateral vocal fold paralysis is surgical trauma during thyroidectomy or parathyroidectomy. However, in the elderly there is an increased incidence of bilateral paralysis of unknown etiology.

Most patients with gradual onset of unilateral paralysis compensate for it with increased motion of the contralateral, normal vocal cord; little change in vocal quality and little or no aspiration result. With acute loss of function, as in surgical trauma to the recurrent laryngeal nerve, the patient notices an acute change in vocal quality with mild-to-severe aspiration. The treatment of these symptoms depends on the integrity of the vagus and recurrent laryngeal nerves. Permanent paralysis, as in total disruption of the recurrent nerve, is treated with an irreversible therapy, whereas temporary paralysis is treated with a reversible therapy.

When the recurrent laryngeal nerve is intact, implying the possibility of slow reinnervation and laryngeal functional recovery, no permanent treatment should be offered. Likewise, patients with vocal cord paralysis of <12 months' duration should be treated with reversible medialization therapy. For vocal cord paralysis that results in poor vocal quality and mild-to-severe aspiration, Gelfoam injection is a rapid, reversible therapeutic option. Gelfoam paste is injected into the paraglottic space under direct laryngoscopy and local anesthesia in the operating suite or via transcervical injection with flexible laryngoscopic guidance in the otolaryngologist's office [29]. The paste is slowly resorbed from the injection site over a 4- to 5-week period; if after this period the recurrent nerve remains paralyzed, then the treatment may be repeated until the contralateral vocal cord is able to compensate for the deficit. If there is no return of function, atrophy of the ipsilateral, paralytic vocal cord occurs, resulting in glottal incompetence and necessitating a permanent solution to the vocal cord paralysis [29].

If the vagus or recurrent laryngeal nerve is sacrificed at operation, completely severed by trauma, or the paralysis remains symptomatic after 1 year in the case of an intact nerve, then permanent medialization procedures are indicated. Options for permanent therapy include Teflon injection, autologous fat injection, and medialization laryngoplasty with Silastic (MLS or phonosurgery). Teflon paste is injected into the paraglottic space in a similar manner to Gelfoam and was for many years a popular treatment. It has recently fallen out of favor due to many problems with its use and due to the availability of other successful treatments. Ossoff et al. described the difficulty in treating patients with complications of Teflon medialization including the "irreversibility of the procedure, narrow margin for error in location and quantity of injection, risk of migration and granuloma formation, and chance of return of recurrent nerve function" [24]. For these reasons Teflon injection should not be considered if there is possibility of return of laryngeal nerve function. The procedure of choice for patients with permanent, unilateral vocal cord paralysis is MLS of the nonfunctional cord. The technique has been described elsewhere by Netterville [25,29]. A block of Silastic is inserted between the inner table of the thyroid cartilage and its perichondrium; this results in moving the free edge of the vocal fold toward the midline without instrumentation of the vocal cord substance [25,29]. Primary MLS is performance of the procedure at the time of sacrifice of the laryngeal nerve; secondary MLS is performed in cases of preexistent vocal cord paralysis. In 1993, Netterville et al. reported a series of 116 patients undergoing both primary and secondary medialization thyroplasty with Silastic implants for treatment of glottal incompetence [26]. The results were good in terms of vocal quality and prevention of aspiration, with only one complication, a laryngocutaneous fistula in a patient previously treated with cervical irradiation. Other advantages of this technique in elderly patients include reversibility (implants can be removed should normal function return), performance under local anesthesia, low rate of implant extrusion (0 in 116), and decreased use of perioperative tracheotomy in primary MLS procedures [25,26,29]. For patients who do not wish to undergo MLS, autologous fat injection appears to be a viable, semipermanent medialization option [24]. Autologous fat harvested from the periumbilical area or abdomen is injected into the paraglottic space in a fashion similar to Gelfoam medialization. Atrophy of the fat is a possible outcome, in which case the procedure may be repeated. If the fat is to be harvested away from the umbilicus, it should be taken from the left lower quadrant to prevent confusion with an appendectomy scar.

Bilateral vocal cord paralysis in elderly patients is often idiopathic in etiology and has an increased incidence compared with other groups. The treatment of bilateral paralysis is a compromise between providing an adequate airway and allowing the patient to protect the airway and have serviceable vocal quality. In acute bilateral paralysis, tracheotomy is usually necessary to maintain an adequate airway. To successfully decannulate these patients, lateralization of one of the vocal cords is necessary to enlarge the glottic airway. This is most commonly accomplished by surgical resection or laser obliteration. In 1985, Ossoff et al. described CO_2 laser arytenoidectomy for treatment of bilateral vocal cord paralysis [30]. This method allows adequate lateralization of one of the affected cords with fair residual vocal quality and little surgical morbidity [30]. This therapy has become the standard therapy for bilateral paralysis.

Treatment of laryngeal incompetence, decreased vocal quality and aspiration, has seen great advances in recent years. The mode of therapy chosen depends on the integrity of the recurrent laryngeal nerves and the medical condition of the patient. Early otolaryngologic and speech pathology consultations are recommended.

Cranial Nerve Rehabilitation

The lower cranial nerves function together as a complex team to orchestrate the function of the upper aerodigestive tract. In young patients, loss of nerves IX, X, XI, and XII presents less of a rehabilitation challenge than in elderly patients. The major etiologies of cranial nerve loss in elderly patients are cerebrovascular accidents and extirpative skull base resection. The primary dysfunctions seen in elderly patients with loss of the lower cranial nerves are alterations in speech, swallowing, and airway protection. Rehabilitation of cranial nerve X has been discussed under aspiration and vocal paralysis; in this section we add arytenoid adduction to the list of therapies for glottal incompetence. In addition, we touch briefly on rehabilitation of nerves IX and XII.

Brain stem strokes may adversely affect multiple cranial nerve nuclei. In elderly patients this may result in dysphagia when nuclei IX, X, and XII are affected. Rehabilitation of deglutition is difficult in elderly patients, especially when more than one cranial nerve nucleus is affected. Speech therapists are quite helpful in this regard and can teach patients to swallow on the contralateral sensate side of the upper aerodigestive tract.

Lesions of the vagal nuclei may result in glottal incompetence and velopharyngeal incompetence. We have previously discussed vocal paralysis and aspiration. One technique not discussed previously for aspiration is arytenoid adduction. Arytenoid adduction is performed under local anesthesia and is an adjunct therapy to MLS. Arytenoid adduction is performed after medialization laryngoplasty when the posterior glottis cannot be adequately closed by the implant. A full description of this technique can be found elsewhere [26]. Patients with velopharyngeal insufficiency find the symptoms of nasal regurgitation and extreme nasality of speech quite bothersome. Unilateral palatal adhesion has been used in these patients with good results [31]. In this technique the nasopharyngeal surface of the soft palate is sewn to the posterior pharyngeal wall down to the prevertebral fascia. The resultant adhesion obliterates the incompetent nasopharynx, allowing normal palatal function on the contralateral side. Palatal adhesion can be performed primarily at the time of extirpative skull base resection or secondarily following objective documentation of incompetence in cases of brain stem stroke [31].

Rehabilitation of cranial nerves in elderly patients requires the various talents of otolaryngologists, speech therapists, occupational therapists, and others. Success in treating these patients requires a flexible, team-oriented approach.

LARYNGEAL NEOPLASMS

As humans age, the integrity of the immune system declines, resulting in an increased incidence of neoplastic disease [5]. Likewise, many years of smoking tobacco and consuming alcohol take a toll on the mucosa of the upper aerodigestive tract. It is estimated that at least half of all patients with head and neck cancer are age 60 or older when the diagnosis is first made [32]. The vast majority of tumors of the larynx are epidermoid carcinomas. Other less common benign and malignant tumors are not discussed. The actual events in carcinogenesis of the larynx are not well understood. It is clear, however, that it is a multistep process of exposure to carcinogens and promoters superimposed on a background of declining natural immunosurveillance [32]. The association between tobacco products and laryngeal cancer is widely accepted. Alcohol consumption increases the incidence of laryngeal cancer in all sites but particularly in the supraglottic larynx. However, another major component in this process is the age-related gradual decline in immunocompetency [32], marked by changes in the number and types of T- and B-lymphocytes and immunoglobulins, deficits in T-cell function, involution of the thymus, and defects in the quality of the immune response [5]. Other factors that have been implicated in laryngeal carcinoma include radiation exposure, industrial chemicals, chronic exposure to wood dust, asbestos exposure, some types of dietary deficiencies, malnutrition, gastroesophageal reflux, and chewing Pan, which is an admixture of pan leaf, betel nuts, tobacco, and slaked lime [33].

Squamous cell carcinoma of the larynx arises from three anatomic sites: supraglottic, glottic, and subglottic sites. Some tumors arising in one site may cross these anatomic borders, becoming transglottic. The underlying importance of this classification is that tumors arising from these various sites have different behavior and 5-year survival rates. A description of the relevant anatomy has been provided previously; the reader may wish to briefly review that section before continuing here.

Supraglottic Tumors

Small tumors of the supraglottic region metastasize early in the course of the disease via the ipsilateral thyrohyoid membrane along the course of the superior laryngeal vessels. The rich lymphatic network draining the supraglottic larynx results in frequent bilateral metastasis with any supraglottic tumor. Two important anatomic spaces serve to direct tumor extension in the supraglottis: the pre-epiglottic space and the paraglottic space. The pre-epiglottic space is a fat-filled space located between the anterior surface of the epiglottic cartilage and the thyrohyoid membrane just inferior to the vallecula. Supraglottic tumors gain access to this space through small fenestrae in the epiglottic cartilage. Once in this space, a tumor can readily spread to the neck through the thyrohyoid membrane or down to the anterior commissure and the paraglottic space laterally. The paraglottic space is located lateral to the quadrangular membrane and the conus elasticus on the deep surface of the false and true vocal cords within the thyroid cartilage and pyriform sinus. Tumors involving this space rapidly become transglottic and extend into the neck, thyroid cartilage, and thyroid gland through the cricothyroid membrane.

Two distinct growth patterns have been observed in supraglottic tumors. Neoplasms with "pushing margins" are found more often in the supraglottic region. These tumors spread with raised, well-defined margins. The surrounding bulky margins encircle the raised exophytic mass, which resides superficially, usually without deep invasion. These lesions have a better prognosis than infiltrating lesions. The latter smaller ulcerative-type lesion tends to be less differentiated than the former and presents with infiltrating obscure margins and a deeply penetrating central ulcer. These lesions can rapidly invade the pre-epiglottic and paraglottic spaces with an apparently small tumor as seen at laryngoscopy. The American Joint Committee on Cancer TNM staging of supraglottic tumors is shown in Table 13-5.

TABLE 13-5. *American Joint Committee on Cancer TNM classification of laryngeal cancer*

Primary tumor (T)
- TX Minimum requirements to assess the primary tumor cannot be met
- T0 No evidence of primary tumor
- Tis Carcinoma in situ
- Supraglottis
  - T1 Tumor confined to site of origin with normal mobility
  - T2 Tumor involves adjacent supraglottic site(s) or glottis without fixation
  - T3 Tumor limited to larynx with fixation or extension to involve postcricoid area, medial wall of pyriform sinus, or pre-epiglottic space
  - T4 Massive tumor extending beyond larynx to involve oropharynx, soft tissues of neck, or destruction of thyroid cartilage
- Glottis
  - T1 Tumor confined to vocal cords with normal mobility (including involvement of anterior or posterior commissures)
  - T2 Supraglottic or subglottic extension of tumor with normal or impaired mobility
  - T3 Tumor confined to larynx with cord fixation
  - T4 Massive tumor with thyroid cartilage destruction or extension beyond the confines of the larynx, or both
- Subglottis
  - T1 Tumor confined to subglottic region
  - T2 Tumor extension to vocal cords with normal or impaired mobility
  - T3 Tumor confined to larynx with cord fixation
  - T4 Massive tumor with cartilage destruction or extension beyond the confines of the larynx, or both

Nodal involvement (N)
- NX Minimum requirements to assess the regional nodes cannot be met
- N0 No clinically positive nodes
- N1 Single clinically positive ipsilateral node ≤3 cm in diameter
- N2 Metastasis in a single ipsilateral node >3 cm but not >6 cm in greatest dimension, or in multiple ipsilateral nodes, none >6 cm in greatest dimension, or in bilateral or contralateral nodes, none >6 cm in greatest dimension
- N2a Metastasis in a single ipsilateral node >3 cm but not >6 cm in greatest dimension
- N2b Metastasis in multiple ipsilateral nodes, none >6 cm
- N2c Metastasis in bilateral or contralateral nodes, none >6 cm in greatest dimension
- N3 Metastasis in a node >6 cm in greatest dimension

Distant metastasis (M)
- MX Minimum requirements to assess the presence of distant metastases cannot be met
- M0 No (known) distant metastasis
- M1 Distant metastasis present

Stage groupings

Stage	T	N	M
Stage 0	Tis	N0	M0
Stage I	T1	N0	M0
Stage II	T2	N0	M0 (Stage 0–II "Early")
Stage III	T1	N1	M0
	T2	N1	M0
	T3	N0	M0
	T3	N1	M0
Stage IV	T4	N0, N1	M0
	Any T	N2, N3	M0
	Any T	Any N	M1

Patients with supraglottic laryngeal cancer usually present with a later stage of disease than patients with glottic tumors. Supraglottic tumors tend to be silent until they reach 2 to 3 cm. By then they usually involve structures outside the supraglottic area. The seven cardinal symptoms of head and neck cancer—dysphagia, odynophagia, referred otalgia, hoarseness, "hot potato" speech (speech disorder), stridor, and globus pharyngeus (sensation of a lump in the throat)—should be sought in the history [34]. Other possible manifestations include sore throat and neck mass. All too often a neck mass is the first sign of supraglottic cancer. Referred otalgia is an ominous symptom in an elderly patient and should be presumed to be caused by cancer until proven otherwise. The symptom of otalgia in supraglottic tumors is caused by referred pain through the vagus nerve and auricular nerve of Arnold to the external auditory canal [19].

Staging procedures are similar for all forms of laryngeal cancer. These include indirect laryngoscopy using either a laryngeal mirror or 90-degree rigid pharyngoscope, flexible nasopharyngolaryngoscopy, CT scanning with contrast media enhancement and/or MRI before biopsy, direct laryngoscopy with biopsy in the operating suite, and chest roentgenography [19]. Preoperative workup is otherwise similar to other surgical patients. Evaluation of the alkaline phosphatase level is helpful in the rare instance of liver metastasis.

Treatment options for supraglottic squamous cell carcinoma include primary radiation therapy, endoscopic laser excision of early tumors, horizontal supraglottic laryngectomy, supracricoid laryngectomy, total laryngectomy, and combined modality treatment with chemotherapy and irradiation. Conservation laryngeal surgery refers to surgical treatment that preserves the patient's voice. In the past, patients >60 years of age were not considered for partial laryngectomy procedures; however, with improvement in postsurgical rehabilitation, this practice has been re-evaluated. We cover treatment of these cancers in a stage by stage fashion. The decision to include neck dissection with the aforementioned therapies is individualized for each patient.

T1 lesions of the supraglottic larynx may be treated with either external beam irradiation or surgery, with comparable 5-year survival rates in the range of 65% to 85% [19]. Surgical options include endoscopic CO_2 laser resection or conventional open supraglottic laryngectomy [34]. For patients with T1 suprahyoid epiglottic tumors, wide endoscopic excision with close postoperative follow-up is adequate; treatment of the neck is usually not indicated in this subset of patients [35]. T1 carcinomas of the infrahyoid supraglottis may be treated with open or endoscopic resection. However, even with necks classified as N0, some form of neck therapy is usually indicated. Bilateral selective neck dissections with postoperative radiation for histologic extracapsular spread or multiple metastatic nodes is a common regimen [35]. Alternatively, patients unwilling to undergo neck dissection may be treated with irradiation to both the primary site and both sides of the neck [35]. Surgical salvage is an option for those who choose radiation and experience a recurrence.

Supraglottic T2N0 tumors can likewise be treated with radiation or conservation surgery. The 5-year survival rates vary from 55% to 80% in various studies, with a slight survival advantage for those treated surgically [19]. Endoscopic supraglottic laryngectomy may be attempted for small T2 tumors [35]. Supraglottic laryngectomy has its greatest use in patients with T2 lesions. The epiglottis, false cords, aryepiglottic folds, pre-epiglottic space, a portion or all of the hyoid bone and thyroid cartilage, and, in extended cases, part of one arytenoid are resected in this operation. This leaves the airway unprotected while the patient learns to swallow. For this reason adequate preoperative pulmonary reserve must be present for the patient to tolerate this insult. Pulmonary reserve may be assessed with arterial blood gas analysis, chest radiography, pulmonary function tests, and a pulmonary stress test (e.g., walking the patient up two flights of stairs) [19]. Radiation is arguably the treatment of choice for elderly patients with little pulmonary reserve, with surgery as an alternative for postradiation recurrence. Select patients with T2 tumors may be candidates for supracricoid laryngectomy as described by Laccourreye et al. [36]. This includes patients with supraglottic tumors involving the glottis or anterior commissure, invading the ventricle, or presenting with transglottic lesions—those who have marked limitation of true vocal cord mobility [36].

Most otolaryngologists would also recommend bilateral selective neck dissection for T2N0 disease. As with T1 tumors, multiple positive nodes or extracapsular spread are indications for postoperative radiotherapy. Modified radical or radical neck dissection is recommended for N1 to N3 disease.

When the patient presents with a clinical stage T3 or T4 lesion of the supraglottis, the tumor has extended beyond the supraglottic larynx and therefore is no longer amenable to conservative surgical procedures. There are basically three options for treatment in these patients: (1) total laryngectomy with postoperative radiation, (2) radical radiotherapy, and (3) chemotherapy plus irradiation. Radiation alone produces a 5-year survival rate of 33% for T3 tumors and 14% for T4 tumors. Total laryngectomy with postoperative radiation improves the survival to 64% and 48%, respectively, at 5 years [19]. Surgery plus radiation is the treatment of choice in elderly patients with T3 or T4 tumors, if they are acceptable operative candidates. Patients who are not appropriate candidates for surgery because of unacceptable risks may be treated with chemotherapy and radiation. In a randomized, prospective trial, the Department of Veterans Affairs Laryngeal Cancer Study Group demonstrated 64% organ preservation with similar 2-year survival rates in patients undergoing induction chemotherapy followed by definitive radiation when compared with standard surgery and radiation [36].

Supraglottic tumors that present as T3 or T4 lesions without palpable neck disease still have a high likelihood of harboring occult metastatic disease in the jugular chain nodes. Many authors have debated the efficacy of postoperative radiotherapy for T3 and T4 lesions with N0 necks. Most believe that the likelihood of occult nodal metastases necessitates some form of treatment directed toward this area. If nodal dissection is not performed at surgery, then radiation of the neck is probably indicated prophylactically. The neck can be accurately staged by performing bilateral selective neck dissections at the time of laryngectomy. If no occult metastatic neoplasm is present or the neck is a pathologic stage N1 without extracapsular spread, then the patient can be observed safely without postoperative radiotherapy. When there is N2 or N3 nodal disease of the neck, either a modified radical neck dissection sparing cranial nerve XI (spinal accessory nerve) or standard radical neck dissection, depending on the findings at surgery, should be performed en bloc with the laryngectomy specimen. Postoperative radiotherapy is usually recommended in these cases to decrease the incidence of local and regional recurrence.

Glottic Carcinoma

Glottic carcinoma is the most common laryngeal tumor and outnumbers supraglottic squamous carcinoma by approximately 3 to 1 [19]. Glottic carcinoma usually occurs as a well-differentiated epidermoid carcinoma. Patients with glottic tumors tend to present earlier than their supraglottic counterparts because of the changes that occur in vocal quality even with very small lesions. The overall prognosis with glottic cancer is quite good due to early detection and delayed metastasis: The reader will recall that the lymphatic network that drains the glottis is quite sparse, which results in delayed spread to regional nodes until an advanced stage of tumor growth has been reached. The history and workup is otherwise similar to that for supraglottic tumors. Treatment options for glottic cancer include primary radiotherapy, chemoradiation, endoscopic laser excision, cordectomy, conservation laryngeal procedures such as vertical hemilaryngectomy, near total laryngectomy, and finally total laryngectomy. The staging of glottic tumors is shown in Table 13-5.

Primary radiation has historically been the mainstay of treatment for T1 glottic lesions. This therapy results in 95% 5-year survival with fair-to-good voice quality following treatment. Recently, however, Ossoff et al. and several other authors have demonstrated a 5-year survival of 98% with endoscopic laser excision of T1 tumors in selected patients [38]. These patients also enjoy good vocal quality after treatment. This is an attractive surgical alternative because endoscopic procedures are well tolerated in elderly patients overall. Patients with T1 lesions who are initially treated with radiation and fail can be treated with salvage surgery. The procedure of choice in this instance is the vertical hemilaryngectomy [39]. This is one of the oldest laryngeal operations, is technically easy to perform, has little postoperative mobility, and is well tolerated by the elderly unless the entire ipsilateral arytenoid must be resected. This leaves the laryngeal introitus unprotected and may lead to significant aspiration and its attendant morbidity in elderly patients. Cure rates of 90% or better are reported with this procedure [39]. The postoperative vocal quality is poor, however. Standard or extended vertical hemilaryngectomy may also be used as primary therapy for patients who refuse radiotherapy or in patients with tumor extending to the vocal process of the arytenoid or to the anterior commissure. In these patients, surgical therapy may be more effective in controlling tumor locally.

Controversy exists for optimal treatment of T2 lesions of the glottis with different trends at various institutions. T2 lesions remain within the realm of early glottic cancer, and thus are amenable to radiotherapy with 5-year survival rates of 70% to 80%; salvage surgery for T2 lesions results in a 5-year survival of approximately 70% [19]. With vertical tumor spread of a glottic lesion, the rich lymphatics of the supraglottis and the subglottis cause these tumors to have an increased incidence of cervical metastasis; most otolaryngologists would recommend adding neck dissection to the surgical treatment of T2N0 patients. There are several surgical options for these patients. For small T2 lesions confined to one side of the larynx without subglottic extension, vertical hemilaryngectomy may be feasible if the surgical margins are well examined at the time of surgery and frozen sections are done to detect deep occult extension [19]. Supracricoid partial laryngectomy is appropriate therapy for selected glottic cancers with extension into the supraglottis [40]. Likewise, near total laryngectomy has been proposed by Tucker et al. for treatment of T2 lesions with good functional results, with respect to respiration, deglutition, and phonation, and minimal morbidity [41]. All 48 patients in the series by Tucker et al. were successfully decannulated postoperatively. T2 tumors with subglottic extension >10 mm anteriorly or 5 mm posteriorly significantly reduces survival when partial laryngectomy is used as therapy; therefore, total laryngectomy is the procedure of choice in these cases. Supraglottic extension of glottic tumors opens the paraglottic space for possible tumor dissemination; these lesions are termed *transglottic*. For those cases not amenable to near total or supracricoid laryngectomy, total laryngectomy is indicated. As with supraglottic cancer, clinically detectable neck disease is treated with modified radical or radical neck dissection in combination with surgical treatment of the primary focus. Absolute 5-year survival for surgically treated patients with T2 lesions is 70% to 82%; cause-specific survival for these same patients is 85% to 96% [19]. Neck metastasis lowers this rate significantly.

Advanced glottic tumors are classified as stage T3 and T4 by the American Joint Committee on Cancer. T3 lesions deeply invade the intrinsic laryngeal musculature and T4 lesions invade the thyroid cartilage or extend outside the larynx into surrounding neck structures. Primary radiotherapy for these cancers results in poor 5-year survival in the range of 20% to 30%; this figure increases to 50% with radical irradiation and salvage total laryngectomy for those who fail treatment. Most otolaryngologists recommend aggressive surgical therapy with total laryngectomy, neck dissection, and postoperative radiation when indicated. Survival at 5 years with this regimen is 58% to 71% for T3 lesions and 30% to 55% for T4 lesions [19]. Metastatic neck disease decreases these figures to approximately 20% to 30%. For poor surgical candidates or patients who desire treatment with vocal preservation, induction chemotherapy radiation is effective without compromising overall survival [37].

Subglottic Carcinoma

Primary subglottic tumors are quite rare. Most subglottic cancers represent extensions of glottic primary cancers. Staging of subglottic tumors is shown in Table 13-5. These cancers are very aggressive with early direct spread to the cricoid cartilage, cricothyroid membrane, and paraglottic space with vocal cord fixation. They may also spread posteriorly to involve the postcricoid esophagus. Nearly one-half of these lesions spread to paratracheal lymph nodes. The only surgical alternative is total laryngectomy with paratracheal node dissection and postoperative radiotherapy. Survival with this therapy has improved over the last 20 years and may be as high as 77% at 5 years, with ranges commonly reported in the literature between 40% and 60% [19].

Vocal Rehabilitation

Since the first laryngectomy was performed over 100 years ago by Billroth, aggressive efforts have been underway to find ways to rehabilitate the verbal communication of laryngectomized patients. The current options available to patients who have had laryngectomies include standard esophageal voice, artificial larynx, nonverbal communication, and tracheoesophageal speech fistulas. Esophageal voice has not been a successful option, with only 40% of patients mastering this technique [42]. In 1957, Bell Laboratories introduced the electrolarynx, which opened the door to transoral communication for many patients who could not use standard esophageal voice successfully. A major breakthrough in speech rehabilitation was made with the advent of speech prostheses. The reported success rates with these devices is 65% to 90% [43]. The critical factor in successful tracheoesophageal speech is not the age or mental capacity of the patient, but the efforts of a dedicated speech pathologist teamed with a surgeon who can motivate these patients and train them in the care and use of their stoma and prosthesis. Careful selection of candidates is essential to prevent needless frustration to the patient and rehabilitative team. Patients with limitations in dexterity resulting in the inability to occlude the stoma with a finger, or with poor visual acuity that prevents the necessary care of the prosthesis or stoma are unlikely to become successful tracheoesophageal speakers. Other relative contraindications include small tracheostomas, esophageal stenosis, tracheal hypersensitivity, general debility, and chronic alcoholism.

SUMMARY

Elderly patients commonly suffer from diseases affecting the nose and larynx. Many of these afflictions can be successfully treated by surgical therapy. Often these problems are compounded by comorbid conditions. For this reason, successful care of these patients is necessarily multidisciplinary. Cooperation between internists, surgeons, otolaryngologists, and other health care workers is essential in elderly patients.

REFERENCES

1. McMahan JT. Paranasal sinusitis: geriatric considerations. Otolaryngol Clin North Am 1990;23:1169–1177.
2. Bailey BJ. Geriatric Otolaryngology. In Bailey BJ (ed), Head and Neck Surgery—Otolaryngology (Vol I). Philadelphia: Lippincott, 1993.
3. Amedee RG. Sinus Anatomy and Function. In Bailey BJ (ed), Head and Neck Surgery—Otolaryngology (Vol I). Philadelphia: Lippincott, 1993.
4. Facer GW, Kern EB. Sinusitis: Current Concepts and Management. In Bailey BJ (ed), Head and Neck Surgery—Otolaryngology (Vol I). Philadelphia: Lippincott, 1993.
5. Miller RA. Age-Related Immune Deficiency. In Goldstein JC, Kashima HK, Koopmann CF Jr (eds), Geriatric Otorhinolaryngology. Philadelphia: Decker, 1989.
6. Schuller DE, Schleuning AJ II. Nose and Paranasal Sinuses. In DeWeese DD, Saunders WH (eds), Otolaryngology—Head and Neck Surgery (8th ed). St. Louis: Mosby–Year Book, 1994.
7. Stankiewicz JA, Newell DJ, Park AH. Complications of inflammatory diseases of the sinuses. Otolaryngol Clin North Am 1993;26: 639–655.
8. Zeifer BA. Sinus Imaging. In Bailey BJ (ed), Head and Neck Surgery—Otolaryngology (Vol I). Philadelphia: Lippincott, 1993.
9. Lanza DC, Kennedy DW. Endoscopic Sinus Surgery. In Bailey BJ (ed), Head and Neck Surgery—Otolaryngology (Vol I). Philadelphia: Lippincott, 1993.
10. Gustafson RO, Bansberg SF. Sinus Surgery. In Bailey BJ (ed), Head and Neck Surgery—Otolaryngology (Vol I). Philadelphia: Lippincott, 1993.
11. Stankiewicz JA. Complications of Sinus Surgery. In Bailey BJ (ed), Head and Neck Surgery—Otolaryngology (Vol I). Philadelphia: Lippincott, 1993.
12. Montgomery WW. Controversies in Surgery for Chronic Frontal Sinusitis. In Bailey BJ (ed), Head And Neck Surgery—Otolaryngology (Vol I). Philadelphia: Lippincott, 1993.
13. Wurman LH. Epistaxis. In Gates GA (ed), Current Therapy in Otolaryngology—Head and Neck Surgery (5th ed). St. Louis: Mosby–Year Book, 1994.
14. Lepore ML. Epistaxis. In Bailey BJ (ed), Head and Neck Surgery—Otolaryngology (Vol I). Philadelphia: Lippincott, 1993.
15. Klotch DW. Otolaryngology in the geriatric patient. Primary Care 1982;9:167–168.
16. Schuller DE, Schleuning AJ II. Epistaxis. In DeWeese DD, Saunders WH (eds), Otolaryngology—Head and Neck Surgery (8th ed). St. Louis: Mosby–Year Book, 1994.
17. Rood SR, Parnes SM, Myers EN, et al. The Management of Epistaxis: A Self-Instructional Package. Alexandria, VA: American Academy of Otolaryngology—Head and Neck Surgery, 1977.
18. Coleman JA Jr. Laser techniques in the management of epistaxis. Operative Techniques Otolaryngol Head Neck Surg 1992;3:117–119.
19. Million RR, Cassisi NJ, Mancuso AA. Larynx. In Million RR, Cassisi NJ (eds), Management of Head and Neck Cancer: A Multidisciplinary Approach (2nd ed). Philadelphia: Lippincott, 1994.
20. Sasaki CT, Isaacson G. Functional anatomy of the larynx. Otolaryngol Clin North Am 1988;21:595–612.
21. Kirchner JC, Sasaki CT. Surgery for aspiration. Otolaryngol Clin North Am 1984;17:49–56.
22. Aviv JE, Martin JH, Jones ME, et al. Age-related changes in pharyngeal and supraglottic sensation. Ann Otol Rhinol Laryngol 1994;103: 749–752.
23. Blitzer A, Krespi YP, Oppenheimer RW, et al. Surgical management of aspiration. Otolaryngol Clin North Am 1988;21:743–750.
24. Ossoff RH, Koriwchak MJ, Netterville JL, Duncavage JA. Difficulties in endoscopic removal of teflon granulomas of the vocal fold. Ann Otol Rhinol Laryngol 1993;102:405–412.
25. Wanamaker JR, Netterville JL, Ossoff RH. Phonosurgery: silastic medialization for unilateral vocal fold paralysis. Operative Techniques Otolaryngol Head Neck Surg 1993;4:207–217.
26. Netterville JL, Stone RE, Luken ES, et al. Silastic medialization and arytenoid adduction: a review of 116 phonosurgical procedures. Ann Otol Rhinol Laryngol 1993;102:413–424.
27. Dunham ME, Holinger LD. Stridor, Aspiration, and Cough. In Bailey BJ (ed), Head and Neck Surgery—Otolaryngology (Vol I). Philadelphia: Lippincott, 1993.
28. Lindeman RC. Diverting the paralyzed larynx: a reversible procedure for intractable aspiration. Laryngoscope 1975;85:157–180.
29. Netterville JL, Aly A, Ossoff RH. Evaluation and treatment of complications of thyroid and parathyroid surgery. Otolaryngol Clin North Am 1990;23:529–552.
30. Ossoff RH, Sisson GA, Duncavage JA, et al. Endoscopic laser arytenoidectomy for the treatment of bilateral vocal cord paralysis. Laryngoscope 1985;94:1293–1297.
31. Netterville JL, Civantos FJ. Rehabilitation of cranial nerve deficits after neurotologic skull base surgery. Laryngoscope 1993;103:45–54.
32. Wolf GT. Aging, the Immune System, and Head and Neck Cancer. In Goldstein JC, Kashima HK, Koopmann CF (eds), Geriatric Otorhinolaryngology. Philadelphia: Decker, 1989.
33. Cantrell RW. Etiologic Factors in the Development of Cancer. In Goldstein JC, Kashima HK, Koopmann CF (eds), Geriatric Otorhinolaryngology. Philadelphia: Decker, 1989.
34. Moloy PJ. How To (and How *Not* To) Manage the Patient with a Lump in the Neck. In Common Problems of the Head and Neck Region: A Manual and Guide for Management of Diseases and Injuries in Otolaryngology—Head and Neck Surgery. Philadelphia: Saunders, 1988.

35. Davis RK. Supraglottic Carcinoma. In Gates GA (ed), Current Therapy in Otolaryngology—Head and Neck Surgery (5th ed). St. Louis: Mosby–Year Book, 1994.
36. Laccourreye H, Laccourreye O, Weinstein G, et al. Supracricoid laryngectomy with cricohyoidopexy: a partial laryngeal procedure for selected supraglottic and transglottic carcinomas. Laryngoscope 1990; 100:735–741.
37. Anonymous. Induction chemotherapy plus radiation compared with surgery plus radiation in patients with advanced laryngeal cancer. The Department of Veterans Affairs Laryngeal Cancer Study Group [see comments]. N Engl J Med 1991;324:1685–1690.
38. Ossoff RH, Sisson GA, Shapshay SM. Endoscopic management of selected early vocal carcinoma. Ann Otol Rhinol Laryngol 1985;94: 560–564.
39. Vaughn CW. Glottic Carcinoma. In Gates GA (ed), Current Therapy in Otolaryngology—Head and Neck Surgery (5th ed). St. Louis: Mosby–Year Book, 1994.
40. Laccourreye H, Laccourreye O, Weinstein GS, et al. Supracricoid laryngectomy with cricohyoidopexy: a partial laryngeal procedure for glottic carcinoma. Ann Otol Rhinol Laryngol 1990;99:421–426.
41. Tucker HM, Benninger MS, Roberts JK, et al. Near-total laryngectomy with epiglottic reconstruction: long-term results. Arch Otolaryngol Head Neck Surg 1989;115:1341–1344.
42. Sanders AD, Blom ED, Singer MI, et al. Reconstructive and rehabilitative aspects of head and neck cancer in the elderly. Otolaryngol Clin North Am 1990;23:1159–1168.
43. Singer MI, Blom ED, Hamaker RC. Vocal rehabilitation after laryngectomy. Otolaryngol Clin North Am 1985;18:605–611.

Surgical Care for the Elderly, 2nd ed., edited by
R. Benton Adkins, Jr., and H. William Scott, Jr.
Lippincott–Raven Publishers, Philadelphia © 1998.

CHAPTER 14

Otology and Neurotology

Michael E. Glasscock, III, David S. Haynes, Ian S. Storper, and Pamela S. Bohrer

Estimated life expectancy jumped to a record high of 75.9 years in 1996 [1]. As such, the physician must be prepared to deal with the physiologic and psychological changes that occur with aging. For example, cardiovascular and pulmonary function, in general, decline with aging. Renal function also declines and therefore may affect medication dosing. Arthritic conditions of the neck, back, and shoulders may impede necessary surgical positioning. Therapy should be determined based on the natural history of the disease process and weighed against the morbidity and mortality of the treatment options. This simple premise takes on added significance in the elderly because life expectancy is a special consideration in this population and should influence treatment options. The quality of life after surgery, radiation, or chemotherapy must also be considered.

Neuro-otologic changes such as auditory or vestibular disorders occur to a significant degree in the elderly population. A large proportion of the elderly experience hearing loss or dysequilibrium. It is important to investigate and treat these disorders rather than just attribute these symptoms to a normal aging process. Many of these disorders are managed the same as they would be in a younger individual. Certain considerations, such as those listed previously, may alter the treatment course in the elderly. This chapter reviews some of the more common otologic disorders encountered in the elderly and how the course of therapy may differ between young and elderly patients.

EXTERNAL EAR

The external auditory canal is 2.5 cm long and extends from the conchal cartilage to the tympanic membrane. The lateral one-third of the external auditory canal is cartilaginous, and the medial two-thirds of the canal are bony. The skin overlying the cartilaginous canal is thicker, with a diameter of 0.5 to 1.0 mm. This skin has well-developed subcutaneous and dermal layers containing numerous hair follicles and sebaceous and ceruminal glands. The skin overlying the bony portion of the canal is extremely thin (0.2 mm) and lacks subcutaneous elements.

Two types of hair are found in the external auditory canal: fine villus hairs that cover the entire length of the canal, and larger, coarser hair found in the lateral (tragal) part of the canal. These tragal hairs are found only in men, and become larger and more noticeable in the elderly. These tragal hairs may entrap cerumen and lead to an increased incidence of cerumen impaction in the elderly man.

Ceruminal glands located in the lateral part of the external canal tend to atrophy and decrease in activity with age. The sebaceous glands of the external canal also atrophy and can lead to drying. Dryness of the skin of the external canal can result in pruritus, a frequent complaint of the elderly population, especially in those who wear hearing aids. These normal changes seen in the external canal as a result of aging can lead to dry, itchy skin exacerbated by dry accumulations of cerumen. These changes also can result in frequent irritation and even development of infection. Although otitis externa is not solely a disease of the elderly, it is more common secondary to the previously mentioned anatomic changes and more frequent use of hearing aids.

Removal of cerumen impaction in the elderly should be performed carefully. Attempts at removal with cotton-tipped swabs may further impact cerumen and traumatize thin skin that may become secondarily infected. Water or peroxide irrigation may drive water through an undiagnosed tympanic membrane perforation or vigorous irrigation may actually cause a perforation. This introduction of water into the middle air space may result in infection, leading to purulent otorrhea, which is especially detrimental in the ear that hears better or the only hearing ear. Removal of cerumen is performed under direct vision in the office with the operative microscope. Dry, itchy ears are best treated with the application of hydrocortisone cream applied topically at the meatus.

Bacterial otitis extima is a common infection in all age groups; however, the predisposing factors mentioned previously make it a common problem in the elderly. Other contributory factors include maceration of the skin from prolonged water exposure or high humidity (environmental or secondary to hearing aid occlusion of the canal), trauma, or contamination or obstruction of glands by cerumen or keratin debris. Hearing aids, especially those with a poorly fitting or occlusive mold, may predispose to infection.

The mainstay in the management of external otitis is primarily frequent and thorough cleaning of the canal. Manual suctioning under the binocular microscope with acetic acid rinses is indicated. Topical otic or ophthalmic drops that provide coverage against *Pseudomonas* species should be instilled in the canal. Systemic antibiotics are not used initially. Strict water precautions are undertaken as water in the canal can exacerbate the infection and slow healing. The hearing aid in the affected ear should be left out and not worn until resolution of symptoms.

Persistent infections should be cultured, and the offending organisms identified and treated with the appropriate antibiotic. It is not unusual for chronic infections to require months of close follow-up before resolution. Chondritis, a rare but serious complication, should be treated aggressively. The patient should be admitted for intravenous antibiotics effective against *Pseudomonas, Staphylococcus,* and *Streptococcus* species, in addition to daily cleaning and topical therapy with antibiotic drops. Cultures should be performed to identify the offending organism and sensitivities obtained.

An unusual, but particularly dangerous type of infection of the external canal is malignant external otitis or osteomyelitis of the skull base. This infection, usually caused by *P. aeruginosa,* results in a necrotizing process involving the temporal bone, skull base, cranial nerves, arteries and veins of the skull base, meninges, and brain. Susceptible individuals tend to be elderly with associated microvascular disease, diabetes, or immune deficiency [2]. A high index of suspicion must be maintained in susceptible individuals with persistent external ear infections not responsive to medical management. Workup should include audiometric testing and high-resolution computed tomographic (CT) scanning of the temporal bone, which may demonstrate erosion of the bony external canal, skull base, or temporomandibular joint. Technetium 99 scanning in patients with osteomyelitis shows increased uptake on the involved side. Gallium scanning may be useful in predicting clinical resolution [3].

Therapy in osteomyelitis of the skull base is primarily medical. The role of surgery in this disease is limited to local debridement and removal of sequestrum. Debrided material should be sent for pathologic evaluation to rule out malignancy, a diagnosis that is often elusive. The mainstay in therapy has been control of serum glucose levels and intravenous antibiotics for a duration of 4 to 8 weeks. Generally accepted agents include an aminoglycoside (e.g., tobramycin) with a beta-lactam antibiotic (e.g., piperacillin or ticarcillin) or cephalosporin (ceftazidime) effective against *P. aeruginosa.* Efficacy with an oral regimen of ciprofloxacin has also been demonstrated [4,5].

Auditory Dysfunction

Twenty-five percent of people between the ages of 65 and 74 and 50% of people aged 75 or older have hearing difficulty [6]. Hearing loss in the elderly should never be assumed to be attributable to old age; full evaluation and audiometric testing is indicated in any type of hearing loss. Causes of hearing loss in the elderly may be conductive, sensorineural, or mixed.

Conductive losses, simply put, result when sound does not reach the cochlea and auditory nerve. Causes of conductive hearing loss include serous otitis media secondary to eustachian tube dysfunction, tympanic membrane perforation, ossicular discontinuity, ossicular fixation, otitis media, and otosclerosis. These disorders are not exclusively found in the elderly but are commonly found in patients of all age groups. The middle ear does undergo age-related changes, however, primarily involving the ossicular joints. The ossicular articulations have been shown to develop arthritic changes and calcification that increase with age. These changes, however, have been studied audiometrically and have been shown to have no effect on sound transmission through the middle ear [7,8]. Otitis externa and cerumen impaction are frequent causes of conductive hearing losses.

Eustachian Tube Dysfunction

The eustachian tube performs three functions: (1) regulation of ear pressure, (2) drainage of middle ear secretions, and (3) protection of the inner ear from intense sound. The ventilatory function of the eustachian tube is affected by body position and becomes less efficient as the body is positioned horizontally. The tensor veli palatini and the levator veli palatini are the two muscles directly responsible for eustachian tube function. Human temporal bone studies have shown atrophy of these muscles (primarily the tensor muscle) with advancing age. This would suggest that the function of the eustachian tube performed by the tensor probably deteriorates with age [9].

These muscle changes as well as changes in mucociliary action may contribute to tubal dysfunction in the elderly. The bedridden patient has poor opening due to positioning and resulting venous engorgement. Chronic eustachian tube dysfunction may lead to serous otitis media that may require ventilation with pressure-equalizing tubes. A full head and neck evaluation should be performed in the adult presenting with serous otitis media, especially unilateral serous otitis media. Mechanical obstruction of the tube such as an oropharyngeal tumor or a nasopharyngeal carcinoma must be ruled out. CT scanning or magnetic resonance imaging (MRI) may also be required in confirming the diagnosis. Otalgia, with or without effusion, must also be aggressively worked up. Tumors of the larynx, hypopharynx, oropharynx, and nasopharynx may present initially with referred pain to the ear, indicating the need for full head and neck evaluation for these patients.

Chronic Otitis Media

Eustachian tube dysfunction can lead to development of chronic otitis media, with or without cholesteatoma formation. Considerations for etiology and treatment are no different from that of any other age group. Investigation of the draining ear should begin with examination under the binocular microscope and cleaning of debris. Tympanic membrane perforation, retraction, granulation tissue, cholesteatoma formation, and status of the external auditory canal should be documented. Topical therapy includes irrigation of debris with 1.5% acetic acid solution, instillation of antibiotic drops, dry ear precautions, and not using the hearing aid during the draining period. Antibiotic therapy may not be indicated in initial treatment but should be instituted in refractory cases after the offending organism is cultured and sensitivities are obtained.

The draining ear that has not responded to conservative therapy requires surgery. Tympanoplasty should be considered in patients who have recurrent drainage that can clear with treatment, but is a recurrent nuisance that may prevent normal hearing aid use. Elective tympanoplasty may be considered even in nondraining ears to improve hearing. The presence of cholesteatoma always indicates surgical disease. Medical disease may prevent the use of general anesthesia, but tympanoplasty may be performed under local anesthesia if necessary. Cholesteatoma may be opened and cleaned of accumulated squamous debris when more extensive surgical procedures are contraindicated. Frequent and close observation is indicated in these patients as the mainstay in both medical and surgical therapy of the draining ear to prevent potentially life-threatening complications. The following is a list of complications resulting from infections, both acute and chronic, of the ear [10]:

- Aural complications
  - Ossicular and tympanic membrane destruction
  - Mastoiditis and bone destruction
  - Subperiosteal abscess
  - Petrositis with bone destruction
  - Facial paralysis
  - Labyrinthitis (serous, suppurative, or chronic)
- Intracranial complications
  - Extradural abscess
  - Lateral sinus thrombosis
  - Subdural abscess
  - Meningitis
  - Brain abscess
  - Otitic hydrocephalus

Otosclerosis

Otosclerosis is a disease process in which the stapes is fixed from movement by a union of new bone growth at the oval window, leading to a conductive hearing loss. Hearing loss usually becomes apparent between puberty and 30 years and is bilateral in more than 90% of those seeking therapy. Other causes of conductive hearing loss must be considered in the differential diagnosis, such as malleus or incus fixation, and attic cholesteatoma. In addition to the conductive hearing loss, there may also coexist a cochlear otosclerosis producing a sensorineural component so severe as to limit useful amplification.

Surgical correction of otosclerosis consists of removal of the fixed stapes with reconstruction of the sound-conducting mechanism with a prosthesis. There are few contraindications to surgical correction of stapes fixation. The procedure is commonly performed under local anesthesia. Age in general is not a contraindication as long as there is sufficient cochlear reserve to provide a useful increase in auditory acuity. There are studies that demonstrate that postoperative improvements in hearing following stapedectomy decline with advancing age [11]. Even profoundly deaf patients can benefit from surgical correction if their hearing can be restored to a level that is useful with amplification [12,13].

Conductive hearing loss in the elderly should be evaluated and treated just as in the younger population. Careful history is indicated and should include onset and progression of loss, family history of hearing loss, presence of otorrhea, prior operative procedures, dysequilibrium, and other systemic illness. Repair of a conductive hearing loss is an elective procedure.

Amplification is often a safe and effective alternative to surgery and should always be offered to the patient.

INNER EAR

Presbycusis is a gradually progressive, symmetric sensorineural hearing loss due to the aging process that is otherwise unexplained. Other etiologies for sensorineural hearing loss must be excluded. Other etiologies include ototoxic drugs [14,15], occupational and recreational noise exposure [16], family history of hearing loss [17], head trauma [18], and postoperative sequelae. Factors that suggest presbycusis are bilateral symmetric hearing loss, a conductive hearing loss of <10 dB, and age >65 years [19]. Hearing loss in the elderly, much like other organ systems in the body, is determined both by genetic susceptibility and physical stress endured over the course of a lifetime. Using the Framingham Heart Study Cohort [20], a multivariate analysis showed that age, sex, illness, family history, Ménière's disease, and noise exposure were significant risk factors for development of hearing loss. This study demonstrated that age was by far the most critical risk factor for development of hearing loss.

Standard tests for hearing should include evaluation of pure-tone thresholds and speech discrimination scores.

Speech discrimination is the ability to hear and understand phonetically balanced monosyllabic words. Pure-tone thresholds may actually reflect the activity of only a few auditory nerve fibers. As much as 75% of nerve fibers can be lost without a change noted in pure-tone thresholds [21]. However, the extent of cochlear neuronal loss in the region where speech frequencies reside corresponds directly with the loss of speech discrimination [22]. Studies have shown that there is a progressive loss of cochlear neurons with age at a rate of approximately 2,000 neurons per decade [23].

There are four types of presbycusis identified by selected degeneration of morphologic structures of the cochlea and audiometric profile. These types of presbycusis have been well defined by Schuknecht [24] as sensory, neural, strial, and cochlear conductive. Sensory presbycusis develops following degeneration of the organ of Corti, resulting typically in an abrupt high-tone hearing loss. Neural presbycusis is caused by a loss of cochlear neurons leading to a severe loss of word discrimination. Strial presbycusis results from strial degeneration leading to a flat pure-tone threshold loss with preservation of word discrimination. Cochlear conductive presbycusis is manifested by gradually sloping high-tone losses and loss of word discrimination. Combinations of these patterns of presbycusis may produce complex patterns of hearing loss.

Rehabilitation of presbycusis and other hearing losses focuses on amplification of sound with a hearing aid, which compensates for loss of sensitivity. Counseling of the patient and family is essential to provide realistic expectations and achieve full benefit from amplification. Manual dexterity, visual acuity, and other health problems must be assessed because they may affect the ability to use and adjust the hearing aid. Cochlear implants are surgically implanted electrical devices that provide auditory input to those individuals who are profoundly deaf and receive no benefit from conventional amplification [25]. This procedure is well tolerated in the elderly and has provided significant improvement in both auditory performance and quality of life in these individuals [26].

For the hearing impaired, using the telephone, listening to the radio and television, awakening to alarm clocks, hearing a baby cry, and hearing the doorbell may require special assistive listening devices in addition to a hearing aid. Assistive listening devices enhance listening in specific situations and may take the place of full-time hearing aid use, especially in those with mild impairments. Most hearing heath care professionals can be of assistance in determining the patient's needs and obtaining the appropriate assistive listening devices [27].

Vestibular Dysfunction

Dysequilibrium, including dizziness, lightheadedness, falling, and fainting, is common in the elderly. The potential causes of dysequilibrium in the elderly are diverse, and the key to diagnosis is a comprehensive and systematic evaluation. In addition to evaluation of the vestibular system, comprehensive evaluation of visual acuity, neurologic status, cardiovascular status, and musculoskeletal strength and coordination should be performed. Although age-specific changes have been defined in the vestibular system, no specific correlation to balance function has been noted. Dysequilibrium should never be attributed just to old age. In fact, a specific cause of dysequilibrium can be found in up to 85% of patients [28].

As in the cochlea, age-related morphologic changes take place in the vestibular neuroepithelia. Johnsson [29] studied temporal bones of 24 patients with presbycusis and found severe degeneration of the saccular nerve network. These changes were not seen in patients under 30 years of age. Rosenhall [30], in a study of vestibular hair cell population, found a 20% reduction in the hair cell population in the macula and 40% reduction in the cristae of the semicircular canals with increasing age. Bergstrom [31] has shown that there is a considerable reduction in the number of vestibular nerve fibers with advancing age. Richter [32] has shown that both vestibular hair cells and nerve cells in Scarpa's ganglia are reduced in aged individuals.

The most important tool in assessing dysequilibrium in the elderly is the history. Specific details regarding the dysequilibrium should be noted, including onset (sudden or gradual), duration, character (true spinning vertigo as opposed to unsteadiness), and positional changes. Aural symptoms should be noted, including hearing loss (fluctuating or stable), aural fullness, and tinnitus, and may suggest inner ear dysfunction. Vertigo that was initiated at the time of a Valsalva's maneuver, such as lifting or straining, or as a result of trauma, such as a motor vehicle accident or a slap to the ear, may indicate a perilymph fistula [33]. Onset of symptoms associated with neck movements, particularly with neck extension, points to a vertebrobasilar type of vascular problem. Upper respiratory tract infection for several days before onset of vertigo is suggestive of a viral labyrinthitis or vestibular neuronitis. Acute otitis media or chronic draining ear before onset of dysequilibrium may suggest bacterial labyrinthitis. Palpitations, pallor, sweating, and fainting suggest cardiogenic disease or postural hypotension. A medication review is essential because many elderly patients take medications concurrently, which may result in dysequilibrium or postural hypotension.

In addition to the history, several tests are available to evaluate the patient with dysequilibrium. The eighth cranial nerve is divided into vestibular and cochlear divisions; therefore, the evaluation of any disorder of the vestibular portion of the eighth cranial nerve should also include evaluation of the cochlear division. Audiometric examination is used to screen for hearing acuity and speech discrimination. Auditory brain stem response measures the cochlear nerve and central auditory tract's electrical response to sound. Waveform morphologies and conduction latencies can be used to distinguish retrocochlear lesions, such as acoustic neuromas from cochlear hearing losses. Electronystagmography may help differentiate between peripheral or central vertigo and document nystagmus that is not apparent clinically. It is critical that drugs that may affect the vestibular or central nervous system be withheld for 72 hours before testing. Another test called the *Hallpike's maneuver* is useful in the diagnosis of positional vertigo. The patient is placed in a sitting position with the head turned 45 degrees to one side and then placed into a laying head-hanging position. The positional change may elicit vertigo and nystagmus. The test must be performed for each side with the ear turned downward.

MRI with gadolinium enhancement is extremely useful in evaluating the patient with dysequilibrium. In addition to complete cranial, cerebellar, and brain stem examination, attention should be directed to the internal auditory canals. The eighth cranial nerve should be fully visualized bilaterally, preferably in both axial and coronal planes. The addition of gadolinium enhancement has allowed for the detection of extremely small intracanalicular acoustic neuromas.

Ménière's Disease

In 1861, Prosper Ménière [34] described the symptom complex that bears his name, consisting of episodic vertigo, fluctuant hearing loss, tinnitus, and aural fullness. The histologic correlate was defined in 1938 by Hallpike and Cairnes [35] by describing the characteristic distention of the endolymphatic system with minimal effects on the auditory and vestibular neuroepithelia. The etiology of Ménière's disease has not yet been defined; presently the actual causes appear to be multifactorial.

The diagnosis of Ménière's disease is primarily dependent on history. The predominant symptoms are vertigo, fluctuating hearing loss, tinnitus, and aural pressure and fullness. The symptoms are classically unilateral; however, bilateral symptoms may occur in up to 15% of patients. Audiometric testing reveals a predominately low-tone and fluctuating sensorineural hearing loss; later a flat audiometric curve is more characteristic. Electronystagmography testing generally reveals a reduced caloric response on the involved side.

The mainstay in treatment is medical [36]. Initially, patients are placed on a 1,500-mg/day sodium diet. A reduction in caffeine, alcohol, and nicotine consumption is emphasized. The patient is also asked to modify his or her life-style to reduce stress. After a therapeutic trial of this regimen, medications are added if symptoms are not well controlled. Diuretics, usually potassium-sparing diuretics, are instituted initially. Anticholinergic medications and vestibular suppressants such as benzodiazepines are added to the regimen as needed. Antidepressant medications can also be effective in relieving symptoms in refractory cases. The medical regimen should be specifically designed for each individual patient and is generally successful in controlling symptoms in 85% of patients.

Patients whose symptoms are not well controlled on medical therapy are offered surgical intervention. The three predominant current surgical procedures offered for refractory Ménière's disease are the endolymphatic shunt, the vestibular nerve section, and transmastoid labyrinthectomy. Questions regarding the efficacy of the endolymphatic shunt have been raised [37,38]; therefore, vestibular neurectomy and labyrinthectomy have emerged as the most useful treatment modalities. The vestibular nerve section is performed through a suboccipital craniotomy with subsequent exposure of the eighth nerve complex. The vestibular nerve is divided, preserving the cochlear division and the facial nerve. Thus, the vestibular nerve section allows for division of the vestibular nerve while preserving hearing and facial nerve function. Vestibular nerve section is extremely effective in relieving vertigo [39] but less effective in treating dysequilibrium associated with vestibular abnormalities other than Ménière's disease [40]. Labyrinthectomy may be performed in a number of ways but the preferred method is transmastoid complete removal of the bony and membranous labyrinth. Transcanal labyrinthectomy may incompletely destroy the neuroepithelium, resulting in residual vertigo. Labyrinthectomy is an extremely effective procedure in relieving vertigo that is usually reserved for patients with marked loss of hearing because this is a destructive procedure resulting in complete hearing loss. Although this procedure is effective in relieving vertigo, there is a significant incidence of postoperative dysequilibrium. The elderly have an increased incidence of dysequilibrium following labyrinthectomy [41].

Gentamicin instillation into the middle ear to ablate vestibular function is an alternative to surgery. Gentamicin, like streptomycin, is an aminoglycoside antibiotic with known vestibular and cochlear toxicity. Titration of intratympanic application has resulted in control of vertigo with preservation of hearing [42]. Streptomycin is used to treat bilateral Ménière's disease or Ménière's disease in an only hearing ear. Daily injections are given intramuscularly and carefully titrated until vestibular caloric responses have ceased bilaterally [43]. Careful titration is required because streptomycin is also toxic to the cochlea and can cause hearing loss.

The success of vestibular nerve section and labyrinthectomy is also dependent on the patient's ability to compensate following the procedure. The initial clinical change following the procedure is dysequilibrium. The acute stage lasts approximately 6 weeks and is characterized by central inhibition of the contralateral vestibular nucleus to allow realignment to a new lower baseline activity level. During the chronic stage, cerebellar suppression of the vestibular nucleus decreases, and accommodation of the resulting increased activity follows. In younger patients, this equalization process may take up to 3 years. The adaptive mechanisms of central compensation become less effective with advancing age [44]. As noted previously, dysequilibrium is common after labyrinthectomy and has an increased incidence in the elderly. The decision to operate may commit the patient to accepting lifelong dysequilibrium in exchange for relief from incapacitating vertiginous episodes.

Positional Vertigo

Benign positional vertigo (BPV) is the most common cause of vertigo in the elderly. Vertigo and resulting horizontal-rotary nystagmus result when the head is placed in a critical position, usually lying down with the head turned to one side or the other. Other exacerbating conditions are getting out of bed while bending over and looking up at an object on the wall or shelf. The vertigo is troublesome but is generally brief and self-limited. The etiology may be secondary to head trauma, stapedectomy, middle ear or mastoid infections, or as a result of aging.

BPV resolves over a period of weeks to months and therefore the initial management is conservative. Rehabilitation exercises such as the Cawthorne-Cooksey [45] and Brandt-Daroff [46] exercises are recommended. These exercises entail nonspecific general eye and head movements repeated several times daily to aid in the compensation process. To be effective, these exercises must include head movement with vision and should begin as soon as possible after vestibular injury [47]. Interestingly, compliance with these exercises is poor, even in patients with long-standing dysequilibrium, possibly due to the fact that vertigo is often provoked with the position changes [48]. Another method of treatment is the positioning procedure as proposed by Epley [49] and Semont et al. [50]. These treatments are based on the theory that symptoms of BPV are the result of debris that adheres to the cupula of the posterior semicircular canal or is free-floating in the posterior canal. The maneuvers involve head positioning that attempts to move the debris into the vestibule where it would not produce symptoms of dysequilibrium. Single treatments with both the Epley and the Semont maneuvers have proved to be highly effective in relieving vertigo secondary to BPV [51]. Vestibular suppressants are usually not highly effective due to the brief, self-limiting nature of the vertigo. In fact, overall compensation may be inhibited by the use of vestibular suppressants.

Acoustic Neuroma

The most frequent tumor of the cerebellopontine angle is the eighth nerve neurilemmoma or acoustic neuroma. The tumor is a benign, encapsulated, Schwann's cell tumor of the eighth nerve, arising predominantly on the superior division of the nerve. The incidence of these tumors is 9.4 per million population per year [52], although temporal bone studies have shown the incidence of undiagnosed tumors to be 0.970 [53]. Presenting symptoms include unilateral tinnitus, sensorineural hearing loss (primarily a loss in speech discrimination or understanding), aural fullness, and dysequilibrium. Larger tumors may rarely present with facial numbness from fifth nerve involvement and facial nerve weakness and paralysis. Increased awareness as well as improved diagnostic screening, primarily with gadolinium-enhanced MRI, has allowed for the detection of smaller and less symptomatic acoustic tumors.

Early diagnosis and improvements in surgical technique and postoperative care have allowed for the safe removal of these tumors in elderly patients. Several authors have suggested that all acoustic tumors, with relatively few exceptions, should be surgically removed following diagnosis [54,55]. Other authors have proposed a more expectant approach to surgical excision [56–58]. Expectant or nonsurgical management is an alternative in selected groups of patients, including those with significant cardiovascular or pulmonary disease, as well as elderly patients with limited longevity. A conservative or nonoperative approach presumes that surgery poses a greater risk to the patient than the gradual increase in tumor size within the lifespan of the patient.

In a paper published by the otology group [59], 51 patients who received nonoperative management were studied. Advanced age (55%) and advanced age and a medical condition (25%) were the predominate reasons for choosing nonoperative therapy. The mean annual tumor growth rate for the entire study group was 0.11 cm per year. The range of tumor growth was 0 to 1.1 cm per year, with 16 patients demonstrating no growth during the entire study period. There was no statistically significant difference between tumor growth rate and the age of the patient. Based on the previously mentioned growth rates, patients over the age of 70, who are not candidates for hearing-preservation surgery, or those with significant medical problems should be managed conservatively. If sequential MRIs with gadolinium scanning reveal increased tumor growth or if progressive neurologic symptoms occur, surgery should be considered.

Facial Nerve Paralysis

In the temporal bone, the facial nerve travels through the longest bony enclosure of any nerve in the body. The facial nerve innervates the muscles of facial expression, lacrimal and submandibular glands, and taste to the anterior two-thirds of the tongue through the chorda tympani nerve. Thus, the facial nerve is important not only for facial animation but for corneal protection and prevention of exposure keratitis, as well as mastication without drooling.

When an elderly patient presents with facial paralysis, a systematic approach to evaluation is required. All too often the patient is given the diagnosis of Bell's palsy and dismissed. There are multiple etiologies for facial nerve paralysis; however, Bell's palsy implies idiopathic paralysis with no known etiologic agent. A full head and neck evaluation should be performed in all patients presenting with facial nerve paralysis. Systematic otologic examination begins with the auricle for evidence of vesicles consistent with herpes zoster oticus (Ramsay Hunt syndrome). The external canal should be examined for ulceration indicative of carcinoma or inflammation or granulation tissue suggestive of malignant external otitis. The postauricular region should be examined for erythema or fluctuance suggesting mastoiditis or subperiosteal abscess as a possible etiologic cause of the facial paralysis. The tympanic membrane should be inspected for both acute otitis media and chronic otitis media with or without cholesteatoma, both of which may cause facial nerve paralysis. The tympanic membrane should also be inspected for a vascular mass behind the intact membrane indicative of a paraganglioma (glomus tympanicum, vagale, or jugulare). The peripheral course of the nerve should be carefully examined as paralysis or paresis may be the result of a benign or malignant parotid tumor.

An audiogram should be performed on every patient with facial nerve paralysis. A conductive hearing loss may suggest a middle ear mass, facial nerve neuroma, or cholesteatoma as the etiology. A sensorineural loss may be seen in Ramsay Hunt syndrome or in cerebellopontine angle tumors such as an acoustic neuroma. Other diagnostic tests such as electroneuromyography may be indicated to assess neuronal integrity and degeneration. Other ancillary tests may be appropriate when clinically indicated, such as thin-cut temporal bone CT scanning for evaluation of traumatic facial nerve palsies, and Lyme titers if paresis as a result of Lyme disease is suspected. MRI may be helpful to rule out cerebellopontine angle tumors; however, the presence of an enhanced facial nerve with gadolinium has no prognostic significance [60]. Topognostic testing is time-consuming and generally not indicated [61] as the site of the lesion in idiopathic paralysis has been shown to be the labyrinthine segment at the meatal foramen of the fallopian canal [62].

The natural history of idiopathic facial nerve paralysis has been determined by Peitersen [63] in his study of 1,011 patients over a 15-year period. In 85% of patients the first signs of remission were observed within 3 weeks of onset, and the remaining 15% had remission 3 to 6 months later; 71% recovered normal function, 13% had insignificant sequelae, and the remaining 16% had permanently diminished function. This study demonstrated no sex predilection or seasonal variation. The incidence was less common before age 15 and after age 60. Interestingly, the influence of age on prognosis is highly significant. After age 60, only one-third of the patients had normal recovery.

Treatment consists initially of care of the eye to prevent exposure keratitis. In addition to the increased exposure secondary to poor closure, the eye is at risk from decreased tearing. A strict regimen is used, consisting of saline drops during the day, lubricating ointment during the night, and the use of an eye bubble or moisture chamber. Specific etiologies should be treated as clinically indicated. Acyclovir is used to treat patients with Ramsay Hunt syndrome [64,65] as these patients tend to have a poor outcome. Corticosteroids have been the mainstay in treating patients with idiopathic facial nerve paralysis. Patients treated with prednisone have less denervation and significant improvement in facial grade at recovery than patients not given corticosteroid therapy [66].

Paragangliomas of the Ear

Paragangliomas, commonly called *glomus tumors*, are highly vascular tumors that may arise in the temporal bone and skull base where paraganglia are found. They may be found in the middle ear space (glomus tympanicum), the jugular bulb (glomus jugulare), and the skull base at the jugular foramen (glomus vagale). These tumors tend to follow a course of slow continuous growth and are locally destructive [67]. In a study from the otology group [68], the most common presenting symptoms are pulsatile tinnitus, hearing loss, aural pressure, facial weakness, vertigo, hoarseness, and otalgia. Other than cranial nerve deficits, the most common presenting signs in patients with glomus jugulare are vascular middle ear mass in 72% of patients. Similarly, in patients with glomus vagale, the most common presenting sign is a palpable neck mass (41%). Sixty percent of the patients had no cranial nerve deficits. The most common presenting cranial nerve deficits were cranial nerves VIII, IX, X, and XII. A high level of suspicion is required in diagnosing these patients because early diagnosis in these patients has a positive impact on postoperative outcome [69].

In general, patients aged 65 or older are not candidates for neurotologic skull base surgery required for excision of glomus jugulare or vagale tumors. Because these lesions are slow growing, it is unlikely that these lesions would cause any significant concern in an elderly patient in the remaining years of his or her life [70]. It is generally believed that surgical morbidity likely exceeds potential surgical benefit as well as the risk of the tumor itself. The elderly patient who is asymptomatic is followed by serial scanning. It should be noted that in a younger patient, surgical excision of these paragangliomas is the treatment of choice because this is the only option that offers a definitive cure.

REFERENCES

1. Peters KD, Martin JA, Ventura SJ, Maurer JD. Births and deaths: United States, July 1995–June 1996. Monthly Vital Stat Rep 1997;45(10):4.
2. Rubin J, Yu VL. Malignant external otitis: insights into pathogenesis, clinical manifestations, diagnosis, and therapy. Am J Med 1988;85: 391–398.
3. Parisier SC, Lucente FE, Hirshman SZ, et al. Nuclear scanning in necrotizing progressive "malignant" external otitis. Laryngoscope 1982;92:1016–1020.
4. Levinson MJ, Parisier SC, Dolitsky J, Bindra G. Ciprofloxacin: drug of choice in the treatment of malignant external otitis (MEO). Laryngoscope 1991;101:821–824.
5. Rubin JR, Stoehr G, Yu VL, et al. Efficacy of oral ciprofloxacin plus rifampin for treatment of malignant external otitis. Arch Otolaryngol Head Neck Surg 1989;115:1063–1069.
6. Patt BS, Meyerhoff WI. Aging and the Auditory and Vestibular System. In Bailey BJ (ed), Head and Neck Surgery—Otolaryngology. Philadelphia: Lippincott, 1993.
7. Etholm B, Belal A. Senile changes of the middle ear joints. Ann Otol Rhinol Laryngol 1974;83:49–54.
8. Wolff D, Bellucci RJ. The human ossicular ligaments. Ann Otol Laryngol Rhinol 1956;65:895–910.
9. Tomoda K, Morji S, Yamashita T, Kumazowa T. Histology of human eustachian tube muscles: effects of aging. Ann Otol Laryngol Rhinol 1984;93:17–24.

10. Harris JP, Darrow DH: Complications of Chronic Otitis Media. In Nadol JB, Schuknecht HF (eds), Surgery of the Ear and Temporal Bone. New York: Raven, 1993.
11. Wengen DF, Pfaltz CR, Uyar Y. The influence of age on the results of stapedectomy. Eur Arch Otorhinolaryngol 1992;249:1–4.
12. Sheehy JL. Surgical correction of far advanced otosclerosis. Otolaryngol Clin North Am 1978;11:121–123.
13. Wiet RJ, Morganstern SA, Zwolan TA, Pircon SM. Far-advanced otosclerosis. Arch Otolaryngol Head Neck Surg 1987;113:299–302.
14. Matz GJ. Aminoglycoside ototoxicity. Am J Otolaryngol 1986;7: 117–119.
15. Griffin JP. Drug-induced ototoxicity. Br J Audiol 1988;22:195–210.
16. Consensus Conference, Noise and hearing loss. JAMA 1990;263: 3185–3190.
17. Grundfast KM, Lalwani AK. Practical approach to diagnosis and management of hereditary hearing impairment (HHI). Ear Nose Throat J 1992;71:479–493.
18. Kamerer DB. Middle Ear and Temporal Bone Trauma. In Bailey BJ (ed), Head and Neck Surgery—Otolaryngology. Philadelphia: Lippincott, 1993.
19. Sataloff J, Vassallo L, Menduke H. Presbycusis: air and bone conduction thresholds. Laryngoscope 1965;75:889–901.
20. Moscicki EK, Elkins EF, Baum HM, McNamara PM. Hearing loss in the elderly: an epidemiologic study of the Framingham Heart Study cohort. Ear Hear 1985;6:184–190.
21. Schuknecht HF, Woellner RC. Hearing losses following partial section of the cochlear nerve. Laryngoscope 1953;63:441–465.
22. Pauler M, Schuknecht HF, Thornton AR. Correlative studies of cochlear neuronal loss with speech discrimination and pure tone thresholds. Arch Otorhinolaryngol 1986;243:200–206.
23. Otte J, Schuknecht HF, Kerr AG. Ganglion cell populations in normal and pathological human cochleae. Implications for cochlear implantation. Laryngoscope 1978;88:1231–1246.
24. Schuknecht HF. Pathology of Presbycusis. In Goldstein JC, Kashima HK, Koopman CF (eds), Geriatric Otorhinolaryngology. Philadelphia: Decker, 1989.
25. Glasscock NE, Haynes DS. Cochlear Implants in Children: The surgeon's Role in Educational Management. In Barnes J, Franz D, Wallace B (eds), Cochlear Implants in Children: An Overview of the Alternatives in Education and Rehabilitation. Washington, DC: AG Bell, 1994.
26. Waltzman SB, Cohen NL, Shapiro WH. The benefits of cochlear implantation in the geriatric population. Otolaryngol Head Neck Surg 1993;108:329–333.
27. De Chicchis AR, Bess FH. Hearing Aids and Assistive Learning Devices. In Bailey BJ (ed), Head and Neck Surgery—Otolaryngology. Philadelphia: Lippincott, 1993.
28. Sloane PD, Baloh RW, Honrubia V. The vestibular system in the elderly: clinical implications. Am J Otolaryngol 1989;10:422–429.
29. Johnsson L. Degenerative changes and anomalies of the vestibular system in man. Laryngoscope 1971;81:1682–1694.
30. Rosenhall U. Degenerative patterns in the aging human vestibular neuroepithelia. Acta Otolaryngol 1973;76:208–220.
31. Bergstrom B. Morphology of the vestibular nerve U. The number of myelinated vestibular nerve fibers in man at various ages. Acta Otolaryngol 1973;76:173–179.
32. Richter E. Quantitative study of human Scarpa's ganglion and vestibular sensory epithelia. Acta Otolaryngol 1980;90:199–208.
33. Meyerhoff WL. Spontaneous perilymphatic fistula: myth or fact. Am J Otol 1993;14:478–481.
34. Ménière MP. Maladies de l'oreille interne. Gaz Med Paris 1861;16:55.
35. Hallpike CS, Cairnes H. Observations on the pathology of Ménière's syndrome. J Laryngol Otol 1938;53:625–655.
36. Schuknecht HF, Brackman DE, Glasscock ME, Jenkins H. Difficult decisions: Ménière's disease. Operat Technique Otolaryngol Head Neck Surg 1991;2:47–53.
37. Glasscock ME, Jackson CG, Poe DS, Johnson CD. What I think of sac surgery in 1989. Am J Otol 1989;10:230–233.
38. Silverstein H, Smouha E, Jones R. Natural history vs. surgery for Ménière's disease. Otolaryngol Head Neck Surg 1989;100:6–16.
39. Glasscock ME III, Thedinger BA, Cueva RA, Jackson CG. An analysis of the retrolabyrinthine vs. the retrosigmoid vestibular nerve section. Otolaryngol Head Neck Surg 1991;104:88-95.
40. Kemink JL, Telian SA, El-Kashlan H, Langman AW. Retrolabyrinthine vestibular nerve section: efficacy in disorders other than Ménière's disease. Laryngoscope 1991;101:523–528.
41. Kemink JL, Telian SA, Graham MD, Joynt L. Transmastoid labyrinthectomy: reliable surgical management of vertigo. Otolaryngol Head Neck Surg 1989;101:5–10.
42. Monsell EM, Cass SP, Ryback LP. Therapeutic use of aminoglycosides in Ménière's disease. Otolaryngol Clin North Am 1993;26: 737–746.
43. Glasscock ME, Johnson GJ, Poe DS. Streptomycin in Ménière's disease: a case requiring multiple treatments. Otolaryngol Head Neck Surg 1989;100:237–241.
44. Norre ME, Forrez G, Beckers A. Vestibular dysfunction causing instability in aged patients. Acta Otolaryngol 1987;104:50–55.
45. Cooksey FS. Rehabilitation in vestibular injuries. Proc R Soc Med 1946;39:273–275.
46. Brandt T, Daroff RB. Physical therapy for benign paroxysmal positional vertigo. Arch Otolaryngol 1980;106:484–485.
47. Konrad HR, Tomlinson D, Stockwell CW, et al. Rehabilitation therapy for patients with dysequilibrium and balance disorders. Otolaryngol Head Neck Surg 1992;107:105–108.
48. Keim RJ, Cook M, Martini D. Balance rehabilitation therapy. Laryngoscope 1992;102:1302–1307.
49. Epley JM. The canalith repositioning procedure: for treatment of benign paroxysmal positional vertigo. Otolaryngol Head Neck Surg 1992;107:399–404.
50. Semont A, Freyss G, Vitte E. Curing the BPPV with a liberatory maneuver. Adv Otorhinolaryngol 1988;42:290–293.
51. Herdman SJ, Tusa RJ, Zee DS, et al. Single treatment approaches to benign paroxysmal positional vertigo. 1993;119:450–454.
52. Tos M, Thomsen J, Samih C. Incidence of acoustic neuromas. Eye Nose Throat J 1992;71:391–393.
53. Stewart TJ, Liland J, Schucknecht HF. Occult schwannomas of the vestibular nerve. Arch Otolaryngol 1975;101:91–95.
54. House JW, Nissen RL, Hitselberger VVE. Acoustic tumor management in senior citizens. Laryngoscope 1987;97:129–130.
55. Brackmann DF, Kivostler JA. A review of acoustic tumors 1983–1988. Am J Otol 1990;11:216–232.
56. Silverstein H, McDaniel A, Norrell H, et al. Conservative management of acoustic neuroma in the elderly patient. Laryngoscope 1985;95:766–770.
57. Wiet RJ, Yog NM, Monsell EM, et al. Age consideration in acoustic neuroma surgery: the horns of a dilemma. Am J Otol 1989;10:177–180.
58. Samjii M, Tatagiba M, Matthies C. Acoustic neuroma in the elderly: factors predictive of postoperative outcome. Neurosurgery 1992;31: 615–620.
59. Strasnick B, Glasscock ME, Haynes DS, et al. The natural history of untreated acoustic neuromas. Laryngoscope 1994;104:1115–1119.
60. Schwaber MK, Larson TC, Zealear DL, Creasy J. Gadolinium-enhanced magnetic resonance imaging in Bell's palsy. Laryngoscope 1990;100:1264–1269.
61. Hughes GB. Practical management of Bell's palsy. Otolaryngol Head Neck Surg 1990;102:658–663.
62. Jackson CG, Hyams VJ, Johnson GD, Poe DS. Pathologic findings in the labyrinthine segment of the facial nerve in a case of facial paralysis. Ann Otol Rhinol Laryngol 1990;99:327–329.
63. Peitersen E. The natural history of Bell's palsy. Am J Otol 1982;4: 107–111.
64. Dickens JRE, Smith JT, Graham SS. Herpes zoster oticus: treatment with intravenous acyclovir. Laryngoscope 1988;98:776–779.
65. Greenberg UN, Meyer W, Kitzes-Cohen R. Herpes zoster oticus: treatment with acyclovir. Ann Otol Rhinol Laryngol 1992;101:161–162.
66. Austin JR, Peskind SP, Austin SC, Rice DH. Idiopathic facial nerve paralysis: a randomized double blind controlled study of placebo versus prednisone. Laryngoscope 1993;103:1326–1333.
67. Culya AJ. The glomus tumor and its biology. Laryngoscope 1993; 103:7–15.
68. Woods CI, Strasnick B, Jackson CG. Surgery for glomus tumors: the Otology Group experience. Laryngoscope 1993;103:65–69.
69. Jackson CG, Cueva RA, Thedinger BA, Glasscock ME. Conservation surgery for glomus jugulare tumors: the value of early diagnosis. Laryngoscope 1990;100:1031–1036.
70. Jackson CG. Diagnosis for treatment planning and treatment options. Laryngoscope 1993;103:7–22.

Surgical Care for the Elderly, 2nd ed., edited by
R. Benton Adkins, Jr., and H. William Scott, Jr.
Lippincott–Raven Publishers, Philadelphia © 1998.

CHAPTER 15

Ophthalmic Diseases

James H. Elliott and Stephen S. Feman

The surgical diseases of the eye can be divided, conveniently, into two main areas. This chapter first discusses surgical aspects of the anterior segment of the eye and then the problems related to the posterior segment of the eye.

A few general principles about surgical diseases of the eye in the elderly are appropriate to consider. In the 1970s, when eye procedures were considered in the elderly, the age of the patient and the status of his or her general health were the paramount considerations in the decision to operate. This applied equally to elective, urgent, and emergency eye operations. Today, this has changed: The patient's age and systemic disease status remain factors to be considered, but at a much lower level of importance in surgical decisions. Now, elective surgical procedures are common in patients who are renal transplant recipients, those who have end-stage renal disease, and in those who require dialysis. Patients with the most severe and most fragile forms of insulin-dependent diabetes mellitus are operated on frequently.

The principal reasons for this change are the low mortality and morbidity that have resulted from improved general anesthesia and local anesthetic techniques. The primary improvement in the use of local anesthesia for eye procedures has been the development of longer-acting infiltrative anesthetics that do not require supplemental use of epinephrine compounds to achieve satisfactory durations of anesthesia, for example, bupivacaine (Marcaine). The standard local anesthetic agents used for eye procedures consist of 0.75% Marcaine and 2% lidocaine (Xylocaine) mixed 50% to 50%. Hyaluronidase (Wydase) is added to facilitate dispersion. Usually a total of 5 ml of this mixture is used for akinesia and 3 ml for retrobulbar anesthesia. There are many variations to this local anesthesia method currently in use in the United States today. With these local anesthetic blocks, one can achieve anesthesia and akinesia of the eye and the periorbital tissues for periods up to 3 hours. Some surgeons now perform cataract surgery under topical anesthesia only, without a retrobulbar or peribulbar injection. Usually this is done with topical 4% Xylocaine, one drop applied every 5 minutes for 30 minutes before surgery. After sterile preparation and draping and placement of lid retractors, a cellulose sponge saturated in 4% Xylocaine is placed over the site of the corneal, limbal, or scleral incision. Surgical procedures are no longer canceled for hypertensive patients and those with cardiovascular disease who have a risk of hypertensive crises or severe arrhythmias for fear of some impending disaster.

Another factor that positively affects the surgical approach in older patients is the increased longevity and better general health and nutrition of our elderly. Elderly patients have gradually developed a philosophy of responsibility for their own health. In the 1960s, the average age of a patient needing a cataract extraction for restoration of vision and responsibility for his or her own hygiene and health care and a degree of independence was 64 to 65 years. Today, the average age of a patient needing cataract extraction for occupational indications or to improve or maintain a desirable life-style is 76 to 80 years.

Today, surgical procedures of the eye are considered so safe that health maintenance organizations, managed care companies, third-party insurers, Medicare, and state Medicaid carriers have regulations requiring that all cataract extractions and lens implants be performed on an ambulatory basis. Even patients who have significant life-threatening disorders, such as liver and renal transplant recipients, bone marrow transplant recipients, and others requiring systemic immunosuppressive agents, have eye surgery performed on a same-day ambulatory basis. This guideline applies to patients with brittle diabetes mellitus and to patients on chronic or acute hemodialysis. In fact, many patients have extensive eye surgery, which can include multiple separate ocular procedures, performed at the same time on an outpatient basis. The most common example of this is a penetrating keratoplasty, combined with a cataract extraction, intraocular lens implantation, and glaucoma filtering procedure, all performed at the same sitting. Same-day eye surgery is so commonplace that there has to be a special set of circumstances that makes it necessary to admit the patient for a postoperative hospitalization. One special circumstance would be a severe, disabling systemic medical condition.

Despite many of the unique health and social and financial challenges with which the elderly present to the eye surgeon, elderly patients deserve our best efforts to preserve the optimal quality of care and assist the elderly to maintain and enjoy the valuable sense of sight.

SURGICAL PROCEDURES OF THE ANTERIOR SEGMENT OF THE EYE

Surgical Diseases of the Eyelid

Chalazion

Chalazion is a pyogenic granuloma that forms in the meibomian glands of the eyelid. It is an infectious process within the tarsus of the upper and lower eyelids and is caused by the obstruction and subsequent infection of the meibomian gland openings. It is not necessarily age related and can be treated successfully by surgical means if conservative medical therapy fails. Conservative medical therapy consists of moist, hot compresses and topical antibiotic drops or ointment. If these measures fail, the residual hard lump may be resolved by surgical incision and curettage. The contents of all chalazions should be submitted for microscopic pathologic examination because occasionally an early sebaceous cell carcinoma has the clinical features of a chalazion.

Essential Blepharospasm

Essential blepharospasm is a morbid and disabling condition characterized by involuntary spasms of the orbicularis muscle in the periorbital area. It occurs principally in the population over age 50, and it is usually bilateral. The cause of blepharospasm is unknown and may be functional, or it may be the result of repetitive involuntary discharges from the higher cortical centers of the central nervous system. When ocular, psychological, and neurologic causes have been ruled out and conservative treatment regimens of muscle relaxants, neurologic drugs, or facial nerve blocks have failed, invasive surgical intervention is indicated. Many surgical procedures are used, including differential section of the seventh cranial nerve, total avulsion of the roots of the seventh nerve where it exits in the preauricular area, and the coronal flap methods for extirpation of segments of the orbicularis muscle. Each of these techniques is associated with considerable complications and, even in the best surgeon's hands, with variable results. The 5-year success rate for all of these operations is <50% in eliminating the condition for which the procedure was performed [1].

Since 1988, a new therapy has emerged for control of this disabling malady. Botulinum toxin A injection has been shown to be safe, simple, repeatable, and effective in controlling the symptoms of blepharospasm. Because of decreased morbidity and excellent therapeutic benefit, as compared with invasive surgical methods previously used (*vide supra*), botulinum toxin A has become the treatment of choice for this condition [2].

Ectropion

Ectropion may be cicatricial and noncicatricial. The noncicatricial form (senile) is the most common lid condition that occurs in the elderly and with few exceptions occurs universally on the lower lids. It is caused by an excessive horizontal length of the tarsal plate. It occurs as an eversion of the lid, mainly during sleep or at the time of tight lid closure.

The correction is nearly always surgical and may be performed on an ambulatory basis. The most common method of correction is the Kuhnt-Szymanowski procedure or one of its modifications [3]. A neglected ectropion of the lower lid results in a chronic blepharoconjunctivitis, constant tearing, drying and keratinization of the usually moist palpebral conjunctival mucous membranes, and eventual corneal ulceration (exposure keratitis). The last complication occurs because of chronic exposure to air and drying of the lower third of the cornea during sleep, and it may result in corneal perforations and loss of the eye.

Occasionally an elderly person develops an ectropion that involves only the punctum of the lower lid (nasal one-third of the lower lid). The rotation of the punctum away from the lacrimal lake results in epiphora. The surgical correction requires a different approach than do the senile ectropion procedures. The usual methods for this condition are the lazy T procedure described by Byron Smith and the Z-T plasty, which is basically a modification of the lazy T procedure [4]. Another method used for correction of medial ectropion is effected by use of the medial canthal ligament for suture plication. All of these procedures turn the eyelid back to a near normal position.

Cicatricial ectropion is caused by secondary scarring of the lids following trauma, infection, irradiation, tumor removal, or previous eyelid procedures. Removal of all scar tissue and replacement of skin using grafting procedures are usually required.

Entropion

Entropion is a term applied to the inversion or turning of the eyelid margin. As a result, the lashes of the lower or upper lid rub the cornea and conjunctivae and may cause corneal ulceration. Entropions may be congenital, involutional, or cicatricial. Involutional entropion of the lower lids is the most common type seen in the elderly.

Cicatricial entropions are caused by shrinkage of the tarsal conjunctival surface. The main causes include trauma, chemical injuries (principally alkali burns of the adnexa), chronic infections (trachoma), ocular cicatricial pemphigoid, and other inflammatory conditions (e.g., Stevens-Johnson syndrome, dermatomyositis, and scleroderma).

Involutional entropion in the elderly occurs because atrophy of the orbital fat results in changes that alter the apposition of the lid to the globe. Three or four highly successful methods of surgical correction have been described, each of which has its enthusiastic advocates [5–10].

Ptosis

Ptosis following ocular surgical procedures, a common sequela (10% to 15% of cases) of cataract surgery, is a slight ptosis or drooping of the upper lid. The exact cause is unclear but may be related to placement of a bridle suture beneath the superior rectus muscle for control of ocular motility. When this occurs, it is believed to be caused by a dehiscence or disinsertion of the levator muscle of the upper lid. This type of ptosis needs to be differentiated from the temporary and reversible type caused by topical corticosteroid medication and ocular inflammations associated with photophobia. The ptosis that follows cataract surgery is quite amenable to surgical correction.

Surgical Treatment of Glaucoma

Glaucoma is a blinding eye disease that is progressive, insidious, and relentless. There are many forms of glaucoma, and all forms tend to be most severe in the elderly. For convenience of discussion and for therapeutic reasons, glaucoma is divided into narrow angle and open angle types. This is an anatomic classification based on the width of the anterior chamber angle, which is measured with a gonioscopic contact lens examination. There are many secondary types of glaucoma classified under the primary types, and on occasion, some patients suffer from a combination of both primary narrow angle and open angle glaucoma.

The most common type of glaucoma in the elderly is the chronic primary open angle glaucoma (POAG). The onset of this type of glaucoma is insidious; the patient is almost totally asymptomatic until it is far advanced. It affects 2% of all patients aged 40 years and over and fully 8% to 10% of all patients who have insulin-dependent diabetes mellitus [11]. It is a genetically inherited disease with autosomal recessive transmission. It has a multifactorial inheritance pattern as judged by human lymphocytic antigen studies and family studies done using topical corticosteroid responsiveness [12–14].

POAG is principally a medically treatable, chronic, incurable disease that must be appropriately managed to prevent visual loss. Medical treatment relies on topical drops and orally administered carbonic anhydrase inhibitors. Topical medications include a variety of drugs with disparate pharmacologic mechanisms of action. These agents include beta blockers, epinephrine compounds, various miotics, alpha-adrenergic agonists, and, more recently, a group of topical carbonic anhydrase inhibitors and a prostaglandin F_2 alpha analogue (Latanaprost). Unfortunately, each of these medications can cause multiple and predictable side effects in a significant percentage of elderly patients. When this occurs, one needs to compare the risk-to-benefit ratio of such medical therapy to alternative surgical procedures.

Surgical intervention may be necessary in the management of POAG when progression of the disease despite maximum tolerated medical therapy is documented. The best parameters to determine progression of glaucoma are progressive loss of vision determined by successive visual field examinations. This loss must be correlated with the progression of the pathologic cupping of the optic nerve. Pathologic cupping of the optic nerve can be documented by stereoscopic photographs that allow the ophthalmologist to view the height, width, and depth of the cup in three-dimensional stereoscopic viewing. Maximum tolerated medical therapy usually entails the combined use of a beta blocker, miotic and adrenaline compounds, an adrenergic agonist, and either a topical or systemic carbonic anhydrase inhibitor. The patient must also be compliant in the use of the prescribed medications. A noncompliant patient frequently requires earlier surgical intervention than a compliant patient. If a patient has significantly documented vision loss (progression of visual fields and pathologic optic cupping), then the patient should be evaluated for a surgical procedure.

Noninvasive Surgical Procedures for Glaucoma

Argon laser trabeculoplasty (ALTP) was popularized and evaluated by Wise as a noninvasive ambulatory procedure. It has high efficacy with few complications and with relatively few side effects [15,16]. It is now the procedure of choice for a patient with progressive POAG despite maximum tolerated medical therapy. It consists of placing 50-µm–argon laser burns through a slit-lamp delivery system with a gonioscopic contact lens along the anterior border of the trabecular pigment band in the anterior chamber angle. The mechanism of action by which intraocular pressure is lowered is thought to be an increase in the rigidity of the wall of the trabecular spaces, which increases the size of the porous outflow channels. Approximately 140 individual spot burns are placed and evenly distributed throughout the 360-degree circumference of each eye for optimal therapy. According to most studies and in our experience, this produces a predictable lowering of the intraocular pressure by 8 to 12 mm Hg in 85% of eyes, no change in pressure in 12% of eyes, and slightly increased pressure in 3% of eyes [15–18].

The beneficial effect of ALTP on POAG has been shown in clinical studies to last an average of 5 years. Repeat ALTP above the optimal amount stated is of questionable value. Some surgeons prefer to treat only 180 degrees of the eye at each sitting. If an adequate response is obtained, the other 180 degrees can be saved for ALTP at a later time. This may extend the length of time the glaucoma can be controlled from 5 years to 6 to 10 years. Following ALTP, some patients are able to reduce their topical and oral medications and maintain adequate control of their POAG and others still require maximum tolerated medication.

Some of the complications of ALTP include synechiae formation from the peripheral iris to the cornea in the area of the burns, short-term corneal abrasions from the contact lens, mild inflammation (iritis), and a short-term increase in intraocular pressure in the first 24 to 48 hours postoperatively.

Laser iridotomy may be done with the yttrium-aluminum-garnet (YAG) or argon laser or with a combination of the two. Not every YAG laser has a thermal mode to control microscopic hemorrhage during the performance of a laser iridotomy. Laser iridotomy is the treatment of choice in any patient with acute or potential angle closure glaucoma. This technique has permitted the surgeon to avoid the many complications previously seen with surgical (invasive) peripheral iridectomy, which was the treatment of choice before the development of laser techniques [19].

Cyclocryotherapy is also a noninvasive method used to destroy or ablate the ciliary body by freezing the tissue. A cryoprobe is centered approximately 3 mm posterior to the limbus, and applications are made for 50 to 60 seconds after the probe tip temperature reaches –79°C. This results in some pain and discomfort postoperatively and requires lid akinesia and retrobulbar anesthesia for the procedure. It is indicated in various far-advanced and difficult cases, in cases of chronic open angle and angle closure types of glaucoma, or when a combination of the two types exists that has failed to respond to the usual conventional medical and surgical procedures [20–22].

Argon laser of ciliary processes is also used to destroy ciliary body processes by a physical, rather than chemical, method. The problem so far has been in the ability to focus the laser beam optically onto the ciliary body processes because of the difficulty, even with the maximally dilated pupil, of visualizing the ciliary body processes. They remain hidden from view even when the various mirrored contact lens currently available are used. Under special conditions (e.g., a patient with a full iridectomy) this technique has a place in the overall management of difficult cases. It also has the appeal of being noninvasive. Another term for this procedure is *transpupillary argon cyclophotocoagulation* [23,24]. This method has largely fallen into disuse but may be a modality to use in special circumstances.

Neodymium:YAG transcleral cyclophotocoagulation is another technique to destroy the ciliary body noninvasively at the site of aqueous humor formation. Two techniques have been developed: One consists of direct contact of the eye with a fiberoptic probe, and the other is a noncontact method where the laser energy is transmitted through a contact lens.

More recently, an adaptation of the contact laser technique, called *contact diode laser cyclophotocoagulation*, appears to be more efficacious. This method has fewer complications and facilitates a more controlled decrease in intraocular pressure. It also provides greater convenience and economy than the other methods of cyclophotocoagulation.

Therapeutic transcleral ultrasound ablation of the ciliary body is another expensive, high-tech method that makes use of sophisticated instrumentation to destroy ciliary processes of the eye where the aqueous is produced. Therefore, it is similar to cyclocryotherapy but uses a different physical method to accomplish the destruction of tissue that produces aqueous humor in the eye. The clinical efficacy of this method has not been ascertained. It does have the advantage of being noninvasive and can be used when the media of the eye is opaque—for example, with dense cataract or corneal scarring. It is applied with an appropriate ultrasound probe transclerally [25].

All of the previously mentioned procedures may be complicated by uveitis, hypotony, blindness, transient but rapid and large increase in the intraocular pressure, phthisis bulbi, flat anterior chamber or vitreous, hemorrhage, choroidal detachment, cystoid macular edema of the retina, and scleral thinning. The transpupillary argon cyclophotocoagulation technique is probably associated with the fewest complications of all the procedures, but it also has the most limited clinical indications and the least effectiveness.

Invasive Surgical Procedures for Glaucoma

Cyclodiathermy has largely been abandoned, but at one time was principally indicated for the treatment of glaucoma in patients who had previous cataract extraction. The procedure consists of reflecting a conjunctival flap in one quadrant of the eye to expose the bare sclera. Then, fine penetrating diathermy needles are passed through the sclera into the ciliary body. The appropriate amount of radiofrequency diathermy is applied to destroy the ciliary body. Multiple puncture sites are required and must be made under sterile operating room conditions. The procedure has largely fallen into disuse, but may still be useful in rare selected cases or in underdeveloped countries [26,27].

Trabeculectomy is the most popular, widely used method for the treatment of medically uncontrolled glaucoma. It creates an opening and pathway for aqueous humor to drain from the anterior chamber to an area beneath the conjunctiva (filtering bleb). All procedures of this type are called *filtering procedures*.

The goal of filtering procedures is to create a pathway for the aqueous humor to flow from the anterior chamber into the subconjunctival and sub-Tenon's spaces. In the past, this path was created by burning, trephining, or punching a hole through the full thickness of the sclera. The advantage of such procedures is that they allow rapid and constantly maintained lowering of the intraocular pressure. The disadvantage is that they may lower the pressure too much and result in hypotony, flat anterior chamber, and cataract. In more recent years, the trabeculectomy operation has become popular because it serves all the desired filtering activities while leaving a partial thickness of sclera as a residual tissue to restrain the aqueous outflow. For this reason, although its pressure-lowering activity is less than a full-thickness filter, it has significantly reduced the surgical complication rate, especially late-onset bacterial endophthalmitis.

The trabeculectomy procedure consists of reflecting an outer scleral flap, which is reflected over the cornea under a conjunctival flap. Then an inner scleral flap that is usually rectangular is mobilized and excised and includes a 3-mm arc of trabecular meshwork anterior to the scleral spur. The outer scleral flap is then resutured at the posterior corners with fine sutures, and the conjunctival mucous membrane is resutured in its normal anatomic position. Aqueous humor then flows from the anterior chamber, through the opening in the excised inner scleral flap, and through the three sides of the rectangle of the outer scleral flap that covers the "trap door" to be absorbed beneath the conjunctiva. A filtering bleb is then formed. Other glaucoma-filtering procedures are based on the same basic principles and tenets just described. Each of the alternative methods has its advocates. These methods include the sclera iridectomy with scleral lip cautery, trephination procedures, iridencleisis, and posterior lip or anterior lip scleral punch procedures [28].

Since the first edition of this book, improved success rates for trabeculectomy have been reported, with the use of antimetabolites in conjunction with the filtering surgery. The antimetabolites used have been 5-fluorouracil (5-FU) and mitomycin C (MMC), each of which has its advantages and disadvantages. Although some eye surgeons reserve use of these ancillary agents for resistant, failed, refractory, or poor prognostic cases of glaucoma, others use them almost routinely. Over time, the dosages used have been reduced because comparable results are obtained with fewer side effects. MMC has an advantage over 5-FU because it can be used intraoperatively, whereas 5-FU requires daily subconjunctival injections from postoperative days 0 to 14 on average.

With the passage of time and further studies, it is likely that other agents or the optimal dose of 5-FU and MMC will be found that will have comparable results and a decreased number of undesirable side effects [29].

In difficult and resistant cases of glaucoma, filtrating procedures using setons, implants, or valves may be necessary. Several ophthalmic centers in the United States are using alloplastic materials fabricated to create permanent lumens or canals for aqueous humor to drain out of the anterior chamber to beneath the conjunctiva. These setons are sutured in place. They have limited usefulness and many complications are associated with their use. Since the 1970s, a total of eight aqueous shunt devices have been evaluated. The two most popular in use at present are the Molteno (IOP Inc., Costa Mesa, CA) and Baerveldt (Pharmacia Iovision, Irvine, CA) implants and have a success rate of approximately 50% to 75% of cases, depending on the type of glaucoma [30,31].

Several invasive filtering procedures used in congenital glaucoma but not indicated in the treatment of glaucoma in the elderly are goniotomy, goniopuncture, and trabeculotomy. Another invasive filtering procedure frequently used during the 1930s, 1940s, and 1950s but since discarded is the cyclodialysis procedure. This is an internal, rather than an external, filtration procedure used in glaucoma occurring in aphakia (patients with previous cataract extraction) [32].

Surgical Treatment of Cataracts

A cataract is any opacity in the lens. Although cataracts may be classified by time of development (congenital or age related) or by anatomic location within the lens (cortical or nuclear), cataracts are most effectively classified by whether they influence vision. There are many cataracts that do not interfere with visual function and do not require extraction; in others, the clinical judgment of the surgeon is needed to determine if the visual impairment is enough to warrant the associated surgical risks. In such a situation, the surgeon needs to ask two major questions. The first is whether the patient's functional ability is reduced by the cataract to a level that satisfies the risk-to-benefit ratio. The second is whether the visual function can be sufficiently improved by the operation. In dealing with an elderly population, the second question becomes more important. The coexistence of cataract with glaucoma and retinal degeneration becomes more common with increasing age. A successful cataract operation is of no value to a patient who has a coexisting disorder that prohibits visual improvement. The evaluation of the visual potential of an eye in the presence of a cataract may be extremely difficult. In such a situation, a series of tests to evaluate physiologic responses may be needed. Such tests allow the surgeon to establish the percentage of visual impairment caused by coexisting optic nerve disease, glaucoma, retinal degeneration, and cataract. It is only with this knowledge that the surgeon can determine whether the planned procedure will offer enough benefit to overcome the surgical risks.

Cataract Extraction Procedures

The current state-of-the-art cataract operations to restore visual acuity have become highly skilled and safe invasive procedures. These procedures are usually divided into two distinct types: intracapsular cataract extraction and extracapsular cataract extraction (ECCE). Engineering achievements since the 1970s have made ECCE a procedure with a high success rate, a low complication rate, and such superb technical control that >95% of all cataract extractions in the United States are now of this variety.

The extracapsular operation involves the removal of the lens nucleus and cortex through an opening in the anterior lens capsule. This leaves the posterior capsule in place, which eliminates complications associated with vitreous adherence to the iris, cornea, and incision. It also provides for fixation of an artificial intraocular lens if the surgeon plans to add that step to the operation. The posterior capsule acts as a barrier to the exchange of molecules between aqueous and vitreous; studies have suggested that this lowers the incidence of macular edema, retinal detachment, and corneal edema.

Extracapsular extraction is best performed in the presence of a dilated pupil. An anterior capsulotomy <7 mm wide is performed. At the same time, the anterior chamber is prevented from collapsing by the infusion of a viscoelastic substance, such as sodium hyaluronate. The lens nucleus can be removed manually or emulsified through a 3-mm incision. Successful ECCE requires the use of an operating microscope with coaxial illumination. With the use of more recent technical refinements, the procedure can be performed under topical or local anesthesia in an ambulatory surgical center in <1 hour of operating room time.

The most common problem of ECCE is late opacification of the residual posterior capsule. This is reported to occur in >25% of cases within 1 to 3 years. However, the YAG laser can be used to manage the opacified posterior capsule without repeated surgical invasion of the eye. The YAG laser shock wave, produced by optical breakdown, results in a predictable and controlled disruption of the opaque posterior capsule.

Posterior Chamber Lens Implantation Technique

The most commonly used technique for cataract extraction over the last 5 years has been phacoemulsification, a form of ECCE that requires a smaller incision (3 mm) and frequently can be done without sutures (sutureless). Phacoemulsification uses a high-frequency ultrasonic vibrator pencil that fragments and removes the hard central core of the cataract called the *nucleus*. For this procedure to be safe, a continuous curvilinear capsulorrhexis is required to open and remove 5.5 to 6.5 mm of the anterior capsule of the lens and leave a peripheral residual anterior capsule with smooth borders. Otherwise, the capsule may tear peripherally into the capsular-zonular zone, resulting in undesirable complications that include vitreous loss and loss of the nucleus or other cataract remnants into the vitreous body posteriorly. When indicated, a trabeculectomy may be combined with small-incision cataract surgery using phacoemulsification techniques. Sutureless cataract surgery has been made possible by technical improvements of posterior chamber lenses, which are made of silicone or acrylic materials. This facilitates the placement of these intraocular lenses through a 3.0- to 3.5-mm surgical incision because these materials facilitate folding of the lens before inserting it into the eye and unfolding it inside the eye so that it is anchored securely in the capsular bag. The surgical incision itself may be within the cornea at the limbus or in the sclera, depending on the surgeon's preference. Many ophthalmic surgeons are performing sutureless cataract surgery procedures. The advantages of sutureless cataract surgery are decreased postoperative morbidity, a shortened period of optimal visual acuity to days rather than weeks or months (due to decreased amounts of astigmatism), and patient comfort. Visual rehabilitation is shortened considerably, and the patient may return more rapidly to full physical activity without limitations.

The more standard technique of ECCE is described because, in certain situations, the eye surgeon must use this technique as opposed to the phacoemulsification method. On occasion during phacoemulsification, the surgeon has to convert to the more standard technique for safety reasons. In other instances, the surgeon may prefer to use the standard ECCE technique because of inadequate pupil dilation. A total mature cataract in which a surgeon cannot obtain an ideal red reflex for performing a continuous curvilinear capsulorrhexis may be another reason to use the standard ECCE technique. Another reason is pseudoexfoliation of the lens, which is associated with lax zonules supporting the lens. The ECCE procedure, which is always performed under an operating microscope, consists of elevating a conjunctival flap in the superior 180 degrees of the eye. A small incision is made to introduce a bent 25-gauge needle attached to a continuous irrigating cannula. The needle is used to perform a circular 6.5- to 7.0-mm diameter anterior capsulotomy in the "can-opener" style. The irrigation solution contains balanced salt solution with added glutathione and 0.5 ml of 1:1,000 aqueous solution of adrenaline per 500 ml solution. The adrenaline is vital to maintaining the dilations of the pupil during the procedure. After the anterior capsulotomy is completed, the corneal-scleral incision is enlarged to 11.5 mm long (chord tangent of a circle). The nucleus of the lens is then delivered after installation of sodium hyaluronate (Healon) to protect the corneal endothelium (posterior layer of cornea). The nucleus is usually expressed by pressure on the globe inferiorly at the limbus and counterpressure superiorly on the globe 4 mm posteriorly to the corneal-scleral incision.

There are four stages or elements to the planned ECCE and posterior chamber lens implant: (1) the anterior capsulotomy, (2) delivery or expression of the nucleus of the lens, (3) cleanup of the cortex of the lens, and (4) implantation of the posterior chamber lens.

Following delivery of the nucleus, the cortical cleanup can be done with either automated or manual techniques. At our institution, we favor the automated technique for irrigation and aspiration of the residual lens material that remains after delivery of the nucleus of the lens. With the automated technique, almost 100% of the residual lens cortex fibers can be removed. The irrigation solution attached to the irrigation-aspiration unit is the same one used for the anterior capsulotomy.

After completion of the cortical lens cleanup, the posterior capsular bag left behind is distended with Healon. This distension of the bag creates a cocoon or pocket into which the posterior chamber lens is inserted. When in the bag, the new artificial lens floats inside the eye. One of the reasons the posterior chamber lens has been so well tolerated by human eye tissues is that it does not touch or attach to any moving part of the eye (e.g., the iris).

Approximately 1 to 3 years following a planned ECCE and posterior chamber lens implant, some 25% of patients experience reduction of visual acuity due to clouding of the posterior capsular membrane. This is easily diagnosed by the ophthalmologist, and the vision can be restored by a simple, safe, effective noninvasive method. It is for this indication that a YAG laser is used as a "cold knife" to cut through the posterior capsule membrane and create a new opening to allow for clear vision. A YAG Abraham contact lens (Ocular Instruments, Inc., Bellevue,WA) applied to the eye facilitates the procedure [33].

Anterior Chamber Lens Implantation

Because of late postoperative complications, the anterior chamber lens is used almost exclusively today for backup purposes. In 2% to 5% of cases, it is technically impossible to remove all of the cortical lens material without rupturing the posterior capsule. In these situations, if the patient wants an intraocular lens implant, it must be of the anterior chamber lens style, which fits anterior to the iris. This is because with rupture of the posterior capsule there is no support for the posterior chamber lens implant. Complications that occur late after anterior chamber lens implant include hyphema, glaucoma, loss of clarity of the cornea (corneal edema), and uveitis (sterile inflammation of the eye).

The incidence of postcataract extraction bacterial endophthalmitis is now only 1 in 1,000 operations. This is a low incidence, but this complication destroys all useful vision in over 50% of the cases.

With the current highly skilled and refined cataract extraction procedure described, an elderly patient can reasonably expect better vision after the operation in >95% of cases. If the vision is not better after the procedure, it is almost always due to some underlying retinal pathology (macular degeneration) [34].

Other Cataract Procedures

Occasionally, the older standard procedure of intracapsular cataract extraction might be the procedure of choice. In this technique, all the lens is removed with a cryoextractor after the zonules are lysed with alpha-chymotrypsin [35]. There are other instances in which a retinal surgeon may remove a cataract during a vitrectomy procedure through the pars plana of the eye. This is called a *pars plana vitrectomy-lensectomy*.

In rare instances a secondary anterior or posterior chamber lens implant is performed. A secondary lens implant procedure is one in which there is an interval of 6 to 8 months to years between the cataract extraction and the lens implant procedure [35]. Also in selected rare instances an intraocular lens implant may be exchanged for another one, called a *lens exchange*.

Surgical Correction of Corneal Conditions

Certain corneal procedures are performed in the elderly. The most common of these is the penetrating keratoplasty procedure (PKP). This procedure needs to be differentiated from a lamellar keratoplasty where only a partial thickness corneal transplant is done. The most common sizes for a penetrating keratoplasty are an 8.0-mm donor into a 7.5-mm diameter recipient bed. Also common is an 8.5-mm donor into an 8.0-mm diameter host cornea.

The main indication for PKP is to restore visual acuity. This decrease in visual acuity is usually a result of corneal scarring or edema or a combination of the two. If this opacification of the cornea cannot be corrected by medical or a simpler surgical operation, PKP is indicated. The diseases that result in opacification and vascularization of the cornea and are amenable to surgical correction by PKP are herpes keratitis, corneal dystrophies, keratoconus, trauma, aphakic and pseudophakic bullous keratopathy, and corneal degenerations.

The PKP procedure is always performed under the operating microscope, and the most common suture is a 10-0 monofilament nylon. After trephination of the diseased corneal button from the recipient, the new donor button is sutured onto the host. The donor button is placed on a bed of Healon during the suturing. This protects the vital layer of donor corneal endothelium from damage caused by rubbing the iris or cornea of the host. At one time, a 360-degree continuous running suture was favored to anchor the donor to the host cornea. More recently, surgeons are returning to the use of 16 to 24 direct radial sutures. By cutting the sutures at selected times during the postoperative period, the development and prevention of corneal astigmatism can be regulated during the postoperative period. All knots are buried in the corneal tissue so they will not irritate the upper lids and the patient will be more comfortable. Overall, the PKP procedure has approximately a 90% chance of success as judged by an optically clear and functioning donor cornea. Approximately 75% of these patients will obtain a Snellen visual acuity result of 20/40 or better [36].

When a PKP is combined with a planned ECCE and posterior chamber lens implant it is called a triple procedure [37]. Sometimes a trabeculectomy is performed for control of glaucoma with either or both of the PKP and cataract procedures [38,39].

A procedure called *epikeratophakia* was described in the first edition but has lost its popularity and fallen into disuse. Epikeratophakia used a donor-lyophilized human donor corneal lenticule that was sutured on top of the patient cornea. It was used in cases of aphakia when an intraocular lens was contraindicated. It was originally designed for patients who did not like or could not tolerate a thick spectacle lens or contact lens and who did not have an intraocular lens inserted at the time of the cataract procedure. Today, nearly all patients get some type of intraocular lens because of their increasing safety. Therefore, the donor lenticule ceased to be commercially profitable for the company lathing the donor corneas to a precise optical power for the recipient.

SURGICAL TREATMENT OF DISORDERS OF THE POSTERIOR SEGMENT OF THE EYE

Surgical Procedures of the Vitreous

During the past decade, vitreous surgical procedures have been developed for many different eye disorders. In the older population, these procedures are most often used to remove vitreous opacities and transvitreous traction fibrous bands. The most common medical disorder associated with this is diabetes mellitus. However, additional causes of vitreous opacification in this population are retinal branch vein occlusions [40] and trauma, which includes the surgical trauma of cataract removal.

The general principles of vitreous surgery have become well established. In most situations, a closed system to maintain the ocular volume is required. This prevents the collapse of the globe and anatomic distortion during surgery. Several microscopic instruments can be inserted into the eye through the pars plana to manipulate intraocular tissues; at the same time, an optically clear solution can be infused into the globe to maintain ocular volume. Current surgical techniques use instruments designed to cut vitreous free from its attachment to the retina and remove it from the globe. Bleeding sites within the eye can be coagulated with intraocular diathermy, laser, or both. Retinal breaks may be identified and closed. Optically clear vitreous replacement agents (both gases and liquids) have been developed to assist this surgery. The interface between these agents and the retina creates a surface tension that results in the temporary closure of any breaks in the retinal surface. This has become a common intraocular technique for the prevention of retinal detachment during intravitreal surgery [41–43].

Retinal Detachments

There are many different kinds of retinal detachments. The most common variety in the older population, and the one for which surgical techniques offer the most benefit, is the rhegmatogenous retinal detachment. This term is derived from the Greek word *rhegma,* which means *a break.* The rhegmatogenous retinal detachment is characterized by a break in the contiguity of the retina, which allows fluid vitreous to pass into the subretinal space. The surgical correction of this disorder is designed primarily to close the holes in the retina. More than one-half of all patients operated on for rhegmatogenous retinal detachments in the United States are >60 years of age. Many of these detachments are found in individuals >70 years of age. The majority of such problems develop in male patients; this high incidence is thought to be related to a preexisting history of trauma. However, most investigators believe that some patients have a developmental predilection for this disorder that becomes apparent only as the patient matures. Almost 20% of individuals with a retinal detachment in one eye will develop a detachment in the other eye at some time [44].

The concept that a retinal break produces a retinal detachment has been known since 1930 and has been the key to reattachment surgery. However, improvements in surgical techniques have allowed the anatomic reattachment rate to approach 96% in the United States. These procedures close the breaks in the retina, and the retina reattaches itself when the retinal pigment epithelium removes the residual subretinal fluid. Most often, scleral buckling techniques are used to close the holes in the retina [45]. In addition, various methods have been developed to create an inflammatory response to surround the retinal breaks; this results in scar formation that creates permanent closure of the retinal defects and reattachment.

Age-Related Macular Degeneration

Age-related macular degeneration is one of the major causes of new blindness in the older population in the United States [46]. In addition, it is the most common cause of new blindness in patients >65 years of age in Canada, Australia, and the United Kingdom [47,48]. This disorder can be divided into two varieties. The first, atrophic age-related macular degeneration, does not benefit from any of the surgical procedures available at this time; however, transplantation techniques are being investigated. The other form of the disease, exudative age-related macular degeneration, occurs in only 10% of the patients with age-related macular degeneration. However, the exudative variety is the cause of blindness in 90% of the eyes affected by age-related macular degeneration [49]. In the past few years a vast literature has developed in regard to the etiology and surgical treatment of this exudative variety.

Age-related macular degeneration originates from preexisting abnormalities in the retinal pigment epithelium. These are localized, microscopic, retinal pigment epithelial detachments. With time, these progress to form (1) areas of geographic atrophy of the retinal pigment epithelium, (2) serous fluid detachments of the retinal pigment epithelium, (3) choroidal neovascularization growing under the retina, or (4) all of these conditions [50].

Several epidemiologic studies have demonstrated features associated with the blinding changes of age-related macular degeneration. This disorder reaches its peak in the decade between age 75 and 85. Almost one-third of the asymptomatic individuals with good vision within this age range have some manifestation of this disorder [51–53]. There does not appear to be a sex predilection for this problem. Although epidemiologic surveys have failed to show a difference between racial groups, several studies have reported that decreased pigmentation of the eye, such as reduced iris color, and chronic photic exposure, are associated with an increased risk of blindness [49]. Of special note has been the recent discovery that certain forms of this disorder may appear in a familial hereditary pattern. If there is a genetic predisposition for a disorder that does not demonstrate clinical manifestations until age 70, it may be difficult to evaluate chromosomal studies [54].

Surgical procedures to prevent this loss have benefited many patients. A nationwide treatment trial has found that, in those with the progressive form of this disorder, laser photocoagulation surgery can maintain vision. Although visual improvement is not achieved in all cases, the prevention of additional vision loss is of great benefit to such patients [55,56]. This surgical procedure consists of using laser photocoagulation to destroy areas of neovascularization whenever they are discovered. However, this treatment does not influence the underlying cause of this disorder. For this reason, new areas and recurrent problems are not uncommon in these patients. Nevertheless, treatment that results in the complete obliteration of the neovascular complex is effective in these patients, and untreated eyes are twice as likely to have progressive vision loss as compared with treated eyes.

Malignant Melanoma of the Choroid

Malignant melanoma of the choroid is the most common cancer of the eye. In the United States, it is found at a frequency of 1 new case per 200,000 each year. The peak incidence of this tumor is age 70 [57]. The size of a choroidal melanoma is the single most important criterion for making a judgment regarding therapy. Lesions measuring <2 mm thick, with a base diameter of <10 mm, are difficult to differentiate by clinical techniques from benign lesions. For this reason, current methods recommend that these be followed carefully to demonstrate growth before any form of treatment is recommended. It has been found that there is a critical threshold size for such tumors; when the total volume is >1,400 mm^3, there is a great risk of metastatic disease. It is estimated that the typical choroidal melanoma has a slow growth pattern and takes almost 5 years to double in volume. For this reason, in most cases it is safe to follow suspicious lesions before recommending any form of intervention. For tumors that are <10 mm in greatest diameter and contain predominately spindle cells, the 5-year survival rate is 95%. With an increase in the percentage of epithelioid cells within the tumor, the survival rate drops to 80%. Larger tumors and the greater frequency of epithelioid cells within them are associated with a gradual reduction in survival rates.

For centuries, surgeons have believed that removing a cancer can prolong the life expectancy of a patient. However, with this particular tumor of the eye, there has been great controversy regarding this concept. Some reports indicate that there may be an increased risk of promoting metastasis when the standard surgical procedure of enucleation is performed in such patients [58]. This has prompted research into new treatment techniques that do not require enucleation. The most well-known study of this variety is the Collaborative Ocular Melanoma Study and involves more than 30 major eye centers throughout the United States. The results of that project are not yet available. However, preliminary reports from similar studies have not demonstrated which therapy is best [59,60]. For this reason, all surgeons who care for older patients are waiting for the results of this treatment trial.

CONCLUSION

Since 1985, there has been a change in the average age of patients undergoing ophthalmic surgery. Although the field of ocular surgery extends for the full range of human potential, from premature infants to the most senior of citizens, the increased numbers of elderly undergoing eye procedures has shifted the average age data. Many patients in the past were thought to be too old or too ill to undergo surgical correction of their disorders; this concern is now rare. The age and health status of a patient remain factors, but at a lower level of significance in the surgical decision-making process.

Many types of ocular disorders (e.g., cataract formation, retinal degeneration) occur most often in the elderly population. Because of increased longevity and the better health and nutrition of our elderly population, more people are alive and aware of their ophthalmic problems. One surprise is that some eye problems that were rare in the past have been found to represent dominantly inherited disorders that were first identified in the older population. If clinically significant features do not develop until a person is >75 years of age, one needs to reexamine the standard methods used for patient counseling for hereditary disease.

As our population matures, the surgical care of the elderly will become the most common type of surgical care. Patients in this age range have developed a philosophy of responsibility for their own health. For this reason, they want more and better care. In addition, they have the knowledge and ability to demand the best that our society can produce. As social and financial pressures are brought to bear on these unique challenges, ophthalmic surgeons will participate in an ever-evolving improvement in care, which will help the elderly enjoy their vision into the future.

REFERENCES

1. Wesley RE. Coronal Flap in Treatment of Blepharospasm. In Wesley RE (ed), Techniques in Ophthalmic Plastic Surgery. New York: Wiley, 1986;413–416.
2. Kohn R. Essential Blepharospasm. In Kohn R (ed), Textbook of Ophthalmic Plastic and Reconstructive Surgery. Philadelphia: Lea & Febiger, 1988;279–285.
3. Leone CR Jr. Plastic Surgery. In Spaeth GH (ed), Ophthalmic Surgery: Principles and Practice. Philadelphia: Saunders, 1982;547–652.
4. Wesley RE. 2-T Plasty for Medial Entropion. In Wesley RE (ed), Techniques in Ophthalmic Plastic Surgery. New York: Wiley, 1986;145–146.
5. Leone CR Jr. Plastic Surgery. In Spaeth GH (ed), Ophthalmic Surgery: Principles and Practice (2nd ed). Philadelphia: Saunders, 1990;545–552.
6. Kohn R. Entropion. In Kohn R (ed), Textbook of Ophthalmic Plastic and Reconstructive Surgery. Philadelphia: Lea & Febiger, 1988;167–175.
7. Wesley RE. Combined Procedure for Entropion Repair. In Wesley RE (ed), Techniques of Ophthalmic Plastic Surgery. New York: Wiley, 1986;118–121.
8. Wesley RE. Marginal Rotation Procedure for Correction of Upper Lid Entropion. In Wesley RE (ed), Techniques of Ophthalmic Plastic Surgery. New York: Wiley, 1986;104–107.
9. Shaefer AJ. Imbrication of the Lower Lid Retractors for Correction of Senile Entropion. In Wesley RE (ed), Techniques of Ophthalmic Plastic Surgery. New York: Wiley, 1986;108–113.

10. Hecht SD. Bowlegs Procedure for Senile Entropion. In Wesley RE (ed), Techniques of Ophthalmic Plastic Surgery. New York: Wiley & Sons, 1986;106–107.
11. Epstein DL. Primary Open Angle Glaucoma. In Chandler PA, Grant WM (eds), Chandler and Grant's Glaucoma (3rd ed). Philadelphia: Lea & Febiger, 1986;129–180.
12. Becker B. The genetic problem of chronic simple glaucoma. Ann Ophthalmol 1971;3:351.
13. Damgaard-Jensen L, Kissmeyer-Nielsen F. HLA histocompatibility antigens in open-angle glaucoma. Acta Ophthalmol Scand Suppl 1978; 56:384–388.
14. Ritch R, Podos SM, Henley W, et al. Lack of association of histocompatibility antigens with primary open-angle glaucoma. Arch Ophthalmol 1978;96:2204–2206.
15. Wise JB, Witter SL. Argon laser therapy for open angle glaucoma, a pilot study. Arch Ophthalmol 1979;97:319–322.
16. Wise JB. Long-term control of adult open angle glaucoma by argon laser treatment. Ophthalmology 1981;88:197–202.
17. Wilensky JT, Jampol LM. Laser therapy for open angle glaucoma. Ophthalmology 1981;88:213–217.
18. Schwartz AL, Whitten ME, Bleiman B, Martin D. Argon laser trabecular surgery in uncontrolled phakic open angle glaucoma. Ophthalmology 1981;88:201–212.
19. Moster MR, Schwartz LW, Spaeth GL, et al. Laser iridectomy, a controlled study comparing argon and neodymium:YAG. Ophthalmology 1986;93:20–24.
20. Bellows AR, Grant WM. Cyclocryotherapy in advanced inadequately-treated glaucoma. Am J Ophthalmol 1973;75:679–684.
21. DeRoetth A Jr. Cryosurgery for the treatment of advanced chronic simple glaucoma. Am J Ophthalmol 1968;66:1034–1041.
22. Burton TC. Cyclocryotherapy. In Becker B, Drews RC (eds), Current Concepts in Ophthalmology. St. Louis: Mosby, 1974.
23. Zimmerman TJ, Worthen DM, Wickham G. Argon laser photocoagulation of ciliary process and pigmented pupillary membrane in man. Invest Ophthalmol 1973;12:622–623.
24. Lee PF. Argon laser photocoagulation of the ciliary processes in cases of aphakic glaucoma. Arch Ophthalmol 1979;97:2135–2138.
25. Stewart WC, Brindlye GO, Shields MB. Cyclodestructive Procedures. In Ritch R, Shields MB, Krupin T (eds), Glaucoma Therapy (2nd ed). New York: Mosby, 1996;1605–1620.
26. Stocker FW. Response of chronic simple glaucoma to treatment with cyclodiathermy puncture. Arch Ophthalmol 1945;34:181–186.
27. Walton DS, Grand WM. Penetrating cyclodiathermy for filtration. Arch Ophthalmol 1970;83:47–48.
28. Shields MB. Textbook of Glaucoma (2nd ed). Baltimore: Williams & Wilkins, 1987.
29. Parrish RK II, Folberg R. Wound Healing in Glaucoma Surgery. In Ritch R, Shields MB, Krupin T (eds), Glaucoma Therapy (2nd ed). New York: Mosby, 1996;1633–1651.
30. Lloyd ME, Baerveldt G, Heuer DK, et al. Initial clinical experience with the Baerveldt implant in complicated glaucomas. Ophthalmology 1994;101:640–650.
31. Heuer DK, Lloyd ME, Abrams DA. Which is better? One or Two? A randomized clinical trial of single plate versus double plate Molteno implantation for glaucomas in aphakia and pseudophakia. Ophthalmology 1992;99:1512–1519.
32. O'Brien CS, Weih J. Cyclodialysis. Arch Ophthalmol 1949;42:606.
33. Stark WJ, Worthen DM, Holladay JJ, Murray G. Neodymium:YAG lasers. Ophthalmology 1985;92:209–212.
34. Stark WJ, Worthen DM, Holladay JJ, et al. The FDA report on intraocular lenses. Ophthalmology 1983;90:311–317.
35. Jaffe NS. Cataract Surgery and its Complications (3rd ed). St. Louis: Mosby, 1981.
36. Brightbill FS. Corneal Surgery: Theory, Technique, and Tissue. St. Louis: Mosby, 1986.
37. Crawford GJ, Stulting RD, Waring GO III, et al. The triple procedure. Analysis of outcome, refraction, and intraocular lens power calculation. Ophthalmology 1986;93:817–824.
38. Savage JA, Thomas JV, Belcher D, Simmons RJ. Extracapsular cataract extraction and posterior chamber intraocular lens implantation in glaucomatous eyes. Ophthalmology 1985;92:1506–1516.
39. Praeger DL. Combined procedure: sub-scleral trabeculectomy with cataract extraction. Ophthalmic Surg 1983;14:130–134.
40. Branch Vein Occlusion Study Group. Argon laser scatter photocoagulation for prevention of neovascularization and vitreous hemorrhage in branch vein occlusion. Arch Ophthalmol 1986;104:34–41.
41. Bourgeois JE, Machemer R. Results of sulphur hexafluoride gas in vitreous surgery. Am J Ophthalmol 1983;96:405–406.
42. Chang S, Lincoff HA, Coleman DJ, et al. Perfluorocarbon gases in vitreous surgery. Ophthalmology 1985;92:651–656.
43. McCuen VW, DeJuan E, Landers MB, Machemer R. Silicone oil in vitreoretinal surgery. Retina 1985;5:189–205.
44. Hilton GS, McClean EB, Norton EWD. Retinal Detachment. San Francisco: American Academy of Ophthalmology, 1981.
45. Williams GA, Aaberg TM. Techniques of Scleral Buckling. In Ryan SJ (ed), Retina. St. Louis: Mosby, 1989;111–149.
46. Bressler NM, Bressler SB, Fine SL. Age related macular degeneration. Surv Ophthalmol 1988;32:375–413.
47. Segato T, Midenam E, Blarzino MC. Age related macular degeneration. Aging Clin Exp Res 1993;5:165–176.
48. Vinding T. Age related macular degeneration: macular changes, prevalence, and sex ratio. Acta Ophthalmol 1989;67:609–616.
49. Hyman LG, Lilienfeld AN, Ferris SL, Fine FL. Senile macular degeneration: a case controlled study. Am J Epidemiol 1983;118: 213–227.
50. Ferris SL, Fine SL, Hyman LG. Age-related macular degeneration and blindness due to neovascular maculopathy. Arch Ophthalmol 1984; 102:1640–1642.
51. Tso MOM. Pathogenetic factors of aging macular degeneration. Am J Ophthalmol 1985;92:628–635.
52. Bressler NM, Bressler SB, Seddon TM, et al. Clinical characteristics of drusen in patients with exudative versus non-exudative age-related macular degeneration. Retina 1988;8:109–114.
53. Sarks SH. Drusen and their relationship to senile macular degeneration. Aust J Ophthalmol 1980;8:117–130.
54. Meyers SM, Zachary AA. Monozygotic twins with age related macular degeneration. Arch Ophthalmol 1988;106:651–653.
55. Macular Photocoagulation Study Group. Argon laser photocoagulation for senile macular degeneration. Arch Ophthalmol 1982;100: 912–918.
56. Macular Photocoagulation Study Group. Argon laser photocoagulation for neovascular maculopathy: three year results from randomized clinical trials. Arch Ophthalmol 1986;104:694–701.
57. Jakobiec SA, Levinson AW. Choroidal Melanoma: Etiology and Diagnosis. Clinical Modules for Ophthalmologists. San Francisco: American Academy of Ophthalmology, 1985.
58. Zimmerman LE, McLean IW. Evaluation of enucleation in the management of uveal melanomas. Am J Ophthalmol 1979;87:741–760.
59. Gass JDM. Comparison of prognosis after enucleation versus cobalt-60 radiation of melanomas. Arch Ophthalmol 1985;103:916–923.
60. Gragoudas ES, Goitein M, Verhey L. Proton beam radiation of uveal melanomas. Results of 5½-year study. Arch Ophthalmol 1982;100: 928–934.

Surgical Care for the Elderly, 2nd ed., edited by
R. Benton Adkins, Jr., and H. William Scott, Jr.
Lippincott–Raven Publishers, Philadelphia © 1998.

CHAPTER 16

Surgery of Thyroid and Parathyroid Disorders in the Aged

Geoffrey B. Thompson and Oliver H. Beahrs

Disorders of the thyroid and parathyroid glands requiring surgical intervention occur among all age groups. However, the incidence and pathology from young to old varies. As we approach the twenty-first century, there will be an ever-increasing population of individuals over the age of 60. This will undoubtedly increase the number of patients with endocrinologic disorders of potential surgical import.

Thyroid and parathyroid disorders in the elderly are common [1,2] but may remain unrecognized for a number of reasons. The clinical manifestations of these disorders may be quite subtle and attributable to normal aging. The coexistence of other medical problems (cardiovascular, pulmonary, neuropsychiatric, etc.) and the use of polypharmacy in the aged may further cloud an already confusing clinical picture [2–10].

When considering surgical intervention in the elderly, one must analyze a number of factors including comorbid conditions, the biological (not just the chronologic) age of the patient, and the potential life expectancy of the individual as perceived by both physician and patient. Studies have already defined the safety and efficacy of thyroid and parathyroid surgery in the hands of experienced surgeons [11–13], and therefore age alone should not deter the patient from undergoing such procedures when the potential benefits outweigh the relatively low surgical risks.

This chapter reviews the more common surgical thyroid and parathyroid disorders seen in the elderly and outlines a reasonable approach for their evaluation and treatment, taking into consideration other alternatives when appropriate.

DISORDERS OF THE THYROID GLAND

Autopsy studies have demonstrated increasing nodularity of the thyroid gland with age. Fibrosis and lymphocytic infiltration of the thyroid gland also increase with time. Despite these morphologic changes, the overall gland size and weight remain fairly constant. Although controversy exists, this holds true for thyroid function as well [8]. With increasing age and cervical kyphosis, the thyroid gland tends to be displaced posteriorly and inferiorly, making its clinical assessment (i.e., by palpation) more difficult.

Nodular goiter, thyroid neoplasia, thyrotoxicosis, and thyroiditis are the main clinical entities of concern to the thyroidologist at any age. Differences exist with regard to their incidence, presentation, and management in the elderly population.

Nodular Goiter and Thyroid Neoplasms

Clinically apparent thyroid nodules occur in upward of 7% of U.S. adults. Nodules are more commonly seen in women and their frequency increases throughout life. Thyroid nodules are also more frequently seen when the thyroid is examined at autopsy (>70% of older individuals), during surgery, or by ultrasonography [14]. Even though one-half of all clinically detected nodules are perceived as solitary by physical examination, most of these are dominant nodules in an otherwise multinodular gland. Greater than 95% of all clinically detected thyroid nodules are benign. Approximately 12,000 new cases of thyroid cancer were diagnosed in the United States in 1995 with fewer than 1,000 associated cause-specific deaths. Many of these deaths, however, occurred in elderly patients more prone to the subtypes of anaplastic, follicular, and the more biologically aggressive forms of papillary carcinoma. It therefore behooves physicians caring for elderly patients to actively evaluate a palpable thyroid mass.

In the selection of patients with nodular goiter for surgery, risks other than cancer must be considered. Cosmesis may be a factor in some older patients, but this is more often an isolated indication in a young patient with a large goiter or nodule. A goiter might enlarge to such a degree as to cause deviation of the trachea or esophagus, resulting in respiratory embarrassment or dysphagia. These symptoms may be more often attributed to other comorbid conditions (e.g., cardiopulmonary or gastrointestinal), and the role of the goiter may therefore be easily overlooked in the older patient. When a goiter is suspected, flow-volume loops, computed tomography (CT) scans, barium studies, and endoscopy may be helpful. The enlarged gland may become impinged at the thoracic inlet or may migrate into the mediastinum causing further symptoms. Spontaneous hemorrhage into a substernal goiter can lead to life-threatening airway compromise in rare situations [15]. Older patients on long-term aspirin therapy or anticoagulants may be at increased risk for this phenomenon. Hyperthyroidism occurring in association with a nodular goiter is much less common now with the overall decline of endemic goiter in this country. If left untreated for several years, however, 10% to 50% of nodular goiters give rise to clinical thyrotoxicosis, a potentially life-threatening problem in the aged that has a more subtle and confusing presentation in this age group [16].

The decision of how to manage a nodular goiter is complex and based on a number of factors, including the overall health of the patient and his or her projected well-being over time.

Selection of Patients for Thyroidectomy

The selection of patients for thyroidectomy is dependent, in part, on the history, physical examination, overall health status, thyroid function, and in many instances, the results of fine-needle aspiration cytology (FNAC).

A history of ionizing radiation to the head or neck, rapid growth of an existing nodule or a previously quiescent goiter, dysphagia, and dysphonia can be worrisome features suggestive of malignancy. Solitary nodules; firm, irregular, or fixed nodules; or nodules associated with adenopathy are more likely to be associated with malignancy. On the other hand, a painful, tender thyroid associated with systemic features (e.g., fever) is usually an indication of thyroiditis, although patients with anaplastic carcinomas can have similar features. Patients with thyrotoxicosis and a dominant nodule are likely to have a benign condition, although cancers can occur (<3%) in the setting of Graves' or Plummer's disease [17].

A family history of endocrinopathy (multiple endocrine neoplasia II [MEN II] or familial medullary thyroid carcinoma [MTC]) should prompt suspicion in a patient with a nodular goiter. MTC, as an inherited disorder, will more likely present in children and young adults. The aggressive, sporadic form is more likely to present in older patients. In the familial setting, specific screening tests would include basal and pentagastrin-stimulated calcitonin levels, 24-hour urine studies for metanephrines, and calcium-parathyroid hormone (PTH) levels in suspected MEN IIa patients. The demonstration of the RET proto-oncogene mutation is diagnostic of patients at risk for MTC in MEN IIa and familial MTC kindreds known to have this mutation [18].

All patients under evaluation for thyroid disorders should have a sensitive thyroid-stimulating hormone (sTSH) level checked. Abnormal values should be followed up with free or total thyroxine (T_4) levels. When T_4 levels are normal and sTSH is fully suppressed, serum triiodothyronine (T_3) levels should be ordered. T_3 thyrotoxicosis is not uncommon in the elderly.

Although not a surgical disorder, surgeons need to be aware of the so-called euthyroid sick syndrome [5], an entity frequently seen in hospitalized patients with severe illness, particularly among the elderly. It is characterized by low T_3 levels, normal or low T_4 levels, and variable TSH levels. It is seen in patients with sepsis, advanced neoplasia, liver failure, renal failure, and major trauma. Overzealous attempts at exogenous hormone replacement can have disastrous consequences, particularly in the elderly cardiopath. Awareness of this entity is essential, and treatment is directed at the associated cause, rather than the abnormal thyroid function test results per se.

Patients with large, benign nonfunctioning goiters associated with compressive symptoms are best managed surgically. In younger patients, near total thyroidectomy is preferred to prevent future recurrence. In older patients, bilateral subtotal thyroidectomy is quite reasonable to alleviate symptoms and minimize the risk of postoperative hypoparathyroidism.

In the past, thyroid scintigraphy, high-resolution real-time ultrasonography, and trials of L-thyroxine (LT_4) suppression therapy were used in the evaluation of thyroid nodules. Thyroid scans and ultrasonography are neither useful nor cost-effective in evaluating thyroid nodules for cancer [19]. We do not advocate LT_4 suppressive therapy, because our own double-blind randomized trial using ultrasonography for accurate measurement failed to show a significant difference in nodule size among treated and placebo groups [20].

FNAC has become the diagnostic modality of choice in patients with nodular thyroid disease [21]. In the 1970s, between 500 and 600 thyroid operations were performed each year at the Mayo Clinic. Due in large part to the introduction of FNAC in the early 1980s, this number has decreased to about 250 thyroidectomies per year. Despite this overall reduction, the total number of cancer operations has remained constant at approximately 100 per year. FNA biopsy is safe, reliable, and inexpensive ($150 to $200) when performed by an experienced team.

More than 65% of FNACs are benign (colloid nodule, lymphocytic thyroiditis) and thus eliminate the need for surgery unless other factors, such as compressive symptoms or thyrotoxicosis, warrant it. False-positive and false-negative rates have been reported at <1% [14,21]. Five percent of FNACs are malignant. These tumors, most of which require operation, are discussed under their individual headings.

Ten percent of FNACs are considered suspicious or indeterminate for malignancy. These are primarily follicular or Hürthle cell neoplasms that require histology, as opposed to cytology, for the detection of capsular and vascular invasion necessary to confirm the diagnosis of malignancy. This category may also include some papillary cancers associated with chronic lymphocytic thyroiditis, a particularly troublesome combination for the cytopathologist. Overall, 20% of suspicious fine needle aspirates turn out to be malignant. Another 10% to 30% of these nodules are either autonomously functioning at presentation or will become so, with the risk of thyrotoxicosis in the years ahead. We therefore advocate surgery for all patients in the suspicious category, assuming the patient has a reasonable life expectancy and a relatively low operative risk.

Fifteen percent to 20% of aspirates are inadequate for diagnosis. This number can be reduced by one-half with a repeat FNAC or with an ultrasound-guided FNAC. The remaining 7% to 10% of patients are then treated according to less reliable criteria, including physician and patient concern, once again taking the patient's overall general health into consideration.

Thyroid Cancer

Thyroid cancers account for <5% of all thyroid nodules. Ninety percent to 95% of all thyroid cancers are of the so-called well-differentiated type (i.e., papillary, follicular variant of papillary, and follicular). In our overall practice, 90% are papillary cancers. Follicular cancer, MTC, anaplastic carcinomas, and primary lymphomas account for the remaining 10%. Metastatic disease from breast cancer, renal cell carcinoma, and melanoma is not uncommon. These figures reflect our overall experience, but our experience in older patients is definitely slanted away from the small, low-grade, papillary cancers seen in younger patients to the higher-grade, aggressive, papillary cancers, follicular cancers, sporadic medullary carcinomas, and anaplastic cancers seen more often in older patients. Most anaplastic cancers occur in older patients, with few if any long-term survivors [22].

In a large Mayo Clinic study of >14,000 patient-years' experience, a multivariate analysis revealed four factors that were statistically significant in predicting death from papillary thyroid cancer (PTC). These are age (>50 years), tumor grade (over grade 1), tumor extent (local invasion of contiguous structures or distant metastases), and tumor size (>2 cm). Surprisingly, regional nodal metastases appear to have little bearing on overall prognosis. On the basis of the regression coefficients obtained, a scoring system was devised (age, grade, extent, size [AGES]), assigning patients to various risk groups [23]. From this calculated Mayo score, rational decisions can be made with regard to therapy. Hay et al. have recently modified the AGES system to improve its clinical utility. Completeness of surgical resection has replaced grade because the overwhelming majority of PTC is grade 1. This new scoring system, used routinely at our institution, is referred to as MACIS (metastases, age, completeness of surgical resection, invasion, and size) [24]. A formula exists from which a score can be derived. A MACIS score of <6.0 is associated with a 0.9% mortality at 20 years, whereas a score of ≥8.0 is associated with a 76.5% 20-year mortality. Although most patients fall into the low-risk categories, there is a preponderance of older patients in the less common, high-risk groups. Information gained from these scoring systems can be applied to follicular carcinomas as well. DNA ploidy has some prognostic value in patients with papillary carcinoma, but adds little to the information gained from the MACIS system [19].

Papillary Thyroid Cancer

PTC is the most commonly seen thyroid cancer. The follicular variant of PTC behaves like a papillary cancer, more so than a follicular carcinoma. Other histologic subtypes of PTC have been described; they are more aggressive and seem to occur more frequently in older patients [2]. Assuming the patient is in reasonable health with a reasonable life expectancy, surgery should be undertaken because it offers the only chance for cure as well as the best palliation. The operation for a malignant or suspicious thyroid nodule should be an ipsilateral total thyroid lobectomy and isthmectomy. With frozen-section confirmation of a PTC, we generally advocate a total or near total resection of the contralateral lobe to facilitate remnant ablation and future whole body scans, reduce the risk of local recurrence, and allow the use of serum thyroglobulin levels as a marker of recurrence. Every attempt should be made to maintain some viable parathyroid tissue. Thus, if two parathyroid glands are sacrificed on the tumor side, a small remnant of thyroid should be left behind on the contralateral side to prevent permanent hypoparathyroidism. This can always be ablated with radioiodine (RAI). Because papillary cancers spread via the lymphatic system, all patients should undergo a central compartment node dissection along the anterior trachea and tracheoesophageal grooves. Clearing these nodes at the initial operation reduces the chance of having to return to the scarred central compartment (with its attendant risks of recurrent nerve and parathyroid injury) should positive nodes develop in the future. A modified neck dissection is performed only in the setting of gross, palpable disease in the lateral neck. Unilateral lobectomy alone is probably sufficient treatment for incidentally discovered micropapillary carcinomas.

Postoperatively, all patients require lifelong T_4 replacement in suppressive doses [25]. This clearly has been shown to reduce recurrence from well-differentiated thyroid cancer. Patients at high risk for recurrence or death from PTC (based on their MACIS score) are selected for remnant ablation with RAI, follow-up whole body scans, and when metastases are present, therapeutic RAI [26]. As previously stated, older age is an independent risk factor for death from PTC and close follow-up is warranted in these patients, including chest radiography, neck ultrasound, whole body scans, and thyroglobulin level measurements. External beam radiation may be useful in patients with locally advanced disease unresponsive to surgery or RAI. We have, on occasion, in select patients, performed concomitant tracheal resections and reconstructions for contiguous involvement of the airway.

Follicular Carcinoma

The incidence of this cancer has decreased, accounting for only 5% of thyroid cancers now treated at the Mayo Clinic. Its differentiation from a follicular adenoma is dependent on the demonstration of capsular or vascular invasion. Poor prognostic indicators for follicular carcinoma include age >45 years, local invasion of contiguous neck structures, marked vascular invasion, and distant metastases (e.g., lung, bone) [27]. These tumors are more aggressive than PTC and tend to spread hematogenously, the exception being the Hürthle cell variant, which also spreads via lymphatics. Treatment includes total or near total thyroidectomy followed by RAI and lifelong LT_4 suppression. When considering T_4 replacement in suppressive doses, special care must be taken in the elderly to adjust the dose precisely to avoid cardiovascular sequelae (i.e., arrhythmia, angina, congestive heart failure, myocardial infarction) and accelerated osteoporosis [19].

Medullary Thyroid Carcinoma

MTC is a more aggressive cancer than its well-differentiated counterparts. These cancers arise from the stromal C cells and thus immunoreactive calcitonin (iCT) serves as an excellent and sensitive biochemical marker for both the diagnosis and follow-up of patients treated for MTC. Eighty percent of cases are sporadic and 20% familial. The familial variety more commonly presents in children and young adults; therefore, further discussion of this subclassification is left to other reviews.

The elevation in iCT level may be evident in the unstimulated (basal) state or following stimulation with pentagastrin or calcium. Because, unlike well-differentiated thyroid cancers, the tumor cells do not take up RAI and because of a high incidence of multicentricity, total thyroidectomy is the operation of choice for MTC. MTC has the propensity to spread to regional nodes, so that a central compartment node dissection should always be performed. Modified neck dissections are performed for biopsy-proven, positive, lateral neck nodes. Once nodal disease has occurred, the chance for cure is at best remote. Aggressive surgical debulking has been the mainstay of treatment of this disease. Factors correlated with a poor outcome include TNM stages III or IV, tumor unresectability, male gender, negative tissue amyloid staining, three or more positive nodes, nondiploid or high S-phase tumors, and low preoperative iCT levels [28–30]. Carcinoembryonic antigen levels, when high, may actually provide a better indicator of disease bulk than do iCT levels. MTC has been shown to secrete a variety of bioactive amines and peptides including adrenocorticotropic hormone, vasoactive intestinal peptide, serotonin, and somatostatin [31]. Following seemingly successful surgery for MTC, persistent hypercalcitoninemia appears to be the rule rather than the exception. In the absence of radiographic or clinically apparent disease, 5- and 10-year survival rates of 90% and 86%, respectively, have been reported [28]. With the liberal use of neck ultrasound, CT, magnetic resonance imaging (MRI), venous sampling, and OctreoScans (these detect tumor cells rich in specific somatostatin receptors), resectable disease confined to limited regions is being identified with increasing frequency. Only long-term follow-up will tell whether an aggressive surgical approach will prolong survival and achieve more cures.

Anaplastic Carcinoma

Anaplastic carcinomas occur in several cellular types, all of which are undifferentiated [22]. They grow rapidly, often arising in a preexisting lifelong goiter, spread to tissues both adjacent to and distant from the thyroid gland, and result in the demise of their victims in a short period of time. Although this entity accounts for the smallest number of primary thyroid cancers, the majority of anaplastic cancers occur in older patients. Most patients die of the disease in 12 months, and almost all die within 36 months. Controversy may exist as to whether surgical intervention is justified. Even though surgery is not curative, debulking the tumor may have some value in freeing up the trachea, protecting the airway, and allowing for the establishment of a tracheostomy, if indicated. This might also permit more effective use of external beam radiation. Multidisciplinary approaches, combining surgery, radiotherapy, and chemotherapy, are under investigation, but no major breakthroughs have occurred with regard to this subgroup of tumors with such a dismal prognosis.

Thyroid Lymphoma

Primary lymphomas of the thyroid gland are generally of the large cell, non-Hodgkin's type [32]. They are rarely localized to the thyroid parenchyma itself and are often associated with regional lymphadenopathy. The role of the surgeon is primarily to establish the diagnosis. FNAC results may be suspicious for lymphoma, but it can be very difficult to differentiate lymphoma from chronic lymphocytic thyroiditis, thereby necessitating an open biopsy to obtain sufficient tissue for histology and lymphocyte tumor markers. Once the diagnosis has been established, treatment involves radiation, chemotherapy, or both, depending on the stage of the disease. Rare localized thyroid lymphomas can be successfully treated by total thyroidectomy alone.

Metastatic Disease to the Thyroid

Metastases from breast cancer, renal cell carcinoma, and melanoma are common to the thyroid gland, particularly during the late stages of the disease. Diagnosis can often be confirmed by FNAC, with surgery reserved for the rare isolated metastasis or in selected individuals with acute airway compromise.

THYROTOXICOSIS (GRAVES' DISEASE AND PLUMMER'S DISEASE)

There are numerous causes of thyrotoxicosis including factitious, iatrogenic, and drug-induced (amiodarone) causes; pituitary problems; ovarian processes; and molar pregnancy. Obviously iatrogenic causes must be avoided or minimized by careful attention to sTSH levels in older patients on exogenous LT_4. The thyrotoxicosis associated with amiodarone is worthy of mention [33]. Amiodarone is a potent third-line drug in the management of intractable ventricular arrhythmias, a problem not uncommon in the elderly. It is thyrolytic and ultimately causes hypothyroidism. In the early stage of this process, patients may become thyrotoxic. If the drug cannot be stopped, and usually it cannot, surgery is the only effective treatment (bilateral near total thyroidectomy). These patients are among the highest risk endocrine patients we see, but our experience has been that of very low perioperative mortality and morbidity. Careful anesthetic and fluid management is essential. These patients are at risk for amiodarone pulmonary toxicity as well, so high FiO_2 levels must be avoided perioperatively.

Far and away, the two most important causes of hyperthyroidism are Graves' disease and Plummer's disease. Graves' disease, or exophthalmic goiter, is the most common cause of thyrotoxicosis in this country. Plummer's disease (toxic multinodular goiter or toxic adenoma) is the most common cause of hyperthyroidism in older patients.

The clinical presentation of hyperthyroidism in the elderly is often quite different from the hypermetabolic state seen in young patients and characterized by anxiety, nervousness, sweating, and hyperactivity. In contrast, older patients are often depressed, lethargic, or apathetic. Eye findings are usually not apparent. The increased appetite; heat intolerance; moist, warm skin; and increased stool frequency seen in younger patients are often replaced with anorexia, cold intolerance, dry skin, and constipation thought to be a consequence of old age and not hyperthyroidism. Associated illnesses and prescription drugs (e.g., beta blockers) may mask some of the more common manifestations. This clinical scenario, often seen in the elderly is best termed *apathetic* or *masked hyperthyroidism* [1]. Older patients are more likely to present with congestive heart failure, refractory atrial fibrillation, angina pectoris, digitalis toxicity, and rarely with systemic emboli (Table 16-1). Thyroid function tests (including T_3 levels) should be checked routinely in these patients.

TABLE 16-1. *Typical manifestations of thyrotoxicosis in young versus old subjects*

Young	Old
Anxiety	Depression
Nervousness	Lethargy
Sweating	Dry skin
Hyperactivity	Apathy
Eye findings present	Eye findings absent
Increased appetite	Anorexia
Heat intolerance	Cold intolerance
Moist, warm skin	Constipation
Increased stool frequency	Congestive heart failure
	Refractory atrial fibrillation
	Refractory angina pectoris
	Digitalis toxicity
	Systemic emboli
	Worsening diabetes
	Abdominal pain

Patients with Graves' disease can be treated with surgery or RAI after appropriate preparation with beta blockers, Lugol's iodine, and, on occasion, antithyroid drugs. RAI has become the treatment of choice for Graves' disease in this country except in pregnant women requiring definitive treatment and patients refusing its use. RAI avoids surgery and its associated risks, albeit low, and is quite effective for managing patients with small- to medium-sized glands. This is true for older patients as well, and in frail elderly patients with mild Graves' disease, RAI is our choice as well. On the other hand, surgery is the most rapid way to alleviate the hyperthyroid state in patients with severe disease and large gland disease. Surgery is also the treatment of choice for Graves' disease associated with a hypofunctioning nodule when the risk of malignancy is increased [1]. Whereas the hypothyroidism associated with RAI treatment is often insidious (a potential problem in the elderly) its occurrence after surgery is far more predictable, a potential advantage for surgery in the elderly. Thyroidectomy for Graves' disease is technically challenging. The gland is firm, less mobile, and of increased vascularity. Preoperative preparation with Lugol's iodine reduces this vascularity, but not entirely. Such glands typically are associated with several enlarged, firm paratracheal nodes that make identification of parathyroid glands and recurrent nerves more difficult. Experienced surgeons, however, can perform this procedure with acceptable morbidity. We currently favor total lobectomy on one side and subtotal resection on the opposite side, in contrast to the bilateral subtotal resections performed in the past. The operation is less bloody, parathyroid function is preserved, hypothyroidism generally ensues rapidly, and thyroid hormone replacement can be regulated early when the patient is still under observation during recuperation from surgery. Hypothyroidism should no longer be considered a complication of surgery.

At the other end of the spectrum are patients with solitary toxic adenomas. These too can be treated surgically or with RAI. Our preference is surgery (i.e., unilateral lobectomy) in patients with an acceptable anesthetic risk [12]. Surgery is curative, eliminates the nodule, is low risk, and is associated with a low incidence of postoperative hypothyroidism. In a recent study from the Mayo Clinic comparing the two treatment modalities for solitary toxic nodules, no surgically treated patient had nodule recurrence or required re-treatment [12]. Over 40% had persistence of the nodule after RAI and 9% required re-treatment. No surgical complications occurred, and the incidence of hypothyroidism was lower in the surgically treated group (22% versus 35%).

Toxic multinodular goiters can be managed with surgery (similar to Graves' patients) or RAI as well [11]. Surgical complication rates are quite acceptable in experienced hands. Toxic multinodular glands often display low uptake of RAI as compared with Graves' disease patients. The probability of success by 1 and 5 years after surgery is significantly better than with RAI (64% vs. 95%, 70% vs. 97%, respectively). The probability of requiring re-treatment by 1 year is 0% for surgery and 24% with RAI. Post-treatment hypothyroidism is similar in both groups (16%). Our preference is to render the patient hypothyroid with a total lobectomy on one side and a subtotal or near total resection on the opposite side. Obviously, patients too frail to undergo anesthesia should be given RAI. Patients with acceptable anesthetic risks, large glands, severe symptomatology, compressive symptoms, or associated nodules suspicious for malignancy should be treated surgically.

THYROIDITIS

Fibrous Thyroiditis or Riedel's Struma

Fibrous thyroiditis or Riedel's struma occurs infrequently, but when it does, it is almost always in the elderly. Actually, it is seen once in approximately 2,000 thyroidectomies carried out for all causes. On palpation, it appears as a firm to hard thyroid gland that is somewhat fixed to adjacent tissues. Because of its physical characteristics, it is impossible to rule out the presence of a cancer. Even though needle or aspiration biopsy might be considered, often the gland is so hard that in this condition, like in so many others, this diagnostic approach is unsuccessful. For this reason, and in particular, to rule out the chance that a cancer is present, thyroidectomy is indicated. At the time of the operation when fibrous thyroiditis is found, it is reasonable to resect a part of the lesion and to free up the trachea. It is not essential that the total thyroid gland be removed, and no adjacent tissues that might be involved need be removed. Following the surgical procedure, in certain incidences, corticosteroids might be given with the hope that they will further reduce the fibrous and inflammatory process.

Subacute Granulomatous Thyroiditis or de Quervain's Thyroiditis

Subacute granulomatous thyroiditis, or de Quervain's thyroiditis, usually starts in one area of the thyroid gland as a painful, tender mass and then gradually involves other parts of the thyroid gland. Most often, this thyroiditis can be identified and diagnosed by its historical and physical characteristics. FNAC is usually confirmatory. Surgical treatment is not necessary. Actually, given a short period varying from a few weeks to several months, the process will "burn" itself out. Corticosteroids may be of some benefit in the treatment of the worst symptoms and appear to have a beneficial effect on reducing the pathologic process.

Hashimoto's Thyroiditis or Chronic Lymphocytic Thyroiditis

Hashimoto's thyroiditis, or chronic lymphocytic thyroiditis, is seen in older age groups much more frequently than in the young. This autoimmune disorder is the most common cause of hypothyroidism in the United States. In Hashimoto's thyroiditis, the thyroid gland can vary considerably in size. Some patients have glands that are normal size and weight, and others with this disease will have glands that weigh 100 g or more. The gland is rubbery and often has a bosselated surface. This can be appreciated on physical examination, and the process is often suspected. Most often, the entire gland is involved. When this condition is suspected, a needle biopsy will usually substantiate the diagnosis. Serum thyroid antibodies are typically present.

Unless there are symptoms related to the presence of a goiter, surgical treatment is not indicated. However, all patients with suspected Hashimoto's thyroiditis should be placed on T_4 therapy using replacement doses of exogenous T_4. These patients should then be followed carefully because, in a certain number of glands with lymphocytic thyroiditis, coexisting neoplasms occur. Clark et al. have stated that patients with Hashimoto's thyroiditis can be separated into those at low risk and those at high risk for cancer. Those glands having a dominant cold nodule have a 25% chance of having cancer [34]. In 605 cases of lymphocytic thyroiditis operated on at our institution, papillary cancer coexisted in 3% of the cases and lymphoma coexisted in another 3% [35]. Because of this experience, we believe that it is essential for a patient with Hashimoto's thyroiditis who is being treated medically to be followed very carefully. If the gland does not significantly reduce or if it becomes apparent that a discrete nodule is present or developing, then FNAC, thyroidectomy, or both should be carried out and the underlying pathology treated appropriately. If a malignant lesion is not found to be present at the time of the surgical exploration, a subtotal thyroidectomy only is indicated. These patients should then be placed again on thyroid replacement therapy in euthyroid doses.

Complications of Thyroidectomy

The complications of thyroidectomy can be divided into those that are specific and nonspecific in nature.

Bleeding, infection, and anesthetic complications occur in <1% of all cases. Cervical hematoma can be a life-threatening complication resulting in rapid asphyxiation if left untreated. In the emergency setting, the incision should be reopened at the bedside to alleviate tracheal obstruction. In less severe situations, the patient can be returned to the operating room with proper control of the airway, evacuation of the hematoma, and control of the bleeding site(s).

With proper attention to detail, recurrent laryngeal nerve injury rarely occurs. Exposure of the nerve throughout its course in the neck is the best way to avoid injury. Stretching injuries are sometimes difficult to avoid, especially when dealing with large tumors or immobile glands. This type of injury (neuropraxia) almost always resolves with time. Occasionally, a nerve has to be sacrificed when involved by tumor. Unilateral cord paralysis is not life-threatening, but can result in significant hoarseness and dysphagia to liquids. Bilateral cord paralysis results in airway obstruction from the adducted position of both cords. This often requires tracheostomy. Most neuropraxias resolve with time, and many unilateral cord paralyses go unnoticed as a result of contralateral cord compensation. Preoperative vocal cord examinations should always be performed in the reoperative setting. If improvement does not occur within 6 to 8 months, Teflon augmentation or type I thyroplasty can be performed with reasonable success.

More often than we would like to admit, the external branch of the superior laryngeal nerve is probably damaged where it approximates the superior pole vessels on its way to innervate the tensor muscle (cricothyroideus) of the cords. Although these patients' voices sound normal, public speakers and singers may have significant difficulty raising their voices. The best way to avoid injury to this delicate slender nerve is to individually ligate the superior pole vessels on the thyroid capsule, avoiding mass ligation of the superior pedicle.

Permanent hypoparathyroidism is probably the most troublesome complication following extensive thyroidectomy. This occurs in 2% to 4% of patients. Temporary hypoparathyroidism is much more common, lasting only a few weeks to months following thyroidectomy. This can usually be managed with oral calcium and vitamin D supplementation. The best way, however, to avoid this problem is careful identification of these glands and preservation of their delicate blood supply by avoiding unnecessary handling. Although these glands can obtain collateral blood flow from tracheal and esophageal arterial tributaries, it is probably better to ligate the terminal branches of the inferior thyroid artery beyond the parathyroid branches, rather than ligate the proximal inferior thyroid artery. In select cases, total thyroidectomy is appropriate, provided the surgeon can be sure that at least one or two viable parathyroid glands can be left in situ.

When, because of their location, parathyroid glands must be removed, they can be minced into 1-mm pieces (provided tumor is not involved) and autotransplanted into small muscular pockets within the sternocleidomastoid muscle. Over 80% of these grafts function in time [36]. Before autotransplantation, a tiny confirmatory biopsy should be performed.

In the early postoperative period, we reserve treatment of hypoparathyroidism for those patients with serum calcium levels <7.5 mg/dl and for those patients with symptoms (e.g., numbness, tingling, muscle twitching, and irritability). Seizures and tetany are the most dreaded complications. Most patients can be managed with oral calcium supplementation. For those who cannot, intravenous calcium gluconate given slowly or by continuous infusion, via a well-established intravenous site, is the preferred route. Chronic hypoparathyroidism is managed by oral calcium, vitamin D, phosphate binders, and a low phosphorus diet.

Summary

Thyroid cancer, nontoxic multinodular goiters, and hyperthyroidism all occur in the elderly population. The spectrum of thyroid cancer seen in older patients is different and more often biologically aggressive. The symptoms of a large compressive goiter may be mistaken for other conditions in the aged population. The early manifestations of hyperthyroidism may be masked in the elderly and written off as signs and symptoms of general old age. The sequelae of such a missed diagnosis can be more profound in the elderly with the development of congestive heart failure, refractory angina, arrhythmia, myocardial infarction, or stroke. The evaluation of the thyroid gland is similar at all ages, but special attention must be given to all other major systems in the elderly patient facing thyroid surgery. With current anesthetic management, thyroid surgery can be carried out safely and effectively with low morbidity and mortality. Adequate preparation, fine tuning techniques, and meticulous attention to detail are imperative for success. Chronologic age alone should not be a deterrent for older patients who may derive the same benefits from successful thyroid surgery as their younger counterparts.

PRIMARY HYPERPARATHYROIDISM

Incidence and Prevalence

Primary hyperparathyroidism is a common endocrine disorder in the elderly. Its overall prevalence is 0.1% in the population as a whole, with female subjects outnumbering male subjects by approximately two to one [10]. Older women show an annual incidence of 188 per 100,000 compared with only 25 per 100,000 for the entire population. The prevalence of the disorder among women over the age of 60 has been estimated to be as high as 1.5%.

Etiology and Pathogenesis

The etiology of primary hyperparathyroidism has not been established. Familial forms of the disease, namely familial hyperparathyroidism and hyperparathyroidism associated with MEN types I and IIa have been well described. This genetic disorder may be caused by defective enzymes regulating transcription or translation of hormone synthesis. Because chronic hypocalcemia appears to be the stimulus for the development of secondary hyperparathyroidism in patients with chronic renal failure and long-standing osteomalacia, one can hypothesize that primary hyperparathyroidism as seen in the elderly may somehow be related to prolonged parathyroid stimulation resulting from decreased intestinal absorption of calcium over time [10]. These theories, however, remain just that.

Pathology

Eighty-five percent to 90% of patients with primary hyperparathyroidism have single-gland disease [10,37,38]. The remaining patients have primary hyperplasia (10%) involving all four glands symmetrically or asymmetrically, double adenomas (2% to 5%), or parathyroid carcinoma (<1%). Patients with familial, non-MEN, and MEN causes of hyperparathyroidism have multigland disease, but the vast majority of cases of primary hyperplasia remain sporadic. Because virtually all familial cases present with hypercalcemia at a young age, no further attempt is made to discuss these specific subgroups.

Clinical Presentation

The clinical presentation of patients with primary hyperparathyroidism is varied and protean. In the past, cases of primary hyperparathyroidism tended to be more severe, with the classic description of "bones, stones, groans, and psychic moans." With the advent of serial blood chemistry screening, the cases seen today usually have far less pronounced symptoms. In the elderly population, fatigue, muscle weakness, and various central nervous system disturbances, all manifestations of hyperparathyroidism, may be confused with normal aging. Constipation, anorexia, nausea, dyspepsia, weakness, and generalized aches and pains are more common presentations in symptomatic elderly persons. Kidney stones are noted in only a minority of elderly patients as compared with their younger counterparts [10]. Declining renal function, however, may be a manifestation of hyperparathyroidism in the elderly. The classic bone changes termed *osteitis fibrosa cystica* are unusual except in severe long-standing cases of the disease. On the other hand, severe osteopenia and accelerated osteoporosis are common manifestations among the elderly with the increased risk of vertebral compression fractures [10]. In elderly patients, depression, personality changes, or impaired cognition may be caused by primary hyperparathyroidism. The diagnosis should always be considered in the elderly demented patient [37]. Typical manifestations of hyperparathyroidism in the elderly are presented in Table 16-2.

TABLE 16-2. *Typical manifestations of hyperparathyroidism*

Fatigue
Muscle weakness
Constipation
Anorexia
Nausea
Dyspepsia
Weakness
Generalized aches and pains
Declining renal function
Severe osteopenia, osteoporosis
Vertebral crush fractures
Depression
Personality changes
Impaired cognition
Kidney stones (rare)

Other Causes for Hypercalcemia in the Elderly

In the elderly patient, the workup for suspected primary hyperparathyroidism generally revolves around the exclusion of other causes of hypercalcemia. In the aged population, two common causes for hypercalcemia must be excluded before focusing on the diagnosis of primary hyperparathyroidism [2,10]. These two causes are the ingestion of thiazide diuretics and malignancy-associated causes with or without metastatic disease. Thiazide diuretics, commonly used for the treatment of hypertension, decrease urinary excretion of calcium, thereby raising serum calcium levels to a modest degree. Cessation of thiazide diuretics for a brief period results in the normalization of the serum calcium level in otherwise healthy patients.

Malignancy-associated causes include solid tumors (e.g., of the breast, lung, kidneys, and ovaries) as well as hematologic malignancies (multiple myeloma and lymphoma). Hypercalcemia can be caused from lytic bone metastases typically associated with breast and lung cancer, as well as with multiple myeloma. Lymphomas produce an osteoclast-activating factor responsible for the hypercalcemic state and still other tumors produce PTH or a PTH-related peptide capable of causing hypercalcemia (squamous cell carcinoma of the lung, islet cell tumors, and renal cell carcinoma).

Asymptomatic hypercalcemia is generally not associated with malignancy. It is rarely if ever the first manifestation of an underlying cancer. On the other hand, a long-standing history of hypercalcemia is more often associated with primary hyperparathyroidism. Chest radiography, skeletal surveys, and bone scans are all useful in ruling out underlying malignancy as is the serum protein electrophoresis for ruling out multiple myeloma. However, the most important clue for ruling in malignancy-associated hypercalcemia is an antecedent history of an underlying malignancy. Other less common causes for hypercalcemia include vitamin A and D intoxication, milk-alkali syndrome, sarcoidosis, prolonged immobilization, lithium therapy, and hyperthyroidism.

Laboratory Studies

The typical laboratory findings in patients with primary hyperparathyroidism include hypercalcemia and hypophosphatemia because of the physiologic effects of PTH at the skeletal and renal level. The availability of an immunochemoluminescent assay capable of measuring the intact PTH molecule has made the diagnosis of primary hyperparathyroidism highly accurate and relatively easy. All other causes of hypercalcemia are associated with low or undetectable PTH levels because of normal negative feedback mechanisms. In patients with primary hyperparathyroidism, hypercalcemia is associated with inappropriate levels of intact PTH. Although the diagnosis is secure with elevated levels of intact PTH, the diagnosis can also be made when the PTH level is in the high normal range. Benign familial hypocalciuric hypercalcemia (BFHH) patients can have calcium, phosphorus, and PTH levels similar to those in patients with primary hyperparathyroidism. This rare inherited disorder results from faulty end-organ responsiveness to calcium and is not subject to the same sequelae as patients with primary hyperparathyroidism. Surgery is neither successful nor indicated in patients with BFHH. Before operating on someone with primary hyperparathyroidism, a 24-hour urine calcium collection should be obtained because patients with BFHH typically have a low urine calcium excretion, whereas patients with primary hyperparathyroidism typically have elevated 24-hour urine calcium levels. If in doubt, screening of first-degree relatives for hypercalcemic hypocalciuria may be indicated. Once the diagnosis of primary hyperparathyroidism has been established, a kidney, ureter, and bladder screen with renal tomography and occasionally bone mineral densitometry are performed to complete the assessment of the patient with primary hyperparathyroidism.

Indications for Surgery

The next major issue is the need for surgery. At present, surgery is the only cure for primary hyperparathyroidism. Numerous medical therapies exist for the management of hypercalcemia [2,10], but these are, at best, temporizing, not without risk, and unable to completely reverse all of the manifestations of primary hyperparathyroidism. These medical therapies are best suited for the control of malignancy-associated hypercalcemia or in primary hyperparathyroidism patients with a limited life expectancy from other causes.

The selection criteria for surgery are controversial. Because of exceedingly high cure rates and low reported morbidity from centers specializing in the care of patients with primary hyperparathyroidism, one school of thought favors surgical intervention for all patients with a clear-cut biochemical diagnosis of primary hyperparathyroidism, regardless of whether the patient is seemingly asymptomatic [13]. The foremost conclusion of the National Institutes of Health consensus conference was that surgery is the best treatment for primary hyperparathyroidism [39]. However, the panel thought that there is a population of patients with primary hyperparathyroidism who can be safely followed and managed medically. Patients with only mildly elevated serum calcium levels (<12 mg/dl), no prior episodes of severe hypercalcemia, and normal renal and bone status are eligible for nonoperative management. In a report from the Mayo Clinic, 384 consecutive patients with primary hyperparathyroidism were surgically treated during a 2-year period. The overall cure rate was 99.5% with an operative mortality of 0.3% and a complication rate of <1% [13]. Because there is no effective medical therapy that can cure this condition, surgery, in our opinion, is the only viable option in patients with a reasonable life expectancy and an acceptable anesthetic risk. In addition, many patients deemed asymptomatic are, in fact, not without symptoms. These patients may have subtle symptoms including memory loss, personality changes, inability to concentrate, excessive fatigue, and nonspecific musculoskeletal pains that may improve following successful surgery. This is particularly true in the elderly population. We also consider surgery as a good form of preventive medicine that is more cost-effective than long-term medical follow-up. There is also evidence that even patients with mild hyperparathyroidism are at increased risk for premature death. Surgery may benefit these patients as well.

Localization Studies

Once the diagnosis has been established and the decision has been made to proceed with surgery, another area of controversy centers on the role of preoperative localization studies. In experienced hands, successful localization and cure of the patient occurs in >95% of patients without the aid of preoperative localization studies in first-time cervical explorations. Preoperative localization studies include ultrasonography, CT scanning, sestamibi scans, MRI, and venous sampling [40]. None of these studies has been as successful at identifying abnormal parathyroid pathology when compared with an experienced parathyroid surgeon, nor do they shorten the time of cervical exploration [40]. We would therefore not recommend the routine use of preoperative localization in first-time neck explorations. There are, however, some exceptions. Patients on lithium therapy for bipolar affective disorders can have a biochemical picture compatible with primary hyperparathyroidism. If cessation of lithium therapy is not a viable option, the use of two confirmatory localization studies is helpful in deciding whether to embark on a cervical exploration (ultrasonography and sestamibi scan). Another situation in which preoperative localization is appropriate is in the patient who arrives in the emergency room comatose from a hypercalcemic crisis. Bedside ultrasonography in the emergency room can confirm the diagnosis of primary hyperparathyroidism because patients with this degree of hypercalcemia, in general, have a large cervical adenoma. After rapid rehydration, emergent cervical exploration and excision of the involved parathyroid gland will restore calcium homeostasis in the most effective and rapid manner.

In reoperations where tissue planes are scarred and the risks of recurrent nerve injury and permanent hypoparathyroidism are increased, the liberal use of preoperative localization studies becomes much more important [41]. In general in the reoperative setting, we like to have an ultrasound-guided FNAC of the lesion in question or combined positive ultrasound and sestamibi scan results, thus facilitating a direct approach to the abnormal area of concern without disturbing other areas in the neck.

Surgical Management

The surgical management of primary hyperparathyroidism is usually fairly straightforward but can be technically challenging. To be a successful parathyroid surgeon, one must have a clear-cut understanding of the embryology and anatomy of the parathyroid glands and their relations. The superior parathyroid glands arise from the fourth branchial pouch and are generally located on the posteromedial aspect of the thyroid capsule near its superior pole. Superior glands, however, can migrate into the posterior mediastinum such that abnormal glands may be found along the tracheoesophageal groove, behind the esophagus, or well down in the posterior mediastinum. The inferior parathyroid glands originate from the third branchial pouch in association with the thymus gland. When they overdescend, they may end up along the trachea or within the anterior mediastinum adjacent to or within the thymus gland. Occasionally, they will not descend in association with an undescended thymus gland and will be in a position near the angle of the jaw, carotid bifurcation, and hyoid bone. Other locations for aberrant parathyroid tissue include the carotid sheath and within the thyroid substance itself, usually just below the thyroid capsule. It has been our experience that only 2% to 3% of patients with primary hyperparathyroidism have tumors out of the reach of the collar incision, deep within the mediastinum. Mediastinal parathyroid glands are usually located within the thymus, posterior to the thymus along the aortic arch, along the tracheobronchial tree, or rarely within the aorticopulmonary window. These tumors are generally approached through a median sternotomy, but successful removal of these tumors can sometimes be achieved through a limited thoracotomy or thoracoscopy.

We strongly advocate bilateral cervical exploration to view all four glands and to rule out the possibility of a double adenoma or asymmetric hyperplasia. In patients with single-gland disease, the solitary adenoma is excised after identifying three other normal parathyroid glands. A biopsy of one normal parathyroid gland is acceptable but not necessary. Excessive handling of the normal parathyroid glands can lead to unnecessary prolonged postoperative hypoparathyroidism. In patients with multigland disease, a subtotal parathyroidectomy is performed (3.5 glands) with maintenance of a 50-mg remnant of viable parathyroid tissue. A portion of the excised tissue should be cryopreserved should the remaining remnant fail and the patient develop persistent postoperative hypoparathyroidism. The cryopreserved tissue can be minced into 1-mm cubes and transplanted into the forearm musculature with reasonable success rates. Patients with multigland disease must understand that the risk for recurrent hyperparathyroidism is in the range of 20% because the tissue left behind remains hyperplastic. A transcervical thymectomy should also be performed in patients with multigland disease because 10% to 15% of patients have a fifth gland within the mediastinal soft tissue.

The use of an intraoperative PTH assay may be especially helpful in patients with multigland disease and in those undergoing reoperations for confirming the adequacy of tissue ablation [41]. In patients having undergone numerous unsuccessful operations or in patients too frail to undergo anesthesia, ultrasound-guided alcohol ablation of abnormal parathyroid glands has been performed with low complication rates and reasonable success [19].

Functioning parathyroid cysts should be excised in a similar fashion to functioning adenomas. Nonfunctioning parathyroid cysts, with their characteristic clear and colorless fluid and calcium richness, can be diagnosed and treated by FNAC. Carcinomas of the parathyroid gland are exceedingly rare but highly lethal [42]. Appropriate management includes parathyroidectomy with an ipsilateral thyroid lobectomy and concomitant central node dissection. Modified neck dissection is performed only in the presence of biopsy-proven metastatic disease in lateral cervical nodes. Patients generally succumb to the local complications of recurrent parathyroid carcinoma as well as from the sequelae of uncontrolled hypercalcemia.

Complications of Parathyroid Surgery

Postoperative hypocalcemia following successful parathyroidectomy is the rule rather than the exception. In most cases, it is mild and the serum calcium level returns to the low normal range within 48 to 72 hours. This initial low serum calcium level is reassurance that the patient has been cured. In some cases, however, the hypocalcemia is more profound (<7.0 mg/dl). Two possibilities exist: hypoparathyroidism or bone hunger. Patients with hypoparathyroidism develop a high serum phosphorus level, whereas patients with the hungry bone syndrome maintain a low serum phosphorus level. Patients with preexisting bone disease, elevated alkaline phosphatase, and large adenomas are at greater risk for bone hunger postoperatively. Significant hypoparathyroidism following parathyroidectomy is usually a result of excessive handling of the remaining normal parathyroid glands. This should be avoided if at all possible. Permanent hypocalcemia following initial cervical exploration should be <1% to 2% of all cases. The other complications of parathyroidectomy are similar to those seen with thyroidectomy and should be exceedingly low. In the elderly, symptoms of postoperative hypocalcemia may be less pronounced [10] (perioral or digital numbness and tingling); therefore, special attention should be paid to twice daily (or more often) monitoring of serum calcium levels to avoid undue complications (tetany). Ionized calcium levels may be of greater value in the elderly, hypoalbuminemic patient.

Summary

Primary hyperparathyroidism is relatively common in the elderly, particularly among women. Many of its clinical manifestations may be subtle and confused with normal aging. Surgery, however, remains the only chance for cure, and the benefits derived from successful surgery are as important in the aged as they are in the young. The success of surgery and postoperative recovery is not as dependent on the age of the patient as it is on the experience of the surgeon.

REFERENCES

1. Kabadi UM. Thyroid disorders and the elderly. Compr Ther 1989;15:53–65.
2. Whitman ED, Norton JA. Endocrine surgical disease of elderly patients. Surg Clin North Am 1994;74:127–144.
3. Sawin CT. Thyroid dysfunction in older persons. Adv Intern Med 1992;37:223–248.
4. Francis T, Wartofsky L. Common thyroid disorders in the elderly. Postgrad Med 1992;92:225–236.
5. Bartuska DG. Thyroid disease in the elderly. Hosp Pract 1991; 26:85–107.
6. Levy EG. Thyroid disease in the elderly. Med Clin North Am 1991; 75:151–167.
7. Feit H. Thyroid function in the elderly. Clin Geriatr Med 1988;4: 151–161.
8. Mokshagundam S, Barzel US. Thyroid disease in the elderly. J Am Geriatr Soc 1993;41:1361–1369.
9. Gambert SR. Atypical presentation of thyroid disease in the elderly. Geriatrics 1985;40:63–69.
10. Kochersberger G. Primary hyperparathyroidism in the elderly. Compr Ther 1988;14:24–29.
11. Jensen MD, Gharib H, Naessen JM, et al. Treatment of toxic multinodular goiter (Plummer's disease): surgery or radioiodine? World J Surg 1986;10:673–680.
12. O'Brien T, Gharib H, Suman VJ, van Heerden JA. Treatment of toxic solitary thyroid nodules: surgery versus radioactive iodine. Surgery 1992;112:1166–1170.
13. van Heerden JA, Grant CS. Surgical treatment of primary hyperparathyroidism: an institutional perspective. World J Surg 1991;15: 688–692.
14. Gharib H, Goellner JR. Fine-needle aspiration biopsy of the thyroid: an appraisal [see comments]. Ann Intern Med 1993;118:282–289.
15. Katlic MR, Wang CA, Grillo HC. Substernal goiter. Ann Thorac Surg 1985;39:391–399.
16. Blum M, Shenkman L, Hollander CS. The autonomous nodule of the thyroid: correlation of patient age, nodule size and functional status. Am J Med Sci 1975;269:43–50.
17. Beahrs OH, Pemberton JJ, Black BM. Nodular goiter and malignant lesions of the thyroid gland. J Clin Endocrinol 1951;11:1157–1165.
18. Tsai MS, Ledger GA, Khosla S, et al. Identification of multiple endocrine neoplasia, type II gene carriers using linkage analysis and analysis of the RET proto-oncogene. J Clin Endocrinol Metab 1994;78:1261–1264.
19. Thompson GB, Beahrs OH. Surgery of the Thyroid and Parathyroid Glands. In Thawley SE, Panje WR (eds), Comprehensive Management of Head and Neck Tumors. Philadelphia: Saunders, 1997.
20. Gharib H, James EM, Charboneau JW, et al. Suppressive therapy with levothyroxine for solitary thyroid nodules. A double-blind controlled clinical study. N Engl J Med 1987;317:70–75.
21. Grant CS, Hay ID, Gough IR, et al. Long-term follow-up of patients with benign thyroid fine-needle aspiration cytologic diagnoses. Surgery 1989;106:980–986.
22. Demeter JG, De Jong SA, Lawrence AM, Paloyan E. Anaplastic thyroid carcinoma: risk factors and outcome. Surgery 1991;110:956–963.
23. Hay ID, Grant CS, Taylor WF, McConahey WM. Ipsilateral lobectomy versus bilateral lobar resection of papillary thyroid carcinoma: a retrospective analysis of surgical outcome using a novel prognostic scoring system. Surgery 1987;102:1088–1095.
24. Hay ID, Bergstralh EJ, Goellner JR, et al. Predicting outcome in papillary thyroid carcinoma: development of a reliable prognostic scoring system in a cohort of 1779 patients surgically treated at one institution during 1940 through 1989. Surgery 1993;114:1050–1057.
25. Clark OH. TSH suppression in the management of thyroid nodules and thyroid cancer. World J Surg 1981;5:39–47.
26. McHenry C, Jarosz H, Davis M, et al. Selective postoperative radioactive iodine treatment of thyroid carcinoma. Surgery 1989;106:956–959.
27. Harness JK, Thompson NW, McLeod MK, et al. Follicular carcinoma of the thyroid gland: trends and treatment. Surgery 1984;96:972–980.
28. van Heerden JA, Grant CS, Gharib H, et al. Long-term course of patients with persistent hypercalcitoninemia after apparent curative primary surgery for medullary thyroid carcinoma. Ann Surg 1990;212:395–401.
29. Hay ID, Ryan JJ, Grant CS, et al. Prognostic significance of nondiploid DNA determined by flow cytometry in sporadic and familial medullary thyroid carcinoma. Surgery 1990;108:972–980.
30. Pyke CM, Hay ID, Goellner JR, et al. Prognostic significance of calcitonin immunoreactivity, amyloid staining, and flow cytometric DNA measurements in medullary thyroid carcinoma [see comments]. Surgery 1991;110:964–971.
31. Tiede DJ, Tefferi A, Kochhar R, et al. Paraneoplastic cholestasis and hypercoagulability associated with medullary thyroid carcinoma. Resolution with tumor debulking. Cancer 1994;73:702–705.
32. Rasbach DA, Mondschein MS, Harris NL, et al. Malignant lymphoma of the thyroid gland: a clinical and pathologic study of twenty cases. Surgery 1985;98:1166–1170.
33. Brennan MD, van Heerden JA, Carney JA. Amiodarone-associated thyrotoxicosis (AAT): experience with surgical management. Surgery 1987;102:1062–1067.
34. Clark OH, Greenspan FS, Dunphy FE. Hashimoto's thyroiditis and thyroid cancer: Indications for operation. Am J Surg 1980;140:65–71.
35. Woolner LB, McConahey WM, Beahrs OH. Struma lymphomatosa and related thyroidal disorders. J Clin Endocrinol Metab 1959;9:53–83.
36. Edis AJ, Linos DA, Kao PC. Parathyroid autotransplantation at the time of reoperation for persistent hyperparathyroidism. Surgery 1980;88:588.
37. Sier HC, Hartnell J, Morley JE, et al. Primary hyperparathyroidism and delirium in the elderly. J Am Geriatr Soc 1988;36:157–170.
38. Uden P, Chan A, Duh QY, et al. Primary hyperparathyroidism in younger and older patients: Symptoms and outcome of surgery. World J Surg 1992;16:791–798.
39. Potts JT, Ackerman IP, Barker CF, et al. Diagnosis and management of asymptomatic primary hyperparathyroidism: consensus development conference statement. Ann Intern Med 1991;114:593–597.
40. Krubsack AJ, Wilson SD, Lawson TL, et al. Prospective comparison of radionuclide, computed tomographic, sonographic, and magnetic resonance localization of parathyroid tumors. Surgery 1989;106: 639–646.
41. Thompson GB, Mullan BP, Grant CS, et al. Parathyroid imaging utilizing technetium-99m-sestamibi: an initial institutional experience. Surgery 1994;116:966–973.
42. Anderson BJ, Samaan NA, Vassilopoulou-Sellin R, et al. Parathyroid carcinoma: features and difficulties in diagnosis and management. Surgery 1983;94:906–915.

Surgical Care for the Elderly, 2nd ed., edited by
R. Benton Adkins, Jr., and H. William Scott, Jr.
Lippincott–Raven Publishers, Philadelphia © 1998.

CHAPTER 17

Breast Disease in Elderly Women

D. Michael Rose and R. Benton Adkins, Jr.

The appropriate management of breast disease in the elderly population can be difficult to define. Although the standards of surgical and medical intervention of breast disease remain relatively constant, the appropriate modifications due to age and rapidly changing technical advances must be considered. The extent of operative therapy, the indications for systemic chemotherapy or hormonal therapy, the impact of comorbid conditions, and the biology of breast tumors in the elderly are all controversial issues. However, the basic tenets of management of breast disease, including early detection, locoregional control, and prevention of distant disease, hold equally for all ages. With all the other factors being equal, the elderly patient with breast disease should receive the same care and surgical treatment as her younger counterpart.

PHYSIOLOGY

The female breast is a dynamic organ that gradually changes over the course of a woman's lifetime. Following embryologic development of a mammary ductal system, glandular changes begin with puberty, continue during the child-bearing years with menstruation and lactation, and are seen to regress in later years as mammary involution occurs.

Mammary involution begins with the termination of ovarian function. Two separate phases of this process have been described. The first phase occurs in women aged 35 to 45 and consists of a moderate decrease in glandular mammary epithelium, combined with a gradual disappearance of acinar and lobular tissue. A loss of elasticity of the supporting connective tissue of the breast is also noted at this time. Between the ages of 45 and 75, most markedly at the time of menopause, the second phase of involution occurs. A simultaneous reduction in the remaining glandular and adipose tissues is noted throughout the breast. The amount of connective tissue increases and becomes increasingly firm and fibrous. The remaining ductal elements continue to regress until only small islands of epithelial parenchyma remain surrounded by a fibrous connective tissue stroma [1].

BENIGN BREAST DISEASE

The incidence of benign breast lesions in the elderly woman is common; however, these lesions rarely achieve clinical significance and are less common than breast cancer. An autopsy study of 70 women aged 70 or greater revealed a majority of specimens to have either microcysts or ductal hyperplasia [2]. In addition, ductal atypia was noted in 10% of the examined specimens. Fibrocystic change, although also frequently present, is rarely of clinical concern in the elderly. The management of the majority of benign lesions, including macrocysts, mastodynia, fat necrosis, abscesses, and benign tumors, should be identical in all age groups. The suspicion for cancer must always be higher as the age of the patient increases.

EPIDEMIOLOGY OF BREAST CANCER IN THE ELDERLY

An overall increase in the incidence and mortality of breast cancer has been noted in Western countries. These negative trends are augmented within the elderly population. The American Cancer Society estimates that 181,600 new cases of breast cancer will be diagnosed in 1997 with 44,190 estimated deaths due to the disease. It is the leading cause of death from malignancy in women aged 55 to 74 years, and the second leading cause over age 75. The overall lifetime probability of contracting breast cancer is estimated to be 12.64%, increasing from 0.5% in patients <40 years to 7% in patients between ages 60 and 79 [3]. According to the Surveillance, Epidemiology, and End Results (SEER) database, a 40% increase in the incidence of breast cancer has been noted in patients over the age of 65 from 1975 to 1995 [4]. An incidence of 333 cases per 100,000 population was noted in women >50 years compared with 32 cases per 100,000 population in patients <50 years. An 85-year-old woman is twice as likely to have breast cancer as a 50-year-old woman [5]. Mortality from breast cancer has also increased from 1975 to 1995 in the elderly patient, with an increase of 6% for women >50 years compared with a decrease in mortality of 11% in women <50 years. Therefore, breast cancer will be an increasingly common occurrence in the aging population in the United States.

Infiltrating ductal carcinoma is the most common histologic subtype of breast cancers across all age groups, including the elderly, accounting for approximately 75% of all lesions [6,7]. Lobular carcinoma occurs in approximately 7% of elderly patients, comparable with the incidence in younger age groups [7]. Mucinous, papillary, and medullary carcinomas also occur in the elderly; however, these subtypes account for <10% of all lesions.

CHARACTERISTICS OF BREAST CANCER IN THE ELDERLY WOMAN

The specific characteristics that may distinguish breast cancer in the elderly patient as compared with her younger counterpart have been controversial. The definition of tumor biology as a function of age is a subject of great interest. The stage at presentation, incidence of nodal disease, and natural history of breast cancers in this population continues to be a rich field for study. The majority of reports agree that the elderly patient does have an increased delay in diagnosis and treatment of breast disease. An average delay in diagnosis of 18 months has been noted in patients >65 years of age presenting with breast cancer [8]. The reason for this delay is uncertain, although some authors have suggested that screening may be less aggressive in the elderly population [9].

The stage of disease at presentation in the elderly woman appears to be inconsistent, with several authors supporting a more advanced presentation in the elderly [7,10], whereas others have not noted this correlation [8,11,12]. The extended follow-up of the Breast Cancer Detection Demonstration Project showed no difference in incidence of stage, T status, or N status among 3,654 women, including 980 women aged 60 to 69 [13]. A cohort of patients examined at Case Western Reserve University [14] also found no difference in the size of the lesion at the time of presentation; however, a significant difference was seen in the number of patients with positive node results, with those <65 years having a greater incidence of nodal disease. The number of patients with unknown stage, however, is higher in the older woman [11] and may unfortunately represent a trend toward less aggressive local surgical intervention in the elderly.

The appropriate management of breast cancer in the elderly patient remains the primary concern for the clinician. The goals of locoregional and systemic control of breast disease are equally paramount in the elderly population and should remain the primary focus in any algorithms defined for these patients.

ESTROGEN RECEPTOR STATUS

In 1971, Jensen et al. [15] reported the importance of the level of cytosolic estrogen receptor sites as a predictor of the clinical response to endocrine treatment of breast cancer. This determination has been widely used in treatment planning since that time. Several authors have observed that breast carcinoma in elderly patients is more often responsive to hormonal manipulation than it is in younger women [16–19]. Most investigators have concluded that patients who are postmenopausal are more likely to have tumors that are positive for estrogen receptors than are premenopausal women. Raynaud et al. [16], Hawkins et al. [20], and Allegra et al. [21] have all found that estrogen receptor levels of the tumor have a significant correlation to the menopausal status of the patient. Others, however, have determined that a more significant relationship exists between estrogen receptor levels and age [19,22]. McCarty and his coworkers [19] at Duke University studied 1,037 primary mammary carcinomas and found that cytosolic estrogen receptor activity steadily increases with age from the third through the tenth decades (Fig. 17-1). They found that age further correlates with estrogen receptor levels even after menstrual status has been considered. Their report supports the earlier work of Elwood and Godolphin [22] that proposed the notion that there is a close correlation between estrogen receptor status and age, and that this relationship is statistically more significant than the association between estrogen receptor levels and the patient's menopausal status. Rochman et al. [23] have reported similar findings. They found that one-sixth of patients <age 29 had tumors that were positive for estrogen receptor, 27% of patients aged 40 to 49, 46% of patients aged 70 to 79, and 62% of patients 80 years or older.

The explanation for the age and estrogen receptor status relationship is probably multifactorial. Theve et al. [24] and Nagai et al. [25] suggest an inverse relationship between the *serum* estrogen levels and the estrogen receptor levels in the developing and growing breast carcinoma. Another suggested theory is that the cyclic levels of serum progesterone in premenopausal women inhibit or limit the formation of estrogen receptor sites in the tumor [26]. Indeed, variations of estrogen receptor levels have been found to be affected by the menstrual cycle in normal human endometrium [27,28] and in the normal human breast [19]. Hormonally dependent tumors are likely to behave in a manner similar to normal breast and endometrium. Finally, the pituitary-ovarian axis also is linked to age [29]. As the reciprocal influence of the aging ovary on the pituitary is diminished and lost, perhaps the breast tumor is stimulated by the uninhibited pituitary to develop more estrogen receptor sites. The elderly woman, in whom cyclic ovarian function no longer exists, may have consistent levels of adrenal and ovarian androgen that can be converted to estrogens peripherally. It is likely that a combination of all of these factors results in the increased likelihood of tumors that are positive for estrogen receptor developing in older patients. If this is the case, one would expect that the older the patient, the more likely the tumor will be receptor positive, and this is being seen as the population ages.

Estrogen receptor status also has been studied in terms of its relationship to the other pathologic characteristics of breast carcinoma. It has been found that tumors with a high degree of nuclear content and low histologic grades, absence of necrosis, and presence of marked tumor elastosis and tumors in older patients are all significantly associated with increased levels of positive estrogen receptor sites. Statistical analysis also has shown that those tumors that are well differentiated are more frequently associated with positive estrogen receptor status in older women than are similar tumors found in younger women [30].

Chabon et al. [31] studied 350 cases of breast cancer to investigate the interrelationships among histopathologic characteristics, estrogen receptor status, and age of the patient. They determined that three variables—estrogen receptor positivity, nuclear grade, and lymphocytic infiltration—are interdependent in their function. When the level of lymphocytic infiltration was intermediate, there appeared to be a steady percentage of estrogen receptor positivity, regardless of the nuclear grade. When lymphocytic infiltration was at a minimum, however, estrogen receptor positivity increased with the worsening of the nuclear grade. In the women over age 50, the percentage of cases of estrogen receptor positivity decreased gradually as the nuclear features approached normal. Among the elderly, they found a high percentage of cases that were positive for estrogen receptor regardless of the degree of nuclear atypia when the degree of lymphocytic infiltration was at a low level.

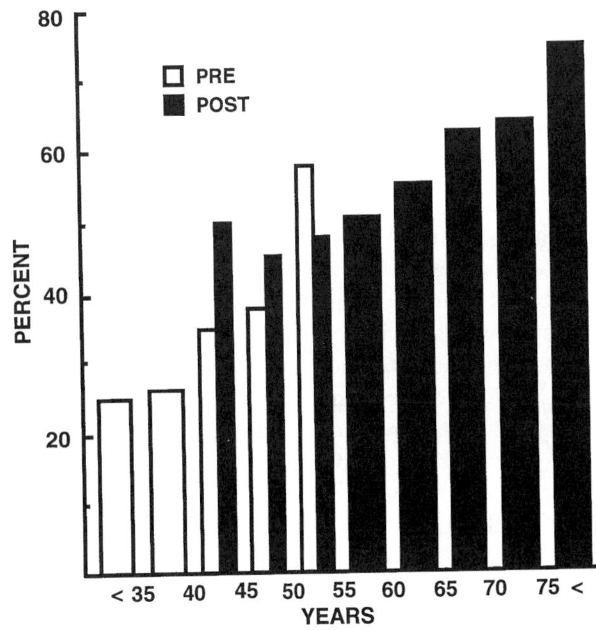

FIG. 17-1. Percentage of patients with estrogen receptor values <10 mol/mg protein are shown for each 5-year increment (premenopausal patients, *open bars;* postmenopausal patients, *solid bars).* (Reprinted with permission from McCarty KS, Silva JS, Cox EB, et al. Relationship of age and menopausal status to estrogen receptor content in primary carcinoma of the breast. Ann Surg 1983;197:123–127.)

HISTOPATHOLOGY OF BREAST CANCER

Invasive Ductal Carcinoma

Approximately 70% to 75% of cases of breast cancer in all age groups are classified by pathologists as invasive ductal carcinoma [6]. Schottenfeld and Robbins [7] found this to be true in the population of women aged 65 and older as well. Clinically, these tumors are hard to palpation and are usually poorly circumscribed. Grossly, they often have yellowish, chalky streaks on the cut surface that represent sclerotic elastic tissue. Generally, these tumors do not grow to a large size before lymph node metastases are present. Microscopically, there are strands and columns of various sizes of tumor cells growing in an abundant, densely collagenous stroma. The size and shape of the tumor cells are not uniform, and glandular formation varies with the degree of differentiation of the tumor. Areas of necrosis are seen in approximately 60% of these lesions. Multiple foci of origin in these kinds of tumors are more common in younger women than in older patients. The prognosis for patients with these tumors is the least favorable of all types of breast cancer [6].

Intraductal Carcinoma

True intraductal carcinoma is not frequently seen in any age group. In these in situ lesions, the tumor cells are confined to the ducts and are not invasive. The incidence of multicentricity in these lesions is relatively high, whereas bilaterality is unusual [6]. They are likely to be centrally located in the breast. Three common patterns of cell growth have been identified: solid, papillary, and cribriform [6,32]. These types are generally clinically occult and rarely, if ever, associated with nodal metastases.

In contrast, another form that is often a clinically palpable, more aggressive type of intraductal carcinoma has been aptly named *comedo carcinoma.* The gross appearance of these tumors is characterized by thick-walled ducts, and often, worm-like necrotic substance extrudes from the cut surface of the tumor. Microscopically, the involved ducts are distended, with proliferating cells that are much more atypical than those found in papillary or cribriform carcinomas. Areas of necrosis are common within the ducts. Haagensen has found that rare nodal metastases with intraductal carcinoma occurred in the comedo carcinoma type [32]. The importance of intraductal and lobular carcinoma in situ lies in the increased risk of subsequent invasive cancer.

Lobular Carcinoma

Lobular carcinoma accounts for 6% to 14% of breast cancer occurring in all age groups [6]. Schottenfeld and Robbins [7] found a comparable incidence of 7% in older women, whereas in the experience of Rosen et al. [33], lobular carcinoma occurred largely in the elderly. Lobular carcinoma arises from the lobules and terminal ducts of the breast and may evolve from lobular carcinoma in situ, which is commonly multifocal and bilateral. Although in situ lobular carcinoma is seen occasionally in younger women, it is rare in women aged 65 and older. In lobular carcinoma, the breast lobules are filled and expanded with cells that are uniform in size and shape and are minimally atypical. Infiltration is characterized by the haphazard cell growth that is most often in single file arrangements. Alternatively, infiltrative lobular carcinomas can form nests of cells with or without single filing. Lobular carcinoma is widely accepted as an especially aggressive form of cancer and should be treated as such in all age groups [6].

Epidermoid Cancer

Epidermoid carcinoma occurs almost solely in elderly women, but it is rare even among the aged. The gross appearance is not characteristically different from other breast carcinomas. Microscopically, areas of squamous metaplasia occur in what must be assumed to be long-standing ductal adenocarcinoma or hyperplasia. Malignant squamous foci are also sometimes found in the lining of the wall of an area of cyst formation within an adenocarcinoma. Within the areas of squamous carcinoma, intercellular bridges are often seen, and the stroma may be abundant. The prognosis is similar to that of ductal adenocarcinoma without squamoid areas [6].

Inflammatory Carcinoma

Inflammatory carcinoma is characterized by a reddened, warm, and edematous breast. These lesions are usually undifferentiated carcinomas with widespread involvement of the dermal lymphatic vessels. These tumors are associated with a poor prognosis [6,30]. In a report from the Mayo Clinic, Knight et al. [34] support modified radical mastectomy after irradiation and chemotherapy to reduce residual tumor burden. They reported on 18 patients treated by this protocol, three of whom were alive without evidence of disease 19 to 21 months after onset of symptoms.

Paget's Disease

Paget's disease of the breast occurs in 1% to 4% of all patients with breast cancer [30]. In these cases, a crusted lesion of the nipple is usually the presenting sign, but an underlying carcinoma is always present. Other nipple changes, such as bleeding and itching, have usually been present for some time. Microscopically, there is involvement of the nipple's epidermis, hair shafts, and sweat glands by numerous large tumor cells with clear cytoplasm and atypical nuclei. A connection between the nipple lesion and the underlying lesion can be found in most cases. The management and prognosis of these lesions depend largely on the nature of the underlying carcinoma [6,30].

Medullary Carcinoma

Medullary carcinomas make up 5% to 7% of reported breast cancers, but are more uncommon in older women. Patients are usually over age 50, and only 2% to 3% of women 65 and older who have cancer of the breast have medullary carcinoma [6]. These lesions are well circumscribed and can grow to be quite large with low-grade histologic qualities. The cells of a medullary tumor are large and pleomorphic with numerous mitotic figures. Glands are not usually formed. A prominent infiltration of small lymphocytes is a usual characteristic. The prognosis for patients of all ages with this tumor is better than for most other breast cancers [6]. Ridolfi et al. [35] found that 84% of their patients with these tumors who had adequate treatment survived at least 10 years.

Papillary Carcinoma

Papillary carcinoma is found more commonly in the older age groups than is medullary carcinoma. Schottenfeld and Robbins [7] found papillary carcinoma in 3% to 5% of older women with breast cancer. Papillary carcinomas arise from the duct epithelium or from preexisting intraductal papillomata and can present as a well-circumscribed mass or involve an entire segment of breast tissue. In contrast to benign papillary lesions that may have numerous cellular variations, the cells of a papillary carcinoma are usually quite uniform in size and shape. The nuclei are elongated and are usually perpendicular to the duct lumen. A cribriform growth pattern with little stroma is usually indicative of malignancy. These lesions tend to test positive for estrogen receptors and are not associated with a high incidence of lymph node metastases [33]. If completely excised, survival for patients of all age groups with these malignant breast tumors can be expected to reach 100% [7].

Mucinous Carcinoma

Schottenfeld and Robbins [7] found mucinous carcinoma in 3% of older women with breast cancer. These tumors present as well-circumscribed lesions that are occasionally crepitant or fluctuant to palpation. These tumors are often referred to as *colloid* tumors, which is a misnomer because the tumors are filled with mucin, rather than colloid. Grossly, they appear as a jelly-like mass with delicate connective tissue support. Hemorrhage into the mass is not uncommon. Microscopically, mucin is the prominent feature. Islands of tumor cells appear to be floating in a sea of mucin, and the tumor cells usually form well-defined acini. The prognosis for patients with these tumors is good, but recurrences can occur many years after primary treatment. This is in contrast to the mucinous tumors that occur in the gastrointestinal tract, which usually portend a more dismal outcome than other gastrointestinal tract tumors. Mucoid breast tumors reportedly occur most often in older women and rarely metastasize [6]. Recent observers have found that many mucinous tumors contain argyrophilic cells and neurosecretory granules, leading to the speculation that these tumors somehow may be related to the rare primary carcinoid tumors found in the breast [6].

Tubular Carcinoma

Tubular carcinomas are favorable lesions. These tumors are grossly suggestive of carcinoma because of their poorly circumscribed margins and hard consistency. Microscopically, however, they are very well differentiated and resemble sclerosing adenosis. Necrosis, mitotic figures, and cytologic atypia are generally absent. The diagnostic features are those of neoplastic cells forming well-defined tubular gland structures, a stellate growth pattern, and isomorphic nuclei. There is usually minimal, if any, lymph node involvement. The prognosis for patients with this lesion is excellent. The lesion occurs approximately equally in all age groups.

Lymphoma and Sarcoma

Lymphoma and sarcoma of the breast are rare, but occur more often in postmenopausal women than in the younger age groups. Malignant lymphoma grows rapidly, although it does not produce skin changes. The tumors are soft and occur in the right breast more often than in the left. Sarcomatous tumors are large, firm, and often necrotic. In young women, the most commonly occurring lesion of this type is cystosarcoma phyllodes. Lymphosarcoma is more usual in the elderly woman. Microscopically, breast sarcomas lack an epithelial component, and most have the characteristic features of fibrosarcoma. The prognosis for older women with either of these lesions is thought to be better than that for young women with similar tumors [36–39]. Excision of the lesion is the only effective treatment regardless of tumor size [40].

SURGICAL INTERVENTION FOR BREAST CANCER

Modified radical mastectomy or segmental mastectomy with axillary node dissection and radiation remain the current standards of care for the surgical management of invasive breast carcinoma. However, the extent of surgical therapy has been controversial in the elderly, with many authors advocating less aggressive approaches. The need for axillary lymph node dissection and the applicability of breast-conserving techniques are still being debated in the literature; however, the validity of less than standard therapy for breast carcinoma has yet to be defined by prospective trials. This is equally applicable for all age groups and as mentioned previously, breast cancer tends to be especially aggressive in the very young and the very old.

It has been our experience, and that of others, that the surgical treatment of breast cancer should be at least as aggressive in the very young and the very old, as it is for women in the mid range of age [41].

Mastectomy and Segmental Mastectomy

Total mastectomy is historically the gold standard of local control, against which other treatment modalities are compared. The operative mortality in elderly patients undergoing total mastectomy has been reported as between 1% and 3% in multiple studies [6,42–44]. Therefore, total mastectomy appears to be a safe and viable option for disease eradication and local control in most elderly women. The need for total mastectomy in all patients in this age group is unlikely, however, because patients may equally benefit from standard breast-conservation techniques. Unfortunately, the option of breast-conserving surgery may be less frequently offered due to the age of the patient. The review by Samet et al. of the SEER database [45] revealed that age was a strong predictor of type of surgery. Newcomb and Carbone also noted that women >65 years of age were less likely to receive conservative therapy [46]. Age as an isolated factor may unduly influence decision making in the extent of resection and the application of breast-conserving therapy in the elderly. This bias is not supported by substantial survival data, perhaps because in the very young and the very old the tumor is more aggressive.

Multiple studies have demonstrated the efficacy of segmental mastectomy with the addition of radiotherapy compared with total mastectomy [47–49]. Of note, older women as a group may even have an improved local control rate following segmental mastectomy and radiation compared with younger women [50,51]. The likelihood of receiving radiation as part of a standard protocol in the elderly population, however, traditionally has been significantly less than in younger patients [46,52]. The omission of radiotherapy leaves this population of patients susceptible to a fourfold increased chance of local recurrence in the ipsilateral breast following segmental mastectomy [53]. The cause for omitting radiotherapy is unclear because studies have shown that this modality of treatment is well tolerated in the elderly without undue complications [52,54,55]. Overall, elderly women should be offered the same surgical radiotherapeutic

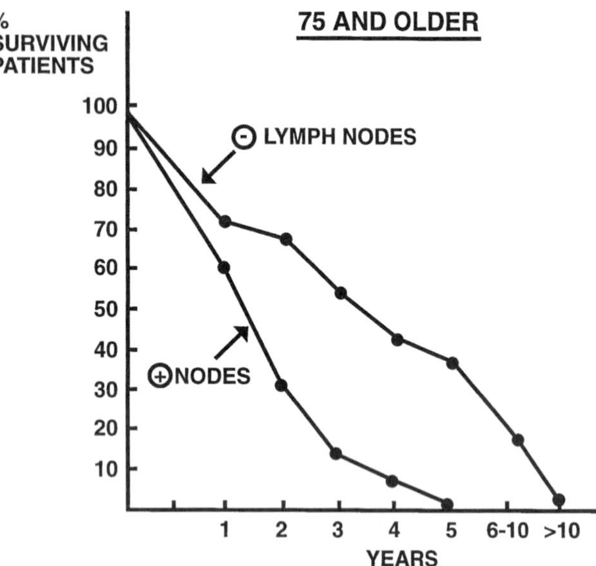

FIG. 17-2. This comparison of survival in a group of elderly patients who had lymph nodes negative for cancer at the time of initial treatment with those who had axillary metastases shows ominous implications of this positive finding. (Reprinted with permission from Adkins RB, Whiteneck JM, Woltering E. Carcinoma of the breast in the extremes of age. South Med J 1984;77:553–559.)

and chemotherapeutic options as their younger counterparts, and all aspects of the disease and treatment, including the cosmetic and psychosocial issues, should be thoroughly discussed and considered. For more discussion of chemotherapy for the elderly breast cancer patient see Chapter 8.

Axillary Lymph Node Dissection

Standard of care dictates the need for axillary lymph node dissection in the surgical management of invasive breast carcinoma whether as a part of a modified radical mastectomy or segmental mastectomy with subsequent radiation. The necessity for node dissection for the elderly patient, however, is becoming increasingly controversial. The two rationales for node dissection are staging and as a local control measure. The determination of nodal status was previously of paramount importance because this was used in part to determine the need for adjuvant therapy. Increasing trends to treat all postmenopausal women with hormonal adjuvant therapy, regardless of nodal status, brings into question the need for routine axillary dissection. The decision to use adjuvant cytotoxic chemotherapy, however, should be based on the presence of nodal disease, justifying the role of axillary dissection as a staging procedure.

Based on the National Surgical Adjuvant Breast Project data [53], survival is not affected by the addition of axillary node dissection to mastectomy, and only 20% of patients require subsequent therapeutic node dissection for clinically positive disease. As noted by Singletary et al. at M.D. Anderson, mastectomy under local anesthetic without nodal dissection may be appropriate in high-risk elderly patients [56]. Wazer et al. followed 73 patients aged 65 or greater for a median of 54 months following segmental mastectomy and radiation without axillary node dissection and noted local control rates of 92% and 8-year breast cancer–specific survival rates of 94% [57]. Therefore, the omission of axillary dissection has been retrospectively demonstrated to have little impact in certain series in the elderly; however, this cannot be considered standard therapy for breast carcinoma. Nodal metastases continue to have a strong prognostic role as noted by Adkins et al. in the elderly population [41] (Fig. 17-2). This information may be very important in planning further treatment protocols and can be extremely important for the elderly patient's treatment plan.

Overall, axillary node dissection remains the standard for the management of breast carcinoma in the elderly population. Whether this portion of the surgical procedure can be safely eradicated in the elderly has not yet been answered and awaits analysis by randomized prospective data. The appropriate utility of newer techniques, such as sentinel node biopsy, in the management of the axilla will also require further definition before widespread acceptance.

HORMONAL THERAPY

Hormonal therapy, most commonly with the antiestrogen agent tamoxifen, is a common modality in the therapy of breast cancer in the postmenopausal patient. Tamoxifen has been used as both a primary agent as an alternative to surgical intervention and as an adjunct to surgical resection.

In an attempt to avoid the morbidity and mortality of surgical treatment, tamoxifen has been proposed as a primary treatment for breast cancer in the elderly. Studies comparing tamoxifen as primary therapy to surgical therapy alone have demonstrated no difference in overall survival; however, local failure rates have been significantly higher in the tamoxifen-treated groups when compared with the surgical groups [58–60]. A recent study by the Group for Research on Endocrine Therapy in the Elderly compared tamoxifen alone with resection plus tamoxifen in 473 patients with a median follow-up of 36 months [61]. A significant decrease in 6-year disease-free survival was noted in the tamoxifen alone group compared with the surgical arm. Bergman et al. have reviewed their recent experience with tamoxifen as primary treatment for breast cancer in patients >75 years of age [62]. Their results led to the recommendation that primary treatment by tamoxifen only delays definitive surgical treatment. As a primary treatment modality, the data suggest that tamoxifen has an unacceptably high failure rate and should be reserved for high-risk elderly patients unable to undergo any type of surgical resection.

The utility of tamoxifen as an adjuvant agent following surgical resection for breast cancer has been well documented. Data from the Early Breast Cancer Trials Collabo-

TABLE 17-1. *Guidelines for adjuvant therapy in women 70 years or older in good general health*

Tumor size (cm)	Number of positive nodes	Approximate 10-year recurrence risk	Treatment
<1	None	10	None[a]
≥1–5	None	20–30	Tamoxifen
Any	1–3	50	Tamoxifen ± chemotherapy[b]
Any	4+	80	Tamoxifen ± chemotherapy[b]

[a] Tamoxifen use may be considered in these patients to decrease the risk of contralateral breast cancer, decrease the risk of cardiovascular events, and maintain bone density. Risks, benefits, and costs must be considered.

[b] Chemotherapy selection is dependent on renal, hepatic, and cardiac function. Full doses of standard regimens should be used whenever possible. Low-dosage treatment is probably of little or no benefit.

Source: Reprinted with permission from Muss HB. The role of chemotherapy and adjuvant therapy in the management of breast cancer in older women. Cancer 1994;74:2165–2171.

rative Group [63] revealed a decrease in the risk of breast cancer recurrence and breast cancer death in patients receiving tamoxifen. These benefits were seen regardless of nodal status. A benefit was maintained in estrogen receptor–negative postmenopausal patients, although this was less striking than that noted for estrogen receptor–positive patients. Cummings et al. have reported their results with adjuvant tamoxifen and have demonstrated a significant increase in disease-free survival [64]. As an adjunctive modality, tamoxifen appears to be beneficial in the majority of patients, although the benefit is less notable in the receptor-negative patient.

SYSTEMIC CHEMOTHERAPY

The utility of adjuvant chemotherapy is even more controversial than adjuvant hormonal therapy in the elderly patient. The overview analysis performed by the Early Breast Cancer Trials Collaborative Group [64] revealed a decreased breast cancer recurrence and death rates in postmenopausal patients receiving adjuvant cytotoxic therapy. The conventional conservative approach to the use of cytotoxic agents in the elderly population is frequently due to the desire to avoid greater toxicities in this age group. Previous studies have demonstrated no significant difference in drug toxicities based on age [65]; therefore, the hesitancy to provide maximal treatment with the addition of cytotoxic therapy appears misplaced. Muss points out that adjuvant chemotherapy has only been minimally studied in the elderly and further trials are needed to clarify the role of chemotherapy [66]. He does present a proposed protocol for adjuvant chemotherapy based on presence of nodal metastases removed by dissection (Table 17-1). The decision to use adjuvant systemic chemotherapy must be individualized with each patient and take into account tumor biology and comorbid conditions of the patient. When indicated, studies suggest that cytotoxic therapy can be tolerated in the elderly with no more toxicity than in younger patients. We would agree with this approach and continue to be aggressive with adjuvant chemotherapy whenever it is indicated in the elderly patient with breast cancer.

CONCLUSIONS AND RECOMMENDATIONS

Breast cancer incidence and mortality progressively increases with age. As the Western population ages, a larger percentage of those with breast cancer will be within the elderly population. The appropriate management of breast disease in this subgroup is becoming progressively more important and will pose a continuous challenge to the active clinician.

Surgical intervention in breast cancer in the elderly should mirror approaches used in younger patients. Total mastectomy is well tolerated in elderly patients, with operative mortalities of <1%. While providing excellent local control, no benefit is seen when mastectomy is compared with the selective use of segmental mastectomy and radiotherapy. The issues of cosmesis and breast conservation are equally applicable to the elderly population, and there is no apparent biological reason to forgo breast-conserving techniques in the older breast cancer patient. Radiotherapy significantly decreases recurrence rates after segmental mastectomy and does not increase morbidity in this elderly population. Axillary node dissection should be included in standard surgical management of invasive breast carcinoma, especially in the elderly breast cancer patient.

Tamoxifen as a primary treatment modality in the place of surgical intervention should only be offered to those patients with unacceptably high surgical risk or comorbid conditions. The utility of tamoxifen as an adjuvant agent in the treatment of postmenopausal patients with breast cancer is well established, although this benefit is somewhat less in estrogen receptor–negative patients. The use of adjuvant systemic cytotoxic therapy has been shown to increase disease-free and overall survival and can be well tolerated in the healthy elderly patient.

Overall, breast cancer algorithms should be similar in all age groups. The management plan for each patient must be individualized; however, management decisions should not be based on chronologic age alone. Physiologic factors of tumor biology, patient status, and comorbid conditions should mandate the degree of surgical and adjuvant therapy offered to any individual patient. The elderly woman with breast cancer deserves an approach to her disease that is at least as thoughtful and aggressive as that which would be offered to her younger sisters in society.

REFERENCES

1. Reyniak JV. Physiology of the Breast. In Gallagher HS, Leis HP, Snyderman RK, Urban JA (eds), The Breast. St. Louis: Mosby, 1978;23–32.
2. Kramer W, Rush B. Mammary duct proliferation in the elderly: a histopathologic study. Cancer 1973;31:130–137.
3. Cancer statistics, 1997. CA Cancer J Clin 1997;47:5–22.
4. Sondik EJ. Breast cancer trends. Cancer 1994;74:995–999.
5. Holmes FF. Aging and cancer. Recent Results Cancer Res 1983;87:9–13.
6. Rosai J (ed). Ackerman's Surgical Pathology (6th ed). St. Louis: Mosby, 1981;1087–1149.
7. Schottenfeld D, Robbins GF. Breast cancer in elderly women. Geriatrics 1971;26:121–131.
8. Hunt KE, Fry DE, Bland KI. Breast carcinoma in the elderly patient, an assessment of operative risk, morbidity, and mortality. Am J Surg 1980;140:339–342.
9. Morrow M. Breast disease in elderly women. Surg Clin North Am 1994;74:145–161.
10. Schaefer G, Rosen PP, Lesser ML, et al. Breast cancer in elderly women: pathology, prognosis, survival. Pathol Annu 1984;19: 195–219.
11. Mueller CB, Ames F, Anderson G. Breast cancer in 3558 women: age as a significant determinant in the rate of dying and causes of death. Surgery 1978;83:123–132.
12. Yancik R, Ries L, Yates J. Breast cancer in aging women: a population-based study of contrasts in stage, surgery, and survival. Cancer 1989;63:976–981.
13. Byrne C, Smart CR, Chu KC, Hartmann WH. Survival advantage differences by age: evaluation of the extended follow-up of the breast cancer detection demonstration project. Cancer 1994;74:301–310.
14. Crowe JP, Gordon NH, Shenk RR, et al. Age does not predict breast cancer outcome. Arch Surg 1994;129:483–488.
15. Jensen EV, Block GE, Smith S, DeSombre E. Estrogen receptors and breast cancer response to adrenalectomy. Natl Cancer Inst Monogr 1971;34:55–70.
16. Raynaud JP, Ojasoo T, Delarue JC, et al. Estrogen and Progestin Receptors in Human Breast Cancer. In McGuire WL, Raynaud JP, Baulieu EE (eds), Progesterone Receptors in Normal and Neoplastic Tissue. New York: Raven, 1977;171–191.
17. Kleinfeld G, Haagensen CD, Cooley E. Age and menstrual status as prognostic factors in carcinoma of the breast. Ann Surg 1963;157:600–605.
18. Block GE, Jensen EV, Polley TZ. The prediction of hormonal dependence of mammary cancer. Ann Surg 1975;182:342–352.
19. McCarty KS, Silva JS, Cox EB, et al. Relationship of age and menopausal status to estrogen receptor content in primary carcinoma of the breast. Ann Surg 1983;197:123–127.
20. Hawkins RA, Roberts MM, Forrest APM. Oestrogen receptors and breast cancer, current status. Br J Surg 1980;67:153–169.
21. Allegra JC, Lippman ME, Thompson EB, et al. Distribution, frequency, and quantitative analysis of estrogen, progesterone, androgen, and glucocorticoid receptors in human breast cancer. Cancer Res 1979;39:1447–1454.
22. Elwood JM, Godolphin W. Oestrogen receptors in breast tumours, associations with age, menopausal status, and epidemiological and clinical features in 735 patients. Br J Cancer 1980;42:635–644.
23. Rochman H, Conniff ES, Kuk-Nagle KT. Age and incidence of estrogen receptor positive breast tumors. Ann Clin Lab Sci 1985;15:106–108.
24. Theve NO, Carlstrom K, Gustafsson JA, et al. Oestrogen receptors and peripheral serum levels of oestradiol-17 beta in patients with mammary carcinoma. Eur J Cancer 1978;14:1337–1340.
25. Nagai R, Kataoka M, Kobayashi S, et al. Estrogen and progesterone receptors in human breast cancer with concomitant assay of plasma 17 β–estradiol, progesterone, and prolactin levels. Cancer Res 1979; 39:1835–1840.
26. Saez S, Martin PM, Chouvet CD. Estradiol and progesterone receptor levels in human breast adenocarcinoma in relation to plasma estrogen and progesterone levels. Cancer Res 1978;38:3468–3473.
27. Levy C, Robel P, Gautray JP, et al. Estradiol and progesterone receptors in human endometrium, normal and abnormal menstrual cycles and early pregnancy. Am J Obstet Gynecol 1980;136:646–651.
28. Pollow K, Schmidt-Gollwitzer M, Nevinny-Stickel J. Progesterone Receptors in Normal Human Endometrium and Endometrial Carcinoma. In McGuire WL, Raynaud JP, Baulieu EE (eds), Progesterone Receptors in Normal and Neoplastic Tissues. New York: Raven, 1977;313–338.
29. Baird DT, Guevara A. Concentration of unconjugated estrone and estradiol in peripheral plasma in nonpregnant women throughout the menstrual cycle, castrate and postmenopausal women and in men. J Clin Endocrinol 1969;29:149–156.
30. Somers AR, Fabian DR. The Geriatric Imperative. New York: Appleton-Century-Crofts, 1981;3–6.
31. Chabon AB, Goldberg JD, Venet L. Carcinoma of the breast. Hum Pathol 1983;14:368–372.
32. Haagensen CD. The Clinical Classification of Carcinoma of the Breast and the Choice of Treatment. In Diseases of the Breast (2nd ed). Philadelphia: Saunders, 1971;617–668.
33. Rosen PP, Lesser ML, Senie RT, Duthie K. Epidemiology of breast carcinoma. IV. Age and histologic tumor type. J Surg Oncol 1982;19:44–47.
34. Knight CD, Martin JK, Welch JS, et al. Surgical considerations after chemotherapy and radiation therapy for inflammatory breast cancer. Surgery 1986;99:385–391.
35. Ridolfi RL, Rosen PP, Port A, et al. Medullary carcinoma of the breast: a clinicopathologic study with 10 year follow-up. Cancer 1977;40:1365–1385.
36. Sonnenblick M, Abraham AS. Primary lymphosarcoma of the breast: review of the literature on occurrence in elderly patients. J Am Geriatr Soc 1976;24:225–227.
37. Lawler MR, Richie RE. Reticulum cell sarcoma of the breast. Cancer 1967;20:1438–1444.
38. Lattes R. Sarcoma of the breast. JAMA 1967;201:531–532.
39. Yoshida Y. Reticulum cell sarcoma of the breast. Cancer 1970;26:94–99.
40. Case TC. Bilateral lymphosarcoma of the breast. J Am Geriatr Soc 1975;23:330–332.
41. Adkins RB, Whiteneck JM, Woltering E. Carcinoma of the breast in the extremes of age. South Med J 1984;77:553–559.
42. Shapiro S, Venet W, Strax P, et al. Periodic Screening for Breast Cancer: The Health Insurance Plan Project and Its Sequelae, 1963–1986. Baltimore: Johns Hopkins University Press, 1988.
43. Kessler H, Seton J. The treatment of operable breast cancer in the elderly female. Am J Surg 1978;135:664–666.
44. Davis S, Karrer F, Moor B, et al. Characteristics of breast cancer in women over 80 years of age. Am J Surg 1985;150:655–658.
45. Samet JM, Hunt WC, Farrow DC. Determinants of receiving breast-conserving surgery: the surveillance, epidemiology, and end results program, 1983–1986. Cancer 1994;73:2344–2351.
46. Newcomb PA, Carbone PP. Cancer treatment and age: patient perspectives. J Natl Cancer Inst 1993;85:1580–1585.
47. Fisher B, Redmond C, Poisson R, et al. Eight year results of a randomized clinical trial comparing total mastectomy and lumpectomy with or without irradiation in the treatment of breast cancer. N Engl J Med 1989;320:822–828.
48. Veronesi U, Banfi A, Salvadori B. Breast conservation is the treatment of choice in small breast cancer: long term results of a randomized trial. Eur J Cancer Clin Oncol 1990;26:668–670.
49. Sarrazin D, Le M, Arrigada R. Ten year results of a randomized trial comparing a conservative treatment or mastectomy in early breast cancer. Radiother Oncol 1989;14:177–184.
50. Veronesi U, Salvadori B, Luini A, et al. Conservative treatment of early breast cancer: long term results of 1232 cases treated with quadrantectomy, axillary dissection and radiation. Ann Surg 1990;211:250–259.
51. Fourquet A, Campana F, Zafiani B, et al. Prognostic factors of breast recurrence in the conservative management of early breast cancer: a 25 year follow-up. Int J Radiat Oncol Biol Phys 1989;17:719–725.
52. Kantorowitz D, Poulter C, Sischy B, et al. Treatment of breast cancer among elderly women with segmental mastectomy or segmental mastectomy plus postoperative radiotherapy. Int J Radiat Oncol Biol Phys 1988;15:263–270.
53. Fisher B, Redmond C, Fisher E. Ten year results of a randomized trial comparing radical mastectomy and total mastectomy with or without radiation. N Engl J Med 1985;312:674–681.
54. Toonkel L, Fix I, Jacobsen L, et al. Management of elderly patients with primary breast cancer. Int J Radiat Oncol Biol Phys 1988;14:677–681.
55. Wyckoff J, Greenberg H, Sanderson R, et al. Breast irradiation in the older woman: a toxicity study. J Am Geriatr Soc 1994;42:150–152.
56. Singletary SE, Shallenberger R, Guinee VF. Breast cancer in the elderly. Ann Surg 1993;218:667–671.
57. Wazer DE, Erban JK, Robert NJ, et al. Breast conservation in elderly women for clinically negative axillary lymph nodes without axillary dissection. Cancer 1994;74:878–883.

58. Gazet J, Markopoulos C, Ford H. Prospective randomized trial of tamoxifen versus surgery in elderly patients with breast cancer. Lancet 1988;1:679–681.
59. Bates T, Riley D, Houghton J, et al. Breast cancer in elderly women: a cancer research campaign trial comparing treatment with tamoxifen and optimal surgery with tamoxifen alone. Br J Surg 1991;78:591–594.
60. Robertson J, Ellis I, Elston C, et al. Mastectomy or tamoxifen as initial therapy for operable breast cancer in elderly patients: 5-year follow-up. Eur J Cancer Clin Oncol 1992;28A:908–910.
61. Mustacchi G, Milani S, Pluchinotta A, et al. Tamoxifen or surgery plus tamoxifen as primary treatment for elderly patients with operable breast cancer: the G.R.E.T.A. trial. Anticancer Res 1994;14:2197–2200.
62. Bergman L, van Dongen JA, van Ooijen B, van Leeuwen FE. Should tamoxifen be a primary treatment choice for elderly breast cancer patients with locoregional disease? Breast Cancer Res Treat 1995; 34:77–83.
63. Early Breast Cancer Trialists Collaborative Group. Systemic treatment of early breast cancer by hormonal, cytotoxic or immune therapy. Lancet 1992;339:1–15, 71–85.
64. Cummings F, Gray R, Tormey D, et al. Adjuvant tamoxifen versus placebo in elderly women with node positive breast cancer: long term follow-up and causes of death. J Clin Oncol 1993;11:29–35.
65. Begg C, Cohen J, Ellerton J. Are the elderly predisposed to toxicity from chemotherapy? Cancer Clin Trials 1980;3:369–374.
66. Muss HB. The role of chemotherapy and adjuvant therapy in the management of breast cancer in older women. Cancer 1994;74:2165–2171.

Surgical Care for the Elderly, 2nd ed., edited by
R. Benton Adkins, Jr., and H. William Scott, Jr.
Lippincott–Raven Publishers, Philadelphia © 1998.

CHAPTER 18

Cardiac Surgery

Walter H. Merrill

The population of the United States is aging. The number of people >65 years of age has increased from approximately 3,000,000 in 1900 to approximately 28,000,000 in 1985. This group constitutes approximately 12% of the population. It is anticipated that the number of persons in this age group will increase to 64,000,000, or roughly 20% of the population of this country, by the year 2020. An unprecedented demographic change will occur as the baby-boom population continues to mature. The most rapidly growing segment of our population is aged 80 years and older. Also, 65% of 80-year-old people will live for at least 5 more years [1].

In addition to the problems imposed by demographic changes, previously fatal diseases are now much more successfully treated, if not cured, a fact that allows the elderly to live on but become subject to other disease processes. This may eventually result in the need for increased custodial care due to the increasing frailty of the elderly [2]. Older persons use health care resources to a greater extent than do other groups of the population. Frequently, the resources they consume are increasingly complex, high-technology services. The appropriateness of this consumption is beginning to be questioned because 15% of the population is using approximately 70% of the health care resources.

Furthermore, it has been estimated that as much as 15% of health care dollars are currently being spent on the last 6 months of life. This is a complex societal issue with great potential for conflict because a large number of our citizens are uninsured and receive little, if any, health care. As a society we will have to make some difficult decisions about the nature of aging: Is it a disease process to be fought with unchecked health care spending, or is it an evolving social process attended by the inevitable consequences of increasing illness, frailty, and death [2]?

Fries has stated that the increasing number of older persons is secondary to an increase in average life expectancy and is not due to an increase in the maximum length of life [3]. According to his data, the average maximum length of life in this century has remained steady at approximately 85 to 87 years of age. However, the average length of life has increased over the past 100 years from 47 to 75 years of age.

Part of the difficulty in analyzing an elderly population is the fact that there is great heterogeneity among the elderly. Many of them are physiologically intact and self-sufficient, although considerable numbers of them are not so healthy. Another factor complicating analysis is that chronology shows a poor correlation with biology and physiologic function [1].

PATHOPHYSIOLOGY OF AGING

Certain pathophysiologic factors occur frequently in the aging cardiovascular system. These include decreased aortic elasticity and mild left ventricular hypertrophy. This is accompanied by diminished myocardial relaxation and a decreased sensitivity to beta-agonists. In addition, there is a gradual loss of pacemaker cells and Purkinje's fibers, plus a decreased reaction to chemoreceptor and baroreceptor reflexes. Additional findings include an increased vagal tone and heightened sensitivity to vagal stimulation. Fibrosis and calcification of the cardiac skeleton and important alterations in pharmacokinetics occur as well.

There is some controversy, but it is generally agreed that the heart weight increases between 1 and 1.5 g per year between the ages of 30 and 90 years [4]. With time there is a diminution in the left ventricular chamber size because of increased septal thickness and a decrease in the base-to-apex dimension. Part of the aging process results in relatively mild, slight hypertrophy and an increase in the connective tissue matrix. The rigid form of collagen increases, which may be responsible for the greater stiffness of the senescent heart [5].

Changes in the aorta include decreased elasticity and distensibility. Dilatation and elongation of the aorta occur independent of the presence or absence of atherosclerosis and hypertension. Endothelium-derived relaxation factor is not elaborated as effectively in the older aorta. There is a loss of diastolic contraction of the aorta, an increase in systolic pressure, and an increase in pulse pressure. Changes that occur in the aorta due to aging result in an increased afterload, which leads to thickening of the left ventricle and an increase in left ventricular muscle mass. Changes due specifically to aging may be modified by genetics and disease.

There is general agreement that the systolic function of the heart is well preserved during aging. However, older individuals have increased levels of catecholamines secondary to stress, and the heart has a diminished chronotropic and inotropic response to the circulating catecholamines.

The diastolic function of the heart diminishes with aging. The most notable changes are secondary to prolonged duration of relaxation, which is caused by a decreased velocity of intracellular calcium handling and by prolongation of the action potential duration.

INTEGRATED CARDIOVASCULAR PERFORMANCE

The integrated response to stress is altered by age-related changes in the heart and peripheral blood vessels. It can be difficult to differentiate between changes due to disease and life-style and changes due to aging. Many studies have shown a decline in maximum oxygen consumption with increasing age, but this may be due to a decrease in muscle mass that occurs with aging and not due to a reduction in overall cardiovascular performance or cardiac output [6]. The decreased responsivity of the myocardium to beta-adrenergic stimulation results in decreased contractility during stress and exercise.

Healthy subjects without evidence of cardiovascular disease demonstrate that cardiac output is maintained during exercise even with advancing age. In careful exercise studies carried out by Rodeheffer et al., there was an age-related decrease in heart rate, an age-related decline in the increased contractility expected to occur with exercise, and an increase in impedance to ejection. These changes were offset by an increase in end-diastolic volume [7].

Data provided by the study by Rodeheffer et al. and other studies indicate that cardiac output can be maintained in healthy, physically fit older persons. However, increases in cardiac output are achieved by mechanisms that are different from those mechanisms used in younger persons. Importantly, some data demonstrate that older people, like younger people, can successfully undergo physical training and can develop increasing exercise tolerance and muscle mass [3].

VALVULAR HEART DISEASE

The most frequent cause of important valvular heart disease in older persons is calcific aortic stenosis. The most frequent cause of calcific aortic stenosis until the sixth decade of life is a congenitally bicuspid aortic valve with acquired calcification and stenosis. However, by the seventh decade of life, aging-related changes to the aortic valve result in calcific deposits and stenosis of what was an initially normal trileaflet valve, and senile aortic valve stenosis begins to predominate.

In older patients, aortic regurgitation is much less common than is aortic stenosis, and it is usually trivial in amount. When present, it generally is caused by hypertension or atherosclerotic valvular deformity.

Minor degrees of mitral regurgitation caused by papillary muscle dysfunction are common. Some patients with mitral valve prolapse go on to develop progressive valvular regurgitation. In older age, these patients may develop chordal rupture and marked mitral regurgitation. This process is always associated with myxomatous degeneration of the mitral valve. Mitral annular calcification may be associated with mild-to-moderate regurgitation and is usually seen only in elderly patients.

CORONARY ARTERY DISEASE

Coronary arteriosclerosis is found with increasing frequency in older persons. In persons over the age of 60, 50% to 80% have coronary arteriosclerosis at postmortem examination [8]. Ischemic manifestations of coronary arteriosclerosis are less frequently seen. However, the frequency with which coronary heart disease is diagnosed is directly related to the methods used to detect it [3]. It is important to remember that a substantial proportion of older persons have silent myocardial ischemia.

Silent and atypical presentations of myocardial ischemia are more frequent with increasing age. It is estimated that approximately one-third of myocardial infarction presentations in older persons are atypical or painless [3]. The mortality of myocardial infarction in the elderly is quite high and not closely related to the clinical presentation. Complications of myocardial infarction such as cardiogenic shock and congestive heart failure occur frequently in older persons. It is possible that age per se may constitute a major risk factor in older persons with myocardial infarction [3].

Atypical symptomatology is common in elderly persons with stable and unstable angina pectoris. There have been no systematic evaluation studies done in older persons to develop standard diagnostic methods of exercise testing [3]. The ability to exercise and the duration of exercise are important prognostic features in the elderly.

Coronary arteriosclerosis is not an inevitable consequence of increasing age; however, there is clearly an increasing incidence associated with increasing age. The most significant identified risk factor for the occurrence of coronary artery occlusive disease is increasing age [9]. Generally, when elderly patients present with coronary artery disease, it is more advanced than that of their younger counterparts. This is manifested by an increased incidence of three-vessel disease, left main coronary artery narrowing, previous myocardial infarction, and so forth.

Healed myocardial infarctions may eventually lead to clinically significant congestive heart failure. Patients may have localized ventricular scars or aneurysms, or ventricular dysfunction may be more diffuse. Long-standing coronary artery disease may be associated with scattered focal areas of degeneration or scarring throughout the myocardium in the elderly.

HETEROGENEITY

The heterogeneous nature of the population of elderly patients must be addressed more objectively to select patients, particularly octogenarians, most appropriate for interventional procedures. An assessment of long-term benefit requires a comprehensive review of the total health status of the patient. This involves not only angiographic and other cardiac findings, but also an assessment of comorbidity and the patient's overall status with reference to aging [10]. It must be kept in mind that chronology is a poor guide to the biology of aging and the diminishing physiologic reserve that accompanies the aging process. An estimate of biological and physiologic age must be factored into the severity of a patient's cardiovascular disease and comorbidity to develop a risk assessment. This is particularly important because older patients with advanced coronary artery disease and other forms of cardiac dysfunction in whom it is feasible to perform interventions will certainly become more numerous in the future. Physician decisions regarding octogenarians with cardiac disease and how they will be treated must be based on improved understanding of the aging process, its interaction with coronary artery disease and comorbidity, and more specific information about long-term functional outcomes of various procedures [10].

The increased availability and understanding of outcome data are critical to assist in the choices that physicians and patients must make regarding therapeutic decisions. Patients need to be fully informed and participate in decision making to the fullest extent possible. Physicians, patients, and patients' families should be involved in philosophic discussions and decision making, with particular attention devoted to attitudes about aging and therapeutic intervention and end-of-life decisions. More data will be required to facilitate highly individualized, thoughtful clinical decisions. Ultimately, these decisions will have to include careful consideration of patient preferences.

GENERAL PRINCIPLES OF CARDIAC SURGERY IN THE ELDERLY

In the not too distant past, advanced age was considered a relative contraindication to cardiac surgery. As surgical techniques and preoperative and postoperative management have improved, however, perioperative mortality has diminished. In recent years elderly patients have been increasingly accepted as candidates for cardiac surgery [11].

Older patients referred for revascularization tend to have more severe angina and a higher incidence of left main and three-vessel coronary artery disease. These patients are more likely to have hypertension, diabetes, peripheral vascular disease, and previous cerebral events. They have a higher incidence of bleeding complications requiring reoperation. Operative mortality is particularly high in older patients who undergo emergency operation or in patients who have complications following a myocardial infarction. However, operative mortality remains reasonably low for older patients who undergo elective cardiac surgery [11].

The preoperative evaluation of an elderly patient is essentially the same as that of a younger patient. A careful estimate of the physiologic status of the patient is required, along with thoughtful consideration of comorbid conditions. Before a final decision is made to proceed with operative intervention, it should be clear to all involved that the patient will likely benefit from the proposed surgical procedure.

The preoperative assessment of the overall physical and mental condition of the older patient is critical to help determine whether a given patient will have significant improvement in exercise capacity postoperatively or whether the postoperative status will be only minimally improved because of comorbid conditions. Properly selected older patients who were physically active before the development of disabling cardiac symptoms may achieve a marked recovery and restoration of a full and productive life-style [12]. This seems to be especially true if the period of cardiac disability has been of relatively short duration before operation.

Elderly patients have tissues that are more friable and more calcified than those of younger patients. These considerations sometimes require alteration in surgical techniques. Careful attention to maintenance of adequate blood pressure and cardiac output is essential. Because of physiologic limitations, surgical procedures may need to be tailored such that they will be less extensive in the elderly patient. Frequently, older patients require a longer stay in an intensive care unit and greater nursing attention per patient as well. The duration of recovery is prolonged, both in the hospital phase and in the subsequent out-of-hospital phase. Typically, the length of postoperative hospital stay increases with increasing age.

OVERVIEW OF CARDIAC SURGERY IN THE ELDERLY

Many cardiovascular system changes that occur in elderly patients do not require surgical intervention. However, there are a number of patients who present with symptomatic coronary artery occlusive disease, significant valvular dysfunction, and other cardiac conditions. These patients may well be candidates for surgical therapy. In some patients operative intervention may be lifesaving, and it may lead to increased long-term survival and improved quality of life.

Multiple studies have shown that cardiac surgical procedures in elderly patients carry a high risk for morbidity and mortality. Because of the increased risk of operation in older patients, it is particularly important that the risk-to-benefit ratio of operative intervention be carefully weighed and compared with the risk-to-benefit ratio of alternative nonoperative management.

Elderly patients who require cardiac surgery may present a number of technical challenges to the operating surgeon. Prominent among these difficulties is marked calcification of the coronary arteries and ascending aorta. Manipulation of the diseased aorta may result in an increased incidence of embolism of atherosclerotic debris. This may lead to either temporary or permanent postoperative neurologic deficits. Many patients who require cardiac surgery have important atherosclerosis of the peripheral vasculature, as well as of the abdominal and thoracic aorta. Consequently, difficulties with femoral artery cannulation or insertion of the intra-aortic balloon pump can occur. A common problem in elderly patients is advanced osteoporosis. This may make secure closure of the sternum difficult, which may result in an increased incidence of postoperative sternal dehiscence. Furthermore, elderly patients frequently present with preexisting impairment of the pulmonary, urinary, gastrointestinal, and other organ systems.

Important involvement of peripheral arteries with atherosclerosis may result in difficult decision making and may present certain technical challenges. The frequent association of important carotid artery disease with coronary atherosclerosis must always be kept in mind.

Coronary Artery Bypass Procedures

As a general rule, the key issue in coronary artery bypass procedures is appropriate selection of patients. Older patients who are otherwise healthy have an excellent prognosis after coronary artery bypass operation. The presence of associated medical diseases is an important factor that helps, in part, to determine the mortality [13].

In a report from St. Louis University 23 patients aged 80 years or older underwent coronary artery bypass between 1980 and 1986 [14]. Of 14 patients undergoing simple elective coronary artery bypass, none died. Three of four patients undergoing emergency procedures died, as did four of six patients who required insertion of an intra-aortic balloon. The operative survivors improved by at least one New York Heart Association class, with a mean classification improvement from 3.7 preoperatively to 1.6 postoperatively. Thirteen of 16 long-term survivors were in class I or II at the most recent follow-up. Actuarial survival at 1 and 2 years was 94% and 82%, respectively. The authors noted three reasons for greatly increased morbidity and mortality in older patients:

1. Older patients have a greater incidence of multiple chronic medical diseases of a noncardiac nature.
2. The elderly have more cardiovascular-related problems including hypertension, diabetes, and peripheral and cerebral vascular disease.
3. Octogenarian patients have an increased risk of primary cardiac risk factors. They commonly present with three-vessel disease, left main disease, or left ventricular dysfunction.

In the opinion of the authors, operative indications for cardiac surgery remain the same in the elderly as they do in younger patients. They also note that appropriate patient selection plays a major role in the results of operative treatment.

A report from the Johns Hopkins Hospital included 228 consecutive patients aged 70 or greater who underwent isolated coronary artery bypass grafting between 1980 and 1984 [15]. These patients were compared with a younger group of patients having operation at the same time. The older patients were more often women and had more extensive preexisting cerebral vascular disease, peripheral vascular disease, and unstable angina and longer mean bypass time. Older patients had a higher hospital mortality (9.3% versus 2.2%), suffered more complications, and had a longer mean postoperative hospital stay. These authors concluded that patient age at operation significantly influenced hospital mortality and morbidity, which seemed to be a consequence of a greater frequency of risk factors found in patients >70 years of age. Following discharge, late mortality was similar, as was the frequency of recurrence of symptoms and the degree of rehabilitation in older and younger patients. Late follow-up at a mean of 30 ± 16 months failed to demonstrate any significant difference based on age alone in survival or functional status.

Edmunds et al. reported on 100 consecutive patients 80 years of age or older who underwent open heart procedures between 1976 and 1987 [16]. Ninety patients had class IV symptoms preoperatively. Twenty-nine patients died perioperatively. Variables associated with early death were New York Heart Association class IV, previous myocardial infarction, cachexia, and emergency operation. There were 17 late deaths. Actuarial survival was 59% at 3 years and 54% at 5 years. Of the 54 patients still alive at the time of follow-up, 53 were in New York Heart Association class I or II.

In the opinion of the Edmunds group, preoperative selection of patients was more important than perioperative management in determining operative mortality. This article points out that mortality can be improved by refusing to operate on patients at high risk. It also indicates that proper prescription of cardiac surgery requires careful assessment of benefits and risk. High-risk patients are often the ones who derive the greatest benefit from operation because non-operative treatments are frequently unsuccessful.

A report from Vanderbilt University included 40 patients aged 80 years or older, with a mean age of 82.4 years, who underwent cardiac surgery [17]. There were 28 patients who underwent coronary artery bypass and 12 who underwent valve replacement(s) with or without coronary artery bypass. The operative mortality was 10%, and postoperative hospitalization averaged 14 days. There were three late cardiac deaths and one late noncardiac death. At a mean follow-up of 20 months, all patients experienced sustained improvement in functional status and minimal late morbidity. All patients were in New York Heart Association class I or II.

O'Keefe et al. reported a group of 390 patients with a mean age of 75 years [18]. This group had a 30% mortality at 5 years whether percutaneous transluminal coronary angioplasty or coronary artery bypass had been performed. Their report emphasized that quality of life and functional improvement are more important considerations than increased longevity because marked increase in longevity is unlikely to be achieved through therapeutic intervention in octogenarians.

Jollis et al. analyzed the Medicare database for more than 37,000 coronary artery bypass grafts performed between 1987 and 1992 in octogenarians [19]. The 1-year outcome demonstrated a mortality of 18.4% in coronary artery bypass patients and a mortality of 16.1% in patients who underwent percutaneous transluminal coronary angioplasty. The influence of increased age is demonstrated by the fact that younger patients had a much lower 1-year mortality.

Surgery for Aortic Stenosis

One of the largest series of patients operated on for aortic stenosis includes 675 patients who were 75 years of age or older, with a mean age of 78.5 ± 3 years [20]. Concomitant procedures were performed in 133 patients. Overall hospital mortality was 12.4% (84 deaths). Multivariant analysis identified age, left ventricular failure, lack of sinus rhythm, and emergency status to be independent predictive factors of mortality. This article suggested that careful attention must be paid to the technique of myocardial protection and cardiopulmonary bypass.

Unfortunately, there are no good alternatives to surgical treatment in symptomatic older patients, because medical treatment remains largely ineffective in the face of symptomatic aortic stenosis, and balloon valvuloplasty generally does not provide successful results and cannot be considered comparable with aortic valve replacement. Logeais et al. mention that, in the overall experience from their unit, 2,871 patients with aortic stenosis were operated on [20]. Those <60 years of age had a mortality between 2.2% and 2.9%, those between 60 and 70 years had a mortality of 6.2%, and those >70 years had a mortality of 11.2%. Myocardial failure and digestive and abdominal complications were the major causes of death in the older patients.

An earlier paper by the same group included 355 patients >70 years of age, with a mean age of 73.7 years, who underwent isolated aortic valve replacement, primarily for pure calcified aortic stenosis [21]. There was a 10.1% mortality. Thirty-six percent of the deaths were related to cardiac causes and 14% were due to cerebral damage. These patients were followed an average of 3.2 years. Eighteen percent of the patients died late; 26% due to cardiac causes and 20% due to cerebral accidents. At 5-year follow-up, the probability of survival was 70% for the entire series, including the operative deaths. This survival result is similar to that of a normal population of the same age. The functional status of these patients was dramatically improved by operation. Virtually all of the patients were in New York Heart Association class I or II at the time of most recent follow-up.

A retrospective analysis from the Brigham and Women's Hospital of Boston included 717 patients at least 70 years of age who underwent aortic valve replacement alone or combined with coronary artery bypass grafting between 1980 and 1992 [22]. The mean age was 77 years. The overall operative mortality was 6.6%, with a 4.2% mortality for aortic valve replacement and 8.8% mortality for aortic valve replacement combined with coronary artery bypass grafting. Coronary artery bypass grafting and New York Heart Association class IV were significant predictors of operative mortality in women. The significant predictors in men were New York Heart Association class IV, atrial fibrillation or flutter or heart block, and the use of a mechanical prosthesis. The authors concluded that advanced stage of disease represented by New York Heart Association class IV was a significant predictor of mortality for the whole group, and they stressed the need for earlier referral of patients for operative intervention.

A review of results of valvular surgery in the elderly from the Toronto General Hospital included 469 patients >70 years of age with a mean age of 74.0 ± 3.4 years [23]. These patients underwent single or multiple valve repair or replacement with or without concomitant coronary artery bypass operation. Left ventricular dysfunction defined as a left ventricular ejection fraction <40% was present in 33.5% of patients. Significant coronary artery disease was present in 54.5% of patients, and urgent operation was required in 15.6%. Concomitant coronary artery bypass grafting was required in 46.4% of patients. The overall operative mortality was 10%. Risk factors that were identified included urgent operation, mitral or double valve operation, coronary artery disease, especially when it was not corrected by simultaneous bypass grafting, female gender, and left ventricular dysfunction. These authors concluded that elderly patients in good risk categories should be offered surgical intervention for correction of valvular lesions and associated coronary artery disease as appropriate. They suggested that alternative therapy might be indicated in patients with multiple risk factors.

The results of cardiac operation in octogenarians have been reported by the Mayo Clinic [24]. Their report examined 191 consecutive patients 80 years of age or older having cardiac surgery between 1982 and 1986. The overall mortality was 18.8% and the mean postoperative hospital stay was 16.4 ± 13.3 days. Urgent operations were performed in 20% of patients with a mortality of 35.9%. An increased perioperative mortality was associated with clinical evidence of left ventricular failure, functional class IV, left ventricular ejection fraction <50%, mitral valve repair or replacement for severe mitral regurgitation, and urgent operation. Follow-up at 22.6 ± 15.8 months documented significant improvement in symptomatic status in the great majority of patients. There was an overall late mortality of 11.6%. The majority of these late deaths was due to noncardiac causes. The actuarial survival rate of the group was significantly better than that of age- and gender-matched control subjects.

The Texas Heart Institute has reported a consecutive series of 171 patients aged 80 to 91 years, with a mean age of 82.6 years, who underwent aortic valve replacement between 1975 and 1991 [25]. Ninety-four patients had concomitant surgical procedures. The overall 30-day mortality was 17.5%. The early mortality was 5.2% for patients with aortic valve replacement only, and it was 27.7% for those with concomitant surgical procedures. The overall actuarial survival at 1, 3, and 5 years was 90.8%, 84.2%, and 76.0%, respectively. These authors concluded that aortic valve replacement can be performed with acceptable operative risk in elderly patients.

As the population ages, the presence of senile calcific aortic stenosis has increased to the point at which a common clinical problem seen in the elderly patient is symptomatic aortic stenosis. The long-term benefit of percutaneous aortic balloon valvuloplasty has not been established [26]. The results from the Massachusetts General Hospital with regard to aortic valve replacement for aortic stenosis in octogenarians have been presented in a retrospective study of 64 patients who underwent aortic valve replacement between 1974 and 1987 [26]. Concurrent coronary artery bypass grafting was performed in 29 patients, mitral valve replacement in two, and both procedures in two. The hospital mortality was 9.4%. Late follow-up at 28 ± 5 months documented four cardiac and seven noncardiac deaths with actuarial 1- and 5-year survival rates of 83% ± 5% and 67% ± 10%, respectively. In most cases survivors were free of cardiac symptoms. In this series, patients with aortic stenosis who were otherwise healthy had a generally favorable outcome even in the presence of preoperative left ventricular systolic dysfunction. Patients who required concurrent cardiac surgery were at higher risk of perioperative mortality and morbidity.

Valve Selection

Selection of the proper type of prosthesis for implantation during valve replacement operations remains somewhat controversial. This is particularly true in older patients. Several authors have noted a significantly increased mortality and morbidity in patients with mechanical prostheses requiring anticoagulation with warfarin in the late postoperative period. This has led some authors to suggest that implantation of a tissue valve may be the most beneficial option to obviate the requirement for anticoagulation in patients aged >70 years [27].

Alternatively, other authors have reported excellent results using mechanical prostheses in older patients. In a study from South Africa of 213 patients aged 65 years and older, with a mean age of 70.4 years, results were obtained that were similar to those in younger patients with regard to survival, thrombotic obstruction, thromboembolism, and freedom from valve-related mortality and morbidity and from valve failure [28]. This study concluded that mechanical prostheses performed well in elderly patients. The concern about an increased incidence of thromboembolic and hemorrhagic complications in the elderly proved unfounded. In addition, this series did not confirm the belief that thromboembolic and hemorrhagic complications are accompanied by higher morbidity and mortality in older patients.

Borkon et al. analyzed 141 patients >70 years who underwent isolated aortic valve replacement at the Johns Hopkins Hospital [29]. In this study patients were followed an average of 4.3 years. No patient required reoperation or experienced structural valve failure whether or not a mechanical or tissue prosthetic valve was used. Anticoagulant-related hemorrhage was more frequent in recipients of mechanical valves, but it did not result in death or lead to permanent disability. There was no difference in freedom from any valve-related complication at 5 years. However, when all morbid events were considered, recipients of biological prosthetic valves experienced fewer valve-related complications than patients receiving mechanical valves. These authors suggested that the reduced incidence of anticoagulant-related hemorrhage and the infrequent need for warfarin anticoagulation favor selection of a tissue prosthetic heart valve in patients >70 years of age.

Additional information on the performance of biological prostheses in the elderly comes from a report of Jamieson and colleagues [30]. They reported on 1,127 patients aged 65 years or older who underwent 1,223 valve replacements with porcine valve prostheses between 1975 and 1987. Operative mortality was 9.5%. It was 7.3% for those 65 to 69 years old, 10.7% for those 70 to 79 years old, and 15.4% for those 80 years old and older. Late mortality was 5.5% per patient year. It was 4.2% per patient year for the 65- to 69-year-old group, 6.3% per patient year for the 70- to 79-year-old group, and 14.1% per patient year for the group 80 years and older. The overall rate of valve-related complications was 5.0% per patient year. Freedom from structural valve deterioration was 80.8% ± 8.1% at 12 years. It was 71.7% ± 11.0% at 12 years for the 65- to 69-year-old group, 97.9% ± 1.2% at 10 years for the 70- to 79-year-old group, and 100% at 12 years for the group 80 years old and older. These authors concluded that the clinical performance of porcine valve prostheses in elderly patients was excellent. It was noted that early mortality increases in patients 70 years of age or older. Importantly, structural valve deterioration was essentially nonexistent in porcine prostheses 12 years postoperatively in patients 70 years of age or older at the time of implantation.

PREOPERATIVE NUTRITION IN THE ELDERLY

The importance of adequate preoperative nutrition was assessed in a study of 92 patients >75 years of age who underwent a variety of major cardiac surgical procedures at the Jewish Hospital at Washington University [31]. Those patients with a serum albumin <3.5 g/dl had an increased frequency of confusion, congestive heart failure, low cardiac output, renal dysfunction, and gastrointestinal complications. In addition, the mean postoperative length of stay was markedly prolonged compared with those patients with a serum albumin >3.5 g/dl.

NEUROLOGIC OUTCOME

Major neurologic injury such as stroke or coma or lesser neuropsychological disturbances may occur following cardiac operations. A number of studies in which neuropsychological tests have been used to measure the impact of cardiac procedures on brain function have found brain impairment during the early postoperative period. Controversy remains, however, concerning the degree and duration of this impairment. Some studies have suggested long-term problems, but others have suggested that there is improvement in neuropsychological testing following operation. Investigators from the University of Washington studied 90 patients undergoing various types of cardiac procedures [32]. The patients were tested before operation, before discharge, and 7 months later. At long-term follow-up testing there was no evidence of residual impairment among surgically treated patients as a whole. A small number of patients demonstrated a decline in their overall status at long-term follow-up testing. The only predictor of a negative outcome was advanced age.

Stroke is an important cause of death and morbidity after cardiac surgery, especially in the elderly. There may be several causes for stroke, but there has been an observed association between high-grade carotid artery occlusive disease and stroke after cardiac procedures. The appropriate treatment of patients with coexisting carotid and cardiac disease undergoing cardiac surgery or cardiopulmonary bypass remains unclear and controversial. A prospective study from Washington University included 1,087 patients 65 years of age and older who underwent cardiac surgical procedures [33]. These patients were evaluated before operation with carotid duplex ultrasonography. Seventeen percent of patients had 50% or greater stenosis and 5.9% had 80% or greater carotid artery stenosis. Carotid endarterectomy combined with cardiac surgical procedures was performed on 46 patients. The overall stroke rate for the 1,087 patients was 2.0%. The stroke rate after carotid endarterectomy was 6.5% (all patients with stroke had severe bilateral disease). Whether improved results could have been obtained by performing cardiac surgery and carotid surgery as separate procedures is unknown.

POSTOPERATIVE IMPROVEMENT

Although cardiac surgery can be performed relatively safely in elderly patients, questions remain as to whether functional capacity of these patients can be improved sufficiently to justify the performance of the procedure. It is important to keep in mind that comorbidity may limit the capacity for improvement in functional performance even after a successful operation has dealt with the cardiac abnormality. A prospective study from several hospitals in northern California enrolled 199 patients with a mean age of 75.8 ± 4.6 years who were to undergo cardiac surgery [34]. Median stay in the intensive care unit was 3 days, and mean total length of hospital stay was 12.7 days. There was a 5% mortality and a 25% morbidity. Follow-up data at 1 year were available for 176 of the 199 patients. One year after operation most patients improved substantially in functional capacity. Eighty-two percent of patients were functional class I. Medication use significantly decreased compared with preoperative medication use. There was a substantial improvement in self-reported functional capacity after operation. The improvement was equivalent to a significantly higher exercise performance allowing moderate exertion. Twenty-six percent of the patients had a diminished activity status 1 year postoperatively. Six preoperative factors were independent predictors of less improvement in functional capacity: smoking, female gender, higher preoperative comorbidity, syncope, previous cardiac operation, and older age. The authors of this study concluded that the majority of older patients achieved meaningful improvement in functional capacity after cardiac surgery, and they noted that clinical factors appeared to modify the degree of improvement attainable.

The authors noted an overall improvement in functional capacity, even for those patients >80 years of age [34]. The degree of improvement attained, however, diminished with advancing age. Postoperative complications were noted to have an important determination on the functional capacity at 1 year of follow-up. The occurrence of postoperative complications may help to explain the postoperative outcome, but this information is, of course, not available for clinical decision making preoperatively. The authors concluded that cardiac surgery procedures in selected elderly patients who have otherwise good physical and mental health can substantially increase functional status and quality of life.

CONCLUSION

Advanced age and its associated comorbidity may provide daunting challenges for physicians and surgeons caring for symptomatic patients with significant cardiac disease. Increasing numbers of elderly patients are presenting with important symptoms and serious cardiac disease, and these patients have conditions that warrant consideration of cardiac surgery.

To say the least, considerable controversy exists regarding whether health care resources expended on the increasing proportion of elderly patients represents a cost-effective and reasonable approach to maintain both quantity and quality of life. Considerations such as these can be resolved only through the examination of data regarding late survival and functional outcome following therapeutic interventions. Careful consideration must be given to early morbidity and mortality as well.

One of the important tasks facing those who care for elderly patients in the future will be to obtain more precise and specific information regarding the outcome of various treatments in older patients [35]. It is anticipated that the problems related to the diagnosis and management of heart disease in the elderly population will greatly increase in frequency during the next several decades. Methods by which older patients are treated should be based not only on improved understanding of the aging process and its interaction with various forms of heart disease, but should also be influenced by the evolution of society's improved philosophy toward aging. Whenever possible, an important part of this philosophy should include choices made by the older patients themselves.

REFERENCES

1. Friesinger GC, Gravanis MB. Aging and the Cardiovascular System: Implications in Health and Disease. In Gravanis MB (ed), Cardiovascular Disorders: Pathogenesis and Pathophysiology. St. Louis: Mosby, 1993;299–316.
2. Matloff JM. The practice of medicine in the year 2010. Ann Thorac Surg 1993;55:1311–1325.
3. Fries JF. Aging, natural death, and the compression of morbidity. N Engl J Med 1980;303:130–135.
4. Kitzman DW, Scholz DG, Hagen PT, et al. Age-related changes in normal human hearts during the first 10 decades of life, Part II (Maturity). A quantitative anatomic study of 765 specimens from subjects 20 to 99 years old. Mayo Clin Proc 1988;63:137–146.
5. Burns RT, Klima M. Morphometry of the aging heart. Mod Pathol 1990;3:336–342.
6. Fleg JL, Lakatta EG. Role of muscle loss in the age-associated reduction in VO_2 max. J Appl Physiol 1988;65:1147–1151.
7. Rodeheffer RJ, Gerstenblith G, Becker LC, et al. Exercise cardiac output is maintained with advancing age in healthy human subjects: cardiac dilatation and increased stroke volume compensate for a diminished heart rate. Circulation 1984;69:203–213.
8. White NK, Edward JE, Dry TJ. Relationship of degree of coronary atherosclerosis with age, in men. Circulation 1950;1:645–654.
9. Fleg JL. Alterations in cardiovascular structure and function with advancing age. Am J Cardiol 1986;57:33C–44C.
10. Friesinger GC. Coronary angiography in octogenarians: problems and possibilities. Am J Med 1995;99:13–15.
11. Keller KB, Lemberg L. Interventional coronary therapy in the elderly. Heart Lung 1991;20:696–697.
12. Buckley MJ, Cheitlin MD, Goldman L, et al. Cardiac surgery and non-cardiac surgery in elderly patients with heart disease. J Am Coll Cardiol 1987;10(2 Suppl A):35–37.
13. Adler DS, Goldman L, O'Neil A, et al. Long-term survival of more than 2000 patients after coronary artery bypass grafting. Am J Cardiol 1986;58:195–202.
14. Naumheim KS, Kern MJ, McBride LR, et al. Coronary artery bypass surgery in patients aged 80 years or older. Am J Cardiol 1987;59: 804–807.
15. Horneffer PJ, Gardner TJ, Manolio TA, et al. The effects of age on outcome after coronary artery bypass surgery. Circulation 1987;76:V6–12.
16. Edmunds LH Jr, Stephenson LW, Edie RN, Ratcliff EMB. Open-heart surgery in octogenarians. N Engl J Med 1988;319:131–136.
17. Merrill WH, Stewart JR, Frist WH, et al. Cardiac surgery in patients age 80 years or older. Ann Surg 1990;211:772–775.
18. O'Keefe JH Jr, Sutton MB, McCallister BD, et al. Coronary angioplasty vs. bypass surgery in patients >70 years old matched for ventricular function. J Am Coll Cardiol 1994;24:425–430.
19. Jollis JG, Peterson ED, Bebchuk JD, et al. Coronary angioplasty in 20,006 patients over age 80 in the United States. J Am Coll Cardiol 1995;25(Suppl A):47.
20. Logeais Y, Langanay T, Roussin R, et al. Surgery for aortic stenosis in elderly patients: A study of surgical risk and predictive factors. Circulation 1994;90:2891–2898.
21. Rioux C, Logeais Y, Leguerrier A, et al. Valvular replacement for aortic stenosis in patients over 70 years: immediate risk and long-term results (from a consecutive series of 355 patients). Eur Heart J 1988;9(Suppl E):121–127.
22. Aranki SF, Rizzo RJ, Couper GS, et al. Aortic valve replacement in the elderly. Effect of gender and coronary artery disease on operative mortality. Circulation 1993;88:II17–23.
23. Fremes SE, Goldman BS, Ivanov J, et al. Valvular surgery in the elderly. Circulation 1989;80:I77–90.
24. Freeman WK, Schaff HV, O'Brien PC, et al. Cardiac surgery in the octogenarian: perioperative outcome and clinical follow-up. J Am Coll Cardiol 1991;18:29–35.
25. Elayda MAA, Hall RJ, Reul RM, et al. Aortic valve replacement in patients 80 years and older. Operative risks and long-term results. Circulation 1993;88:II11–16.
26. Levinson JR, Akins CW, Buckley MJ, et al. Octogenarians with aortic stenosis. Outcome after aortic valve replacement. Circulation 1989;80:I49–56.
27. Pifarré R. Open heart operations in the elderly: changing risk parameters. Ann Thorac Surg 1993;56(5 Suppl):71–73.
28. Antunes MJ. Valve replacement in the elderly. Is the mechanical valve a good alternative? J Thorac Cardiovasc Surg 1989;98:485–491.
29. Borkon AM, Soule LM, Baughman KL, et al. Aortic valve selection in the elderly patient. Ann Thorac Surg 1988;46:270–277.
30. Jamieson WR, Burr LH, Munro AI, et al. Cardiac valve replacement in the elderly: clinical performance of biological prostheses. Ann Thorac Surg 1989;48:173–184.
31. Rich MW, Keller AJ, Schechtman KB, et al. Increased complications and prolonged hospital stay in elderly cardiac surgical patients with low serum albumin. Am J Cardiol 1989;63:714–718.
32. Townes BD, Bashein G, Hornbein TF, et al. Neurobehavioral outcomes in cardiac operations. J Thorac Cardiovasc Surg 1989;98:774–782.
33. Berens ES, Kouchoukos NT, Murphy SF, Wareing TH. Preoperative carotid artery screening in elderly patients undergoing cardiac surgery. J Vasc Surg 1992;15:313–321.
34. Jaeger AA, Hlatky MA, Paul SM, Gortner SR. Functional capacity after cardiac surgery in elderly patients. J Am Coll Cardiol 1994;24:104–108.
35. Friesinger GC. Coronary heart disease in the elderly: management considerations. Am J Geriatr Cardiol 1994;3(6):42–50.

Surgical Care for the Elderly, 2nd ed., edited by
R. Benton Adkins, Jr., and H. William Scott, Jr.
Lippincott–Raven Publishers, Philadelphia © 1998.

CHAPTER 19

Vascular Surgery in the Elderly Patient

C. Keith Ozaki and Lazar J. Greenfield

The clinical practice of contemporary surgeons is changing rapidly due to population and economic dynamics. The U.S. elderly population (persons 65 years or older) numbered 32.8 million in 1993, or approximately one in every eight Americans. The U.S. Department of Health and Human Services reports that this group accounted for a disproportionally high 36% of total health care expenditures and 46% of all days of care in hospitals in 1992. Looking ahead, the U.S. Bureau of the Census projects that the number of Americans 65 or older will more than double by the year 2030 (70.2 million) and represent 20% of the U.S. population [1].

This heterogeneous older population itself is getting older. Data, again from the U.S. Bureau of the Census, indicates that the 1993 65- to 74-year-old group was eight times larger than in 1900, but the 75- to 84-year-old group was 14 times larger, and the older than 85 group was 27 times larger. Average life expectancy for a person reaching the age of 65 has now risen to an additional 17.5 years.

The prevalence of major vascular disease and overall mortality from major vascular reconstruction [2] correlates directly with age. Thus, against this backdrop, the modern clinician faces more vascular disease in an aging population with limited societal resources. Fortunately, the efficiency and safety of the therapeutic armamentarium has expanded to meet these challenges. Medical and public health interventions have steadily pushed cardiovascular mortality downward over the last few decades [3–5].

Physicians tend to overestimate the morbidity and mortality of vascular surgical operations in the elderly, probably leading to unnecessary complications and costs of vascular disease in this often frail population. Each individual patient with vascular disease should be informed about the natural history of his or her disease, longevity outlook, therapeutic alternatives, procedure durability, operative risk, and quality of life considerations (i.e., daily function, pain relief). As recognized for decades in vascular surgery [2,6–10], individual risk-benefit analyses change continually with increased life expectancy, expanded treatment options, and cost-containment considerations. There are data assisting these decisions in the general population, but the elderly stand as a special subset. Results of interventions in younger patient populations are not directly extrapolative to the elderly. By age 65, many patients with more malignant forms of atherosclerosis (e.g., severe type I diabetes, familial lipid disorders) have succumbed. Additionally, the cost-to-benefit ratio of risk factor modification and some medical therapies is increased because of limited life expectancies.

To assist in these difficult clinical decisions, this chapter begins with a review of the biology and general considerations when managing the elderly patient with vascular disease. It then focuses on the more common and clinically challenging types of extracardiac vascular disease seen in elderly patients: atherosclerotic peripheral occlusive, carotid artery disease, and abdominal aortic aneurysms (AAAs). This chapter mentions many excellent references available on general vascular surgery, and the reader is referred to them for more detailed discussions of related topics and further references [11–13].

VASCULAR BIOLOGY OF AGING

Many older persons can and do maintain high degrees of health and functioning, even into very late years [14]. The aging process affects all organ systems, usually with no baseline functional impairment. However, with stress, the elderly patient's response to increased demand is greatly impaired owing to a diminished reserve capacity [15]. At the cellular and molecular level, age-related changes include modified rates of transcription for certain genes, altered protein synthesis rates, and changes in post-translational protein modifications, including glycation and oxidation [16]. Additionally, the elderly population carries significant comorbid disease, including hypertension (36%), heart disease (32%), and diabetes (11%), and they all affect the individual patient's ability to respond to stress.

Atherosclerosis is the most common significant vascular disease that affects the elderly. With aging, there is a longer exposure to risk factors and a diminished ability to cope with them, resulting in a doubled incidence of cardiovascular sequelae at any level of risk factors. In the arteries, increasing age correlates with alterations in the elastin fibers and elastic lamellae, together with an increase in wall thickness. This leads to an increased wall stiffness [15,17]. Atherosclerotic changes also alter the properties of the vessel wall, again leading to less distensible conduits.

APPROACH TO THE ELDERLY VASCULAR PATIENT

The surgical care of the geriatric patient with vascular disease follows classic routes of diagnosis and therapy, but several points deserve emphasis. Any elderly patient who presents with signs or symptoms of vascular disease should undergo a thorough history, physical, and appropriate testing with special attention to associated vascular and heart disease. The following approaches, and several fundamental aspects of perioperative care, are constant whether the patient presents with atherosclerotic occlusive disease of the lower extremities or carotid, or an AAA.

When interviewing the geriatric patient, ensure that the patient can see and hear you by directly facing the patient in a well-lit, quiet environment. The patient should be wearing glasses and hearing aids if needed. Communication can be enhanced by speaking clearly and directly to the patient. Ensure that the elderly patient has understood what was asked or explained, and allow time for him or her to respond fully.

The complete geriatric medical history documents a patient's living situation, functional status, and detailed medication list, in addition to the usual history of the present illness, past medical, surgical, and family histories, allergies, social habits, and review of systems. Diabetic and sedentary patients may give a falsely benign review of systems and may harbor significant occult cardiovascular disease. Has there been significant recent weight loss? What are the patient's dietary, sexual, urinary, and bowel habits? How physically active is the patient? Also, determine the patient's legal status: Is there a guardian or durable power of attorney for medical affairs and advanced care directives?

Clear documentation of the physical examination is critical. Start with vital signs, including weight. Make note of the patient's mental and nutritional status. In addition to the usual physical examination, a complete examination in the patient with vascular disease should include pulse rates, blood pressure in both arms, and notation of the presence of bruits, thrills, or aneurysms. Is there funduscopic evidence of long-standing hypertension or nervous system embolism? The cardiac examination includes auscultation and assessment of jugular venous distention and peripheral edema. Screen for evidence of pulmonary disease with chest auscultation and percussion. Is there evidence of peripheral arterial insufficiency, such as ulcers, or atrophic skin changes? What is the status of upper and lower extremity veins, and is there evidence of deep venous thrombosis, venous insufficiency, or varicose veins? Rectal examination can screen for occult gastrointestinal blood losses and prostatic hypertrophy. Finally, many elderly patients have significant degenerative joint diseases and this should be documented.

Further testing to better assess cardiovascular risk and for general health maintenance can then proceed as warranted. Consideration should be given to blood tests such as a complete blood count, platelet count, electrolyte status, blood urea nitrogen and creatinine levels, blood sugar level, liver function tests, coagulation tests, glycosylated hemoglobin count, and drug levels. Screening for hypercoagulable states is probably more useful in young patients with aggressive vascular disease complications, unless there are signs or symptoms of coagulation disorders. Physicians must strive to minimize costs, iatrogenic anemia, and duplication; thus, tests should only be obtained when their results will alter clinical behavior. Microscopic urinalysis can determine the presence of a urinary tract infection and assist in the workup of renal insufficiency. An electrocardiogram and chest radiograph assist in screening for cardiopulmonary disease, but, again, should not be repeated if there have been recent ones and no clinical changes. Plain radiography can help determine the presence of osteomyelitis under soft-tissue lesions. Preoperative room air arterial blood gases and pulmonary function test results identify patients who require special postoperative pulmonary care.

Most elderly patients with clinical extracardiac vascular disease have coronary vascular disease, and a significant rate of reconstructible coronary artery disease has been demonstrated in patients with vascular disease [18]. This cardiac disease stands as the major cause of significant perioperative complications, including death, but the overall risk is quite low, even in the elderly. Theoretically, definition and treatment of this cardiac disease should affect long-term survival positively, although this effect is diminished in the elderly. Clinical assessment followed by selective noninvasive screening for at-risk myocardium has been recommended in recent reviews. Yet it is not clear that preprocedure definition and treatment of cardiac disease beyond a complete history, physical examination, and intense perioperative monitoring with myocardial protection eventually lead to better outcomes in the elderly. Testing and treatments that have not been shown to substantially affect outcome make suboptimal use of our limited societal resources. For those facing major vascular reconstructions, cardiac workup is therefore reserved for geriatric patients with reasonable life expectancy and signs, symptoms, radiographic, or electrocardiographic evidence of significant heart disease. These patients are then subjected to testing for myocardium at risk by exercise tolerance, dipyridamole thallium scintigraphy, or dobutamine stress echocardiography. If significant viable myocardium becomes ischemic with these provocative tests, cardiology consultation for cardiac catheterization should be obtained. Theoretically, interventions such as angioplasty or other revascularization techniques in the elderly before major vascular procedures will decrease perioperative complications and enhance long-term quality and quantity of life, but these extra procedures expose patients to substantial risks [19]. Coronary angiography and possible revascularization must therefore be reserved for patients with very high expected preprocedural mortality yet potential long-term longevity.

Because few will proceed to revascularization, clinicians should use several relatively low-cost adjuncts that assist with minimizing perioperative cardiac risk in the elderly undergoing major vascular surgery. Invasive monitoring lines (arterial lines and central venous or pulmonary artery catheters) should be placed preoperatively and baseline hemodynamic parameters recorded before induction of anesthesia. These also ensure adequate hydration status, which optimizes hemodynamics for oxygen delivery. Volume monitoring lines should be left in place until the patient is stable and has successfully mobilized the third-space fluids postoperatively. Pharmacologic agents such as nitroglycerin and beta blockers can optimize myocardial oxygen delivery to demand ratios. The physiologic reserve in these patients is often quite limited, and judicious use of diuretics for postoperative intravascular volume overload may lessen cardiopulmonary stress. Unless contraindicated, long-term, low-dose aspirin therapy should be prescribed for protection against cardiac events.

Several general perioperative techniques to minimize other complications deserve mention. Adequate hydration at the time of contrast medium infusion can minimize the nephrotoxicity of these agents. Those with pulmonary disease should cease smoking and undergo medical therapy and aggressive pulmonary toilet. Blood sugar control around the time of operation minimizes intravascular volume depletion due to osmotic diuresis and probably prevents the impaired immune function associated with hyperglycemia. The rigid elderly arterial tree does not tolerate hypotension or hypertension well, and blood pressure control in this population is pivotal for prevention of complications.

Postoperatively, accurate monitoring of weight and input and output volumes can assist in following total body volume status. The elderly patient often faces clinical disease and interventions with limited nutritional reserve, and this issue needs close attention in the hospital. The patient may need assistance with oral feedings or a short course of supplemental enteral feedings. In-hospital constipation should be avoided by using stool softeners prophylactically. Use of psychoactive drugs should be minimized to avoid iatrogenic altered mental status.

Discharge planning begins on admission to the hospital. The family must be updated on the patient's progress, and the nursing staff should educate and train the family if they will be assisting with the patient's rehabilitation after discharge. As indicated, the surgeon should enlist the assistance of the patient's primary care provider, geriatric consultants, physical therapists, and social workers. Before discharge, needed equipment should have arrived, and support, such as visiting nurses, arranged. On the day of discharge, clear written instructions for care and medicine administration and follow-up appointments are given, and the patient's family and primary care provider are also included in the discussions. In view of the chronic nature of vascular disease, the surgeon should follow the patient for the patient's whole life. Strict attention to holistic patient care will not only ensure minimal overall morbidity and mortality, but also optimal clinical outcome and individual comfort, dignity, and independence.

PERIPHERAL ARTERIAL OCCLUSIVE DISEASE

The prevalence of intermittent claudication, one of the first symptoms of peripheral vascular disease, has been estimated at 0.3% to 14.4% [20], with an increasing incidence with age. Approximately 5% to 10% of the population >70 has symptomatic lower-extremity ischemia. Women tend to have approximately a decade lag in the development of symptoms. If noninvasive testing is used to screen for lower-extremity occlusive disease, the rate increases to two- to fivefold higher, with the same age and sex trends [20]. Despite this high prevalence, only 100,000 operations are performed each year in this country for lower-extremity revascularization [21]. This small numerator with such a large denominator implies that most patients with peripheral vascular disease do not come to operation. The following discussion centers on chronic lower-extremity ischemia. Acute ischemia, often from an embolus or dissection, is covered extensively in standard textbooks [11–13].

Obstructions to blood flow to the lower extremities usually result from atherosclerosis, and the most common sites of involvement are bifurcations—for example, the terminal aorta and its branches and the common femoral artery bifurcation. The distal superficial femoral artery is also frequently involved. Approximately two-thirds of patients have significant disease in both the in-flow aortoiliac segment and infrainguinal outflow tract. Diabetic patients tend to have greater tibial vessel involvement [22] and a higher risk of amputation. Major risk factors include cigarette smoking, diabetes, hypertension, dyslipidemias, male sex, age, genetic factors, android obesity, and physical inactivity. Possible protective effects include high-density lipoprotein cholesterol, estrogens, and moderate alcohol intake.

Because the incidence of patients with lower-extremity peripheral vascular disease (as defined by noninvasive testing) is higher than estimates based on clinical signs and symptoms, a significant proportion (at least two-thirds) of patients with this disease are asymptomatic. Symptoms usually begin when collateral blood flow cannot meet tissue metabolic demands, leading to a cramping pain in affected muscle groups with exercise (intermittent claudication). It can progress to pain at rest and, finally, tissue necrosis when flow is so limited that the basal requirements are not met. Embolism and acute thrombosis may hasten the progression of disease and can account for acute clinical exacerbations.

Early symptomatic occlusive disease is a clinically stable problem in 75% of people as they age [20]. Less than 10% require arterial reconstruction, and amputation will be required in fewer than 5% [23]. The need for arterial revascularization and amputation correlate inversely with the ankle brachial index. Continued smoking promotes this clinical deterioration.

Occlusive peripheral vascular disease also stands as a strong predictor of mortality, especially from ischemic heart disease [24]. Overall 5-year survival is >95% in patients with claudication treated nonoperatively, 80% in those requiring operation for claudication, 50% after operation for limb-threatening ischemia, and only 12% for patients requiring reoperation for limb-threatening ischemia.

The usual initial symptom of lower-extremity occlusive disease is intermittent claudication. Next, rest pain begins in the toes or forefoot, is worse with recumbency or elevation, and relieved by placing the foot in a dependent position. Associated related symptoms include impotence, anorexia, and weight loss. The clinician must rule out nonvascular causes of leg pain including neurologic problems (e.g., neuropathy or herniated intervertebral disk), arthritis, primary muscle cramps, and venous claudication.

The physical examination in the elderly patient with peripheral vascular disease begins with an assessment of pulses as outlined previously. Additionally, the physician must look for pallor of the limb with elevation, dependent rubor, shiny atrophic skin changes, signs of arterial emboli, and extremity ulcers. Ischemic ulcers tend to be located distally on the foot or toes, whereas stasis lesions are on the lower third of the leg, and neurotrophic lesions are under calluses or pressure points. The ankle brachial index should be calculated by dividing the systolic blood pressure in each lower limb by the highest arm pressure.

Confirmation of the diagnosis of peripheral vascular disease is initially achieved using noninvasive testing. This testing should include segmental pressure measurements and arterial waveform tracings recorded at the high thigh, above and below knee, and ankle levels. Patients with calcified, noncompressible vessels (such as diabetics) should have pressures and waveforms recorded by plethysmography from the toes. A drop in the leg pressure by at least 20% at the point of claudication with exercise indicates significant occlusive disease. Duplex scanning is used in some centers for assessment of abdominal arterial occlusive disease [25].

If invasive therapeutic interventions are contemplated, and the patient is an acceptable risk, arteriography is performed next. Angiography is useful to define a precise anatomic "roadmap" to identify anatomic variants and the exact location of the patient's obstructing atherosclerotic lesions. The systolic pressure on both sides of these lesions in larger arteries should be measured to determine their hemodynamic significance. Runoff views to the foot with digital subtraction techniques are mandatory before reconstructions involving the distal circulation.

Magnetic resonance angiography may eventually assist in the workup of these patients, although its role had yet to be precisely defined [26,27]. Some advocate carotid artery disease screening in all patients with lower-extremity occlusive disease because >25% have asymptomatic carotid lesions [28]. Carotid artery screening in the elderly population should proceed on an individual basis.

In view of the favorable natural history of claudication, the initial therapy is nonoperative for patients with claudication without threatened tissue loss. Exercise training has been acknowledged as an effective treatment, although data are primarily from younger patients. Patients should be told to exercise to the point of claudication, then rest, and repeat this cycle for defined time periods, such as 1 hour. Risk factor modification such as cessation of smoking, control of hypertension and hyperglycemia, dietary and pharmacologic manipulation of blood lipid levels, weight loss, and exercise probably modify progression of symptoms and perhaps atherosclerosis in selected populations. It is unclear what role such modifications have in the older patient with advanced lesions and limited life expectancy.

For drug therapy, pentoxifylline is the only agent in the United States approved for the treatment of intermittent claudication. It probably exerts its beneficial effects by increasing the deformability of the red blood cell membrane, and therefore decreasing blood viscosity. Blood flow to the ischemic limb thus increases. Approximately one-third of patients experience a clinically significant (doubling) improvement in treadmill walking distance. The drug should be given for a minimum of 6 to 8 weeks before its effectiveness is judged.

Endovascular techniques successfully relieve obstructions in selected disease distributions. Percutaneous transluminal angioplasty (PTA) of the iliac vessels has the best record, with 90% initial success and 50% to 80% 5-year patency. Popliteal artery PTA rates are much worse: 80% initially, with 20% to 70% 5-year patency. PTA patency rates for tibial arteries and bypass grafts are universally low [29]. While PTA is attractive in the elderly in view of the lessened tissue trauma compared with open reconstruction, it is not without risk. Complication rates of 6% to 13% include hemorrhage, pseudoaneurysm, thrombosis, embolization, and arteriovenous fistula. Contrast loads are usually higher than conventional angiography. PTA can, however, be combined with open procedures. Balloon dilation has for years been used as an adjunct to open surgical therapy in populations that included a high proportion of elderly, high-risk patients [30].

Several other endovascular or minimally invasive techniques (e.g., atherectomy, laser angioplasty, stents) have been applied to patients with peripheral vascular disease [29]. None is as well established as balloon angioplasty of the iliacs, and they should be used only for selected indications by those familiar with the devices. Catheter-directed intra-arterial fibrinolysis can be used in the management of acute and subacute limb ischemia and planning of revascularization procedures [31]. Major complication rates (including bleeding and renal failure) occur in up to 20% of patients. Endovascular ultrasound is a technology that may assist in the completion of these and other more invasive procedures.

As for surgery, patients with a useless extremity, severe irreversible dementia, or others who will never be able to ambulate or use a prosthesis are best considered for primary amputation. Indications for surgical intervention include ischemic rest pain, tissue necrosis, or claudication that fails nonoperative therapy and impairs the life-style of an acceptable risk and anatomically appropriate patient. Reconstruction is dependent on the patient's operative risk and the extent and distribution of occlusive disease. In active centers around the country, aggressive attempts at limb preservation in the face of critical ischemia have pushed primary amputation rates to 2% to 3%.

Direct aorta-iliac reconstruction should be considered in low-risk patients who are expected to survive at least 10 years. Acceptable procedures that may have less surgical stress include unilateral iliofemoral bypass via a retroperitoneal approach. Nonanatomic bypasses, such as the axillobifemoral bypass, are associated with less local tissue trauma, but also lower long-term patency. If an iliac occlusion is unilateral, then femorofemoral bypass may be carried out, even under local anesthesia. Moving more distally, femoral endarterectomies and profundoplasty can be performed under local anesthesia if necessary in the geriatric, high-risk patient.

If bypass of lesions is necessary, autologous saphenous vein is the conduit of choice, with no clear benefit for reversed or nonreversed techniques. Other vein sources include arm veins, lesser saphenous veins, and superficial femoral veins. Prosthetic conduits may be used in selected settings, such as bypasses to the above-knee popliteal artery, or when no autologous conduit is available. Cryopreserved vein allografts fare poorly [32]. The role of anticoagulants and antiplatelet drugs in promoting graft patency in the elderly is currently not known, but they may offer overall health benefits to selected patient groups [33], although there is also an increase in complications from anticoagulation in the elderly woman. At this time, it is difficult to state whether aggressive postoperative graft surveillance with preemptive intervention is efficacious and cost-effective in the elderly.

These reconstructive vascular procedures can be performed with acceptable morbidity and mortality in selected patients, although these rates tend to be higher in the geriatric patient. In 1985, the Cleveland Vascular Surgery Society reported a retrospective series of operations performed on a large number of patients [2]. Mortality of 2.9% and 12.3% for elective aortic reconstructions for occlusive disease, 1.8% and 16.2% for femorofemoral bypass grafts, and 2.2% and 6.7% for femoropopliteal-tibial reconstructions were found for patients <75 years old or 75 and greater, respectively. They suggest nonanatomic reconstructions in high-risk patients. More recent overall reconstructive operative mortalities for the elderly range from 0% to 4.6% [7,34]. Ekman et al. have reported using expanded polytetrafluoroethylene (ePTFE) grafts in lower-extremity revascularization in 68 elderly patients aged 70 to 88 years. Postoperative mortality was 3%, whereas 1- and 2-year limb salvage rates were 75% and 55%, respectively [35]. Up to 30% of patients have some type of wound complication. Other problems include mild postoperative edema, pain, and paresthesias. Expected outcomes are equivalent in diabetic and nondiabetic patients [28,34].

In general, long-term patency for direct aortoiliac reconstruction is approximately 90% at 5 years and 75% at 10 years. Axillobifemoral grafts maintain approximately a 50% 5-year primary patency, and femorofemoral grafts have approximately an 80% 5-year patency. As for more distal reconstructions, factors such as quality of the conduit and site of distal anastomosis affect infrainguinal bypass patency. Primary 5-year patency rates for grafts to the popliteal are approximately 80% for claudication [36]. Bypass to infrageniculate outflow vessels results in an overall patency rate of 75% to 80%.

When faced with critical ischemia, the geriatric patient can expect durable benefit from aggressive attempts to restore lower-extremity blood flow. Scher et al. [37] reviewed 168 consecutive patients over 80 years of age with limb-threatening ischemia. They used the traditional vascular surgery armamentarium to achieve limb salvage rates of 84% and 71% at 1 and 3 years, respectively, with a 6% procedural mortality. A recent review estimates limb salvage at 50% to 87% at 3 to 5 years in the elderly [7].

As noted previously, each patient's cost-to-benefit ratio must be calculated; however, when considering nonrevascularization therapy for critical ischemia, the clinician must also include the morbidity, mortality, and cost of amputation. Patients requiring amputation face mortality of 10% and 15% for below and above knee amputations, respectively. About one in three elderly patients is unable to ambulate satisfactorily after a below knee amputation [7], and many amputees go on to bilateral amputation. Realistically, amputation often leads to institutionalization and loss of independence in the elderly population with the increased costs of dependent care. Traditional reconstructions, coupled with a commitment to optimal perioperative care, offer durable benefit to selected geriatric patients. Although these reconstructions have some morbidity and mortality, the rates compare favorably with the outcomes of the alternatives, such as primary amputation.

CAROTID ARTERY DISEASE

Cerebrovascular disease stands as the third most common cause of death in the United States, and the remaining stroke survivors suffer substantial long-term physical and psychological disability. Stroke incidence, mortality, and societal financial costs increase with age [7,38]. An annual incidence of almost 2% per year has been reported in the elderly [39].

Carotid endarterectomy stands as the most commonly performed peripheral vascular operation in the United States [40].

Although the etiologies of cerebral ischemia and infarction are varied, the majority of strokes are the result of extracranial cerebrovascular disease at the carotid bifurcation extending into the internal carotid artery. This location holds true for the geriatric patient, although the elderly also tend to have more intracerebral disease. The mechanisms of cerebrovascular accidents include low flow through atherosclerotic stenoses or embolism of thrombus, plaque, or fibrin, often from a plaque ulcer. Vasospasm may be superimposed on these events. Cardioembolic strokes can also occur in the elderly.

The duration of symptoms ranges from the brief transient ischemic attack (TIA; <24 hours), to reversible ischemic neurologic dysfunction, and finally permanent infarction or stroke [41]. Patients with symptomatic carotid artery disease classically complain of contralateral paresis, paresthesias, sensory changes, or ipsilateral amaurosis fugax and, if the dominant hemisphere is involved, aphasia. Nonhemispheric symptoms (e.g., ataxia, dizziness, vertigo) can result from global ischemia or vertebrobasilar insufficiency. Brain tumors, seizures, heart disease, migraines, and metabolic disorders such as hyperglycemia and hypoglycemia can all mimic cerebrovascular disease and should be included in the differential diagnosis of an elderly patient presenting with these symptoms. Syncope, presyncope, incontinence, confusion, amnesia, and seizures are unlikely to be caused by TIAs.

The annual stroke event rate for asymptomatic patients with hemodynamically significant carotid artery stenosis ranges from 2% to 5% [42]. Although cerebral infarction may be the initial event in many patients with carotid artery disease, TIAs occur in 25% to 50% of patients before atheroembolic infarcts. In patients who have TIAs, one-third will have had a stroke after 5 years. Antiplatelet therapy decreases this rate by 14% and carotid endarterectomy by 66%. The diagnostic evaluation of a patient with a recent TIA should be completed within a week or less [43].

Cervical bruits are an indicator of systemic atherosclerotic disease and much less of an indicator for significant carotid pathology. When examining a patient with suspected carotid artery disease, in addition to a complete examination with special consideration for the cardiovascular system, a careful neurologic examination is warranted.

Color duplex scanning, which combines real-time B-mode ultrasound imaging with Doppler assessment of blood flow, is the initial study of choice. It provides an accuracy of 90% to 95% for identifying hemodynamically significant carotid artery disease. Contrast angiography (either conventional or digital subtraction) remains the gold standard for defining anatomic detail, but it is associated with ionizing radiation and carries a significant incidence of stroke. In the recent Asymptomatic Carotid Atherosclerosis Study there was at least a 1.2% incidence of stroke from arteriography [42]. For this reason, some centers recommend operation based on a strong clinical history and a quality duplex study [44]. Magnetic resonance angiography has been used to confirm duplex findings [45], although it provides less detail than angiography. Computed tomography (CT) and magnetic resonance imaging (MRI) may be useful to detect ischemic brain parenchyma, especially in recent infarcts.

Treatment of carotid artery disease is medical for all patients and surgical in defined subsets. In the patient with carotid artery disease, all reversible risk factors for atherosclerosis should be addressed, including treatment of hypertension, cessation of smoking, elimination of excessive alcohol consumption, and treatment of heart disease and lipid disorders. Discontinuation of postmenopausal estrogen is not recommended [43]. Aspirin is often prescribed for cerebrovascular disease as an antiplatelet agent, although its primary benefit is a reduction of cardiac morbidity and mortality. This effect is independent of age [43]. The antiplatelet agent ticlopidine hydrochloride, which is more expensive than aspirin and associated with side effects (e.g., diarrhea, reversible neutropenia), can be used in patients who cannot take aspirin. Warfarin and dipyridamole are also prescribed occasionally. Warfarin certainly has a role for stroke prevention in patients with atrial fibrillation and prosthetic heart valves [46]. Neither warfarin nor dipyridamole has been demonstrated to have a clinically significant impact on the natural history of carotid artery disease, and there is no evidence to support their use in patients with TIAs. Falls in the elderly quickly unmask the downside of warfarin therapy in this population.

Angioplasty of the internal carotid artery is still in experimental stages and should be avoided unless performed as part of a thoughtful, formal experimental protocol.

Carotid artery endarterectomy is the primary surgical therapy for carotid artery disease. It is performed to decrease the risk of cerebral infarction and rarely in the acute phase of a stroke. Recent large trials have demonstrated clear benefit from carotid endarterectomy in patients with hemispheric or retinal TIAs or nondisabling stroke within 120 days who had 70% to 99% stenosis in the appropriate carotid artery [47]. The results of the Asymptomatic Carotid Atherosclerosis Study demonstrate that patients with asymptomatic carotid artery stenosis of ≥60% whose general health makes them good candidates for elective surgery have a reduced 5-year risk of ipsilateral stroke if carotid endarterectomy is performed, with <3% morbidity and mortality [42]. Endarterectomy may be performed safely under general, regional, or local anesthesia. Likewise, no difference has been demonstrated between routine or selective use of intraoperative shunts or no shunts. In patients with significant coexisting carotid and coronary disease, the lesion representing the major immediate threat should be addressed first. In the rare instances when both are critical, simultaneous procedures can be performed.

Carotid artery endarterectomy is in essence a superficial operation and has repeatedly been documented to be a safe, durable operation in the elderly [2,38,42,48–52]. Plecha et al. found no difference in perioperative stroke rates or operative mortality between patients grouped by age using a 75-year-old age division [2], as have others [48,49]. Data indicate a combined overall arteriography and surgery morbidity and mortality of 2.7% [42]. By combining several series, Perler estimates perioperative stroke and death rates at 2.8% and 2.4%, respectively, for the elderly population. A combined perioperative mortality and stroke rate of 1.3% has been reported in patients 80 years old or greater in an institution where 76% of the procedures were performed under local anesthesia [51].

Long-term results are good in the elderly. In a cohort of patients with a minimum age of 75 after carotid artery endarterectomy, cumulative stroke-free rates were 92% at 2 years and 80% at 5 and 10 years of follow-up. Although an estimated 10% of patients may develop recurrent stenosis after endarterectomy, few have clinical sequelae requiring intervention.

ABDOMINAL AORTIC ANEURYSMS

An aneurysm is a dilation of a vessel to 1.5 times its normal diameter. Aneurysmal disease of the abdominal aorta stands as a significant health problem in the elderly of Western societies. In community screening, approximately 2.8% of men aged 65 to 79 have aortic aneurysms by ultrasound, and in a Swedish study there was a peak incidence of 5.9% at the age of 80 [53]. The incidence seems to be increasing, probably as a result of both an aging population and greater diagnostic awareness.

Aneurysms can be lethal. They are the thirteenth leading cause of death in the United States. Data from Great Britain indicate that one in 70 men between 60 and 84 years of age dies from a ruptured AAA [54]. Men are affected more often than women by a ratio of four to one.

A first-degree relative with an aortic aneurysm, cigarette smoking, and hypertension are all positive risk factors for aneurysms. Ninety-five percent of AAAs arise below the renals, and 10% to 25% are associated with significant arterial vascular occlusive disease. Only 2% to 4% of patients with AAAs have synchronous femoral or popliteal aneurysms. However, approximately two-thirds of patients with either femoral or popliteal aneurysms have an AAA. Medical problems such as atherosclerosis, chronic obstructive pulmonary disease, or hypertension are present in over one-half of patients with AAAs.

Most AAAs (>90%) are associated with atherosclerosis. It is not clear if these atherosclerotic changes are primary or secondary, and thus these aneurysms are referred to as *nonspecific aneurysms*. Disorders that cause cystic medial necrosis, dissections, Ehlers-Danlos syndrome, syphilis, and infection can also lead to aneurysms. Biochemically, the aneurysm wall has decreased elastin and collagen, and laminated thrombus can line the luminal side of this wall.

Aneurysms progressively enlarge, leading to rupture in a significant percentage of cases. On average, AAAs enlarge at a rate of 0.4 cm per year. Aneurysm rupture risk correlates directly with size, although even small aneurysms can rupture. The yearly risk of rupture for aneurysms <5 cm in diameter is approximately 4%. Ranges for published 5-year rupture rates by size include <5 cm, 9% to 20%; 5 to 7 cm, 20% to 42%; and >7 cm, 59% to 95%. Chronic obstructive pulmonary disease and hypertension are also risk factors for rupture [55]. Rupture is usually a lethal complication of AAAs. In general, up to 50% of patients with a ruptured aneurysm die in the field [56]. Another 24% die in the hospital before operation, and of those who make it to the operating room, only 50% survive [57,58].

Approximately one-third of elderly patients with multiple medical problems who do not have elective aneurysm repair will die of a ruptured aneurysm [59,60]. Mortality from AAA rupture for patients over the age of 80 remains high [61]. Although rupture is the primary concern with AAAs, they can lead to other complications, such as embolism or rarely thrombosis.

The clinical presentation of an AAA ranges from no symptoms to hypovolemic shock. Three-fourths of all infrarenal AAAs are asymptomatic when diagnosed and usually found on an imaging study performed for another reason or on routine physical examination. Aneurysm expansion, rupture, distal embolism, or thrombosis can all cause symptoms. Severe back, flank, or abdominal pain should alert the clinician to possible acute aneurysm expansion or rupture. Inability to palpate an aneurysm does not rule it out, because small aneurysms are difficult to palpate in obese patients.

Several radiographic studies are useful in the patient with suspected AAA. Plain abdominal and lateral radiographs demonstrate calcium in the aneurysm wall in approximately two-thirds of cases and can assist in defining aneurysm size. Chest radiographs should be performed to screen for cardiopulmonary disease and intrathoracic aneurysmal disease. Real-time B-mode ultrasound accurately defines infrarenal aneurysm size without ionizing radiation, and its sensitivity approaches 100%.

CT scans permit measurement of aneurysm size, location, and associated soft-tissue and vascular anomalies, such as a horseshoe kidney or retroaortic left renal vein. CT scans should be performed with enteral and intravenous contrast when possible. Recent advances in CT technology allow three-dimensional reconstructions from the data acquired. In general, CT scans are more expensive than abdominal ultrasound studies and are associated with ionizing radiation.

MRI is a relatively new modality for aneurysms. This study in general costs more than CT or ultrasound and is not associated with ionizing radiation. Early results indicate that MRI has excellent agreement with ultrasound and CT, but the role of MRI in evaluating the patient with an AAA remains to be defined.

Although ultrasound and CT scans with intravenous contrast can define external aneurysm size and luminal thrombus, angiography only gives a projection of contrast in the portion of the vessel lumen that is carrying blood. Therefore, it should only be used in aneurysm patients where there is suspected mesenteric or renal artery disease, a horseshoe kidney, or significant peripheral vascular disease that is being considered for therapeutic intervention. Aortography is associated with ionizing radiation, significant financial cost, bleeding, thrombosis, embolization, and contrast-induced nephrotoxicity.

Prosthetic graft replacement of the abdominal aorta remains the only effective treatment for AAAs. The most common cause of death among patients with AAA is rupture. Elective surgical repair prevents rupture and is associated with improved survival [60]. Aneurysm repair should be undertaken in all patients with an acceptable operative risk with either symptomatic aneurysms or asymptomatic aneurysms >5 cm in diameter and an estimated life expectancy of at least 2 years. If expansion of ≥0.5 cm in 1 year is documented, operation should be considered seriously. The benefits of early operation decrease with increasing age [62], and thus the size threshold for repair in the elderly with 4- to 5-cm aneurysms tends to be pushed more toward the upper end.

Exposure and repair of an AAA results in significant tissue trauma and fluid shifts. The retroperitoneal rather than transperitoneal approach offers some theoretical advantages in the elderly patient [7,58], but small randomized prospective studies have not demonstrated substantial outcome differences in variously aged patient groups [63]. Transluminal repair with an endovascular prosthesis is currently under investigation and may offer greatly reduced surgical stress [64,65].

Operative mortality for elective aortic aneurysm repair has declined substantially over the past two decades for all patients, including the elderly [7,57]. Several factors have probably contributed to this trend. Improved monitoring and anesthetic techniques have allowed better perioperative management. The need for homologous blood transfusions is now decreased due to preoperative autologous donation and intraoperative blood salvage. On the other hand, operative mortality for repair of ruptured aneurysms in the elderly remains high, almost 60% on average [7].

Recent overall mortality for elective AAA repair ranges from approximately 1.6% to 5.6%, with a mean of approximately 4% [56–58]. Age correlates positively with mortality. In 1985, Plecha et al. [2] retrospectively noted a twofold increased mortality in patients 75 or older (11.3%) compared with those younger than 75 (5.6%) for elective AAA surgery. A Canadian series combining nonruptured asymptomatic and symptomatic patients reported mortality for the age groups <60, 60 to 80, and >80 years at 0%, 5.0%, and 9.3%, respectively; multivariate analysis indicated that the higher mortality could be explained by other risk factors associated with advancing years [66]. A recent review that included all Michigan hospitals reported mortality of 4.2% and 10.7% for patients aged 69 or less and 70 or older, respectively [57]. There was a trend toward lower rates in the elderly group in the 1980s. Summarizing several series, a recent review estimates mortality for abdominal aneurysm repair in the elderly at 6.6% [7].

Higher morbidity and mortality is associated with cardiac disease, renal insufficiency, and pulmonary disease, all of which can be present in the elderly. The most common cause of postoperative mortality is myocardial dysfunction, and postoperative myocardial infarction has been reported in approximately 7% of patients. Overall, complications include hemorrhage, renal failure (4% to 7%), pulmonary dysfunction (20% to 40%), cardiac dysfunction (20% to 37%), ileus, intestinal ischemia (1%), paraplegia, distal embolism, and infection. A 50% incidence of nonlethal complications in octogenarians undergoing elective aneurysm repair has been reported [60], including arrhythmias (20%), atelectasis (11%), pneumonia (9%), congestive heart failure (15%), oliguric azotemia (2%), nonoliguric azotemia (11%), myocardial infarction (7%), respiratory failure (4.5%), bleeding (4%), and wound infection (2%). Sexual dysfunction data are limited [56].

Late complications such as graft occlusion, infection, aortoenteric fistula, and anastomotic aneurysms add an additional 2% to overall mortality [56]. Long-term survival is >90% at 1 year, 67% at 5 years, and better in subsets without evidence of coronary artery disease [58]. Additionally, the quality of life is maintained. In a study before many recent advances in the care of aneurysm patients, 86% of octogenarians reported better or equal physical status by the first year postoperatively [67].

SUMMARY

Although vascular interventions carry significant morbidity and mortality in the elderly patient, the clinician must weigh these slightly higher risks against each individual's risks and potential benefits. In general, with increasing life expectancy and use of less invasive, safer therapeutic interventions, the risks are shrinking and benefits increasing [7] for this population. The literature repeatedly emphasizes that chronologic age is not a contraindication to vascular surgery, but rather physiologic age and comorbid disease must be considered in calculating operative risk [6,7,15,59]. Careful selection and aggressive therapy when appropriate can lead to significantly increased quality and quantity of life for the geriatric patient with vascular disease.

REFERENCES

1. Administration on Aging. A Profile of Older Americans. Washington, DC: U.S. Department of Health and Human Services
2. Plecha FR, Bertin VJ, Plecha EJ, et al. The early results of vascular surgery in patients 75 years of age and older: an analysis of 3259 cases. J Vasc Surg 1985;2:769–774.
3. Kannel WB. Epidemiology of Cardiovascular Disease in the Elderly: An Assessment of Risk Factors. In Brest AN (ed), Cardiovascular Clinics, Cardiovascular Disease in the Elderly. Philadelphia: Davis, 1992;9–22.
4. Manton KG, Vaupel JW. Survival after the age of 80 in the United States, Sweden, France, England, and Japan. N Engl J Med 1995;333: 1232–1235.
5. Thomas TJ, Kannel WB. Downward trend in cardiovascular mortality. Annu Rev Med 1981;32:427–434.
6. Weisz GM, Erlik D, Schramek A. Vascular surgery in elderly patients. Geriatrics 1970;25:166–176.
7. Perler BA. Vascular disease in the elderly patient. Surg Clin North Am 1994;74:199–216.
8. Atnip RG. Vascular Surgery in the Elderly. In Katlic MR (ed), Geriatric Surgery Comprehensive Care of the Elderly Patient. Baltimore: Urban & Schwarzenberg, 1990;513–540.

9. Adkins RB, Scott HW (eds). Surgical Care for the Elderly. Baltimore: Williams & Wilkins, 1988.
10. Rhodes RS, Hutton MC, Baele HR, et al. Vascular Surgery in the Elderly. In Meakins JL, McClaran JC (eds), Surgical Care of the Elderly. Chicago: Year Book, 1988;414–433.
11. Ernst CB, Stanley JC (eds). Current Therapy in Vascular Surgery (3rd ed). St. Louis: Mosby–Year Book, 1995.
12. Moore WS (ed). Vascular Surgery: A Comprehensive Review (4th ed). Philadelphia: Saunders, 1993.
13. Rutherford RB (ed). Vascular Surgery (4th ed). Philadelphia: Saunders, 1995.
14. Williams TF. Demographics of Aging. In Brest AN (ed), Cardiovascular Clinics, Cardiovascular Disease in the Elderly. Philadelphia: Davis, 1992;3–7.
15. Evers BM, Townsend CM, Thompson JC. Organ physiology of aging. Surg Clin North Am 1994;74:23–39.
16. Cristofalo VJ, Gerhard GS, Pignolo RJ. Molecular biology of aging. Surg Clin North Am 1994;74:1–21.
17. Hertzer NR, Beven KG, Young JR, et al. Coronary artery disease in peripheral vascular patients. Ann Surg 1984;199:223–233.
18. Koruda MJ, Sheldon GF. Surgery in the Aged. St. Louis: Mosby–Year Book, 1991;293–331.
19. Mason JJ, Owens DK, Harris RA, et al. The role of coronary angiography and coronary revascularization before noncardiac vascular surgery. JAMA 1995;273:1919–1925.
20. Vogt MT, Wolfson SK, Kuller LH. Lower extremity arterial disease and the aging process: a review. J Clin Epidemiol 1992;45:529–542.
21. Taylor LM, Porter JM, Winek T. Femoropopliteal and Infrapopliteal Occlusive Disease. In Greenfield LJ (ed), Surgery Scientific Principles and Practice. Philadelphia: Lippincott, 1993;1656–1668.
22. LoGerfo FW, Pomposelli FB, Freeman DV, et al. Peripheral vascular disease in diabetes mellitus: implications for surgical management. Surg Rounds 1991;14:1055–1060.
23. Dormandy J, Mahir M, Ascandy G, et al. Fate of the patient with chronic leg ischemia. J Cardiovasc Surg 1989;30:50–57.
24. Criqui MH, Langer RD, Fronek A, et al. Mortality over a period of 10 years in patients with peripheral arterial disease. N Engl J Med 1992;326:381–386.
25. Zierler RE. Noninvasive detection of abdominal arterial occlusive disease. Surg Rounds 1991;14:1055–1060.
26. Baum RA, Rutter CM, Sunshine JH, et al. Multicenter trial to evaluate vascular magnetic resonance angiography of the lower extremity. JAMA 1995;274:875–880.
27. Owen RS, Carpenter JP, Baum RA, et al. Magnetic resonance imaging of angiographically occult runoff vessels in peripheral arterial occlusive disease. N Engl J Med 1992;326:1577–1626.
28. Gentile AT, Taylor LM, Moneta GL, et al. Irrelevance of asymptomatic carotid stenosis in patients undergoing infrainguinal bypass surgery. Arch Surg 1995;130:900–903.
29. Ahn SS, Eton D, Moore WS. Endovascular surgery for peripheral arterial occlusive disease. Ann Surg 1992;216:3–16.
30. Pfeiffer RB, Strong ST. Adjunctive use of the balloon dilatation catheter during vascular reconstructive procedures. J Vasc Surg 1986;3:841–845.
31. STILE Investigators. Results of a prospective randomized trial evaluating surgery versus thrombolysis for ischemia of the lower extremity. Ann Surg 1994;220:251–268.
32. Martin RS, Edwards WH, Mulherin JL, et al. Cryopreserved saphenous vein allografts for below-knee lower extremity revascularization. Ann Surg 1994;219:664–672.
33. Kretschmer G, Herbst F, Prager M, et al. A decade of oral anticoagulant treatment to maintain autologous vein grafts for femoropopliteal atherosclerosis. Arch Surg 1992;127:1112–1115.
34. Shah DM, Darling C, Chang BB, et al. Long-term results of in situ saphenous vein bypass. Ann Surg 1995;222:438–448.
35. Ekman C. Claes G, Carlsson I. Use of polytetrafluoroethylene grafts in elderly and high risk patients. South Med J 1982;75:1553–1555.
36. Kent KC, Magruder MC, Attinger CE, et al. Femoropopliteal reconstruction for claudication. Arch Surg 1988;123:1196–1198.
37. Scher LA, Veith FJ, Ascer E, et al. Limb salvage in octogenarians and nonagenarians. Surgery 1986;99:160–165.
38. Perler BA, Williams GM. Carotid endarterectomy in the very elderly: is it worthwhile? Surgery 1994;116:479–483.
39. Matsumoto N, Whisnant JP, Kurland LT, et al. Natural history of stroke in Rochester, Minnesota, 1955 through 1969: an extension of a previous study, 1945 through 1954. Stroke 1973;4:20–29.
40. Pokras R, Dyken ML. Dramatic changes in the performance of endarterectomy for disease of the extracranial arteries of the head. Stroke 1988;19:1289–1290.
41. Baker WH. Cerebrovascular Occlusive Disease. In Greenfield LJ (ed), Surgery Scientific Principles and Practice. Philadelphia: Lippincott, 1993;1597–1608.
42. Executive Committee for the Asymptomatic Carotid Atherosclerosis Study. Endarterectomy for asymptomatic carotid artery stenosis. JAMA 1995;273:1421–1428.
43. Feinberg WM, Albers GW, Barnett HJM, et al. Guidelines for the management of transient ischemic attacks. Circulation 1994;89:2950–2965.
44. Mattos MA, Hodgson KJ, Faught WE, et al. Carotid endarterectomy without angiography: is color-flow duplex scanning sufficient? Surgery 1994;116:776–783.
45. Kent KC, Kuntz KM, Patel MR, et al. Perioperative imaging strategies for carotid endarterectomy. JAMA 1995;274:888–893.
46. Barnett HJM, Eliasziw M, Meldrum HE. Drugs and surgery in the prevention of ischemic stroke. N Engl J Med 1995;332:238–248.
47. North American Symptomatic Carotid Endarterectomy Trial Collaborators. Beneficial effects of carotid endarterectomy in symptomatic patients with high-grade carotid stenosis. N Engl J Med 1991;325:445–453.
48. Treiman RL, Wagner WH, Foran RF, et al. Carotid endarterectomy in the elderly. Ann Vasc Surg 1992;6:321–324.
49. Ouriel C, Penn TE, Ricotta JJ, et al. Carotid endarterectomy in the elderly patient. Surg Gynecol Obstet 1986;162:334–336.
50. Pinkerton JA, Gholkar VR. Should patient age be a consideration in carotid endarterectomy? J Vasc Surg 1990;11:650–658.
51. Coyle KA, Smith RB, Salam AA, et al. Carotid endarterectomy in the octogenarian. Ann Vasc Surg 1994;8:417–420.
52. Meyer FB, Meissner I, Fode NC, et al. Carotid endarterectomy in elderly patients. Mayo Clin Proc 1991;66:464–469.
53. Bengtsson H, Bergqvist D, Sternby NH. Increasing prevalence of abdominal aortic aneurysms: a necropsy study. Eur J Surg 1992;158:19–23.
54. Goldstone J. Abdominal Aortic Aneurysms. In Greenfield LJ (ed), Surgery Scientific Principles and Practice. Philadelphia: Lippincott, 1993;1711–1722.
55. Cronenwett JL, Murphy TF, Zelenock GB, et al. Actuarial analysis of variables associated with rupture of small abdominal aortic aneurysms. Surgery 1985;98:472–483.
56. Ernst CB. Abdominal aortic aneurysm. N Engl J Med 1993;328: 1167–1172.
57. Katz DJ, Stanley JC, Zelenock GB. Operative mortality rates for intact and ruptured abdominal aortic aneurysms in Michigan: an eleven-year statewide experience. J Vasc Surg 1994;19:804–817.
58. Kiell CS, Ernst CB. Advances in Management of Abdominal Aortic Aneurysm. In Frykberg ER, Bland KI (eds), Advances in Surgery. St. Louis: Mosby–Year Book, 1993;73–98.
59. Meacham PW. Management of the Elderly Atherosclerotic Patient. In Adkins RB, Scott HW (eds), Surgical Care for the Elderly. Baltimore: Williams & Wilkins, 1988;421–435.
60. Treman R, Levine K, Cohen J, et al. Aneurysmectomy in the octogenarian: a study of morbidity and quality of survival. Am J Surg 1982; 144:194–197.
61. Kannel WB. Epidemiology of cardiovascular disease in the elderly: an assessment of risk factors. Cardiovasc Clin 1992;22(2):9–22.
62. Katz DA, Littenberg B, Cronenwett JL. Management of small abdominal aortic aneurysms. JAMA 1992;268:2678–2686.
63. Cambria RP, Brewster DC, Abbott WM, et al. Transperitoneal versus retroperitoneal approach for aortic reconstruction: a randomized prospective study. J Vasc Surg 1990;11:314–325.
64. Moore WS, Vescera CL. Repair of abdominal aortic aneurysm by transfemoral endovascular graft placement. Ann Surg 1994;229:331–341.
65. Marin ML, Veith FJ, Cynamon J, et al. Initial experience with transluminally placed endovascular grafts for the treatment of complex vascular lesions. Ann Surg 1995;222:449–469.
66. Johnston KW, Scobie TK. Multicenter prospective study of nonruptured abdominal aortic aneurysms. I. Population and operative management. J Vasc Surg 1988;7:69–81.
67. O'Donnell TF, Darling RC, Linton RR. Is 80 years too old for aneurysmectomy? Arch Surg 1976;111:1250.

Surgical Care for the Elderly, 2nd ed., edited by
R. Benton Adkins, Jr., and H. William Scott, Jr.
Lippincott–Raven Publishers, Philadelphia © 1998.

CHAPTER 20

Pulmonary Disease and Mediastinal Surgery

Richard M. Peters and James B.D. Mark

In this chapter we address the disorders of the lungs and the mediastinum and nonvascular cardiac diseases that occur in the mediastinum. Aging has important effects on the function of the lungs and the chest cage that compromise the ability of elderly patients to tolerate surgical procedures. These effects of aging are severely aggravated by deleterious noxious agents, such as smoking, asbestos, and other environmental pollutants. The integrity of the lungs in the elderly has often been compromised by infections that leave residual damage to the lungs. These include such diseases as tuberculosis, bronchiectasis, and other pulmonary infections that may lead to fibrosis and destruction of lung tissue.

Conditions in the elderly for which surgical management may be indicated are carcinoma of the lung, asbestosis and mesothelioma, lymphoma, empyema, lung abscess, destruction of lung by infection, and emphysema and its complication pneumothorax. In this age group, metastatic carcinoma to the chest, which is often complicated by malignant pleural effusions, is not uncommon. Unfortunately, the elderly are victims of trauma, particularly vehicular injury, that results in fractured ribs, pneumothoraces, and hemothoraces. Among the common complications of other diseases is loss of control of the swallowing mechanism, which can lead to lung abscesses, pneumonia, and their complications, pleural effusion and empyema. The most common disease of the elderly that needs surgical management is carcinoma of the lung. This used to be predominantly a disease of men, but with the marked increase in cigarette smoking by women during and since World War II, the incidence of carcinoma of the lung in women is increasing; in much of the United States it is now a more common cause of death than carcinoma of the breast. The incidence of chronic infection such as tuberculosis has gone down and is now seen most commonly in patients who have compromised immune function or those unfortunate elderly people who are homeless. Because carcinoma of the lung is the most common disease seen in the elderly patients, it is used in this chapter to illustrate many of the problems of surgery on intrathoracic disease in the elderly. The treatment of carcinoma of the lung requires resection of the lung. Therefore, it is important to understand the effects of aging on the chest cage and lung.

EFFECTS OF AGING ON CHEST CAGE AND LUNG

With aging, height decreases due to some narrowing of the invertebral spaces and vertebral bodies that usually leads to a progressive kyphosis. This change in the geometry of the chest is associated with a decrease in the chest wall compliance. The chest wall becomes stiffer. In emphysema, where the elastic tissue of the lungs breaks down, the inward pull of the lungs is less and the chest wall tends to expand, so the elderly patient has a larger anteroposterior diameter than a 20-year-old patient. As the elastic elements of the lung deteriorate [1–3], the number of alveoli decreases, which leads to a decrease in the capillaries. In addition, there is an increase in thickness of the small arteries, which results in increased pulmonary artery pressure and pulmonary vascular resistance [4].

These structural changes are associated with a decrease in the vital capacity and the expiratory reserve volume. At the same time, the functional residual volume increases from 30% of the total lung capacity at age 20 to 55% of the total lung capacity at age 70. The closing volume, or that volume at which the small airways are collapsed, increases so that at functional residual volume, a number of the small airways, particularly in the bottom of the lungs, may be closed. The consequence is an increasing mismatch between ventilation and perfusion and inefficiency of the lungs as gas exchangers. The ventilation-perfusion mis-

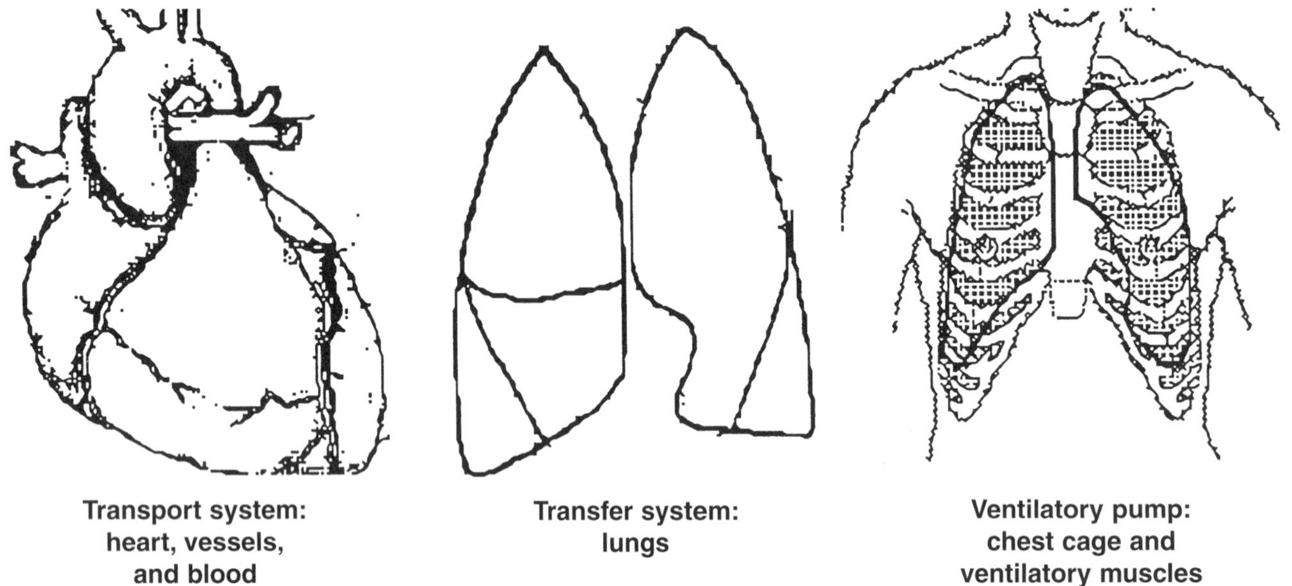

FIG. 20-1. The elements necessary for gas exchange: heart and circulation, lungs, ventilatory pump, and chest cage and its muscles. The surgeon must appraise both their individual and integrated functions. The laboratory data most specific to failure of each component are described in the text. (Reprinted with permission from Peters RM. Routine Respiratory Care and Support. In Hardy JD [ed], Hardy's Textbook of Surgery [2nd ed]. Philadelphia: Lippincott–Raven, 1988.)

match results in a decline in Pao_2 from 95 at age 20 to 75 at age 70, and the increase in the physiologic shunt from approximately 5% at age 20 to 15% at age 70. In terms of the patient's total ability to respond to stress, the maximal oxygen consumption decreases 35% between the ages of 20 and 70.

There have been and continue to be many efforts to develop accurate ways of predicting the reserve required for the patient to tolerate a pulmonary resection. These efforts have not met with complete success because the important function of the gas exchange is dependent on three elements (Fig. 20-1): (1) the heart and circulation, (2) the lungs, and (3) the chest cage. These integrated functions must be tested. If one uses criteria for adequate function of only one of these three systems, the prediction may be inaccurate. A patient with coronary artery disease or other cardiac disease will require better lung function, and a patient with compromised lung function will be less tolerant of compromise of the function of the chest cage and heart. The interaction of these three systems means it is important to evaluate all of them in predicting the outcome of an operative procedure and also in designing safe and effective postoperative care for patients undergoing thoracic surgical procedures.

The two most commonly used methods for assessing the adequacy of pulmonary reserve are spirometry and, often mistakenly, arterial blood gases. Spirometry depends on the patient's ability to cooperate and perform at a maximum to test the reserve. A well-done study includes a slow vital capacity to measure the maximum amount of air that the patient can breathe, and a forced vital capacity in which the patient makes a maximum effort to expel air as fast as possible after a maximum inspiration. These two simple studies are the major useful measurements. In patients who have interstitial lung disease such as sarcoidosis or pulmonary fibrosis, some additional information may be gained by measuring diffusion capacity. The first second forced expired volume (FEV_1) of the lungs is a measure of the speed with which the patient can force air out. FEV_1 and forced vital capacity both decrease with age. This decrease in FEV_1 is due to the changes in the lung and probably to a decrease in muscle strength of the respiratory muscles as patients age.

Spirometry results should include the absolute value for each measurement and the percent of predicted normal value, which are related both to the size and age of the individual. The unwary surgeon may make serious errors when dealing with elderly patients because as age increases, calculations of normal values predict a decrease in FEV_1 and forced vital capacity. If percentage of normal is used to assess operability as the patient ages, the progressively smaller absolute reserve will be missed.

Unfortunately, as a person ages he or she does not necessarily need less reserve to function, nor is it easier to have a pulmonary resection. Therefore, particularly in patients in the eighth decade of life, one must not use prediction formulas to decide whether the functional reserve is adequate but use the absolute figures. Perhaps more useful would be to use the predicted normal reserve at age 45 regardless of the age of the patient. Table 20-1 gives some of the values that have been suggested as setting the limits for pulmonary resection. For the patient undergoing pulmonary resection, the amount of function that will be left after resection is critical. To provide this essential information, it was necessary to develop a methodology to allow prediction of function remaining after pulmonary resection.

Spirometry should always be interpreted in association with evaluation of chest radiography. By assessing what segments of the lung need to be removed, the portion of lung that will remain can be predicted from figures of normal percent of total tissue in each segment [5]. This type of prediction may overestimate the decrease in function if the diseased portion of the lung is essentially nonfunctional, as it might be in a patient with central carcinoma obstructing the bronchus.

A more sophisticated way of predicting postpulmonary resection function is to perform a quantitative perfusion scan. With such a scan, one can predict how much of the function is going to the portions of the lung to be resected. By simple algebra, subtracting that percentage from the total gives the prediction of the remaining function [6]. An accepted rule of thumb is that a patient needs a postoperative FEV_1 of 800 ml. The 800-ml FEV_1 is a rough approximation that should not be used alone as an absolute criterion.

Some studies have suggested, as one might expect because the function of gas exchange involves the heart, lung, and chest cage, that the best predictor would be exercise testing and measurement of the maximum oxygen uptake. This particular method of testing is not so useful in patients who have intermittent claudication or skeletal disease that limit their exercise capacity. A study done in Sweden [7] showed that exercise testing was a superior predictor because it integrates the function of all three critical components: the chest wall, heart, and lungs. They studied 82 patients >70 years old and found the maximum oxygen consumption was reached at a mean level of 83 W of exercise during 6 minutes. Patients whose work capacity fell below 83 W had an operative mortality of 22%; those above it, none. This study supports an important principle: The risk factors defined by spirometry must not be considered alone but in conjunction with the assessment of the general health of the patient. The factors most important to evaluate are (1) evidence of muscle wasting, (2) the activity level the patient was able to achieve before the acute illness, (3) whether the patient continues to smoke, (4) evidence of chronic bronchitis and whether it has been maximally treated with a full and carefully planned medical regime, and (5) whether the patient is overweight.

In patients who show evidence of compromised pulmonary function, preoperative blood gases are important. If the patient has a PCO_2 >45, it is evidence that the patient already has ventilatory insufficiency. The patient is not a candidate for pulmonary resection unless there is clear evidence that at operation, something can be done that will improve function.

The significance of change in PO_2 is more difficult to predict. Resection of an atelectatic perfused area of the lung may improve PO_2. No set figure for a lower limit on PO_2 is appropriate. The PO_2 must be evaluated in terms of the abnormality of the lung.

TABLE 20-1. *Risk for pulmonary resection*

Test	High risk	Moderate risk	Low risk
Vital capacity (liters)	<1.85	1.85–3.00	>4.0
First second forced expired volume (liters)	<1.2	1.2–3.0	>3.2
Maximum voluntary ventilation (liters/min)	<28.0	>30<80	>80.0
Maximum midexpiratory flow (liters/sec)	<1.0	>1.0<2.0	>2.0

Source: Reprinted with permission from Peters RM. The Lung. In Peters RM, Peacock EE Jr, Benfield JR (eds), The Scientific Management of Surgical Patients. Boston: Little, Brown, 1983.

A history of angina requires careful workup to evaluate the degree of abnormality with exercise testing and isotope studies. If these test results are positive, one must define the coronary anatomy with coronary angiography. For patients who have significant coronary disease, the critical decision is the feasibility of an angioplasty or coronary artery bypass graft, followed usually at a later date by pulmonary resection [8]. A report by Miller et al. indicates that the late survival of patients undergoing a simultaneous coronary bypass graft and pulmonary resection is severely compromised [9]. The final and important consideration in dealing with elderly patients who are going to require a thoracotomy is their mental status. Patients who are unable to cooperate postoperatively, cannot cough effectively, are hard to mobilize, and are likely to pull out chest tubes will have a significantly increased morbidity and mortality. The increased morbidity and mortality must be considered in deciding the social and ethical issues inherent in advising operation on patients who cannot cooperate.

With the exception that one does not have to anticipate that the lung will be removed, the same set of criteria is applicable to patients requiring other forms of intrathoracic operations.

CHARACTERISTICS OF CARCINOMA OF THE LUNG IN THE ELDERLY

Thirty percent of carcinoma of the lung is squamous, 50% is adenocarcinoma, 15% small cell carcinoma, and 5% undifferentiated large cell carcinoma [10]. Squamous carcinoma is more often proximal, occurring in the larger bronchi, and likely to produce bronchial obstruction. It tends to metastasize late. Adenocarcinoma usually presents as a peripheral coin lesion, and is more likely to have blood-borne metastases than the squamous cell type. Small cell carcinoma, like squamous carcinoma, is more commonly proximal. It tends to metastasize early and can produce hormones that result in many types of endocrine abnormalities. Large cell undifferentiated carcinomas tend to be large, often with central necrosis. Fifty percent of patients at the time the diagnosis of carcinoma of the lung is made have stage HIB or IV tumor, which is not amenable to resection.

Carcinoma of the lung in the elderly behaves differently than in younger patients [11–13]. A number of studies have shown that older patients are more likely to have earlier stages of carcinoma of the lung. Huang et al. [14] suggest that older patients have a lower DNA protein content in their tumors that may explain slower tumor growth and less frequent metastases. In contrast to virtually every other site of carcinoma, there is an inverse relationship between age and stage in carcinoma of the lung. The incidence of carcinoma is greater in older patients, but it is more likely to be confined to the lung. Carcinoma of the lung also has a short time course if not effectively treated. In most cases, survival for 2 or 3 years after surgical treatment signifies confidence for a cure. Five-year survival has a high incidence of cure. This is in contrast to breast or colon cancer, where recurrences may occur in significant numbers for 5 and 10 years. There are those who have written off those in the 70-year age group as candidates for pulmonary resection. Both the biological nature and the effectiveness of modern thoracic surgery make this attitude insupportable. The recent trend toward adjuvant chemotherapy and radiation therapy for stage IIIB and IV lung carcinoma adds a significant risk to the operation when performed on elderly patients.

An important problem in carcinoma of the lung is that the carcinogen that induces the carcinoma, whether cigarette smoke or other pollutants, affects the entire lung parenchyma. Therefore, if one is successful in treating a first carcinoma of the lung and the patient survives, the incidence of second carcinomas increases. The thoracic surgeon must keep in mind the possibility of a second carcinoma of the lung when planning any lung resection. Removal of more lung than is essential for a first carcinoma may preclude successful surgical treatment of the second carcinoma. This is particularly important in the elderly, where carcinomas are likely to be local, and resection of a second cancer can be successful if pulmonary reserve is adequate. Patients who have had carcinoma of the head and neck are likely to have either synchronous or metachronous carcinoma of the lung [15]. These patients can present difficult clinical decisions.

Most stage I and II cancers of the lung are asymptomatic, and first suspicion starts with a routine chest radiograph. The value of routine chest radiography to detect cancer of the lung in high-risk patients is controversial. Central carcinomas that cause bronchial obstruction, hemoptysis, and pneumonia are most likely to produce symptoms. Symptomatic cancers for which the patient seeks help fail to get the correct diagnosis due to an incomplete workup. In caring for all patients who develop pneumonia, and particularly for smokers over age 45, the physician should consider bronchial obstruction as a cause of the pneumonia. Three to 4 weeks after treatment for the pneumonia, the physician should order radiography to check that there is complete resolution of the infiltrate. Incomplete resolution indicates the need for further study, in particular bronchoscopy, to rule out an obstructing lesion and obtain appropriate cytologic and biopsy specimens. Hemoptysis is an indication for bronchoscopy at the earliest possible time. The hemoptysis caused by a central carcinoma usually occurs at the time of respiratory infection, when cough is increased. Patients with lung cancer usually have only blood streaking in their sputum; they do not cough up significant amounts of blood.

Peripheral lesions are more often picked up in the early stages by the routine chest film. In high-risk patients, those with a history of heavy smoking or toxic chemical exposures, the physician should obtain periodic chest films. Controversy persists on this subject and good cost-benefit studies that equate the risk factors to the life years saved are needed. Routine cytology on sputum for discovery of early carcinoma of the lung is generally not cost-effective.

A patient suspected of having carcinoma of the lung, peripheral or central, should have fiberoptic bronchoscopy and chest computed tomography (CT) at the earliest possible time. In the central cancers, the lesion will be viewed and direct biopsy or brushings will provide a cytologic diagnosis. Obtaining cells for cytologic diagnosis of peripheral lesions requires fluoroscopic directed brushings and transbronchial biopsy, a transthoracic fine-needle biopsy, or both. Bronchoscopy provides other information. For a central cancer, bronchoscopy allows evaluation for resection and estimates of how much lung will have to be removed. A widened and blunted carina strongly suggests metastases to the subcarinal nodes. Transcarinal needle biopsy is a useful method of verifying the involvement of subcarinal nodes [16].

Some comment is in order about the value of transthoracic needle biopsy. In a patient with a coin lesion and a negative needle biopsy result, only thoracotomy and excisional biopsy can assure that the carcinoma is not missed. It is our experience that in 95% of our patients we obtain a preoperative diagnosis with the use of transbronchial and fine-needle biopsy. A preoperative diagnosis shortens and simplifies the operative procedure and allows us to emphasize to the patient the importance of undertaking the risk of thoracotomy. We have found the morbidity of fine-needle biopsy to be low and the mortality negligible. The major morbidity, pneumothorax, in most circumstances responds to the placement of a small catheter for closed suction drainage, if any treatment is needed at all.

When the cytologic diagnosis is established, it is essential to determine the extent of the tumor. Studies of ours and others [17,18] have shown the futility of obtaining routine bone, liver, and brain radionucleotide scans to assess the extent of tumor in patients who have no neurologic symptoms, a normal alkaline phosphatase level, and no evidence of bone pain. The evidence is unclear about whether routine head CT scans or magnetic resonance imaging (MRI) might pick up a significant number of patients (particularly for those with adenocarcinoma) with silent brain metastases. Today, the CT scan, MRI, and ultrasound have replaced the radionucleotide scan for evaluating the liver.

For assessment of the extent of tumor in the chest, we have used the CT scan [19]. CT evidence of mediastinal lymph nodes >1 cm indicate the need for a mediastinoscopy. If the nodes are <1 cm, we proceed with a thoracotomy without mediastinoscopy. Because some patients with CT scan nodes <1 cm have intranodal disease, in a poor-risk patient we are much more inclined to do a mediastinoscopy regardless of the finding of the CT scan. It is extremely important to point out that nodes >1 cm may not be carcinoma. The false-positive rate is >20%. Node enlargement requires a mediastinoscopy to determine whether the nodes are involved with carcinoma. Stage IV mediastinal node involvement makes complete resection unlikely.

Precision of TNM staging is an essential part of the workup of a patient with carcinoma of the lung. Carcinomas are best staged by the anatomic TNM system. At present, stages I, II, and III correlate the anatomic system with outcome. The presence or absence and location of lymph node metastases has become a major determinant of survival [20]. Using a lymph node map based on the anatomic structures within the mediastinum provides not only more accurate but also extra information. We use the map effectively for two purposes: (1) as an anatomic guide to accurate nodal mediastinoscopy [21], and (2) to identify the location of the excised nodes to permit correlation of positive nodes at various locations to the prognosis of disease.

Differential diagnosis of coin lesions always raises the question of whether the tumor is primary in the lung or might be metastatic from colon, breast, or another area. In the older age group with no history of primary tumor elsewhere, the overwhelming likelihood is that the tumor is primary in the lung. However, it is important to perform some simple clinical tests to minimize the chance of missing a metastatic lesion. These include, of course, the careful history of any prior carcinomas, sarcomas, or melanomas and evaluation of the likelihood of a metastatic lesion, careful examination of the breast and skin for evidence of melanoma or other obvious surface carcinoma, and evaluation of the important source of metastatic disease, the colon. We always take a careful history of change in bowel function and ascertain that patients have no occult blood in their stools.

SURGICAL TREATMENT OF CARCINOMA OF THE LUNG

Complete surgical resection offers the patient the best chance for cure; therefore, the workup should determine the likelihood that surgical resection will control the cancer. The stage of disease, more than the size of the tumor, particularly whether the patient has distant metastases or mediastinal node involvement, predicts a curative resection. Equally important is whether the patient can tolerate removal of a portion of the lung or lung and chest cage to remove all of the cancer. Until the early 1950s, total pneumonectomy was the accepted treatment for all patients with carcinoma of the lung.

Because not all patients can withstand this extensive resection, a number of patients received lesser resections. A classic paper by Churchill et al. [22], presenting results of lobectomy for cancer of the lung, evoked one of the most interesting discussions by the pioneers of cardiothoracic surgery. Their contemporaries complimented Churchill et al. on their presentation and then declared their own convictions that pneumonectomy, if suitable for one patient, was the preferred treatment for any size carcinoma of the lung. However, following this presentation by Churchill et al., there was a progressive change. The accepted form of treatment for cancer of the lung became a lobectomy where possible and pneumonectomy only if the tumor could not be removed with a lesser procedure. With this change, history repeated itself and patients who had limited pulmonary function and could not tolerate a lobectomy started to have lesser resections.

There have been a number of reports that parallel the experience with lobectomy versus total pneumonectomy [23–26]. These reports indicate that the standard by which all treatments of carcinoma of the lung must be measured is a lobectomy, a form of therapy that has never been subjected to any controlled studies that would justify this assumption. There are a number of studies of series of patients that show that limited resection gives acceptable results and, most important, lowers the operative mortality and immediate operative morbidity [23–25]. The difficulty in evaluating these various methods is that a rational basis of comparing the effects of various resections has not been worked out. There are no good studies of the incidence of local recurrence; the effects of operative mortality on group survival are disregarded [27]. The quality of life, namely how short of breath the patient is, whether he or she is able to play golf and do the other things that make life enjoyable, is completely neglected. Finally, no consideration is given in these studies to the fact that the incidence of second carcinoma is increasing as treatment success occurs. The more conservative the primary resection, if it removes any of the primary cancer, the greater chance that the patient can tolerate resection of a second carcinoma should that prove necessary.

In these authors' opinion, experience with resection tailored to the functional reserve of the patient and the extent of the cancer will force the conclusion that the correct pulmonary resection removes the smallest amount of the lung that provides an adequate margin to encompass all tumor. Even studies of large numbers of elderly patients to determine the importance of local recurrence with limited resection versus lobectomy cannot provide a definitive answer [28]. All thoracic surgeons should carefully correct prospective data on their patients and evaluate whether limited resections have smaller operative mortality and morbidity and a recurrence rate that is acceptable. At present, we use wedge or segmental resections to preserve function in a large portion of our elderly patients with limited pulmonary functions. In elderly patients with T3 tumors and chest wall invasion that requires a pulmonary resection and chest cage resection, the risks are very high. In a study of pulmonary resections in patients >70 years of age, Wilcox et al. reached the conclusion that combined pulmonary and chest wall resection carried a very high risk [29]. Also, as patients pass the 70th year, the risks of pneumonectomy begin to escalate almost logarithmically with age.

In patients with carcinoma of the lung, there should not be just one operative approach—pneumonectomy, lobectomy, or wedge resection. Both the amount of lung removed and the surgical incision used for this resection should be carefully tailored to the patient's needs. Unfortunately, most surgeons still use complete posterolateral thoracotomy incision for major pulmonary resections. The major cause of morbidity with pulmonary resection is not the operation itself, but the effects of the operation on the chest cage. Videothoracoscopy is another alternative for performing wedge resections. Procedures that limit damage to the chest cage can improve the prognosis of patients significantly. For wedge resections, a short thoracotomy that is carefully designed to overlay the area of lung to be removed allows the rib spreader to be opened less, sparing the patient the disruption of the chest cage. Videotherapy is another alternative for performing wedge resections. In patients who require a lobectomy, we usually use a posterolateral thoracotomy, but leave the serratus anterior intact. The group in Chicago under Faber and Jensik [30] has advocated the axillary incision without division of the latissimus or the serratus. In selected patients, Urschel and Razzuk [31] have advocated the use of a midline thoracotomy incision. The midline thoracotomy is the least painful incision and least disruptive to the chest wall unless the rib spreader has been markedly elevated and posterior ribs have been fractured. When the sternum is reapproximated and is immobile, the point of incision does not have to move so the pain is far less. With an incision in the posterolateral chest, every cough and every breath cause muscles to distort the closure and produce pain. If a double-lumen tube is used to ventilate the patient and the retractor is carefully positioned, all lobes, except perhaps the left lower lobe, can be resected through a sternotomy without great difficulty. It is neither appropriate nor feasible to present details of these various incisions in this chapter, but we urge the thoracic surgeon who performs thoracotomies on the elderly to recognize that the posterolateral thoracotomy incision is only one of the methods of entering the chest. The place of videothoracoscopy is discussed in the last section of this chapter.

Appropriate Anesthesia and Perioperative Respiratory Care of Elderly Patients Requiring Thoracotomy

A major factor in the increasing safety of thoracotomy and pulmonary resection in elderly patients has been the progress in anesthesiology, such as one-lung anesthesia and the cardiac anesthetic techniques for patients requiring coronary artery bypass. The most common cause of death following pulmonary resection is a coronary occlusion. This might be expected because patients who have carcinoma of the lung may have the risk factors for coronary artery disease, such as heavy smoking, little exercise, and other risky behaviors. The safety of thoracotomies can be enhanced by careful, controlled anesthetic that avoids transient hypotension or hypertension and compromise of cardiac function. Prevention of periods of hypotension and hypertension also requires careful control of perioperative fluids and anesthetics and analgesics.

The double-lumen tube is required for videothoracoscopy and also has a number of advantages for open thoracotomy. The double-lumen tube allows collapse of lung undergoing resection, decreases the manipulation of the lung, and allows the surgeon to resect through a smaller incision or through an incision that might otherwise give poorer exposure, such as the sternal splitting incision. The double-lumen tube is necessary to prevent spillage into the good lung in patients who have sepsis or bleeding. However, classic double-lumen tubes are stiff and have small internal diameters. Later designs provided a lumen of sufficient diameter to accommodate a balloon and a fiberoptic bronchoscope for manipulation in the major bronchus of the lung.

Fluid Therapy

In the preoperative preparation, it is important to make sure that elderly patients, and particularly those with emphysema, are not dehydrated. Physician orders may specify nothing by mouth on the evening before the operation. If the operation is not scheduled early in the morning, the patient will continue to be without fluids until the time of the operation, which may add up to 14 to 18 hours without fluid intake. In elderly patients with emphysema and bronchitis, this results in thickening of the secretions and an inability to cough up sputum. The dehydration also results in relative hypovolemia. The induction of anesthesia leads to hypotension that the anesthesiologist tries to correct, and infusion of balanced salt solution in turn leads to excessive intraoperative fluid infusion. A much safer regimen is to give patients a liter of intravenous 5% glucose in water early in the morning of the operation to keep hydration normal when the patient goes to the operating room.

During induction of anesthesia and the operative procedure, replace fluid and blood loss by precise administration of adequate but not excessive amounts of fluid. Patients who undergo pulmonary resections rarely require transfusions. Careful opening of the chest with a cautery and precise dissection usually can limit the blood loss to <500 ml, and at the most 700 ml, amounts that do not warrant a transfusion in the nonanemic patient. If crystalloid or colloid solutions are infused in adequate quantities to maintain blood volume, a hematocrit >25 is usually adequate. Removing a unit of blood or arranging for patient predonation can provide a backup to avoid the risks of banked blood. In patients with coronary disease, the decreased blood viscosity resulting from a decrease in hematocrit results in increasing blood flow to areas of the myocardium served by narrowed vessels [32]. Lower hematocrit may also act to lower the incidence of pulmonary emboli. The use of unnecessary transfusions adds other known risks, particularly those of non-A, non-B hepatitis and what is still a possibility, induction of acquired immunodeficiency syndrome.

It is essential to recognize that, after pulmonary resection, patients have a decrease in the size of the pulmonary vascular bed, and to maintain preoperative cardiac output, an increase in the blood flow through the remaining capillary bed is needed. Increase in flow in any capillary bed results in increased mean capillary pressure and the area of capillary bed opened. Both these factors increase fluid filtration. The removal of filtered fluid depends on the pulmonary lymphatics. Removal of a portion of the lung includes the pulmonary lymphatics. Following pulmonary resection more fluid is filtered through the remaining lung with a lower lymph pump capacity to remove the filtered fluid. The remaining lung is vulnerable to postoperative pulmonary congestion and edema. In our laboratories, we have made some studies of this problem [33]. Excessive intraoperative fluid infusion, which usually results in a large urine output in the immediate postoperative period, correlates with postresection pulmonary edema.

The surgeon should monitor carefully the quantity of intraoperative fluid given. Patients who receive a large amount of intraoperative salt solution and have high urine output are vulnerable to post–pulmonary resection pulmonary edema. The pulmonary edema becomes clinically manifest after the first 24 hours, usually 36 to 48 hours postoperatively. From the time of lung removal, the lymphatic pump progressively falls behind in fluid removal, until clinical edema manifests. The accumulation of fluid within the interstitium of the lungs overflows into alveoli to produce clinical pulmonary edema. Careful postoperative monitoring of patients at risk for pulmonary edema can provide the only chance for preventing this complication, which is induction of early diuresis. The complication of postpneumonectomy pulmonary edema is usually lethal. Any evidence of respiratory difficulty indicates the need for immediate intubation and assisted ventilation until pulmonary function is clearly back to normal and pulmonary congestion has resolved. Aggressive diuresis and ventilatory support are essential.

After pulmonary resection, minute ventilation and insensible water losses increase. In the postoperative period, care should begin to be taken not to overhydrate, but also to avoid underhydration. If all intravenous fluids are stopped in the morning after surgery, the patient will be dehydrated by the evening. It is better to give a modest amount of intravenous fluid throughout the first day until the patient has shown that he or she can sustain an oral intake adequate to avoid postoperative dehydration and thick secretions that cannot be coughed up. Patients should continue to have a minimum of 1,200 to 1,400 ml free water (5% glucose in water or oral salt-free fluids) in the first and second postoperative days to replace the insensible and renal water losses.

Postoperative Pain Control

The most common postoperative complication for all patients is respiratory. Thoracotomy amplifies the incidence and severity of postoperative pulmonary complications. Postoperative pulmonary complications result from malfunction of the chest bellows, principally resulting from pain. The usual manner of controlling this pain is to administer parenteral narcotics. In the elderly patient the level of narcotics necessary for control of pain frequently results in central respiratory depression and underventilation. Most elderly patients requiring pulmonary resection have emphysema and so have inefficient lungs. Inefficient chest bellows added to inefficient lungs, commonly cause respiratory insufficiency. Compromise of the chest bellows is not relieved but rather prolonged by postoperative use of the ventilator. The use of a ventilator increases the risk of disruption of bronchial closure and weakening of ventilatory muscles by disuse. It is important to use an analgesia technique that allows early spontaneous breathing and deep breaths and coughing and controls the pain of getting out of bed to encourage early ambulation. The goals of postoperative care depend on a method of controlling pain that does not require systemic narcosis [34]. We introduce an epidural catheter in the high lumbar or the thoracic region and use a continuous infusion of fentanyl or other short-acting narcotic for anesthesia.

The protocol that we use for this infusion is as follows: The epidural catheter can be put in just before or just after surgery. The catheter is inserted, carried all the way up the back, and taped along the spine, with the entry port for injection in the shoulder. The entry port (at the shoulder) and the connection are well secured. Strict sterile procedure is essential. After the anesthesiologist puts in the epidural catheter, he or she gives a test dose of lidocaine (Xylocaine) to ensure that the placement is accurate. The fentanyl solution contains 1,250 μg in 250 ml normal saline, 5 μg/ml, and is administered with an infusion pump at the rate of 10 to 20 ml per hour. *It is imperative that no sedatives or narcotics other than the specifically ordered fentanyl infusion run into the epidural catheter.* If the dressing becomes loose or wet or the catheter disconnects, the anesthesiologist checks the system immediately. The epidural catheter fluid pathway must be handled with strict sterile technique. Absolutely no other narcotics are to be given to the patient by any route. The infusion is discontinued if the patient develops evidence of central depression. If the patient exhibits profound respiratory depression (i.e., respiratory rate <6), oxygen is administered by mask at 6 liters per minute; naloxone (Narcan), 0.2 mg intravenously, is administered; and the patient is encouraged to take deep breaths. The minor side effects of epidural fentanyl (i.e., itching, urinary retention, and nausea) can usually be controlled and do not require cessation of the narcotic infusion. We have administered this range of fentanyl without difficulty in the intensive care unit and after discharge from the intensive care unit. We usually continue the epidural fentanyl for 2 or 3 days, although in some cases we have kept it up for considerably longer (in one case for as long as 2 weeks). The risk of the cumulative effects of epidural narcotics leading to acute respiratory depression increases if epidural and systemic narcotics are administered simultaneously.

Patients who have had this form of analgesia have moderate euphoria at the low dose of fentanyl and superior pain control. They cough effectively. To control pain in this manner for these few days cuts down on the need for narcotics later. If it appears that the acute immediate perioperative pain is well handled with the epidural analgesia, it is discontinued and the mobility and cough are kept up with moderate use of oral narcotics or analgesics. The result is quick re-expansion of the lungs, early administration of oral fluids, and a low incidence of atelectasis. It is hard to overemphasize the salutary effect of this form of postoperative pain control. Its value is most apparent in the elderly or patients who have evidence of emphysema.

Care of Chest Drainage

A few words should be given about the care of chest tubes in these patients. For lobectomy or segmental or wedge resection of lung, a right-angle chest tube is inserted through the fifth or sixth interspace in the posterior axillary line and placed into the posterior gutter and a short anterior tube is placed through the third or fourth interspace in the midaxilla, positioned into the apex of the chest. The exact type or site of insertion of the tube is not the critical factor. One tube should drain the posteroinferior chest to remove dependent fluid and one more anterior and superior to remove any air that leads from the lung. The tubes are connected to closed drainage and 20 cm of suction until the air leak is small, when they are put on gravity drainage. Most patients are gotten out of bed the night of the operation if the operation was done in the morning and asked first to sit on the side of the bed, then in a chair next to the bed, and progress to walking by the end of 36 hours. The chest tube devices are placed in a small cart, usually the type used for laundry bags, so the patient can wheel the cart about and ambulate not later than 48 hours after operation. For ambulation, it is reasonable to disconnect the chest tube suction for a short time, even if the patient still has a leak. If the air leak stops and fluid effusion is <80 to 100 ml per day, it is our practice to remove the chest tubes. It is important not to leave chest tubes in for fear that the leak may recur. Chest tubes have a negative effect as well as a therapeutic effect. They decrease the patient's mobility and cause pain, which inhibits cough. Chest tubes should only be left in as long as there is significant fluid and air egress. A limited apical air cap that is not increasing is a benign space that will usually absorb itself within the first 3 postoperative weeks.

With a regimen of double-lumen tube, careful control of fluids, epidural anesthesia, and early effective cough and ambulation, the duration of chest tube insertion and hospitalization has decreased for patients requiring thoracotomy.

Arrhythmias

A common complication of thoracotomy and pulmonary resection is a supraventricular tachycardia, atrial fibrillation, or flutter. This is usually adequately treated by digitalization to increase the atrioventricular (AV) block, but if the high ventricular rate is poorly tolerated, one of the calcium channel blockers should be given to control the rate. Digitalis should be maintained for 4 to 6 weeks to produce an adequate AV block to control tachycardia should the atrial fibrillation or flutter recur. There is a difference of opinion about the advisability of preoperative digitalization in patients over age 60. With more skill in the handling of cardiac drugs by cardiothoracic surgeons, the indications for preoperative digitalis have decreased. We now confine its use to those patients for whom digitalis is indicated on the basis of existing heart disease.

Infections

Surgical therapy is never a primary treatment for infections. Surgery is the treatment for the complications of infection. The complications can be divided into those that occur in the pleura, those that occur within the lungs and by etiologic agent, those due to pyogenic bacteria, and those due to fungus and tuberculous infections. The pyogenic infections occur as complications of pneumonia, lung abscesses, trauma, and operations within the chest.

The most common infections within the chest are infections of the pleura—empyema. An empyema is an abscess of the pleural cavity. The diagnosis of empyema is made by an appropriately placed thoracentesis and a culture to identify organisms. These abscesses require drainage. The difference in the treatment of pleural infections compared with infections in other areas of the body is that open drainage leads to collapse of the lung and a sucking chest wound. Until such time as the lung is adherent to the parietal pleura, the primary treatment of an intrapleural infection is early closed chest drainage [35]. Particularly in the elderly, for an infected pleural effusion >150 to 200 ml, it is advisable to put in a chest tube to avoid the complications of a chronic empyema. Of course, the patient should simultaneously have appropriate antibiotics. If drainage fails to remove all the fluid, one must determine whether the fluid is loculated and another procedure is necessary. In a healthy, vigorous individual with a loculated empyema and effective antibiotics to control the spread of infection, choices include an open thoracotomy for decortication and evacuation of the empyema. In most elderly patients, this more radical form of therapy is not indicated. Videothoracoscopy or open thoracostomy drainage to break down loculations and drain the fluid are safer and more appropriate therapy. Open drainage can, if necessary, be done under local anesthesia with resection of a short portion of one rib, preferably in the dependent portion of the empyema, usually the sixth or seventh rib in the posterior axillary line.

To determine whether the patient will withstand open drainage, two methods are available. Consider the type of drainage. If fluid sedimentation is >50% cellular mass, open drainage will almost certainly be tolerated because the lung will be stuck to the chest wall. If, after opening the chest, it is found that the lung tends to collapse, a large tube can be placed and attached to a water seal until such time as the lung does stick and open drainage becomes safe.

If before any tap there is any air-fluid level, then there is a bronchopleural fistula. It is urgent to drain the lung in these patients because the bronchopleural fistula provides a route for the infected pus to flood the tracheobronchial tree and drown the good dependent lung. When doing this drainage, it is important not to put the healthy lung downward during the operation, but rather to sit the patient up. To prevent fluid spilling from the diseased lung into the dependent lung, a well-placed double-lumen tube is essential before putting the patient with the good lung in the down position.

Pyogenic lung abscesses occasionally require surgical therapy. Pyogenic lung abscesses are principally the result of aspiration and therefore appear in the posterior portions of the lungs, superior segment of the lower lobe, and posterior segment of the upper lobe. Lung abscesses require vigorous antibiotic therapy, usually large doses of penicillin, and the patient should receive bronchoscopy to remove any aspirated material and ascertain whether the abscess is actually a complication of an endobronchial tumor. With appropriate antibiotic therapy and postural drainage, most lung abscesses resolve. Many abscesses are complicated by pleural effusions, and occasionally the abscess ruptures into the pleural cavity, a complication that demands immediate pleural drainage to prevent flooding of tracheobronchial tree with pleural fluid.

Abscesses that persist in a sick, toxic patient may require drainage or removal. With modern interventional radiology we have found that introducing a small catheter under radiologic control into the abscess is a conservative, often successful, and definitive method of drainage. If a small catheter is not effective in the elderly, very sick patient, emergent surgical drainage may be necessary. Drainage is best done by localizing the area on the chest wall where the cavity abuts the parietal pleura and resecting a portion of rib right over this area. With a chronic lung abscess, the area over the abscess will usually be adherent to the pleura so that the abscess can be entered without contaminating the pleura. If there are no pleural adhesions, it is best to pack the wound for a few days and allow some adhesions to develop before draining the cavity. One of the problems of pyogenic abscesses is hemorrhage. Therefore, hard tubes that might erode a vessel should not be put into the lung. If the patient is a good risk, resection of the cavity may be warranted.

Other infections of the lung in the elderly that occasionally require resection are the complications of tuberculosis or fungus, or a combination of the two. With modern chemotherapy for tuberculosis, it is rare that the elderly patient is a candidate for resection. Tuberculosis is rarely a fatal disease if treated with effective antibiotics and the patient's immune system is intact. Most chronic pulmonary disease that warrants resection is far advanced, for which resection is rarely indicated in the elderly patient [36]. Surgical treatment is reserved for life-threatening complications such as hemorrhage. One of the common combinations that leads to hemorrhage in the patient with tuberculous cavities is the colonization of the cavity with *Aspergillus* organisms. These patients develop a fungus tumor within the cavity, which then erodes vessels and results in significant hemorrhage [37]. Complications of chronic pulmonary cavities require balancing the threat of exsanguinating hemorrhage and the usually compromised pulmonary function. If bleeding is uncontrollable, conservative methods may be most appropriate. These can include the introduction of a Fogarty catheter into the bronchus of the bleeding area and blowing up the balloon to occlude the bronchus and tamponade hemorrhage. Some advocate interventional radiologic embolization of the bronchial arteries, which may give only temporary respite, and, particularly in the elderly, carries the risk of the material blocking vessels to the spinal cord and producing neurologic damage.

It is impossible to provide one treatment plan for elderly patients with hemoptysis. The surgeon must make the difficult judgment of what pulmonary function the patient will have left after resection. In patients with chronic abscesses and bleeding, it is essential to use a double-lumen tube or some method to isolate and tamponade the bleeding area of the lung. The destroyed area of the lung usually has dense adhesions to the chest and mediastinum, and it is a slow and difficult process to get down to the hilar vessels. In the elderly, the principal caveat in the treatment of the complications of pulmonary infections is conservatism. Be certain that the proposed surgery is going to improve the patient's condition, not threaten his or her life.

Pleural Malignancies

Pleural malignancies have two principal etiologies, mesotheliomas and metastatic malignancies to the pleura. For half a century, asbestos was a widespread pollutant of construction industries, and over the next few decades, many more of the elderly will fall victim to the careless use of this material. Asbestos exposure can cause the relatively benign disease asbestosis, manifest as some fibrotic changes within the lung and pleural plaques that inhibit pulmonary function, but without surgical implications. The surgeon must not confuse asbestosis with mesotheliomas. Benign mesotheliomas are usually pedunculated tumors that arise from visceral pleura often in an interlobar fissure. They are not associated with asbestos exposure. Usually they are picked up on routine chest radiography.

Malignant mesotheliomas may be localized or diffuse with effusion and encasement of the lung [38]. The most common symptoms are pain and dyspnea. The peak incidence is between the ages of 70 and 79. The malignant form can have two cytologic patterns: fibrosarcomatous or epithelial. The localized form is usually fibrosarcomatous and appears as a mass on radiography. The diffuse form is more often epithelial. The fibrosarcomatous form is less common but should be excised with an adequate margin. The role of surgery in the diffuse form is more controversial. Eighty-five percent of patients have pleural effusion on presentation. Unfortunately, the problem of mesotheliomas, whether benign or malignant, is that the pathologic diagnosis is difficult. Without a large tissue biopsy, histologic characteristics make a definitive diagnosis difficult. Cytology is usually nonproductive.

However, the radiographic and clinical picture of mesothelioma is quite distinctive: pleural effusions and intrapleural sheets of tumor. The accompanying history of asbestos exposure is important in establishing the diagnosis. In most cases the diagnosis can be made with the radiologic evidence alone. To satisfy our demands for a definitive diagnosis and often for medicolegal reasons, a tissue biopsy is necessary. Videothoracoscopy or a conservative thoracotomy should excise at least a 2 × 2–cm piece of tissue taken for pathologic study. Therapy of diffuse mesotheliomas is controversial; some consider surgery useless.

Pleurectomy and radical extrapleural pneumonectomy may have some place in vigorous patients, but not in the elderly. En bloc resection of tumor in the lung together with diaphragm has been unrewarding even in young patients and has no justification in the elderly. Pleurectomy is justified in good-risk patients, although better survival may be due to treatment of earlier stage disease. One of the major complications of mesothelioma is pleural effusion, which responds only marginally well to chest drainage. Mesothelioma results in progressive restrictive pulmonary disease with pain and dyspnea due to tumor within the chest and extension to surrounding chest wall, diaphragms, and mediastinum. Unfortunately, the treatment of mesothelioma is purely symptomatic: drainage of pleural effusion, achievement of pleural symphysis, and pain control.

Pleural effusion from metastatic malignancy is most commonly seen in association with carcinoma of the colon, breast, or lung. If the effusion compromises the patient's pulmonary reserve, closed chest drainage is advisable. In perhaps 50% of the patients, effective closed chest drainage leads to obliteration of the pleural space and to continued control of the effusion. If the effusion is large, it is important not to try to drain the fluid all at once. It is best to let the fluid out in increments of 500 to 1,000 ml, stopping when the patient has any symptoms of cough. If a patient's lung does not expand rapidly, the mediastinum will be displaced toward the side of the effusion and the patient will develop severe cough and difficulty in getting a breath due to overexpansion of the contralateral lung. In some patients, the lung will be so involved with the carcinoma that re-expansion is not possible. In these patients, drainage will have little effect. Whether to introduce sclerosing agents at the first drainage to increase the likelihood of pleural symphysis is controversial. The most commonly used sclerosing agent was tetracycline, which is no longer available. At the present, talc, doxycycline, and bleomycin are the most common agents used. Talc is the most effective agent, and the theoretic contraindications of possible carcinogenesis do not apply to elderly patients.

Pneumothorax

In the elderly patients with emphysema, pneumothorax is a dreaded and not uncommon problem. In the elderly it is best treated by introduction of a large-bore chest tube. We usually put the chest tube either in the second anterior interspace or high in the axilla, just below the axillary hair. The chest drainage is connected to 20 cm of suction. It is important to manage the chest tubes of patients with spontaneous pneumothorax the same as postresection patients: control the pain and get them out of bed and coughing. If the leak is not too big, at times the patient can be disconnected from suction and encouraged to ambulate. When the leak is large, long pieces of tubing can be used to connect the chest drainage to the suction apparatus, which is maintained while the patient wanders around the room. Confining such patients to bed leads to chronic leak or other complications of immobilization. To get the expanded lung to stick to the parietal pleura requires coughing and moving, as well as suction on the chest tubes.

In a young patient with pneumothorax, if a leak persists for 2 to 3 days, thoracoscopic repair is the therapy of choice. The risks are greater in elderly patients. Recent experience treating emphysema patients may indicate that a similar approach to that of a young patient is warranted in an elderly patient with emphysematous lungs.

Elderly patients with emphysema need tube drainage for longer periods, and some may go home with a Heimlich-type valve for control of small pneumothorax. Some advocate the use of strong sclerosing agents in these patients; however, sclerosing agents used in a patient with pneumothorax result in far more pain than in a patient with an already inflamed pleura from an effusion. We advise that if sclerosing agents are to be used, the patients should have epidural analgesia. If the sclerosing agents obliterate the space, the leak will seal and prevent further pneumothoraces. In elderly patients, the use of talc for inducing pleurodesis can produce severe pleuritic pain, so it should be a therapy of last resort.

Mediastinal Tumors

Mediastinal tumors are often diagnosed by routine chest film or when a chest film is taken for symptoms as diverse as vague discomfort to pain and the effects of superior vena caval obstructions. Preoperative CT of the chest is essential. In most instances, a good indication of the type of mediastinal tumor is possible with CT scanning. Histologic diagnosis of mediastinal tumors in most instances requires a generous biopsy. Differentiating between a lymphoma, thymoma, or germ cell tumor may tax a pathologist even with a generous biopsy. Current specific treatment requires a generous amount of tissue for precise definition, using both cytologic and immunologic techniques.

Thymoma and Myasthenia Gravis

Thymoma is more frequently associated with myasthenia gravis in the elderly [39]. Two peaks in the incidence of non-thymoma myasthenia gravis are between 10 and 30 years and 60 and 70 years of age. Following resection of the thymus, the remission rates are the same for both elderly and young patients. A short duration of myasthenia usually has earlier and more complete remission. The remission rate increases over at least 3 years to between 50% and 60%. Elderly patients undergoing surgery for myasthenia gravis should have the same preparation as younger patients, optimal drug control of the myasthenia gravis including, if necessary, corticosteroids. Three approaches to operation are presently advocated for thymectomy: a cervical incision without opening the sternum [40,41], a sternal splitting incision, and videothorascopic removal. The transcervical method is criticized by some for being likely to leave portions of the thymus in the mediastinum. Sternal splitting incision is mandatory in the patient with a tumor of the thymus. Determination of whether a thymoma is malignant or benign depends on the surgeon identifying whether the tumor has remained within the capsule or has invaded outside the capsule of the gland. Attempts should be made to excise all of the tumor even if it requires resection of the pericardium. In elderly patients, resection of a phrenic nerve is almost certainly unwarranted because they may be unable to sustain ventilation with even unilateral phrenic paralysis.

Diseases of the Esophagus

Diseases of the esophagus have peak incidence in the >65 age group. The principal problems are motor disorders, the results of incompetence of the gastroesophageal sphincter mechanism, and carcinoma of the esophagus.

Carcinoma of the esophagus peaks in the seventh and eighth decades. The incidence of carcinoma of the esophagus has wide geographic variations. In the United States, it is an uncommon carcinoma and is usually seen late. The case finding method of brushing for cytology used in China and Japan is not cost-effective in the United States except in high-risk patients such as those with Barrett's esophagus or achalasia. These patients should have annual esophagoscopies with biopsy of suspicious areas. Patients presenting with a history of difficulty swallowing have a symptom that signifies organic disease. They should have a barium swallow and esophagoscopy with biopsy if an area of abnormal mucosa is present.

Controversy characterizes the indications for and type of surgical therapy and the use of adjuvant radiation or chemotherapy for carcinoma of the esophagus [42]. At the time of diagnosis, most patients have advanced stages of the disease and are relatively poor risks due to age and associated diseases. Carcinoma of the esophagus is staged by tumor length (T1 <5 cm; T2 >5 cm), absence of penetration through the wall of the esophagus (T1 and T2), penetration through the wall (T3), movable unilateral nodes (N1), movable bilateral nodes (N2), and fixed nodes (N3). M1 is often manifest as nodes in the celiac area. Carcinoma of the esophagus spreads for extended distances in the submucosal lymphatics. This propensity for extension has led many to advocate total thoracic esophagectomy for all patients. To reconstruct the esophagus, most surgeons now use the stomach. The accepted method of esophagectomy with esophagogastrostomy is to mobilize the stomach through a laparotomy and remove the esophagus through a right thoracotomy. For total esophagectomy, a cervical incision is needed for the anastomosis. Orringer [43] has championed the removal of the esophagus by mobilization through the hiatus and cervical incisions—nonthoracotomy esophagectomy. This approach decreases the operative stress but results in more blood loss. For selected cases Skinner [44] advocated radical esophagectomy with extensive removal of perigastric and periesophageal lymph nodes. He used laparotomy and right thoracotomy with cervical esophagogastric anastomosis. The 2- to 5-year survival rate after resection of esophageal carcinoma is only approximately 5%, so in most patients the operation is palliative. Swallowing is restored and usually maintained for the duration of life. Radiation is used as definitive treatment and as adjunctive therapy preoperatively and postoperatively, and adjunctive preoperative and postoperative chemotherapy has been tried. There are no clinical trials comparing concurrent groups of comparable patients. The only constant is high recurrence rate and a significant population of patients who have unresectable disease at time of presentation.

At this time, we advocate total removal of thoracic esophagus with cervical esophagogastric anastomosis to prevent local recurrence at the anastomosis and change the anastomotic leak from a life-threatening to a minor complication. The choice of transhiatal or right thoracotomy depends largely on the experience of the surgeon. The transhiatal approach can lead to intraoperative hemorrhage but avoids the trauma of simultaneous laparotomy and thoracotomy. If nodes about the celiac axis or extension to the liver are found on CT or exploratory laparotomy, resection is not justified except in good-risk patients with the inability to swallow. Radical esophagectomy, as advocated by Skinner, has yet to be proved efficacious and is applicable only to a small percent of patients, even in Skinner's hands.

The complication of tracheoesophageal fistula, spontaneous or after radiation therapy, can justify bypass of the esophagus without thoracotomy by closing the esophagus in the neck and at the hiatus, bringing the stomach up without removal of the esophagus. For patients who cannot swallow and are not candidates for esophageal resection, insertion of one of the Silastic splints can provide significant palliation. If there is a good shelf to hold the tube, it can be inserted endoscopically. The alternative is to do a small laparotomy and gastrotomy to permit the tube to be pulled through the narrowed area of the esophagus and sutured to fascia to prevent migration. The esophageal splints permit the patient to swallow saliva, liquids, and often soft foods. The tubes may block a tracheoesophageal fistula and prevent aspiration.

The choice of appropriate therapy for carcinoma of the esophagus requires careful assessment of the extent of the cancer, physiologic state of the patient, and procedure that will provide the greatest comfort at a reasonable risk. In the occasional patient with early-stage disease, we need more information to know if radical resection will improve survival. Preoperative radiation can make local resection easier. Whether it improves longevity is not clear.

Motor disorders of the esophagus are more frequent as patients age. Achalasia and the uncommon entity, diffuse esophageal spasm, are disorders of coordination and neurotransmission. In achalasia, the peristaltic wave does not progress in an orderly manner, so the lower esophageal sphincter fails to relax. The esophagus becomes distended, and patients often aspirate the foul contents of the megaesophagus. The radiologic picture is distinctive, but the patient should have esophagoscopy after the esophagus has been cleaned out to inspect the mucosa for ulceration. Attempts can be made to burst the muscle of the sphincter with an inflatable dilator. The surgical approach is transthoracic myotomy extending from the stomach to at least the inferior pulmonary vein. The edges of the myotomy incision must be separated by dissecting the mucosa from the muscle. Controversy rages over the advisability of performing an antireflux procedure and whether it should be a complete or partial wrap [45]. The advocates cite a late high incidence of regurgitation and peptic esophagitis. If the wrap is used, it should be loose and short. Patients with achalasia have increased risk of carcinoma. Careful follow-up with annual brushing of the esophagus for cytology, esophagoscopy, or both are indicated.

Diffuse esophageal spasm is, fortunately, uncommon. Diagnosis is made from both radiography and manometry. Treatment must focus on symptoms. The most conservative manipulative treatment is dilatation. In patients with intractable symptoms, a long myotomy from the stomach to the upper third of the esophagus, which has striated muscle, can relieve symptoms. Henderson [46] advocates a myotomy all the way to the neck.

Hiatus Hernia

Hiatus hernia is common in the elderly patient. Surgical repair should be reserved for patients with complications of the hernia, peptic esophagitis, or bleeding from gastric ulceration, usually at the point the diaphragm compresses the stomach. Peptic esophagitis should be evaluated with 24-hour pH monitoring, esophageal manometry, and esophagoscopy. If symptoms are associated with an increase in esophageal pH and cannot be controlled with a medical regimen of antacids and H_2 blockers, elevation of the bed, and abstinence from food or drink for 2 to 3 hours before bedtime, operative repair of hernia and an antireflux procedure are indicated. If esophagoscopy shows evidence of Barrett's esophagus, stricture, or ulceration, preoperative biopsy is essential to rule out cancer. Most strictures respond to intraoperative dilatation. If sphincter competency is restored, the stricture and ulcerations regress.

Each type of operative approach and sphincter-restoring procedure has its advocates. Belsey, Nissen, and Hill's methods are effective in preventing regurgitation. If the wrap is too tight or too long, the patient cannot burp or vomit and gas bloat results. Care must also be taken to suture the wrap to the stomach and to fix the stomach in the abdomen to prevent the wrap from migrating into the chest where the sphincter will be ineffective. The surgeon should be conservative about indications for hiatal hernia repair in the elderly. If the patient requires operation, all the principles described for preoperative, postoperative, and intraoperative care for thoracotomy patients are essential.

Pneumectomy

Since the publication of the first edition of this book, Cooper has resurrected an operative procedure first done by Brantigan to palliate the symptom of dyspnea for patients with advanced chronic obstructive pulmonary disease (COPD). Cooper et al. [47] named the procedure *pneumectomy*. The symptom dyspnea arises when the effort to breathe taxes the reserve of the ventilatory muscles. The efficiency of the lungs as gas exchangers and the chest bellows and ventilatory muscles that pump air in and out of the lungs determine the level of ventilatory effort that induces dyspnea.

Patients with COPD have lungs with diminished alveolocapillary surface area, expiratory airway obstruction, and loss of elastic recoil. The combination of these factors results in an increase in the end-expiratory lung volume. The chest bellows and its muscles operate as a suction pump. Ventilatory muscles act during inspiration to stretch the elastic elements of the lungs and chest cage and overcome the resistance of inspiratory airflow. Expiration is a passive event driven by the elastic recoil of the lungs and chest cage. Like the myocardial fibrils, the ventilatory muscles need an adequate preload force to stretch them to function efficiently. Ventilator muscles are stretched some, even at small lung and chest cage volume. The COPD patient's inefficient lungs make the chest cage muscles inefficient. Emphysematous lungs have a low elastic recoil and high airway resistance that leads to a high end-expiratory volume. At high end-expiratory lung volumes the chest cage muscles have inadequate stretch to initiate a strong efficient inspiratory force.

Lung transplant for COPD raised questions of how to determine the appropriate size of the donor lung, the normal lung volume, or the expanded chest volume. Cooper et al. [47] reported that after lung transplant the chest cage adapted to the size of the lungs as appropriate to a normal volume for the patient. The less compliant transplanted lungs with more elastic recoil pulled the chest to a normal end-expiratory volume. The mechanics of the lung were the major determinant of end-expiratory volume and preload of the inspiratory muscles. Brantigan et al. [48] resected portions of the lung in a series of patients with COPD to reduce the lung volume. They reported great symptomatic improvement for the patients, but there was a high operative mortality. Brantigan's operation failed to gain popularity because of the high operative mortality and failure to develop objective measures of increased respiratory function.

Cooper et al. [47] studied a large number of patients with COPD awaiting donor lungs for transplant, and their experience with adaptation of chest cage volume to transplanted lung size reasoned that reducing the lung volume in patients with COPD might relieve dyspnea by making the chest cage more efficient. They selected a group of patients from the waiting list to undergo his standard pretransplant ventilatory training before having a pneumectomy. Cooper et al. used a median sternotomy approach and one-lung anesthesia technique to resect the peripheral hyperexpanded and bullous lungs sequentially. Cooper et al. soon learned that reinforcing the staples with bovine pericardium diminished postoperative air leaks and greatly improved the postoperative course of the patients.

Wakabayashi et al. [49] have used thoracoscopy and laser ablation for lung reduction. Fortunately, the peripheral portions of the lungs are the most dysfunctional and so the lung reduction does not sacrifice intolerable amounts of gas-exchange surface. The relief of dyspnea in the COPD patients occurs despite loss in marginal functional lung because the lung resection reduces both the volume and compliance of the lungs. The chest cage volume decreases to the point that the ventilatory muscles have an adequate preload at end expiration. The increased preload makes the muscles more efficient, which relieves the sensation of dyspnea and allows the patients to increase their activity levels. A more subatmospheric intrapulmonary pressure holds the airways open during expiration and also increases the filling pressure of the heart. The system operates at more optimal pressures and volumes.

This operation has gained wide acceptance without developed criteria for patient selection or methods of objectively evaluating its success. All studies have centered common measurements of lung volume, air flow rates, and blood gases. The results documented by these tests have proved inconsistent with the clinical results. The problem arises because the tests used do not measure the effectiveness of chest cage mechanics. Cooper et al. [47] have shown using dynamic MRI that higher end-expiratory pressure increased diaphragmatic excursion. This methodology is a research tool. A simpler method, measurement esophageal pressures before and after pneumectomy, can objectively document improvement in diaphragmatic and chest wall function. A COPD patient who is a candidate for pneumectomy should have high (near atmospheric) end-expiratory esophageal pressures and low delta pressures with respiration. Postoperatively, the end-expiratory pressure should decrease (become more subatmospheric) and the delta pressures increase. Maximum inspiratory pressure measurement is a simpler test to determine if the patient can create better ventilatory force. Another explanation of symptomatic improvement is better cardiac muscle mechanics. The filling pressure of the heart is the difference between the intracardiac pressure and the pleural pressure. The more subatmospheric pleural pressure increases the cardiac filling pressure and should increase myocardial efficiency. The change in pleural pressure may alter pulmonary vascular mechanics also, but this seems an unlikely source of relief of symptoms. Patients who are candidates for pneumectomy are very sick and require careful selection, preoperative preparation, operative technique that minimizes postoperative air leaks, and excellent postoperative pain control and respiratory care. In a discussion of pneumectomy, Miller et al. cautioned that patients with significantly elevated $PaCO_2$ were high risks and had poor outcomes. They also emphasized that these patients have complex systemic complications that are difficult to manage [9].

ROLE OF VIDEOTHORACOSCOPY

The use of thoracoscopy for various intrathoracic diagnostic and therapeutic purposes is not new. In 1910, Hans Christian Jacobaeus, a Swedish internist, used a cystoscope to view the pleural cavity and to divide adhesions with cautery in patients with pulmonary tuberculosis for whom collapse therapy was advised [50]. The need for thoracoscopy diminished as other forms of collapse therapy became popular, drugs for tuberculosis were found, and resectional surgery developed. Until recently, the inherent disadvantage of single-viewer observation remained.

In 1989, Reddick and Olsen reported the therapeutic utility of videolaparoscopy [51]. It was not long before the video technique was adapted to the more receptive thoracic cavity. Videothoracoscopy for both diagnostic and therapeutic purposes has grown rapidly [52,53]. Its major advantage over nonvideothoracoscopy is that many people can view the field simultaneously on television screens. The development of instruments specifically suited for videothoracoscopy has been helpful as well. The major advantage for the patient is that there is less pain following videothoracoscopy than following thoracotomy. This allows some intrathoracic diagnostic and therapeutic procedures to be carried out safely in elderly, poor-risk patients who would be unable to tolerate standard thoracotomy. The inherent disadvantage of two-dimensional viewing remains, although three-dimensional systems are under development.

Solitary Pulmonary Nodules

It is not unusual for asymptomatic, peripheral, solitary pulmonary nodules to be discovered in elderly patients when chest radiographs are taken for other purposes or as part of a routine examination. Unless the patient has had previous chest radiography, the age of the lesion is unknown. If the lesion does not contain stippled or concentric or heavy calcification and especially if the patient is or has been a cigarette smoker, lung cancer usually leads the diagnostic list. In many such elderly patients, it is clear that even lobectomy, let alone pneumonectomy, would be accompanied by high or even prohibitive risk. However, unless there are strong and specific reasons to the contrary, accurate diagnosis of the lesion should be established and the best available treatment should be carried out. Although fine-needle aspiration (FNA) of the lesion can be carried out, it has several disadvantages in this setting. The FNA result is positive in approximately nine instances out of 10 if the mass is malignant, but it is positive in less than one-half of the instances of benign lesions [54,55]. Even if it is accurate in establishing a diagnosis, FNA alone has no therapeutic value. Additionally, complications of FNA, specifically pneumothorax and bleeding, are likely to occur more frequently in older patients and be more troublesome and dangerous when they do occur. In contrast, videothoracoscopy with wedge resection of suitably situated lesions of appropriate size is both the best diagnostic tool and best available treatment. The disadvantages of general anesthesia and hospitalization and the inherent risk and discomfort are associated with the procedure. However, whereas further treatment, radiotherapy, or less likely chemotherapy, will be necessary following the diagnosis of cancer by FNA, thoracoscopic wedge resection may well be sufficient treatment for a stage I non–small cell lung cancer (NSCLC) [56].

If a peripheral pulmonary nodule proves to be a granuloma, hamartoma, typical carcinoid, or other less life-threatening lesion, video-assisted thoracic surgery (VATS) with wedge resection is in many instances an ideal operation for elderly patients [57–59]. In the rare instance of small cell lung cancer (SCLC) in a coin lesion, VATS wedge resection provides solid diagnostic information and the opportunity to determine the advisability of adjuvant therapy. The diagnosis of SCLC by FNA alone is frequently erroneous. Atypical carcinoid and other neuroendocrine or mixed tumors may be confused with SCLC on the basis of cytologic examination alone.

Carcinoma of the Lung

The standard pulmonary resection with curative intent is lobectomy with removal of regional lymph nodes. Pneumonectomy is carried out only if lobectomy is not adequate for complete resection of the tumor. Lesser resections, although appealing in many ways, have not been shown to result in cure rates as high as those following lobectomy [28,60]. However, in elderly patients whose cardiopulmonary reserve may be limited, lesser resections become the procedure of choice for many stage I NSCLCs. For those lesions suitably located in the lung periphery, videothoracoscopy is the ideal surgical approach. Because videothoracoscopy causes less early postoperative pain than thoracotomy [61], it permits more elderly patients to be candidates for tumor resection, provided that adequate resection of the tumor can be carried out by this technique. Although lobectomy with lymph node dissection and even pneumonectomy have been carried out using VATS [62,63], these are neither widely applied nor universally safe uses of videothoracoscopy. The major advantage of VATS in the treatment of lung cancer is for removal of stage I NSCLC in instances when a standard or even limited thoracotomy approach would be riskier.

Thoracoscopic resection of lung tumors and other uses of videothoracoscopy require the use of double-lumen endobronchial tubes, a technique now widely available. One concern with this technique is whether the elderly patient with poor pulmonary reserve and poorly compliant lungs would be able to tolerate one-lung anesthesia. In our experience this has not been a problem. Using FiO_2 of 1.0 and relatively high tidal volumes as long as inspiratory pressures are not high, older patients seem to tolerate single-lung anesthesia well. High inspiratory pressures are avoided to decrease the possibility of secondary pneumothorax, which might occur in the nonoperated side if respiratory pressures are excessive. Although cure is not assured and probably not as likely as it would be following lobectomy, wedge resection may result in 5-year cures of 40% to 75% [56]. Wedge resection of accessible stage I NSCLC is not the treatment of choice in patients of any age who are able to tolerate lobectomy with low risk. Local recurrence rates of >20% have been reported even in open wedge resection [28]. Recurrence rates are higher with T2 tumors removed by wedge resection than with T1 lesions [60]. Nonetheless, when the risk of open thoracotomy is too great, or when the patient chooses the lesser procedure after carefully weighing the options, wedge resection of stage I NSCLC using VATS is a reasonable option.

Pleural Disease

Videothoracoscopy is the ideal way to secure a diagnosis and, in many instances, to institute treatment in a wide variety of pleural diseases [52,53]. Unilateral or even bilateral pleural effusion may occur with some frequency in older patients. The causes are varied. Primary or secondary malignancy, heart failure, and various types of infections are but a few of the possible causes. Thoracentesis and, if necessary, needle biopsy of the pleura provide diagnostic material in most instances. In those pleural effusions, particularly unilateral ones, that remain undiagnosed after thoracentesis and needle biopsy, thoracoscopy with biopsy provides diagnostic material almost every time. In cases of malignant pleural effusion, there is the opportunity for insufflation of talc at the time of thoracoscopy to accomplish pleural symphysis and prevent the recurrence of fluid. We have found this to be the most effective method for ensuring control of malignant pleural effusions. It is better in our hands than talc slurry, bleomycin, or doxycycline instilled through a thoracostomy tube. During videothoracoscopy for undiagnosed pleural effusion the opportunity exists to lyse adhesions, widely visualize the visceral and parietal pleural surfaces, and biopsy any abnormalities directly and safely.

Other pleural diseases are quite suitable for thoracoscopic diagnosis and treatment, particularly in elderly patients. Individuals with incompletely evacuated empyema or hemothorax may be helped by thoracoscopy in circumstances when thoracotomy may be too risky. Similarly, some benign pleural tumors may be removed thoracoscopically in patients in whom thoracotomy would be less likely to be recommended. The major advantages of thoracoscopy over thoracotomy are better visualization of the pleural cavity in most instances and less postoperative morbidity due to less postoperative pain. Although pain following thoracotomy is generally well managed by use of epidural narcotics and analgesics [64], the fewer the drugs and the smaller the doses used in elderly patients, the better.

Metastatic Tumors to the Lungs

VATS would seem to be an appealing way to approach pulmonary metastases in older patients. However, the role of videothoracoscopy in the treatment of metastatic tumors to the lungs has yet to be established with certainty [65]. FNA is quite accurate for diagnosis, so VATS is usually not necessary for that purpose. If the pulmonary metastases seen on CT seem to be accessible for removal by VATS, this procedure would seem to offer definite advantages over thoracotomy for single-stage treatment of bilateral metastases. The advantages of VATS over unilateral or staged thoracotomies are even greater. Bilateral VATS wedge resections can be done in one or two stages as indicated. One major shortcoming of VATS remains, the inability of the surgeon to carry out thorough, systematic bidigital or bimanual palpation of the lungs, searching for additional lesions undetected on preoperative chest radiography and CT (McCormack P, personal communication, 1995). Although imaging techniques are becoming more sensitive, albeit at the loss of some specificity, it is not uncommon for more metastases to be detected at thoracotomy than were apparent on preoperative imaging studies. The decision for or against VATS for resection of pulmonary metastases will remain highly individualized depending on the circumstances of the case and the skill of the surgeon. The number and location of the lesions are important. More lesions in difficult locations are better approached by open techniques. If the lesions are truly resectable by VATS, the advantages of the technique will have to be weighed against the inability to thoroughly evaluate the rest of the lung. Long-term data comparing the two techniques are not available at this time.

Pneumothorax

VATS is well suited, perhaps ideally suited, for the treatment of pneumothorax in the elderly [66,67]. Its safety and efficacy allow earlier intervention than would be possible if thoracotomy were the treatment and more direct and effective treatment than is possible with tube thoracostomy alone. Although the occurrence of pneumothorax secondary to emphysematous blebs and bullae is relatively more frequent in the elderly than is pneumothorax due to rupture of a single apical bleb, secondary pneumothorax of this nature can usually be well managed by VATS techniques alone. Visualization of the leaking point or points, their excision or control by VATS stapling or suturing, and then effective pleurodesis by one of a number of methods, if needed, is usually effective in solving the problem. Relatively early use of VATS for the treatment of pneumothorax in the elderly may result in shorter and safer hospitalizations than were possible when the alternative to tube thoracostomy was open thoracotomy. The willingness to intervene earlier in the patient in whom tube thoracostomy alone is not enough to control the leak is the most appealing aspect of VATS treatment of pneumothorax. We have found that the use of ventilation lung scans using technetium aerosol [68] may be helpful in identifying the leaking point or points and therefore guide VATS treatment of these patients. There will still be those with particularly complex problems who will require thoracotomy, but VATS techniques for the treatment of pneumothorax in the elderly is an important addition to our armamentarium.

Bullous or Diffuse Emphysema

Surgical treatment by any method of pulmonary emphysema is a controversial topic. Decisions are easier to make and results are better when the bullae are large and localized and cause compression of relatively normal remaining lung. Excision of these bullae using open techniques yields satisfying results in properly selected patients, even, or maybe even especially, those who are severely disabled preoperatively. The use of VATS in these patients is controversial. Wakabayashi and his colleagues [69,70] have championed laser treatment using VATS for both localized and diffuse disease.

The wisdom of any surgical treatment of diffuse emphysema is still undecided. Cooper et al. [71] and others (Mack MJ, personal communication, 1995) have reported favorable results using sternotomy for lung volume reduction surgery in selected patients with diffuse emphysema, initially as an alternative to transplantation. VATS techniques for treating these patients have also been used (Little AG, personal communication, 1995) and are even more controversial. Criteria for patient selection, operative techniques, and perioperative care are all in a state of flux. Early postoperative mortality may be 10% or more, even in expert hands. Long-term results are unknown.

Many patients with diffuse emphysema have reached a level of maximal benefit on medical treatment that still leaves them severely disabled. If surgical treatment—VATS or open, laser, or mechanical—could offer these patients significant relief for reasonable periods at acceptable levels of safety, such treatment might descend on the scene with all the fanfare of coronary artery bypass grafting. It is most important to note that the jury is still out on the applicability of these procedures by any technique. (See section on Pneumectomy.)

Pulmonary Infiltrates

It is not unusual in the hospital setting for lung biopsy to be necessary or at least desirable for the diagnosis of localized or diffuse pulmonary infiltrates. These infiltrates are generally interstitial and have defied diagnosis by noninvasive or even invasive methods, including, in most instances, bronchoscopy. Because the differential diagnosis may include literally scores of disease entities, appropriate treatment is possible only if a proper diagnosis has been established.

The surgical approach to lung biopsy in such patients in the past has been open biopsy through a limited thoracotomy incision adjacent to the area of infiltrate. The increased accuracy and decreased morbidity possible using VATS biopsy has resulted in better acceptance of lung biopsy by both patients and physicians. This leads to earlier biopsy in many instances with resultant earlier diagnosis and treatment. In the absence of adhesions, the entire lung surface can readily be visualized and an appropriate area or areas chosen for biopsy [72]. Elderly patients, particularly, are excellent candidates for VATS biopsy when biopsy is indicated. Avoiding delay in diagnosis may be especially beneficial in older patients. VATS lung biopsy is usually carried out as an elective diagnostic procedure but sometimes is necessary urgently on a patient already in the hospital and may even be done on some patients who are on ventilators.

Other Uses of Videothoracoscopy

Abnormalities in the mediastinum including cysts, neoplasms, and lymph nodes may be removed or biopsied using videothoracoscopy [73–76]. Thymectomy for myasthenia gravis using videothoracoscopy has been described [77]. Again, if these procedures can be carried out equally accurately by thoracoscopy as by thoracotomy, older patients are likely to be afforded the opportunity for safer, more comfortable invasive procedures. The same is true for Heller's myotomy [78] and removal of esophageal leiomyomas. Although VATS esophagectomy has been described [79], it is a procedure not as well suited for videothoracoscopy. The length of the operation, the extensive use of auxiliary incisions, the absolute necessity for relatively prolonged single-lung ventilation, and the relatively prolonged learning curve limit the applicability of VATS esophagectomy. VATS is well suited for carrying out dorsal sympathectomy [80,81], which may be indicated in patients with hyperhidrosis or sympathetic dystrophy. Although these diseases do not occur frequently in older people, the technique is highly suitable when they do occur. Chylothorax, another problem infrequent in older patients, may be controlled by VATS in many instances [82]. The same is true for pericardial effusion [83].

Summary

To summarize the important factors in general thoracic surgery in the elderly patient: Carefully assess the patient's heart, lungs, chest cage function, and general health to ascertain that the operation chosen is appropriate to the reserves of your patient. There are no absolute figures or rules that can be used because the reserves are dictated by the integrated cardiac function, lung function, chest wall function, central nervous system function, and even functions of the organs within the abdominal cavity. Carcinoma of the lung is the most common noncardiac thoracic surgical disease of the elderly, and one that can have both synchronous cancers of different parts of the lung and, as treatment is successful, metachronous cancers are likely to develop. The likelihood of second cancers of the lung dictates that lung resection of each cancer should conserve as much function as possible. Aging in itself reduces reserve. The etiologic agents producing carcinoma of the lung, or mesothelioma, restrict lung function, as do acute and chronic infection. Patients who are candidates for thoracic surgery have limited respiratory reserve and will have less postoperatively. The criterion for a well-conceived intrathoracic operation is conservation of as much normally functioning lung as possible. In the perioperative period, control of pain and early mobilization are essential to avoid pulmonary complications and deep venous thrombosis.

The use of videothoracoscopy for various intrathoracic diagnostic and therapeutic endeavors has increased rapidly in just a few years. Approximately one-third of the intrapleural operations carried out in our service use videothoracoscopy and approximately one-fourth are accomplished by VATS alone without the necessity for rib-spreading thoracotomy. The safety and efficacy of VATS depend on proper instruments and surgeon skills, both of which are still improving at a relatively rapid rate. When carried out for the proper indications by skilled thoracic surgeons, VATS can be a boon to older patients by providing a safe, relatively comfortable operation and ultimately a better quality and length of life.

REFERENCES

1. Levitzky MG. Effects of aging on the respiratory system. Physiologist 1984;27:103–107.
2. Peters RM. The Lung. In Peters RM, Peacock EE Jr, Benfield JR (eds), The Scientific Management of Surgical Patients. Boston: Little, Brown, 1983.
3. Campbell JC. Detecting and correcting pulmonary risk factors before operation. Geriatrics 1977;32:54–57.
4. Mackay EH, Banks J, Sykes B, Lee G. Structural basis for the changing physical properties of human pulmonary vessels with age. Thorax 1978;33:335–344.
5. Nakahara K, Monden Y, Ohno K, et al. A method for predicting postoperative lung function and its relation to postoperative complications in patients with lung cancer. Ann Thorac Surg 1985;39:260–265.
6. Tisi GM. Pulmonary Physiology in Clinical Medicine (2nd ed). Baltimore: Williams & Wilkins, 1983.
7. Berggren H, Ekroth R, Malmberg R, et al. Hospital mortality and long-term survival in relation to preoperative function in elderly patients with bronchogenic carcinoma. Ann Thorac Surg 1984;38:634–636.
8. Peters RM, Swain JA. Management of the patient with emphysema, coronary artery disease, and lung cancer. Am J Surg 1982;143: 701–705.
9. Miller DL, Thomas AO, Pairolero PC, et al. Combined operation for lung cancer and cardiac disease. Ann Thorac Surg 1994;58:989–994.
10. Matthay RA, Balmes JR. Lung cancer: a persistent challenge. Geriatrics 1982;37:109–112.
11. Holmes FF. Aging and cancer. Recent Results Cancer Res 1983;87:9.
12. Holmes FF, Hearne EM III. Cancer stage-to-age relationship: implications for cancer screening in the elderly. J Am Geriatr Soc 1981;29:55–57.
13. Ershler WB, Socinski MA, Greene CJ. Bronchogenic cancer, metastases, and aging. J Am Geriatr Soc 1983;31:673–676.
14. Huang MS, Kato H, Konaka C, et al. Quantitative cytochemical differences between young and old patients with lung cancer. Chest 1985;88:864–869.
15. Shankar PS. Laryngeal carcinoma with synchronous or metachronous bronchogenic carcinoma. J Am Geriatr Soc 1981;29:370–372.
16. Shure D, Fedullo PF. The role of transcarinal needle aspiration in the staging of bronchogenic carcinoma. Chest 1984;86:693–696.
17. Ramsdell JW, Peters RM, Taylor AT Jr, et al. Multiorgan scans for staging lung cancer. Correlation with clinical evaluation. J Thorac Cardiovasc Surg 1977;73:653–659.
18. Gutierrez AC, Vincent RG, Bakshi S, Takita A. Radioisotope scans in the evaluation of metastatic bronchogenic carcinoma. J Thorac Cardiovasc Surg 1975;69:934–941.
19. Friedman PJ, Feigin DS, Liston SE, et al. Sensitivity of chest radiography, computed tomography, and gallium scanning to metastasis of lung carcinoma. Cancer 1984;54:1300–1306.
20. Mountain CF. A new international staging system for lung cancer. Chest 1986;89:223S–233S.
21. Tisi GM, Friedman PJ, Peters RM, et al. Clinical staging of primary lung cancer. Am Rev Respir Dis 1987;127:659.
22. Churchill ED, Sweet RH, Soutter L, et al. The surgical management of carcinoma of the lung. J Thorac Surg 1950;20:340.
23. Hoffman TH, Ransdell HT. Comparison of lobectomy and wedge resection for carcinomas of the lung. J Thorac Cardiovasc Surg 1980; 79:211–217.
24. Jensik RJ, Faber LP, Kittle CF. Segmental resection bronchogenic carcinoma. Ann Thorac Surg 1973;28:475.
25. Stair JM, Womble J, Schaefer RF, Read RC. Segmental pulmonary resection for cancer. Am J Surg 1985;150:659–664.
26. Ginsburg RJ, Rubenstein LV. Randomized trial of lobectomy versus limited resection for T1 N0 non–small cell lung cancer. Lung Cancer Study Group. Ann Thorac Surg 1995,60:615–623.
27. Martini N, Bains MS, Burt ME, et al. Incidence of local recurrence and second primary tumors in resected stage I lung cancer. J Thorac Cardiovasc Surg 1995;109:120–129.
28. Landrenau RJ, Sugarbaker DJ, Mack MJ, et al. Wedge resection versus lobectomy for stage I (T1 N0 M0) non–small cell lung cancer. J Thorac Cardiovasc Surg 1997;113:691–700.
29. Keagy BA, Pharr WF, Bowes DE, Wilcox BR. A review of morbidity and mortality in elderly patients undergoing pulmonary resection. Am Surg 1984;50:213–216.
30. Breyer RH, Zippe C, Pharr WF, et al. Thoracotomy in patients over age seventy years. J Thorac Cardiovasc Surg 1981;81:187–193.
31. Urschel HC Jr, Razzuk MA. Median sternotomy as a standard approach for pulmonary resection. Ann Thorac Surg 1986;41:130–134.
32. Shah DM, Gottlieb MA, Rahm RL, et al. Failure of red blood cell transfusion to increase oxygen transport or mixed venous Po_2 in injured patients. J Trauma 1982;22:741–746.
33. Zeldin RA, Normandin D, Landtwing D, Peters RM. Postpneumonectomy pulmonary edema. J Thorac Cardiovasc Surg 1994;87: 359.
34. Staren ED, Cullen ML. Epidural catheter analgesia for the management of postoperative pain. Surg Gynecol Obstet 1986;162:389–404.
35. Bell RC, Andrews AP. Pleural effusions: meeting the diagnostic challenge. Geriatrics 1985;40:101–108.
36. Nagami PH, Yoshikawa TT. Tuberculosis in the geriatric patient. J Am Geriatr Soc 1983;31:356–363.
37. Daly RC, Pairolero PC, Piehler JM, et al. Pulmonary aspergilloma. Results of surgical treatment. J Thorac Cardiovasc Surg 1986;92:981–988.
38. Martini N, McCormack PM, Bains MS, et al. Pleural mesothelioma. Ann Thorac Surg 1987;43:113–120.
39. Monden Y, Nakahara K, Fujii Y, et al. Myasthenia gravis in elderly patients. Ann Thorac Surg 1985;39:433–436.
40. Slater G, Papatestas AB, Kornfeld P, Genkins G. Transcervical thymectomy for thymoma in myasthenia gravis. Am J Surg 1982;144:254–256.
41. Miller JI, Mansour KA, Hatcher CR Jr. Median sternotomy T incision for thymectomy in myasthenia gravis. Ann Thorac Surg 1982;34:473–474.
42. Little AG. Tumors of the Esophagus. In Moossa AR, Robson MC, Schimpff SC (eds), Comprehensive Textbook of Oncology. Baltimore: Williams & Wilkins, 1986.
43. Orringer MB. Technical aids in performing transhiatal esophagectomy without thoracotomy. Ann Thorac Surg 1984;38:128–132.
44. Skinner DB. Enbloc resection for neoplasms of the esophagus and cardia. J Thorac Cardiovasc Surg 1983;85:59–71.
45. Ellis FH Jr, Crozier RE, Watkins E Jr. Operation for esophageal achalasia. Results of esophagomyotomy without an antireflux operation. J Thorac Cardiovasc Surg 1984;88:344.
46. Henderson RD. Diffuse esophageal spasm. Surg Clin North Am 1983; 63:951.
47. Cooper JD, Trulock EP, Triantafillou AN, et al. Bilateral pneumectomy (volume reduction) for chronic obstructive pulmonary disease. J Thorac Cardiovasc Surg 1995;109:106–119.
48. Brantigan OC, Kress MB, Mueller EA. The surgical approach to pulmonary emphysema. Dis Chest 1961;39:485–501.
49. Wakabayashi A, Brenner M, Kayaleh RA, et al. Thoracoscopic carbon dioxide laser treatment of bullous emphysema. Lancet 1991;337: 881–883.
50. Jacobaeus HC. Possibility of the use of the cystoscope for investigation of serous cavities. Munch Med Wocheushr 1910;57:2090–2092.
51. Reddick EJ, Olsen DO. Laparoscopic laser cholecystectomy: a comparison with minilap cholecystectomy. Surg Endosc 1989;3:131–133.
52. Kaiser LR. Video-assisted thoracic surgery: current state of the art. Ann Surg 1994;220:720–734.
53. Mack MJ. The first international symposium on thoracoscopic surgery. Ann Thorac Surg 1993;56:609–806.

54. Michel RP, Lushipan A, Ahmed MN. Pathologic findings of transthoracic needle aspiration in the diagnosis of localized pulmonary lesions. Cancer 1983;51:1563–1572.
55. Sagel SS, Ferguson TB, Forrest JV, et al. Percutaneous transthoracic aspiration needle biopsy. Ann Thorac Surg 1978;26:399–404.
56. Shennib HAF, Landreneau R, Mulder DS, et al. Video-assisted thoracoscopic wedge resection of Tl lung cancer in high-risk patients. Ann Surg 1993;218:555–560.
57. Allen MS, Deschamps C, Lee RE, et al. Video-assisted thoracoscopic stapled wedge excision for indeterminate pulmonary nodules. J Thorac Cardiovasc Surg 1993;106:1048–1052.
58. Mack MJ, Hazelrigg SR, Landreneau RJ, et al. Thoracoscopy for the diagnosis of the indeterminate solitary pulmonary nodule. Ann Thorac Surg 1993;56:825–832.
59. Schwarz CD, Lenglinger F, Eckmayr J, et al. VATS (video-assisted thoracic surgery) of undefined pulmonary nodules: preoperative evaluation of videoendoscopic resectability. Chest 1994;106:1570–1574.
60. Warren WH, Faber LP. Segmentectomy versus lobectomy in patients with stage I pulmonary carcinoma. J Thorac Cardiovasc Surg 1994;107:1087–1094.
61. Landreneau RJ, Hazelrigg SR, Mack MJ, et al. Postoperative pain-related morbidity: video-assisted thoracic surgery versus thoracotomy. Ann Thorac Surg 1993;56:1285–1289.
62. Kirby TJ, Mack MJ, Landreneau RJ, et al. Initial experience with video-assisted thoracoscopic lobectomy. Ann Thorac Surg 1993;56: 1248–1253.
63. McKenna RS. Lobectomy by video-assisted thoracic surgery with mediastinal node sampling for lung cancer. J Thorac Cardiovasc Surg 1994;107:879–882.
64. Lubenow TR, Faber LP, McCarthy RJ, et al. Postthoracotomy pain management using continuous epidural analgesia in 1,324 patients. Ann Thorac Surg 1994;58:924–930.
65. Liu HP, Lin PJ, Hsieh MJ, et al. Application of thoracoscopy for lung metastases. Chest 1995;107:266–268.
66. Inderbitzi RGC, Leiser A, Furrer M, et al. Three years' experience in video-assisted thoracic surgery (VATS) for spontaneous pneumothorax. J Thorac Cardiovasc Surg 1994;107:1410–1415.
67. Waller DA, Forty J, Morritt GN. Video-assisted thoracoscopic surgery versus thoracotomy for spontaneous pneumothorax. Ann Thorac Surg 1994;58:372–377.
68. Nielsen KRK, Blake LM, Mark JBD, et al. Localization of bronchopleural fistula using ventilation scintigraphy. J Nucl Med 1994;35:867–869.
69. Wakabayashi A. Thoracoscopic partial lung resection in patients with severe chronic obstructive pulmonary disease. Arch Surg 1994;129: 940–944.
70. Brenner M, Kayaleh RA, Milne EN, et al. Thoracoscopic laser ablation of pulmonary bullae: radiographic selection and treatment response. J Thorac Cardiovasc Surg 1994;107:883–890.
71. Cooper JD, Trulock EP, Triantafillou AN, et al. Bilateral pneumectomy (volume reduction) for chronic obstructive pulmonary disease. J Thorac Cardiovasc Surg 1995;109:106–119.
72. Krasna MJ, White CS, Aisner SC, et al. The role of thoracoscopy in the diagnosis of interstitial lung disease. Ann Thorac Surg 1995;59: 348–351.
73. Landreneau RJ, Hazelrigg SR, Mack MJ, et al. Thoracoscopic mediastinal lymph node sampling: useful for mediastinal lymph node stations inaccessible by cervical mediastinoscopy. J Thorac Cardiovasc Surg 1993;106:554–558.
74. Roviaro G, Rebuffat C, Varoli F, et al. Videothoracoscopic excision of mediastinal masses: indications and technique. Ann Thorac Surg 1994;58:1679–1684.
75. Urschel JD, Horan TA. Mediastinoscopic treatment of mediastinal cysts. Ann Thorac Surg 1994;58:1698–1701.
76. Vaflieres E, Findlay JM, Fraser RE. Combined microneurosurgical and thoracoscopic removal of neurogenic dumbbell tumors. Ann Thorac Surg 1995;59:469–472.
77. Sugarbaker DJ. Thoracoscopy in the management of anterior mediastinal masses. Ann Thorac Surg 1993;56:653–656.
78. Pelligrini C, Wetter LA, Patti M, et al. Thoracoscopic esophagomyotomy: initial experience with a new approach for the treatment of achalasia. Ann Surg 1992;216:291–299.
79. Cuschieri A, Shimi S, Banting S. Endoscopic esophagectomy through a right thoracoscopic approach. J R Coll Surg Edinb 1992;37:7–11.
80. Chen HJ, Shih DY, Fung ST. Transthoracic endoscopic sympathectomy in the treatment of palmar hyperhidrosis. Arch Surg 1994; 129:630–633.
81. Shachor D, Jedeikin R, Olsfanger D, et al. Endoscopic transthoracic sympathectomy in the treatment of primary hyperhidrosis. Arch Surg 1994;129:241–244.
82. Graham DD, McGahren ED, Tribble CG, et al. Use of video-assisted thoracic surgery in the treatment of chylothorax. Ann Thorac Surg 1994;57:1507–1512.
83. Liu HP, Chang CH, Lin PJ, et al. Thoracoscopic management of effusive pericardial disease: indications and technique. Ann Thorac Surg 1994;58:1695–1697.

Surgical Care for the Elderly, 2nd ed., edited by R. Benton Adkins, Jr., and H. William Scott, Jr. Lippincott–Raven Publishers, Philadelphia © 1998.

CHAPTER 21

Surgical Diseases of the Esophagus

Robert W. Youngblood

Esophageal problems in the elderly differ from those in the general population in that congenital lesions are no longer seen and there is an increased incidence of neoplasia. As physical limitations and tribulations such as degenerative arthritis, osteoporosis, cardiovascular problems, and diminishing sexual functions reduce the joys of living for the elderly, eating assumes an increasingly important role in social interaction and pleasure. Thus, the efficient management of esophageal disorders is important for the elderly.

The anatomic location and physiologic function of the esophagus render endoscopic and surgical procedures a serious risk, especially for individuals who have respiratory and cardiac problems [1]. However, age alone is not a contraindication to necessary surgical therapy, and the risks involved are warranted to re-establish normal swallowing function [2].

It is important to briefly describe the normal anatomy and physiology as they relate to esophageal disease and discuss the diagnosis and management of some of the common diseases of the esophagus in the elderly. These abnormalities include motility disorders, esophageal injuries, diverticular disease, inflammatory diseases, gastroesophageal reflux, and tumors both benign and malignant. In addition, some of the newer diagnostic and therapeutic techniques such as the laser and minimally invasive procedures are discussed.

ANATOMY

Varying in length with the patient's height, the esophagus is a 25- to 35-cm long muscular tube that extends from the hypopharynx to the stomach and lies immediately anterior to the vertebral column. The mucosal lining of stratified squamous epithelium is encased in an inner circular and outer longitudinal layer of muscle. This outer layer of longitudinal muscle is surrounded by mediastinal connective tissue. Thus, there is no serosal surface.

The three divisions of the esophagus are defined by body cavity: the cervical, thoracic, and abdominal segments. A narrowing is located at each extremity of the esophagus. The superior narrowing consists of the pharyngoesophageal constrictors. The inferior narrowing at the level of the diaphragm consists of the diaphragmatic sling and thickening of the circular muscle fibers to form the lower esophageal sphincter. There is also a narrowing at the junction of the upper and middle third of the esophagus at a point where the left main stem bronchus and the aorta abut the esophageal wall. A point of potential weakness in the posterior cervical esophagus between the oblique inferior pharyngeal constrictor and the transverse cricopharyngeus muscle is the site of Zenker's diverticulum. This area is at risk of injury during esophagoscopy.

The innervation of the esophagus consists of a parasympathetic supply from the vagus via the superior laryngeal nerve and the recurrent laryngeal nerve for the upper esophagus and branches from the vagal plexus for the remaining portion of the esophagus [3]. The sympathetic innervation to the cervical esophagus is from the superior and inferior cervical sympathetic ganglion, and in the chest it is from the thoracic and splanchnic sympathetic nerves. An intrinsic autonomic nervous system is located in the plexus of Meissner and Auerbach, the former being situated in the submucosa and the latter between the circular and longitudinal muscle fibers. The vagus nerves lie to each side of the upper esophagus. They diverge into a plexus of small nerves over the subcardinal esophagus and coalesce above the diaphragm to form the vagal trunks that pass through the diaphragmatic hiatus to supply innervation to the liver, stomach, and pylorus [4].

The blood supply to the esophagus is segmental. It arises from numerous small vessel branches of the superior and inferior thyroid arteries in the neck. Small branches from the aorta, intercostal, and bronchial arteries supply the intrathoracic esophagus. Subphrenic branches of the aorta and coronary twigs from the left gastric arteries in the abdomen supply the abdominal esophagus [5].

All of these vessels divide into small branches before they enter the esophageal wall; therefore, blunt dissection of the esophagus is not usually associated with major bleeding if the dissection is performed in the areolar tissue closely adjacent to the outer layer of longitudinal esophageal muscle. The venous drainage is also segmented and drains into small adjacent veins of the mediastinum. Some of the names of the vessels are *pharyngeal, hemiazygos, intercostal,* and in the abdomen, *small branches of the coronary vein.*

The lymphatic drainage of the esophagus originates in submucosal and muscular plexus that intercommunicate and run within the esophageal wall for considerable distances before draining into mediastinal lymph nodes. The lymphatic flow from the distal third of the esophagus drains into the lower mediastinum and infradiaphragmatic nodes along the lesser curvature of the stomach. The upper two-thirds of the esophagus tend to drain into the nodes of the superior mediastinum and to the internal jugular and supraclavicular nodes of the neck. Some of this drainage from the upper third flows directly into the thoracic duct, which lies immediately behind the esophagus. After entering the chest through the aortic hiatus, the thoracic duct continues superiorly on the anterior surface of the vertebrae, crossing to the left at T4 level under the aortic arch, and proceeds along the left side of the posterior esophagus into the neck where it empties into the venous system at the junction of the internal jugular and subclavian veins [6].

Anatomic findings unique to the esophagus become important when surgical procedures are considered. The loose submucosal areolar tissue and the lack of an external serosa demand careful anastomotic technique. The segmental vascular anatomy and division of vessels away from the esophageal wall allow blunt dissection in the transhiatal (Orringer) resection. Additionally, the extensive intramural lymphatic communications necessitate wide resection of malignant neoplasms. Thus, considerable anatomic knowledge and surgical experience are prerequisites for the success of surgical procedures on the esophagus.

PHYSIOLOGY

The physiologic function of the esophagus in its simplest form is to serve as a passage for food from the mouth and pharynx into the stomach while preventing aspiration into the larynx and bronchial tree proximally and serving as a barrier to reflux of digestive juices from the stomach distally. The swallowing mechanism begins as a voluntary action with the tongue pressing cranially and posteriorly propelling the food into the hypopharynx and upper esophagus while the larynx is elevated against the epiglottis to prevent aspiration. The pharyngeal constrictors relax and then contract as the bolus of food is forced into the esophagus and pushed downward toward the stomach by an involuntary contraction of the circular muscles, whose elliptical configuration produce a rotational or screwlike motion [6]. The lower esophageal sphincter undergoes reflex relaxation, allowing passage of the bolus into the stomach.

This action is initiated by muscles of the tongue, pharynx, and upper esophagus that are under voluntary control in the upper third of the esophagus, but as the bolus passes downward, usually assisted by gravity, reflex contraction and relaxation of sphincters are involuntary. Diseases such as achalasia and diffuse esophageal spasm result from failure of coordination and integration of the previously described processes [7]. Failure of coordination of the swallowing mechanism between the oblique fibers of the inferior pharyngeal constrictors and the transverse fibers of the cricopharyngeus at the esophageal inlet posteriorly may be the cause of the bulge that results in a pharyngoesophageal (Zenker's) diverticulum. Abnormalities in the delicately balanced reflex mechanism of the esophageal motility and sphincter tones may result in esophageal disease that requires surgical correction whether this be excision of diverticulum, division of sphincters, or procedures to enhance reflux control [8].

Modern techniques of manometry can define the altered physiologic processes that affect normal esophageal function. pH measurements in the distal esophagus can also assess the results of pathologic anatomy and physiologic dysfunction that may lead to gastroesophageal regurgitation and failure of normal esophageal clearing.

MOTILITY DISORDERS

Esophageal motility disorders are caused by lack of coordination in the normal neurologic processes of swallowing. These disorders in the elderly can be caused by degenerative changes in the parasympathetic supply of the vagus nerve and in the ganglia of Auerbach's plexus or may be secondary to collagen vascular diseases, such as scleroderma or lupus erythematosus, generalized neuromuscular diseases, or endocrine disorders [9,10].

ACHALASIA

Achalasia is the most common esophageal motility disorder in the elderly. It has an insidious onset but leads to progressive dysphagia without anatomic obstruction. There is an initial failure of the distal esophageal sphincter to open on swallowing, associated with loss of peristalsis in the intrathoracic esophagus. Gradual dilatation of the thoracic esophagus occurs, and it becomes elongated and tortuous, presenting as a smooth dilated aperistaltic esophagus ending in a tapered narrowing at the level of the lower esophageal sphincter [11–13].

Achalasia may be treated by careful balloon dilatation, but if this is unsuccessful, distal esophageal myotomy

(Heller's procedure) may be necessary [14]. The advantage of balloon dilatation for the elderly patient is that it can be done on an outpatient basis under local anesthesia, but there is a risk of perforation. Although division of the lower esophageal sphincter allows the emptying of the esophagus by gravity, it fails to restore the normal peristaltic wave and may result in gastroesophageal regurgitation. Individual consideration must be given to the length and distal extent of the myotomy. If the myotomy must be extended onto the stomach, a fundoplication should be considered to prevent gastroesophageal reflux [15–17].

ESOPHAGEAL SPASM

Esophageal spasm is another motor disorder that may either be diffuse or segmental. This disease may be characterized by substernal pain or dysphasia and can sometimes be confused with coronary artery disease in the elderly. The diagnosis can be confirmed by manometric abnormalities that are most often seen in the distal esophagus.

Esophageal spasm differs from achalasia in that it may be intermittent, it is more likely to be associated with pain, and some normal or abnormal peristaltic activity in the esophagus usually persists [18]. The management of esophageal spasm in severe cases may require identification of the area of the esophagus involved and long myotomies in these areas of spasm [19].

The most notable of these esophageal motility disorders secondary to systemic disease is scleroderma, but esophageal involvement may be seen in other collagen vascular diseases as well [20]. As the esophagus becomes more involved and rigid, there is gradual loss of peristalsis and diminished tone in the lower sphincter. This results in gastroesophageal regurgitation with inflammation and scarring of the distal esophagus. Scarring and stricture obviously compound the problem. Poor esophageal peristalsis may also result in regurgitation and aspiration. The management of these disorders for all age groups is treatment of the underlying disease and management of the distressing symptoms with antacids, H_2 blockers, postural therapy, and, on occasion, multiple small feedings.

ESOPHAGEAL DISRUPTIONS

Esophageal integrity can be interrupted in a variety of ways: foreign body or iatrogenic perforation, injuries from penetrating trauma, or from spontaneous rupture due to abrupt intraluminal pressure changes. The diagnosis of esophageal injury may, on occasion, be difficult, but prompt recognition and management are critical because contamination of the mediastinum and rapid spread of virulent infection may ensue. The acute inflammatory process in response to this infection or the spillage of saliva and digestive juices may result in rapid third spacing of fluid in the chest with loss of intravascular volume, hypotension, and respiratory distress, often leading to the acute respiratory distress syndrome. Additionally, the digestive juices in the saliva, gastric juice, and bile may cause rapid dissolution of the esophageal wall and mediastinal tissues. Therefore, chest pain, fever, dysphagia, or respiratory distress following esophageal instrumentation, external trauma, retching, or vomiting must be investigated carefully and esophageal perforation ruled out [21]. To diagnose esophageal perforation, there must be a high index of suspicion, and when in doubt, a contrast swallow radiographic study should be performed. The morbidity from esophageal injury is directly proportional to the time lapse between injury and diagnosis. The diagnosis may be suspected on anteroposterior and lateral radiographs of the chest, but a contrast radiographic study is essential to rule out such an injury [22–24].

Spontaneous rupture of the esophagus (Boerhaave's syndrome) is almost always associated with retching or vomiting. The suddenly elevated intra-abdominal pressure associated with violent retching is transmitted to the distal esophagus and may cause it to tear. The defect is most frequently longitudinal and is located along the left lateral esophagus in 80% of instances. Extravasation may be below or above the diaphragm, but if above the diaphragm, it may extend through the mediastinum and into the pleural space [25].

The symptom of severe substernal pain is frequently confused with myocardial infarction, and indeed, there may be, on occasion, some confusing changes on the electrocardiogram. The episode usually starts with a sudden onset of severe pain that often immediately follows retching or vomiting. The pain may radiate to the back or into the upper chest and shoulders. The patient may show signs of cardiovascular collapse that also may be attributed to an acute cardiac episode. Important points to remember in the diagnosis are to think of the possibility of esophageal rupture, inquire about retching, and immediately request the radiologic studies that will confirm the diagnosis.

Clues to the diagnosis on physical examination may include crepitus in the neck, mediastinal crunch on auscultation, hypotension associated with dyspnea, and, on chest radiography, air in the mediastinum, a pneumothorax, or fluid accumulation in the pleural space. Abdominal examination may reveal no dramatic findings, but if there is peritoneal soilage, the abdominal findings include exquisite tenderness, upper abdominal rigidity, and absence of bowel sounds, all of which suggest a perforation.

Boerhaave's syndrome is of particular importance in the elderly because approximately two-thirds of patients with this disease are over age 50, and one-third are over age 65. The mortality also is directly related to the age of the patient. Another critical factor in mortality is the time lapse between the time of injury and definitive treatment [26].

The ideal management for spontaneous rupture of the esophagus is early diagnosis and immediate resuscitation and repair. Debridement of devitalized tissue and copious irrigation is essential. Appropriate antibiotics should be administered immediately on diagnosis, and parenteral and subsequent enteral alimentation should be addressed at the time of the surgical procedure.

PERFORATION

Perforation of the esophagus may occur from within due to swallowing of foreign bodies or from iatrogenic perforation secondary to esophagoscopy, dilatation, or intubation. In the elderly, the most frequent foreign body perforation is due to swallowed dentures. An injury may occur during attempts at removal of the foreign body. Extraction should be done with great care by an endoscopist skilled in this procedure. Any patient who has fever, chest pain, dyspnea, or dysphagia following esophageal instrumentation should have immediate evaluation for esophageal perforation [27].

Any person who has had a penetrating injury of the neck or chest should be suspected of having an esophageal injury and the appropriate diagnostic studies undertaken. If possible, esophagography should be obtained preoperatively, but if the acuity of the patient's injuries does not allow this, the esophagus can be inspected at the time of neck exploration or thoracotomy to determine whether there is an injury [28]. On occasion, the installation of a dye such as methylene blue via a nasal catheter may help evaluate the integrity of the esophageal wall. Knife and gunshot wounds of the esophagus are rather uncommon in the elderly, but the general principles of diagnosis and repair are similar to those in the younger age group.

MANAGEMENT

The successful management of esophageal injuries requires a high index of suspicion and the vital importance of early diagnosis and operative repair should be emphasized. If at all possible, sites of esophageal closure should be reinforced with viable structures having a good blood supply, the ideal reinforcement being muscle flap, omentum, or adjacent structures. In case there has been a delay in surgical treatment and tissue necrosis or the extent of injury renders primary repair impossible, the area of injury should be excluded [29]. This can be done with cervical esophagostomy and the distal esophagus can be stapled with absorbable staples. When large amounts of devitalized tissue are found, emergency esophagectomy may be necessary. If possible, plans for long-term enteral therapy should be instituted at the time of the initial procedure if a long time before esophageal reconstruction seems likely. Extensive debridement, copious irrigation, and appropriate antibiotic therapy are all important in the management of this condition.

Diverticula

Esophageal diverticula usually occur at one of the three locations in the esophagus. They are classified by their locations as pharyngoesophageal, peribronchial, and epiphrenic; their etiologic mechanism, that is, pulsion or traction; and the degree of involvement of the esophageal wall. False diverticula are composed only of esophageal mucosa, and true diverticula are composed of the entire thickness of the esophageal wall.

Zenker's Diverticulum

The most common esophageal diverticulum in the elderly is the pharyngoesophageal or Zenker's diverticulum. This outpouching projects dorsally between the fibers of the inferior pharyngeal constrictors and the transverse fibers of the cricopharyngeus and the more oblique fibers of the thyropharyngeus muscles. Although difficult to document, there seems to be incoordination of constriction and relaxation in the swallowing mechanism with increased cricopharyngeal tone during deglutition, resulting in a false diverticulum of esophageal mucosa bulging between the two previously described muscles [30,31].

The symptoms consist of dysphagia and delayed regurgitation of contents from the diverticulum. As the diverticulum becomes larger and descends posterior to the esophagus, the esophageal channel may be displaced anteriorly. The resultant dysphagia is manifested by weight loss, choking, and episodic aspiration. As the esophagus is displaced further and the opening of the diverticulum becomes enlarged, the danger of perforation due to instrumentation increases.

Surgical management of Zenker's diverticulum should include a myotomy of the cricopharyngeus muscle, which, in the case of a small diverticulum, may be the only therapy necessary. However, in case of a large diverticulum displacing the esophagus, removal or suspension of the redundant mucosa may be indicated [32,33].

Midesophageal Diverticulum

The peribronchial or midesophageal diverticulum is most often caused by a granulomatous process with enlarged adherent nodes in the region of the tracheal carina, which may exert traction on the esophageal wall. The incidence of this abnormality has decreased with more effective control of tuberculosis and is now infrequently seen. The diverticulum usually causes no symptoms, and the presence of such a diverticulum is most often an incidental finding seen either at endoscopy or on contrast study. Unless the rare complication of inflammatory tracheal esophageal fistula occurs, no surgical therapy is indicated.

Epiphrenic Diverticulum

The etiology of the epiphrenic diverticulum is similar to that of the pharyngoesophageal diverticulum. It is frequently related to mechanical obstruction of the esophagus at the diaphragmatic hiatus, resulting in a pulsion diverticulum involving only bulging mucosa. Appropriate surgical therapy for this lesion must take into account elevated pressure due to distal obstruction or from uncoordinated relaxation of the distal esophageal sphincter during swallowing. Therefore, a myotomy may be indicated and in the presence of hiatus hernia, gastroesophageal reflux must be considered and treated appropriately as part of the procedure for the cure of an epiphrenic diverticulum [34].

Inflammatory Diseases

In the elderly population, fungal infections must be differentiated from other diseases and neoplasms of the esophagus for appropriate management. Although surgical treatment is not indicated in the management of these conditions, it is a condition frequently seen in surgical patients. It is usually associated with antibiotic therapy, corticosteroid administration, chemotherapy, and any condition that alters immunologic response. The early symptom of monilial esophagitis is painful swallowing, and there may be associated oral and pharyngeal manifestations. If untreated, this may progress to a pseudomembrane formation and ulceration, which produces a characteristic pattern seen on contrast studies and by endoscopy. The endoscopic appearance is usually that of a cheesy exudate that may be confluent, giving the appearance of a pseudomembrane. Progressive ulceration may cause interference with esophageal peristalsis, and scarring may lead to stricture formation.

Fungal esophagitis should always be suspected in patients who have been on antibiotics or who have altered immunologic states, and early treatment with antifungals such as nystatin should be instituted.

Another inflammatory process in the esophagus seen frequently in the elderly is the inflammatory reaction associated with irradiation therapy. This may be seen with irradiation treatment of numerous neoplasms in such areas as the lung, larynx, mediastinal lymph system, and so forth. The associated dysphagia often results in poor nutrition, which may compound the patient's primary illness. The best management is prevention by careful monitoring and shielding the esophagus during radiation.

Other rare inflammatory lesions of the esophagus include histoplasmosis, tuberculosis, sarcoidosis, blastomycosis, actinomycosis, and Crohn's disease. These diagnoses are made by culture and endoscopic biopsy. Treatment consists of managing the underlying disease.

Gastroesophageal Reflux

The most common esophageal malady in the elderly is gastroesophageal reflux. This is usually associated with hiatus hernia. A wide variety of symptoms and a number of interrelated causes exist for gastroesophageal reflux. The severity of the symptoms is related to the acidity and concentration of digestive enzymes in the regurgitated gastric contents, the frequency and duration of the regurgitation, and the ability of the esophageal clearing mechanism to rid the esophagus of the irritating material. The causes of gastroesophageal reflux are related to abnormalities in anatomy and physiology discussed previously [35]. The configuration of the esophageal hiatus, tone of the lower esophageal sphincter, increased intra-abdominal pressure, effectiveness of esophageal peristalsis, and mucosal sensitivity all affect the severity of abnormalities associated with reflux [36].

The initial symptoms of reflux consist of heartburn and water brash. There may be associated pulmonary symptoms from nocturnal aspiration and anemia from chronic blood loss at the sites of ulceration. The end stage of the peptic esophagitis is a stricture that can be prevented by control of the reflux and treated with esophageal dilatation. Persistent chronic reflux may result in histologic alterations of the esophageal mucosa, leading to Barrett's esophagus, a premalignant condition [37].

Techniques to diagnose esophageal reflux include manometric evaluation of esophageal peristalsis and strict evaluation of the lower esophageal sphincter. pH monitoring allows a quantitative evaluation of the degree of acidity and frequency of reflux episodes [38].

Medical management is the initial treatment of gastroesophageal reflux: Control of the hyperacidity with H_2 blockers and acid neutralizers is most important. Postural therapy such as elevating the head of the bed and avoiding bending and straining is also helpful in the management of reflux. If medical management fails, surgical therapy is indicated, especially when the reflux is associated with hiatus hernia. Repair of the hiatus hernia associated with a partial or complete plication of the gastric fundus around the distal esophagus is necessary. This gives support for the lower esophageal sphincter and secures the gastroesophageal junction beneath the diaphragm. Should esophageal strictures progress to the point that they cannot be controlled by dilation, either with balloon or bougie, resection may be necessary. Progression to Barrett's esophagus with atypical mucosal cells may require esophageal resection as a prophylaxis against the development of esophageal cancer [39].

Esophageal Tumors

Neoplasms of the esophagus in the elderly may be benign or malignant. Benign tumors of the esophagus are quite rare, accounting for <1% of all esophageal neoplasms. The most common benign esophageal tumor is a leiomyoma, which usually occurs in the middle aged rather than the elderly. The characteristic appearance of a leiomyoma on barium swallow is a smooth bulge into the esophagus. If large enough, it may cause obstructive symptoms. Such lesions rarely undergo malignant degeneration and can usually be observed. Resection is indicated only if obstructive symptoms or bleeding occurs. These tumors can be peeled from their submucosal location either with open thoracotomy or thoracoscopic techniques. Wide resection is not necessary, and leiomyomas can frequently be removed without transgressing the esophageal mucosa.

Other benign lesions of the esophagus are exceedingly rare. They consist of lipomas, polyps, hemangiomas, and so forth. Esophageal cysts are congenital and rarely present in the elderly age group.

Malignant Tumors

There are two main types of carcinoma of the esophagus: squamous cell carcinoma, which is more frequent, and adenocarcinoma. The latter arises in the distal esophagus from the junctional columnar epithelium, aberrant rests of gastric mucosa, or in Barrett's esophagus [40]. It may be difficult to differentiate an adenocarcinoma of the fundus of the stomach with esophageal invasion from an adenocarcinoma arising in the distal esophagus. Statistics have shown an increasing incidence of adenocarcinoma. However, approximately 95% of these neoplasms are still squamous cell, especially those arising in the main body of the esophagus. Esophageal carcinoma is two to five times more prevalent in men than in women, and in the United States it is more prevalent in black individuals than in whites. More than half of the esophageal cancers occur at age 60 and older.

There are localized areas throughout the world where esophageal carcinoma is prevalent: in northeastern Iran, the Transkei in South Africa, Hunan Province in northern China, and areas of southern Russia along the Caspian Sea. This suggests that there are local dietary habits or genetic factors involved. These areas have an instance of carcinoma that is tenfold greater than that seen in the United States. Epidemiologic studies in the United States suggest a relationship between esophageal cancer and excessive use of tobacco and alcohol, especially in combination. There is an increased prevalence of the disease along the eastern seaboard of the United States.

The most common presenting symptom for esophageal carcinoma is dysphagia. It is present in >90% of cases. Other presenting complaints are pain, anorexia, weight loss, aspiration, hoarseness, or a left cervical mass. The diagnosis should be made when a barium swallow shows an early lesion with an irregularity of the mucosa. This progresses to marked narrowing, shelf formation, "apple core" appearance, and then esophageal obstruction with moderate proximal dilatation. The diagnosis can be confirmed with esophagoscopy and biopsy. On occasion, shoulder formation from submucosal extension may make visualization and biopsy of the ulcerated tumor difficult.

Patients frequently suffer from weight loss and negative nitrogen balance due to anorexia out of proportion to their obstructive symptoms. As esophageal occlusion becomes more severe and the patient is unable to swallow saliva, hypokalemia may occur. Aspiration may lead to fever, bronchitis, and pneumonia.

The treatment of esophageal cancer in the past has had poor results. The three modalities of treatment—surgery, irradiation, and chemotherapy—used singly have all failed to produce significant improvement in survival [41]. The anatomic location of the esophagus is an important consideration. It is in the posterior mediastinum immediately anterior to the vertebral column behind the trachea superiorly and the heart inferiorly, and bordered laterally on either side by the mediastinal pleura. This renders wide en bloc resection impractical. The extensive submucosal lymphatic network of the esophagus results in early longitudinal spread within the wall of the esophagus. Although the possibility of curative surgical excision always exists with early lesions, the majority of patients have advanced disease at the time of presentation.

Studies now underway in a number of centers using multimodal therapy of preoperative irradiation and chemotherapy followed by resection have considerably improved palliation [42,43]. Whether this combined therapy will improve mortality and long-term cure has yet to be determined, but early results have been encouraging.

The common surgical approaches for carcinoma of the esophagus consist of a left thoracotomy for disease in the distal esophagus and cardia. The Ivor-Lewis procedure is done by the combination of an epigastric incision and a right thoracotomy. It is used for diseases of the middle third of the esophagus [44] and for total esophagectomy. The Ivor-Lewis procedure uses either gastric pull-up or colonic interposition with an anastomosis in the neck. The transhiatal esophagectomy without thoracotomy as proposed by Orringer has gained increased acceptance since 1985 [45]. The advantages of this procedure are that a near total esophagectomy can be performed, avoiding an intrathoracic anastomosis and avoiding the morbidity of thoracotomy. Orringer uses the gastric pull-up for esophageal replacement, whereas some individuals favor the colon interposition. This latter procedure, although satisfactory, is more time-consuming and technically demanding than the gastric pull-up. The disadvantage of the procedure is the inability to do a wide field dissection and assay the paraesophageal nodes. When combined with preoperative irradiation and chemotherapy, however, excellent palliation has been obtained.

Other means available for palliation of an obstructing esophageal carcinoma consist of transesophageal laser ablation of tumor and placement of stents through the area of obstruction. These have not met with great success. On occasion, intensive radiation may temporarily relieve obstruction, and a variety of surgical procedures have been used to bypass the lesion. These palliative procedures, however, are of considerable magnitude and have a relatively high morbidity and mortality.

Carcinoma of the esophagus is a miserable disease for which the ideal management has not yet been found. Patients are unable to eat, and they lose their dignity and independence while drowning in their own secretions. Carefully managed combined therapy using radiation, chemotherapy, and surgery significantly improve palliation, but as in most malignant diseases, efforts at prevention and early diagnosis offer the best hope for management.

NEW THERAPEUTIC MODALITIES

Several new techniques for the diagnosis and management of esophageal disease have been developed. Of the new diagnostic tools, the use of a transesophageal echo has aided in the visualization of the extent of neoplasms and improved the accuracy of clinical staging [46]. Radioisotope clearance studies using technetium 99m have helped to assess gastric emptying, and technetium HIDA (hepatic 2,6–dimethyliminodiacetic acid) dynamic biliary imaging has assisted in the evaluation of duodenal gastric bile reflux. Better pH monitors have also improved the evaluation of gastrointestinal reflux.

The use of the neodymium:yttrium-aluminum-garnet laser endoscopically has been effective in the treatment of esophageal webs and especially the management of esophageal obstruction in patients with carcinoma of the esophagus [47].

The use of the minimally invasive surgical technique of thoracoscopy in managing esophageal disease is also being investigated. This technique can be used for mobilization of the esophagus under direct vision, removal of benign tumors of the esophageal wall, evaluating and staging the extent of malignant disease, and treating gastroesophageal reflux by hiatus hernia repair and fundoplication [48].

SUMMARY

A wide range of diseases of the esophagus, from aggravating to life-threatening, is seen in the elderly. These problems affect the joy of living, nutrition, independence, and occasionally the lives of the elderly. Knowledge of the early diagnosis and successful management of these diseases by the physician will make the life of the elderly more pleasant.

REFERENCES

1. Friedman LS. Gastrointestinal disorders in the elderly. Gastroenterol Clin North Am 1990;19:227–257.
2. Pelemans W, Vantrapper G. Oesophageal disease in the elderly. Clin Gastroenterol 1985;1:635–656.
3. Shackelford RT. Surgery of the Alimentary Tract (2nd ed). Philadelphia: Saunders, 1978;16–19.
4. Rothberg M, DeMeester TR. Surgical Anatomy of the Esophagus. In Shield TW (ed), General Thoracic Surgery (3rd ed). Philadelphia: Lea & Febiger, 1989;76–86.
5. Hermann JD, Murugasu JJ. The blood supply of the esophagus in relation to esophageal surgery. Aust N Z J Surg 1966;35:195–201.
6. Postlethwait RW. Surgery of the Esophagus (2nd ed). Norwalk, CT: Appleton-Century-Crofts, 1986.
7. Hurwitz AL, Duranceau A. Normal Esophageal Motility. In Hurwitz AL, Duranceau A, Haddad JK (eds), Disorders of Esophageal Motility. Philadelphia: Saunders, 1979;14–26.
8. Henderson RD. Normal Esophageal Motor Activity: Function and Control. In The Esophagus—Reflex and Primary Motor Disorders. Baltimore: Williams & Wilkins, 1980;11–21.
9. Khan TA, Shragge BW, Crispit JS, et al. Esophageal motility in the elderly. Dig Dis 1977;22:1049–1054.
10. Cohn S. Motor disorders of the esophagus. N Engl J Med 1979;301: 184–192.
11. Goldblum JR, Whyte RI, Orringer MB. Achalasia: a morphological study of 42 resected specimens. Am J Surg Pathol 1994;18: 327–337.
12. Lock JR, Ellis H. Achalasia of the cardia in elderly patients. Postgrad Med J 1978;54:538–540.
13. Orringer MB. The treatment of achalasia: controversy resolved? Ann Thorac Surg 1979;28:100–102.
14. Heller E. Extramucosal cardioplasty in chronic cardiospasm with dilatation of the esophagus. Grenzgeb Med Surg Chir 1913;27:141–148.
15. Belsey R. Functional disease of the esophagus. J Thorac Cardiovasc Surg 1966;52:164–171.
16. Ellis FH, Payne WS. Motility disturbances of the esophagus and its inferior sphincter: recent surgical advances. Adv Surg 1965;1: 79–184.
17. Murray GF, Battaglini JW, Keagy BA, et al. Selective application of fundoplication in achalasia. Ann Thorac Surg 1984;37:185–188.
18. Orringer MB, Orringer JS. Esophagectomy: definitive treatment for esophageal neuromotor dysfunction. Ann Thorac Surg 1982;34:237–248.
19. Henderson RD, Pearson FG. Reflux control following extended myotomy in primary disordered motor activity (diffuse spasm) of the esophagus. Ann Thorac Surg 1976;22:278–284.
20. Henderson RD, Pearson FG. Surgical management of esophageal scleroderma. J Thorac Cardiovasc Surg 1973;66:686–692.
21. White RD, Morris DM. Diagnosis and management of esophageal perforations. Am Surg 1992;58:112–119.
22. Michel L, Malt RA, Grillo HC. Operative and non-operative management of esophageal perforation. Ann Surg 1981;194:57–63.
23. Orringer MB, Stirling MB. Esophagectomy for esophageal disruption. Ann Thorac Surg 1990;49:35.
24. Sawyers JL, Lane CE, Foster JH. Esophageal perforation: an increasing challenge. Ann Thorac Surg 1975;19:233–238.
25. Patton AS, Lawson DW, Shannon JM, et al. Re-evaluation of the Boerhaave syndrome. A review of 14 cases. Am J Surg 1979;137: 560–565.
26. Grillo HC, Wilkins EW. Esophageal repair following late diagnosis of intrathoracic perforation. Ann Thorac Surg 1975;20:387–399.
27. Barber GB, Peppercorn MA, Ehrlich C, et al. Esophageal foreign body perforation: report of an unusual case and review of literature. Am J Gastroenterol 1984;79:509–511.
28. Splener CW, Benfield JR. Esophageal disruption from blunt and penetrating external trauma. Arch Surg 1983;118:663–668.
29. Brewer LA, Carter R, Malder GA, et al. Options in the management of perforations of the esophagus. Am J Surg 1986;52:62–69.
30. Cook IJ, Gabb H, Panagopouols V, et al. Zenker's diverticulum: a defect in upper esophageal sphincter compliance. Gastroenterology 1989;96:A98–A99.
31. Knuff TE, Benjamin SB, Castell DO. Pharyngoesophageal (Zenker's diverticulum): a reappraisal. Gastroenterology 1982;82:734–736.
32. Altorki NK, Sunagawa N, Skinner DB. Thoracic esophageal diverticula. Why is operation necessary? J Thorac Cardiovasc Surg 1993; 105:260–264.
33. Maglione M, Payne H, Jeyasingham K. Pathophysiological basis for operation on Zenker's diverticulum. Ann Thorac Surg 1994;57: 1616–1620.
34. Evander A, Little AG, Ferguson MK, et al. Diverticula of the mid and lower esophagus: pathogenesis and surgical management. World J Surg 1986;10:820–828.
35. Dent J, Holloway RH, Toouli J, et al. Mechanisms of lower esophageal sphincter incompetence in patients with symptomatic gastroesophageal reflux. Gut 1988;29:1020–1028.
36. Dodds WJ. The pathogenesis of gastroesophageal reflux disease. Am J Radiol 1988;151:49–56.
37. Bernstein IT, Kruse P, Anderson ID. Barrett's oesophagus. Dig Dis 1994;12:98–105.
38. Timmer R, Breumelhof R, Nadorp JH, et al. Ambulatory esophageal pressure and pH monitoring in patients with high-grade reflux esophagitis. Dig Dis Sci 1994;39:2084–2089.
39. Demeester TR, Attwood SE, Smyrk TC, et al. Surgical therapy in Barrett's esophagus. Ann Surg 1990;212:528–542.
40. Rusch VW, Levine DS, Haggitt R, et al. The management of high-grade dysplasia and early cancer in Barrett's esophagus: a multidisciplinary problem. Cancer 1994;74:1225–1229.
41. Sugimachi K, Watanabe M, Sadanoga N, et al. Recent advances in the diagnosis and surgical treatment of patients with carcinoma of the esophagus. J Am Coll Surg 1994;178:363–368.
42. Carey RW, Hilgenberg AD, Wilkins EW, et al. Long term follow-up of neoadjuvant chemotherapy with 5-fluorouracil and cisplatin with

surgical resection and possible postoperative radiotherapy and/or chemotherapy in squamous cell carcinoma of the esophagus. Cancer Invest 1993;11:99–105.

43. Fordstiere AA, Orringer MB, Perez-Tamayo C, et al. Concurrent chemotherapy and radiation therapy followed by transhiatal esophagectomy for local-regional cancer of the esophagus. J Clin Oncol 1990;8:119–127.
44. Lewis I. The surgical treatment of carcinoma of the esophagus with special reference to a new operation for growths of the middle third. Br J Surg 1946;34:18–31.
45. Orringer MB. Transhiatal esophagectomy without thoracotomy for carcinoma of the esophagus. Ann Surg 1984;200:282–288.
46. Dancygier H, Classen M. Endoscopic ultrasonography in esophageal disease. Gastrointest Endosc 1989;35:220–225.
47. Isaac JR, Sim EK, Ngoi SS, et al. Safe and rapid palliation of dysphagia for carcinoma of the esophagus. Am Surg 1991;57:245–249.
48. Bumm R, Holscher AH, Feussner H, et al. Endodissection of the thoracic esophagus—technique and clinical results in esophagectomy. Ann Surg 1993;218:97–104.

Surgical Care for the Elderly, 2nd ed., edited by
R. Benton Adkins, Jr., and H. William Scott, Jr.
Lippincott–Raven Publishers, Philadelphia © 1998.

CHAPTER 22

Diseases of the Stomach and Duodenum

Benjamin B. Peeler, R. Benton Adkins, Jr., and H. William Scott, Jr.

Gastrointestinal complaints often become more frequent with advancing age and may become increasingly nonspecific. The expectation of more frequent vague gastrointestinal complaints by the elderly patient may delay presentation with significant illness and diagnosis. Alterations in gastric physiology once thought to be a natural consequence of the aging process have been shown to be largely associated with pathologic conditions. For elderly patients free of gastritis or other conditions, gastroduodenal function is generally well preserved. Although some complaints may be functional in the elderly, the preservation of normal anatomy and physiology in healthy aged patients as well as the tendency of the elderly to present with vague symptom complexes mandates a heightened awareness on the part of the clinician and an aggressive approach to the evaluation of elderly patients with upper gastrointestinal complaints.

ANATOMY AND PHYSIOLOGY

Changes in gastroduodenal anatomy and physiology that accompany aging have been studied extensively. For many years it was thought that aging caused a general decrease in gastric acid production. It is now known that in normal healthy volunteers in whom chronic gastritis and atrophic gastritis have been excluded, gastric acid production may actually increase with age or at least remain stable [1,2]. Hypochlorhydria in the elderly, as in the younger population, is usually associated with the gastritises. The increased prevalence of gastritis in the elderly led to the generalization that a degree of hypochlorhydria was a normal part of the aging process. This is now known to be inaccurate. Age-related differences in gastric acid secretion are more pronounced in men but are also present in women. Age-related impairment in the secretion of intrinsic factor is also related to the increased incidence of atrophic gastritis in the elderly. In the absence of gastritis, and even in the presence of mild-to-moderate gastritis, vitamin B_{12} absorption should be unimpaired. Additionally, calcium bioavailability and ferric iron absorption are dependent on the acid environment of the stomach and should be relatively normal in the absence of gastritis. Basal serum gastrin levels are slightly higher in older subjects as are serum gastrin levels in response to a meal. Serum pepsinogen levels are also higher in older subjects [1].

Several investigators have shown that the effects of trophic factors on the stomach, factors known to stimulate gastric mucosal growth and maturation as well as to maintain gastric integrity, may become relatively impaired with aging. In animal models a reduction in proliferative response to gastrin and epidermal growth factor, known trophic factors for the stomach, has been documented. Other studies have shown that the cellular response of stomachs to noxious stimuli in aging animals is more severe mucosal and submucosal damage and reduced proliferative activity as compared with younger control subjects. These factors may play an important role in the development of gastroduodenal ulcerations and their impaired healing [3]. At least in the case of gastrin, the decreased trophic effects could be related to a reduction in gastrin receptor number, binding affinity in the stomach, which in fact has been documented, or both [4].

The study of gastric motility in the elderly has also been difficult secondary to confounding factors in the study populations. Several methods have been used, including antral manometry, antral myoelectric recording, and studies using a radionuclide-labeled meal, to study changes in gastric emptying with age [5]. Many early studies failed to report the association or the control with normal subjects for disease entities known to be associated with delayed gastric emptying, such as Parkinson's disease and hypothyroidism [6]. Additionally, the use of medications known to delay gastric emptying were not reported in many studies [6,7]. Better controlled studies indicated that there is no difference in solid food emptying rates between the young and old. Delays in liquid emptying have been noted, however [8,9]. In the study by Kao et al. [9], the half-time of radiolabeled liquid emptying was 45% longer in subjects >60 years old as compared with those 60 or younger. It has been proposed that the delay in liquid emptying in elderly subjects may be due to a diminished ability to generate gastric fundal pressures, a property ascribed to the oblique muscle of the fundus [8,10]. It is unlikely that these significant increases in liquid emptying time are clinically important, however, because the participants in the study groups who had delayed liquid emptying times denied gastrointestinal complaints.

Effects of Long-Term Acid Suppression

In the past few years, medical suppression of gastric acid production has replaced surgical treatment of peptic ulcer disease, largely relegating surgical procedures to the treatment of ulcer complications. Among the elderly population, the use of pharmacologic agents to block gastric acid secretion is common. As a result, a significant number of patients are encountered who have been on long-term suppressive therapy with H_2 antagonists and increasingly with omeprazole. The long-term effects of H_2 blockade on gastric physiology have been studied extensively, and as more clinical experience has been gained with omeprazole, its long-term effects are also being elucidated.

Long-term maintenance blockade of gastric acid secretion using H_2 antagonists has been shown generally to be safe [1–14]. Some concern existed regarding chronic alterations in gastric pH leading to bacterial overgrowth, nitrosation, and carcinogenesis. No increase in gastric cancer has been seen with long-term cimetidine use, however [15,16]. Fasting serum gastrin levels increase only slightly with H_2-blocker therapy, whereas 24-hour gastrin levels increase greater than twofold. Problems related to hypergastrinemia have not been seen with H_2 blockers, including no predisposition to gastric carcinoid tumors. Although abundant data are not yet available for H_2 blockers, when compared with omeprazole, gastric endocrine cell hyperplasia is usually not a significant problem with H_2 blockers [15]. Another investigation has supported the concept of immune system enhancement with H_2-blocker therapy in certain clinical conditions [16].

Omeprazole causes greater increases in serum gastrin levels than H_2 blockade. In patients on long-term omeprazole therapy for resistant peptic ulcer disease, pronounced hypergastrinemia can be seen. Generally, long-term omeprazole therapy results in an initial increase in serum gastrin levels that levels off after several months. Reduction in dosage is usually not associated with reduction in gastrin levels. A number of follow-up studies have been done on patients treated with omeprazole for periods up to 7.4 years. In these studies regular gastric biopsies were performed. In a review of these studies [17], involving a total of 744 patients, it was found that 7% of these patients had histologic evidence of gastric endocrine cell hyperplasia, whereas 91% exhibited no change in mucosal histology. No evidence of adenomatous change, metaplasia, dysplasia, or neoplasia was seen.

Helicobacter pylori and Aging

The discovery of *Helicobacter pylori* in the human stomach has dramatically altered the way we think about and treat several gastroduodenal conditions. *H. pylori* was first characterized and cultured by Warren and Marshall, the first reports occurring in 1984, after observing these organisms in a high proportion of patients with gastritis and peptic ulcer disease [18,19]. Since that original description, much has been learned about this organism and its relation to gastrointestinal disease. Along with causative links to gastritis and peptic ulcer disease, a strong association between chronic *H. pylori* infection and gastric cancer has been found [20–22].

On exposure to *H. pylori,* which is spread by the fecal-oral route, there is a period of bacterial proliferation in the stomach, which results in inflammation. Upper gastrointestinal symptoms may develop, and the initial immune response develops during the initial weeks. The inflammatory process results in intense gastritis and hypochlorhydria. After the initial inflammation subsides, the infected person may become asymptomatic for a period of decades. In a subset of patients, peptic ulceration develops during this period, and in a smaller proportion, gastric lymphoma may develop. In many more hosts, however, over a period of three to four decades atrophic gastritis develops as a consequence of chronic low-grade inflammation. Atrophic gastritis and concurrent intestinal metaplasia serve as premalignant lesions to distal gastric carcinoma. *H. pylori* infection is yet to be related to malignancies of the cardia or esophagogastric junction. Several studies in 1991 showed a link between chronic *H. pylori* infection and distal gastric cancer. These cohort studies showed that groups of patients with proven infections with *H. pylori* for multiple decades had significantly higher rates of gastric cancer than age-matched seronegative individuals [22].

At least one-third of the world's population is infected with *H. pylori,* and infection usually occurs early in life. The clinical manifestations of infection are generally not seen until decades after the infection is acquired. In developed countries, children rarely become infected, whereas in undeveloped countries, 60% to 70% of children acquire the infection by age 10 [22]. The prevalence of infection continues to increase in the developed countries with age, such that by the seventh decade, 67% are seropositive. No significant gender difference exists. Prevalence rates plateau beyond the seventh decade, which suggests that in developed nations most of the transmission of the infection occurs during the third through sixth decades of life. In developed countries, the prevalence of detectable antibodies remains stable in persons aged 60 to 99 years. This suggests that *H. pylori* infection persists for many years, even for life, in infected individuals, and that infection results in continued antigenic stimulation [23]. All patients with peptic ulcer disease and *H. pylori* infection should receive therapy with an appropriate antimicrobial regimen in addition to acid-reduction therapy. The currently recommended regimens for *H. pylori* eradication are usually tolerated well, regardless of age.

Chronic Gastritis

Chronic gastritis is linked to several other pathologic processes occurring in the stomach, including peptic ulcer disease, pernicious anemia, and gastric neoplasia. Although there has been considerable debate regarding the classification of chronic gastritis, Correa's classification scheme has gained wide acceptance in the United States [24]. He divides chronic gastritis into five types based on morphology and etiology:

1. Superficial gastritis
2. Diffuse antral gastritis
3. Reflux gastritis
4. Diffuse corporal atrophic gastritis
5. Multifocal atrophic gastritis

As reported by Correa, superficial gastritis may be a precursor to other forms of chronic gastritis. This entity is also morphologically similar to acute gastritis and may be associated with ingestion of certain foods, as well as alcohol and nonsteroidal anti-inflammatory drugs (NSAIDs). An association with *H. pylori* has also been seen.

Diffuse antral gastritis is often associated with peptic ulcer disease and is usually associated with acid hypersecretion [25] and often with *H. pylori* infection. Diffuse antral gastritis is not associated with gastric atrophy or cancer.

Reflux gastritis is a well-known postgastrectomy syndrome, resulting from bile reflux into the gastric remnant [26]. The presence of bile salts on the gastric mucosal barrier permits back-diffusion of hydrogen ions resulting in mast cell release of serotonin, histamine, and other vasoactive amines. Capillary dilatation, mucosal hemorrhage, and superficial mucosal ulceration result. Medical management of reflux gastritis has generally been unsatisfactory, requiring a remedial gastric procedure for relief of symptoms [26].

Atrophic gastritis is a particularly important pathophysiologic process in the elderly. The prevalence of atrophic gastritis increases with age. A study in one major city showed that approximately 40% of the population over the age of 80 years had proven atrophic gastritis [27]. Diffuse corporal atrophic gastritis is associated with pernicious anemia and shows a progressive pattern from initial superficial gastritis to advanced intestinal metaplasia [24]. The presence of autoantibodies against parietal cells is characteristic of diffuse corporal atrophic gastritis.

Multifocal atrophic gastritis is the most common form of atrophic gastritis. Multifocal atrophic gastritis results in decreased production of gastric acid, pepsinogen, and intrinsic factor, as does diffuse corporal atrophic gastritis in many cases [24,28]. Additionally, detrimental effects on calcium bioavailability and iron absorption have been shown to occur with atrophic gastritis. This form of chronic gastritis has been associated with diets high in salt and a deficiency in fresh fruits and leafy vegetables.

HYPERPLASTIC GASTROPATHY

Hyperplastic gastropathy is a term introduced by Ming in 1973 to designate a group of uncommon conditions that are characterized by gross and sometimes gigantic enlargement of the rugal folds of the gastric mucosa [29]. Ming's term replaced the older term, *hypertrophic gastritis,* which is considered a misnomer because rugal enlargement is caused neither by inflammatory gastritis nor hypertrophy, but by hyperplasia of the mucosal epithelial cells.

Fieber and Rickert [30] have strongly endorsed the pathologic classification of hyperplastic gastropathy suggested by Ming in 1973, in which three types are defined:

1. *Mucous cell type.* Hyperplasia involves the mucous surface and the foveolar cells. The glands are normal or atrophic. Systemic dilatation of glands can frequently be observed, and occasionally intestinal metaplasia is found.
2. *Glandular cell type.* Hyperplasia involves the gastric glands with an increase in the numbers of parietal and chief cells. Often the foveae are shortened, and the number of mucous cells may be reduced.
3. *Mixed mucous-glandular type.* According to Ming, hyperplasia involves both the mucous and the specialized cells.

In 50 cases selected from the literature by Fieber and Rickert [30], the incidence by Ming's pathologic type was (1) 33 cases of mucous cell hyperplasia, (2) 11 cases of glandular cell hyperplasia, and (3) six cases of mixed mucous-glandular cell hyperplasia.

The 33 cases of mucous cell hyperplasia seem to be cases of Ménétrier's disease both with and without protein losses [30]. In our opinion, the Zollinger-Ellison syndrome is the most frequently encountered clinical manifestation of Ming's glandular cell hyperplasia, and gastrinomas of pancreas or duodenum are the specific cause [31].

Ménétrier's disease may occur in the very young and in the elderly. Its etiology is no better known today than when described by Ménétrier in 1888 [17]. On pathologic examination, the enlarged rugal folds of Ménétrier's disease are caused by enormous hyperplasia of the mucous cells of the gastric epithelium. There is a concomitant atrophy with disappearance of the parietal and chief cells of the gastric mucosa. In Fieber and Rickert's collected series, the average age was 40 years, with a range from 5 to 87 years. The ratio of male to female subjects was 39 to 11. Radiographic studies show the enlarged rugal folds in the upper part of the stomach with sparing of the antrum, which may be quite small. Gastroscopy shows massive enlargement of rugal folds, and on gross examination differences between mucous-glandular forms of hyperplasia cannot be determined. Ménétrier's disease must be differentiated from the mucosal hyperplasia of the Zollinger-Ellison syndrome and from the forms of hyperplastic gastropathy to which Schindler gave the name *hypertrophic glandular gastritis* and which Stempien classified as hypertrophic hypersecretory gastritis. These are all known to be possible conditions

TABLE 22-1. *Factors adversely affecting peptic ulcer prognosis in old age**

1. Inadequate finances and access to health care
2. Atypical or absent symptoms and signs of disease
3. Delayed, advanced-stage presentations of disease
4. Decline in mental function (of many causes) leading to
   a. Poor comprehension of questions (possible deafness)
   b. Poor recall of salient history
   c. Difficulty cooperating with tests or procedures
   d. Difficulty complying with treatment regimens
   e. Failure or inability to seek needed help
5. Comorbidity with serious diseases in other vital organs (e.g., heart, lungs, kidneys, liver, brain)
6. Need to take drugs with gastrointestinal side effects (e.g., aspirin, nonsteroidal anti-inflammatory drugs, potassium chloride, theophylline, chemotherapy)
7. Polypharmacy and drug errors (some from poor sight)
8. Malnutrition and immunodeficiency
9. Poor outcomes of anesthesia or surgery
10. High incidence of iatrogenic illness and institutional neglect

*Items 2, 3, 4a, 5, 6, and 9 have major effects on ulcer disease.

Source: Reprinted with permission from McCarthy DM. Acid peptic disease in the elderly. Clin Geriatr Med 1991;7:231–254.

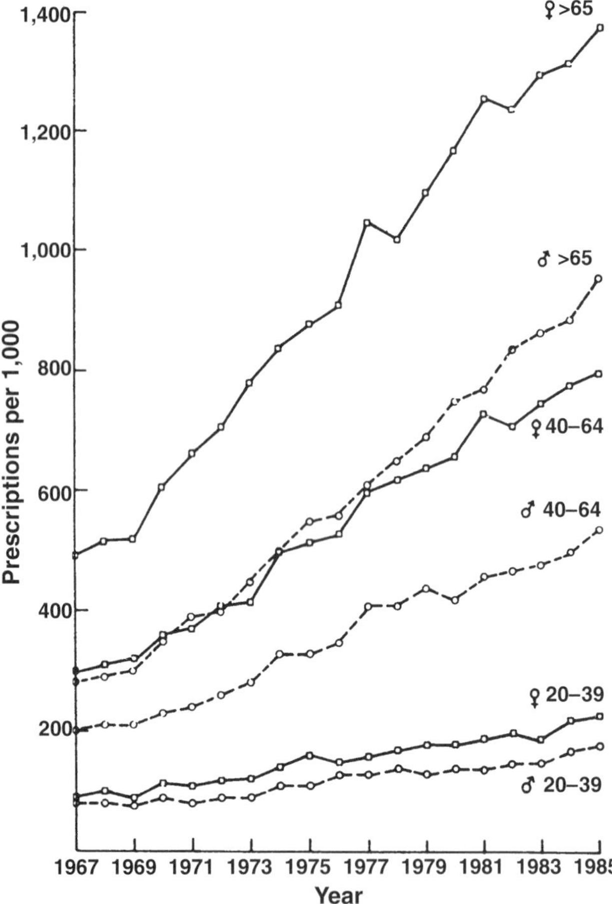

FIG. 22-1. Age-specific nonsteroidal anti-inflammatory drug prescription rates in the United Kingdom, 1967 to 1985. (Reprinted with permission from Walt R, Logan R, Katschinski B, et al. Rising frequency of ulcer perforation in elderly people in the United Kingdom. Lancet 1986;1:489–492.)

in the elderly patient. A carefully done endoscopy with multiple biopsies is mandatory when any of these abnormalities is discovered on radiographic studies of elderly patients.

Peptic Ulcer Disease

Peptic and gastric ulcer disease is responsible for a significant portion of the presentations of the elderly with gastrointestinal complaints. The increased difficulty in the diagnosis and treatment of peptic ulcer disease in the elderly contributes to the increased morbidity and mortality associated with its treatment. A number of factors adversely affect the prognosis of peptic ulcer disease in the elderly (Table 22-1).

The formerly quoted tenet that peptic ulcer "burns out" in the elderly [32] has been disproved by several studies [33,34]. Physician visits for treatment of peptic ulcer disease increase with age, paralleling increasing incidence rates for peptic ulceration in the elderly. Hospitalization rates for treatment of ulcer disease are greater in the elderly, especially for women. The reason for this increased incidence of hospital admissions is mainly for treatment of complications. Age-specific duodenal ulcer perforation rates have been shown to increase sharply after the age of 75, as has the age-specific mortality for all elderly peptic ulcer disease patients since the early 1980s. This increase in mortality from peptic ulcer disease in the elderly has occurred with the increased use of newer and more effective antiulcer medications. Much of this increase in mortality can be attributed to the delay in surgical treatment of elderly patients being treated medically; when complications occur they are in an older, higher risk group [35]. With less physiologic reserve and a higher prevalence of comorbid conditions, the morbidity and mortality for surgical treatment of the complications of peptic ulcer disease in the elderly are higher. As other chapters of this book have discussed, this is especially true when the situation has become urgent or an emergency condition develops (see Chapter 1).

Several factors contribute to the increased incidence of peptic ulcer disease in the elderly. The increased use of NSAIDs by the elderly places them at significant risk. The use of prescription NSAIDs has tripled over the last 20 years. This statistic does not take into account the use of over-the-counter agents, such as aspirin and ibuprofen, the use of which is also prominent in the elderly. Increases in prescription rates of these drugs have been more dramatic in the elderly (Fig. 22-1).

It is estimated that 40% of these medications being sold today are used by patients >60 years old. Although it has not been clearly shown that the potential of NSAIDs to cause mucosal injury is increased in the elderly, the elderly tolerate complications of NSAID therapy less well than younger patients. The risk of significant ulcer bleeding in all NSAID-treated patients is increased four to eight times. In the Aspirin and Myocardial Infarction Study, 1 g per day of aspirin increased the risk of hospitalization for duodenal ulcer 10.7-fold, and for gastric ulcer, 9.1-fold [36]. A dose-dependent relationship between NSAID dose and bleeding risk has also been demonstrated [5,37]. The use of parenteral NSAIDs has likewise been shown to cause an increased risk of gastrointestinal bleeding in the elderly. In the study by Strom et al. [38] involving patients administered 10,272 courses of parenteral NSAID therapy, patients ≥75 years old were nearly three times as likely to have gastrointestinal bleeding events as patients aged 15 to 64 years. Patients aged 65 to 74 were nearly twice as likely as their younger counterparts to have gastrointestinal bleeding events. NSAID use is also related to the risk of ulcer perforation. A number of studies have shown a correlation between NSAID use and the risk of mortality from peptic ulcer disease. The risk of NSAID use is sometimes difficult to separate from the risk of age itself. However, it is clear that NSAIDs contribute significantly to the danger of peptic ulcer disease in the elderly.

H. pylori infection has been firmly established as an important etiologic contributor in peptic ulcer disease. As mentioned previously, the prevalence of *H. pylori* infection increases with age in developed countries. The increase in prevalence is such that by the seventh decade, 67% are infected. *H. pylori* infection has been shown to be an important pathophysiologic mechanism in peptic ulcer disease by its ability to impair mucosal defenses and thereby increase susceptibility to noxious stimuli. As a result of the National Institutes of Health Consensus Development Panel on *Helicobacter pylori* in Peptic Ulcer Disease, treatment of *H. pylori* with a triple-drug regimen has been recommended in addition to antisecretory drugs whether at the time of the first presentation of the illness or with its recurrence [21].

Smoking increases the prevalence of peptic ulcer disease in all age groups. In addition to the adverse effects of smoking on prognosis in patients who require operation for peptic ulcer disease, smoking also adversely affects disease severity, recurrence, and complication rates.

Clinical Features of Peptic Ulcer Disease in the Elderly

Uncharacteristic presentations are more common in elderly peptic ulcer disease patients. In fact, >50% of elderly patients present with a complication as their first symptom [35]. Pain is less commonly a presenting feature in the elderly. Additionally, some presentations, such as weight loss, may mimic other conditions also seen more frequently in the elderly, further clouding the diagnostic picture. Melena is generally the most frequent presentation of peptic ulcer disease in patients >50 years old. Given the higher incidence of complications in the elderly and their tendency to have a paucity of typical symptoms, the diagnosis of peptic ulcer disease in the elderly requires heightened clinical suspicion and aggressive pursuit.

Gastric Ulcer

A majority of gastric ulcers occur in patients later in life. It must be remembered that certain pathophysiologic trends in the disease occur as the age of the patient increases. Trends in location, size, outcome, and cancer incidence are all related to age. These factors must be kept in mind both by surgeons and gastroenterologists participating in the care of elderly patients.

More proximal locations along the lesser curvature are seen in gastric ulcers in the elderly. More proximal location is associated with a higher incidence of achlorhydria as well as a higher risk of cancer. Gastric ulcers often have a more severe course in the elderly. Despite the availability of improved medications, the proportion of patients older than 65 requiring hospitalization for the treatment of gastric ulcer complications has risen because of the increased complication rates [39]. Since 1981, the rate of hospitalization for gastric ulcer hemorrhage has increased dramatically [40]. The majority of gastric ulcers >3 cm in diameter occur in patients older than 50. Generally, these ulcers are located higher along the lesser curvature, and bleeding from these sites is more difficult to handle endoscopically. The rate of malignancy in gastric ulcers >3 cm (10.7%) is five times greater than that in smaller ulcers [41]. Endoscopic evaluation with ulcer biopsy is absolutely necessary in all elderly patients. Endoscopic assessment of the more proximal gastric lesions is technically more difficult, however, and resection is more often necessary. Initial therapy for gastric ulcer in the elderly following successful endoscopic evaluation consists of a 12-week course of acid reduction therapy along with the elimination and control of other risk factors. Repeat evaluation is then necessary at 12 weeks. If ulcer healing or near healing has not occurred, resection is then recommended. If at least 50% healing of an ulcer >3 cm has occurred, medical therapy may be continued. The continued judicious use of medical therapy in patients with slowly healing gastric ulcers and who require continued NSAID therapy is also appropriate [35].

Duodenal Ulcer

The characteristics of duodenal ulcer unique to the elderly population include an increased incidence of bleeding and an increased tendency to erode into adjacent organs with relatively mild initial symptoms. Age-specific ulcer perforation rates for patients >75 years old have increased, reflecting the greater tendency for older patients to present with complications [35]. These factors are partly responsible for the increasing age-specific death rates seen in elderly patients when compared with the decreasing age-specific death rates seen from duodenal ulcer in younger patients (Fig. 22-2).

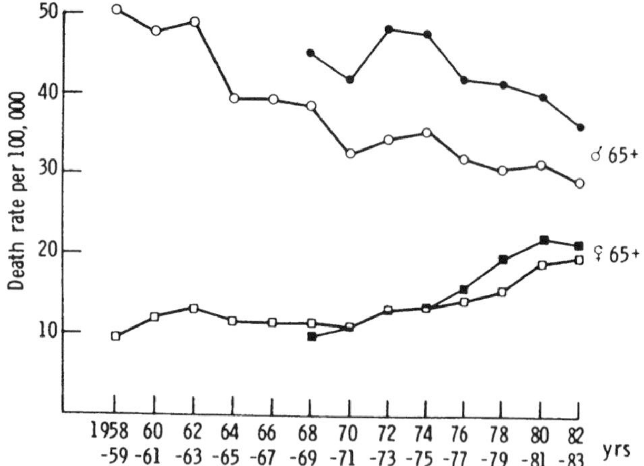

FIG. 22-2. Age-specific death rates from duodenal ulcer in England and Wales (*open symbols*) and Scotland (*closed symbols*) for men and women aged 65 years and older. (Reprinted with permission from Walt R, Logan R, Katschinski B, et al. Rising frequency of ulcer perforation in elderly people in the United Kingdom. Lancet 1986;1:489–492.)

Initial duodenal ulcer therapy includes blockade of acid production. Eradication of *H. pylori* is often beneficial, given the higher prevalence of the infection in the elderly. Compliance with the multidrug regimen required to combat the rapid organism resistance is more difficult in the elderly, however. At a minimum, those elderly patients who test positive for *H. pylori* and with duodenal ulcer recurrence or complications, as well as those patients in poor physical condition, should receive antibacterial therapy.

COMPLICATIONS OF PEPTIC ULCER DISEASE

Hemorrhage

Age is an important prognostic indicator in bleeding peptic ulcer disease. More than 75% of ulcer operations in the elderly are performed as an emergency [34,42]. In many of these cases there have been no preceding symptoms. While bleeding, duodenal ulcer, already a frequent cause of upper gastrointestinal hemorrhage in younger patients, becomes an important etiologic factor for upper gastrointestinal bleeding in the elderly, because the incidence of bleeding gastric ulcer increases among the elderly (Table 22-2).

Clearly, elderly patients tolerate the hemodynamic stress of hemorrhage less well than younger patients. A clear positive correlation between volume of upper gastrointestinal hemorrhage and mortality was shown by Kaplan et al. [43]. In this study, patients bleeding >5,000 ml had mortality four times greater than patients who bled <3,000 ml.

Prospective studies have shown that early surgical intervention for elderly patients with peptic ulcer disease results in lower mortality [40]. Morris et al. [44] randomized 142 patients with bleeding peptic ulcer disease into either early

TABLE 22-2. *Sources of upper gastrointestinal bleeding in young and old subjects*

Source	Young (%)	Old (%)
Duodenal (ulcer, duodenitis)	20–56	17–25
Gastric ulcer	15	25–30
Gastric erosions	7–25	17–20
Esophageal varices	4–36	1–12
Esophagitis, esophageal ulcer	0–12	12–13
Mallory-Weiss tears	0–18	0–2
Vascular malformation (including Dieulafoy's erosion)	0–4	?
Neoplasm	0–4	2–8

Source: Reproduced with permission from Miller DK, Burton FR, Burton MS, Ireland GA. Acute upper gastrointestinal bleeding in elderly persons [clinical conference]. J Am Geriatr Soc 1991;39:409–422.

surgical therapy or initial nonoperative therapy groups. In the early surgical therapy group patients underwent operation if 4 U blood were required in a 24-hour period, if they rebled, or if certain ominous endoscopic findings were seen. In the initial nonoperative therapy group the patients were operated on only if they required 8 U blood within 24 hours, 12 U within 48 hours, 16 U within 72 hours, or if they rebled twice. At 15 months there was no difference in mortality between the two groups for patients <60 years. For patients >60, however, mortality was 4% for the early surgical therapy group versus 15% in the initial nonoperative therapy group. Subsequent management protocols have been evaluated and have confirmed that a policy of early surgical intervention for bleeding peptic ulcer disease in the elderly patient results in disease-specific mortality similar to that in younger patients, who can better tolerate delayed operation [45]. The adage that the physiologic stress of a well-executed operation for ulcer disease is less than that of repeated ulcer hemorrhage holds especially true for elderly patients [46].

For elderly patients with upper gastrointestinal hemorrhage, early endoscopy is advocated. The endoscopic finding of active arterial bleeding, a visible bleeding vessel in the ulcer crater, or an adherent clot should lower the threshold for early operation in the elderly. Additionally, lower volumes of blood loss should be allowed before surgical intervention is undertaken. In elderly patients requiring an operation to control hemorrhage, we have traditionally used truncal vagotomy and pyloroplasty for duodenal ulcer. For elderly patients with bleeding gastric ulcer, vagotomy and antrectomy to include the ulcer is favored whenever possible. Ulcer oversewing and biopsy with proximal gastric vagotomy (PGV) should be used only rarely in this population in our experience and that of others [47,48].

Perforation

Since Crisp's description in 1843 [49], the epidemiology and pathophysiology of perforated peptic ulcer has changed significantly. Perhaps most importantly, perforated peptic ulcer has become, more and more, a complication affecting older patients (Fig. 22-3).

In their excellent review of 1,483 patients with perforated peptic ulcer treated between 1935 and 1990, Svanes et al. [50] observed a shift in the median age of patients from 41 years in 1935 to 62 years in 1990. Additionally, the proportion of women treated for perforated peptic ulcer increased fourfold during the second half of the study. Other investigators reporting large Western series have shown similar trends [51–53]. The reasons for this trend have not been definitively explained. Most likely, a combination of host and environmental factors is responsible. Decreased physiologic resilience as well as patterns of NSAID use and smoking in the elderly are likely contributing factors [53]. It is unlikely that the large increase in peptic ulcer perforation among the elderly can be attributed to increased recognition. Delayed presentation or recognition along with age, coexisting medical conditions, ulcer location, hemodynamic instability, degree of peritoneal contamination, large ulcer size, delay in operation, and nonoperative versus operative therapy have all been shown to correlate with mortality from perforated peptic ulcer [54–58]. A lethal outcome is 3.6 times as likely with perforated gastric ulcer when compared with perforated duodenal ulcer [54]. Patients ≥50 years of age are nearly four times as likely to have a fatal outcome from perforated peptic ulcer as are patients <50 years. With each decade of life after 50, the relative risk of having a fatal outcome from a perforated peptic ulcer doubles [54]. Higher mortality seen in older patients, because of their decreased physiologic reserve and more frequent associated comorbidities, is likely related to the delayed presentation or recognition with a more frequent lack of antecedent complaints. The more frequent occurrence of proximal perforations also contributes to higher mortality in the elderly.

Historically, resection with or without vagotomy, vagotomy and drainage, closure with PGV, simple closure, and nonoperative therapy have all been advocated for the treatment of perforated peptic ulcers [57–59]. The experience of Jordan and Thornby [60,61], as well as others [55], with perforated duodenal ulcers treated by omental patch closure and PGV has established this as the procedure of choice in this situation. The method of PGV and patch closure has also been applied to pyloric channel and prepyloric ulcers, but is associated with an approximate 30% recurrence rate versus 9% to 10% recurrence for perforated duodenal ulcers [61]. Thus, in the case of juxtapyloric ulcers, selective vagotomy and antrectomy to include the ulcer is the preferred method. For perforated acute or chronic gastric ulcer, primary gastric resection with or without vagotomy has been shown to be much superior to patch closure [58]. For perforations closer to the esophagogastric junction, modified resectional procedures, such as the Pauchet procedure, or biopsy and simple closure are sometimes used [60]. Although elderly patients may in some circumstances require modifications of these general principles of operative treatment for perforated gastroduodenal ulcers, the majority of elderly patients should be treated by the same principles that have been shown by vast experience to maximize survival and disease control and at the same time minimize the recurrence of the ulcer in the younger patient.

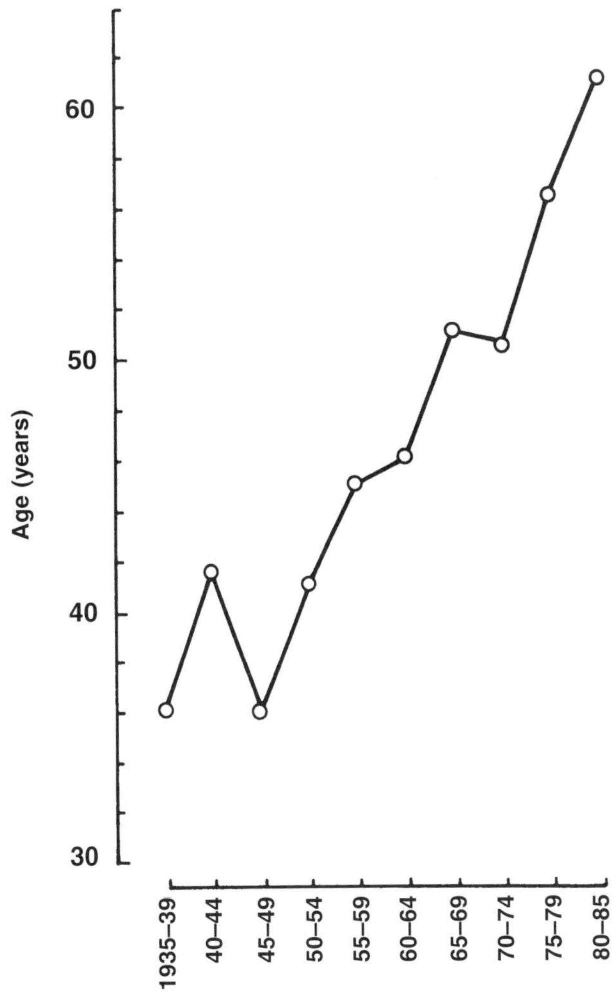

FIG. 22-3. Median age of 1,128 patients admitted to Haukeland Hospital, Bergen, Norway, for treatment of perforated peptic ulcer, 1935 to 1985. (Reprinted with permission from Svanes C, Salvesen H, Espehaug B, et al. A multifactorial analysis of factors related to lethality after treatment of perforated gastroduodenal ulcer, 1935–1990. Ann Surg 1989; 209:418–423.)

GASTRIC POLYPS

Gastric polyps occur in 5% to 10% of patients, as has been reported in endoscopic series [62]. Nearly 60% of gastric polyps removed or biopsied occur in patients >60 years of age. Gastric polyps can be of various histologic types

TABLE 22-3. *Age distribution and average age of patients with various polyps*

	Average age (years)	Age (%)						
		<30	30–39	40–49	50–59	60–69	70–79	≥86
Tumor-like lesions								
Glandular cysts	57	4.1	7.9	21.1	24.5	20.7	18.0	3.5
Hyperplasiogenous polyps	72	0.1	0.2	2.0	13.2	31.0	39.5	13.5
Inflammatory polyps	64	0.7	2.0	10.6	20.5	27.2	32.5	6.6
Brunner's gland heterotopia	60	6.1	8.2	12.2	18.4	32.7	20.4	2.0
Pancreatic heterotopia	45	26.3	15.8	31.6	31.2	7.9	5.3	0.0
Peutz-Jeghers polyps	33	25.1	25.0	31.3	6.3	6.3	0.0	6.3
Juvenile polyps	39	14.3	57.1	28.6	0.0	0.0	0.0	0.0
Cronkhite-Canada polyps	64	0.0	0.0	0.0	50.0	50.0	0.0	0.0
Total		**2.8**	**4.8**	**13.3**	**19.7**	**25.0**	**26.8**	**7.7**
Neoplasias								
Tubular adenomas	70	0.0	1.4	4.1	11.0	25.1	40.2	18.3
Tubulopapillary adenomas	70	0.0	0.0	0.0	2.0	14.3	38.8	44.9
Papillary adenomas	70	0.0	0.0	0.0	0.0	20.0	80.0	0.0
Carcinomas	69	0.0	0.9	2.3	11.2	28.4	42.8	14.4
Carcinoid tumors	64	3.7	1.2	7.4	17.3	25.9	30.9	13.6
Pyloric gland adenomas	80	0.0	0.0	0.0	0.0	0.0	0.0	100.0
Total		**0.3**	**1.1**	**3.5**	**11.1**	**25.8**	**40.5**	**17.7**

Source: Reprinted with permission from Stolte M, Sticht T, Eidt S, et al. Frequency, location, and age and sex distribution of various types of gastric polyp. Endoscopy 1994;26:659–665.

[63]. These histologic types, their frequency, and age distribution are shown in Table 22-3.

The presence of gastric polyps has been shown to be associated with higher risk for the development of gastric cancer either within the polyp itself or in different areas within the stomach. In a study of 3,914 patients undergoing endoscopy, the presence of gastric polyps was associated with a relative risk of 2.43 for the eventual development of gastric cancer [64]. Adenomatous polyps show the greatest association with malignancy. Kato et al. [64] found that the proportion of adenomatous polyps among total polyps was higher in subjects who developed stomach cancer (50%) when compared with those who did not develop cancer (9%). Eight percent of gastric adenomas are associated with coexistent gastric cancer. Such cancers occur predominately in men and most commonly in the eighth decade. Additionally, 11% of gastric adenomas followed endoscopically undergo malignant degeneration [65]. Given the fact that gastric polyps seen in the elderly are more likely to be malignant, they should always be removed when technically feasible, and all that are removed should be closely examined histologically.

GASTRIC CANCER

Gastric cancer is currently the second most common form of cancer worldwide, ranking only behind cancer of the lung. In the United States, gastric cancer was the most common form of cancer in adults up through the 1930s, when its incidence began to decline [66–68]. The decline in the incidence of gastric cancer in the United States continued over the next several decades and then plateaued. From 1976 to 1986, the incidence rose by 8% in the United States from 22,900 to 24,700. The incidence remains at this level. The male-to-female ratio is 1.6 to 1 [66,68]. Gastric cancer is predominately a disease of older people now, with two-thirds of cases occurring in patients >65 years of age. No further change in the age distribution of the disease has occurred in the last several decades. The median age in men diagnosed with gastric cancer is 68.4 and in women it is 71.9.

Gastric adenocarcinoma accounts for 95% of gastric cancer [69]. Two main types of gastric adenocarcinoma have been described: intestinal and diffuse. The diffuse type is predominant in populations at low risk and is becoming more frequent, especially in populations experiencing a decline in the intestinal type of gastric adenocarcinoma. The pathophysiologic and etiologic processes underlying the diffuse type are largely unknown. The intestinal type of gastric adenocarcinoma resembles other intestinal carcinomas and usually arises in areas of the gastric mucosa that have previously become "intestinalized." This is the type of gastric adenocarcinoma that has been decreasing in incidence in the industrialized nations. The intestinal form of gastric cancer is thought to be the end result of a process that unfolds over a period of decades, as described by Correa [69]. The process involves the appearance of an ordered series of lesions culminating in gastric adenocarcinoma. In order of their progression, these lesions are superficial gastritis, atrophy, small intestinal metaplasia, colonic metaplasia, dysplasia, and finally invasive carcinoma. The sum of

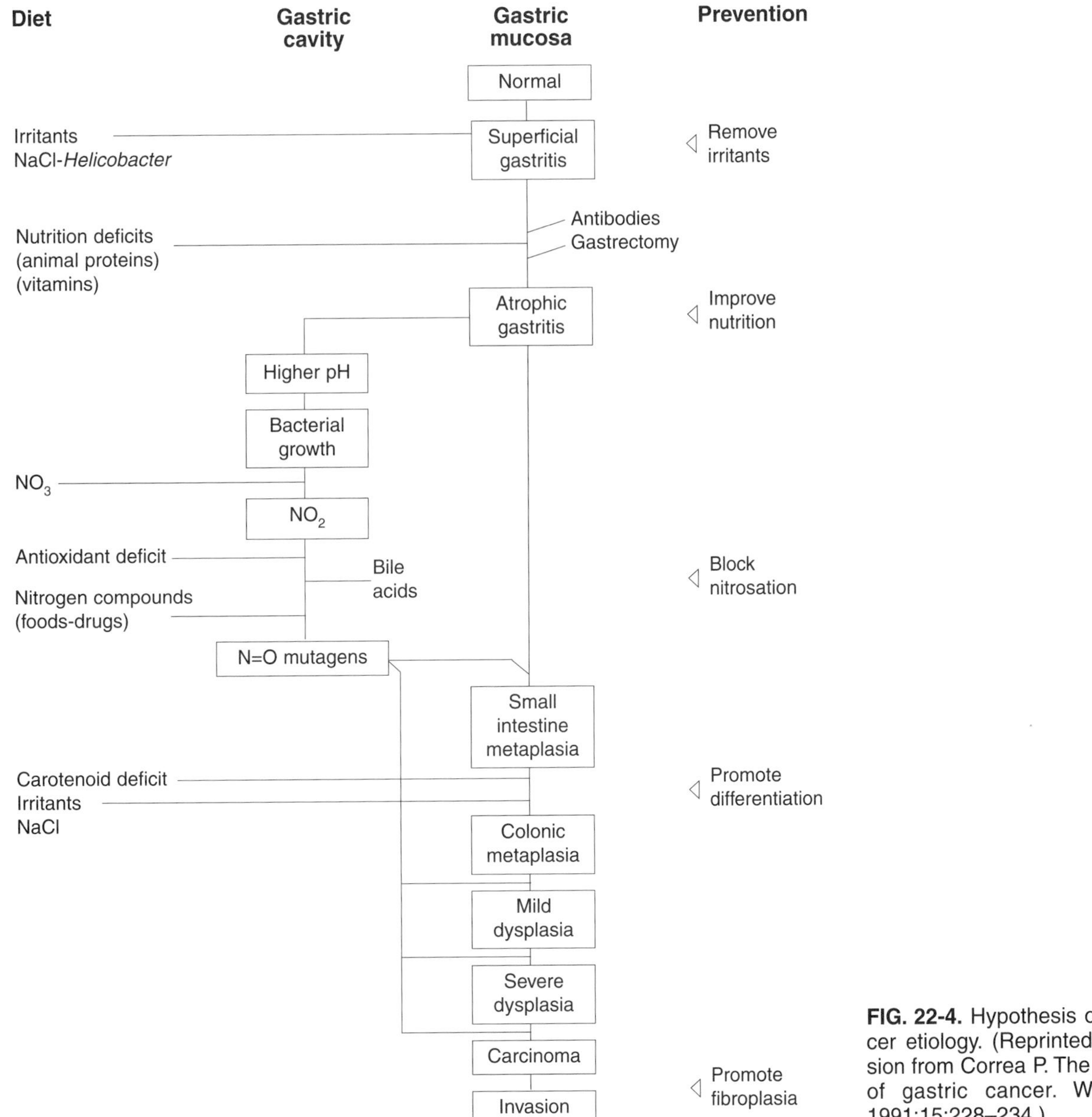

FIG. 22-4. Hypothesis of gastric cancer etiology. (Reprinted with permission from Correa P. The epidemiology of gastric cancer. World J Surg 1991;15:228–234.)

the work of many investigators studying gastric cancer, along with oncogenesis in general, has led to the development of an etiologic hypothesis for the development of the lesion in gastric cancer (Fig. 22-4).

The established risk factors for gastric cancer function, in this hypothesis, as gastric irritants. Excessive salt intake leads to gastritis. Salt-induced gastritis is accompanied by excessive cell replication and enhances the effects of other gastric carcinogens [70]. *H. pylori* induces the migration of polymorphonuclear leukocytes from the capillaries to the stroma and to the glands of the gastric mucosa, especially into the epithelium of the glandular neck cells, where the bacteria are located close to the replicating cells. Polymorphonuclear leukocytes give rise to oxidative bursts in the presence of *H. pylori,* which may give rise to DNA damage and mutagenesis in replicating gastric epithelium. Recently, it has been found that certain strains of *H. pylori,* containing the cytotoxin-associated gene A (cagA gene), are associated with enhanced induction of intestinal metaplasia within the gastric mucosa. The cagA gene encodes for a high molecular weight immunodominant antigen, and cagA-positive *H. pylori* strains are associated with enhanced induction of acute gastric inflammation leading to atrophic gastritis and a higher incidence of gastric cancer [71].

Other dietary and environmental factors associated with the increased incidence of gastric cancer, such as smoked foods, aflatoxin exposure, and smoking, also produce gastric inflammation and gastritis. Dietary factors thought to protect the stomach from the development of cancer include vitamin C and carotene. Vitamin C is thought to be protective by preventing the formation of *N*-nitroso compounds within the gastric juice. Carotene is protective by its antioxidant function [66].

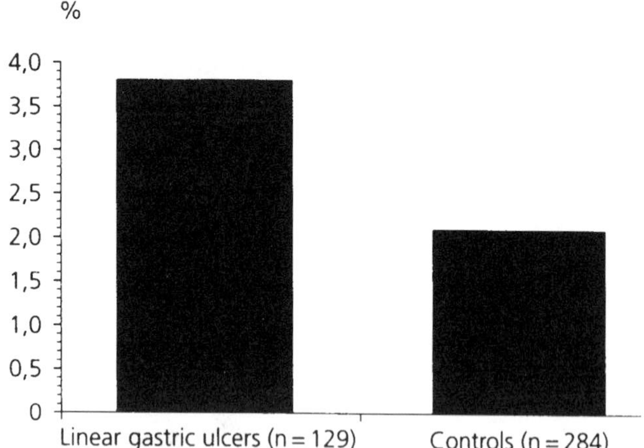

FIG. 22-5. Incidence of gastric cancer in patients with linear gastric ulcer and control subjects. (Reprinted with permission from Shimizu S, Tada M, Kawai K. Early gastric cancer: its surveillance and natural course. Endoscopy 1995;27:27–31.)

Several other clinical conditions have been shown to be associated with gastric cancer. As described previously, adenomatous gastric polyps are associated with increased rates of gastric cancer occurrence. Carcinoma develops in a low percentage of preexisting gastric benign ulcers, a percentage not significantly different from controls [66,72] (Fig. 22-5). However, gastric malignancy may first appear as gastric ulceration and if not biopsied, it may be missed in this early stage. Of patients diagnosed with gastric cancer, 25.5% have a history of gastric ulcer [68]. An aggressive approach to endoscopy with four-quadrant ulcer biopsy should be taken with all elderly patients with gastric ulcer, who may present with vague complaints. It is for this reason that an aggressive surgical approach is indicated for all patients whose gastric ulcers do not show prompt healing with medical therapy [66]. In the elderly patient with an unhealed, partially healed, or recurrent gastric ulcer, the ulcer must be assumed to be malignant until proven otherwise.

Diagnosis and Staging

In the West, the diagnosis of gastric cancer traditionally has been dependent on the development of symptoms, which are often vague. As a result, a high proportion of gastric cancers are advanced at the time of diagnosis. The symptoms often mimic those of other, more common, benign gastrointestinal conditions, and this contributes to delayed diagnosis (Table 22-4).

In the elderly, the more frequent occurrence of a vague symptom complex may compound the problem of delayed diagnosis. This mandates heightened awareness on the part of clinicians caring for elderly patients with gastrointestinal complaints. Early investigation is necessary to maximize early-stage diagnosis. Physical findings and laboratory evaluation have not been particularly valuable in the diagnosis of early gastric cancer.

Conversely, air-contrast, thin barium upper gastrointestinal series have a >90% accuracy in the diagnosis of advanced cancer and have been used in mass gastric cancer screening programs in Japan, where the disease is endemic. The detection of early gastric cancer has been made possible by the development of increasingly sophisticated endoscopic technology [66,72] (Fig. 22-6).

The current endoscopic capabilities used in Japan, including use of the videoendoscopy and dye-spraying methods, have led to the increased detection of smaller tumors and multiple synchronous tumors [66,72,73]. The development of the endoscopic Congo red–methylene blue test led to an 88.9% rate of detection for coexisting lesions compared with 28.3% with endoscopy alone. In Japan, multiple synchronous gastric cancers have been found to occur most frequently in elderly men [73].

The use of dynamic computed tomographic (CT) scanning and endoscopic ultrasound has led to improved staging of known gastric cancer. Endoscopic ultrasound is most useful in determining depth of tumor invasion and perigastric lymph node involvement and thus is most valuable in characterizing early disease. CT scanning is more valuable in characterizing advanced disease and determining resectability. The application of laparoscopy to the staging of gastric cancer may also prove beneficial in determining resectability.

Treatment

The treatment of gastric cancer has been primarily surgical, because resection provides the most effective therapy in terms of both cure and palliation. Resection has been the initial mode of therapy in 77% of cases in the United States as reported by Wanebo et al. [68] in 1993. Adjuvant chemotherapy, radiation, or both was used in 34.7% of cases reported in this series of 18,365 patients treated up to 1987. Surgical experience in the United States has included various degrees of gastric resection based on tumor location [68]. Based on the Vanderbilt experience with gastric cancer as well as his review of the current literature, Sawyers [66] indicates that a general consensus regarding the extent of gastric resection based on tumor location has developed. He states that radical distal subtotal gastrectomy of approximately 80% to 85% is indicated for antral-pyloric tumors and small midcorpus tumors. Total gastrectomy is indicated for patients with large cancers in the midstomach and fundus. Cancers in the cardia should be treated by total gastrectomy with excision of the distal 10 cm of esophagus.

The Japanese experience with gastric cancer, a byproduct of the endemic nature of the disease in that country, has more clearly highlighted the importance of regional lymph node dissection in the control of the disease process. Their detailed classification of regional nodes and more aggressive approach to lymph node dissection has allowed more accurate tumor staging. Although there is a lack of randomized prospective trials reported in the Japanese experience with

TABLE 22-4. *Symptoms present at initial diagnosis in 18,365 patients diagnosed with gastric cancer*

Symptom	
Weight loss	61.6%
Abdominal pain	51.6%
Nausea	34.3%
Anorexia	32.0%
Dysphagia	26.1%
Melena	20.2%
Early satiety	17.5%
Ulcer-type pain	17.1%
Swelling of lower extremities	5.9%
Previous history	
Gastric ulcer	25.5%
Duodenal ulcer	7.5%
Pernicious anemia	5.9%
Gastric polyps	3.5%
Polyps in large bowel	3.0%
Achlorhydria	1.8%
Polyposis of small bowel	1.4%

Source: Reprinted with permission from Wanebo HJ, Kennedy BJ, Chmiel J, et al. Cancer of the stomach: a patient care study by the American College of Surgeons. Ann Surg 1993;218:583–592.

lymphadenectomy [66], it is likely that their more extensive use of R2 resection is therapeutic and has contributed significantly to the superior survival rates reported in their series as compared with U.S. series [68,74] (Table 22-5).

In 70% to 80% of cases, gastric cancer recurs despite resection. Given this high rate of recurrent disease, adjuvant forms of therapy could potentially make a large impact on the treatment of the disease. The results of adjuvant chemotherapy and radiation protocols reported to date have been disappointing, however. No adjuvant treatment for gastric cancer has been consistently shown to prolong survival. Protocols involving polychemotherapy as well as multimodality therapy currently being investigated will be directed toward improving survival for the large proportion of patients who have metastatic or recurrent disease [75].

Survival

Improvements in surgical technique and perioperative care have led to improved survival following surgical treatment of gastric cancer. Operative mortality for all ages has decreased from 16.2% in series reported up to 1970 [76] to 7% to 8% more recently [68,76]. A review of the English literature showed that 5-year survival rates in the United States after resection have improved from 20.7% before 1970 to 28.4% as of 1990. This is largely due to improved patient selection and preoperative staging. The 5-year survival rate after curative or radical resection has risen from 37.6% to 55.4% over the same period [77].

Advanced age is not a contraindication to aggressive surgical treatment of gastric carcinoma. Numerous studies have shown operative mortality for elderly patients similar to that of younger age groups after gastric resection for cancer [78–83]. Surgical morbidity is higher in some studies involving elderly patients [79,82], whereas other studies show no significant difference [78,80,81]. In the studies showing higher morbidity for the elderly patient, complications more frequently involve the cardiopulmonary system and seem to occur even more frequently in the >80 age group. However, the quality of life of elderly patients undergoing gastric surgery is generally good [84], and therefore aggressive surgical treatment is justified in cases in which the overall physical status of the patient is acceptable.

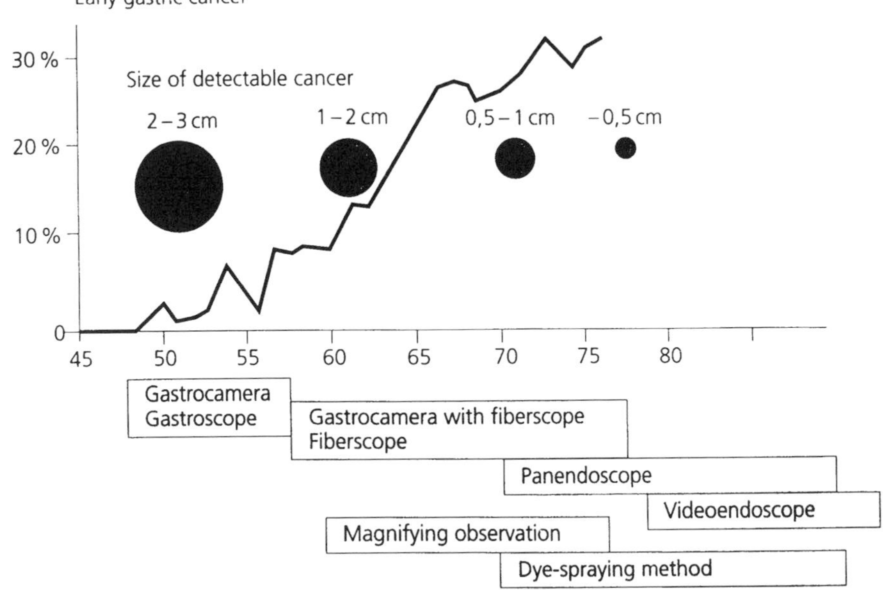

FIG. 22-6. Relationship between the percentage of early gastric cancer cases detected among total gastric cancer cases detected in Japan and the development of endoscopy. (Reprinted with permission from Shimizu S, Tada M, Kawai K. Early gastric cancer: its surveillance and natural course. Endoscopy 1995;27:27–31.)

TABLE 22-5. *U.S. and Japanese 5-year survival rates in gastric cancer*

	Percent survival					
Country	Stage IA	Stage IB	Stage II	Stage IIIA	Stage IIIB	Stage IV
United States (n = 10,237)	59	44	29	15	9	3
Japan (n = 11,845)	99	88	71	48	22	10
Japan (n = 7,513)	95	84	67	47	23	3

Source: Reprinted with permission from Hundahl SA, Stemmermann GN, Oishi A. Racial factors cannot explain superior Japanese outcomes in stomach cancer. Arch Surg 1996;131:170–175.

EARLY GASTRIC CANCER

As defined by the Japanese Gastroenterological Society in 1962 and the Japanese Research Society for Gastric Cancer in 1963, early gastric cancer was defined as cancer of the stomach in which invasion was limited to the submucosa, regardless of size and lymph node status. As of 1985, the Japanese national records on gastric cancer showed that with mass screening protocols, the percentage of early gastric cancers among resected cases had reached 40%. In addition, the proportion of tumors ≤2 cm had increased to 15% of total cases [72]. More recent series report that over one-half of gastric cancers diagnosed in Japan are now in the early stage [85].

In Western countries, where mass screening is not performed, the proportion of early gastric cancer is much less. From our institution, a report of 23 years' experience with gastric carcinoma revealed that only 3.6% of patients had early gastric cancer, whereas the remainder had more advanced lesions [86]. When screening protocols similar to those used in Japan are used in Western countries, the percentage of early gastric cancer increases from 15% to 20% [66].

Early gastric cancer has a relatively high rate of multicentricity as well as an unusually frequent association with other neoplasms. Rates of lymph node metastases in patients with early gastric cancer are surprisingly high, occurring in 10% to 11% of cases. In lesions confined to the mucosa, lymph node metastases occur in 2.5% to 5% of cases, whereas for lesions extending into the submucosa, the rate of lymph node metastases is 16% to 21% [85,87].

For early gastric cancer, 5-year survival rates exceed 90%. The 5-year survival rate is 94.5% for mucosal cancers and 91.3% for submucosal cancers [85]. The 5-year survival rate for node-negative patients is 97.1% and for node-positive patients it is 83.3%. Ten-year survival rates are 94.1% and 52.8%, respectively [87]. In the healthy, vigorous elderly patient with any complaint that could be from gastric ulcer, gastritis, or gastric cancer, screening protocols should be used to rule out early cancer.

GASTRIC LYMPHOMA AND SARCOMA

Gastric lymphoma and sarcoma are infrequent tumors, accounting for <5% of gastric malignancies [88,89]. Gastric lymphoma accounts for two-thirds of gastrointestinal lymphomas. Our approach to gastric lymphoma has traditionally been aggressive surgical resection [31]. As more experience has been gained with primary chemotherapy and radiation, favorable results have been seen. Some centers currently approach gastric lymphoma with primary chemotherapy, reserving radiation and resection for patients who have recurrence or who do not achieve a complete response with primary therapy, whereas other centers continue to advocate surgical resection as the primary modality [75,89]. Resolution of this controversy will likely await results of randomized, prospective trials.

At the time of diagnosis, gastric sarcoma is often shown to involve adjacent organs. When resection with wide 10- to 12-cm margins is feasible, as occurs in two-thirds of cases, a significant prolongation of survival is seen. In cases of advanced disease precluding curative resection, tumor debulking, chemotherapy, and radiation generally do not prolong survival significantly [31]. We currently recommend wide 10-cm resection and lymph node dissection in all healthy elderly patients with gastric sarcomas [31]. This general subject of lymphoma and sarcoma of the stomach has been covered by Scott and Sawyers [90].

EFFECTS OF GASTRIC RESECTION IN THE ELDERLY

Improved medical therapy for peptic ulcer disease has greatly reduced the need for surgical treatment and thus the number of patients followed long-term after gastric resection continues to decline. Currently, however, a great number of elderly patients are seen who have undergone gastric resection for benign and malignant gastroduodenal conditions in previous decades. Patients currently undergoing gastric resection for complications of peptic ulcer disease and gastric cancer will continue to be seen for some time.

The effect of procedures for peptic ulcer surgery on life expectancy has been debated in the literature. Shortened life expectancy is reported in some series [91,92], but is refuted in others [93,94]. Increased rates of gastric cancer have been seen in some studies 20 to 40 years following vagotomy and acid-reductive resections [95]. This has been postulated to be related to alterations in the gastric milieu that result from increased gastric remnant pH and the effects of bile salts on the gastric mucosa [16]. Increased rates of smoking-related deaths have also been seen in post–ulcer surgery cohorts [92]. Increased smoking-related mortality has been seen in patients treated with H_2 antagonists. Smoking cessation therefore takes on an even greater importance in this patient population.

Several physiologic effects of gastric resection have been observed. A Swedish study [93] compared long-term physiologic changes in elderly men following partial gastrectomy with age-matched nonoperated controls. Patients between the ages of 70 and 75 showed weight reduction compared with controls, which was thought to be due to impaired digestion. Osteoporosis, bone fractures, as well as B_{12} and iron-deficiency anemia were also seen more frequently following gastrectomy. There was no difference in functional status between the two groups.

Investigations show that elderly patients followed long term after partial gastric resections generally fare well [82,85,95]. Several areas, including overall nutritional status, tobacco use, bone mineral content, and iron and B_{12} levels are areas that require increased attention in patients after gastric resection. The favorable functional status of elderly patients after most types of gastric resections supports the use of operative therapy when necessary in this population.

REFERENCES

1. Goldschmeidt M, Barnett CG, Schwarz BE, et al. Effect of age on gastric acid secretion and serum gastrin concentrations in healthy men and women. Gastroenterology 1991;101:977–979.
2. Keeki M, Samloff IM, Ihamaki T, et al. Age and sex related behavior of gastric acid secretion at the population level. Scand J Gastroenterol 1982;17:737–743.
3. Atillasoy E, Holt PR. Gastrointestinal proliferation and aging. J Gerontol B Sci Soc Sci 1993;48:43–49.
4. Singh P, Rae-Venter B, Townsend CM Jr, et al. Gastrin receptors in normal and malignant gastrointestinal mucosa: age-associated changes. Am J Physiol 1985;249:G761–G769.
5. Anuras S, Loening-Baucke V. Gastrointestinal motility in the elderly. J Am Geriatr Soc 1984;32:386–390.
6. Evans MA, Triggs EJ, Cheung M, et al. Gastric emptying rate in the elderly: implications for drug therapy. J Am Geriatr Soc 1981;29: 201–205.
7. Van Liere EJ, Northup DW. The emptying time of the stomach of old people. Am J Physiol 1941;134:719.
8. Moore JG, Tweedy C, Christian PE, Datz FL. Effect of age on gastric emptying of liquid-solid meals in man. Dig Dis Sci 1983;28:340–344.
9. Kao CH, Lai TL, Wang SJ, et al. Influence of age on gastric emptying in healthy Chinese. Clin Nucl Med 1994;19:401–404.
10. Kekki M, Samloff IM, Ihamaki T, et al. Age and sex-related behaviour of gastric acid secretion at the population level. Scand J Gastroenterol 1982;17:737–743.
11. Walan A, Bianchi PG, Hentschel E, et al. Maintenance treatment with cimetidine in peptic ulcer disease for up to 4 years. Scand J Gastroenterol 1987;22:397–405.
12. Bardhan KD for the Anglo-Irish Cimetidine Long-Term Study Group. Six years of continuous cimetidine treatment in peptic ulcer disease: efficacy and safety. Aliment Pharmacol Ther 1988;2:395–402.
13. Wade AG, Rowley-Jones D. Long-term management of duodenal ulcer in general practice. How best to use cimetidine. BMJ 1988;296:971–974.
14. Penston J, Wormsley KG. Efficacy and safety of long-term maintenance therapy of duodenal ulcers. Scand J Gastroenterol 1989; 24:1145–1152.
15. McCloy RF, Arnold R, Bardhan KD, et al. Pathophysiological effects of long-term acid suppression in man. Dig Dis Sci 1995;40(Suppl):96–120.
16. Soybel DI, Modlin IM. Implications of sustained suppression of gastric acid secretion. Am J Surg 1992;163:613–620.
17. McCloy RF. Implications of a review of long-term safety of omeprazole and management strategies for peptic disease. Hepatogastroenterology 1992;39:90–91.
18. Marshall BJ, Royce H, Annear DI, et al. Original isolation of *Campylobacter pyloris* from human gastric mucosa. Microbios Lett 1984;25:83–88.
19. Marshall BJ, Warren JR. Unidentified curved bacilli in the stomach of patients with gastritis and peptic ulceration. Lancet 1984;1:1311–1315.
20. Blaser MJ, Parsonnet J. Parasitism by the "slow"' bacterium *Helicobacter pylori* leads to altered gastric homeostasis and neoplasia. J Clin Invest 1994;94:4–8.
21. NIH Consensus Development Panel. *Helicobacter pylori* in peptic ulcer disease. JAMA 1994;272:65–69.
22. Blaser MJ. The bacteria behind ulcers. Sci Am 1996;274:104–107.
23. Perez-Perez GI, Marrie T, Inouye H, et al. The effect of age and occupation on the seroprevalence of *Helicobacter pylori* infection. Can J Infect Dis 1992;3:134–138.
24. Correa P. Chronic gastritis: a clinico-pathological classification. Am J Gastroenterol 1988;83:504–509.
25. Correa P. The gastric microenvironment determines *Helicobacter pylori* colonization. Am J Gastroenterol 1995;90:1379–1381.
26. Sawyers JL. Management of postgastrectomy syndromes. Am J Surg 1990;159:8–14.
27. Krasinski SD, Russell RM, Samloff IM, et al. Fundic atrophic gastritis in an elderly population. J Am Geriatr Soc 1986;34:800–806.
28. Russell RM. Changes in gastrointestinal function attributed to aging. Am J Clin Nutr 1992;55(Suppl):1203–1207.
29. Ming SC. Tumors of the Esophagus and Stomach. Washington, DC: Armed Forces Institute of Pathology, 1973.
30. Fieber SS, Rickert RR. Hyperplastic gastropathy: analysis of 50 selected cases 1955–1980. Am J Gastroenterol 1981;76:321–329.
31. Adkins RB, Scott HW, Sawyers JL. Gastrointestinal lymphomas and sarcomas: a case for aggressive search and destroy. Ann Surg 1987; 205:625–633.
32. Fry J. Peptic ulcer: a profile. BMJ 1964;2:809–812.
33. Elashoff JD, Van Deventer G, Ready TJ, et al. Long-term follow-up of duodenal ulcer patients. J Clin Gastroenterol 1983;5:509–515.
34. Gilinsky NH. Peptic ulcer disease in the elderly. Gastroenterol Clin North Am 1990;19:255–271.
35. McCarthy DM. Acid peptic disease in the elderly. Clin Geriatr Med 1991;7:231–254.
36. Soll AH, Weinstein WM, Kurata J, et al. Non-steroidal anti-inflammatory drugs and peptic ulcer. Ann Intern Med 1991;114:307–319.
37. Griffin MR, Piper JM, Daugherty J, et al. Non-steroidal anti-inflammatory drug use and hospitalization for peptic ulcer in elderly persons [abstract]. Gastroenterology 1990;98:A4.
38. Strom BL, Berlin JA, Kinman JL, et al. Parenteral ketolorac and risk of gastrointestinal and operative site bleeding. JAMA 1996;275:376–382.
39. Commission on Professional and Hospital Activities. Length of Stay by Diagnosis and Operation, United States, 1987. Ann Arbor, MI: CPHA Publications, 1988;98–100.
40. Cochran TA. Bleeding peptic ulcer: surgical therapy. Gastroenterol Clin North Am 1993;22:751–758.
41. Wenger J, Brandborg LL, Spellman FA. The Veteran's Administration Cooperative Study on Gastric Ulcer, part I. Gastroenterology 1971; 61:598–621.
42. Permutt RP, Cello JP. Duodenal ulcer disease in the hospitalized elderly patient. Dig Dis Sci 1982;27:1–6.
43. Kaplan MS, List JW, Stemmer EA, Connolly JE. Surgical management of peptic ulcer disease in the aged patient. Arch Surg 1972; 104:667–671.
44. Morris DL, Hawker PC, Brearley S, et al. Optimal timing of operation for bleeding peptic ulcer: prospective randomized trial. BMJ 1984;288:1277–1280.
45. Wheatley KE, Snyman JH, Brearley S, et al. Mortality in patients with bleeding peptic ulcer when those aged 60 or over are operated on early. BMJ 1990;301:272.
46. Bonnevie O. Changing demographics of peptic ulcer disease. Dig Dis Sci 1985;30:85–145.
47. Pulvertaft CN. Comments on the incidence and natural history of gastric and duodenal ulcer. Postgrad Med J 1968;44:597–602.
48. Herrington JL, Scott HW, Sawyers JL. Experience with vagotomy-antrectomy and Roux-en-Y gastrojejunostomy in surgical treatment of duodenal, gastric, and stomal ulcers. Ann Surg 1984;199:590–597.

49. Crisp E. Cases of perforation of the stomach. Lancet 1843;2:639–649.
50. Svanes C, Salvesen H, Strangeland L, et al. Perforated peptic ulcer over 56 years. Time trends in patients and disease characteristics. Gut 1993;34:1666–1671.
51. MacKay C. Perforated peptic ulcer in the west of Scotland: a survey of 5343 cases during 1954–1963. BMJ 1966;1:701–705.
52. Cohen MM. Perforated peptic ulcer in the Vancouver area: a survey of 852 cases. Can Med Assoc J 1971;104:201–205.
53. Walt R, Logan R, Katschinski B, et al. Rising frequency of ulcer perforation in elderly people in the United Kingdom. Lancet 1986;1: 489–492.
54. Svanes C, Salvesen H, Espehaug B, et al. A multifactorial analysis of factors related to lethality after treatment of perforated gastroduodenal ulcer, 1935–1990. Ann Surg 1989;209:418–423.
55. Horowitz J, Kukora JS, Ritchie WP. All perforated ulcers are not alike. Ann Surg 1989;209:693–697.
56. Svanes C, Lie RT, Svanes K, et al. Adverse effects of delayed treatment of perforated peptic ulcer. Ann Surg 1994;220:168–175.
57. Bodner B, Harrington ME, Kim U. A multifactorial analysis of mortality and morbidity in perforated peptic ulcer disease. Surg Gynecol Obstet 1990;171:316–320.
58. McGee GS, Sawyers JL. Perforated gastric ulcers: a plea for management by primary gastric resection. Arch Surg 1987;122:555–561.
59. DeBakey ME. Acute perforated gastroduodenal ulceration. Surgery 1940;8:852–884, 1028–1076.
60. Jordan PH, Thornby J. Perforated pyloroduodenal ulcers: long-term results with omental patch closure and parietal cell vagotomy. Ann Surg 1995;221:479–488.
61. Jordan PH, Thornby J. Twenty years after parietal cell vagotomy or selective vagotomy antrectomy for treatment of duodenal ulcer: final report. Ann Surg 1994;220:283–296.
62. Jarvinen HJ. Other gastrointestinal polyps. World J Surg 1991;15: 50–56.
63. Stolte M, Sticht T, Eidt S, et al. Frequency, location, and age and sex distribution of various types of gastric polyp. Endoscopy 1994;26: 659–665.
64. Kato I, Tominaga S, Ito Y, et al. A prospective study of atrophic gastritis and stomach cancer risk. Jpn J Cancer Res 1992;83:1137–1142.
65. Kamiya T, Morishita T, Asakura H, et al. Long-term follow-up study on gastric adenoma and its relation to gastric protruded carcinoma. Cancer 1982;50:2496–2503.
66. Sawyers JL. Gastric carcinoma. Curr Probl Surg 1995;32:103–178.
67. Longmire WP. A current view of gastric cancer in the US. Ann Surg 1993;218:579–582.
68. Wanebo HJ, Kennedy BJ, Chmiel J, et al. Cancer of the stomach: a patient care study by the American College of Surgeons. Ann Surg 1993;218:583–592.
69. Correa P. The epidemiology of gastric cancer. World J Surg 1991;15: 228–234.
70. Correa P. Is gastric carcinoma an infectious disease? N Engl J Med 1991;325:1170–1171.
71. Kuipers EJ, Perez-Perez GI, Meuwissen SGM, Blaser MJ. *Helicobacter pylori* and atrophic gastritis: importance of cagA status. J Natl Cancer Inst 1995;87:1777–1780.
72. Shimizu S, Tada M, Kawai K. Early gastric cancer: its surveillance and natural course. Endoscopy 1995;27:27–31.
73. Lishi H, Tatsuta M, Okuda S. Diagnosis of simultaneous multiple gastric cancers by the Congo red-methylene blue test. Endoscopy 1988; 20:78–82.
74. Hundahl SA, Stemmermann GN, Oishi A. Racial factors cannot explain superior Japanese outcomes in stomach cancer. Arch Surg 1996;131:170–175.
75. Staley CA. Gastric Carcinoma. In Berger DH, Feig BW, Fuhrman GM (eds), The MD Anderson Surgical Oncology Handbook. Boston: Little, Brown, 1995;120–141.
76. Macintyre IMC, Akoh JA. Improving survival in gastric cancer: review of operative mortality in English language publications from 1970. Br J Surg 1991;78:773–778.
77. Akoh JA, Macintyre IMC. Improving survival in gastric cancer: review of 5-year survival rates in English language publications from 1970. Br J Surg 1992;79:293–299.
78. Maehara Y, Oshiro T, Oiwa H, et al. Gastric carcinoma in patients over 70 years of age. Br J Surg 1995;82:102–105.
79. Korenaga D, Moriguchi S, Baba H, et al. Surgery for gastric carcinoma is feasible for patients over 80 years of age. World J Surg 1991;15:642–648.
80. Bandoh T, Isoyama T, Toyoshima H. Total gastrectomy for gastric cancer in the elderly. Surgery 1991;109:136–142.
81. Hioki K, Nakane Y, Okamura S, et al. Evaluation of surgical treatment of gastric cancer in the aged. Japan J Ger 1994;31:23–28.
82. Fujimoto S, Takahashi M, Ohkubo H, et al. Clinicopathologic characteristics and survival of elderly patients with gastric cancer. Anticancer Res 1994;14:1405–1408.
83. Coluccia C, Ricci EB, Marzola GG, et al. Gastric cancer in the elderly: results of surgical treatment. Int Surg 1987;72:4–10.
84. Pannella A, Laboranti F, Zambianchi M, et al. The quality of life of the elderly after a surgical intervention. II. Gastric carcinoma. Minerva Chir 1994;49:15–19.
85. Nishi M, Ishihara S, Nakajima T, et al. Chronological changes of characteristics of early gastric cancer and therapy: experience in the Cancer Institute Hospital of Tokyo, 1950–1994. J Cancer Res Clin Oncol 1995;121:535–541.
86. Scott HW Jr, Adkins RB Jr, Sawyers JL. Results of an aggressive surgical approach to gastric carcinoma during a twenty-three-year period. Surgery 1985;97:55–59.
87. Habu H, Takeshita, Sunagawa M, Endo M. Lymph node metastases in early gastric cancer. Int Surg 1986;71:244–247.
88. Carson W, Karakousis C, Douglass H, et al. Results of aggressive treatment of gastric sarcoma. Ann Surg Oncol 1994;1:244–251.
89. Frazee RC, Roberts J. Gastric lymphoma treatment: medical versus surgical. Surg Clin North Am 1992;72:423–431.
90. Adkins RB, Johnson D, Gray GF. Gastric Lymphomas, Sarcomas, and Carcinoids. In Scott HW, Sawyers JL (eds), Surgery of the Stomach, Duodenum, and Small Intestine (2nd ed). Boston: Blackwell, 1992;361–375.
91. McLean Ross AH, Smith MA, Anderson JR, Small WP. Late mortality after surgery for peptic ulcer. N Engl J Med 1982;307:519–522.
92. Tersmette AC, Offerhaus GJA, Giardiello FM, et al. Long-term prognosis after partial gastrectomy for benign conditions. Gastroenterology 1991;101:148–153.
93. Mellstrom D, Rundgren A. Long-term effects after partial gastrectomy in elderly men: a longitudinal population study of men between 70 and 75 years of age. Scand J Gastroenterol 1982;17:433–439.
94. Stemmerman GN, Heilbrun L, Nomura A, et al. Late mortality after partial gastrectomy. Int J Epidemiol 1984;13:299–303.
95. Elder JB, Knight T. Surgical suppression of gastric acid secretion: lessons from long-term follow-up studies. Scand J Gastroenterol Suppl 1991;188:26–32.

Surgical Care for the Elderly, 2nd ed., edited by
R. Benton Adkins, Jr., and H. William Scott, Jr.
Lippincott–Raven Publishers, Philadelphia © 1998.

CHAPTER 23

Liver, Gallbladder, and Biliary Tract Disease

Kim U. Kahng and Joel J. Roslyn

The number of elderly patients undergoing major abdominal surgical procedures has been increasing since the mid part of the century [1]. This finding, coupled with the observation that hepatobiliary procedures account for over one-third of all abdominal operations performed in this age group [2], underscores the importance of a clear understanding of diseases affecting the liver, gallbladder, and bile ducts as they occur in the geriatric population. Although the pathogenesis and pathology of these disorders are similar in young and old alike, the clinical manifestations and sequelae vary appreciably in the different age groups, thereby necessitating different treatment strategies.

A revolution in technologic advances has facilitated both the diagnosis and management of individuals with either benign or malignant diseases of the liver and extrahepatic biliary tract. The emergence of skilled interventional endoscopists and radiologists has promoted and fostered original areas of investigation, which in turn have provided the clinician with new information and insight, and, perhaps more importantly, innovative options for patient care. The widespread application of laparoscopy has been a significant advance in the surgical approach to biliary disease. The net effect is that a multidisciplinary approach to complicated hepatobiliary disorders now offers nonoperative and surgical therapeutic options.

The formulation of a management strategy for the elderly patient with hepatobiliary disease requires the consideration of several issues unique to geriatric surgery. The presence of concurrent disease is an important factor in choosing among treatment options. Several studies show that the most significant determinant of mortality in elderly patients after cholecystectomy is the presence of cardiovascular or cerebrovascular disease [3,4]. The relationship between hyperbilirubinemia and renal dysfunction [5] is a factor that may be critical in elderly patients, many of whom already have an element of renal insufficiency. The development of cholangitis may be particularly life-threatening in elderly patients because of an increased susceptibility to the consequences of systemic hypoperfusion.

Perhaps most challenging to the clinician are the ethical and philosophical issues that must be considered with malignancies arising in the hepatobiliary tree. Given the grave prognosis, the surgeon must weigh the relative merits and risks of a curative resection versus a palliative procedure. This decision is particularly difficult when dealing with geriatric patients. Chronologic age alone, however, cannot justifiably be used to preclude a curative approach. Average life expectancy has increased to the extent that the average 75-year-old individual can be expected to live another 10 years. In addition, careful consideration must be given to such social issues as quality of life, the ability of the patient and the family to recognize the prognosis, the ability to provide long-term care, and the potential for rehabilitation.

The purpose of this chapter is to review the surgical management of disorders affecting the liver, gallbladder, and biliary tract as they occur in the elderly patient. Prior to discussing specific diseases, the effects of aging on the hepatobiliary tract are considered.

PHYSIOLOGIC CHANGES OF AGING

Liver

Morphologic and physiologic changes occur in the liver with advancing age. The liver gradually becomes smaller in both absolute size and size relative to body weight. By age 90, the liver accounts for only 1.6% of total body weight, compared with 2.5% prior to age 50 [6]. Molding of the liver to adjacent structures becomes more pronounced with increasing age [7]. Although the factors that regulate hepatic blood flow are not well defined, hepatic blood flow diminishes 0.3% to 1.5% per year, resulting in 40% less total liver blood flow in those >60 years of age compared with those <25 years of age [8]. The decrease in liver size may be due to an actual reduction in the number of hepatocytes, even though individual liver cells increase in mean volume [9]. In addition to these changes in hepatocyte number and size, bile duct proliferation occurs with increasing age [10].

Despite these changes that occur with aging, the effect on hepatic function appears to be minimal. Standard liver function test results, such as total bilirubin, alkaline phosphatase, and serum glutamic-oxaloacetic transaminase levels, are unaltered, and biliary excretion as determined by retention of sodium sulfobromophthalein and rose bengal scan remains normal in elderly patients [11]. Furthermore, hepatic metabolism of most drugs is normal in elderly patients [12].

Although these general measures of overall liver function may remain normal, subtle changes in subcellular function may occur with aging. Considerable clinical data have documented a higher incidence of cholesterol gallstones associated with aging in both men and women [5]. This is most likely due to alterations in biliary metabolism that result in a greater degree of cholesterol saturation of bile. Aging has been shown to affect the activities of specific hepatic enzymes critical to cholesterol biosynthesis. The activity of 7-α-hydroxylase is decreased, whereas the activity of HMG-CoA reductase is increased [13]. The net effect of these changes is an increase in the degree of cholesterol saturation of bile. The mechanism leading to these age-induced modifications in hepatic enzyme activity is unclear although investigations have implicated alterations in the ratios of androgen to estrogen.

Gallbladder

The effects of aging on overall gallbladder function have not been well defined. Most investigative efforts have centered on the changes in motility that occur with aging. Animal studies have demonstrated an aged-related diminution in gallbladder sensitivity to cholecystokinin (CCK), the primary hormonal stimulus for gallbladder contraction [14]. Furthermore, the increased incidence of gallbladder stones associated with aging in cholesterol-fed guinea pigs was prevented by treatment with exogenous CCK [15]. These animal studies suggest that gallbladder dysmotility secondary to age-induced changes in gallbladder sensitivity to CCK may contribute to the higher incidence of gallbladder stones observed with aging. In humans without gallstones, ultrasonographic studies suggest that gallbladder sensitivity to CCK decreases with aging. A compensatory increase in circulating CCK, however, results in gallbladder contraction that is similar in older and younger individuals [16]. It is tantalizing to speculate that humans who develop gallstones do so because of lower levels of CCK or greater gallbladder insensitivity to CCK. Unfortunately, the limited clinical information available about gallbladder motility in those with gallstones is not as straightforward. A bimodal distribution of fat-stimulated gallbladder contraction has been described, with one group having normal gallbladder contraction with increased sensitivity to CCK and the other group having slow or absent gallbladder contraction [17]. Thus, the role of alterations in CCK-mediated gallbladder motility in gallstone formation remains unclear.

The serum concentrations of pancreatic polypeptide, a hormone that inhibits choleresis and gallbladder motility, has been shown to increase with aging [18]. This may be due to an increase in pancreatic secretion [19]. Pancreatic polypeptide has been shown to inhibit gallbladder emptying [20] and to enhance postcontractile gallbladder filling [21]. Further studies are needed to clarify the effect of CCK, pancreatic polypeptide, and other peptides on hepatobiliary function in the elderly.

LIVER DISEASE

Malignant Tumors

Metastatic Cancer

In the elderly, malignant tumors of the liver are considerably more frequent than benign lesions. Therefore, the finding of a filling defect on ultrasonography or liver scan is reason for grave concern. Metastatic cancer is 20 times more common than primary tumors in the liver. Although carcinomas of the breast, lung, kidney, and ovary can metastasize to the liver, the overwhelming majority of hepatic metastases arise from a gastrointestinal primary cancer. The correlation between the incidence of gastrointestinal malignancy and increasing age underscores the importance of metastatic neoplasms of the liver in the geriatric population.

Elderly patients with hepatic metastases may have vague symptoms or no symptoms referable to the liver lesions. Usually, however, these patients have constitutional symptoms of weight loss, anorexia, and fatigability. Right upper quadrant pain, jaundice, and ascites indicate advanced disease in which much of the liver has been replaced by tumor. Abnormal liver test results (bilirubin, alkaline phosphatase, serum glutamic-oxaloacetic transaminase) may be the only indicator of liver involvement in an otherwise asymptomatic patient. These findings should prompt further evaluation, particularly in the elderly patient. Although there are currently no data that define the frequency with which the initial manifestation of malignancy is metastases to the liver, our experience suggests that this is not unusual in elderly patients.

The surgical management of colorectal metastases to the liver has become increasingly important because resection of isolated liver metastases is associated with a significant chance for long-term survival [22–24]. Routine surveillance, improved preoperative and intraoperative assessment of resectability, and growing experience with segmental resections and liver-conserving procedures have promoted early detection of isolated liver metastases, better selection of patients who would benefit from resection, and decreased morbidity and mortality after hepatic resection. Several factors that influence long-term survival after resection of hepatic metastases have been identified and include the presence or absence of extrahepatic disease, extent of the margin of resection, number and distribution of the metastases, and initial stage of the primary tumor. Although the effect of age has not been well defined, the patient's overall medical condition and factors related to the malignancy are more important considerations than chronologic age.

Obstruction of the major bile ducts can occur in the presence of metastatic cancer and may be due to tumor debris [25] or extrinsic compression. Intubation of the biliary tract usually provides good palliation for these patients and can generally be achieved without significant morbidity or mortality.

Primary Hepatic Malignancy

Hepatocellular Carcinoma

Hepatocellular carcinoma (HCC) is the most common primary liver malignancy. Its prevalence varies widely around the world and even within countries. Hepatoma is the most common cancer in Taiwan and the third most common in China. In contrast, it ranks twenty-second among cancers treated in the United States [26]. HCC develops more frequently in men than women, and its incidence increases with age, although the incidence appears to plateau in the elderly. The strong association between HCC and chronic hepatitis B, as well as cirrhosis, has resulted in screening programs to identify small, potentially curable lesions. Several prospective studies indicate that ultrasonography is more sensitive than serial serum α-fetoprotein levels for screening purposes [27,28].

The diagnosis of HCC may be suggested by ultrasonography, computed tomography (CT), or magnetic resonance imaging (MRI) with varying degrees of accuracy [29–32]; all three studies may give useful information with regard to extent of disease and resectability. CT portography is superior to conventional dynamic CT in the detection of small lesions [33,34]. Ultrasonography is particularly useful in detecting portal venous thrombosis. The combination of CT and MRI detects most lymph nodes >1 cm in diameter [35]. Visceral angiography differentiates the typical hypervascular HCC from other lesions and may give useful information about the anatomy of the hepatic vasculature if resection is anticipated [30]. Ultrasonography or CT-guided percutaneous needle aspiration or core needle biopsy can be performed, although the risk of rupture, tumor seeding, and bleeding from these hypervascular lesions must be considered. Establishing a tissue diagnosis by percutaneous biopsy may be necessary in patients who are not resectable or who will be receiving neoadjuvant therapy. In patients who are surgical candidates, definitive resection may be undertaken for both diagnosis and therapy, thus avoiding percutaneous biopsy.

Although surgical resection has been the primary treatment for cure, recurrence rates are high. Poor prognostic indicators include lymph node involvement, vascular invasion, tumor thrombus, the diffuse spreading type of HCC, the absence of a capsule, size >5 cm, and multiple or bilobar tumors [36]. The mortality of hepatic resection for HCC depends on the extent of resection and the functional reserve of the remaining liver. The presence of cirrhosis limits the extent of resection that can be tolerated. Morbidity and mortality after hepatic resection for hepatoma are comparable for elderly and young patients, indicating that surgery should not be avoided on the basis of age alone [37,38].

Alternative approaches that have been gaining acceptance include ultrasound-guided ethanol injections and intra-arterial chemoembolization. In addition, intra-arterial neoadjuvant chemotherapy is being investigated as a means of preoperative cytoreduction. Liver transplantation has shown promise in providing better long-term survival than resection, but its role in the treatment of HCC has not been clearly delineated.

Cholangiocarcinoma

Cholangiocarcinomas account for approximately 15% of all primary hepatic tumors. The clinical presentation of cholangiocarcinomas is similar to that of HCC, although associated cirrhosis is far less common. Intrahepatic metastases and extension within the biliary tree are typical of cholangiocarcinoma. Regional lymph node involvement is also common [39]. As a result of both diffuse involvement of the liver and lymph node metastases, surgical resection is rarely feasible.

Benign Tumors and Hepatic Cysts

Hemangiomas, hepatic adenomas, focal nodular hyperplasia, and solitary cysts constitute the majority of benign liver lesions. Of these, hemangiomas and cysts are more likely to be encountered in the elderly patient. The major clinical significance of both of these lesions in the elderly is the importance of distinguishing them from metastases. The complementary use of ultrasonography and CT can help characterize the filling defects as simple cysts [40]. ^{99m}Tc-labeled red blood cell scanning is useful for confirming the presence of hemangiomas.

Although solitary cysts are congenital, their pattern of slow growth makes their presentation in later life not uncommon. Most of these lesions are located in the right lobe, and they typically contain clear fluid. Although solitary cysts are generally asymptomatic, large ones may extrinsically compress surrounding viscera, resulting in early satiety, obstructive jaundice, or respiratory symptoms. Infection and hemorrhage are rare complications. Cyst decompression relieves symptoms quickly, once they occur. After biopsy of the cyst wall to exclude cyst adenocarcinoma, operative drainage can be easily accomplished by unroofing the cyst and allowing free intraperitoneal drainage. Roux-en-Y cystojejunostomy is performed if the cyst contains bile. Percutaneous aspiration is not recommended as definitive therapy because of the high recurrence rate.

TABLE 23-1. *Cholelithiasis prevalence by age group*

	Percentage with stones	
Age (yrs)	Women	Men
10–39	5.0	1.5
40–49	12.0	4.4
50–59	15.8	6.2
60–69	25.4	9.9
70–79	28.9	15.2
80–89	30.9	17.9
90+	35.4	24.4

Source: Reprinted with permission from Bateson MC. Gallbladder disease and cholecystectomy rates are independently variable. Lancet 1984;2:621–624.

Hepatic Abscess

The epidemiology of abscesses involving the liver has changed appreciably during recent years. In the past, appendicitis and diverticulitis were the primary infectious sites, but biliary tract disease has become much more prominent [41]. In approximately 10% to 50% of the patients, no antecedent infection can be identified; these have been termed *cryptogenic abscesses*. Although hepatic abscesses may be parasitic, fungal, or bacterial, the majority of such lesions in the United States are pyogenic. The clinical course may be indolent, with the only symptoms being low-grade fever and generalized malaise, or the course may be fulminant with significant toxicity, high fever, jaundice, and right upper quadrant pain. Often the liver is enlarged, and the pain may be severe. Jaundice is unusual in the absence of significant biliary obstruction, multiple abscesses, or rapid deterioration.

Chest radiography may provide clues to the diagnosis of liver abscess. Findings may include basilar atelectasis, pleural effusion, and when the process involves the right lobe of the liver, an elevated right hemidiaphragm. Ultrasonography and CT are the most useful diagnostic tests. Percutaneous drainage has become well accepted as a means of both confirming the diagnosis and achieving drainage [42,43]. Operative drainage may be required if percutaneous drainage is incomplete because of viscous pus or a multiloculated abscess cavity. Multiple liver abscesses are usually secondary to biliary obstruction from either benign or malignant causes. Therapy should be aimed at relieving the obstruction, draining the infection, and treating the underlying cause of obstruction if possible.

GALLBLADDER DISEASE

Cholelithiasis

Incidence

In the elderly, abdominal surgery is most commonly performed for gallstone disease [44]. Numerous studies [44–46] have demonstrated an almost linear increase in the prevalence of gallstones with advancing age (Table 23-1). The actual frequency with which gallstones are found in any given ethnic group or country varies considerably and is dependent on multiple factors. Nonetheless, there appears to be a direct correlation between gallstone prevalence and increasing age, regardless of locale. In the United States, the incidence of gallstones in white women increases from 5% at age 20 to 10% at age 40 and up to 25% by age 60 [47]. In Scandinavia, the incidence of stones is higher, with >40% of women between the ages of 60 and 69 having stones [48]. Perhaps most impressive is the 20% incidence of gallstones among Pima (American Indian) women aged 15 to 24, which increases to >60% by 35 years of age [49]. In 1931, an autopsy study indicated that gallstones were present in more than 50% of individuals over the age of 70 [50]. More recent autopsy studies confirm these earlier observations [51]. Similar age-related trends exist for men, although the prevalence remains less than in women at any given age.

Natural History

The basis for decision making in the treatment of the elderly patient with gallstones should be a clear understanding of the natural history of this disease. Unfortunately, there are few prospective data that address this issue. Considerable evidence suggests, however, that gallstone disease in the elderly may be more virulent than in a younger population. This is based on clinical observations of an increased percentage of elderly patients who develop choledocholithiasis [52,53], emphysematous cholecystitis [54], perforation of the gallbladder [55], and septic complications of cholecystitis [56,57]. Whether these increased complications result from differences in the evolution of the disease process or delayed diagnosis and treatment remains unclear. We suspect that a major contributing factor is the reluctance on the part of many physicians and surgeons to recommend early elective surgery in the elderly patient with cholelithiasis. In actuality, studies suggest that elective cholecystectomy can be safely performed in elderly patients with minimal morbidity and mortality [29,58]. In contrast, the mortality increases by at least 10-fold when emergency cholecystectomy is performed in this same population. Although it is becoming increasingly clear that a more aggressive attitude is warranted in the elderly patient with symptomatic gallstone disease, a critical question remains unanswered: What are the chances that a patient over age 65 with asymptomatic gallstones will develop symptoms in the future and require cholecystectomy?

Treatment of Asymptomatic Stones in the Elderly

Despite continued interest in the prevention and dissolution of gallstones, cholecystectomy remains the gold standard of treatment for patients with cholelithiasis. Nonetheless, the selection of elderly patients for operative intervention and the timing of the procedure itself continue to be controversial. Reliable, definitive data to resolve these issues are not currently available. Those recommending watchful waiting point to the frequency with which gallstones are found at autopsy, suggesting that many patients live with silent gallstones. They also point to a prospective study of male university faculty with initially asymptomatic gallstones discovered by oral cholecystography [59]. In this study, Gracie and Ransohoff reported that the likelihood of developing complications requiring cholecystectomy was 7%. These authors concluded that routine prophylactic cholecystectomy for asymptomatic gallstone disease is unnecessary.

Can these data, derived from an all male university faculty, be extrapolated to the geriatric population? We strongly believe that the complexity of biliary disease in the elderly necessitates an individualized and rational approach. The distinction between asymptomatic and symptomatic stones is difficult to define in the elderly. A variety of seemingly nonspecific and common complaints in the elderly such as dyspepsia, vague epigastric discomfort, or even increased flatulence may be the primary manifestations of gallstone disease, and significant benefit may be derived from cholecystectomy [60]. The subtlety of these symptoms may explain the repeated observation that the initial presentation of biliary disease in the elderly is a major complication of gallstone disease without antecedent symptoms of chronic cholecystitis [3,55,61,62]. Emergency surgery for biliary disease in the elderly has a mortality ranging from 5% to 19% [63]. In addition to the influence of comorbidities, the high mortality of emergency procedures may be related to the greater severity of gallstone disease in the elderly, as indicated by the higher prevalence of empyema, gangrene, and perforation of the gallbladder [44–46]. In contrast, the mortality was 0.5% for elective cholecystectomy in patients older than 65 during a 1-year period [40]. Similar data have been reported from Europe, indicating a mortality of 0.4% after elective cholecystectomy in the elderly [64]. Elective laparoscopic cholecystectomy may be particularly advantageous in the elderly, as suggested by lower mortality when compared with open cholecystectomy [65].

Ultimately, the decision to treat an elderly patient with either asymptomatic or symptomatic stones must be based on a number of individual patient-specific factors. Although we do not advocate routine prophylactic cholecystectomy in the elderly patient with truly asymptomatic gallstones, cholecystectomy is appropriate when laparotomy is required for other indications. A number of studies have demonstrated the safety of incidental cholecystectomy in patients having major abdominal surgery [55,66]. The value of this approach is underscored by the recognition that postoperative cholecystitis can be a potentially lethal complication of an otherwise routine procedure [67]. For geriatric patients with symptomatic gallstone disease, the primary physician and surgeon need to weigh the potential risks versus benefits of an elective procedure based on each individual patient profile. The desire to avoid surgery must be tempered by the realization that emergent cholecystectomy in the elderly is associated with a significant increase in postoperative mortality.

TABLE 23-2. *Incidence of acute cholecystitis*

Age (yrs)	1970–1977 Number	1970–1977 Percent	1980–1987 Number	1980–1987 Percent
1–69	216	84.4	143	55.0
70–79	32	12.5	74	28.5*
80+	8	3.1	43	16.5

*P <0.001 versus 1970 to 1977.

Source: Modified from Reiss R, Nudelman I, Gutman C, Deutsch AA. Changing trends in surgery for acute cholecystitis. World J Surg 1990;14:567–571.

Complications of Gallstone Disease

Acute Cholecystitis

Clinical Presentation

The incidence of acute cholecystitis in the elderly has significantly increased over the past two decades (Table 23-2), becoming one of the more common indications for emergency admissions of elderly patients to a surgical service. Acute cholecystitis is often a more complex disease in the elderly than in the young. A study from Israel demonstrates that patients needing cholecystectomy for acute cholecystitis are not only increasingly older but are also more likely to be diabetic men who have a greater incidence of choledocholithiasis, acalculous cholecystitis, or gangrene [68].

Although the classic triad of right upper quadrant pain, fever, and leukocytosis may be present in some elderly patients with acute cholecystitis, the clinical presentation is often atypical. A high index of suspicion for the diagnosis of acute cholecystitis is essential when an elderly patient presents with abdominal pain or signs of sepsis. Abdominal pain is the predominant complaint in more than 70% of elderly patients with documented acute cholecystitis [69]; however, fever, nausea, and emesis may be the only signs of an intra-abdominal process. A palpable mass is noted in approximately 20% of these patients. Even in the absence of choledocholithiasis, jaundice may be a significant finding in elderly patients with acute cholecystitis. Although the mechanism by which it occurs is not clear, altered mental status may be the primary manifestation of hepatobiliary disease in the elderly patient [70]. Of great concern is a report that 12% of 131 patients over the age of 70 who presented with acute cholecystitis were in septic shock at the time of admission [71].

TABLE 23-3. *Cholecystectomy: preoperative laboratory evaluation*

	Patients age (yrs)		
	<49 (%)	50–69 (%)	70+ (%)
Number	235	392	98
Acute cholecystitis	13 (5.5)	14 (3.6)	8 (8.1)[a]
Abnormal liver function test result	91 (38.7)	191 (48.7)	50 (60.2)[a]
Anemia	42 (17.9)	73 (18.6)	39 (39.8)[b]
Hypoproteinemia	6 (2.6)	15 (3.8)	15 (9.2)[b]
Abnormal renal function	2 (0.9)	6 (1.5)	9 (9.2)[b]

[a] P <0.05 versus 50–69 years.
[b] P <0.01 versus 50–69 years.
Source: Modified from Shinagawa N, Mahita K, Yura J. The operative risk factors of cholelithiasis in the elderly. Jpn J Surg 1992;22:29–34.

Diagnosis

The diagnosis of acute cholecystitis must be considered in any elderly patient who has right upper quadrant pain of >12 hours' duration, with or without a significant fever or an elevated white blood cell count. Furthermore, the diagnosis of acute cholecystitis must be entertained in the elderly patient who presents with sepsis of undetermined cause [71]. Regardless of the manner in which the evaluation is conducted, the goal is rapid diagnosis and prompt implementation of appropriate therapy.

Other than white blood cell count, useful laboratory evaluation includes liver function tests. Choledocholithiasis is common in elderly patients with gallstones; however, liver function tests are frequently abnormal with acute cholecystitis alone. Data from Japan indicated that significant alterations in liver function test results occurred more often in older patients who had cholecystectomy than in their younger counterparts (Table 23-3) [72].

Oral cholecystography has no role in the evaluation of patients with suspected acute cholecystitis. This test has been replaced by abdominal ultrasonography, which can be rapidly performed in an acutely ill patient. Aside from the detection of gallstones, for which ultrasonography is the most sensitive study available, findings that support the diagnosis of acute cholecystitis include gallbladder distention, a thickened gallbladder wall, and pericholecystic fluid collections. These signs are particularly important when stones are not present because acalculous acute cholecystitis is not infrequent in the elderly. Additional information that is often provided by ultrasonography includes the presence or absence of dilatation of the intrahepatic and extrahepatic biliary tree or abnormalities of the pancreas. If the presence of gallstones has been established, biliary scintigraphy may be superfluous in the patient presenting with a straightforward clinical picture of acute cholecystitis. With atypical symptoms, however, the additional demonstration of cystic duct occlusion by biliary tract scintigraphy may be necessary to confirm the diagnosis of acute cholecystitis.

Biliary scintigraphy is an important diagnostic test in the elderly patient with suspected acute cholecystitis. Its reported accuracy and specificity approaches 98% [67]. One of the primary advantages of radionuclide imaging is its ability to demonstrate cystic duct obstruction despite serum bilirubin levels >15 dl. Significant information regarding focal hepatic masses, parenchymal function, and gallbladder motor activity can be obtained using this imaging technique. In most patients with biliary disease, the intrahepatic bile ducts, gallbladder, common bile duct, and duodenum can all be visualized within 30 to 60 minutes. It should be emphasized that radionuclide imaging is not a suitable diagnostic test for cholelithiasis. However, these scans are the most accurate tool for diagnosing cystic duct obstruction, which is the sine qua non for acute cholecystitis. False-positive results have been reported in patients fasting for prolonged periods as well as those being given morphine analgesics.

Whether to obtain an abdominal ultrasound or a hepatobiliary scan in a patient with right upper quadrant symptoms continues to be debated. It is important to emphasize that although abdominal ultrasonography is the best means of diagnosing cholelithiasis, its ability to accurately diagnose acute cholecystitis is limited. In contrast, radionuclide imaging, as currently used, is an accurate test for acute cholecystitis, but in turn it does not detect gallstones per se. In many clinical situations, however, knowledge of the presence of gallstones is all that is needed. We believe that there are advantages to both ultrasonography and biliary scintigraphy and that the decision to proceed with one or the other should be based on the individual clinical situation. Previous scintigraphy may delay ultrasonography of the gallbladder due to possible radiation exposure to ultrasound technicians.

Management

Regardless of age, cholecystectomy combined with antibiotic therapy remains the preferred treatment for acute cholecystitis. Initial management includes volume resuscitation with invasive monitoring if necessary; evaluation and control of concurrent disease such as diabetes, arrhythmias, or pulmonary dysfunction; and correction of any associated coagulopathy due to warfarin. Broad-spectrum antibiotic therapy covering enteric organisms is begun while diagnostic studies are being obtained. Because the incidence of positive bile culture results increases from 30% in patients younger than 50 to >50% in those older than 70 [73], a full therapeutic course of antibiotics is advisable. Antibiotic therapy alone is insufficient treatment, especially because acute cholecystitis in the elderly is often complicated by gangrene or perforation.

It is generally accepted that early cholecystectomy is preferable to delayed operation in patients with acute cholecystitis [74,75]. The reluctance of physicians to adhere to this principle in the treatment of elderly patients may be responsible in part for the increased morbidity and mortality that have been previously reported for this age group. Glenn [76] reported that patients 65 years of age and older accounted for 70% of all deaths resulting from acute cholecystitis at the New York Hospital. In that study, the two most common causes of death were sepsis and cardiovascular disease. Similarly, the overall mortality in a series of 88 elderly patients undergoing cholecystectomy was 7% [77], nearly 10 times the rate for younger patients. The importance of the timing of treatment in the elderly patient with acute cholecystitis is underscored by a more careful analysis of these data. Medical therapy consisting of intravenous fluids and antibiotics was attempted in 44% of these 88 patients with cholecystitis. Emergency cholecystectomy became necessary in 97% of this subgroup because of failure to respond to conservative, supportive treatment. The morbidity and mortality were 44% and 10%, respectively, in patients who required emergency cholecystectomy. In contrast, the morbidity and mortality were only 22% and 2%, respectively, in the group of patients who underwent semiurgent operation. In our experience, elderly patients with acute cholecystitis are best managed by timely diagnosis, early stabilization, and semiurgent cholecystectomy.

For more than 100 years, cholecystectomy has been the treatment of choice for patients with acute cholecystitis. The procedure remains the primary and only curative treatment for cholelithiasis and acute cholecystitis [78]. The emergence of laparoscopic cholecystectomy has provided an alternative to open cholecystectomy for acute cholecystitis. Growing experience suggests that the procedure can be performed safely even with acute inflammation. Zucker et al. [79] reported their experience with laparoscopic cholecystectomy for acute cholecystitis in 83 patients over a 3-year period. Conversion to open laparotomy occurred in 27% of these cases. No mortality and no bile duct or major vascular injury occurred. The overall morbidity for the entire group was 16.9%. Similar outcomes in smaller series have been reported as well [80,81]. These experiences make it clear that expertise with routine, elective laparoscopic cholecystectomy must be acquired before undertaking laparoscopic cholecystectomy for acute cholecystitis. In particular, there must be little hesitancy to convert to an open procedure. No data are available that focus on laparoscopic cholecystectomy for acute cholecystitis in the elderly as a specific subpopulation. It is reasonable to assume, however, that minimally invasive surgery may be perfectly appropriate and even desirable when it can be performed for acute cholecystitis without any additional risk or mortality. It is important to re-emphasize that the determining factor in outcome following cholecystectomy is not the biliary disease per se but the underlying cardiovascular status of the patient.

Although cholecystectomy remains the standard treatment for acute cholecystitis, cholecystostomy may be a safer option for the critically ill patient with severe hepatic or cardiopulmonary disease. The use of local anesthesia to perform the cholecystostomy is particularly advantageous in these patients [82]. Cholecystostomy, however, is not feasible when the gallbladder has become gangrenous. Drainage of the gallbladder in combination with systemic antibiotic therapy allows acute nongangrenous cholecystitis to resolve. Despite the efficacy of this approach, the mortality ranges between 25% and 40%. This high mortality reflects patient selection rather than difficulties with the procedure itself. When performing a cholecystostomy in a geriatric patient, the high incidence of choledocholithiasis must be considered. The discovery of nonobstructing common bile duct calculi at the time of cholecystostomy may not necessarily mandate common bile duct exploration. Patency of the cystic duct may be restored by either resolution of the acute cholecystitis or mechanical extraction of stones occluding the cystic duct. This may provide sufficient access to the remainder of the biliary tree and common duct stones using radiologic or endoscopic techniques. Although the issue of subsequent elective cholecystectomy after cholecystostomy has yet to be definitively addressed, this is probably less of a concern in the geriatric patient, who usually remains at significant operative risk because of concurrent disease.

Alternatives to operative cholecystostomy are ultrasound-guided percutaneous transhepatic cholecystostomy [83] and endoscopic transpapillary drainage of the gallbladder [84]. As in any percutaneous transhepatic procedure, complications include bile leaks and hemorrhage. In reviewing >200 patients from anecdotal reports of percutaneous transhepatic cholecystostomy, however, only 13 major complications were seen: four bile leaks, two occurrences of significant hemorrhage, and seven instances of catheter dislodgment. In one report, the majority of these percutaneous procedures was performed in the intensive care unit, stressing the acute nature of illness in these patients. These nonoperative approaches may have particular application in the elderly; however, their safety and efficacy require further definition.

Cholecystitis and Diabetes

A significant percentage of elderly patients has diabetes mellitus. In addition, it has long been suggested that there is an increased incidence of cholesterol gallstone disease among diabetic patients [45] and that these patients are more likely to develop acute cholecystitis and its associated complications [85]. However, in a prospective review of 175 diabetic and nondiabetic patients undergoing cholecystectomy, the incidence of gallbladder perforation, wound infection, and overall morbidity and mortality was not significantly different between the two groups [86]. The conclusion that diabetes itself is not a significant risk factor for severe biliary tract disease should be tempered because the study cited was not controlled for the timing of operation. Nonetheless, we continue to recommend aggressive preoperative evaluation and treatment with early operation in the elderly diabetic patient with presumed acute cholecystitis.

Choledocholithiasis

The reported incidence of common bile duct stones in elderly patients having cholecystectomy ranges from 20% to 54%. In contrast, common duct stones are found far less frequently in younger patients. The reasons for this discrepancy are not fully understood, although reluctance to treat cholelithiasis when patients are younger may be a contributing factor. A similar contrast exists in mortality after common bile duct exploration. In those younger than 50 years, the mortality is 0.4% [87], whereas in patients older than 70 years, the mortality ranges from 7% to 29% [88].

Two major issues are related to the management of common duct stones in the elderly: the role of protective prophylactic biliary-enteric bypass and the role of preoperative endoscopic retrograde cholangiopancreatography (ERCP) and sphincterotomy. Routine choledochoduodenostomy has been advocated for the elderly patient with common bile duct stones [89]. The rationale for this proposal is to avoid re-exploration when stone extraction cannot be achieved by nonoperative means, particularly because choledochoduodenostomy can be performed with low morbidity and mortality. In view of the current expertise of invasive radiologists and endoscopists, however, we believe that choledochoduodenostomy should be done only for specific indications, such as numerous stones, especially in the hepatic duct system, recurrent or primary stones, or bile duct stricture. In other words, we prefer to do only what is necessary at the time of laparotomy. In general, a meticulous and expeditious operation provides the greatest chance of cure with the least risk.

Preoperative ERCP and sphincterotomy before open or laparoscopic cholecystectomy have proven useful in the management of patients with suspected common bile duct stones [90,91]. The success of this approach requires an experienced endoscopist who can safely perform ERCP and sphincterotomy with minimal morbidity and mortality. The ability to clear the common bile duct of stones preoperatively may facilitate a laparoscopic cholecystectomy. For those who are not candidates for the laparoscopic approach, preoperative clearance of the common bile duct may be beneficial by minimizing the duration of an open procedure. An additional consideration is that preoperative ERCP and sphincterotomy may be more cost-effective than open cholecystectomy and common bile duct exploration [92]. Endoscopic sphincterotomy alone, leaving the gallbladder in situ, may be the only alternative in the patient who is a prohibitive risk for general anesthesia.

Gallbladder Perforation

It has long been recognized that gallbladder perforation occurs more frequently in the aged population. Although the explanation for this observation is not evident, the presumption is that circulatory changes in the elderly render the wall of the gallbladder more susceptible to ischemia [93]. Gallbladder perforations are categorized into three types: type I is acute perforation with bile peritonitis, type II is subacute perforation with pericholecystic abscess, and type III is perforation resulting in a fistula between the gallbladder and the gastrointestinal tract. Cholecystenteric fistulae are found in the majority of patients with perforation of the gallbladder and are particularly important in the elderly [55,94,95]. Most often, the fistulous communication is between the gallbladder and duodenum, although other areas of involvement have been reported [95]. Depending on the size of the fistulous communication, gallstones may pass through this tract and ultimately cause bowel obstruction.

Gallstone ileus is a relatively rare condition and accounts for <5% of all causes of intestinal obstruction. However, in the elderly population, gallstone ileus accounts for 20% to 25% of all cases of small bowel obstruction [96]. As one would anticipate, this condition is more typically seen in women and represents one of the more common causes of small bowel obstruction in this subset of patients. The stone frequently lodges in the terminal ileum, resulting in a typical distal small bowel obstruction. Occasionally, the diagnosis is suspected preoperatively based on the finding of intrahepatic biliary air noted on abdominal radiography [97]. In most cases the diagnosis is made at the time of laparotomy when a gallstone is palpated at the site of obstruction. The primary therapeutic goals at laparotomy in a patient with gallstone ileus are correction of obstruction and removal of the offending stone. Because most of these elderly patients are quite ill, cholecystectomy and closure of the biliary-enteric fistula probably should not be performed at that time. Although early reports indicated that the mortality associated with this condition approached 40%, more recent studies suggest a mortality of 5% to 15% [97-99]. Our current practice is to correct the bowel obstruction by removing the impacted stone by enterotomy proximal to the impaction site and retrograde extraction of the stone. Cholecystectomy is not done unless there is evidence of acute biliary tract disease. Our experience supports the literature [99] indicating that most of these patients will not require subsequent cholecystectomy for recurrent symptoms.

Emphysematous Cholecystitis

Acute emphysematous cholecystitis is an unusual clinical entity characterized by the radiographic demonstration of gas either within the gallbladder lumen or wall [100]. This entity is more common in elderly men and diabetic patients and is associated with gangrene and perforation of the gallbladder. Clostridial organisms are present in most patients with emphysematous cholecystitis, although other gas-forming organisms may also be found. The pathogenesis of this disorder is not clear because up to 50% of patients may not have associated gallstones. Ischemia has been implicated as a potential etiologic factor in this process. The associated mortality is high and prompt cholecystectomy is indicated.

Biliary Sepsis

Much has been written about biliary sepsis in the aged population, particularly with regard to gallstone disease. Elderly patients, presumed to be asymptomatic, may have septic shock as their initial manifestation of acute cholecystitis [101]. Prospective studies have demonstrated that the incidence of positive bile cultures in patients with acute cholecystitis increases linearly with age. The reported incidence of positive bile cultures in patients <50 years of age is 30% and increases to >50% in patients 70 years or older [75]. Most bacteria are of enteric origin, with *Escherichia coli* being the most common. *Bacteroides fragilis* has been recovered from 28% of elderly patients undergoing biliary tract procedures [102]. In their now classic article, Chetlin and Elliott [103] identified high-risk factors for the development of septic complications following cholecystectomy. Among other factors was age >70 years.

The importance of this observation has been clarified by studies that have looked at the role of prophylactic antibiotic therapy [104,105]. Antibiotic prophylaxis is now an accepted feature of gallstone surgery in the elderly. We administer a broad-spectrum antibiotic (a second-generation cephalosporin) 1 hour preoperatively to all elderly patients undergoing elective cholecystectomy. An intraoperative Gram's stain is generally performed only to identify those patients who may have an anaerobic infection. We generally give one or two doses of antibiotics postoperatively unless there are clinical indications to extend treatment. We tend to be more aggressive in the elderly patient with acute cholecystitis and frequently use a therapeutic regimen with good anaerobic coverage and coverage for enterococcus. In general, septic complications in the elderly can be minimized by the judicious use of appropriate antibiotics.

Gallstone Dissolution in the Elderly

The medical dissolution and prevention of gallstones have been goals of clinicians dating back to ancient times. Two agents, chenodeoxycholic acid and ursodeoxycholic acid, have been shown to be effective in the dissolution of cholesterol gallstones in a limited number of carefully selected patients. These two bile salts dissolve cholesterol stones by decreasing hepatic cholesterol synthesis and expanding the bile acid pool, thereby reducing the degree of cholesterol saturation of bile. In the most complete and comprehensive study of stone dissolution, performed under the supervision of The National Cooperative Gallstone Study, the rate of complete stone disappearance was only 13.5% and partial response was an additional 28% [106]. In addition to this disappointingly low success rate, other problems with the use of these agents, especially in the elderly, include (1) the need for lifetime therapy to prevent the recurrence of stones (50% 5-year recurrence rate), (2) the need for strict compliance, (3) the length of time required to achieve a response, and (4) the potential toxic side effects. Although intuitively the ideal candidate for dissolution therapy would be the elderly, infirm patient with symptomatic gallstones, this is the very individual who will predictably have the least chance of responding to this type of therapy. Currently, we do not believe that dissolution therapy has a role in the management of elderly patients with gallstone disease. Local dissolution of gallbladder stones by percutaneous instillation of specific agents (methyl tert-butyl ether) directly into the gallbladder has been introduced [107]. The efficacy of this procedure and its potential role in the management of elderly patients with asymptomatic or symptomatic gallstone disease remain to be defined.

Colon Carcinoma and Cholecystectomy

Clinical studies have reported conflicting findings about the possibility of an increased risk of colorectal carcinoma following cholecystectomy. The theoretic basis for this proposal is that the relative concentrations of primary and secondary bile acids (deoxycholic and lithocholic acid) seem to be increased among patients with colorectal cancer [108]. The evidence to support this hypothesis is based on retrospective and circumstantial studies [109,110]. A more recent prospective study of >16,000 patients undergoing cholecystectomy suggests that there is no etiologic association whatsoever between cholecystectomy and the subsequent development of colorectal carcinoma [111]. Therefore, we believe that the decision whether to perform cholecystectomy in an elderly patient with symptomatic biliary tract disease should be based on the biliary tract disease process, and not on whether the patient will be at an increased risk for colon carcinoma.

Gallbladder and Bile Duct Cancers

Carcinoma of the gallbladder and extrahepatic biliary tract are uncommon gastrointestinal malignancies in the United States, representing <10% of the total number of patients with colorectal cancer. Although rare, these lesions tend to occur in older patients. Although surgical resection remains the primary approach for cure, curative resection can rarely be achieved. Gallbladder carcinoma classically presents at an advanced stage, and bile duct tumors, although often small at the time of diagnosis, may defy surgical extirpation because of proximity and involvement of vital structures. Because of these characteristics, these lesions are rarely amenable to cure and require a multidisciplinary approach using endoscopic, radiologic, and surgical techniques for diagnosis and palliation. Technical advances in these fields coupled with new knowledge regarding the systemic effects of hyperbilirubinemia and the interrelationships between jaundice, renal dysfunction, and nutritional and immunologic defects have allowed broader insight into the development of a rational approach to the management of elderly patients with these complex lesions.

Gallbladder Cancer

Carcinoma of the gallbladder accounts for approximately two-thirds of all cancers of the extrahepatic biliary tract. The association between cholelithiasis and carcinoma of the gallbladder has been well described [112]. Although the vast majority of patients with carcinoma of the gallbladder has gallstones, the converse is not true; in fact, the incidence of gallbladder cancer is quite low in patients with cholelithiasis. As in cholecystitis, carcinoma of the gallbladder predominates in women, with a female-to-male ratio of 3 to 5:1. The median age at diagnosis is approximately 70 years.

In the absence of jaundice as part of the presentation, the diagnosis of carcinoma of the gallbladder is typically made at the time of cholecystectomy for what was thought preoperatively to be acute or chronic cholecystitis. Although surgical extirpation continues to be the mainstay of treatment for carcinoma of the gallbladder, the extent of the resection remains unclear. Recommendations vary widely, ranging from simple cholecystectomy to cholecystectomy with regional lymphadenectomy and wedge resection of the gallbladder bed to more radical procedures including resection of the right hepatic lobe and medial segment of the left lobe [113–115]. The long-term benefits of such radical procedures continue to be investigated, but such procedures are probably not warranted in elderly patients. This statement is based largely on the realization that the only curable lesions are those removed incidentally during cholecystectomy. It has been our practice to proceed with regional lymphadenectomy and wedge resection of the gallbladder bed for a resectable gallbladder carcinoma that is discovered intraoperatively, provided a definitive histologic diagnosis can be established. The overriding consideration, however, is the general condition of the patient. Any procedure beyond cholecystectomy can be undertaken only in the good-risk patient for whom little additional risk for morbidity or mortality can be expected.

The extent of surgical treatment is a more difficult issue when the diagnosis of carcinoma is made postoperatively after routine histologic examination of the gallbladder. The decision to reoperate is influenced by the depth of penetration through the gallbladder wall and the overall status of the patient. Age by itself should not be a critical factor in the decision process. Stage I disease in which the tumor is intramucosal is probably adequately treated by cholecystectomy alone, and little benefit is derived from re-exploration. In those patients deemed reasonable surgical candidates, lymphadenectomy and limited hepatic resection should be considered for stage II or III disease, in which the tumor has extended to the submucosa or serosa, respectively.

Carcinoma of the Extrahepatic Biliary Tree

Extrahepatic bile duct malignancies are present in <1% of autopsies and are found in approximately 1% of biliary operations [114]. Carcinoma of the bile duct tends to be a disease of the elderly, with the mean age of presentation between 60 and 65 years in most reported series. In a series of 186 patients from the University of California, Los Angeles, with documented bile duct cancers, 23% were over age 70 [117]. The distribution of these carcinomas varies within the biliary tree: 10% are diffuse, 60% are in the upper third, 15% are in the middle third, and 15% are distal [117–119]. These figures differ only slightly when considering the distribution of bile duct carcinomas in the elderly [117]. The clinical presentation is obstructive jaundice, for which biliary drainage is often the initial step. A tissue diagnosis may be established by biliary brushing or percutaneous needle biopsy, but open biopsy or resection is often required for histologic confirmation. The primary curative mode remains surgical resection, which can be performed in roughly 50% of cases [35]. Distal carcinomas usually require pancreaticoduodenectomy, a procedure no longer contraindicated on the basis of age alone. Local hepatic resection for hilar tumors has been advocated, and occasionally formal lobectomy may be required for curative resection of carcinoma arising from one of the hepatic ducts. After curative resection, 5-year survival is best for distal bile duct carcinomas, ranging from 28% to 50%. Upper and middle third lesions are associated with <10% 5-year survival [35]. The efficacy of adjuvant therapy after curative resection remains unclear in the absence of a prospective randomized trial; however, radiation therapy after palliative surgery or biliary drainage has been shown to extend survival. For this reason, a tissue diagnosis is crucial for patients not amenable to curative resection. Alternative palliative approaches being studied include brachytherapy combined with external beam irradiation and intraoperative radiotherapy.

Although surgical extirpation provides the only chance for cure in these patients [120,121], some studies advocate nonoperative palliation of all malignant biliary obstruction using biliary endoprostheses placed either endoscopically or percutaneously [92,122]. Nonoperative rather than surgical biliary drainage has been particularly recommended for the treatment of elderly patients in whom radiographic studies indicate unresectable disease. Advantages of nonoperative management for these elderly patients include shorter initial hospital stays, a lower incidence of procedure-related morbidity, and a 30-day mortality of 9% to 15% [117]. A nonoperative approach has several potential disadvantages that must be considered as well. In approximately 70% of patients, a definitive histologic or cytologic diagnosis cannot be established without an open procedure [123]. Furthermore, evaluating resectability of these often small focal lesions by radiographic means is unreliable. Finally, two studies suggest that nonoperative decompression may be associated with poorer quality of life than operative decompression when factors such as frequency of hospital readmissions, incidence of catheter-related problems, and postprocedural pain and jaundice are taken into account [124,125].

There is little question that a nonoperatively placed biliary prosthesis is preferable to a surgical procedure in the elderly patient with a bile duct carcinoma who is not a surgical candidate because of the degree of comorbid disease. In the patient who is a good surgical risk, albeit older, an aggressive approach including surgery is warranted. Intraoperative evaluation can be expected to establish a diagnosis in 95% of patients and to allow definitive determination of resectability. Either curative resection or palliative biliary drainage can be performed based on these intraoperative findings. At one institution over a 25-year period, the rate of resectability increased, and 1-year survival improved from 21% to 53% [117]. These data suggest that elderly patients with bile duct tumors should not be denied surgical evaluation based solely on age.

MANAGEMENT OF THE JAUNDICED PATIENT

The elderly patient with jaundice often presents considerable diagnostic and therapeutic challenges for even the experienced clinician and surgeon. The differentiation among jaundice secondary to hepatocellular disease, drug-induced cholestasis, or extrahepatic obstruction may be difficult in the geriatric population, especially in those individuals with multiple associated medical problems. The presence of jaundice is associated with increased operative morbidity and mortality, and it is therefore essential that the diagnosis be precise and that nonoperative interventions be considered before the development of a surgical therapeutic plan. Studies from the mid-1970s suggested that the mortality for jaundiced patients over the age of 70 years who underwent operations for gallstone disease was >30%. Although biliary sepsis was a contributing factor, the predominant cause for this high mortality appeared to be renal failure. With our increased awareness of nephrotoxic agents and improved care of the critically ill, the mortality is appreciably less. Nonetheless, the widespread use of nonoperative means, such as endoscopic sphincterotomy, has led to a critical re-evaluation of the need for operative intervention in the jaundiced elderly patient.

Diagnostic Evaluation

The basic question to be answered when confronted with an elderly patient with jaundice is whether this individual has a medical or surgical cause (extrahepatic obstruction) for the jaundice. Although biochemical tests may provide a clue, further evidence to substantiate a clinical impression is often mandated. The typical profile of a patient with extrahepatic biliary obstruction includes elevated levels of total bilirubin and alkaline phosphatase with normal or minimally elevated transaminases. The pattern for a patient with hepatocellular disease or drug-induced cholestasis frequently consists of elevated serum transaminase levels and only mild increases in the alkaline phosphatase levels. Ultimately, the key for differentiating medical versus surgical jaundice lies in diagnostic imaging of the intrahepatic and extrahepatic bile ducts. Ultrasonography has been shown to be a simple, safe, and accurate tool for the identification of dilated intrahepatic and extrahepatic ducts, which may be due either to gallstones or tumor. Once biliary ductal dilatation has been identified, it is essential to define the anatomy and if possible establish a definitive diagnosis before considering laparotomy. This may be greatly facilitated by a CT scan that may show a mass in the head of the pancreas or some other lesion to explain the biliary obstruction. If the diagnosis is still in doubt or if anatomic delineation of the biliary tract is deemed essential, either percutaneous transhepatic cholangiography or ERCP is suggested, depending on local expertise. When a lesion is suspected in the distal common bile duct, ERCP provides certain advantages over transhepatic cholangiography, including the ability to visualize and biopsy the ampulla of Vater. For those lesions believed to be in the mid or proximal bile duct, however, percutaneous transhepatic cholangiography is much more helpful in delineating the intrahepatic anatomy, which will aid in the preoperative decision making.

Management of Obstructive Jaundice

The realization that most causes of extrahepatic jaundice in the elderly patient can be treated without surgical intervention has led to a re-evaluation of therapeutic guidelines in this patient population. Studies from the 1970s suggested that the operative mortality for elderly patients with jaundice who undergo cholecystectomy is considerable [126]. The widespread use of endoscopic sphincterotomy has provided a reasonable alternative for the management of elderly patients with biliary obstruction secondary to calculous disease. The reported mortality in elderly patients who undergo endoscopic sphincterotomy and gallstone removal approaches 2% [80]. In addition, the procedure generally requires minimal hospitalization, and the recovery period is usually shorter than that of a laparotomy. Certainly, cholecystectomy, operative cholangiography, and common bile duct exploration (when indicated) remain the gold standard of treatment. Endoscopic sphincterotomy should be weighed in view of available expertise and the patient's overall condition.

Unfortunately, most studies suggest that malignant tumors are twice as common as gallstone disease as the cause of jaundice in the elderly [15,127]. Although the most common malignant lesion causing jaundice in the elderly patient is carcinoma of the head of the pancreas, the lesions most amenable to surgical treatment are ampullary tumors. Curative resection for ampullary carcinoma is associated with a 5-year survival rate of 25% to 30% [14]. Based on these data, we believe that age alone should not preclude aggressive surgical management in a patient with a potentially resectable tumor. In contrast, tumors that involve the more proximal bile duct and the gallbladder are associated with shorter survival rates, and in these situations good palliation should be the goal.

There are several different methods available for treatment of obstructive jaundice due to malignancy, including surgical resection, biliary enteric bypass, insertion of an endoprosthesis either via the percutaneous or endoscopic route, and endoscopic sphincterotomy. In a report of 180 patients [67], many of whom were elderly, there was no difference in overall survival between the patients who were treated by the biliary enteric bypass and those treated by the placement of biliary stents. Experience with the nonoperative modalities for the management of obstructive jaundice is increasing worldwide. Interventional radiologists have gained considerable experience with the placement of transhepatic tubes for the purpose of internal drainage of an obstructed biliary system. The placement of these tubes often obviates the need for an operation and generally provides excellent palliation. There are, however, certain problems that arise with the use of these tubes. If the tumor is high in the biliary tree, a definitive tissue diagnosis may not be feasible unless a laparotomy is performed; cytologic analysis of biliary drainage is generally not conclusive in establishing a diagnosis of malignancy. Furthermore, these tubes frequently become occluded with debris, leading to sepsis, and in our experience generally require changing every 2 to 4 months. Endoscopically placed prostheses are used with increasing frequency and can generally be placed through a malignant stricture without difficulty. When palliation is contemplated for the jaundiced patient with underlying malignancy, the goal should be internal drainage, rather than the creation of an external biliary fistula. The symptoms associated with jaundice, which include anorexia and pruritus, can be greatly ameliorated by the percutaneous or endoscopic placement of internal biliary stents. As stated previously, the most common tumor causing extrahepatic obstruction is carcinoma involving the head of the pancreas. This is discussed in detail in Chapter 24.

FUTURE OF BILIARY TRACT SURGERY IN THE ELDERLY

The radiologic, endoscopic, and surgical advances already discussed have had a profound effect on the management of diseases of the liver, gallbladder, and biliary tract as they occur in the geriatric population. The indications and applications of this technology will continue to influence the care these patients receive in the future. Endoscopic manipulation of the biliary tract, for either benign or malignant disease, has revolutionized our thinking about disease processes in these patients. The decreased morbidity of laparoscopic versus open biliary procedures may have its greatest impact in the elderly. In addition, our ability to perform radical surgical procedures safely has been greatly improved. Age by itself, therefore, should never preclude the aggressive treatment of a biliary disorder in an elderly patient, either by nonoperative or operative means. The value of our knowledge and capabilities is only as great as our rational ability to apply these principles to individual patients. The problems associated with the elderly patient in particular mandate an overall understanding of the surgical principles as outlined in this and other chapters.

REFERENCES

1. Reiss R. Moral and ethical issues in geriatric surgery. J Med Ethics 1980;6:71–77.
2. Reiss R, Deitsch AA. Emergency abdominal procedures in patients above 70. J Gerontol 1985;40:154–158.
3. McSherry CK, Ferstenberg H, Calhoun WF, et al. The natural history of diagnosed gallstone disease in symptomatic and asymptomatic patients. Ann Surg 1985;202:59–63.
4. McSherry CK, Glenn F. The incidence and cause of death following surgery for nonmalignant biliary tract disease. Ann Surg 1980;191: 271–275.
5. Wait RB, Kahng KU. Renal failure complicating obstructive jaundice. Am J Surg 1989;157:256–263.
6. James OFW. Gastrointestinal and liver function in old age. Clin Gastroenterol 1983;12:671–691.
7. Okuda K, Normura F, Okuda H, Shimokaha Y. Aging and Gross Anatomical Alteration of the Liver. In Kitan E (ed), Liver and Aging. Amsterdam: Elsevier, 1978;159–176.
8. Mooney H, Roberts R, Cooksley WGE, et al. Alterations in the liver with aging. Clin Gastroenterol 1985;4:757–771.
9. Schaffner F, Popper H. Nonspecific reactive hepatitis in aged and infirm people. Am J Dig Dis 1959;4:389–399.
10. Watanabe T, Tanaka Y. Age-related alterations in the size of human hepatocytes. Virchows Arch 1982;39:9–20.
11. Koff RRS, Garvey AJ, Burney SW. Absence of an age effect on sulfobromophthalein retention in healthy men. Gastroenterology 1973; 65:300–302.
12. Woodhouse KW. Drugs and the aging gut, liver, and pancreas. Clin Gastroenterol 1985;14:863–880.
13. Bowen JC, Brenner HI, Ferrante WA, Maule WF. Gallstone disease: pathophysiology, epidemiology, natural history, and treatment of options. Med Clin North Am 1992;76:1143–1157.
14. Poston GJ, Singh P, MacLellan DG, et al. Age related changes in gallbladder contractility and gallbladder cholecystokinin receptor population in the guinea pig. Mech Ageing Dev 1988;46:225–236.
15. Poston GJ, Draviam EJ, Yao CZ, et al. Effect of age and sensitivity on cholecystokinin on gallstone formation in the guinea pig. Gastroenterology 1990;98:993–999.
16. Khalil T, Walker JP, Wiener I, et al. Effect of aging on gallbladder contraction and release of cholecystokinin-33 in humans. Surgery 1985;98:423–429.
17. Thompson JC, Fried CM, Ogden WD, et al. Correlation between release of cholecystokinin and contraction of the gallbladder in patients with gallstones. Ann Surg 1982;195:670–676.
18. Berger D, Crowther RC, Floyd JC Jr, et al. Effect of age on fasting plasma levels of pancreatic hormones in man. J Clin Endocrinol Metab 1978;47:1183–1189.
19. Brunicardi FC, Druck P, Sun YS, et al. Regulation of pancreatic polypeptide secretion in the isolated perfused human pancreas. Am J Surg 1989;155:63–69.
20. Floyd JC Jr, Fajans SS, Pek S, Chance RE. A newly recognized pancreatic polypeptide; plasma levels in health and disease. Recent Prog Horm Res 1976;33:519–570.
21. Conter RL, Roslyn JJ, DenBesten L, Taylor IL. Pancreatic polypeptide enhances postcontractile gallbladder filling in the prairie dog. Gastroenterology 1987;92:771–776.
22. Asburn HJ, Hughes KS. Management of recurrent and metastatic colorectal carcinoma. Surg Clin North Am 1993;73:145–166.
23. Lise M, DaPain PP, Nitti D, et al. Colorectal metastases to the liver: present status of management. Dis Colon Rectum 1990;33:688–694.
24. Registry of Hepatic Metastases. Resection of the liver for colorectal carcinoma metastases: a multi-institutional study of indications for resection. Surgery 1988;103:278–288.
25. Roslyn JJ, Kuchenbecker S, Longmire WP Jr, Tompkins R. Floating tumor debris: a cause of intermittent biliary obstruction. Arch Surg 1984;119:1312–1315.

26. Linsell A. Primary Liver Cancer: Epidemiology and Etiology. In Wanebo HJ (ed), Hepatic and Biliary Cancer. New York: Marcel Dekker, 1987;4.
27. Cattone M, Turri M, Caltagirone M, et al. Early detection of hepatocellular carcinoma associated with cirrhosis by ultrasound and alpha-protein: a prospective study. Hepatogastroenterology 1988;35:101–103.
28. Kanematsu T, Sonoda T, Takenada K, et al. The value of ultrasound in the diagnosis and treatment of small hepatocellular carcinoma. Br J Surg 1985;72:23–25.
29. Sheu JC, Sung JL, Chen DS, et al. Ultrasonography of small hepatic tumors using high resolution linear-array real-time instruments. Radiology 1984;150:797–802.
30. Clouse ME. Current diagnostic imaging modalities of the liver. Surg Clin North Am 1989;69:193–234.
31. Itai Y, Ohtomo K, Furui S, et al. MR imaging of hepatobiliary carcinoma in old age. Clin Gastroenterol 1986;10:963–968.
32. Kuntslinger F, Federle MP, Moss AA, Marks W. Computed tomography of hepatocellular carcinoma. AJR Am J Roentgenol 1980;134: 431–437.
33. Matsui O, Kadoya M, Suzuki M, et al. Work in progress: dynamic sequential computed tomography during arterial portography in the detection of hepatic neoplasm. Radiology 1983;146:721–727.
34. Merine D, Takayasu K, Wakao F. Detection of hepatocellular carcinoma: comparison of CT during arterial portography with CT after intraarterial injection of iodized oil. Radiology 1990;175:707–710.
35. Lotze MT, Flickerger JC, Carr BI. Hepatobiliary Neoplasms. In Devita VT Jr, Hellman S, Rosenberg SA (eds), Cancer: Principles and Practice of Oncology (4th ed). Philadelphia: Lippincott, 1993;895.
36. Ringe B, Bichlmayr R, Wisttekind C, et al. Surgical treatment of hepatocellular carcinoma: experience with liver resection and transplantation in 198 patients. World J Surg 1991;15:270–285.
37. Ezaki T, Yukaya H, Ogawa Y. Evaluation of hepatic resection for hepatocellular carcinoma in the elderly. Br J Surg 1987;74:471–473.
38. Nagasue N, Change Y-C, Takemoto Y, et al. Liver resection in the aged (seventy years or older) with hepatocellular carcinoma. Surgery 1993;113:148–154.
39. Nakajima T, Konda Y, Miyazaki M, et al. A histopathologic study of 102 cases of intrahepatic cholangiocarcinoma: histologic classification and modes of spreading. Hum Pathol 1988;19:1228–1234.
40. Roslyn JJ, Binns GS, Hughes EF, et al. Open cholecystectomy: a contemporary analysis of 42,474 patients. Ann Surg 1993;218:129–137.
41. Gyorffy EJ, Frey CF, Silva J Jr, McGahan J. Pyogenic liver abscess. Ann Surg 1987;206:699–705.
42. Ferrucci JTT, van Sonneberg E. Intra-abdominal abscess: radiological diagnosis and treatment. JAMA 1980;246:2728–2733.
43. Gerzof SG, Johnson WC, Robbins AH, Nabseth DC. Intrahepatic pyogenic abscesses: treatment by percutaneous drainage. Am J Surg 1985;149:487–494.
44. Heaton KW. The epidemiology of gallstones and suggested etiology. Clin Gastroenterol 1973;2:67–83.
45. Lieber MM. The incidence of gallstones and their correlation with other disease. Ann Surg 1952;135:394–405.
46. Friedman GD, Kannel WB, Dawber TR. The epidemiology of gallbladder disease. Observation in the Framingham study. J Chronic Dis 1966;19:273–292.
47. Bateson MC. Gallbladder disease and cholecystectomy rates are independently variable. Lancet 1984;2:621–624.
48. Glambek J, Kvaale G, Arnesjo B, Soreide O. Prevalence of gallstones in a Norwegian population. Scand J Gastroenterol 1987;22:1089–1094.
49. Sampliner RE, Bennett PH, Comess LJ, et al. Gallbladder disease in Pima Indians. Demonstrations of high prevalence and early onset by cholecystography. N Engl J Med 1970;283:1358–1364.
50. Crump C. The incidence of gallstones and gallbladder disease. Surg Gynecol Obstet 1931;53:447–455.
51. Newman HF, Northup JD. The autopsy incidence of gallstones. Abstr Surg 1959;109:1–13.
52. Ibach JR, Hume HA, Erb WH. Cholecystectomy in the aged. Surg Gynecol Obstet 1968;126:523–528.
53. Karup T, Sonderstup J, Kruse-Blinkerberg HO, Schmidt A. Surgery for gallstones in old age: do we operate too late? Acta Chir Scand 1982;148:263–266.
54. Mentzer RM, Golden CT, Chandler JG, Horsley JS III. A comparative appraisal of emphysematous cholecystitis. Am J Surg 1975;129: 10–15.
55. Roslyn J, Busittil R. Gallbladder perforation: pitfalls in management. Am J Surg 1979;137:307–312.
56. Fry DE, Cox RA, Harbrecht JP. Gangrene of the gallbladder. South Med J 1981;74:666–668.
57. Norman DC, Yoshikawa TT. Intraabdominal infections in the elderly. J Am Geriatr Soc 1983;31:677–684.
58. Sullivan DM, Hood TR, Griffen WO Jr. Biliary tract surgery in the elderly. Am J Surg 1982;143:218–220.
59. Gracie WA, Ransohoff DF. The natural history of select gallstones: the innocent gallstone is not a myth. N Engl J Med, 1982;307:798–800.
60. Gilliland TM, Traveso W. Cholecystectomy provides long-term symptoms relief in patients with acalculous cholecystitis. Am J Surg 1990;159:489–492.
61. Lund J. Surgical indications in cholelithiasis: prophylactic cholecystectomy elucidated on the basis of long-term follow-up on 526 non-operated cases. Ann Surg 1960;151:153–162.
62. Wenckhert A, Robertson B. The natural course of gallstone disease. Gastroenterology 1966;50:376–381.
63. Rosenthal RA, Anderson DK. Surgery in the elderly: observation on the pathophysiology and treatment of cholelithiasis. Exp Gerontol 1993;28:459–472.
64. Herzog U, Messmer P, Sutter M, Tondelli P. Surgical treatment for cholelithiasis. Surg Gynecol Obstet 1992;175:238–242.
65. Feldman MG, Russell JC, Lynch JT, Mattie A. Comparison of mortality rates for open and closed cholecystectomy in the elderly: Connecticut Statewide Survey. J Laparoendoscopic Surg 1994;4:165–172.
66. Ouriel K, Ricotta JJ, Adams JT, Deweese JA. Management of cholelithiasis in patients with abdominal aortic aneurysm. Ann Surg 1983;198:717–719.
67. Johnson LB. The importance of early diagnosis of acute acalculous cholecystitis. Surg Gynecol Obstet 1987;164:197–203.
68. Reiss R, Nudelman F, Gutman C, Deutsch AA. Changing trends in surgery for acute cholecystitis World J Surg 1990;14:567–571.
69. Heberer G, Paumgartner G, Saurbruch T. A retrospective analysis of 3 years' experience of an interdisciplinary approach to gallstone disease including shock-waves. Ann Surg 1988;208:274–278.
70. Cobden I, Lendrum R, Venables CW, James OF. Gallstones presenting as mental and physical debility in the elderly. Lancet 1984;1:1062–1064.
71. Madden JW, Croker JR, Beynon GPJ. Septicemia in the elderly. Postgrad Med J 1981;57:502–506.
72. Shinagawa N, Mashita K, Yura J. The operative risk factors of cholelithiasis in the elderly. Jpn J Surg 1992;22:29–34.
73. Reiss R, Eliashiv A, Deutsch AA. Septic complications and bile cultures in 800 consecutive cholecystectomies. World J Surg 1982;6: 195–199.
74. Van der Linden W, Sunzel H. Early versus delayed operation for acute cholecystitis. A controlled clinical trial. Am J Surg 1970;120:7–13.
75. Lahtinen J, Alhava EM, Aukee S. Acute cholecystitis treated by early and delayed surgery. A controlled clinical trial. Scand J Gastroenterol 1978;13:673–678.
76. Glenn F. Trends in surgical treatment of acalculous disease of the biliary tract. Surg Gynecol Obstet 1975;140:877–884.
77. Glenn F. Surgical management of acute cholecystitis in patients 65 years of age and older. Ann Surg 1981;193:56–59.
78. Morrow DJ, Thompson J, Wilson SE. Acute cholecystitis in the elderly. A surgical emergency. Arch Surg 1978;113:1149–1152.
79. Zucker KA, Flowers JL, Bailey RW, et al. Laparoscopic management of acute cholecystitis. Am J Surg 1993;165:508–514.
80. Phillips EH, Carroll BJ, Bello JM, et al. Laparoscopic cholecystectomy in acute cholecystitis. Am J Surg 1992;58:273–276.
81. Wilson RG, Macintyre IMC, Nixin SJ, et al. Laparoscopic cholecystectomy is a safe and effective treatment for severe acute cholecystitis. BMJ 1992;305:394–396.
82. Kaufman M, Weissberg D, Schwartz I, Moses Y. Cholecystectomy as a definitive operation. Surg Gynecol Obstet 1990;170:533–537.
83. McGahan JP, Lindfors KK. Percutaneous cholecystectomy: an alternative to surgical cholecystostomy for acute cholecystitis? Radiology 1989;173:481–485.
84. Feretis CB, Manouras AJ, Apostolidis NS, Golematis BC. Endoscopic transpapillary drainage of gallbladder empyema. Gastrointest Endosc 1990;36:523–525.
85. Turrill FL, McCarron UM, Mikkelsen WP. Gallstones and diabetics: an ominous association. Am J Surg 1961;102:184–190.
86. Walsh DB, Eckhauser FE, Ramsburg SF, Burney RB. Risk associated with diabetes mellitus in patients undergoing gallbladder surgery. Surgery 1982;91:254–257.

87. Haff FC, Butcher HR, Ballinger WF. Biliary tract operations: a review of 1000 patients. Arch Surg 1969;98:428–434.
88. Lygidakis NJ. Operative risk factors of cholecystectomy-choledochotomy in the elderly. Surg Gynecol Obstet 1983;157:15–19.
89. Moesgaard F, Nieson ML, Pedersen T, Hansen JB. Protective choledochoduodenostomy in multiple common duct stones in the aged. Surg Gynecol Obstet 1982;154:232–234.
90. Boulay J, Schellenberg R, Brady PG. Role of ERCP and therapeutic biliary endoscopy in association with laparoscopic cholecystectomy. Am J Gastroenterol 1992;87:837–842.
91. Van Stiegmann G, Pearlman NW, Goff JS, et al. Endoscopic cholangiography and stone removal prior to cholecystectomy. A more cost-effective approach than operative duct exploration? Arch Surg 1989;124:787–789.
92. Shepherd HA, Royle G, Ross AP, et al. Endoscopic biliary endoprosthesis in the palliation of malignant obstruction of the distal common bile duct: a randomized trial. Br J Surg 1988;75:1166–1168.
93. Glenn F, Moore SE. Gangrene and perforation of the wall of the gallbladder. A sequela of acute cholecystitis. Arch Surg 1942;44:677–686.
94. Ramanujam P, Shabeeb N, Silver JM. Unusual manifestations of gallstone migration into the gastrointestinal tract. South Med J 1983;76:30–32.
95. Williams NF, Scobie TK. Perforation of the gallbladder: analysis of 19 cases. Can Med Assoc J 1976;115:1223–1225.
96. Cooperman AM, Dickson ER, ReMine WH. Changing concepts in the surgical treatment of gallstone ileus. Ann Surg 1968;167:377–383.
97. Rigler LG, Borman CM, Nobel JF. Gallstone obstruction: pathogenesis and roentgen manifestation. JAMA 1941;117:1753–1759.
98. Kurtz RJ, Herman TM, Kurtz AB. Gallstone ileus: a diagnostic problem. Am J Surg 1983;146:314–317.
99. Heuman R, Sjodahl R, Wetterfors J. Gallstone ileus: an analysis of 20 patients. World J Surg 1980;4:595–600.
100. Hegner CG. Gaseous pericholecystitis with cholecystitis and cholelithiasis. Arch Surg 1931;22:993–1000.
101. Faber RC, Ibrahim SZ, Thomas DM, et al. Gallstone disease presenting as septic shock. Br J Surg 1978;65:101–105.
102. Shimada K, Inamatsu T, Yamashiro M. Anaerobic bacteria in biliary disease in elderly patients. J Clin Infect Dis 1977;135:850–854.
103. Chetlin SH, Elliott DW. Biliary bacteremia. Arch Surg 1971;102:303–307.
104. Chetlin SH, Elliott DW. Preoperative antibiotics in biliary surgery. Arch Surg 1973;107:319–323.
105. Keighley MRB, Baddeley RM, Burdon DW, et al. A controlled trial of parenteral prophylactic gentamicin therapy in biliary surgery. Br J Surg 1975;62:275–279.
106. Schoenfield LJ, Lachin JM. Chenodiol (chenodeoxycholic acid) for dissolution of gallstones: the National Cooperative Gallstone Study. A controlled trial of efficacy and safety. Ann Intern Med 1981;95:257–282.
107. Allen MJ, Borody TJ, Bugliosi TF, et al. Rapid dissolution of gallstones by methyl tert-butyl ether. Preliminary observations. N Engl J Med 1985;312:217–220.
108. Hill MJ, Draser BS, Williams REO. Faecal bile acids and clostridia in patients with cancer of the large bowel. Lancet 1975;1:535–538.
109. Turunen MJ, Kivalaks EO. Increased risk of colorectal cancer after cholecystectomy. Ann Surg 1981;194:639–641.
110. Turnbull PRG, Smith AG, Isbister WH. Cholecystectomy and cancer of the large bowel. Br J Surg 1981;68:551–553.
111. Lowenfels AB, Domellof L, Lindstrom CG. Cholelithiasis, cholecystectomy, and cancer: a case-control study in Sweden. Gastroenterology 1982;83:672–676.
112. Diehl AK. Gallstone size and the risk of gallbladder cancer. JAMA 1983;250:2323–2326.
113. Nakamura S, Sakaguchi S, Suzuki S, Muro H. Aggressive surgery for carcinoma of the gallbladder. Surgery 1989;106:467–473.
114. Ouchi K, Owada Y, Matsuno S, Sato T. Prognostic factors in the surgical treatment of gallbladder carcinoma. Surgery 1987;101:731–737.
115. Silk YN, Douglass HO Jr, Nava HR, et al. Carcinoma of the gallbladder. The Roswell experience. Ann Surg 1989;210:751–757.
116. Mori W, Nagasato K. Cholangiocarcinoma and Related Lesions. In Okuda K, Peter RL (eds), Hepatocellular Carcinoma. New York: Wiley, 1976;227–246.
117. Saunders K, Tompkins R, Longmire W Jr, Roslyn J. Bile duct carcinoma in the elderly: a rationale for surgical management. Arch Surg 1991;126:1186–1190.
118. Chao TC, Greager JA. Carcinoma of the extrahepatic bile ducts. J Surg Oncol 1991;46:145–150.
119. Reding R, Buard JL, Lebeau G, et al. Surgical management of 552 carcinomas of the extrahepatic bile ducts (gallbladder and preampullary tumors excluded): results of the French Surgical Association Survey. Ann Surg 1991;213:236–241.
120. Bismuth H, Castaing D, Traynor O. Resection or palliation: priority of surgery in the treatment of hilar cancer. World J Surg 1988;12:39–47.
121. Cameron JL, Pitt HA, Zinner MJ, et al. Management of proximal cholangiocarcinomas by surgical resection and radiotherapy. Am J Surg 1990;159:91–97.
122. Speer AG, Cotton PB, Russell RC, et al. Randomised trial of endoscopic versus percutaneous stent insertion in malignant obstructive jaundice. Lancet 1987;2:57–62.
123. Huibregtse K, Katon RM, Coene PP, Tytgat GN. Endoscopic palliative treatment in pancreatic cancer. Gastrointest Endosc 1986;32:334–338.
124. Lai EC, Chu KM, Lo CY, et al. Choice of palliation for malignant hilar biliary obstruction. Am J Surg 1992;163:208–212.
125. Lai EC, Tompkins RK, Mann LL, Roslyn JJ. Proximal bile duct cancer: quality of survival. Ann Surg 1987;205:111–118.
126. Lee E. Obstructive Jaundice. In Truelove SC, Trowell J (eds), Topics in Gastroenterology (2nd ed). Oxford: Blackwell, 1974;255–270.
127. O'Brien GF, Tan CV. Jaundice in the geriatric patient. Geriatrics 1970;25:114–127.

Surgical Care for the Elderly, 2nd ed., edited by
R. Benton Adkins, Jr., and H. William Scott, Jr.
Lippincott–Raven Publishers, Philadelphia © 1998.

CHAPTER 24

Surgical Management of Pancreatic Disease

Keith D. Lillemoe and John L. Cameron

Pancreatic disease is a significant health care problem in the elderly. Although the entire spectrum of benign and malignant disease of the pancreas can occur in the aged, two conditions, acute gallstone pancreatitis and pancreatic carcinoma, are by far the most common pancreatic disorders seen in this age group. As our population ages, these pancreatic diseases are likely to become more common and represent an increased clinical challenge for surgeons. This trend is already apparent, as the incidence of pancreatic carcinoma has clearly risen. Because gallstone disease is also much more common in older patients, many patients may be expected to present with gallstone pancreatitis as a complication of cholelithiasis.

The management of diseases of the pancreas is no different in older patients. Both acute pancreatitis and the surgical management of pancreatic cancer, however, can be associated with significant morbidity and mortality in older patients. Early diagnosis, good supportive care, and aggressive surgical management are key in optimizing the care of the elderly and avoiding complications. The surgical management of patients in the older age group will always be associated with significant risks, but with appropriate care, many of these patients can be restored to a healthy and active state.

CHANGES IN THE PANCREAS WITH AGING

Anatomic Changes

Changes in the anatomy of the pancreas occur with aging. An understanding of these changes is necessary for the accurate interpretation of radiographic imaging studies and the pancreatograms of older patients. First, the duodenal C loop and the pancreas may be displaced inferiorly in older patients. The head of the pancreas is often located as low as the body of the second sacral vertebrae [1]. This low-lying pancreas may lead to difficulty in visualization of the pancreas by imaging studies if they are not projected low enough.

The human pancreas also atrophies after the age of 70 years so that its weight decreases from a normal value of 60 ± 20 g to 40 g or less by 85 years [2]. These atrophic changes in the pancreas may actually improve the ability to diagnose a subtle pancreatic mass that may appear more prominent in the face of an otherwise atrophic gland.

Changes in pancreatic ductal anatomy have also been described. Kreel and Sandin performed retrograde pancreatography at necropsy in 120 patients of whom 107 were at least 60 years of age and 84 were 70 years or older [1]. Pancreatic duct width was noted to increase with age at a rate of 8% per decade. This increase occurs throughout the whole pancreas (head, body, and tail) at proportionally the same rate. The dilated duct in the elderly retains its uniform tapered appearance with smooth margins, with only scattered and intermittent branch dilatation. This is in contrast to the sudden and irregular duct dilatation seen in pancreatic carcinoma. Peripheral, single, or conglomerate tiny cysts were also frequently noted. Cyst formation was most commonly associated with greater duct width, and therefore there was a significant correlation of the presence of cysts with increasing age.

A second autopsy series evaluated 69 pancreatograms in patients without pancreatitis. The studies were interpreted blindly by six experienced endoscopists without knowledge of the histologic findings. Eighty-one percent were interpreted as showing chronic pancreatitis (37% minimal, 33% moderate, 11% severe) [3]. However, when the pancreatograms were correlated with histologic and gross appearance, it became clear that the ductular changes were due to perilobular fibrosis and intraductal epithelial hyperplasia. Whether these changes seen in autopsy series correlate with clinical observations made in patients undergoing endoscopic retrograde cholangiopancreatography (ERCP) is controversial. Differing clinical reports, both confirming [4] and disputing [5] the findings, can be found in the literature. In summary, the morphologic changes in the pancreas from aging may be striking. Endoscopists must be aware of these changes in interpreting ERCP findings and be cautious in the diagnosis of chronic pancreatitis in elderly patients.

Pathologic Changes

Pathologic changes in the pancreas of the elderly are seen in almost all patients. Histologic changes affect both the glandular tissue and pancreatic ducts. The glandular changes most frequently involve fatty infiltration (79%) and fibrosis (60%) [6]. The fatty infiltration appears to be a replacement phenomenon, with small remnants of lobules completely surrounded with adipose tissue. The fibrosis noticed is fine and patchy and not associated with destruction of the exocrine parenchyma as seen in chronic pancreatitis. These changes may account for the increased inhomogeneous and patchy appearance of the pancreas observed on computed tomography (CT) scans in the elderly.

Ductal changes consisting of proliferation and metaplasia of ductal epithelial cells are also noted [7]. This proliferation often leads to the formation of a solid cord of cells, which is followed by lumen formation, expansion, and cavitation. Metaplasia of the pancreatic duct can occur to the extent that ductal epithelium eventually becomes a stratified squamous epithelium in the interlobular ducts. These senescent pathologic changes in the pancreas are not paralleled equally by dramatic alterations in glandular function, because the reserve capacity of the pancreas is enormous and clinical malabsorption is not associated until 90% of a gland is functionally absent [8].

Functional Changes

Pancreatic exocrine function in the elderly patient may also be altered. Studies using secretin stimulation have failed to demonstrate changes in volume and output of bicarbonate and amylase in elderly patients [9,10]. With repeated stimulation, however, the pancreas of older subjects appears to show fatigue and diminished function when compared with that of younger individuals [9]. Analysis of specimens of pure pancreatic juice collected endoscopically has also demonstrated that pancreatic function does diminish with age. Significant decreases in the volume of pancreatic secretion in response to secretin stimulation and pancreatic protein and lipase concentration in response to cholecystokinin stimulation have been observed in subjects >65 years of age [11]. Thus, some physiologic decline in exocrine pancreatic function does indeed occur, but because only 10% to 15% of pancreatic secretion is needed for normal digestion, it is unlikely that these changes are of any clinical significance.

Experimental information suggests a diminished endocrine cell function with aging, although B-cell function has been demonstrated to be normal, elevated, or decreased in various studies. A report by Chen and colleagues has demonstrated both a significant B-cell defect in insulin secretion and diminished peripheral response to insulin in the elderly [12]. Pancreatic endocrine changes may contribute to the pathogenesis of age-related glucose intolerance.

INFLAMMATORY DISEASES OF THE PANCREAS

Acute Pancreatitis

Acute pancreatitis has an incidence of 0.5% in the general population. Aging itself is not associated with an increased risk of acute pancreatitis. It is, however, an important cause of acute abdominal pain in the elderly, accounting for approximately 5% to 7% of cases from collected series [13,14]. Moreover, acute pancreatitis in the elderly is associated with increased morbidity and mortality [15–18].

In large series of patients with acute pancreatitis, the proportion of elderly patients varies considerably. In series in which alcohol is the leading cause of pancreatitis, elderly patients make up a small percentage of the patients. However, in series in which gallstones are the leading cause of pancreatitis, elderly patients make up a much greater proportion. In one such series, 45% of patients with acute gallstone pancreatitis were in their seventh, eighth, or ninth decades [19]. The mean age for patients presenting with acute gallstone pancreatitis was 67 years versus 44 years in a series of patients presenting with alcohol-induced pancreatitis. The sex distribution for elderly patients with acute pancreatitis also reflects a biliary tract etiology, with elderly women affected more often than men.

Etiology

As in younger patients, there are a multitude of causes of acute pancreatitis in the elderly (Table 24-1). Although gallstones and alcohol are etiologic factors in up to 90% of cases in all age groups, gallstones are by far the most common cause of acute pancreatitis in the elderly, with alcohol an infrequent factor. Biliary sludge, a suspension of cholesterol monohydrate crystals and calcium bilirubinate granules, has been implicated as a cause of acute pancreatitis. In one review, 36% of patients presenting with acute pancreatitis were initially classified as idiopathic [19]. Further analysis, with careful ultrasonography and bile sampling, identified biliary sludge in 74% of these patients.

In the elderly patient, external trauma is an uncommon cause of pancreatitis. However, the elderly patient who is undergoing an operation for unassociated conditions appears to be susceptible to postoperative pancreatitis, which is presumably, at least in part, secondary to pancreatic trauma. In a report by Park and colleagues, the second leading cause of pancreatitis in the elderly was operative trauma (12.5%) [20]. Injury to the pancreas can occur during almost any upper abdominal or retroperitoneal operation, but is frequently observed after biliary or gastric operations, splenectomy, or aortic reconstruction. ERCP performed to evaluate the pancreaticobiliary tree is often associated with transient elevation of serum amylase level. However, <5% of patients actually develop clinical pancreatitis. It would appear that elderly patients are at no higher risk for post-ERCP pancreatitis than is the general population [21].

Ischemia has been recognized as an initiating factor in some patients with acute pancreatitis. This etiology would appear to play an important role in the elderly. Acute pancreatitis has been noted in up to 50% of patients with oligemic shock following repair of ruptured abdominal aortic aneurysms [22]. Similarly, 10% to 20% of patients who die following cardiac operations have pathologic evidence of acute pancreatitis [22,23]. These findings are thought to be secondary to ischemic injuries incurred during the low-flow state of hypovolemic shock or cardiopulmonary bypass. There appears to be some disparity in the incidence observed in these autopsy series and the reported incidence of acute pancreatitis following cardiopulmonary bypass, which is generally <0.5% [24].

A multitude of drugs have been suspected of initiating acute pancreatitis [25]. For most of those drugs suspected, the incidence is extremely low and the pathogenic mechanisms are entirely unknown. A list of drugs in which evidence may suggest causation of acute pancreatitis is provided in Table 24-2. Although relatively uncommon, drug-induced acute pancreatitis should be considered in elderly patients with acute pancreatitis because of the incidence of polypharmacy in this population. Whenever such a relationship is suspected, the drug should be withdrawn.

Endocrine and metabolic abnormalities such as hyperlipidemia and hypercalcemia have been associated with acute pancreatitis. Acute pancreatitis has been well documented to occur in hyperlipoproteinemia types I and V. Hypercalcemia should always be considered in the elderly patient with recurrent pancreatitis without evidence of gallstones. A low serum calcium level at the time of presentation, due to pancreatic inflammation, may mask hypercalcemia as an etiologic factor. Finally, diabetes mellitus and uremia have been suggested as etiologic factors. Evidence in support of these latter conditions is weak, and the diagnosis of pancreatitis may be falsely based on elevations of serum amylase levels not associated with pancreatic disease.

Pancreaticobiliary abnormalities such as periampullary duodenal diverticula, papillary stenosis, and pancreatic divisum are rare causes of acute pancreatitis. The most important cause of pancreatic duct obstruction resulting in acute pancreatitis in the elderly patient is pancreatic carcinoma. In a large series of patients with pancreatic carcinoma, clinical pancreatitis occurred in 3% of cases [26] and frequently led to a delay in diagnosis and unfavorable outcome. Although only approximately 1% of cases of acute pancreatitis are secondary to pancreatic cancer, this relationship should not be overlooked in the elderly. Pancreatic carcinoma should be considered in any patient over the age of 60 with a new onset of pancreatitis in which the diagnosis of gallstones or biliary sludge cannot be confirmed.

Finally, in any large series of patients with acute pancreatitis, the etiology in a proportion of patients will remain unknown or idiopathic. In two large series of elderly patients, 20% to 30% of the cases remained idiopathic [20,27]. Furthermore, in the report by Browder and colleagues, those patients without a defined etiology of their pancreatitis tended to have more severe disease with a greater number of Ranson's criteria, higher morbidity and mortality, and more days spent in the intensive care unit [27]. In neither of these series, however, was ERCP routinely performed, and thus anatomic abnormalities of the pancreatic or biliary ductal system or pancreatic sludge

TABLE 24-1. *Causes of acute pancreatitis in the elderly*

Biliary tract disease
Gallstones
Biliary sludge
Alcohol consumption
Trauma
External
Operative
Postendoscopic retrograde cholangiopancreatography
Ischemia
Cardiopulmonary bypass
Drugs
Metabolic and endocrine
Hyperlipidemia
Hypercalcemia
Pancreatic duct obstruction
Tumors
Duodenal diverticula
Papillary stenosis
Pancreas divisum
Idiopathic

TABLE 24-2. *Drugs implicated in the etiology of acute pancreatitis*

Thiazides
L-Asparaginase
Furosemide
Corticosteroids
Azathioprine
Ethacrynic acid
Sulfonamides
Methyldopa
Tetracyclines
Procainamide
Estrogens
Metronidazole
6-Mercaptopurine
Valproic acid
Nonsteroidal anti-inflammatory drugs

TABLE 24-3. *Causes of hyperamylasemia in the elderly*

Intra-abdominal disorders	Extra-abdominal disorders
Pancreatic disorders	Salivary gland disorders
Acute pancreatitis	Parotitis
Chronic pancreatitis	Trauma
Trauma	Surgery
Pseudocyst	Impaired amylase excretion
Pancreatic ascites	Renal failure
Pancreatic carcinoma	Macroamylasemia
Nonpancreatic disorders	Miscellaneous
Biliary tract disease	Cerebral trauma
Peptic ulcer with perforation or penetration	Severe burns
	Diabetic ketoacidosis
Intestinal obstruction	Pneumonia
Mesenteric infarction	Prostate surgery
Acute appendicitis	
Ruptured aortic aneurysm	
Peritonitis	

may have remained undetected. Such abnormalities have been shown to account for 45% of cases previously thought to be idiopathic [28]. Therefore, regardless of a patient's age, a thorough evaluation for the etiology of acute pancreatitis should be completed, including ERCP if necessary, in hopes of identifying a correctable etiology. The morbidity and mortality associated with repeated attacks of acute pancreatitis in this age group would support this philosophy.

Clinical Presentation

The presentation of acute pancreatitis in the elderly is similar to that in younger patients except that the findings may be more subtle than expected in the presence of severe disease. Acute pancreatitis may manifest as a mild illness with pain as the predominant symptom and few abdominal signs. However, it can also present as a full-blown illness with symptoms of shock, respiratory distress, renal failure, coma, hypocalcemia, leukocytosis, and fever. The symptoms of most patients with acute pancreatitis will fall between these two extremes. The most common symptom is pain, which is characteristically located in the epigastrium, radiates to the back, and is occasionally referred to the left shoulder. In the elderly population, in whom gallstones are the likely cause of pancreatitis, the pain may be in the right upper quadrant. The onset of pain is usually gradual, but occasionally may be sudden, mimicking that of a perforated duodenal ulcer. The pain is often steady and severe. Patients with pancreatitis typically seek relief from the pain by leaning forward. Constant agitation and movement are typical, as opposed to the patient with peritonitis who often lies as motionless as possible. Nausea and vomiting almost invariably are present and are often a predominant early feature.

The physical findings can vary widely. The patient may be restless with a rapid pulse and respiratory rate. The temperature is usually elevated in the range of 38°C, but elevations up to 40°C may be seen. The abdomen is usually moderately distended and bowel sounds are diminished or absent. Diffuse tenderness with guarding and rebound is usually most marked over the epigastrium, upper abdomen, and sometimes the flank. True rigidity of the abdomen, however, is uncommon. It is not unusual, especially in elderly patients, for the clinical presentation to be out of proportion with physical findings. Jaundice may be noted, especially in cases of gallstone pancreatitis. However, it is more common for the patients to be anicteric at presentation. Frequently, severe pancreatitis patients present with respiratory distress. Findings of respiratory difficulty, as well as peripheral signs of hypoxemia, may be obvious, especially in the elderly patient.

Diagnosis

The diagnosis of acute pancreatitis is made on the basis of clinical presentation, with laboratory determinations serving to confirm the diagnosis. Serum amylase level elevations can occur from a multitude of causes (Table 24-3), many of which may mimic acute pancreatitis clinically. In one report, only 68% of patients with hyperamylasemia and abdominal pain had acute pancreatitis [29]. The acute extrapancreatic abdominal conditions commonly associated with serum amylase level elevations include perforated peptic ulcer, mesenteric infarction, small bowel obstruction, and acute biliary tract disease. Many of these conditions require urgent operation, and thus, it is of utmost importance to differentiate these conditions from acute pancreatitis. It does not appear that amylase level elevation is a less sensitive indicator of pancreatitis in the elderly. However, elderly patients may be particularly susceptible to other conditions causing hyperamylasemia.

The level of hyperamylasemia is not a reliable indicator of the severity of pancreatic inflammation, but it is often valuable in establishing the etiology of pancreatitis. Biliary pancreatitis is frequently associated with a marked elevation in serum amylase level, often a 5- to 10-fold increase, whereas alcoholics with pancreatitis often have a relatively low degree of hyperamylasemia. Patients with postoperative pancreatitis, an important cause in the elderly, frequently present with only minimal or no elevation of serum amylase level. Hyperlipidemic serum may also result in spuriously low amylase levels.

Other abnormal laboratory measurements in patients with acute pancreatitis include a leukocytosis of 10,000 to 15,000 cells/μl, elevation of the hematocrit secondary to extracellular fluid sequestration, or a low hematocrit due to retroperitoneal bleeding. Hyperglycemia and hypocalcemia may be observed in acute pancreatitis and are uncommon with other acute abdominal conditions.

The radiologic findings associated with acute pancreatitis may include a small left pleural effusion, segmental small bowel ileus (sentinel loop), dilatation of the transverse colon with absence of air in the left colon, the so-called colon cutoff sign, and duodenal ileus. In patients with acute relapsing pancreatitis, calcifications in the region of the pancreas may also be noted. Ultrasonography is especially useful in the diagnosis of elderly patients with acute pancreatitis because of the high incidence of gallstones causing pancreatitis in this age group. Although somewhat difficult because of gaseous distention of the bowel, imaging of the pancreas may also show generalized enlargement, localized swelling or fluid collections, or cyst formation. In a high percentage of patients, however, ultrasonography of the pancreas is normal.

CT scanning is the most useful tool in the assessment of the severity of acute pancreatitis and its complications. The CT scan provides a quick, noninvasive, generally accurate assessment of the pancreas and peripancreatic retroperitoneum. Abnormal CT findings are present in up to 90% of cases [30,31] (Fig. 24-1) and include diffuse pancreatic enlargement, obliteration of peripancreatic fat planes, and inflammation of the anterior perirenal space. Peripancreatic fluid collections can also be visualized. There appears to be a direct correlation between the degree of CT abnormalities and the severity of acute pancreatitis. Ranson and his colleagues have used dynamic contrast-enhanced CT scanning to define and identify groups of patients with increased risk of pancreatic abscess [31] (Table 24-4). CT scanning should be included in both the diagnosis and hospital management of elderly patients with all but mild cases of acute pancreatitis. After the diagnosis of acute pancreatitis is confirmed, serial CT scanning in severely ill patients should be performed in hopes of identifying complications of pancreatitis at an early stage.

Historically, diagnostic exploratory laparotomy played an important role in the diagnosis of acute pancreatitis. At present, the diagnosis of acute pancreatitis can be made based on a careful, nonoperative evaluation in almost all patients. By the aggressive use of CT scanning, the need for diagnostic laparotomy has been almost completely eliminated in the diagnosis of acute pancreatitis. However, the presence of acute pancreatitis does not rule out the presence of coexisting intra-abdominal pathology in elderly patients. Older patients have a higher probability of other intra-abdominal catastrophes such as mesenteric ischemia, gangrenous cholecystitis, or perforated viscus. Diagnostic laparotomy should be used to avoid disastrous complications of nonoperative management of these disorders.

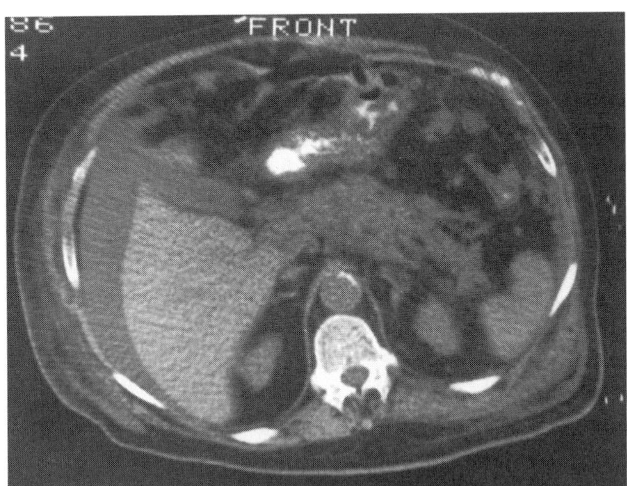

FIG. 24-1. Computed tomography of a 68-year-old man with acute pancreatitis. The scan demonstrates inflammation and edema of the body of the pancreas and the surrounding small bowel mesentery. The presence of ascites is also noted.

TABLE 24-4. *Ranson/Balthazar computed tomographic classification of acute pancreatitis*

Grade	Description	Incidence of pancreatic abscess (%)
A	Normal	0
B	Pancreatic enlargement	0
C	Inflammation of pancreas and peripancreatic fat	12
D	Above and one pancreatic fluid collection	17
E	Above and two or more peripancreatic fluid collections	61

Clinical Course

Because of improvements in supportive care, the overall mortality for acute pancreatitis has decreased to approximately 5%. Moreover, in many series of patients with mild-to-moderate pancreatitis, no hospital mortalities are noted. The clinical course of all patients with acute pancreatitis is highly dependent on the severity of disease. Most patients (approximately 75%) have relatively mild edematous pancreatitis, with improvement noted within 48 to 72 hours of hospitalization. Most of the morbidity and mortality that does occur is in the small group of patients with severe and hemorrhagic pancreatitis.

Elderly patients represent the extreme in the spectrum of patients with acute pancreatitis. Most authors consider age >55 years a significant risk factor for death associated with acute pancreatitis [15–18]. In a large review by Corfield and colleagues, the mortality for patients aged 60 or greater was 28% versus 9% for patients below that age (P <0.001) [15]. In a review of pancreatitis in patients 70 years of age or older, a mortality of 20% was noted, with an average hospital stay >3 weeks [20]. This is significantly higher than the mortality in the general population, but represents an improvement over the mortality of 40% observed by Pollock in his report of pancreatitis in the elderly published in 1959 [32]. Thus, it can be concluded that elderly patients are at significant risk for death from acute pancreatitis, and aggressive supportive care and intensive care monitoring should be instituted early to avoid disastrous outcomes.

TABLE 24-5. *Ranson's early prognostic signs of acute pancreatitis*

At admission
Age >55 years
White blood cell count >16,000/µl
Blood glucose level >200 mg/dl
Serum lactic dehydrogenase >350 IU/liter
Serum glutamic-oxaloacetic transaminase >250 U/dl
During initial 48 hours
Hematocrit decrease >10%
Blood urea nitrogen elevation >5 mg/dl
Serum calcium decrease to <8 mg/dl
Pao_2 <60 mm Hg
Base deficit >4 mEq/liter
Estimated fluid sequestration >6 liters

TABLE 24-6. *Proposed nonoperative measures for the treatment of acute pancreatitis*

Measures to suppress pancreatic secretion or enzyme activity	Supportive measures
Nothing by mouth	IV fluid replacement
Nasogastric suction	Electrolyte replacement
Anticholinergics	Analgesics
Glucagon	Nutritional support
Histamine receptor antagonists	Respiratory support
Aprotinin (Trasylol)	Peritoneal dialysis
Somatostatin analogue (octreotide)	Antibiotics
Cholecystokinin-receptor antagonist (proglumide)	

During the early clinical assessment, those patients with a high risk of complications can be predicted. Perhaps the most important tool in the assessment of the severity of acute pancreatitis early in its course has been described by Ranson and his colleagues [18]. These authors were able to identify 11 early prognostic signs (including age >55) strongly correlated with subsequent occurrence of serious prolonged illness or death (Table 24-5). In a retrospective study [18], and subsequently in a prospective study [33], these authors found excellent correlation between the number of grave prognostic signs and the subsequent clinical course. In almost 80% of patients, fewer than three positive signs were present, and there was an overall mortality of 0.9%. In those patients with three to four positive signs, the mortality rose to 16%; in those with five to six positive signs, it was 40%; in those with seven or more signs, the mortality was 100%. The number of grave prognostic signs also correlates well with the days of intensive care required. These grave signs were initially described in patients with pancreatitis secondary to alcohol abuse, and their value in elderly patients with gallstone pancreatitis has been questioned. Subsequently, however, they have been shown to achieve good prognostic separation of patients with biliary, postoperative, and other forms of acute pancreatitis [34]. The value of these signs is that they may identify, by early assessment, those patients (approximately 25%) at risk for serious, prolonged, and complicated hospitalizations that may result in death. They can be immediately admitted to the intensive care unit and monitored carefully with appropriate supportive care. In this group of patients, nonoperative measures such as peritoneal lavage, broad-spectrum antibiotic coverage, and total parenteral nutrition should be considered. In addition, frequent CT scans should be obtained for early identification of peripancreatic fluid collections or pancreatic abscess so that early aggressive operative management can be instituted.

Treatment

Initial management after the diagnosis of acute pancreatitis consists of resuscitation and correction of fluid and electrolyte deficits. There is little difference in the initial management of patients of any age. Meticulous replacement of fluid and electrolyte losses with adequate maintenance therapy is of utmost importance. Constant attention to urinary output, central venous pressure, and in those elderly patients with evidence of heart disease, pulmonary capillary wedge pressure is mandatory. A urinary catheter and central venous line should be used in all elderly patients with pancreatitis. Replacement of extracellular fluid losses is accomplished by administration of crystalloid solution. In patients with severe hemorrhagic pancreatitis, blood transfusion may be required. In those patients with evidence of glucose intolerance, control must be obtained with administration of insulin. Hypocalcemia should be corrected by intravenous (IV) administration of calcium gluconate.

Several other steps have been advocated through the years in the specific treatment of acute pancreatitis (Table 24-6). These modalities were designed to decrease the severity of pancreatic inflammation by inhibition of pancreatic secretion and enzyme activity. With all these modalities, only the institution of nothing by mouth (NPO) and IV fluids are universally accepted management techniques of patients with acute pancreatitis. The resumption of oral feedings before resolution of pancreatic inflammation is associated with reactivation of the pancreatitis. Thus, patients should remain NPO until there is a complete resolution of abdominal pain, tenderness, fever, and leukocytosis. In addition to NPO, IV fluids, and pain control, elderly patients with gallstone pancreatitis or severe pancreatitis should also receive broad-spectrum antibiotic coverage. Nasogastric suction is recommended for those patients with persistent vomiting or evidence of an ileus. H_2 blockers or antacids should be used in patients at risk for stress ulceration and gastrointestinal hemorrhage. Parenteral nutrition can be provided as a means of nutritional support in selected patients requiring prolonged periods of fasting for pancreatic inflammation.

Finally, peritoneal dialysis may be effective in removing potentially toxic substances from the peritoneal cavity. Two prospective randomized trials of early institution of peritoneal dialysis, within 24 to 48 hours of hospitalization, appear to show favorable influence on the early clinical course of acute pancreatitis by reducing the duration of hyperamylasemia, leukocytosis, and hypocalcemia [33,35]. Peritoneal dialysis did not, however, reduce the incidence of subsequent abscess formation, and thus overall mortality does not appear to be improved with dialysis. A controlled study with a longer period of peritoneal lavage (7 days) has shown a reduction in the prevalence of late infection from 50% to 22% and sepsis-related mortality from 20% to 0% [36].

The management of gallstone pancreatitis is evolving. The vast majority of patients with gallstone pancreatitis do well with conservative treatment. When a stone has passed, there is no need for early intervention. Acosta and colleagues challenged this premise by performing a definitive biliary tract procedure within the first 2 days after presentation [37]. In this series, a gallstone was found to be impacted in the ampulla of Vater in 70% of the cases. By using this approach, they decreased the hospital mortality from 16% to 2%. Hospital stay was also decreased from 25 days to 13 days.

An extension of the principles of early operation to remove an impacted stone have now been advanced by the development of therapeutic ERCP. Two clinical trials evaluated the safety and efficacy of urgent ERCP and endoscopic sphincterotomy in patients with acute gallstone pancreatitis [38,39]. Neoptolemos and colleagues randomized 131 patients to either conventional treatment or urgent ERCP with sphincterotomy and stone extraction if stones were visualized on retrograde cholangiography [38]. The patients were stratified by the Glasgow criteria, similar to Ranson's criteria useful in predicting severity of acute pancreatitis. This study revealed that ERCP could be performed safely during a bout of acute pancreatitis with no increase in the complication rate even in the presence of choledocholithiasis. There was a significant reduction in the morbidity (18% vs. 54%) and time in the hospital in those patients with predicted severe attacks treated with ERCP and sphincterotomy as compared with those treated conservatively. No statistical difference in mortality was shown in this study, although there was a trend in favor of ERCP. In 1993, the group from the University of Hong Kong performed a prospective randomized study in patients suspected of having acute gallstone pancreatitis [39]. Patients were randomized to either conventional therapy or early ERCP and endoscopic papillotomy within 24 hours after admission. Emergency ERCP with or without endoscopic papillotomy resulted in a reduction of biliary sepsis as compared with conservative treatment (0 of 97 patients vs. 12 of 98 patients; $P < 0.001$). The decrease in biliary sepsis occurred in patients predicted to have both mild and severe pancreatitis. There were no major differences in the incidence of local complications or systemic complications of pancreatitis between the two groups, but the hospital mortality was again lower in the group undergoing emergency ERCP with or without endoscopic sphincterotomy. This difference, however, did not reach statistical significance. The results of these two studies support the role of ERCP in the management of patients with gallstone pancreatitis; although it is hard to imagine why patients who underwent ERCP without papillotomy benefited. It could be inferred that this benefit should be extended to most elderly patients with acute gallstone pancreatitis because the potential of this group for increased morbidity and mortality associated with the acute attack warrants an aggressive approach.

The most recent tool in the management of acute gallstone pancreatitis has been laparoscopic cholecystectomy. In the past, 4 to 6 weeks of convalescence was recommended before an elective biliary tract operation was performed for acute gallstone pancreatitis. However, even before introduction of laparoscopic cholecystectomy, it was realized that cholecystectomy performed at the initial hospitalization both eliminates the risk of recurrent pancreatitis during the interval and reduces the overall length of hospital stay. Laparoscopic cholecystectomy, either with preoperative endoscopic retrograde cholangiography or with intraoperative cholangiography, can be performed in almost all patients with gallstone pancreatitis during the same hospital admission without significant increased risk to the patients [40]. It currently represents the management of choice for most patients regardless of age with gallstone pancreatitis.

The role of surgery in patients with acute pancreatitis for the diagnosis and treatment of cholelithiasis is well accepted. Significant controversy, however, exists with respect to a direct operative approach on the inflamed or necrotic pancreas associated with severe acute pancreatitis. The two views differ primarily with respect to the management of pancreatic necrosis not associated with infection. Bradley and Allen identified pancreatic necrosis in 20% of patients with acute pancreatitis [41]. Surgical intervention with pancreatic debridement was used only for patients with infection documented by fine-needle aspiration (71%). The remaining patients were successfully managed without surgery despite associated renal and pulmonary insufficiency.

Rattner and colleagues advocated a more aggressive surgical approach and determined that peripancreatic infection was not a factor in determining outcome following surgical debridement of pancreatic necrosis [42]. This group concluded that infection should not be the sole determinant of intervention, but other clinical factors such as increased APACHE II score, respiratory failure, and shock should lead to an aggressive surgical approach. Unfortunately, this study does not provide data concerning the nonoperative management of noninfected pancreatic necrosis. Until prospective comparison data exist, it cannot be concluded that surgical debridement and drainage should be advocated for noninfected pancreatic necrosis, regardless of extent, severity, or patient age. Aggressive supportive care of associated organ failure and frequent CT scans with needle aspiration looking at secondary infection would appear to be the best approach for those elderly patients with pancreatic necrosis.

Complications of Acute Pancreatitis

Despite optimal management of both simple edematous pancreatitis and hemorrhagic pancreatitis, complications can occur. Elderly patients are not only susceptible to an increased risk of complications, but have a worse prognosis when such complications develop. The older patient, often with preexisting medical conditions, tolerates poorly the significant hemodynamic, respiratory, or septic complications occurring with severe acute pancreatitis. The lack of essential organ reserve often leads to multisystem organ failure and death. The initial therapeutic efforts in the management of acute pancreatitis are designed to resuscitate the patient and prevent the catastrophic outcome related to shock. Elderly patients are sensitive to hypovolemic shock resulting from extensive fluid sequestration or pancreatic hemorrhage. Aggressive fluid resuscitation and blood transfusion are required at the time of presentation during the initial few hours. Acidosis may also occur and should be corrected with bicarbonate administration to avoid cardiovascular dysfunction.

The most serious complications noted in elderly patients with severe pancreatitis are respiratory. Respiratory complications, which occur in up to 60% of all patients, occur more frequently in older patients. Ranson et al. noted such complications in two-thirds of patients >55 years of age as opposed to only 20% of younger patients [43]. Respiratory complications included left-sided pleural effusions, characterized by elevated amylase content due to seepage of pancreatic inflammatory fluid through the diaphragm into the thoracic cavity. Atelectasis and pneumonia may be due to elevation of the diaphragm secondary to abdominal distension, splinting because of abdominal pain, or compression of parenchyma by pleural effusions. The most serious respiratory complication is respiratory failure with resulting hypoxemia. In a series of 116 patients, Ranson et al. were able to associate the development of severe respiratory insufficiency with a number of factors, including age >55 years [43]. Despite the liberal use of intubation and respiratory support, a 25% mortality was noted in this group of patients.

The management of respiratory complications of early pancreatitis includes recognition and intensive respiratory support. Patients with massive fluid requirements, underlying cardiorespiratory disease, or clinical evidence of early respiratory insufficiency require monitoring of oxygen saturation, arterial blood gases, and pulmonary artery pressures with a Swan-Ganz catheter. Aggressive monitoring of elderly patients is necessary because of the likelihood of underlying cardiorespiratory diseases. Hypoxia improves as pancreatitis resolves. If there is progressive respiratory insufficiency or a recent laparotomy, full mechanical ventilation is indicated. Albumen and diuretic therapy have been recommended with monitoring of pulmonary artery pressure to decrease pulmonary capillary fluid sequestration. Using these modalities, Ranson et al. were able to demonstrate diminished need for ventilatory support and hospital mortality [43].

Pancreatic Necrosis and Abscess

One of the most serious life-threatening complications facing patients with severe acute pancreatitis is the development of pancreatic necrosis and abscess. Pancreatic necrosis occurs in up to 30% of patients with pancreatitis. Dynamic CT with bolus vascular contrast medium is the most sensitive method for detection [31]. The patient will most likely experience ongoing pain, low-grade fever, and hyperamylasemia, with a mass effect of the pancreatic phlegmon that may cause biliary, gastroduodenal, or colonic obstruction.

The extensive necrosis of the pancreas and surrounding retroperitoneal fat may provide an excellent culture medium for invading bacteria and the formation of a pancreatic abscess. Abscess occurs in up to 10% of patients and is influenced by both the etiology and severity of the pancreatitis [44,45]. Pancreatic abscess is more common in patients with postoperative pancreatitis than with alcoholic, biliary, or miscellaneous causes. Pancreatic abscess develops in <3% of patients with fewer than three prognostic signs, 32% of patients with three to five Ranson signs, and 50% of patients with more than five prognostic signs. Because age >55 is included in these prognostic signs, advancing age can be expected to be associated with an increased risk of pancreatic abscess. Because postoperative pancreatitis is a relatively more important cause of pancreatitis in the elderly, the aged are again at significant risk for this disastrous complication.

The diagnosis of infected pancreatic necrosis or pancreatic abscess is made by clinical suspicion, CT findings, and the use of percutaneous aspiration of peripancreatic fluid. Between the first and fourth weeks following a severe attack of acute pancreatitis, fever, abdominal pain, and tenderness with persistent ileus may develop. On CT, fluid collection and the demonstration of gas bubbles in the pancreatic and peripancreatic tissue are pathognomonic of pancreatic abscess (Fig. 24-2). In cases in which pancreatic sepsis is suspected but no clear-cut abscess is presence on CT, CT-guided aspiration of peripancreatic fluid can often detect infection of this fluid and lead to prompt surgical intervention before further progression of the infectious response [46].

Once the diagnosis of pancreatic abscess is made, prompt surgical drainage is necessary no matter how old the patient because the mortality of an undrained abscess is 100%. Broad-spectrum antibiotics covering both gram-negative and anaerobic organisms should be instituted. There is no role for conservative management with antibiotics alone. Furthermore, attempts at percutaneous drainage are invariably met with failure [42]. Laparotomy should be performed, the lesser sac entered, and all necrotic pancreatic and peripancreatic tissue debrided by blunt and sharp dissection. Most surgeons now favor an initial aggressive debridement followed by packing the peripancreatic space with antibiotic-soaked gauze pads and returning the patient to the operating room at 24- to 48-hour intervals. At that time, the packs are removed and further blunt and sharp dissection is performed removing all remaining necrotic tissue. The abdominal pads tamponade any hemorrhage and debride necrotic tissue when they are removed. At re-exploration, the tissues are more delineated and further debridement can be performed. Eventually, debridement can be done in the intensive care unit with analgesics alone. This technique was developed for control of hemorrhage that frequently accompanied debridement of pancreatic abscesses, as well as for prevention of recurrent abscess formation. Two series using this technique have reported reduced mortality in the range of 9% to 15% [47,48]. This compares favorably with the previous technique of debridement and placement of multiple drains, which was associated with an incidence of approximately 30% of a recurrent abscess requiring reoperation and mortality ranging from 20% to 50%. Although this technique requires multiple general anesthetics in the elderly and may appear to be extremely aggressive, it may offer the most conservative approach to control sepsis and avert the dreaded complication of recurrent abscess, prolonged sepsis, and multisystem organ failure.

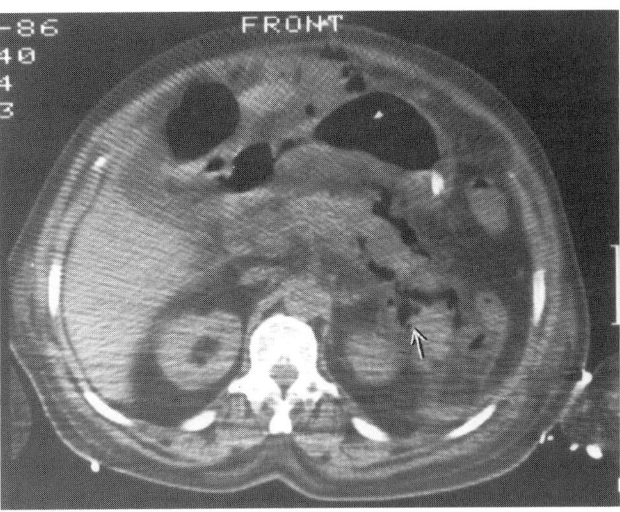

FIG. 24-2. Computed tomography of an 80-year-old man with a pancreatic abscess. The presence of air bubbles (*arrow*) in the inflammatory pancreatic phlegmon is pathognomonic of pancreatic abscess.

Pancreatic Pseudocysts

A pancreatic pseudocyst develops when a pancreatic duct disruption occurs and pancreatic secretions leak and are walled off by the inflammatory adherence of the adjacent structures and the surrounding tissue planes, usually in the lesser sac. The pancreatic pseudocyst persists and enlarges until the pancreatic ductal disruption heals. The pancreatic secretions then resorb and the pancreatic pseudocyst collapses and disappears. Peripancreatic fluid collections occur acutely in approximately 50% of patients with acute pancreatitis [49]. The majority of these are not associated with duct disruption, resolve spontaneously, and are not of clinical concern. Pseudocysts occur in only 5% to 10% of cases of acute pancreatitis. Most are related to alcoholism and are uncommon in the elderly.

Pseudocysts may be asymptomatic or may be detected because of symptoms of persistent pain or amylase level elevation after an episode of acute pancreatitis. A palpable mass or symptoms from extrinsic compression by the enlarging pancreatic mass may also suggest a pseudocyst. Sonography and CT will demonstrate the cystic nature of the mass, distinguishing it from a pancreatic phlegmon or abscess (Fig. 24-3).

If a patient is asymptomatic with a pseudocyst, regardless of size, a conservative approach of observation is warranted in patients of all age groups [50]. Patients with acute pseudocysts should have an initial attempt at conservative management with maintaining the patient NPO with total parenteral nutrition. When the patient is free of pain, attempts at oral intake may be made regardless of the size of the remaining pseudocyst. If no pain recurs, the patient can be advanced to a regular diet and the cyst followed on an outpatient basis. If symptoms persist, drainage of the pseudocyst should be considered.

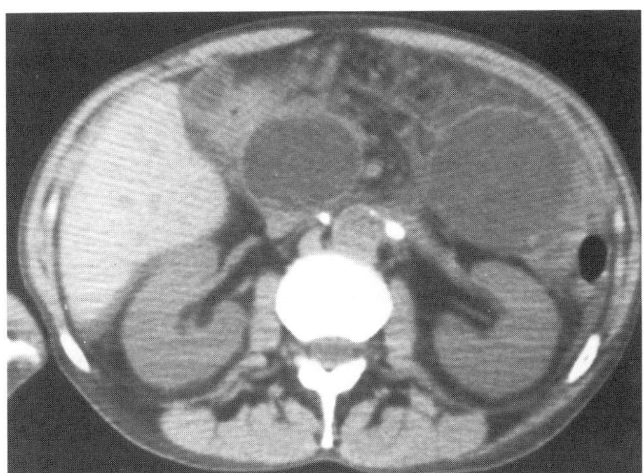
FIG. 24-3. Computed tomography showing two large pancreatic pseudocysts located in the head and body of the pancreas in a 65-year-old man.

A number of options for drainage of pancreatic pseudocysts exist. Optimal surgical management requires a mature fibrous pseudocyst wall suitable for anastomosis to create surgical drainage. Generally, 6 to 8 weeks of observation of a new pseudocyst or CT findings of a well-defined wall in a pseudocyst of undetermined age will allow internal drainage. The specific form of drainage advocated depends on the location of the pseudocyst with respect to adjacent structures. A Roux-en-Y cystojejunostomy allows drainage of the pancreatic fluid into a defunctionalized limb and minimizes the risk of reflux of intestinal contents into the pseudocyst cavity. The Roux loop can be anastomosed at the most dependent portion of the pseudocyst to allow optimal drainage. Cystogastrostomy can be performed in situations in which the pseudocyst is tightly adherent to the posterior gastric wall.

Enthusiasm has been generated for the nonsurgical drainage of pancreatic pseudocysts. Cysts can be drained by percutaneous, radiologic catheter drainage or by creation of an endoscopic cystogastrostomy. There have been favorable results for both techniques [51,52]. A prospective randomized trial is currently underway to ascertain the optimal form of management of pancreatic pseudocysts. Although these techniques offer promise, especially in the management of the rare elderly patient with a pancreatic pseudocyst, it should be emphasized that an asymptomatic pseudocyst warrants no treatment, especially in the elderly patient.

Chronic Pancreatitis

Chronic pancreatitis is usually related to alcohol abuse and generally is a disease of younger patients rather than the elderly. Biliary tract disease, the most common cause of acute pancreatitis in the elderly, rarely progresses to chronic pancreatitis, because after recognition, cholecystectomy usually stops the progression of the disease. Idiopathic senile chronic pancreatitis is an uncommon disorder, with a peak age of onset of approximately 65 years. Despite its uncommon nature, chronic pancreatitis is exceeded only by celiac disease as a cause of steatorrhea in patients >65 years of age [53].

Presentation

Approximately 5% of patients with chronic pancreatitis are asymptomatic, but the majority of patients have chronic abdominal or back pain. The elderly patient, however, with idiopathic chronic pancreatitis may have little or no pain. Symptoms of exocrine and endocrine insufficiency may be a major component of chronic pancreatitis in the elderly. Steatorrhea, malabsorption, and weight loss occur in three-fourths of patients. Diabetes associated with pancreatitis is similar to adult onset diabetes; however, these patients frequently have an unusual sensitivity to insulin.

Diagnosis

Chronic pancreatitis is diagnosed by a history of frequent hospitalizations for pancreatitis with the subsequent development of chronic pain. Amylase levels are infrequently elevated. Pancreatic calcification is pathognomonic of chronic pancreatitis (Fig. 24-4). Endocrine and exocrine insufficiency may be present. Exocrine insufficiency can be determined by measurement of a 72-hour fecal fat collection or by bicarbonate and enzyme concentration. A decrease in the bicarbonate output of the duodenal aspirate is a most characteristic finding of chronic pancreatitis.

CT and sonography are useful in the identification of dilated ducts of the biliary tract and pancreas. However, ERCP is the most useful tool for demonstration of pancreatic ductal abnormalities. A dilated duct, strictures, or the presence of strictures and dilatations (chain of lakes) in the pancreatic ductal system may be seen (Fig. 24-5). ERCP is mandatory for the determination of patients who might benefit from surgical procedures for chronic pancreatitis.

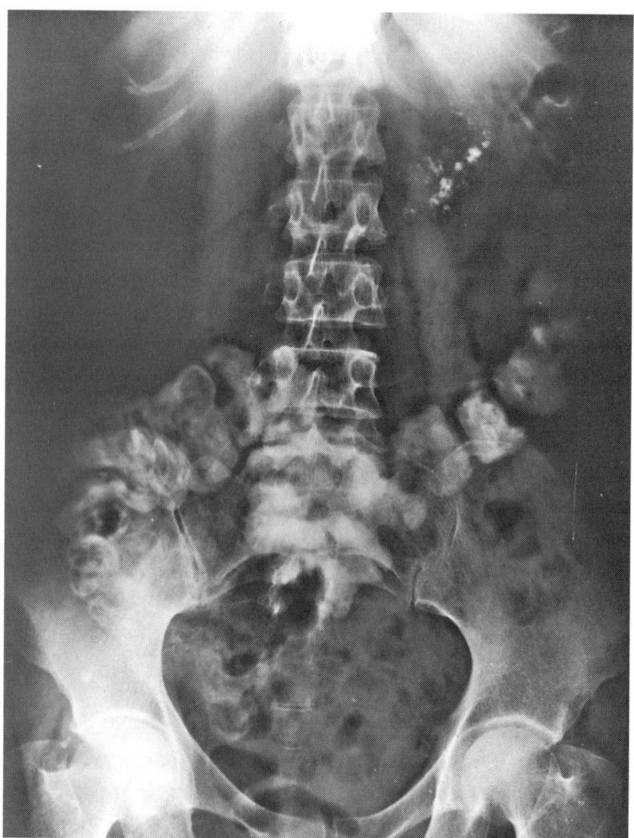

FIG. 24-4. Plain abdominal radiograph demonstrating extensive pancreatic calcification in a patient with chronic pancreatitis.

A major differentiation in the elderly is between chronic pancreatitis and pancreatic cancer (Table 24-7). A number of characteristics such as weight loss, chronic abdominal and back pain, and even jaundice are shared by both diseases. Radiographic studies showing the presence or absence of calcification, ERCP appearance of the pancreatic and biliary ductal system, and CT scan usually differentiate a chronic inflamed gland from a mass in the head of the pancreas [54]. Percutaneous needle aspiration for cytology is helpful, but only if carcinoma is seen on cytology. In many cases a diagnosis cannot be made preoperatively, and even at laparotomy there may be difficulty in distinguishing chronic pancreatitis from pancreatic cancer. Although some believe it is useful to obtain a histologic diagnosis before proceeding with pancreatic resection, it must be remembered that in the most favorable cases of pancreatic carcinoma, obtaining a tissue diagnosis will be most difficult. Therefore, if in the judgment of the surgeon, the clinical and operative findings are consistent with pancreatic carcinoma, proceeding with a pancreaticoduodenectomy may be necessary to provide the absolute differentiation between the two diagnoses.

Management

Medical management of chronic pancreatitis is directed at the precipitating factors such as alcohol or drugs and the complications of pain, diabetes, steatorrhea, and weight loss. Surgical therapy is reserved for persistent jaundice or unrelenting pain. Pancreatic diabetes frequently can be managed by dietary manipulations alone. However, insulin is usually preferred over oral hypoglycemic agents. Steatorrhea and weight loss can usually be managed with the administration of exogenous enzymes. These supplements, given with each meal, decrease the steatorrhea and prevent weight loss as nutritional status improves. H_2 blockers are also useful in increasing gastric pH and therefore increase the delivery of effective enzymes into the duodenum.

The pain of chronic pancreatitis can range from mild discomfort to profound debilitation. Treatment of this chronic pain in the elderly should be of utmost importance to preserve quality of life. In mild or moderate pain, if medical therapy can be maintained long enough, the disease may eventually burn out and subsequently require no therapy. Operative management of chronic pancreatitis for severe pain in the elderly is uncommon. Operative treatment for chronic pancreatitis is ductal decompression. ERCP is essential in determining the form of ductal decompression to be performed. With a dilated ductal system and a single proximal stricture, a retrograde drainage with a pancreatectomy and end-to-side pancreaticojejunostomy (Duvall) procedure will provide ductal decompression. If extensive areas of stricturing and dilatations are present through the entire gland, the side-to-side pancreaticojejunostomy (Peustow procedure) is indicated. In those patients in whom a clear ductal abnormality exists, ductal decompression by either the Duvall or Peustow procedure can provide successful pain relief in up to 80% of cases [55]. Operative mortality is usually low and although postoperative complications are frequent, most are well tolerated. Pancreatic resection may also be necessary in some cases of chronic pancreatitis. In diseases involving the distal gland, resection of anywhere from 70% to 90% of the pancreas can be performed. Distal pancreatectomy may be successful in pain relief with an operative mortality of <5%. In chronic pancreatitis in which extensive changes involve the head of the pancreas or in cases in which is it impossible to rule out pancreatic carcinoma, pancreaticoduodenectomy remains the procedure of choice [56].

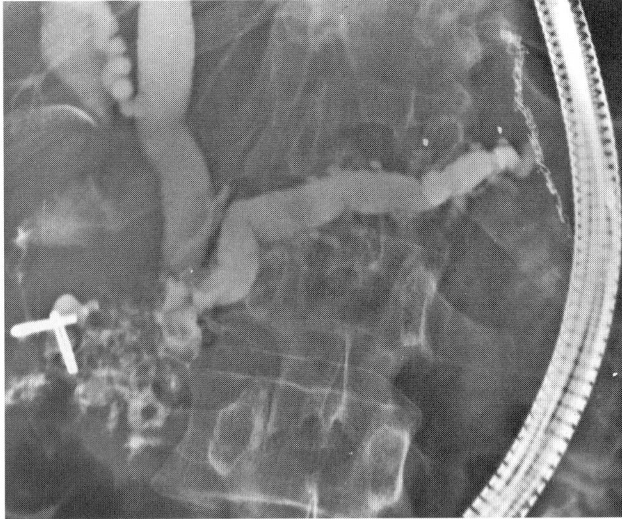

FIG. 24-5. Endoscopic retrograde cholangiopancreatogram in patient with chronic pancreatitis demonstrating dilation of the pancreatic and common bile ducts.

NEOPLASMS OF THE PANCREAS

Pancreatic and Periampullary Carcinoma

Carcinoma of the pancreas has steadily increased in incidence since the 1940s. In the United States, it was estimated that over 28,000 new cases were diagnosed in 1994 [57]. Carcinoma of the pancreas is an extremely lethal disease, with an overall estimated cure rate of <5%. Although it represents only 2% to 3% of all cancers, it results in >6% of can-

TABLE 24-7. *Differential diagnosis of pancreatic cancer and chronic pancreatitis*

Assessment measure	Pancreatic cancer	Chronic pancreatitis
History and physical examination	Jaundice, weight loss, older patients, cigarette smoker, palpable gallbladder (Courvoisier's sign), evidence of metastasis	Alcohol abuse, younger patients, frequent attacks of pancreatitis, steatorrhea
Laboratory data	Elevated bilirubin, liver enzymes, decreased serum albumin	Normal; elevated bilirubin, alkaline phosphatase if biliary obstruction
Plain radiographs	Normal	Pancreatic calcification
Endoscopic retrograde cholangiopancreatography	Ductal cutoff	Chain of lakes appearance, secondary and tertiary ducts, calculi, pseudocysts
Computed tomography/sonography	Mass in pancreas, dilated biliary tree, metastasis	Diffuse enlargement, dilated pancreatic duct, pseudocyst
Angiography	Vessel encasement	Normal
Cytology	Malignant cells	Inflammatory cells

TABLE 24-8. *Relative frequency of periampullary neoplasms*

Location	Percentage
Pancreas	83
Head	70
Body and tail	30
Ampulla of Vater	10
Duodenum	4
Common bile duct	3

cer deaths. Age is one of the principal risk factors for pancreatic cancer. The annual incidence in the age range of 40 to 44 years is approximately 2 per 100,000, increasing thereafter to 100 per 100,000 in the age range of 80 to 84 years, a 50-fold increase [58]. Nearly three-fourths of patients with pancreatic carcinoma are 60 years of age or older. A male-to-female ratio of 1.7 to 1.0 is noted in the overall number, but older patients have an equal sex ratio. Blacks have a higher risk of pancreatic cancer than nonblacks, and it is more common in smokers. Diabetes and chronic pancreatitis are also possible risk factors.

Pathology

Periampullary tumors include tumors of the pancreas, ampulla of Vater, distal bile duct, and duodenum. Adenocarcinoma is by far the most common periampullary tumor, accounting for approximately 85% of tumors in this area. It is, however, difficult to distinguish the primary location of many of these tumors even at laparotomy. Therefore, most large series group all such tumors together. Adenocarcinoma of the pancreas arises from the pancreatic ductal tissue. The most common location for the tumor is the head of the pancreas (65% to 70%) (Table 24-8). Tumors of the head of the pancreas tend to be smaller than tumors in body or tail because they are more apt to be diagnosed earlier by presentation with obstructive jaundice. Nevertheless, the majority of cancers of the pancreas tend to present at an advanced stage. In a large review of >500 cases from the Memorial Hospital in New York, only 14% of tumors were limited to the pancreas, with 21% involving regional lymph nodes. Sixty-five percent had advanced local disease with or without dissemination [59]. These statistics reflect the late presentation seen in the vast majority of patients with pancreatic carcinoma. Adenocarcinomas originating from the distal bile duct and ampulla of Vater usually present with obstructive jaundice earlier in their course, resulting in more localized disease and thus a better chance for cure. Duodenal cancers also have a better prognosis than pancreatic cancer.

Clinical Presentation

Carcinoma of the pancreas often presents in an insidious manner. Screening techniques are not available and the symptoms of pancreatic carcinoma are often vague, nonspecific, and similar to functional gastrointestinal disorders. For tumors arising in the pancreatic head, jaundice eventually leads to the diagnosis. Lesions in the body and tail of the pancreas present with pain, weight loss, and early satiety or nausea. By the time these symptoms have occurred, the disease is almost always locally unresectable or metastatic. The duration of symptoms typically precedes diagnosis by 3 to 6 months, and survival from the time of diagnosis to death is usually <6 months.

Abdominal pain occurs in the majority of patients and is the presenting symptom in up to two-thirds of patients. The pain is most frequently in the midepigastrium or radiating through to the back. Typically, the pain is a dull, boring ache that becomes progressively worse. The pain may be aggravated by food. Weight loss and anorexia occur in almost all patients.

Seventy-five percent of patients with carcinoma of the head of the pancreas develop jaundice that is usually progressive, unremitting, and associated with abdominal pain. The development of jaundice should lead to prompt attempts at diagnosis with a high index of suspicion for an underlying malignancy. In a report of 80 elderly jaundiced patients with a mean age of 75.7 years, malignant obstruction was the most common cause, with pancreatic cancer being the most common neoplasm [60].

A variety of other symptoms including change in bowel habits and abdominal distension may occur, but will contribute little to making an early diagnosis. Early satiety progressing to complete gastric outlet obstruction with nausea and vomiting may occur from duodenal involvement by the tumor, but is usually a late occurrence. Finally, an important historical point that may suggest pancreatic carcinoma in an elderly patient is the new onset of diabetes mellitus or instability of previously well-controlled diabetes. Islet cell injury can result from the obstruction of the pancreatic duct with resultant chronic pancreatitis. Therefore, pancreatic carcinoma should be considered in all such patients.

Diagnosis

There is no screening test currently available for pancreatic carcinoma. To make an early diagnosis of pancreatic cancer, the physician must have a high index of suspicion. The evaluation of any patient with jaundice, regardless of age, should begin with noninvasive imaging studies of the pancreas and biliary tract. CT and ultrasonography of the pancreas and biliary tree are the most sensitive and specific tests for pancreatic disease. CT is probably the better of the two studies in that it will not only demonstrate the presence of biliary duct dilatation but it will also define the presence of a pancreatic mass, pancreatic ductal enlargement, local invasion, and liver metastasis (Fig. 24-6).

If imaging studies demonstrate the presence of biliary obstruction, more invasive techniques to image the biliary system may be indicated. ERCP provides an endoscopic view of the ampulla as well as visualization of the biliary and pancreatic ductal systems (Fig. 24-7). Endoscopic biop-

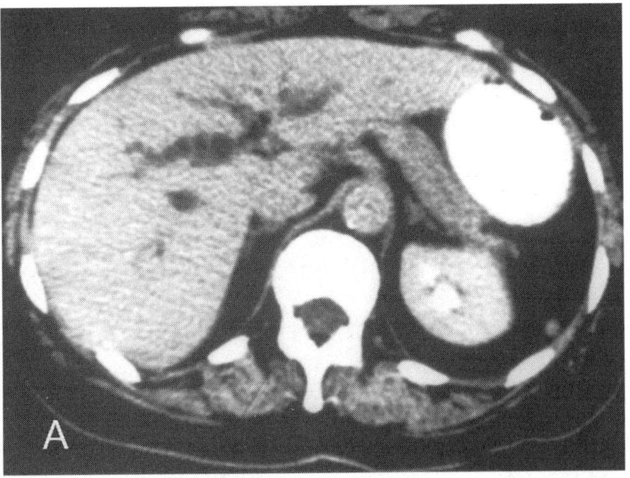

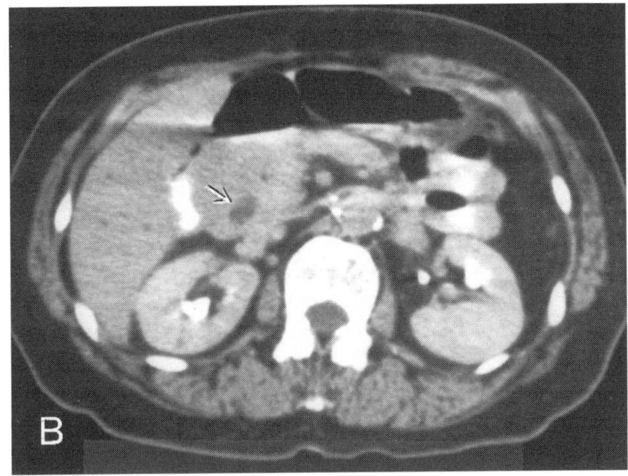

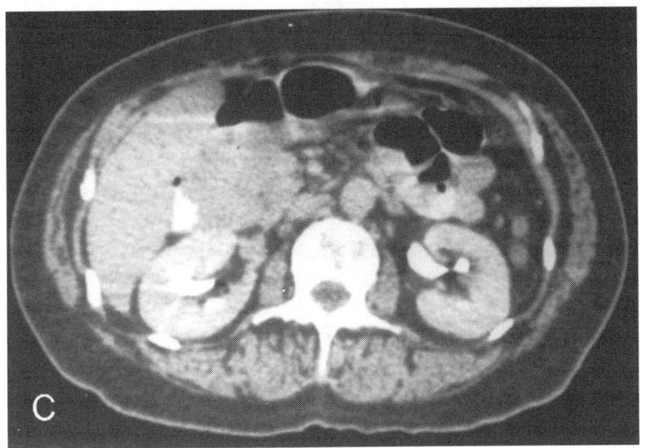

FIG. 24-6. Computed tomography of 73-year-old woman with obstructive jaundice due to pancreatic carcinoma. **(A)** Scan shows dilated intrahepatic bile ducts. **(B)** Scan demonstrates a mass in the head of the pancreas surrounding the dilated common bile duct (*arrow*). **(C)** Scan taken 1 cm inferiorly shows persistence of the pancreatic mass but the absence of the dilated common bile duct, representing complete obstruction of the duct by tumor.

sies of any masses present in the ampulla or periampullary duodenum can be performed. An alternative to ERCP is percutaneous transhepatic cholangiography. The classic cholangiographic finding associated with a pancreatic neoplasm is the tumor meniscus with complete obstruction of the common bile duct at the knee of the biliary tree as it enters the glandular substance of the pancreas (Fig. 24-8). Bile can be aspirated for cytology, as well as brushings taken from the bile duct itself.

Visceral angiography may show vascular involvement suggesting carcinoma but is used primarily as a staging tool in the preoperative investigation of patients thought to be candidates for major pancreatic resection. Major arterial (hepatic, splenic, superior mesenteric) or venous (portal, superior mesenteric, or splenic) encasement is virtually pathognomonic of unresectability (Fig. 24-9). Angiography is primarily a useful technique in avoiding exploration in high-risk patients. In a review from the Johns Hopkins Hospital, if a patient was found by angiography to have major vascular occlusion, the chance of resection was nil [61]. Therefore, appropriate management in an elderly or high-risk patient may be by nonoperative means. Angiography is also useful in detecting anatomic variations such as a replaced right hepatic artery or celiac stenosis, which may alter operative management. Recent information would suggest that contrast-enhanced spiral CT may have similar sensitivity in evaluating patients for resectability.

Management

A number of important risk factors must be considered in the management of carcinoma of the pancreas. These risk factors include the age and life expectancy of the patient, associated medical conditions, extent of the tumor, and the need for palliation of symptoms. It must be stressed, however, that surgical resection offers the only chance for cure with this disease. Although age cannot be an absolute contraindication for surgical management in any patient, in the past it was considered to be a factor in predicting surgical morbidity and mortality. Several decades ago, operative mortality for pancreaticoduodenectomy for periampullary carcinoma was in the range of 15% to 25% for all patients. This rate has decreased significantly in a number of series with mortalities of 5% or less [62–65]. Historically, advanced age was considered a major factor associated with perioperative mortality. Herter et al., noting that major morbidity remained constant in all groups, observed that operative deaths increased from 7.7% in patients 41 to 50 years of age to 25% in patients 61

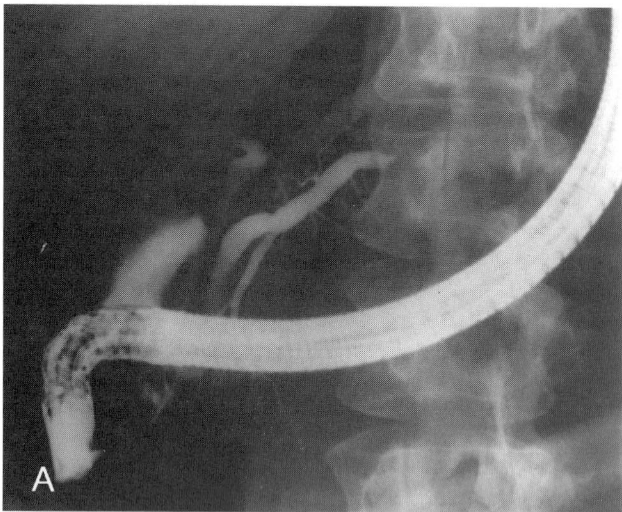

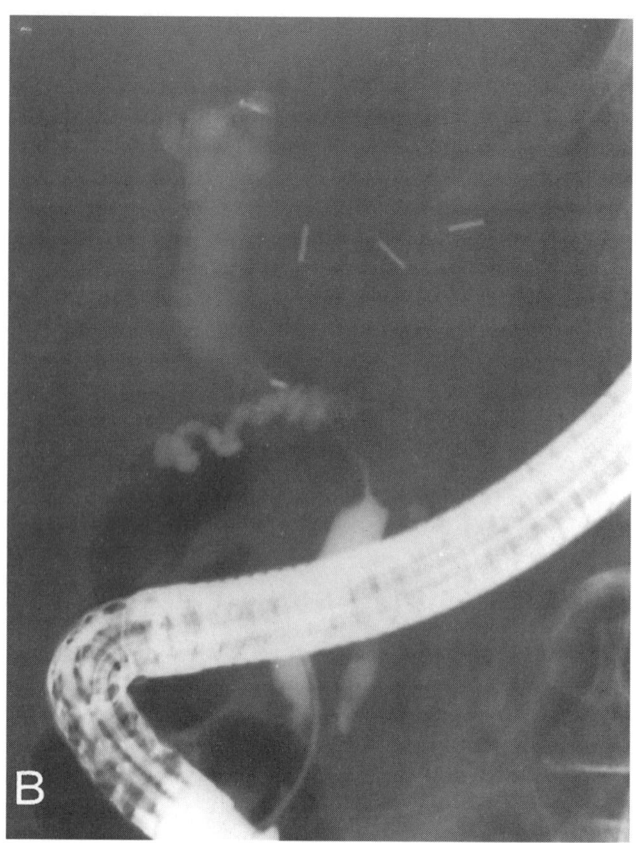

FIG. 24-7. (A) Endoscopic retrograde cholangiopancreatogram demonstrating an abrupt tapering of the pancreatic duct at the pancreatic body due to pancreatic carcinoma in a 72-year-old woman. **(B)** Endoscopic retrograde cholangiopancreatogram of a 71-year-old woman with obstructive jaundice due to pancreatic cancer. The cholangiogram demonstrates a long stricture of the common bile duct just distal to the cystic duct. Dilatation of the proximal bile duct is also seen.

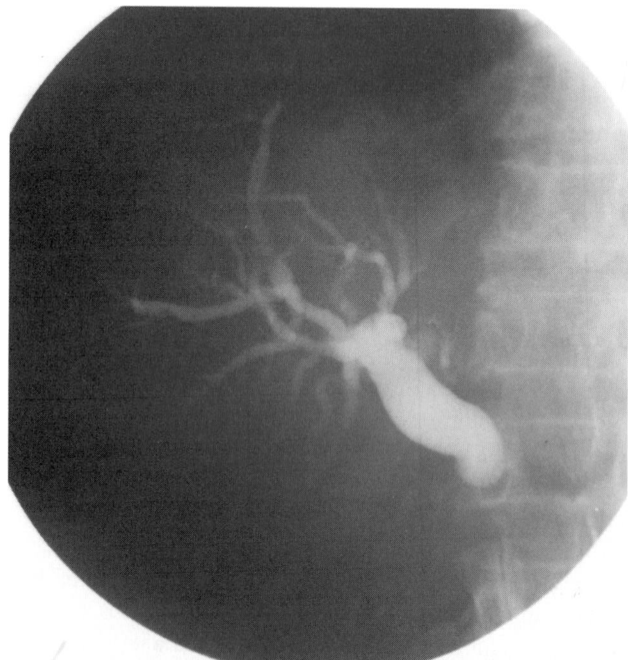

FIG. 24-8. Percutaneous transhepatic cholangiogram demonstrating obstruction of the common bile duct due to pancreatic cancer in a 76-year-old woman. The area of obstruction is at the "knee" of the common bile duct where it enters the glandular substance of the pancreas.

to 70 years of age [66]. Lerut and colleagues also noted a significant increase in mortality (41% vs. 5%, $P < 0.001$) and morbidity (58.8% vs. 16.3%, $P < 0.01$) in patients undergoing pancreaticoduodenectomy over the age of 65 when compared with younger patients [67]. Finally, Obertop and others [68] reported a 33% mortality following pancreaticoduodenectomy in patients >70 compared with 4% in patients <70. In those patients undergoing palliative bypass procedures, there were no deaths in 20 patients <70 years of age. However, two of nine patients >70 (22%) died postoperatively [68].

The view that pancreaticoduodenectomy may be contraindicated in elderly patients has been challenged by data from the Johns Hopkins Hospital [64]. In a report of 145 consecutive pancreaticoduodenectomies performed without a death at our institution, advanced age was not a factor in predicting either morbidity or mortality. In this series, the subgroup of patients 70 years of age or older (n = 37) was compared with those patients 69 years of age and younger (n = 108). No statistically significant differences in preoperative risk factors such as prior myocardial infarction, hypertension, diabetes, chronic obstructive pulmonary disease, peripheral vascular disease, or alcohol use were present in the two groups. No mortalities occurred in either age group nor was there a significant difference in the incidence of postoperative complications. No specific complication was

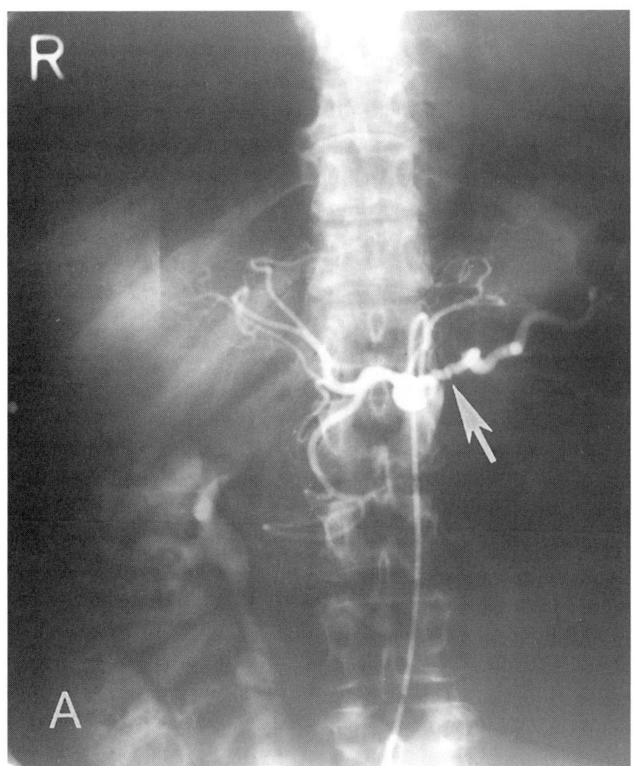

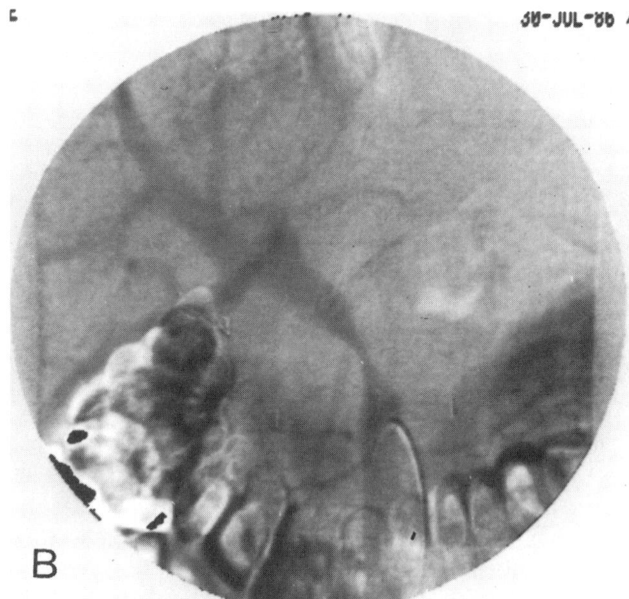

FIG. 24-9. (A) Selective arteriogram of celiac artery demonstrating encasement of splenic artery *(arrow)* in a 72-year-old woman with pancreatic carcinoma. **(B)** Venous phase of selective superior mesenteric arteriogram demonstrating encasement and narrowing of portal vein at the junction of the superior mesenteric vein.

significantly more frequent in the older group, and for many serious complications including intra-abdominal abscess, pancreatitis, and biliary anastomotic leak, patients over the age of 70 actually had a lower incidence (Table 24-9). The hospital courses of the two groups were also similar. Operative time, estimated blood loss, number of transfusions per patient, and the length of hospital stay were not significantly different. This experience suggests that age is no longer even a relative contraindication for pancreaticoduodenectomy of carcinoma of the head of the pancreas.

Similar excellent overall results have also been reported from other centers. Delcore and colleagues reported a series of 42 patients undergoing pancreaticoduodenectomy between the ages of 70 and 80 years [69]. The incidence of major complications was 14%, with two operative deaths (5%). Hannoun and colleagues in Paris reported perioperative morbidity and mortality in 223 patients undergoing pancreaticoduodenectomy for periampullary neoplasms [70]. Forty-four patients were 70 years of age or older. The perioperative morbidity was similar in both groups (35%). The operative mortality was 4.5% in the older patients versus 10% in those patients <70 years of age.

Unfortunately, by the time the diagnosis is made, many patients with carcinoma of the pancreas are surgically unresectable. Thus, optimal palliation of symptoms, to maximize the quality of life, is of primary importance. The three primary symptoms warranting palliation are obstructive jaundice, gastric outlet obstruction, and pain. The palliation of patients with unresectable pancreatic carcinoma has evolved significantly with the introduction of nonoperative palliation of jaundice. Four prospective studies have been completed in which surgical bypass has been compared with nonoperative biliary stenting for malignant obstructive jaundice [71–74] (Table 24-10). The conclusions of these studies are similar, demonstrating that both techniques are equally effective in the relief of jaundice. Nonoperative palliation, however, seems to be accompanied by lower complication rates, lower procedure-related mortality, and a shorter initial period of hospitalization. As a result of these studies, great enthusiasm has been generated for the nonoperative palliation of periampullary carcinoma especially in older patients. Advocates of surgical palliation, however, criticize these studies on two counts. First, 30-day mortality in the surgical arms of these studies ranges from 15% to 24%, much higher

TABLE 24-9. *Postoperative complications after pancreaticoduodenectomy*

Postoperative complication	Age <69 yrs (%, n = 108)	Age >70 yrs (%, n = 37)
Delayed gastric emptying	32	46
Pancreatic fistula	19	22
Intra-abdominal abscess	10	5
Wound infection	6	11
Pancreatitis	7	3
Biliary leak	6	3
Cholangitis	5	5
None	52	38

TABLE 24-10. *Results of randomized comparison of nonoperative versus surgical bypass for palliation of obstructive jaundice*

	Bornman [71]		Shepard [72]		Andersen [73]		Smith [74]	
	Stent	Operation	Stent	Operation	Stent	Operation	Stent	Operation
Success (%)	84	76	82	92	96	88	95	94
Complication (%)	28	32	30	56	36	20	11	29
30-day mortality (%)	8	20	9	20	20	24	3	14
Hospital stay (days)	18	24	5	13	26	27	20	26
Late complications								
Jaundice/cholangitis	38	16	30	0	0	0	35	2
Gastric outlet obstruction	14	0	9	4	0	0	17	7
Survival (wks)	19	15	22	18	12	14	21	26

than in many surgical series. Second, nonoperative palliation is frequently associated with late complications of recurrent jaundice and gastric outlet obstruction. Self-expanding endoprostheses may be associated with a lower incidence of late jaundice.

In a review from the Johns Hopkins Hospital, 118 consecutive patients underwent surgical palliation for unresectable periampullary adenocarcinoma [75]. The most common operative procedure was a combined biliary bypass and gastrojejunostomy performed on 75% of the patients. A gastrojejunostomy either with biliary bypass or alone was performed in 107 of the 118 patients (91%). The hospital mortality was 2.5%. Postoperative complications occurred in 37% of the patients but were seldom life-threatening. During late follow-up, only 4% of the patients had gastric outlet obstruction and only 2% had recurrent jaundice. The mean survival time postoperatively was 7.7 months. This series did not compare morbidity and mortality based on subgroups of age. However, 70% of the patients were 60 years of age or older, 35% were 70 years or older, and 4% were 80 years or older. The three deaths all occurred in patients 60 years of age or older. However, only one death occurred in a patient over the age of 70. This series concluded that surgical palliation of unresectable periampullary carcinoma can be completed with minimal perioperative mortality, acceptable morbidity, and provide good palliation.

The role of prophylactic gastrojejunostomy for palliation in patients with unresectable pancreatic carcinoma is controversial. A review of >8,000 patients reported in the English literature from 1965 to 1970 determined that creation of a gastrojejunostomy did not increase operative mortality [76]. Moreover, if a gastrojejunostomy was not performed, 13% of patients had subsequent duodenal obstruction requiring a gastrojejunostomy before death and nearly 20% of the remaining patients died with symptoms of gastroduodenal outlet obstruction.

Pain is the last feature of pancreatic carcinoma that frequently requires palliation. Epigastric and back pain can become the most incapacitating and disabling of symptoms that a patient can experience. The actual incidence of severe unrelenting pain due to pancreatic carcinoma is probably in the range of 30% to 35% but increases significantly in the advanced stages of disease. In a randomized prospective double-blind study completed at the Johns Hopkins Hospital, intraoperative chemical splanchnicectomy with 50% alcohol was compared with a placebo injection of saline in patients with histologically proven unresectable pancreatic carcinoma [77]. The two groups were similar by all preoperative criteria, with a mean age of patients in both groups of 64 years. Patients were assessed preoperatively and after hospital discharge using a visual analog scale for pain, mood, and disability. The results of this study showed no difference in hospital mortality or complications, time to return to oral intake, or length of hospital stay between the two groups. Mean pain scores were significantly lower in the alcohol group at 2-, 4-, and 6-month follow-up and at the final assessment before the patient's death. Patients were stratified into those patients who had significant pain preoperatively versus those patients without preexisting pain. In patients without preoperative pain, alcohol significantly delayed or prevented the subsequent onset of pain. In patients with significant preoperative pain, alcohol significantly reduced pain. Finally, a surprising observation was that in those patients with significant preoperative pain who received alcohol celiac axis injection, a significant improvement in survival was observed when compared with the controls. Celiac axis chemical splanchnicectomy should therefore be performed in all patients found to have unresectable pancreatic carcinoma undergoing laparotomy. In those patients not undergoing laparotomy, percutaneous celiac axis injection using either fluoroscopic or CT guidance can effectively control pain in the majority of patients.

In conclusion, the management of an elderly patient with suspected periampullary carcinoma must be individualized. If the patient's overall health status does not preclude consideration of surgical management and the spiral CT scan shows no evidence of liver metastases or carcinomatosis, a visceral angiogram should be completed. If major visceral involvement is not present, the patient should undergo exploration for possible pancreaticoduodenectomy. If operative findings preclude resection, a palliative biliary bypass, gastrojejunostomy, and chemical splanchnicectomy should be performed.

In patients with preoperative evidence of unresectability based on CT scan or visceral angiography, the decision to use operative versus nonoperative palliation of obstructive jaundice must also be individualized. Overall medical state, extent of disease with predicted life expectancy, and the presence of symptoms of impending duodenal obstruction are all factors to consider. Age alone should not be a primary factor, although in the elderly debilitated patient with advanced pancreatic cancer, nonoperative palliation offers an attractive option.

Preparation for Operation

If the decision is made to proceed with an operation for periampullary carcinoma in an elderly patient, proper preoperative preparation is required. Thorough assessment of cardiopulmonary status, renal and hepatic function, the state of hydration and nutrition, and anemia and coagulation abnormalities are necessary. All efforts should be made to optimize the patient's overall health before proceeding with operation for either resection or palliation.

A major question is the value of preoperative biliary decompression in these patients. Biliary decompression can be performed by either percutaneous transhepatic drainage or by the placement of an endoscopic stent. Although initially uncontrolled studies showed a benefit for such drainage by decreasing operative morbidity and mortality, a subsequent prospective controlled randomized trial performed by Pitt and colleagues at the University of California, Los Angeles, showed no benefit [78]. The length of hospital stay and hospital costs were significantly increased by preoperative biliary decompression. In both benign and malignant obstruction, there was no difference in the results based on the nature of obstruction, advanced age, level of bilirubin, or other potential risk factors. In contrast, Lyaidakis and his group in Amsterdam, using preoperative endoscopic drainage in patients with cancer of the head of the pancreas, significantly reduced perioperative morbidity and mortality [79]. It appears likely, therefore, although not indicated routinely, that in selected patients with advanced malnutrition, sepsis, or correctable medical conditions, preoperative drainage is useful to improve the patient's overall health status.

Postoperative Care and Complications

Adequate fluid and electrolyte maintenance as well as glucose regulation, pulmonary care, nutritional support, and provision of antibiotics are routine. Biliary contrast examination is done at postoperative day 4 or 5 to demonstrate the biliary anastomosis. A gastrografin upper gastrointestinal series may follow to determine the status of the gastrointestinal anastomosis as well as the return of gastric emptying. If all studies are satisfactory, perioperative drains from the area of the biliary and pancreatic anastomosis can be removed and oral intake can be initiated slowly, watching for potential delays in gastric emptying.

A number of complications can occur following pancreaticoduodenectomy. The leading complication in the Hopkins' experience has been delayed gastric emptying [64]. A randomized prospective study from our institution has found a decrease in this overall complication by the use of perioperative IV erythromycin as a prokinetic agent for gastric motility [80]. Leakage at the pancreatic anastomosis has been particularly disastrous in the past. Experience suggests that although the incidence of anastomotic leak remains at 10% to 20%, adequate placement of perianastomotic drains and improved postoperative management has lessened the severity of this complication [62,64,81]. A prospective study at Hopkins compared the results following the operative techniques of pancreaticojejunostomy and pancreaticogastrostomy [81]. The incidence of anastomotic leak was similar with both techniques (12%). Multivariant analysis revealed that the experience of the surgeon and the texture of the pancreas determined the likelihood of a pancreatic fistula. Age was not a significant factor in predicting anastomotic leak. Although the occurrence of a pancreatic leak significantly prolonged hospital stay, no deaths were observed in those patients.

The incidence of complications after pancreaticoduodenectomy and palliative operations for pancreatic carcinoma continues to be high (35% or greater); however, most of these are not life-threatening. In general, the improvements in the management of these complications have resulted in reports of reduced operative mortality. The elderly patient, however, frequently lacks the reserve to handle such complications, and failure to avoid these complications may be disastrous with ensuing multisystem organ failure and eventual death.

Results of Operation

For many years the operative mortality for pancreaticoduodenectomy at major centers has been in the 10%-to-25% range. As previously noted, significant reductions in perioperative mortality have occurred [62–65]. Although a number of factors may contribute to this reduction, the most likely reason lies in the concentration of more patients in the hands of surgeons in major centers with extensive experience with the procedure. If an elderly patient is thought to be a candidate for surgical resection, consideration of referral to such a center should be made [82].

Despite the improvements in the surgical management, the results for long-term survival remain less than optimum. The best results appear to come from three series in which a 5-year survival of 20% was achieved for pancreatic carcinoma [62,63,83]. Ampullary, distal bile duct, and duodenal carcinoma appear to be associated with a better 5-year survival in the range of 40% to 60%. A number of factors have been identified as prognostic indicators for long-term survival following a pancreaticoduodenectomy [83]. These include tumor size <3 cm, diploid tumor DNA content, negative surgical margin results, negative lymph node states, and the decade of resection. Age is not a predictor of survival.

Cancer of the Body and Tail of the Pancreas

Survival for carcinoma of the body and tail of the pancreas is even more dismal than that for cancer of the pancreatic head. The silent asymptomatic nature of these tumors leads to late presentation, usually too late for consideration for resection. The diagnosis of these tumors can frequently be made by percutaneous techniques because of the advanced size at the time of diagnosis. Because often such tumors are not associated with obstructive jaundice, there is little benefit to proceeding with laparotomy for diagnosis. Preoperative arteriography demonstrating major vessel encasement or occlusion followed by percutaneous biopsy for tissue diagnosis usually eliminates the need for exploratory laparotomy. In patients with significant pain associated with the tumor, percutaneous celiac axis block can provide excellent long-term palliation.

Role of Chemotherapy and Radiation Therapy for Pancreatic Carcinoma

Because of the modest results following resection for patients with pancreatic carcinoma, attention has turned to adjuvant chemotherapy or radiation therapy for this disease. A prospective randomized study has demonstrated a significant improvement with the addition of postoperative radiation therapy and single-agent chemotherapy using 5-fluorouracil [84]. This protocol is reasonably well tolerated by patients and should be recommended for all patients undergoing resection of a pancreatic carcinoma regardless of age if their overall postoperative health status will allow such therapy.

The role of radiotherapy and chemotherapy for unresectable pancreatic carcinoma is limited primarily to palliation and likely offers little benefit to those elderly patients with unresectable pancreatic carcinoma in which palliation for pain and jaundice can be managed by other means.

CYSTADENOMA AND CYSTADENOCARCINOMA

Cystadenoma and cystadenocarcinoma are neoplastic cystic lesions of the pancreas. Cystadenomas account for approximately 10% of nonmalignant cystic lesions of the pancreas, and cystadenocarcinomas represent 1% of the primary pancreatic malignant lesions. Cystadenoma appears primarily in middle-aged women. However, reports of patients in their 70s and 80s have appeared. Cystadenocarcinoma occurs at about the same age as pancreatic exocrine cancers, that is, between 50 and 70 years of age. There is no sex predilection in this group.

The symptoms of cystadenoma and cystadenocarcinoma are virtually identical. Patients usually present with abdominal pain, weight loss, nausea, vomiting, anorexia, weakness, or an enlarging abdominal mass. Jaundice is uncommon with the benign cystadenoma but can occur in up to one-fourth of patients with cystadenocarcinomas [85].

The management of these lesions is surgical excision. Complete excision of the lesion for pathologic examination is important because needle biopsy is not suitable for detecting malignant potential. Cystadenomas are classified as either serous or mucin producing. The serous cystadenomas, or microcystic adenomas, are benign and thought to have little or no malignant potential. The mucinous cystadenomas are often filled with a mucinous material and thought to have malignant potential, with the ability to progress to a cystadenocarcinoma. Surgical resection of either benign lesion is generally considered curable. In a review of cystic tumors from the Johns Hopkins Hospital, 67% of cystadenocarcinomas were resectable at the time of surgical exploration [85]. The 5-year survival in this group was 72%.

ENDOCRINE TUMORS OF THE PANCREAS

Tumors of the endocrine and pancreatic islet cells are relatively unusual, making up only 10% of pancreatic neoplasms. They are of great interest, however, because of the unique clinical syndromes associated with the effects of gastrointestinal hormones that they produce. Although islet cell tumors are uncommon in older age groups, their occurrence has been reported.

Insulinomas, a tumor of the pancreatic B cells, was the first recognized and is the most common endocrine tumor of the pancreas. Insulinomas can occur in all age groups, but the age of presentation is usually in the range of 20 to 75 years, with a mean age in the mid-40s. In two large series, 25% to 33% of patients were >60 years of age [86,87]. Approximately 60% of cases are in women. These tumors produce insulin autonomously, and thus produce symptomatic hypoglycemia with secondary symptoms related to a hypoglycemia-induced surge of catecholamines. These symptoms include tremor, restlessness, irritability, weakness, diaphoresis, and palpitations. Progressive and prolonged hypoglycemic attacks may lead to neuropsychiatric symptoms that may be particularly confusing and hard to diagnose when seen in the elderly.

The diagnosis of insulinoma depends on the documentation of fasting hypoglycemia and inappropriately elevated insulin levels. The classic triad of insulinoma was described by Whipple and Frantz in 1935 [88]: (1) symptoms of hypoglycemia with fasting, (2) blood sugar level <50 mg/100 ml, and (3) relief of symptoms with glucose administration. The addition of a radioimmunoassay for insulin confirms the diagnosis by documenting an insulin level >25 U/ml. The measurement of concomitant serum levels of connecting peptide, which is released by the B cell on a one-to-one basis with endogenous insulin, is valuable to rule out surreptitious insulin administration.

Insulinomas can now be preoperatively localized in many cases. CT scan and ultrasonography are frequently not helpful because of the small size of the tumors, often <2 cm. Arteriography appears to be the most commonly available test for detection of insulinomas, identifying the tumor in up to 75% of the cases (Fig. 24-10). Eighty percent of insulinomas are benign and single, with 10% benign and multiple. Ten percent of insulinomas are malignant. Ninety-eight percent of insulinomas are found in the pancreas, and 2% of ectopic insulinomas are located in peripancreatic or periduodenal sites. The treatment of insulinoma is surgical. If the tumor is identified at operation and found to be located superficially, it can be enucleated without damage to the underlying duct. If the tumor is embedded in the body or tail, a distal pancreatectomy should be performed. In the rare case when the lesion is embedded in the head of the pancreas, pancreaticoduodenectomy may be indicated.

The results of surgical therapy for insulinoma are excellent, with complete cure after resection in 70% to 80% of cases. Ten percent of patients develop diabetes postresection no matter how much pancreas is removed. Approximately 10% to 15% have persistent or recurrent hypoglycemia. In those cases of malignant insulinoma, debulking procedures provide significant palliation in 60% to 70% of cases.

The Zollinger-Ellison syndrome of gastric hypersecretion with virulent peptic ulcer disease, caused by hypergastremia from a non-B islet cell tumor has been recognized since the mid-1950s. As in the other pancreatic endocrine tumors, the discovery of the causative peptide, gastrin, and the development of its radioimmunoassay have improved our understanding of the disease and its diagnosis and management. Gastrinomas are now recognized to occur both in a sporadic form (75%) or as a component of the multiple endocrine neoplasia I. In contrast to insulinomas, the majority (60%) of gastrinomas are malignant, with metastasis in up to 50% of these.

Gastrinomas account for only 0.1% of all peptic ulcer disease in the United States and for 2% of recurrent peptic ulcers after standard ulcer operations. Gastrinomas have been reported in all age groups, but as in other pancreatic endocrine tumors, the usual age of presentation is in patients 40 to 50 years old. Almost every series, however, includes patients over the age of 70.

The clinical presentation for most patients with Zollinger-Ellison syndrome (70% to 95%) is abdominal pain related to peptic ulcer disease. Approximately 20% of patients have diarrhea as the initial symptom either with or without ulcer disease. Another 30% develop diarrhea later during their course. Because the incidence of severe peptic ulcer disease has decreased markedly in this country, consideration of gastrinoma should be given to all cases with severe complications or intractability due to usual medical management.

The diagnosis of Zollinger-Ellison syndrome is based on gastric analysis with a basal acid output of >15 mEq per hour. Such levels of acid secretion are uncommon in elderly patients. Because acid secretion is at or near maximum stimulated state, the pentagastrin-stimulated acid secretion is not much higher than the basal level. A ratio of basal to stimulated acid secretion of 0.6 or greater suggests gastrinoma. The mainstay of diagnosis of gastrinoma is the serum gastrin level. Most patients with gastrinoma have basal gastrin levels >500 pg/ml, with those patients with peptic ulcer disease usually having levels <100 pg/ml. Intermediate levels may require stimulation testing with secretin, which shows elevations in patients with gastrinoma but not in normal patients or those with peptic ulcer disease, antral hyperplasia, or retained antrum.

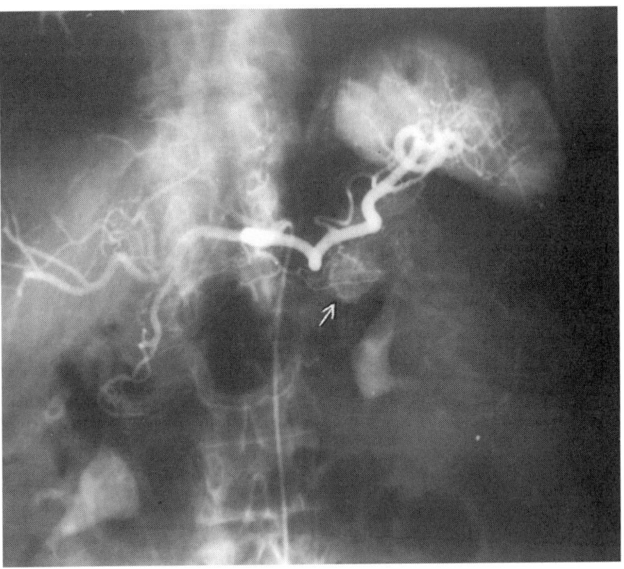

FIG. 24-10. Selective arteriogram of the celiac artery in an 80-year-old woman with an insulinoma. The hypervascular well-circumscribed tumor in the inferior aspect of the pancreas is shown (*arrow*).

The initial management of patients with gastrinoma consists of control of acid secretion by either histamine-receptor antagonists or omeprazole. All patients should undergo evaluation for localization of the gastrinoma using CT scan, selective arteriography, and in rare cases, selective venous sampling. In those good-risk patients including the elderly with localized disease, surgical exploration and attempt at resection are warranted. This is possible in 20% to 30% of patients. The management of those patients who are preoperatively found to have extensive disease or who are found to have unresectable tumors at operation consists of pharmacologic control of acid secretion. This treatment is based on rigid control of acid secretion as determined by measurement of gastric acid output. It appears that nearly all gastrinoma can be controlled by this means, and failure is related to inadequate dosing. Surgical therapy for gastric hypersecretion should be left only for those patients with complications or who fail medical management.

The major benefit of surgical resection of gastrinoma, besides acid control, is the malignant potential of these tumors. Unfortunately, only approximately 30% of patients are found to have localized disease at the time of diagnosis [89]. In those patients, including the elderly who are an otherwise good risk without evidence of liver metastasis, surgical exploration of the pancreas and surrounding viscera and attempted resection are warranted. In most cases, resection can consist of local excision of the gastrinoma including any peripancreatic lymph nodes in the draining area of the gastrinoma, which may be the only method by which it is determined whether the gastrinoma is benign. In the past, it was considered that regional metastasis precluded a cure. However, there is increased evidence that the biological behavior of malignant gastrinomas that have metastasized to the lymph nodes differs from that of tumors that have metastasized to the liver. Surgical excision of both the primary tumor and the involved lymph nodes may cure the disease. Unfortunately, the projected cure rate for gastrinomas is only 25% to 30%. It should be emphasized, especially in the elderly, that gastrinomas are slow-growing tumors, and even without surgical therapy 5- and 10-year survival rates approach 30% to 40%.

A number of other pancreatic endocrine tumors with associated syndromes have been recognized. Such tumors are rare, with only small numbers in reported series. In general, the tumors are uncommon in the elderly. In addition, nonfunctioning islet cell tumors do occur. The majority of these tumors are malignant and frequently do not present until they have reached such a large size that resection for cure is uncommon.

REFERENCES

1. Kreel L, Sandin B. Changes in pancreatic morphology associated with aging. Gut 1973;14:962.
2. Rossle O. Beitrage Zur Kentniss der gesunden und der kranken bauchspeicheldruse. Beitraege zur pathologicshen Anatomie und zur allgemeinen. Pathologie 1921;163:69.
3. Schmitz-Moormann P, Himmelmann GW, Brandes JW, et al. Comparative radiological and morphological study of the human pancreas: pancreatitis-like changes in post-mortem ductograms and their morphological pattern. Possible implication for ERCP. Gut 1985;26:406.
4. Szalaij W, Skwarskil L, Namiot Z, et al. Endoscopic retrograde pancreatography in elderly patients. Mater Med Pol 1991;23:21.
5. Cotton PB. The normal endoscopic pancreatogram. Endoscopy 1974; 6:65.
6. Wallace SA, Ashwarth CT. Histopathology of the senile pancreas. Tex State J Med 1942;37:584.
7. Andrew W. Senile changes in the pancreas of Wistar Institute rats and of man with special regard to the similarity of locule and cavity formation. Am J Anat 1944;74:97.
8. DiMagno EG, Go VLW, Summerskill WHJ. Relations between pancreatic enzyme outputs and malabsorption in severe pancreatic insufficiency. N Engl J Med 1973;288:813.
9. Bartos V, Groh J. The effect of repeated stimulation of the pancreas on the pancreatic secretion in young and aged men. Gerontol Clin 1969;11:56.
10. Rosenberg IR, Friedland N, Janowitz HD, Dreiling DA. The effect of age and sex upon human pancreatic secretion of fluid and bicarbonate. Gastroenterology 1966;50:191.
11. Langier R, Sarles H. The pancreas. Clin Gastroenterol 1985;14:749.
12. Chen M, Bergman RN, Pacini G, et al. Pathogenesis of age-related glucose intolerance in man: insulin resistance and decreased β-cell function. J Clin Endocrinol Metab 1985;60:13.
13. Fenjö G. Acute abdominal disease in the elderly. Am J Surg 1982; 143:751.
14. Ponka JL, Welborn JK, Brush BE. Acute abdominal pain in aged patients: an analysis of 200 cases. J Am Geriat Soc 1983;11:993.
15. Corfield AP, Cooper MJ, Williamson RCN. Acute pancreatitis: a lethal disease of increasing incidence. Gut 1985;26:724.
16. Imrie CW, Benjamin IS, Ferguson JC, et al. A single-centre double-blind trial of Trasylol therapy in primary acute pancreatitis. Analysis of factors influencing survival. Ann Surg 1977;185:43.
17. Jacobs ML, Daggett WM, Civetta JM, et al. Acute pancreatitis: analysis of factors influencing survival. Ann Surg 1977;1285:43.
18. Ranson JHC, Rifkind KM, Roses DF, et al. Prognostic signs and the role of operative management in acute pancreatitis. Surg Gynecol Obstet 1974;139:69.
19. Lee SP, Nicholls JF, Park HZ. Biliary sludge as a cause of acute pancreatitis. N Engl J Med 1992;326:589.
20. Park J, Fromkes J, Cooperman M. Acute pancreatitis in elderly patients. Am J Surg 1986;152:638.
21. MacMahon M, Walsh TN, Brennan P, et al. Endoscopic retrograde cholangiopancreatography in the elderly: a single unit audit. Gerontology 1993;39:28.
22. Warshaw AL, O'Hara PJ. Susceptibility of the pancreas to ischemic injury in shock. Ann Surg 1978;188:197.
23. Feiner H. Pancreatitis after cardiac surgery. Am J Surg 1976;131:684.
24. Lefor AT, Vuocolo P, Paulsen EB, Sillin LF. Pancreatic complications following cardiopulmonary bypass. Factors influencing mortality. Arch Surg 1992;127:1225.
25. Mallory A, Kern F. Drug-induced pancreatitis: a critical review. Gastroenterology 1980;78:813.
26. Gambill EE. Pancreatitis associated with pancreatic carcinoma: a study of 26 cases. Mayo Clin Proc 1971;465:174.
27. Browder W, Patterson MD, Thompson JL, Walters DN. Acute pancreatitis of unknown etiology in the elderly. Ann Surg 1993;217:469.
28. Cooperman M, Ferrara JJ, Carey LC, et al. Idiopathic acute pancreatitis: the value of endoscopic retrograde cholangiopancreatography. Surgery 1981;90:666.
29. Weaver DW, Bouwman DL, Walt AJ, et al. A correlation between clinical pancreatitis and isoenzyme patterns of amylase. Surgery 1982;92:576.
30. Hill MC, Barkin J, Isikoff MB, et al. Acute pancreatitis: clinical vs. CT findings. AJR Am J Roentgenol 1982;139:263.
31. Ranson JHC, Balthazar E, Cacarale R, Cooper M. Computerized tomography and prediction of pancreatic abscess in acute pancreatitis. Ann Surg 1985;201:656.
32. Pollock AV. Acute pancreatitis. Br J Med 1959;1:6.
33. Ranson JHC, Rifkind KM, Turner JW. Prognostic signs and nonoperative peritoneal lavage in acute pancreatitis. Surg Gynecol Obstet 1976;143:209.
34. Ranson JHC. Etiologic and prognostic factors in human acute pancreatitis: a review. Am J Gastroenterology 1982;77:633.
35. Stone HH, Fabial TC. Peritoneal dialysis in the treatment of acute alcoholic pancreatitis. Surg Gynecol Obstet 1980;150:828.
36. Ranson JHC, Berman RS. Long peritoneal lavage decreases pancreatic sepsis in acute pancreatitis. Ann Surg 1990;211:708.
37. Acosta JM, Rossi R, Galli OMR, et al. Early surgery for gallstone pancreatitis: evaluation of a systematic approach. Surgery 1978;83:367.
38. Neoptolemos JP, Car-Locke DL, London NJ, et al. Controlled trial of urgent endoscopic retrograde cholangiopancreatography and endoscopic sphincterotomy versus conservative treatment for acute pancreatitis due to gallstones. Lancet 1988;2:979.
39. Fan ST, Zai ECS, Mok FPT, et al. Early treatment of acute biliary pancreatitis by endoscopic papillotomy. N Engl J Med 1993;328:228.
40. Soper NJ, Callery MP, Brunt LM, et al. The role of laparoscopic cholecystectomy in the management of gallstone pancreatitis. Am J Surg 1994;167:42.
41. Bradley EL, Allen K. A prospective longitudinal study of observation versus surgical intervention in the management of necrotizing pancreatitis. Am J Surg 1991;161:19.
42. Rattner DW, Legermate DA, Lee MJ, et al. Early surgical debridement of symptomatic pancreatic necrosis is beneficial irrespective of infection. Am J Surg 1992;163:105.
43. Ranson JHC, Turner JW, Roses DF, et al. Respiratory complications in acute pancreatitis. Ann Surg 1974;179:557.
44. Beger HG, Bittner R, Block H, Buchler M. Bacterial contamination of pancreatic necrosis: a prospective clinical study. Gastroenterology 1986;1:433.
45. Ranson JHC, Spencer FC. Prevention, diagnosis, and treatment of pancreatic abscess. Surgery 1977;82:99.
46. Gerzof SG, Banks PA, Robbins AH, et al. Early diagnosis of pancreatic infection by computed tomography–guided aspiration. Gastroenterology 1987;93:1315.
47. Bradley El, Fulenwider JJ. Open treatment of pancreatic abscess. Surg Gynecol Obstet 1984;159:509.
48. Stone HH, Strom PR, Mullins RJ. Pancreatic abscess management by subtotal resection and packing. World J Surg 1984;8:340.

49. Siegelman SS, Copeland BE, Saba GP, et al. CT of fluid collections associated with pancreatitis. Am J Radiol 1980;134:1121.
50. Yeo CJ, Bastidas JA, Lynch-Nghan A, et al. The natural history of pancreatic pseudocysts documented by computed tomography. Surg Gynecol Obstet 1990;170:411.
51. Kozarek RA, Patterson DJ, Ball TJ, Traverso LW. Endoscopic placement of pancreatic stents and drains in the management of pancreatitis. Ann Surg 1989;209:261.
52. van Sonnenberg E, Wittich GR, Casola G, et al. Percutaneous drainage of infected and noninfected pancreatic pseudocysts. Experience in 101 cases. Radiology 1989;170:757.
53. Price TL, Gazzard BG, Dawson AM. Steatorrhea in the elderly. Br J Med 1977;1:1538.
54. Mackie CR, Cooper MJ, Lewis MH, Moossa AR. Non-operative differentiation between pancreatic cancer and chronic pancreatitis. Ann Surg 1979;189:480.
55. Frey CF, Suzuki M, Isaji S, Zhu Y. Pancreatic resection for chronic pancreatitis. Surg Clin North Am 1989;69:499.
56. Rossi RL. Pancreatic resection for chronic pancreatitis. Hepatogastroenterology 1990;37:277.
57. Steele GD Jr., Osteen RT, Winchester DP, et al. Clinical highlights from the National Cancer Data Base: 1994. CA Cancer J Clin 1994;44:71.
58. MacMahon B. Risk factors for cancer of the pancreas. Cancer 1982;50:2676.
59. Cubilla AL, Fitzgerald PJ. Surgical Pathology of Tumors of the Exocrine Pancreas. In Moossa AR (ed), Tumors of the Pancreas. Baltimore: Williams & Wilkins, 1980;159.
60. Doll R, Muir M, Waterhous J (eds). Cancer Incidence in Five Continents (Vol 2). Internationalia Contre le Cancer, Geneva, Switzerland, 1970.
61. Dooley WC, Cameron JL, Pitt HA, et al. Is preoperative angiography useful in patients with periampullary tumors. Ann Surg 1992;211:649.
62. Crist DW, Sitzmann JV, Cameron JL. Improved hospital morbidity, mortality and survival after the Whipple procedure. Ann Surg 1987;206:358.
63. Trede M, Schwall G, Saeger H. Survival after pancreaticoduodenectomy. Ann Surg 1990;211:447.
64. Cameron JL, Pitt HA, Yeo CJ, et al. One hundred and forty-five consecutive pancreaticoduodenectomies without mortality. Ann Surg 1993;217:430.
65. Castillo CF, Rattner DW, Warshaw AL. Standards for pancreatic resection in the 1990s. Arch Surg 1995;130:295.
66. Herter FP, Cooperman AM, Ahlborn TN, Antinori C. Surgical experience with pancreatic and periampullary cancer. Ann Surg 1982;195:274.
67. Lerut JP, Gianello PR, Otte JB, Kestens PJ. Pancreaticoduodenal resection: surgical experience and evaluation of risk factors in 103 patients. Ann Surg 1984;199:432.
68. Obertop H, Bruining HA, Schattenkerk ME, et al. Operative approach to cancer of the head of the pancreas and the periampullary region. Br J Surg 1982;69:573.
69. Delcore R, Thomas JH, Hermreck AS. Pancreaticoduodenectomy for malignant pancreatic and periampullary neoplasms in elderly patients. Am J Surg 1991;162:532.
70. Hannoun L, Christophe M, Ribeiro J, et al. A report of forty-four instances of pancreaticoduodenal resection in patients more than seventy years of age. Surg Gynecol Obstet 1993;177:556.
71. Bornman PC, Harries-Jones EP, Tobias R, et al. Prospective controlled trial of transhepatic incurable carcinoma of the head of the pancreas. Lancet 1986;1:69.
72. Shepard HA, Royle G, Ross APR, et al. Endoscopic biliary endoprosthesis in the palliation of malignant obstruction of the distal common bile duct: a randomized trial. Br J Surg 1988;75:1166.
73. Andersen JR, Sorensen SM, Kruse A, et al. Randomized trial of endoscopic prosthesis versus operative bypass in malignant obstructive jaundice. Gut 1989;30:1132.
74. Smith AC, Dowsett JF, Russell RCG, et al. Randomised trial of endoscopic stenting versus surgical bypass in malignant low bile duct obstruction. Lancet 1994;344:1655.
75. Lillemoe KD, Sauter PK, Pitt HA, et al. Current status of surgical palliation of periampullary carcinoma. Surg Gynecol Obstet 1993;176:1.
76. Sarr MG, Cameron JL. Surgical management of unresectable carcinoma of the pancreas. Surgery 1982;91:123.
77. Lillemoe KD, Cameron JL, Kaufman HS, et al. Chemical splanchnicectomy in patients with unresectable pancreatic cancer. A prospective randomized trial. Ann Surg 1993;217:447.
78. Pitt HA, Gomes AS, Louis JF, et al. Does preoperative percutaneous biliary drainage reduce operative risk or increase hospital cost? Ann Surg 1985;201:545.
79. Lyaidakis NJ, Van Der Heyde MN, Lubler MJ. An evaluation of preoperative biliary drainage in the surgical management of pancreatic head carcinoma. Acta Chir Scand 1987;153:665.
80. Yeo CJ, Barry MK, Sauter PK, et al. Erythromycin accelerates gastric emptying following pancreaticoduodenectomy. Ann Surg 1993; 218:229.
81. Yeo CJ, Cameron JL, Maher MM, et al. A prospective randomized trial of pancreaticogastrostomy versus pancreaticojejunostomy after pancreaticoduodenectomy. Ann Surg 1995;222:580.
82. Gordon TA, Burleyson GP, Tielsch JM, Cameron JL. The effects of regionalization on cost and outcome for one general high-risk surgical procedure. Ann Surg 1995;221:43.
83. Yeo CJ, Cameron JL, Lillemoe KD, et al. Pancreaticoduodenectomy for cancer of the head of the pancreas: 201 patients. Ann Surg 1995;221:721.
84. Kalser MH, Ellenberg SS. Pancreatic cancer: adjuvant combined radiation and chemotherapy following curative resection. Arch Surg 1985;120:899.
85. Talamini MA, Pitt HA, Hruban RH, et al. Spectrum of cystic tumors of the pancreas. Am J Surg 1992;10:117.
86. Glickman MH, Hart MJ, White TT. Insulinoma in Seattle: 39 cases in 30 years. Am J Surg 1980;140:119.
87. van Heerden JA, Edis AJ, Service FJ. The surgical aspects of insulinomas. Ann Surg 1979;198:677.
88. Whipple AO, Frantz VK. Adenoma of the islet cell with hyperinsulinism. Ann Surg 1935;101:1299.
89. Wolfe MM, Jensen RT. Zollinger-Ellison syndrome: current concepts in diagnosis and management. N Engl J Med 1987;317:1209.

Surgical Care for the Elderly, 2nd ed., edited by
R. Benton Adkins, Jr., and H. William Scott, Jr.
Lippincott–Raven Publishers, Philadelphia © 1998.

CHAPTER 25

Diseases of the Small Bowel

R. Benton Adkins, Jr., and James G. Drougas

The normal physiologic and functional responses of the small bowel to the general process of aging are still not thoroughly understood. One might expect intestinal function to become sluggish with age, but experimental and clinical evidence does not indicate any major functional abnormalities that occur in the aging intestine. Functional small bowel problems in the elderly are more often the result of systemic disorders and drug ingestion than any measurable effect of aging itself.

NORMAL EFFECTS OF AGING

The small intestine decreases in weight after age 40. The mucosal parenchyma is reported to be replaced to some degree by fibrous tissue, and fewer healthy smooth muscle fibers are seen [1]. However, anatomic and histologic changes in the aging intestine have been difficult to identify as a specific alteration due to the *normal* result of aging. In many of the earlier studies of the aging gut, neither the nutritional state nor the presence or absence of disease in the study group was addressed, although these conditions are known to have a considerable effect on mucosal structure and protein and enzyme content of the small bowel. This should be kept in mind as the literature on the subject is reviewed.

In the mid- and late 1970s, several studies were published that reported abnormal small bowel histology in aged rats. The abnormalities included villus atrophy, decreased villus height, decreased length of the small bowel, disoriented microvilli, and increased collagen and amyloid within the mucosa. None of these reports, however, included mention of the overall health status of these older rats. In 1984, Holt et al. studied the effects of aging on the small bowel in a large group of Fischer 344 rats [2]. These animals were barrier-reared, checked regularly for infections, and maintained since birth on the same diet. They found villus-crypt length and villus height in the duodenum and jejunum in the older rats to be identical to that in the young. Ileal villus height and crypt depth were actually greater in the older rats. Of course, normal histology does not arbitrarily equate with normal function. Holt and his coworkers found that the functional expression of several enzymes in the epithelial cells of the intestinal villus was delayed in aged rats [2]. This supports a paradoxic notion that the epithelial cells in the aged small bowel are more immature than those seen in the young.

Considerable experimental and clinical research has addressed the question of malabsorption in the elderly. The general consensus of most researchers is that aging is accompanied by a component of malabsorption in the small bowel; however, morphologic changes that might account for this malabsorption have not yet been identified. Small bowel bacterial overgrowth is an increasingly recognized phenomenon in the elderly. Researchers have shown that treatment of these patients with cyclic antibiotic therapy is accompanied by increases in weight, body fat, serum protein, and calcium levels [3].

Carbohydrate absorption has been studied by many researchers [4–9]. The results of their studies do not consistently provide evidence for, but are suggestive of, an age-related reduction in carbohydrate absorption by the bowel. Moreover, Feibusch and Holt suggest that a further absorption impairment occurs in elderly subjects aged 75 and older [9]. It has been suggested that this malabsorption in the older elderly is the result of some type of malfunction in the mucosal cells, specifically in the intestinal enzyme production.

The investigations of fat absorption have been hampered by the problems involved with the use of institutionalized subjects. In these elderly individuals, systemic diseases and nutritional deficits have been present and thus may interfere with normal lipid absorption. There are studies demonstrating decreased absorption of lipids with increasing age: Holt and Dominguez found that the intestinal absorption of triolein was reduced in the elderly apparently due to impaired luminal uptake and delayed transintestinal transport [10]. However, one review of the literature actually demonstrated that lipid absorption is well preserved in the elderly [11]. The data remain equivocal due to the uncontrolled variables of systemic diseases, concomitant pharmacotherapy, and baseline nutrition deficits in this patient population.

Little information is available about protein absorption in the elderly, and the studies that have been done have also produced conflicting findings. There is general agreement that overall protein absorption is not diminished by the aging process. There is disagreement, however, in the amount of protein normally required to maintain a positive nitrogen balance in the elderly. Gersovitz et al. have suggested that, in advanced age, the process of albumin synthesis responds less well to altered types and amounts of dietary protein [12].

There is some evidence that fat-soluble vitamins are absorbed as readily, if not more readily, in the elderly individual as they are in younger persons. Vitamin D may be an exception to this general hypothesis. Concentrations of plasma 25-hydroxycholecalciferol are also found to be lower in elderly subjects. Water-soluble vitamins do not appear to be poorly absorbed in the elderly [4].

It appears that calcium absorption may decrease with advancing age. The need for research in this area is great because of the prevalence of osteoporosis and osteomalacia in the elderly. There is strong evidence to support the thesis that the major factor causing these conditions may be an age-related deficiency in vitamin D, which may then prevent or alter normal calcium absorption [4]. However, there are some data that suggest senile hyperparathyroidism is a compensatory mechanism by which the body maintains serum calcium homeostasis [13]. The long-term effects of senile hyperparathyroidism on bone density remain unclear.

Concentrations of serum iron and transferrin are generally expected to decrease with advanced age, but the large number of studies on this subject do not provide absolute proof of this decrease. A host of clinical conditions may also be responsible for the increased incidence of iron-deficiency anemia in the elderly. Intestinal blood loss should be excluded first when iron deficiency or any type of anemia occurs in the elderly.

Intestinal Motility

As the geriatric population base has continued to increase, the amount of research in the area of gut motility has also increased. Human studies evaluating the motility of the small bowel have yielded equivocal results in the past [3,14]; however, more recent data seem to suggest that small bowel motility in healthy elderly subjects is normal when compared with that of younger patients. One study revealed slightly delayed gastric emptying in elderly patients when compared with younger controls, but the study showed no difference in the small bowel transit time [14]. More recent studies evaluating the electrical activity of the gut have demonstrated similar motility patterns throughout the aging process in humans [15,16]. Most often, small intestinal motility is hampered by systemic disease and the multiple medications taken by the elderly patient.

INFLAMMATORY BOWEL DISEASE

Although inflammatory bowel diseases (IBDs) are generally considered to be disorders of the young, they are not that uncommon in the elderly. In many series, a bimodal incidence curve is seen, with a secondary increase in the incidence of IBD in patients between 50 and 80 years old, and most often near age 70 [17]. It has been estimated that approximately 8% to 20% of all patients with IBD are over age 60 [18].

Most reports indicate that recurrence of quiescent IBD is less likely in older patients than in younger age groups. This hypothesis is difficult to prove; however, it is based on the available data. In most reported series, those patients who develop IBD at age 60 or 65 are not separated from those who had the disease before that age [4].

In many series, a distinction is not made between IBD of the small bowel and IBD of the colon. Shapiro et al. describe the experience with IBD in 33 patients over age 60. Eighteen had the disease confined to the small bowel and four others had ileocolitis. The remaining 11 had colonic disease only [19].

The presenting symptoms of IBD in the elderly are much the same as those seen in younger patients. Diarrhea, weight loss, and abdominal cramps are the primary symptoms, with less common symptoms including fever and rectal bleeding. Considering that Crohn's disease is not generally thought of as a diagnosis in the elderly, the diagnosis is even more difficult because of the extensive differential diagnosis entertained in the elderly patient with abdominal cramps, diarrhea, and fever, including diverticular disease, malignancy, tuberculosis, and colitides due to ischemia, infection, or radiation. Shapiro et al. found the differential diagnosis to be difficult in their series from Beth Israel Hospital [19]. Another study showed a fourfold increase in delayed diagnosis of IBD in the elderly population when compared with younger patients [20].

Watts et al. have emphasized the severe morbidity and mortality associated with the initial onset of IBD in elderly patients, and they recommend early operative treatment [21]. Others have pointed out that all inflammatory diseases are more poorly tolerated in older age groups and that postoperative mortality is greater in older patients. These authors call for a more conservative approach to the elderly with IBD [22]. We agree with Watts and his colleagues and suspect that Gupta's group could avoid the complications and postoperative deaths they report if they would begin to treat their cases with early resection when indicated.

The medical treatment of Crohn's disease in the elderly is generally the same as that in younger patients. However, complications of medical therapy are common in the elderly population. One study demonstrated a 40% complication rate in elderly patients on long-term corticosteroid treatment [23]. Osteoporosis, atherosclerosis, diabetes, glaucoma, cataracts, and hypertension may all be worsened by the use of corticosteroids. Metronidazole is often efficacious in the treatment of IBD, but its use may be limited by the occurrence of peripheral neuropathy. Immunosuppressive regimens should also be used judiciously in elderly patients, who may be more sensitive to these agents. We recommend early diagnosis followed by intensive preoperative preparation and early surgical intervention for the elderly patient with IBD.

MESENTERIC ISCHEMIA

Intestinal problems resulting from circulatory disorders are seen almost exclusively in older age groups. In an early study, Brandfondbrener et al. showed that reduced mesenteric flow occurred in the elderly as a result of reduction in resting cardiac output [24]. Another contributing factor may be a reduced responsiveness to physiologic need in the elderly. For example, the shift in blood volume occurring after a meal can produce hypotension in healthy elderly subjects, presumably because of age-associated blunting of sympathetic baroreflex sensitivity. Concomitant diseases, such as congestive heart failure, frequently result in poor intestinal perfusion.

Atherosclerotic vascular disease does not have the dramatic effect on the function of the small intestine that might be expected. Holt points out that the gradual development of complete proximal obstruction of the three major intestinal vessels can be accompanied at times by no symptoms and that a minimum of two vessels must be involved before signs of intestinal ischemia are seen [4].

Acute intestinal ischemia, on the other hand, usually occurs abruptly with the onset of severe abdominal pain. It may be the result of superior mesenteric artery embolism or thrombosis, mesenteric venous thrombosis, or nonocclusive mesenteric ischemia. The mortality for acute occlusive intestinal ischemia is >70% in most series [25,26]. Embolic mesenteric ischemia has a more favorable prognosis than mesenteric artery thrombosis, because most emboli lodge distal to the origin of the middle colic artery. This permits partial perfusion of the midgut through the middle colic artery and its branches. Thrombotic superior mesenteric artery occlusion occurs at its orifice and sacrifices middle colic perfusion. In these cases, the diagnosis is often confirmed by the emergency use of mesenteric arteriography and should be followed by immediate surgical intervention.

Gradual occlusion of abdominal vessels by progressive atherosclerosis occasionally produces pain that may be confused with peptic ulcer disease or cholelithiasis [27]. Bouts of "abdominal angina," or chronic mesenteric ischemia, usually occur with meals. Patients often have a fear of eating and present with significant weight loss, which can be confused with the presence of an occult malignancy. Ischemic ileitis usually occurs in patients >50 years of age when inferior mesenteric artery disease is accompanied by congestive heart failure, hypertension, or other conditions that decrease blood flow to the abdominal vessels. Abdominal pain and bloody diarrhea are the most common symptoms and may occur in varying degrees of severity. If not treated by immediate revascularization, intestinal gangrene can occur that will require operative intervention and resection. Antibiotics and intravenous fluids are appropriate treatment for less serious cases.

Nonocclusive mesenteric ischemia usually is seen in the setting of congestive heart failure, anoxia, shock, or high-dose alpha-adrenergic drugs. This is often a problem in the elderly patient in the intensive care unit with cardiac failure. In these situations, blood is shunted preferentially to the brain and other vital organs, causing intestinal ischemia. The diagnosis is confirmed with mesenteric arteriography, which reveals a patent mesenteric arterial trunk with spastic tapering of its branches. Primary treatment consists of improving cardiac function, but superior mesenteric arterial infusion of papaverine can help vasodilate the small mesenteric vessels as a temporizing measure. It is an ominous finding with poor prognosis. One study reported a 100% mortality in elderly patients who developed nonocclusive mesenteric ischemia after cardiopulmonary bypass [28]. Surgical resection is often necessary due to transmural necrosis and perforation.

DIVERTICULAR DISEASE

Uncommon in patients under age 40, diverticula occur with considerable frequency in older individuals. Approximately 20% to 30% of patients over 60 and >40% of those over 70 have diverticular disease [29]. Moreover, the number of diverticula usually found in a given individual is likely to increase in older persons.

Diverticula may occur singularly in the duodenum. Pearce has reported an incidence of 20.1% of duodenal diverticula in patients in a geriatric hospital (average age, 80.1 years) compared with 6.5% in a general hospital [30]. He found that these lesions are rarely responsible for nutritional deficiencies.

It has been reported that 60% of duodenal diverticula are juxtapapillary [4]. Duodenal diverticula have been associated with biliary calculi in some reports. It has been suggested that patients with juxtapapillary diverticula have an associated choledochoduodenal sphincter dysfunction [4]. We recommend a conservative surgical approach to duodenal diverticula in the elderly. We have tended to treat only those that bleed, perforate, or ulcerate (Fig. 25-1).

Diverticula of the jejunum and ileum are seldom solitary lesions. These false diverticula are acquired lesions that occur on the mesenteric side of the intestine, protrude into the mesentery, and may be hidden by mesenteric fat. Fifty percent of patients with small bowel diverticula have concomitant colonic involvement [31,32]. Most often occurring in the proximal jejunum, they can be asymptomatic for considerable periods; however, perforation, hemorrhage, formation of enteroliths, and bezoars may result in more severe cases. The

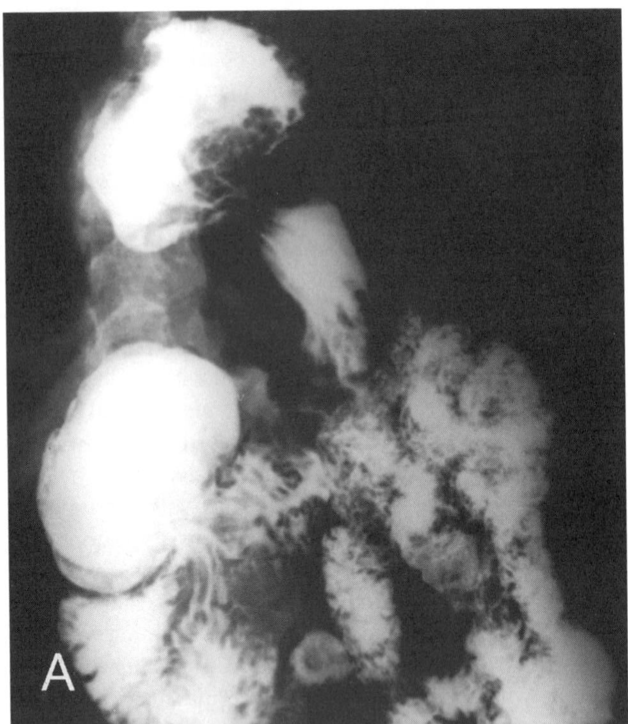

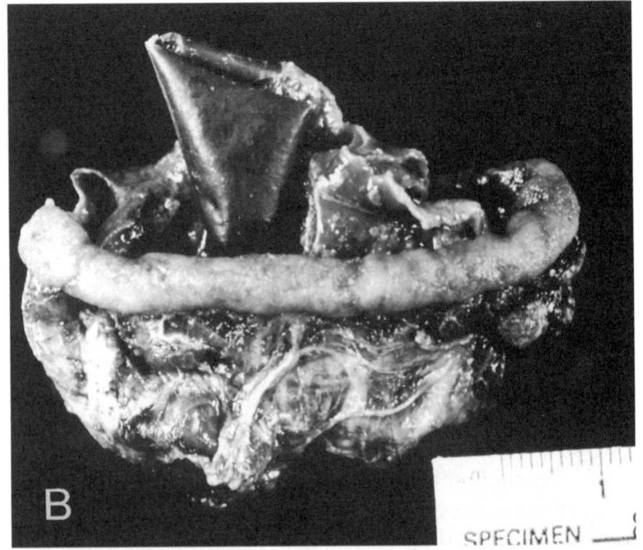

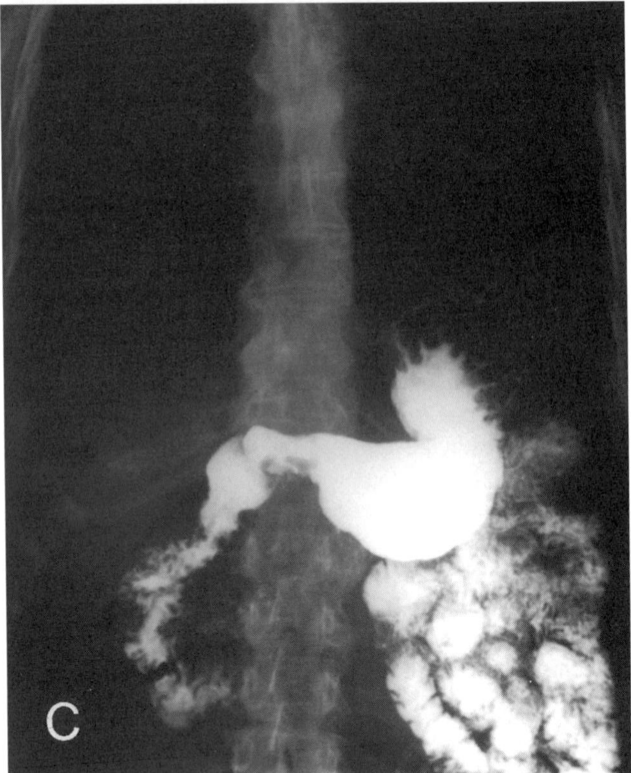

FIG. 25-1. (A) An upper gastrointestinal series done for chronic abdominal complaints and anemia in a 76-year-old woman shows a moderate-sized hiatal hernia and an enormous juxtapapillary duodenal diverticulum. Notice the suggestion of foreign material inferiorly within the diverticulum. **(B)** Resected specimen showing duodenal diverticulum. The opening is 5 cm in diameter with a receptacle-like appearance and contains debris, food particles, and fruit peelings. Notice the rim of ulcerated mucosa secondary to foreign body trauma. **(C)** Postoperative film done 6 weeks after operation showing no evidence of hiatal hernia and absence of the large duodenal diverticulum. The patient remains symptom free with a normal hematologic profile more than 1 year postoperatively at age 78 years.

symptoms resulting from the consequential bacterial overgrowth are more insidious. These may include abdominal cramps, distension, diarrhea, steatorrhea, vitamin B_{12} deficiency, and weight loss. These symptoms occasionally may be treated successfully with antibiotics. Most often, however, surgical intervention and intestinal resection are necessary.

Unlike the acquired false diverticula of the jejunum and proximal ileum, Meckel's diverticula are congenital lesions affecting 2% of the general population [33]. The risk of complications from a Meckel's diverticulum was thought to decrease with increasing age, making its incidental removal at celiotomy in older patients unnecessary. However, a population-based study from the Mayo Clinic demonstrated the lifetime risk of complication to be 6.4% until age 80, without a decrease in the incidence of complications in the elderly [34]. This study also revealed a sixfold and twofold increase in the morbidity and mortality, respectively, for patients undergoing operation for complications of Meckel's diverticulum compared with its incidental removal. We support the notion that routine removal of an incidentally encountered Meckel's diverticulum in most elderly patients is warranted.

SMALL BOWEL OBSTRUCTION

Intestinal obstruction occurs frequently in older age groups. In one reported series, operations for intestinal obstruction were the second most common emergency surgical procedures in patients over age 70 [35]. Characteristically, symptoms include abdominal pain, vomiting, abdominal distention, and obstipation. The etiology can include postoperative adhesions, incarcerated hernia, gallstone ileus, cecal carcinoma, small bowel tumors (primary or metastatic), Crohn's disease, foreign bodies, or even volvulus in the setting of a congenital malrotation. Elderly persons have a higher mortality from intestinal obstruction than is seen in younger patients, making prompt diagnosis and treatment imperative. In 1978, 70% of patients who died from small bowel obstruction were >70 years of age [36]. Usually, however, the mortality from intestinal obstruction resulting from nonmalignant conditions is much lower than in those instances of malignant obstruction (10% vs. 41%). Reiss and Deutsch's work supports this notion; the mortality for their elderly patients with benign obstructive conditions was only 6% [35]. Under elective conditions (i.e., in the absence of sepsis or gangrene), the mortality decreased to 0%. Obviously, early operative treatment of small bowel obstruction is important for a good result. Some authors have reported that elderly patients with intestinal strangulation do not always present with the classic signs of that disorder. Zadeh et al. found this to be true in 35% of the older patients they treated for small bowel obstruction [36]. In one-half of these cases, operative treatment was delayed for some reason for more than 24 hours. In that group, the morbidity increased from 50% to 71%. They have concluded that in the absence of carcinomatosis, Crohn's disease, early postoperative obstruction, and partial small bowel obstruction, operative management of suspected small bowel obstruction should be done expeditiously.

SMALL BOWEL NEOPLASMS

Only 5% of all gastrointestinal tract neoplasms occur in the small bowel. This low incidence is surprising when one considers that the small bowel accounts for >75% of the length and >90% of the absorptive surface of the entire gastrointestinal tract [37,38]. Local factors in the small bowel, such as mild alkalinity or neutral pH and a rapid transit time have been thought to help prevent the development of neoplasms. The incidence of benign and malignant small bowel tumors varies from author to author, but when taken in aggregate, relatively equal rates for benign and malignant small bowel neoplasms are seen [39]. The average age of patients diagnosed as having benign small bowel neoplasms is 62 years, whereas most patients with malignant tumors are slightly younger at diagnosis (57 years) [40]. In some reports, as many as 62% of malignant tumors are seen in patients in their sixth and seventh decades of life [41]. There is a higher incidence of small bowel neoplasms in cases of familial polyposis, Gardner's syndrome, Crohn's disease, and other inherited disorders of the gastrointestinal tract.

Benign Tumors

Almost 50% of all benign tumors of the small bowel are asymptomatic, and approximately one-third are found incidentally at the time of autopsy. When these tumors are symptomatic, pain is usually the presenting complaint. In >50% of these cases, the pain is the result of partial or total obstruction. Intussusception, caused by the tumor, can also result in intestinal obstruction. Mild chronic bleeding resulting from mucosal involvement with the tumor occurs in approximately one-fourth of patients who are symptomatic [42,43]. Benign tumors are usually not large enough to be palpable, but if so, they are generally freely mobile. Rarely do benign tumors cause malabsorption, jaundice, or signs of an acute abdominal condition.

Approximately 35% of all benign small bowel tumors are adenomas [44,45]. These growths are the result of benign proliferation of epithelium from the mucosa or mucosal glands. Most of these lesions are polypoid, but villous adenomas and Brunner's gland adenomas also occur. Although adenomas of Brunner's glands are rare, when present, they may cause symptoms similar to those of peptic ulcer disease, that is, duodenal obstruction and bleeding. Surgical excision is the treatment of choice.

Adenomatous polyps occur in the duodenum more often than in other areas of the small intestine. Generally, they are solitary, but multiple adenomatous polyps can occur. Although usually asymptomatic, these lesions can result in intussusception, obstruction, or chronic intestinal bleeding. If symptomatic or found incidentally at laparotomy, surgical excision is indicated. When intussusception or obstruction has occurred, reduction of the twist or intussusception and segmental resection of the bowel will be necessary. As mentioned earlier, the risk incurred by emergency procedures in older patients is considerable, and the prognosis is improved significantly when elective procedures are possible [46]. Those polyps discovered on routine gastroduodenoscopy should be managed by endoscopic retrieval.

A subset of patients can present with diffuse gastroduodenal polyposis—those patients with familial adenomatous polyposis. It has become increasingly evident that these patients have an increased risk of duodenal carcinoma with increasing age [47]. The incidence of duodenal polyposis in patients with familial adenomatous polyposis is 30% to 60%, and this increases with age [47,48]. Following colectomy, the main cause of death in patients with familial adenomatous polyposis is upper gastrointestinal malignancy, which generally presents 20 years postoperatively. The true risk of duodenal carcinoma remains unclear, but malignant transformation may be in the range of 3% to 5% [49–51]. An aggressive approach to endoscopic surveillance and clear-

TABLE 25-1. *Review of the literature on malignant tumors of the small intestine, 1920 to 1960*

Location	Number
Total cases	
Duodenum	136
Jejunum	184
Ileum	308
Multiple	22
Total	650
Sarcomas	
Duodenum	12
Jejunum	61
Ileum	118
Multiple	17
Total	208
Carcinomas	
Duodenum	113
Jejunum	108
Ileum	98
Multiple	2
Total	321
Carcinoid tumors	
Duodenum	11
Jejunum	15
Ileum	92
Multiple	3
Total	121

Source: Reprinted with permission from Rochlin DB, Longmire WP. Primary tumors of the small intestine. Surgery 1961;50:586–592.

ance in duodenal polyposis is warranted, with operative management reserved for those good-risk patients with dysplasia, carcinoma, or severe polyposis. In those patients considered poor surgical candidates, treatment with sulindac has shown some efficacy in decreasing the number and size of duodenal polyps [52].

Villous adenomas occur rarely in the small bowel and reportedly make up <1% of small bowel neoplasms [53]. Like adenomatous polyps, these lesions are usually asymptomatic unless they have grown to be quite large. Up to one-half of these lesions become malignant if left untreated [54,55]. When symptomatic, crampy intermittent pain and intestinal bleeding are usually present. Mucous diarrhea may rarely occur with large tumors. These lesions produce filling defects radiographically and are successfully diagnosed preoperatively in 75% of cases [56]. Surgical excision is the only treatment for villous adenomas. Large lesions may require segmental resection, and if there is evidence of malignancy, excision with wide margins (10 cm) and including all of the involved mesentery is necessary. For large duodenal lesions with malignant transformation, a pancreaticoduodenal resection should be performed.

Fibromas of the small intestine make up approximately 8% of all benign small bowel tumors. Arising from the subserosa, these tumors usually extend intraluminally. Many of these tumors remain undiagnosed because they do not typically produce symptoms. When symptomatic, intussusception and obstruction usually occur and excision is necessary.

Malignant Tumors

Over 90% of patients with malignant tumors of the small bowel are symptomatic. Weight loss, pain, anemia, and nausea and vomiting account for the vast majority of symptoms [44]. Sawyer and his coworkers described a symptom complex they thought was typical for malignant tumors of the small intestine. The symptom complex consists of consecutive gurgling bowel sounds, a sense of abdominal fullness, cramps, nausea, and vomiting [45]. This series of events occurs intermittently at the same intervals of time following each of three daily meals. This complex of symptoms was more predictable with lesions of the proximal jejunum but occurred with tumors at all small bowel sites.

When studied with upper gastrointestinal radiography, 75% to 80% of malignant tumors of the small bowel can be seen or their presence suspected [42]. In those tumors of the duodenum, nearly 100% should be seen on upper gastrointestinal series [45]. Those in the terminal ileum may be seen more easily with barium enema using reflux of the barium to the midileum [41].

In Rochlin and Longmire's comprehensive review of small bowel tumors, the pertinent literature of the preceding 40 years was carefully reviewed, and the site of occurrence of 650 neoplasms of various types was documented [57]. Carcinomas, sarcomas, carcinoids, and metastatic lesions were found to occur in the small bowel, with a general tendency of distribution of adenocarcinomas proximally and lymphosarcomas distally (Table 25-1). To the authors' knowledge, a review of this magnitude has not since been reported. The current situation, however, continues to reflect this early report. In more recent series, adenocarcinoma occurs primarily in the duodenum, and next most frequently in the jejunum. Carcinoids and lymphosarcoma occur mostly in the ileum, whereas the other types of sarcomas are usually evenly distributed in all parts [41,42,45,57,58].

In an extensive review by Resnick and Cooper, 40% of the cancers of the duodenum were found to be suprapapillary, 40% subpapillary, and only 20% periampullary [59]. Most of these tumors required a major resection, usually a pancreaticoduodenectomy [57].

Ileal and jejunal tumors always require a wide segmental resection including the mesentery all the way to its base. We prefer a 10-cm margin proximally and distally for all small bowel carcinomas or sarcomas [60–62].

Carcinoid tumors are the most common malignant small bowel tumors in most reported series [58,63] and therefore deserve special mention. These are neuroendocrine tumors that most often occur in the ileum and appendix. When metastatic to the liver, they can produce the carcinoid syndrome, which is characterized by flushing, diarrhea, and

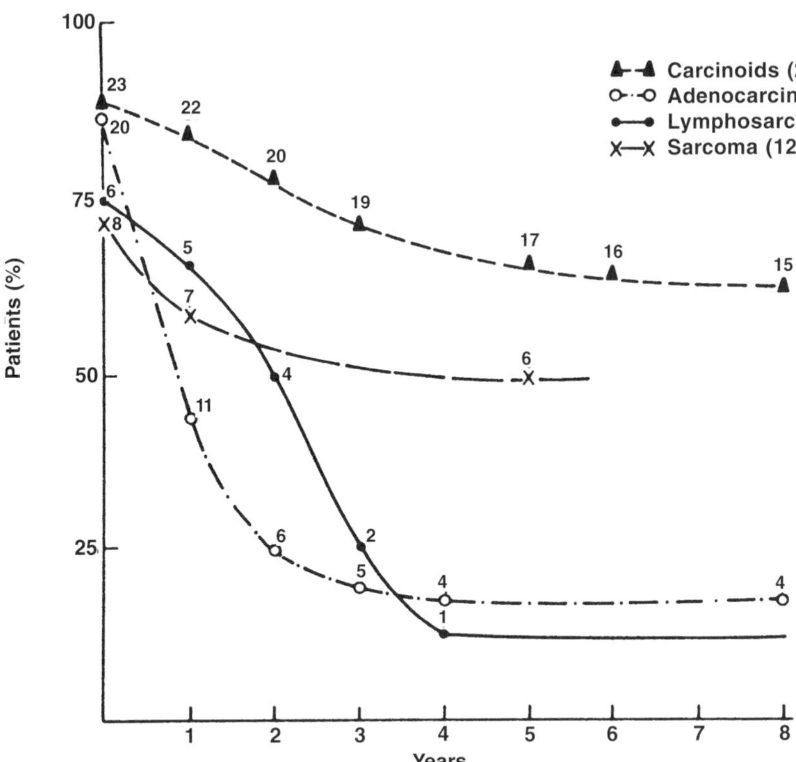

FIG. 25-2. Survival of patients with malignant small intestinal tumors. The curve for sarcomas includes nine leiomyosarcomas, two fibrosarcomas, and one hemangioendothelioma. (Reprinted with permission from Waterhouse G, Skudlarick JL, Adkins RB. A clinical review of small bowel neoplasms. South Med J 1981;74:1201–1203.)

cramps associated with an abdominal mass, enlarged liver, and elevated urinary 5-hydroxyindoleacetic acid level [64].

Resection of the primary carcinoid tumor and metastatic lesions and the administration of drugs to block the neuroendocrine effects of the tumor are indicated. All carcinoid tumors should be treated as malignant tumors whenever and wherever found.

The prognosis for patients with early detected and adequately resected malignant tumors of the small bowel depends on many factors including the length of symptoms, extent of tumor, tumor cell type, and its location within the small bowel (Fig. 25-2).

We continue to recommend the same vigorous diagnostic search in the elderly patient with symptoms attributable to a small bowel neoplasm as we would for a younger patient with the same symptoms. The surgical and adjuvant treatment of these lesions must be tempered by the extent of the disease when discovered and the overall physical condition of the patient. If discovered in a curable stage, the same surgical resection for a small bowel cancer that would be performed in a middle-aged patient should be offered to the elderly patient with a similar tumor.

SUMMARY

The pathologic conditions that commonly lead to surgical treatment of small bowel problems in the elderly tend to be dramatic. Vascular insufficiency, neoplasms (malignant and benign), inflammatory conditions, and various types of mechanical obstruction (Nyhus) attack the elderly population with alarming regularity. As with all surgical conditions in the elderly, if the problem is diagnosed early, the patient prepared at leisure, the condition treated with skill and care, and complications avoided, these problems can be solved for many patients who may seem beyond the hope of cure. It is the elderly patient in need of surgical treatment for one of these conditions who is neglected who will have little hope of survival.

REFERENCES

1. Schuster MM. Disorders of the aging GI system. Hosp Pract 1976; 11:95–103.
2. Holt PR, Pascal RR, Kotler DP. Effects of aging upon small intestinal structure in the Fischer rat. J Gerontol 1984;39:642–647.
3. Haboubi NY, Montgomery RD. Small-bowel bacterial overgrowth in elderly people: clinical significance and response to treatment. Age Ageing 1992;21:13–9.
4. Holt PR. The small intestine. Clin Gastroenterol 1985;14:689–723.
5. Welch JD, Poley JR, Bhatia M, Stevenson DE. Intestinal disaccharidase activities in relation to age, race, and mucosal damage. Gastroenterology 1978;80:94–98.
6. Vinardell P, Bolufer J. Age dependent changes on jejunal sugar absorption by rat invivo. Exp Gerontol 1984;19:73–78.
7. Klimas JE. Intestinal glucose absorption during the lifespan of a colony of rats. J Gerontol 1968;23:529–532.
8. Calingaert A, Zorzoli A. The influence of age on 6-deoxy-D-glucose accumulation by mouse intestine. J Gerontol 1965;20:211–214.

9. Feibusch J, Holt PR. Impaired absorptive capacity for carbohydrates in the elderly. Am J Clin Nutr 1979;32:942–944.
10. Holt PR, Dominguez AA. Intestinal absorption of triglyceride and vitamin D_3 in aged and young rats. Dig Dis Sci 1981;26:1109–1115.
11. Holt PR, Balint JA. Effects of aging on intestinal lipid absorption. Am J Physiol 1993;264:1–6.
12. Gersovitz M, Munro HN, Udall J, Young VR. Albumin synthesis in young and elderly subjects using a new stable isotope methodology: response to level of protein intake. Metabolism 1980;29: 1075–1086.
13. Ravaglia G, Forti P, Maioli F, et al. Calcium regulating hormones in healthy elderly men: relation to intestinal calcium absorption. Boll Soc Ital Biol Sper 1994;70:323–328.
14. Kupfer RM, Heppell M, Haggith JW, Bateman DN. Gastric emptying and small-bowel transit rate in the elderly. J Am Geriatr Soc 1985;33: 340–343.
15. Nishimura N, Hongo M, Yamada M, et al. Gastric myoelectric activities in elderly human subjects—surface electrogastrographic observations. J Smooth Muscle Res 1995;31:43–49.
16. Husebye E, Engedal K. The patterns of motility are maintained in the human small intestine throughout the process of aging. Scand J Gastroenterol 1992;27:397–404.
17. Fleischer DE, Grim IS, Friedman LS. Inflammatory bowel disease in older patients. Med Clin North Am 1994;78:1303–1319.
18. Grimm IS, Friedman LS. Inflammatory bowel disease in the elderly. Gastroenterol Clin North Am 1990;19:361–389.
19. Shapiro PA, Peppercorn MA, Antonioli DA, et al. Crohn's disease in the elderly. Am J Gastroenterol 1981;76:132–137.
20. Foxworthy DM, Wilson JA. Crohn's disease in the elderly: prolonged delay in diagnosis. J Am Geriatr Soc 1985;33:492–495.
21. Watts JM, De Dombal FT, Watkinson G, Goligher JC. Early course of ulcerative colitis. Gut 1966;7:16–31.
22. Gupta S, Saverymuttu SH, Keshavarzian A, Hodgson HJF. Is the pattern of inflammatory bowel disease different in the elderly? Age Ageing 1985;14:366–370.
23. Thomas TP. The complications of systemic corticosteroid therapy in the elderly. A retrospective study. Gerontology 1984;30:60–65.
24. Brandfondbrener M, Londowne M, Shock NW. The relation of age to certain performance of the heart and the circulation. Circulation 1955;12:567–576.
25. Ottinger LW. The surgical management of acute occlusion of the superior mesenteric artery. Ann Surg 1978;188:721–731.
26. Hansen HJ, Oigaard A. Embolization to the superior mesenteric artery. Arteriography and embolectomy in four cases. Acta Chir Scand 1976;142:451–455.
27. Cohen N. Gastroenterology in the aged. Mt Sinai J Med 1980;47: 142–149.
28. Gennaro M, Ascer E, Matano R, et al. Acute mesenteric ischemia after cardiopulmonary bypass. Am J Surg 1993;166:231–236.
29. Bustin MP, Iber FL. Management of common nonmalignant GI problems in the elderly. Geriatrics 1983;38:69–76.
30. Pearce VR. The importance of duodenal diverticula in the elderly. Postgrad Med J 1980;56:777–780.
31. Salomonowitz E, Wittich G, Hajek P, et al. Detection of intestinal diverticula by double-contrast small bowel enema: differentiation for other intestinal diverticula. Gastrointest Radiol 1983;8:271–278.
32. Maglinte DDT, Chernish SM, DeWeese R, et al. Acquired jejunoileal diverticular disease: subject review. Radiology 1986;158:577–580.
33. Haber JJ. Meckel's diverticulum. Am J Surg 1947;73:468–485.
34. Cullen JJ, Kelly KA, Moir CR, et al. Surgical management of Meckel's diverticulum—an epidemiologic, population-based study. Ann Surg 1994;220:564–569.
35. Reiss R, Deutsch AA. Emergency abdominal procedures in patients above 70. J Gerontol 1985;40:154–158.
36. Zadeh BJ, Davis JM, Canizaro PC. Small bowel obstruction in the elderly. Am Surg 1985;51:470–473.
37. Braasch JW, Denbo HE. Tumors of the small intestine. Surg Clin North Am 1964;44:791–809.
38. Schier J. Diagnostic and therapeutic aspects of tumors of the small bowel. Int Surg 1972;57:789–792.
39. Sindelar WF. Cancer of the Small Intestine. In DeVita VT, Hellman S, Rosenberg SA (eds), Cancer Principles and Practice of Oncology. Philadelphia: Lippincott, 1982;616–642.
40. Botsford TW, Crowe P, Crocker DW. Tumors of the small intestine. A review of experience with 115 cases including a report of a rare case of malignant hemangioendothelioma. Am J Surg 1962;103:358–365.
41. Croom RD, Newsome JF. Tumors of the small intestine. Am Surg 1975;41:160–167.
42. Ebert PA, Zuidema GD. Primary tumors of the small intestine. Arch Surg 1965;91:452–455.
43. Schmutzer KJ, Holleran WM, Regan JF. Tumors of the small bowel. Am J Surg 1964;108:270–276.
44. Silberman H, Crichlow RW, Caplan HS. Neoplasms of the small bowel. Ann Surg 1974;180:157–161.
45. Sawyer RB, Sawyer KC Jr, Sawyer KC, Larsen RR. Benign and malignant tumors of the small intestine. Am Surg 1963;29:268–272.
46. Adkins RB, Scott HW. Surgical procedures in patients aged 90 years and older. South Med J 1984;77:1357–1364.
47. Sarre RG, Frost AG, Jagelman DG, et al. Gastric and duodenal polyps in familial adenomatous polyposis: a prospective study of the nature and prevalence of upper gastrointestinal polyps. Gut 1987;28:306–314.
48. Sugihara K, Muto T, Kamiya J, et al. Gardner's syndrome associated with periampullary carcinoma, duodenal and gastric adenomatosis. Dis Colon Rectum 1982;25:766–771.
49. Bulow S, Alm T, Fausa O, et al. Duodenal adenomatosis in familial adenomatosis polyposis. DAF Project Group. Int J Colorectal Dis 1995;10:43–46.
50. Debinski HS, Spigelman AD, Hatfield A, et al. Upper intestinal surveillance in familial adenomatous polyposis. Eur J Cancer 1995;31A: 1149–1153.
51. Adedeji OA, Trescoli-Serrano C, Garcia-Zarco M. Primary duodenal carcinoma. Postgrad Med J 1995;71:354–358.
52. Nugent KP, Farmer KC, Spigelman AD, et al. Randomized controlled trial of the effect of sulindac on duodenal and rectal polyposis and cell proliferation in patients with familial adenomatous polyposis. Br J Surg 1993;80:1618–1619.
53. Kutin ND, Ransom JHC, Gouge TH, Localio SA. Villous tumors of the duodenum. Ann Surg 1975;181:164–168.
54. Shulten MF, Dyasu R, Beal JM. Villous adenoma of the duodenum: a case report and review of the literature. Am J Surg 1976;132:90–96.
55. Bremer EH, Battile WB, Bulle PH. Villous tumors of the upper gastrointestinal tract. Clinical review and report of a case. Am J Gastroenterol 1968;50:135–143.
56. Ring EJ, Ferrucci JT, Eaton SB, Clements JL. Villous adenomas of the duodenum. Radiology 1972;104:45–48.
57. Rochlin DB, Longmire WP. Primary tumors of the small intestine. Surgery 1961;50:586–592.
58. Miles RM, Crawford D, Duras S. The small bowel tumor problem. Ann Surg 1979;189:732–740.
59. Resnick HLP, Cooper DR. Carcinoma of the duodenum; review of literature from 1948 to 1956. Am J Surg 1958;95:946–952.
60. Waterhouse G, Skudlarick JL, Adkins RB. A clinical review of small bowel neoplasms. South Med J 1981;74:1201–1203.
61. Kieffer RW, McSwain B, Adkins RB. Sarcoma of the gastrointestinal tract: a review of 40 cases. Am Surg 1982;48:167–169.
62. Adkins RB, Scott HW, Sawyers JL. Gastrointestinal lymphoma and sarcoma: a case for aggressive search and destroy. Ann Surg 1987; 205:625–633.
63. Rich JD. Malignant tumors of the intestine: a review of 37 cases. Am Surg 1977;43:445–454.
64. Durning P, Galland RB, Nagorney DM, Welbourn RB. Neuroendocrine tumors of the gut. World J Surg 1985;9:348–360.

Surgical Care for the Elderly, 2nd ed., edited by
R. Benton Adkins, Jr., and H. William Scott, Jr.
Lippincott–Raven Publishers, Philadelphia © 1998.

CHAPTER 26

Diagnosis and Management of Intestinal Obstruction and Herniae

Raymond Pollak and Lloyd M. Nyhus

The term *intestinal obstruction* connotes a clinical syndrome in which the contents of the intestine are unable to pass in the usual physiologic way, from proximal to distal, ultimately reaching the rectum. A hernia, on the other hand, may be defined as the protrusion of a viscus through a defect in the musculoaponeurotic structures that enclose that viscus. When this viscus is either the small or large intestine, it is apparent that a hernia may be a contributing cause to acute or chronic intestinal obstruction. As we show in this chapter, both intestinal obstruction and herniae of the abdominal wall are not uncommon in the population as a whole and therefore also affect the elderly, that is, those >65 years of age.

A discussion of the principal factors that result in intestinal obstruction is presented, including herniae of the abdominal wall, and the diagnosis, management, and the ultimate outcome of these conditions in the elderly population.

INCIDENCE

It is estimated that 10% of the population of the United States are >65 years of age. By the year 2000 this number is predicted to approximate 30,000,000 persons [1,2]. In 1985, it was estimated that 20% of surgical beds were occupied by elderly patients with serious and morbid surgical illnesses [3]. The incidence of intestinal obstructions increases progressively with age. There is a sharp increase in incidence after the age of 50 years and again after the age of 70 years [4].

In a large series of 400 elderly Israeli patients admitted for emergency surgical therapy, 25% had symptoms and signs of intestinal obstruction [5]. An updated series from the same group, published in 1992 [6], demonstrated an increase in the number of octogenarians undergoing elective and emergent operative procedures (from 1.1% to 5.1%) during the period 1973 to 1989. From this analysis of 700 patients, 265 (37.8%) required laparotomy and 169 (24.1%) required hernia surgery (15.8% elective and 8.3% emergent).

A series from the United Kingdom described 375 patients, 218 of whom had symptoms and signs related to intestinal obstruction or incarcerated and strangulated abdominal wall hernia [7]. There were 115 strangulated herniae (31% of all patients) and 103 episodes of intestinal obstruction (27.5% of all patients). These large series emphasize that surgical intervention, especially emergency surgical intervention in the elderly, can be expected to increase dramatically in the future.

In the general population the incidence of hernia of the abdominal wall has been estimated to be approximately 15 per 1,000 [8]. The incidence, however, for men in the sixth decade is 50 per 1,000 and increases to 120 per 1,000 for men >75 years of age. Thus, 3.75 million persons in the United States are estimated to suffer from some form of abdominal wall hernia or the complications thereof. Furthermore, approximately 550,000 persons, many of them elderly, undergo herniorrhaphy annually in the United States [9].

ETIOLOGY AND PATHOGENESIS

Traditionally, causes of intestinal obstruction have been classified according to the nature of the obstructing process, that is, the process involves an intraluminal obstruction, a disease of the intestinal wall impinges on the lumen, or a disease process from without compresses and obstructs intestinal transit. Most reviews of intestinal obstruction in elderly persons, however, divide the causes of obstruction into those that involve the large intestine and herniae that result in intestinal obstruction themselves [3,5,7,10]. In the series by Greene in 1969 [10], the large intestine, small intestine, and herniae each accounted for one-third of the number of patients who presented with symptoms and signs of intestinal obstruction. Colonic neoplasms, volvulus of the sigmoid, diverticulitis, fecal impaction, or volvulus of the cecum, in that order, were the major causes of large intestinal obstruction. The small intestine was obstructed for the most part by postoperative adhesions, gallstone ileus, metastatic tumors, mesenteric vascular accidents, regional enteritis, foreign bodies, and volvulus of the entire small intestine. In terms of the frequency of herniae encountered, inguinal herniae were the most common followed by femoral, umbilical, ventral, and internal herniae.

When the entire spectrum of emergency abdominal operations in elderly patients is examined in more detail, however, operations for intestinal obstruction usually account for approximately 25% of the operative procedures, closely following biliary tract operations and surgery for tumors of the colon and rectum [6]. Again the obstructions are caused by incarcerated and strangulated herniae, as well as by mechanical obstruction resulting from adhesions, followed by mesenteric vascular accidents and malignant tumors. A similar series that examined emergency abdominal operations in elderly persons from the United Kingdom found operations for strangulated hernia and intestinal obstruction to be more common than all other forms of emergency abdominal procedures [7]. In the latter series, strangulation was more common, with femoral herniae closely followed by inguinal, incisional, paraumbilical, and obturator herniae. The causes of intestinal obstruction were also divided into those that affected the large and small intestines, with a similar spectrum of etiologic factors as previously mentioned. Conversely, when large series of elderly patients who are operated on for repair of abdominal wall herniae are examined, 16% of these patients present with incarceration, of whom 10% have strangulation [1]. Only 3% of patients operated on electively for abdominal wall hernia have small intestinal obstruction as the presenting disease. In large series of elective repairs of groin herniae, approximately one-half are found to be indirect inguinal herniae, one-third to be direct inguinal herniae, and 10% to be pantaloon herniae. Men outnumber women by 6.5 to 1.0 in terms of the incidence of hernia, whereas the sex incidence is almost equal for patients who present with an acute abdominal surgical emergency or with acute intestinal obstruction [1,3,10].

Despite diverse causes, intraluminal obstructions, disease processes of the intestinal wall, and causes from without, such as postoperative adhesions, all produce a series of common pathologic events that eventually lead to compromise of intestinal viability and ultimate strangulation. These events are elegantly described by Stolar and Randolph in a rabbit model [11]. When the obstructing mechanism causes an increase in the intramural tension of the intestinal wall, initially the low pressure venous and lymphatic flow within the wall becomes obstructed, resulting in engorgement and outpouring of extracellular fluid into the wall itself and into the lumen of the intestine. The proximal intestine makes spasmodic efforts to relieve the obstruction by active peristaltic movements, resulting in nonspecific symptoms of poorly localized abdominal pain, often accompanied by nausea and vomiting. Continued application of the obstructing mechanism results in a further outpouring of extracellular fluid into the intestinal lumen and a further increase in the intramural tension of the intestinal wall. As demonstrated by Stolar and Randolph, this process can continue unabated only for a few hours before a critical point is reached beyond which the intestine is unlikely to recover even though corrective measures are instituted. With increasing intraluminal and intramural tension, the arterial supply to the involved bowel part is jeopardized and strangulation ultimately occurs. Loss of the structural integrity of the intestinal mucosa, as well as stagnation, with absence of prograde intestinal movement, results in the overgrowth of a mixed flora of intestinal bacteria and migration of bacteria through the intestinal wall to involve the visceral peritoneum. Furthermore, the loss of the structural integrity of the intestinal wall, together with continuing intraluminal accumulation of fluid and bacteria and their products, eventually causes intestinal perforation and generalized peritonitis.

A clear understanding of the pathophysiology of intestinal obstruction and the resulting compromise of intestinal viability with strangulation should prompt timely and aggressive diagnostic and therapeutic measures to obviate progression to the state of generalized peritonitis, irreversible loss of portions of the intestine, and a possible threat to the patient's life.

CLINICAL SIGNS AND SYMPTOMS

A classic triad of crampy abdominal pain accompanied by nausea, vomiting, and absolute constipation may not always be present in the elderly patient with intestinal obstruction. In fact, delay in presentation is the factor most commonly seen in a large series of patients, and is related to socioeconomic factors, self-medication, and the minimizing of symptoms and signs by the family, patient, and physician [9]. Up to 4% of such patients in large series with late presentations died in the first few hours after the initial presentation without undergoing surgical treatment [9]. A history of previous operations or treatment for intestinal obstruction may be elicited in up to 11% of patients. It is also important to establish a prior history of carcinoma, Crohn's disease, or the presence of a previously existing hernia. Many herniae in these elderly patients have been present for anywhere from 2 to 36 years [1].

The common presenting symptoms of a herniae in a large elderly population are a mass in the groin or scrotum or localized inguinoscrotal pain. A previous history of hernia may be overlooked, however, in the setting of a seriously ill, toxic elderly patient who is in pain.

Concurrent comorbid diseases, such as severe cardiovascular disease, obstructive chronic pulmonary disease and emphysema, chronic pyelonephritis, and senile dementia, may be present in >18% to 20% of patients [9]. Diabetes mellitus may be present in approximately 6% of these patients [1].

Physical examination reveals a varying picture depending on the time of presentation and progression of the disease.

Thus, when the situation is of several hours' duration, few physical signs are elicited other than that of vague abdominal tenderness. With more advanced disease, signs of extracellular fluid loss and dehydration are readily apparent. The mucous membranes are dry, oliguria is present, and the patient suffers from hypotension and tachycardia. The temperature may be normal or elevated. Hypothermia is an ominous sign and often denotes serious and far advanced disease, with an underlying septic process. Examination of the chest, heart, and lungs may reveal the presence of comorbid cardiovascular and respiratory disease.

Examination of the abdomen should be thorough and include an evaluation from "nipples to knees," with due respect to patient modesty. Localized findings in the abdomen are infrequent apart from vague abdominal guarding and tenderness. Involuntary guarding and rebound tenderness can be expected to be found when the disease process has progressed to a state of generalized peritonitis. Even in elderly patients, however, these signs are often vague and ill defined. Auscultation of the abdomen for bowel sounds initially might reveal the presence of hyperactive rushes and "tinkles," but late in the course of the disease no bowel sounds may be heard. Examination of the inguinal region and hernial orifices and a rectal examination in men and a bimanual pelvic examination in women are all very important. Occasionally, the rare obturator hernia may be appreciated during the pelvic examination in women.

The presence of accompanying neurologic disorders, such as senile dementia and Parkinson's disease, should make one aware fairly soon that the elicitation of classic symptoms and signs may not be possible. Furthermore, these disease processes, together with their attendant forms of therapy, may result in signs and symptoms resembling those of intestinal obstruction, so-called pseudo-obstruction. The latter process, however, is a diagnosis of exclusion and should only be made when all chances of organic intestinal obstruction have been ruled out. Similarly, the presence of surgical abdominal scars, atrial arrhythmias, and jaundice might provide clues as to the nature of the obstruction. When a hernia in the groin is thought to be responsible for the problem, especially in obese persons, examination of the patient in the upright position to more clearly delineate the nature of any mass in the groin is important. The liberal use of proctoscopy, and flexible sigmoidoscopy and colonoscopy if indicated, completes the physical examination.

DIAGNOSTIC MEASURES

Initial radiographic studies of the abdomen and chest are likely to provide much useful information. We routinely recommend the so-called obstructive series, in which an upright chest radiograph, supine and upright films of the abdomen, and decubitus view of the abdomen are all obtained. Depending on the site of the obstructing process, a variety of radiographic findings may be seen. In large intestinal obstruction, massively dilated loops of large and small intestine are visualized. When the ileocecal valve remains competent, only the large intestine is distended with its typical haustral markings. Small intestinal obstruction is characterized by the presence of dilated loops of intestine with characteristic valvulae conniventes accompanied by numerous air-fluid levels in a stepladder manner. Intestinal obstructions that are proximal and in the jejunum may demonstrate a nonspecific gas pattern and a distended stomach only. In situations of colonic pseudo-obstruction, or even with true obstruction of the large intestinal lumen, a low-pressure barium enema provides diagnostic information. In the former situation the barium is seen to precede proximally to the ileocecal valve without hindrance, whereas in obstruction of the lumen the barium does not pass the obstructing process.

When air is noticed in the rectum on plain abdominal films, partial intestinal obstruction may be suspected. Under these circumstances and when there is no question of bowel viability a so-called enteroclysis may be performed. In this procedure, thin barium is given orally, and its passage is followed through the intact intestinal tract to demonstrate the point of partial or complete obstruction in its lumen. Another feature of note in radiography is free air under the diaphragm, which is best seen on upright chest films. Fifty percent of patients with small intestinal obstruction due to gallstones, so-called gallstone ileus, have air in the biliary tree, and in 20% the gallstones may be visualized in a supine view of the abdomen [12]. Few patients with gallstone ileus have the classic triad of air in the biliary tree, ectopic stones, and small intestinal obstruction. Once again the use of thin barium may confirm the diagnosis in these patients by demonstrating barium in the biliary tree or in the fistulous tract between the biliary tree and the intestine. Oral and intravenous cholangiography rarely confirms the diagnosis. Clues from the plain radiographic films allow us to make the diagnosis in one-third of patients, whereas contrast studies increase the rate to 80% to 90% and are important when the patient is stable and the diagnosis of gallstone ileus is suspected [12].

Computed tomography, ultrasonography, and angiography are rarely required to make the diagnosis of bowel obstruction except under exceptional circumstances. When acute mesenteric ischemia is thought to be present, transfemoral abdominal aortography may be performed in the emergency setting. Similarly, abdominal ultrasonography has been successfully used to diagnose occult herniae of the abdominal wall, such as spigelian herniae and other such obscure herniae. Injection of contrast agents into the peritoneal cavity to demonstrate a hernial sac has also been used, especially when bilateral herniae are thought to be present.

For both elective hernia repairs and emergency procedures, important laboratory studies, such as a complete blood count, serum electrolyte values, and studies of the coagulation profile, are required before proceeding to the operating room. The results obtained may reflect the sequelae of some chronic comorbid disease states, such as iron-deficiency anemia, which is characteristic of large intestinal cancer. The values vary with the current clinical disease state and may be grossly abnormal. Thus, with intestinal obstruction, the white cell count may be elevated, reflecting an ongoing inflammatory process. Electrolyte abnormalities are common as a result of the fluid shifts between the intracellular and vascular compartments and the extravascular compartmental space (so-called third space). Although the combination of clinical features, such as an elevated temperature and laboratory values showing grossly elevated white cell counts, has been reported to be predictive of underlying intestinal ischemia and strangulation [13], well-designed prospective studies have failed to confirm these observations [14]. Skillful interpretation, however, of the clinical, laboratory, and radiographic findings should provide accurate information and clues to the diagnosis in >80% to 90% of patients [15].

Other invasive procedures, such as an abdominal tap and peritoneal lavage, occasionally reveal the presence of either purulent material, blood, or the "prune juice" fluid characteristic of mesenteric ischemia with infarction. Occasionally, flexible sigmoidoscopy and colonoscopy reveal the absence of an organic obstructing lesion when the patient is suspected of having intestinal obstruction and is found to have pseudo-obstruction. Colonoscopy might also reveal the cause of large intestinal obstruction and allow for biopsy, reduction of a volvulus, or the alteration of the approach to the planned therapy.

MANAGEMENT AND THERAPY

Preoperative Phase

Rather than proceeding with an emergency surgical procedure, it is often prudent to delay the operation 4 to 6 hours to correct fluid and electrolyte abnormalities and allow for resuscitation of the elderly patient, especially when a number of comorbid conditions exist. Admission to an acute care ward or intensive care unit is often required for these patients, many of whom have been ignored and who have become desperately ill. Immediate measures to relieve nausea and vomiting include the insertion of a nasogastric tube to aspirate air and intestinal contents. A Foley catheter is inserted into the bladder to monitor hourly urine output. Intravenous fluids in the form of dextrose-containing electrolyte solutions should be infused, preferably through catheters placed in large central veins to allow for accurate monitoring of filling pressures within the heart and extracellular intravascular compartmental space.

Assessment of Operative Risk

At this point in the management of these patients, an evaluation of operative risk is important to assess the need for invasive monitoring devices, such as Swan-Ganz catheters and arterial lines [16]. A preoperative evaluation scale of the American Society of Anesthesiologists (grades 1 to 5) has been used to evaluate operative risk in 500 consecutive patients >80 years of age [17]. Mortality increased with increasing grade, and at class 5 (patients with severe life-threatening disorders) 25% of patients died. The studies of DelGuercio and Cohn [18] used an objective preoperative evaluation technique to assess cardiorespiratory risk factors in the elderly and allowed for a more scientific assessment of operative risk and the need for continued invasive monitoring.

There are many age-related morphologic changes found in the heart, including conduction defects and valvular abnormalities, but the functional importance of these changes may vary considerably. Compounding these age-related changes are numerous pathologic conditions, the most serious and prevalent of which is atherosclerosis and its attendant sequelae of myocardial infarction and ventricular dysfunction. A normal decline in respiratory function occurs with aging due to changes in the chest wall, as well as in the lung. Chest wall compliance decreases, often because of increasing kyphosis and perhaps aggravated by vertebral collapse secondary to osteoporosis. Respiratory muscle weakness also is not uncommon and may result in a 50% decrease in maximum inspiratory and expiratory forces generated, with a resulting decrease in the strength of cough. Lung volume and function also change with age as the lung loses its reserve capacity, and many of these physiologic changes caused by increasing age are aggravated by disease processes active in elderly patients [16].

Evaluation and Management of Comorbid Conditions

Because >20% of elderly patients with emergency abdominal conditions have comorbid conditions referable most often to cardiovascular or respiratory symptoms, evaluation and management of these disease processes before proceeding to the operating room may greatly influence the outcome. Thus, treatment of arrhythmias, and when necessary, insertion of a pacemaker, may be important to stabilize pulse and blood pressure. Uncontrolled hypertension may require the placement of an arterial line and the use of such potent agents as nitroprusside.

Because of the work of DelGuercio and Cohn [18], the use of Swan-Ganz catheters preoperatively in elderly patients has now received wide acceptance, and for the most part the catheters should be used routinely in many emergency circumstances. The use of these catheters allows both arterial and mixed venous blood gases to be obtained and the determination of cardiac output. These data allow a ventricular functional curve to be generated, demonstrating left ventricular stroke work as a function of mean pulmonary capillary wedge pressure. On the basis of these data, inotropic agents can be administered to improve contractility and cardiac output, together with volume expansion or depletion to achieve optimal cardiac output. Patients at great risk for postoperative ventilatory failure can be identified early by a number of preoperative pulmonary function tests, of which the forced expiratory volume is the most valuable. When these pulmonary function tests are used with routine arterial blood gas measurements, high-risk patients can be identified and treated appropriately [19].

In elective circumstances, such as routine hernia repairs, patients should be encouraged to cease smoking, and preoperative breathing exercises with emphasis on inspiratory efforts should be performed. Preoperative sputum cultures are often useful, as are humidification of inspired air and nebulized bronchial dilators to keep secretions moist and decrease bronchial spasm.

The appropriate use of modern monitoring equipment and devices should enable appropriate fluid and electrolyte replacement and maximize optimal renal function. Before going to the operating room an elderly patient should be in as close to an ideal state of physiologic balance as possible to tolerate the proposed operative procedure and general anesthesia if such anesthesia is to be used.

Prophylactic Antibiotics

Another measure, perhaps equally important for ensuring a successful outcome, is the use of the appropriate combination of broad-spectrum antibiotics. It is well established that the intestinal microflora undergo dramatic changes in the presence of intestinal obstruction, and this accounts for the so-called feculent vomitus of which patients with long-standing intestinal obstructions often complain. Thus, appropriate broad-spectrum antibiotics, to cover both aerobic and anaerobic intestinal flora, should be given intravenously. Single agents, such as second- and third-generation cephalosporins, appear to be adequate in most cases and are attractive choices in the elderly, especially because they provide a good broad-spectrum coverage without the increased risk of nephrotoxicity. The use of prophylactic antibiotics for elective hernia repairs is rarely justified.

Prophylaxis of Deep Venous Thrombosis

On statistical grounds, all elderly patients, and especially those with an underlying carcinomatosis, are at risk for postoperative morbidity from deep venous thrombosis and possibly pulmonary embolism. In a study of hospitalized patients, those >60 years of age had a 25% incidence of pulmonary embolism as the primary cause of death, compared with a 3% incidence for patients <50 years of age [20]. Because many of these venous thromboses occur during and after operations, it is prudent to provide some form of prophylaxis before, during, and after the operation. A wide variety of prophylactic measures have been reported in the literature, with both mechanical external compression devices and subcutaneous low-dose heparin advocated by various proponents [21]. For many elderly patients, early ambulation is the key to prevention once the operative procedure is completed.

Evaluation of Nutritional and Immune Status

Nutrition and immune function also have a bearing on the ability of elderly ill patients to withstand major operative morbidity. A number of physiologic, psychological, and socioeconomic factors influence the nutritional status of the elderly surgically ill population. Furthermore, it is often difficult to distinguish age-related changes in the immune system from altered immune functions caused by nutritional deficiencies. In otherwise healthy elderly patients undergoing elective hernia repairs, preoperative immune deficiencies have been difficult to demonstrate by mitogen assay, mixed lymphocyte cultures, skin tests, or levels of immunoglobulins when compared with healthy younger control patients [22]. Biochemical measurements of nutritional status do not vary significantly with age. Depressed levels of serum albumin, transferrin, and retinol-binding protein, however, are thought to be accurate indicators of nutritional status. Thus, malnutrition adds an additional burden to a potentially depressed immune system in elderly surgical patients, and malnutrition may well lead to major problems with wound healing and ongoing sepsis postoperatively. When time allows and when operations such as elective herniorrhaphy can be deferred, it is of obvious benefit to improve the patient's nutritional status. When nutritional support is thought necessary, the enteral route is preferred over the intravenous route whenever possible [16]. In emergency situations, however, little time is available to provide satisfactory alimentation to a patient who requires an immediate operation.

Operative Procedure

Anesthesia

It is apparent from large series in which a mix of local, regional, and general anesthetic techniques were used that, for elective operations in the groin, local anesthetic techniques are associated with the lowest incidence of postoperative complications and morbidity [1]. However, skillfully applied general endotracheal anesthesia, using relaxation techniques, with the infusion of potent narcotic agents, should allow successful recovery of even the most ill patient from a major abdominal exploration. As mentioned previously, the liberal use of invasive monitoring devices aids the anesthesiologist in intraoperative management in ensuring that an elderly, seriously ill, surgical patient survives the operation itself, all other factors being equal.

Abdominal Exploration

Exploratory procedures of the abdomen in patients with intestinal obstruction due to postoperative adhesions or causes other than an incarcerated or strangulated inguinal hernia should be done through a generous midline or transverse incision. Our preference is to use a transverse supra-umbilical incision whenever possible, especially when a previous midline incision has been made. The transverse incision allows for adequate exploration of the abdominal cavity and is associated with rapid healing and minimal compromise to respiratory function in the postoperative period. The editors prefer to use a midline incision in most instances.

Careful dissection in the abdominal cavity may be required regardless of the choice of incision, especially when multiple adhesions are found. Proximal dilated loops of intestine should be sought and traced distally to the point of obstruction, where collapsed loops of small and large intestines are encountered. For the most part, gentle handling of the tissue is emphasized; unintentional or even deliberate enterotomies are associated with high postoperative morbidity.

When adhesions are thought to be the obstructing mechanism, simple incision of the adhesive band is usually all that is required. Extensive dissection of other adhesions, techniques to layer the intestine in such a way as to prevent recurrent adhesive obstruction, and long intestinal tubes have not been shown to be of great benefit [23]. However, when proximal decompression of dilated fluid-filled loops of intestine is believed to aid the closure of the abdominal wound of entry, the Nelson-Nyhus long intestinal tube is preferable to making an enterotomy [24]. When prolonged postoperative intubation and nasogastric suction are anticipated, it is prudent to perform a gastrostomy before closure of the abdomen to decompress the proximal intestine and to act later as a route for nutrition.

Numerous techniques have been proposed to evaluate the safety of leaving in situ loops of intestine of questionable viability. These methods include fluorescein studies, Doppler ultrasonic examination, and the injection of radiolabeled microspheres into the mesenteric vasculature [25]. None of these measures, however, has replaced experience and sound surgical judgment as to bowel viability. The presence of peristalsis and pulsatile vessels within the mesentery and the color and turgor of the intestinal wall are still the most reliable guides as to whether resection should be undertaken. The aphorism, "when in doubt, resect," still holds should any doubt exist in the experienced surgeon's mind. These ill, frail patients usually have only one opportunity for survival, and a successful operation should be the goal. The opportunity for the surgeon to perform a second-look procedure often does not present itself because the elderly patient may die of ongoing sepsis and acidosis before it can be done.

If during the abdominal exploration, the entire small intestine is found to be dusky and ischemic, heroic measures at revascularization are required. These efforts can be greatly aided, as mentioned previously, by preoperative aortography and selective mesenteric arteriography at the celiac or superior mesenteric artery. Under these circumstances, revascularization usually consists of a bypass procedure from the aorta to the artery that is predominantly involved, usually the superior mesenteric artery.

Unexpected internal herniae may be encountered at the time of laparotomy, and often only a minimal procedure is required to effect their cure. Most patients with this finding have a satisfactory outcome. This subject has been dealt with extensively elsewhere [26].

Gallstone ileus as a cause of small intestinal obstruction is fairly common in elderly patients and should be suspected in most patients whose preoperative history, physical examination, and diagnostic studies have been appropriate. Incision of the intestine proximal to the obstructed stone should be made and the stone delivered proximally. As a rule, in poor-risk elderly patients, no attempt should be made to correct the biliary-enteric fistula at the first operative procedure [12].

Hernia Repair

For all obstructing and incarcerated herniae of the groin, the preperitoneal technique is to be used routinely [27]. A transverse incision is made approximately 4 to 6 cm superior to the suprapubic ramus and is carried down through the abdominal wall musculature to the preperitoneal space. The hernial sac is seen to be incarcerated in any one of a number of hernial orifices (i.e., inguinal, femoral, or obturator), and skillful sharp dissection is required to reduce the sac and the entrapped viscera back into the abdominal cavity. The peritoneum can then be incised and the contained intestine examined critically for evidence of compromised viability. When the contained viscera do appear normal, no further therapy is necessary, and the peritoneum can be closed with absorbable suture material after incision of the redundant peritoneal sac. When the intestinal viability is thought to be compromised, a small intestinal resection with an end-to-end anastomosis in a single layer usually suffices. After the viscera is returned to the abdominal cavity, attention can be given to the herniorrhaphy to effect a repair.

For nonrecurrent herniae of the inguinal region, approximation of the transversalis fascia to the iliopubic tract from the posterior approach using monofilament nonabsorbable suture material suffices. For femoral herniae, closure of the femoral canal can be accomplished by sutures placed between the iliopubic tract and the tough Cooper's ligament inferiorly. For recurrent inguinal herniae, in addition to the aforementioned closure of the hernial defect, a reinforcing buttress of polypropylene mesh is now used routinely. No recurrences have been noted in long-term follow-up studies [28]. For uncomplicated primary indirect and direct inguinal herniae of the groin, we advocate the anterior approach of Condon to effect a sound repair [29]. All primary uncomplicated femoral herniae, however, should be repaired by the posterior preperitoneal approach.

The availability of minimal access or laparoscopic hernia repair, together with a laparoscopic approach to a number of other intra-abdominal surgical diseases, promises widespread application to surgical problems such as hernia repair and intestinal obstruction in the elderly patient. However, a large reference on this topic [30] and the authors' own

MEDLINE search of >9,000 papers published since 1989 (the beginning of the era of minimal access surgery) have revealed no specific mention or study of the efficacy and safety of laparoscopic surgery in the elderly. Doubtless, many elderly individuals are undergoing laparoscopic hernia repair as well as laparoscopic approaches to intestinal obstruction worldwide with satisfactory outcomes. Soon-to-be-published trials comparing this new technology with standard open operative approaches will undoubtedly establish the role of laparoscopic surgery for a number of surgical disorders, particularly herniae. If the widely promoted benefits of laparoscopic surgery (e.g., less invasive, less surgical trauma, shorter hospital stays, less analgesia required) have both short- and long-term durability with equivalent surgical outcomes, there is likely to be considerable benefit to the growing elderly patient population.

Epigastric, umbilical, incisional, and spigelian herniae may also give rise to intestinal obstruction in the elderly patient, although they do so rarely. Detailed descriptions of the repair of these herniae have been provided elsewhere [31]. In brief, the hernial sac and contained viscera are exposed by sharp dissection, and an attempt is made to define the margins of the fascial defect clearly. After inspection of the contents of the hernial sac and excision of redundant peritoneum, the fascial margins should be closed per primum whenever possible with monofilament nonabsorbable suture. Simple mattress sutures usually suffice, and complex techniques (i.e., vest over pants) and the use of a prosthesis (polypropylene mesh or oxfascia) are rarely required.

Closure of Incision

At the conclusion of the operation, when the operative procedure has not involved spillage of intestinal contents, the wound may be closed in layers per primum. When there has been some contamination, an enterotomy has been made, or frank intestinal gangrene and peritonitis have been encountered, it is prudent to leave the skin and subcutaneous tissues open after the fascial closure. For the most part these patients should have the fascial closure performed with monofilament, long-lasting, absorbable suture material (polydioxan) or nonabsorbable monofilament suture material, such as stainless steel wire or polypropylene.

Treatment of Various Causes of Obstruction

Large intestinal obstructions are largely caused by inflammatory disorders, such as diverticulitis, or malignant disease in the distal colon. When time allows, definitive therapy for these diseases should be undertaken because colostomies are associated with high morbidity and mortality in the elderly population [3]. In the emergency setting, however, there is little choice other than to perform a resection of the diseased colon and create an end colostomy with a Hartmann's procedure. This will immediately relieve the problem at hand. A secondary operation to re-establish intestinal continuity is often not feasible in these elderly patients, especially when widespread carcinomatosis is present at the initial procedure. When the patient makes a satisfactory recovery, however, especially when complications from diverticular disease were the only findings at the initial operation, an attempt to restore intestinal continuity should be made at a later date. The use of the Prasad colostomy technique should greatly facilitate the latter goal [32].

Appendicitis and perforated appendicitis may present in the elderly as a small intestinal obstruction. It is interesting that 72% of elderly patients present with right lower quadrant pain and tenderness, but still have delayed diagnosis and appropriate therapy [33]. The mechanism for the bowel obstruction is largely from the perforation of the appendix, with adherence of the small intestine to the periappendiceal phlegmon. A simple appendectomy with drainage of the right lower quadrant is usually all that is required in these circumstances.

Another rare cause of intestinal obstruction is paracolostomy hernia in the elderly. These herniae should always be repaired by relocation of the colostomy aperture within the rectus sheath itself and a repair or complete closure of the initial fascial defect [34].

Giant herniae of the abdominal wall even with incarceration of bowel rarely undergo strangulation. Liberal use of preoperative pneumoperitoneum allows for closure of these hernias. Optimal respiratory therapy preoperatively and postoperatively is important if these repairs are to be successful [35,36].

Postoperative Complications and Outcomes

The mortality for general surgical procedures in general increases linearly from the fifth to the tenth decades of life from 8.4% to a high of 22.1% overall. The mortality for elective operations increases linearly from a low of 1.3% for patients younger than 60 years of age to >11% for patients older than 89 years of age. The mortality for emergency operations, however, remains at a constant 25% to 28% for all patients between 60 and 90 years of age. This mortality has not decreased significantly in 50 years, unlike the elective operative mortality [16].

In large series of older patients, stratification by risk category has prognostic value [6]. Thus, emergency procedures, age >85 years, presence of peritonitis, presence of malignancy, and the need for laparotomy influence outcome. When none of these risk factors were present, postoperative mortality was 0.8%. With two or more factors, postoperative mortality was 21.6%.

More specifically, large series of patients who have emergency operations for intestinal obstructions do experience serious complications and high mortality. Cardiovascular complications are the most frequent and are observed in 21% of patients. These complications include cardiac arrhythmias, digitalis toxicity, and cerebrovascular accidents. Pulmonary complications constitute 20% of the postoperative incidence of morbidity and include pneumonia, atelectasis, and the need for tracheostomy in some patients. Fever and sepsis are seen in 13.6% of patients, and half of the time these complications are caused by wound infections. Genitourinary disorders are not uncommon (8% of patients) and are largely related to episodes of urinary retention and acute renal failure. Patients unfortunate enough to experience acute renal failure also experience a high mortality, 40% in some series [10].

In one large series of 300 elderly patients with intestinal obstruction, 84 (28%) died [10]. Most of the patients who died were between 70 and 85 years of age. One-third of the deaths were caused by pneumonia alone, 27% were the result of ongoing sepsis, and 22% were the result of cardiovascular morbidity. Pulmonary embolism accounted for 6% of all deaths. Mortality and complication rates also are influenced significantly by the disease process present at the time of the operation. Thus, large intestinal obstructions caused by carcinoma carry a mortality of 40% to 50%, as seen on short-term follow-up studies [3,15]. When palliation or colostomy only is performed for intestinal carcinoma, the mortality may increase to 80% [3]. Far fewer patients, approximately 30%, die of localized and resectable carcinomas of the large intestine. These mortality figures for carcinoma are increased significantly also by increasing age, especially for patients >70 years of age. No deaths were encountered in the absence of peritonitis or gangrenous intestine [3].

Wound infections are far more common when the skin is closed (21% versus 6%) than when the wound is left open. This is especially so in the presence of a contaminated field and when enterotomies have been made during the operative procedure.

The importance of elective repair of groin herniae in the elderly has been stressed previously. In a large series of 1,500 elderly patients who underwent early elective hernia repairs, the complication rate was 2.6%; 14 of these patients died, for a total death rate of 1.3% [1]. Complications encountered included those referable to urinary retention, cardiorespiratory systems, and wound complications in 5% to 10% of instances. When a hernia operation is undertaken for emergency indications or for small intestinal obstruction, 56% of patients experienced complications; 18 of these patients died, for a death rate of 7.5%. Both this large study and those of others emphasize that (1) elective repair of abdominal wall herniae is safe despite the usual comorbid conditions in the elderly, (2) a higher morbidity and mortality can be expected with emergency repairs especially where the obstruction occurs in the femoral hernia position, and (3) the lowest complication rates are associated with the use of local anesthesia.

Attention to the appropriate preoperative preparation should obviate many of the cardiovascular and respiratory complications reported in many historic series. Similarly, postoperative wound complications can be avoided by meticulous technique and the avoidance of accidental and even planned enterotomies [13,15].

Postoperative chest physical therapy, optimization of cardiovascular function using the Swan-Ganz catheter as a guide, and early endotracheal extubation and ambulation all postoperatively reduce the prohibitive morbidity and mortality these elderly patients experience otherwise. Successful application of these newer techniques reduces the mortality from the current 25% to more acceptable levels.

Less frequent and less severe complications can still be a source of some concern in the postoperative period. The most frequent of these troublesome problems is urinary retention, usually consequent on occult urinary bladder outlet obstruction. The measurement of urinary flow rates (<10 ml per second) in men is a good diagnostic screening test for the presence of bladder outlet obstruction [37]. Residual urine estimations are of little value. Thus, urinary retention can be expected to occur in approximately 7% of men undergoing elective hernial repairs. This number is often greatly increased by the use of spinal or regional anesthesia. Conversely, in a large series of men who experienced urinary obstruction due to prostatic hypertrophy (2,810 patients), only 5.4% had associated groin herniae [38]. Other annoying complications included uncontrolled hypertension, constipation, renal dysfunction, and deep venous thrombosis. An aggressive and dedicated nursing staff is often all that is required to obviate some of these postoperative conditions [39].

CONCLUSIONS

Worldwide improvements in health care and living conditions have generated a great increase in the population >65 years of age. These people will become patients who will not only have elective and emergency clinical problems, but also will have numerous degenerative and comorbid conditions that adversely affect the outcome of any surgical endeavor. Sociocultural decisions and ethical and moral issues related to the quality of life, dignity of death, and the expense to society for the care of these persons have not been addressed in this chapter. These are important issues, and though as physicians we may prefer to turn our attention away from them, society and elderly competent patients themselves are forcing these issues on us. Especially troublesome are such cases in which extensive carcinomatosis or other terminal diseases have already manifested. As practicing physicians and surgeons, we can only advocate the earlier detection and surgical correction of any such disease states, including herniae of the abdominal wall and colonic neoplasms, that might result in intestinal obstruction. The application of these principles, together with the skills and use of modern preoperative, intraoperative, and postoperative therapeutic strategies, should result in a gratifying and successful outcome for most elderly patients with these problems.

REFERENCES

1. Nehme AE. Groin hernias in elderly patients. Am J Surg 1983;46: 257–260.
2. Tingwald GR, Cooperman M. Inguinal and femoral hernia repair in geriatric patients. Surg Gynecol Obstet 1982;154:704–706.
3 Reiss R, Deutsch AA. Emergency abdominal procedures in patients above 70. J Gerontol 1985;40:154–158.
4. Gleysteen JJ. Intestinal Obstruction. In Condon RE, Nyhus LM (eds), Manual of Surgical Therapeutics (2nd ed). Boston: Little, Brown, 1985;131–149.
5. Reiss R, Deutsch AA, Eliashiz A. Decision making process in abdominal surgery in the geriatric patient. World J Surg 1983;7:522–526.
6. Reiss R, Deutsch A, Nudelman I. Surgical problems in octogenarians: epidemiological analysis of 1083 consecutive admissions. World J Surg 1992;16:1017–1021.
7. Blake R, Lynn J. Emergency abdominal surgery in the aged. Br J Surg 1976;63:956–960.
8. Gentile A. The incidence of hernia in the United States. Industrial Med Surg 1962;31:19–21.
9. Pollak R, Nyhus LM. Complications of groin hernia repair. Surg Clin North Am 1983;63:1363–1371.
10. Greene WW. Bowel obstruction in the aged patient. Am J Surg 1969;118:541–545.
11. Stolar CJH, Randolph JG. Evaluation of ischemic bowel viability with a fluorescent technique. J Pediatr Surg 1978;13:221–225.
12. Balthazar EJ, Schechter LS. Gallstone ileus. AJR Radium Therm Nucl Med 1975;125:374–379.
13. Stewardson RH, Bombeck CT, Nyhus LM. Critical operative management of small bowel obstruction. Ann Surg 1978;181:189–193.
14. Sarr MG, Buckley GB, Zuidema GD. Preoperative recognition of intestinal strangulation obstruction: prospective evaluation of diagnostic capability. Am J Surg 1983;145:176–182.
15. Zadeh BJ, Davis JH, Canizaro PC. Small bowel obstruction in the elderly. Am Surg 1985;51:470–473.
16. Rosenthal RA, Anderson DK. Surgery in the Elderly. In Andres R, Bierman EL, Hazzard WR (eds), Principles of Geriatric Medicine. New York: McGraw-Hill, 1985;909–932.
17. Djokovic JL, Hedley-Whyte J. Prediction of outcome of surgery and anesthesia in patients over 80. JAMA 1979;242:2301–2306.
18. DelGuercio LRM, Cohn JD. Monitoring operative risk in the elderly. JAMA 1980;243:1350–1355.
19. Hodgkin JE, Dines DE, Didier EP. Pre-operative evaluation of patients with pulmonary disease. Mayo Clin Proc 1975;48:114–118.
20. Morrell MT, Dunhill MS. The post-mortem incidence of pulmonary embolism in a hospitalized population. Br J Surg 1968;55:347–352.
21. Lee BV, Thoden WR, Trainor FS, Kavner D. Noninvasive detection and prevention of deep vein thrombosis in geriatric patients. J Am Geriatr Soc 1980;28:171–175.
22. Linn BS, Jensen J. Age and immune response to a surgical stress. Arch Surg 1983;118:405–409.
23. Pollak R. Miscellaneous Surgical Techniques for the Small Intestine. In Nyhus LM, Baker RJ (eds), Mastery of Surgery. Boston: Little, Brown, 1984;894–900.
24. Nelson RL, Nyhus LM. A new long intestinal tube. Surg Gynecol Obstet 1979;149:581–582.
25. Pollak R. Strangulating External Hernias. In Nyhus LM, Condon RE (eds), Hernia (3rd ed). Philadelphia: Lippincott, 1987.
26. Pollak R, Nyhus LM. The unexpected internal hernia. Probl Gen Surg 1984;1:226–237.
27. Nyhus LM. The Preperitoneal Approach and Iliopubic Tract Repair of Inguinal Hernias. In Nyhus LM, Condon RE (eds), Hernia (4th ed). Philadelphia: Lippincott, 1995;153–174.
28. Nyhus LM, Pollak R. Inguinal and Femoral Hernias. In Beahrs OH, Beart RW (eds), General Surgery Therapy. Media, PA: Harwal Publishing, 1986.
29. Condon RE. Anterior Iliopubic Tract Repair. In Nyhus LM, Condon RE (eds), Hernia (4th ed). Philadelphia: Lippincott, 1995;136–152.
30. Greene FL, Ponsky JL (eds). Endoscopic Surgery. Philadelphia: Saunders, 1994.
31. Pollak R, Nyhus LM. Hernias. In Schwartz SI, Ellis H (eds), Maingot's Abdominal Operations (8th ed). Norwalk, CT: Appleton-Century-Crofts, 1985;297–350.
32. Prasad ML, Pearl RK, Abcarian H. End-loop colostomy. Surg Gynecol Obstet 1984;158:380–382.
33. Smithy WB, Wexner SD, Dailey TH. The diagnosis and treatment of acute appendicitis in the aged. Dis Colon Rectum 1986;29:170–173.
34. Prian GW, Sawyer RB, Sawyer KC. Repair of peristomal colostomy hernias. Am J Surg 1975;130:674–696.
35. Buddee FW, Coupland GAE, Reeve TS. Large abdominal wall herniae: an easy method of repair without prosthetic material, with the induction of pneumoperitoneum. Aust N Z J Surg 1975;45:265–270.
36. Moreno IG. The Rational Treatment of Hernias and Voluminous Chronic Eventrations: Preparation with Progressive Pneumoperitoneum. In Nyhus LM, Condon RE (eds), Hernia (2nd ed). Philadelphia: Lippincott, 1978;536–560.
37. Brugh R, Rous SN. Bladder outlet obstruction and inguinal hernia. Urology 1977;19:550–552.
38. Riches E. Prostatic destruction: the treatment of associated conditions. Proc R Soc Med 1962;55:744–746.
39. Nyhus LM, Vitello JM, Condon RE (eds). Abdominal Pain: A Guide to Rapid Diagnosis. Norwalk, CT: Appleton & Lange, 1995;101–102, 226.

Surgical Care for the Elderly, 2nd ed., edited by
R. Benton Adkins, Jr., and H. William Scott, Jr.
Lippincott–Raven Publishers, Philadelphia © 1998.

CHAPTER 27

Diseases of the Colon and Rectum

John L. Sawyers

This chapter discusses disorders of the intestinal tract extending from the ileocecal valve to the anus, including the appendix, entire colon, rectum, and anal canal (Fig. 27-1). Except for the anal canal, which is of ectodermal origin, this part of the intestine arises from the endoderm.

The anatomic and pathologic changes seen in the aging bowel are similar to those that occur elsewhere in the gastrointestinal tract. Tucker described the anatomic changes of mucosal atrophy, increased connective tissue, and atrophy of the muscular layer in elderly subjects [1]. In 1966, Pace reported that the thickening of the colon wall increased with aging as did the amount of elastin in the wall [2].

There is evidence of an overall weakness predominantly in the circular muscles and that most of the thickening is in the longitudinal layer of the teniae coli. The overall size of the colon increases both in diameter and length as chronic constipation and acquired megacolon develop in those individuals with poor bowel habits.

Several studies have addressed the question of whether bowel habits change as a person ages [3,4]. The major finding from these studies has been that a regular laxative-taking routine develops in most older individuals, especially among older women. Constipation is not more common in the elderly patient than in the younger patient; but in immobile, elderly patients confined to a bed or chair, constipation can be a major problem. Milne and Williamson found that 70% of the elderly population had one bowel movement per day [4]. Transit time through the colon is delayed in elderly people, particularly in those who are immobile. Immobile elderly people develop a condition described as the *terminal reservoir syndrome.* The elderly patient lacks the stimulus of mobility to cause mass propulsion that is usually associated with a gastrocolic reflex combined with morning physical activity. Furthermore, the elderly person frequently depends on assistance to reach the toilet. If the call to stool is ignored, the rectal feces move back into the sigmoid colon, and the urge to defecate passes. Stool softeners and purgatives of the anthracene type are probably the most effective in relieving constipation in the elderly [5]. The excessive use of laxatives may damage the myenteric neurons within the submucosa and intramural layers and result in functional disorders, such as constipation, acquired megacolon, and chronic colon ileus [6]. None of the changes seen in the aging colon seems to affect its absorptive ability.

A study of patients >80 years of age between 1981 and 1986 [7] showed that 82% of those with gastrointestinal tumors had involvement of either the colon or rectum. Only 40% of the patients were free of any systemic disorder other than the tumor before operation. In the elderly, the mortality from operation is directly related to associated disease. In this series the overall postoperative mortality was 17%, but the rate decreased by performing elective operations on well-prepared patients. Over 80% of the deaths were related to systemic organ failures. The authors concluded that surgery is a safe, valid option for treatment of disorders in the elderly.

LOWER GASTROINTESTINAL BLEEDING

Gastrointestinal bleeding is an important and common problem in elderly patients. In a study of 58 patients presenting with massive lower gastrointestinal bleeding, Cathcart et al. found an average age of 67.6 years [8]. Many diseases associated with bleeding, such as diverticulosis, vascular ectasia, and cancer, increase in frequency in the elderly, and therefore the physician must consider a wide range of diseases when evaluating an elderly patient who has lower gastrointestinal bleeding.

Approximately 90% of acute episodes of gastrointestinal bleeding originate from sites proximal to the ligament of Treitz. Bright red bleeding from the rectum is usually indicative of a colonic or rectal bleeding site. A nasogastric tube should always be placed, however, to investigate the presence of upper gastrointestinal bleeding, although a negative aspirate result does not completely rule out this possibility. Upper gastrointestinal endoscopy has been a rapid, accurate method of eliminating the esophagus, stomach, and duodenum as possible bleeding sites.

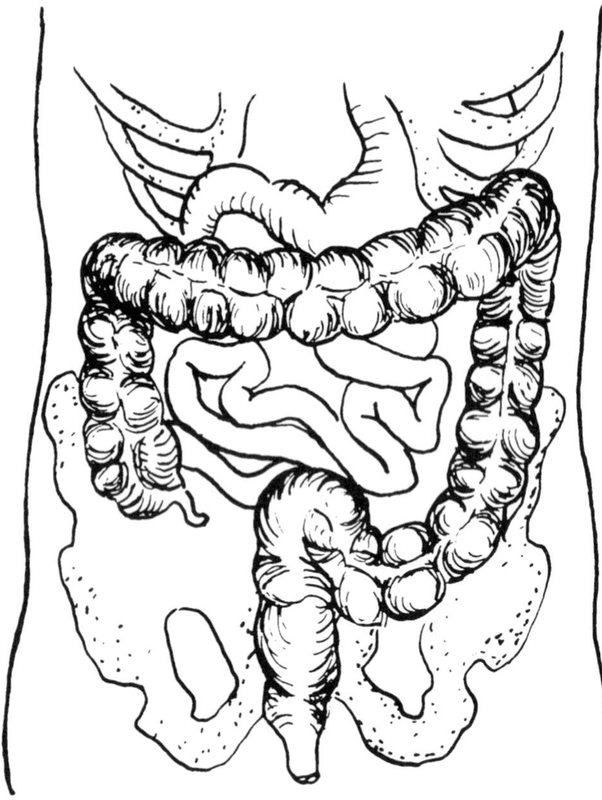

FIG. 27-1. The colon, rectum, and anus are shown in the darker area and extend from the termination of small bowel at the cecum distally to the anal orifice.

TABLE 27-1. *Causes of lower gastrointestinal bleeding*

Common causes
- Hemorrhoids
- Anal fissure
- Cancer of the colorectum
- Polypoid lesions of the colon
- Ulcerative colitis
- Diverticular disease
- Vascular ectasia of the colon

Unusual causes
- Anticoagulants and blood dyscrasia
- Infectious disease such as amebiasis, schistosomiasis, and infectious diarrheas
- Meckel's diverticulum
- Colonic ischemia
- Traumatic lesions
- Crohn's disease
- Duodenal ulcer
- Intussusception
- Idiopathic ulcers of the colon
- Small bowel tumors
- Benign tumors of the colon
- Varices of the colon
- Aortoduodenal fistula from aneurysm or secondary to an aortic graft
- Endometriosis
- Postoperative hemorrhage
- Bleeding from unknown source

The evaluation of lower gastrointestinal bleeding should include a sigmoidoscopy and coagulation studies. Colonoscopy is performed if the rate of bleeding persists. With active lower gastrointestinal bleeding, an urgent angiographic study of the superior mesenteric, inferior mesenteric, and celiac arteries, in that order, is performed. Barium enema and small bowel series are deferred until after angiography [9]. Infusion of technetium-tagged red cells as an initial evaluation in the slowly bleeding patient before the use of angiography may be useful in localizing the bleeding point.

The elderly patient does not tolerate episodes of bleeding as well as younger individuals. Therefore, stabilization and blood loss replacement are even more critical in the elderly patient. Immediate exploratory laparotomy for diagnosis and treatment may be necessary for patients in whom the bleeding continues and is not readily controlled.

If selective arteriography localized the site of the bleeding, vasopressin can be infused at the time of arteriography into the vessels of the bleeding area. This technique is sometimes effective, but its benefit is often temporary. Matolo and Link have suggested the use of transcatheter embolization in selected patients in whom vasopressin infusion has failed or who are poor surgical risks [10]. They have selectively embolized the bleeding vessels using absorbable gelatin sponges (Gelfoam), autologous clot, or coils. They further suggest that operative intervention can then be considered after the patient's bleeding is controlled and the operation can be done electively.

If arteriography demonstrates evidence of a vascular abnormality, such as an angiodysplastic lesion or ectasia, then this area may be removed electively. Such lesions are generally found on the right side of the colon, and right hemicolectomy is the preferred procedure. Even if the patient is not actively bleeding, angiography may identify a vascular ectatic lesion, which can be resected when the patient is brought to an optimal condition for operation. It should be remembered that angiographic changes of the vessels within a cancer of the colon may mimic angiodysplasia. This makes elective resection an even more appropriate method of treatment.

When all study results including the angiography are normal and the patient is still actively bleeding, urgent colectomy is performed with ileoproctostomy as a lifesaving procedure, preferably before transfusion of 10 U of blood. Causes of lower gastrointestinal bleeding are listed in Table 27-1.

HEMORRHOIDS

The incidence of internal hemorrhoids was 72% in 2,000 consecutive proctoscopic examinations [11]. Hemorrhoids are classified into four groups. First-degree hemorrhoids do

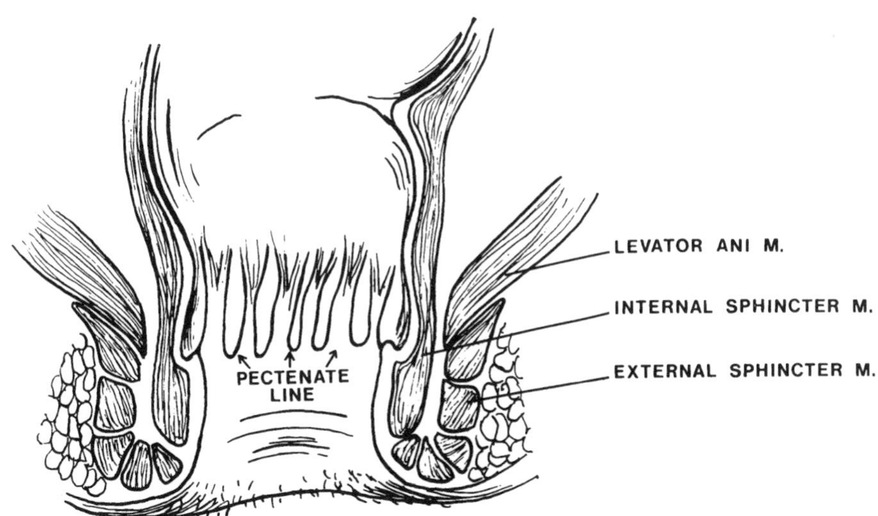

FIG. 27-2. Anatomy of the rectoanal area showing the pectinate (dentate) line and sphincters.

not descend below the pectinate (dentate) line of the rectum (Fig. 27-2) when the patient is instructed to strain as if he or she were attempting to evacuate the bowel. Second-degree hemorrhoids protrude into the lower anal canal on straining, but after defecation or cessation of straining, the protruding hemorrhoids spontaneously return to their normal position above the pectinate line. Third-degree hemorrhoids do not retract spontaneously into the rectum and must be pushed back manually. Fourth-degree hemorrhoids have overstretched submucosal attachments with redundant rectal mucosa, and the internal hemorrhoids are not retained in the rectum, resulting in chronic prolapse.

The most frequent symptom of internal hemorrhoids is painless bleeding of bright red blood per rectum during or after defecation. Other symptoms, depending on the hemorrhoid classification, are prolapse and rarely strangulation. Patients with bleeding hemorrhoids may be treated by conservative medical management after ruling out other causes of bleeding such as cancer or polyps by colonoscopy. First- and second-degree hemorrhoids not responding to hydrophilic bulk laxatives, rectal suppositories, and good anal hygiene may be managed by rubber band ligation [12]. Long-term success with banding internal hemorrhoids has been reported in 94% of patients [13]. Other methods of treatment include CO_2 laser treatment and sclerotherapy, which may be performed on an outpatient basis.

Symptomatic patients with third- and fourth-degree internal hemorrhoids are usually managed by surgical excision. Several surgical techniques are available, but closed hemorrhoidectomy is preferred by most surgeons. Prolapsed hemorrhoids may also be managed by diathermy excision. A prospective randomized trial comparing scissor excision with ligation versus diathermy excision without ligation revealed no statistical difference in severity of postoperative pain or complications. Diathermy excision is faster and accompanied by less bleeding [14].

External thrombosed hemorrhoids cause acute onset of pain that may last for 48 hours and then diminish, leaving a clot in the lower anal canal. Excision of the clot under local anesthetic relieves the pain.

DIVERTICULOSIS

The incidence of diverticulosis steadily increases after age 40 and becomes more common in patients 60 and older [15]. Approximately one-third of the population over age 45 has been estimated to have diverticular disease [16]. Autopsies of patients 80 and older suggest an incidence of >50% in that age group [17].

The incidence of diverticulosis is significantly less in Africa and Asia than it is in the West. Apparently, populations that have a diet high in vegetable fiber are protected from the development of diverticula [18]. Persons on this diet do, however, develop colon volvulus at a high rate.

In most cases (45% to 65%) diverticular disease is confined to the sigmoid colon. Grossly, the colon involved with diverticulosis appears to be shortened and thickened. On examination, both the longitudinal and circular muscle show abnormal thickening, and the diameter of the lumen is decreased. The origin of the diverticula is found to be between the folds of the circular muscle fibers and adjacent to the teniae coli. If the bowel has been inflamed, fibrous tissue is also evident [19].

Most individuals with colon diverticula never experience symptoms from the disorder. Only one in 70 individuals needs hospital care for acute attacks of diverticulitis, and only one in 200 requires surgical treatment [20]. Inflammation may spread along the serosa of the colon and eventually lead to the formation of adhesions in some cases. Other organs that might become adherent to the colon are therefore involved in the inflammatory process. Approximately 12% to 25% of patients with inflammatory diverticular disease develop a fistula, usually a vesicocolic fistula [19]. If repeated episodes of diverticulitis are allowed to continue to recur, the colon eventually becomes obstructed due to increased fibrosis and stricture formation [21].

Bleeding is a common consequence of diverticulosis, because of the proximity of the diverticulum to the blood vessels of the colon. It is likely that inflammation plays a part in this particular complication also. Usually, the bleeding is substantial and always intraluminal [22].

The complications of colonic diverticula include acute peridiverticulitis, hemorrhage, free perforation, obstruction, pericolic abscess, and fistula formation to bladder, vagina, small intestine, adjacent loop of colon, or skin.

The majority of patients with symptoms of diverticulitis complain initially of left lower quadrant pain with tenderness, mild distension, low-grade fever, and leukocytosis. A mass may be palpable in the left lower quadrant by abdominal examination, but in an estimated 15% to 20% of patients a mass can be palpable only on rectal or pelvic examination. Flexible sigmoidoscopy is useful in ruling out colitis or tumors. Mucosal edema is encountered at approximately 15 cm with inability to pass the scope because of patient discomfort that reproduces the pain of diverticulitis. An abdominal computed tomographic scan is helpful in confirming the diagnosis and may show an abscess, fluid, or intra-abdominal air from bowel perforation.

Unless the patient has had a free perforation of a colonic diverticulum into the peritoneal cavity, the initial treatment is nonoperative with bowel rest, intravenous fluids, and antibiotics. After symptoms improve, the patient should be instructed to stay on a high-fiber diet to reduce the frequency of recurrent attacks of acute diverticulitis. A barium enema helps delineate the location and extent of the diverticula, but should be performed only after the patient has recovered from an acute attack.

Patients with perforated sigmoid diverticulitis require emergency operation. Hartmann's procedure, consisting of resection of the sigmoid colon, stapled closure of the rectum, and proximal end colostomy of the descending colon, is consider safer than resection with primary anastomosis. Colorectal continuity is established at a second operation 3 to 6 months later. The end-to-end stapler makes this second operation technically easier.

Patients with large diverticular abscesses are best managed by preoperative percutaneous drainage as initial treatment rather than emergency resection. Sepsis usually resolves rapidly, and drainage is usually not required beyond 3 weeks. Single-stage sigmoid colectomy with primary anastomosis can then be performed usually without complications, avoiding the need for colostomy and multiple-stage operations [23].

Even in the aged patient, resection for diverticular disease can usually be performed with primary anastomosis in uncomplicated and selected complicated cases with a low morbidity and mortality of <5% [24].

COLONIC VOLVULUS

Of all patients in the United States and Western Europe with intestinal obstruction, 3% to 5% have colonic volvulus as the etiologic factor. In Russia, India, and Eastern Europe, the incidence of colonic volvulus increases dramatically and results in 30% to 50% of all cases of intestinal obstruction [6]. This may be due in part to the bulky high-fiber diet common in those geographic regions, which has been called the *volvulus belt* by some.

Colonic volvulus is more common in older people than in younger individuals, and it usually affects the sigmoid colon in the elderly patient. Volvulus occurs at three major sites in the colon: (1) approximately 75% in the sigmoid colon, (2) 20% in the cecum, and (3) 5% in the transverse colon [16]. Many factors leave the elderly patient susceptible to the development of a colon volvulus. Enlargement of the colon, which can lead to volvulus, is not uncommon in the elderly and is the cause of most cases, especially in those patients who are physically inactive or institutionalized.

When managed nonoperatively, colon volvulus will likely recur. Arnold and Nance reported a 55% recurrence rate of sigmoid volvulus in patients seen at the Charity Hospital in New Orleans [25]. They advocate elective resection in the elderly who are at a much higher operative risk with emergency procedures.

Peoples et al., in a review of 54 patients treated for sigmoid volvulus from 1983 to 1987, found that 7.4% required emergency resection for gangrene, with a mortality of 75%. Fourteen of 26 patients managed by nonoperative detorsion required no further treatment. Nonoperative mortality was 0%. Factors associated with poor outcome after operation were patient age and history of previous volvulus. All deaths occurred in patients >70 years presenting with a first episode of volvulus (mortality of 33%). These surgeons advocate nonoperative detorsion alone for patients >70 years presenting with sigmoid volvulus as a first episode or recurrence [26].

Geriatric patients are susceptible to the development of an asymptomatic pseudomegacolon because of swallowing air, laxative abuse, and chronic constipation. The bowel becomes too long for its mesentery. The mesentery itself is then stretched and elongated, and this long, thinned pedicle has a disproportionately short base on which the sigmoid, cecum, or transverse colon can rotate. The pretwisted or partially rotated condition of the bowel usually remains asymptomatic for years until volvulus occurs. The closed loop obstruction leads to gangrene, perforation, and peritonitis if the volvulus is not promptly corrected.

Colonic volvulus is characterized by abdominal distention, tenderness, an abdominal mass, and radiographic evidence of air in a distended loop of colon, which is described as the *bent inner tube sign*. Air-fluid levels may be present in the distended small bowel. Barium enema contrast studies show a narrowing of the proximal rectum at the site of the obstruction, resulting in a bird-beak deformity. Acute volvulus rapidly results in dehydration, fever, and electrolyte problems that progress to shock. The differential diagnosis includes toxic dilation of the colon, pseudo-obstruction (Ogilvie's syndrome), and distal colonic obstruction from tumor or anal stenosis.

Once the diagnosis is suspected, measures to rehydrate, decompress the stomach and bowel, and correct the electrolyte imbalance should be taken. A sigmoid volvulus may be decompressed 70% to 90% of the time by passing a rectal tube through the rigid sigmoidoscope. The rectal tube should be left in place for several days. If reduction of the volvulus is successful, a forceful evacuation of flatus and bowel contents occurs. The operator is best advised to wear a protective gown and consider a face shield. These nonoperative maneuvers should not be tried if there is questionable perforation, vascular compromise, suspected bowel necrosis, or peritonitis. If nonoperative measures are unsuccessful, emergency laparotomy, in spite of age, is indicated as soon as the situation permits.

A review of patients with colonic volvulus at the University of Louisville Hospitals between 1983 and 1988 found 45 patients: Twenty-nine patients had sigmoid volvulus, 17 with cecal volvulus (one had both). Nonoperative decompression was successful in 26 of 29 patients with sigmoid volvulus. Fourteen of 29 patients underwent operation and 50% died following resection. The 15 patients who elected to be treated nonoperatively for recurrent volvulus had no mortality. There was no mortality in patients with cecal volvulus treated by cecopexy alone, but all three patients who had tube cecostomy died [27].

These reports indicate that nonoperative decompression for colonic volvulus should be tried initially and can be performed successfully on successive occasions. If operation is necessary, resection should be done only to excise gangrenous bowel. Mesosigmoidopexy has been reported to be a safe, effective treatment for sigmoid volvulus [28], as is cecopexy for cecal volvulus. However, a study from Africa comparing mesosigmoidopexy with resection and primary anastomosis reported improved results with the latter (90% versus 71.5% success) [29]. In the United States, most surgeons prefer sigmoid resection with primary anastomosis.

CECAL VOLVULUS

Although less common than sigmoid volvulus, cecal volvulus constitutes a surgical emergency because of the danger of cecal perforation. The *rule of nine* has been a standard, meaning that when the diameter of the cecum reaches 9 cm, the possibility of cecal perforation is greatly increased.

Cecal volvulus is generally thought to be due to incomplete fusion of the cecum to the parietal peritoneum. Torsion of the ileocecal intestinal segment usually occurs, with counterclockwise rotation displacing the ileum and upward folding of the cecum in the so-called cecal bascule fashion. The diagnosis can usually be made on presentation of a patient who has abdominal distention and the typical roentgenographic findings. On palpation of the abdomen, the right iliac fossa is generally found to be empty. Bowel sounds are typical of obstruction. A barium enema will help make the diagnosis.

A flexible colonoscope may be used, especially for volvulus of the transverse colon and cecum [30–34]. If not successful, then treatment is urgent laparotomy with detorsion of the cecal volvulus. If the bowel is viable, the colon may be fixed by cecopexy.

INFLAMMATORY BOWEL DISEASES

The usual inflammatory bowel diseases seen in the elderly are granulomatous colitis (Crohn's disease) and ulcerative colitis. Granulomatous colitis and ulcerative colitis have in common many clinical symptoms and pathologic and roentgenographic findings.

Granulomatous colitis is a disease, acute or chronic, involving all layers of the colon and is commonly termed *Crohn's disease of the colon.* Crohn's disease may involve any part of the gastrointestinal tract and is characterized by segmental areas of involvement with normal intervening skip areas. Crohn's disease of the colon frequently extends into the terminal ileum and characteristically spares the rectum. No specific infectious agent has been found in granulomatous colitis.

Ulcerative colitis is an inflammatory disease of the colon, acute or chronic, involving primarily the mucosa and submucosa. The rectal mucosa and varying portions of the more proximal colon are usually involved without skip areas. No infectious agent has been identified.

Differentiation of granulomatous colitis from ulcerative colitis depends primarily on the gross and microscopic findings. Typically, ulcerative colitis begins in the rectum and extends proximally throughout the large intestine. The serosa of the colon is intact in ulcerative colitis, except in the acute fulminating form (toxic megacolon). The inflammation is confined to the mucosa and submucosa, and ulceration is patchy. Areas of intact mucosa within a denuded area may give rise to pseudopolyps. The colon is shortened, with loss of the haustral markings as a result of contraction of the musculature. The ileum may be involved secondarily by "backwash ileitis." Microscopic examination reveals increased vascularity, with loss of goblet cells and a relative lack of fibrosis. Crypt abscesses are common.

The gross pathology of granulomatous colitis is characterized by segmental involvement, with intervening segments of normal intestine. The bowel wall is thickened, owing to transmural inflammation. The serosa is involved and may be studded with tiny tubercles that represent noncaseating granulomas. The mesentery is usually thick, and regional lymph nodes are enlarged. The mucosa may have a cobblestone appearance where intercommunicating fissures surround islands of mucosa elevated by underlying inflammation and edema. Noncaseating granulomas represent a

TABLE 27-2. *Ulcerative colitis versus granulomatous colitis*

	Ulcerative colitis	Granulomatous colitis
Usual location	Rectum, left colon	Ileum and right colon
Diarrhea	Severe	Moderate
Rectal bleeding	Common (almost 100%)	Intermittent (approximately 50%)
Rectal involvement	Almost 100%	Approximately 20%
Perianal disease	Rare	Fistulas and abscesses common
Abdominal wall and internal fistulas	No	Frequent
Sigmoidoscopy	Uniform, diffuse friability with shaggy irregular ulcers	Patchy involvement, linear ulcers (cobblestone mucosa)
Colon roentgenographic findings	Diffuse, tiny serrations (crypt abscess), uniform loss of haustration, shortening of colon	Segmental, skip areas, internal fistulas, no shortening
Carcinoma	10% in 10 years	Rare
Toxic megacolon	Common	Rare
Associated systemic disease (arthritis, uveitis, pyoderma)	Common	Infrequent
Recurrent ileitis after colectomy	No	Frequent
Pathologic		
Gross appearance of colon	Confluent involvement, mesentery normal, pseudopolyps common, bowel wall thin or normal	Segmental involvement, mesentery thickened, lymph nodes enlarged, cobblestone mucosa, bowel wall thickened
Microscopic appearance of colon	Inflammation limited to mucosa and submucosa	Transmural inflammation
	No granulomas	Frequent granulomas
	No serositis	Serositis always present
	Crypt abscesses	Rare crypt abscesses
Surgical treatment	Proctocolectomy with Brooke ileostomy or ileoanal pouch	Subtotal or total colectomy, rectum frequently preserved

typical microscopic feature of granulomatous colitis. These lesions resemble the reaction seen in sarcoidosis. Granulomas may be found in 50% to 70% of patients. Crypt abscesses are less frequent than in ulcerative colitis, but may be present. Fissuring (knifelike clefts into the wall of the intestine) may occur, with development of fistulas into the small intestine, bladder, vagina, or abdominal wall. Table 27-2 lists the typical pathologic findings.

Granulomatous Colitis

Granulomatous disease of the bowel was first recognized in 1932, when Crohn, Ginburg, and Oppenheimer published their description of regional ileitis [35]. According to that report, Crohn thought the disease was confined to the distal small bowel. It is now known that Crohn's disease may involve any portion of the gastrointestinal tract.

The cause of granulomatous colitis is not known. The search for an infectious agent continues. The condition has not been produced experimentally, but immunologic methods are being studied.

The disease may occur in any group and is more serious in children and geriatric patients. There is an increased incidence in families, between parent and child as well as between siblings. Although not recognized as a specific entity until 1960, the disease has been reported in most countries throughout the world. In the United States, approximately 30% of patients with inflammatory bowel disease have granulomatous colitis; ulcerative colitis accounts for approximately 60%. In approximately 10% of patients, inflammatory bowel disease cannot be classified as either granulomatous or ulcerative colitis, but has characteristics of both.

Clinical Manifestations

The onset of symptoms from granulomatous colitis is usually insidious. Abdominal pain and diarrhea are the most prominent symptoms and may be accompanied by weight loss, anorexia, fever, and malaise. Abdominal pain unrelieved by defecation has been described as characteristic of granulomatous colitis. The pain may be generalized or localized to the lower abdomen and is usually constant. Diarrhea is usually less severe than in patients with ulcerative colitis and consists of frequent watery stools without blood. Patients with rectal involvement may complain of tenesmus, but patients seldom have proctitis. Rectal sphincter control is usually not impaired. However, the presence of perianal fistulas or granulomas should suggest the presence of granulomatous colitis.

Symptoms may occur from complications of obstruction in the distal segments of the colon, usually the descending or sigmoid colon. In patients with ileocolitis, obstruction is commonly seen in the terminal ileum from fibrosis and lymphedema. Internal fistulas are common in patients with chronic disease and may occur to adjacent loops of bowel or to ureter, vagina, or bladder. External fistulas may develop through the abdominal wall. Abdominal masses consisting of dilated loops of small bowel or of abscesses may be palpated, usually in the right lower quadrant or deep in the left pelvis.

Surgical treatment for granulomatous colitis is for the complications of the disease—obstruction, bleeding, and fistula formation. Perianal disease manifested by fistulas and recurrent abscesses that does not respond to metronidazole (Flagyl) and other antibiotics may be an operative indication. The majority of patients with Crohn's disease of the anus and perianal area can be managed by meticulous drainage of sepsis with preservation of the anal sphincter.

Carr and Schofield reported that, in their experience, elderly patients with inflammatory bowel disease had an increased incidence of complications and an increased mortality when compared with younger patients [36]. They stressed, therefore, the need for early, elective, surgical management for the complications of the disease. If performed under elective, controlled conditions, the elderly patient tolerates bowel resection and is able to avoid many of the serious complications of neglected Crohn's disease. It has been suggested that patients aged 60 or older who develop Crohn's disease are more likely to respond well to surgical treatment than are younger patients [37,38].

Ulcerative Colitis

The occurrence of ulcerative colitis peaks between the ages of 20 and 40 and again between 60 and 65 years [16]. This disease produces symptoms of severe, often bloody diarrhea and is associated with abdominal pain. Fever, weight loss, tenesmus, and anemia are not uncommon. The diarrhea consists of frequent loose bowel movements (10 to 20 per day) and occurs during the day and at night after the patient has gone to bed. Normal absorption of the colon is impaired, with loose, watery, or mushy stools. Mucus and pus may be abundant. Blood per rectum may be bright red or mixed with the stool and results from the increased vascularity and ulceration of the mucosa. At times, brisk massive rectal hemorrhage may occur.

Lower abdominal cramping is frequently present with urgency. Tenesmus may be a prominent feature if the rectal capacity is reduced by fibrosis. In the later stages of the disease, defecation may occur without warning, leading to the increased anxiety and insecurity so often exhibited by ulcerative colitis patients.

Systemic complications of ulcerative colitis are numerous and may be related to hypersensitivity. These symptoms include iritis, uveitis, arthritis, spondylitis, hepatitis, pyoderma gangrenosum, and erythema nodosum. Dramatic clearing of the symptoms may occur after proctocolectomy.

Medical therapy for ulcerative colitis includes dietary restrictions, corticosteroids, and sulfasalazine (Azulfidine). When conservative management is unsuccessful, colon resection is indicated. Proctocolectomy is curative for ulcerative colitis.

Absolute indications for surgical treatment include perforation, hemorrhage, obstruction, cancer, and acute fulminating disease with or without toxic megacolon. Free perforation of the colon usually occurs in association with toxic megacolon, which is much more common in patients with ulcerative colitis, but can occur in patients with granulomatous colitis. Perforations may be single or multiple. Omentum may be adherent to the colon at the site of an impending perforation and should not be dissected from the bowel wall, but the adherent omentum should be resected along with the colon. In some patients, the signs and symptoms of colonic perforation are present, but no free perforation can be found. The purulent exudate in the peritoneal cavity is probably secondary to the acute, diffuse serosal inflammation.

Repeated and massive hemorrhage may occur in patients with ulcerative colitis, but seldom in patients with granulomatous colitis. Hemorrhage may occur in association with an acute attack of colitis and not necessarily in disease of long duration. In most patients, bleeding may be managed by multiple blood transfusions, but when life-threatening uncontrolled hemorrhage develops, urgent proctocolectomy and ileostomy are necessary. It is a difficult decision to proceed to surgery, but both internists and surgeons should be aware that procrastination while giving multiple blood transfusions will cause the patient to become more debilitated and increase the operative risk.

Obstruction secondary to inflammatory disease of the colon is seldom acute. Chronic obstructive symptoms may develop from stricture formation and occur in patients with granulomatous colitis. Tight stricture formation causing colonic obstruction in patients with ulcerative colitis arouses suspicion of cancer.

Relative indications for surgical treatment include failure to respond to medical management and recurring disease in the elderly. The frequency with which operation is required as an elective procedure varies with the philosophy of the medical-surgical team. Increasing acceptance of a permanent ileostomy because of improved patient education and the availability of trained enterostomal therapists may liberalize the indications for elective surgery in patients with inflammatory bowel disease.

The most frequent indication for elective operation is failure of the patient's symptoms to respond to medical management with Azulfidine, corticosteroids, or both. Azathioprine (Imuran) has also been used for the symptoms of inflammatory colitis before surgical intervention. Intractable diarrhea with its restrictions on the patient's occupation and social life, plus the side effects of anemia, malnutrition, water and electrolyte depletion, and repeated hospitalizations for treatment of exacerbations of the disease, finally forces patient and internist to seek relief by surgical management even though this necessitates a permanent ileostomy. Elderly patients (>60 years of age) with ulcerative colitis have an average annual mortality of almost 5% when managed by medical treatment with operation reserved for life-threatening complications.

Elective operation in the elderly should be considered to reduce the high mortality associated with emergency operation and to prevent the complications of inflammatory colitis that are so difficult and hazardous for the elderly patient.

Ileoanal pull-through with ileal pouch has not been as successful in the older patient who has trouble adjusting to frequent stools. Proctocolectomy with a Brooke ileostomy is preferable in the elderly patient. This is performed as a one-stage procedure. The concept of performing ileostomy and total proctocolectomy simultaneously has been widely accepted as the procedure of choice when surgical intervention is indicated in the management of patients with ulcerative colitis. Despite the magnitude of the operation, this single-stage procedure offers the cardinal advantage to the patient of immediate ablation of all inflammatory bowel disease, thus eliminating the serious complications of persistent or recurrent ulcerative colitis, with the attendant morbidity and mortality.

In patients with ulcerative colitis treated by single-stage proctocolectomy, early postoperative complications occurred only in those patients who had received massive or prolonged preoperative corticosteroid treatment. Accordingly, it is reasonable to raise the question as to the advisability of the use of prolonged or massive corticosteroid therapy in ulcerative colitis.

The complications of perforation and bleeding are poorly tolerated and can be devastating in all patients, especially the elderly [39,40]. Reiss and Deutsch found that the mortality for emergency procedures in which peritonitis was present was 32% compared with 8% in emergency cases in which peritonitis was not present [41]. Therefore, in the older, otherwise healthy patient with ulcerative colitis, an early, aggressive surgical approach may do much to preserve the well-being and life-style of the patient.

An equally important indication for early surgical treatment for patients with inflammatory bowel disease is the risk of colon cancer developing in the presence of ulcerative colitis and Crohn's disease [42,43]. Levinson and coworkers studied the risk of cancer developing in adults with ulcerative colitis [44]. They found that in patients with a 10-year history of the disease, the risk was 5%. This increased to 25% in 20 years and continues to increase as time goes on. Lightdale and Winawer estimate that the risk increases approximately 20% per decade [45]. Although the symptoms of colonic carcinoma and inflammatory bowel disease are similar, there are clinical features that might lead the physician to suspect a carcinoma. These features include abrupt exacerbation of symptoms, new symptoms of bowel obstruction, abdominal pain not associated with defecation, unusual onset of constipation, palpable abdominal mass, and stricture formation [16].

Colonic cancers occurring in association with ulcerative colitis are difficult to recognize. The tumors are often multicentric and small and invade rapidly into the bowel wall. The tumors tend to produce infiltrating lesions that mimic fibrous strictures in the colon. Aggressive surgical management (proctocolectomy with ileostomy) can lead to long-term survival. Colonoscopy with multiple blind biopsies for changes of metaplasia in the mucosa has been advocated to detect early malignant changes in patients with ulcerative colitis.

Other Types of Colitis

A form of granular proctitis occurring in older patients presents with an endoscopic appearance similar to ulcerative colitis. These patients have mild, intermittent symptoms characterized by moderate diarrhea and bleeding. The inflammatory process usually does not extend proximal to the distal sigmoid colon. Rectal biopsies of the diseased areas show a marked increase in cells containing IgE in the lamina propria [46]. These patients usually respond favorably to medical management, such as corticosteroid enemas.

Colitis developing in patients receiving antibiotics has been reported with increasing frequency, but appears to be simply another example of pseudomembranous colitis. Clindamycin, lincomycin hydrochloride monohydrate, ampicillin, tetracycline, and chloramphenicol have been associated with the development of pseudomembranous colitis. Toxic dilatation of the colon may complicate pseudomembranous enterocolitis induced by antibiotics and must be differentiated from the toxic megacolon associated with ulcerative colitis.

Amebiasis is an infection caused by the protozoan *Entamoeba histolytica* and primarily involves the colon. Other body organs may be involved secondarily, the most common manifestation being amebic abscess of the liver. The disease is found worldwide.

Ischemic colitis is not an inflammatory bowel disease, but may cause confusion with the diagnosis of ulcerative colitis, especially in elderly patients.

VASCULAR DISORDERS OF THE COLON

Because atherosclerotic disease is a natural process of aging, it is not surprising that ischemic disease of the colon occurs in the elderly. Both acute and chronic ischemic changes can affect the large bowel.

Mesenteric Vascular Occlusion

Acute Mesenteric Ischemia

Acute mesenteric vascular occlusion is usually secondary to an embolus. With the increased incidence of heart disease in the elderly, mural thrombi from the left ventricle following myocardial infarction or from a left atrium in fibrillation are the most frequent source of the emboli. Dissecting aortic aneurysms and arteriosclerotic occlusion of the superior or inferior mesenteric arteries may also be a precipitating factor of acute mesenteric occlusion. The patient is seized by sudden, severe abdominal pain usually associated with bloody diarrhea and the sudden onset of a shocklike state. A major embolus rapidly results in infarction of the colon and requires emergency operation with surgical resection of the nonviable bowel. Proximal colostomy with later re-establishment of colonic continuity, if possible, is advised.

Acute superior mesenteric artery embolus is the etiologic factor in approximately 50% of the cases of acute intestinal ischemia [47]. Nearly half of these patients admit to having had abdominal pain in the past weeks [48]. These patients then experience severe abdominal pain and rectal bleeding. A generalized abdominal pain then ensues; ileus and peritonitis follow. Death is certain in the absence of aggressive surgical intervention and is a possibility even with surgery [49].

Chronic Mesenteric Ischemia

Chronic mesenteric vascular ischemia occurs when atherosclerotic changes progress and occlusion results, with obstruction of the major intestinal branches from the aorta. A characteristic syndrome known as *abdominal angina* may be seen. This is characterized by the presence of postprandial abdominal pain, usually occurring 20 to 30 minutes after eating and lasting for 2 to 3 hours. Patients dread eating and have weight loss and eventual malnutrition. Diarrhea, nausea and vomiting, and abdominal bloating are nonspecific symptoms. Physical findings are minimal, but occasionally an abdominal bruit may be heard on auscultation. The diagnosis may be confirmed by arteriography, which shows occlusion of at least two of the major visceral vessels. Surgical therapy is indicated to improve blood supply to the intestinal tract, usually by a bypass procedure, but occasionally reimplantation of the artery or arterial endarterectomy may be performed.

Ileus is evident radiographically early in the disease. Barium enema shows spasm, irritability, thickening of the haustra, and submucosal hemorrhage. When necrosis of the mucosa occurs, ulceration follows. As the disease progresses, fibrosis and stricture result.

Mild forms of this disorder may resolve spontaneously and result only in the fibrous stricture. Other cases progress to fulminant gangrene that requires immediate, aggressive surgical intervention. Immediate resection of all affected areas of the colon is mandatory; primary anastomosis is usually not done under these circumstances [49].

A number of patients present with pain or diarrhea without signs of perforation or clinical decline. In these situations, conservative management including intravenous fluids and intestinal decompression may be appropriate. Careful monitoring is extremely important in the elderly patient who might poorly tolerate a complication and emergency operation. If improvement is not evident within 48 hours, surgical management must be used to avoid a lethal situation.

Nonocclusive vascular occlusion occurs from a low-flow state in patients with congestive cardiac failure, anoxia, and shock. Mesenteric blood flow is preferentially shunted to the brain and other vital organs, resulting in ischemic necrosis of the bowel. Angiography shows no occlusion of the vessels, but there may be spasm, narrowing, and irregularity of the vessels. Infusion of vasodilators and correction of the low-flow state are indicated. Surgical intervention is performed only if infarction of the intestine is strongly indicated, thereby requiring resection.

Ischemic Colitis

A clinical syndrome of abdominal pain and rectal bleeding associated with localized areas of colonic ischemia is known as *ischemic colitis*. This is usually seen in elderly patients. The lesion usually involves the splenic flexure and descending colon. The disease is highly variable, depending on the extent of disruption of colonic blood supply. The onset may be acute with abdominal pain and bloody diarrhea, or a gradual onset of symptoms may be seen, leading to a confusing diagnostic dilemma. The vascular lesion primarily involves the small arteries. Barium enema shows a characteristic appearance of intramural edema and hemorrhage. These lesions have been described as *thumb-printing*. The disease is usually mild and subsides with nonoperative treatment, which should be the initial management, consisting of stabilizing the patient and administering appropriate antibiotics. Occasionally, a residual stricture results that requires surgical correction. Patients who develop acute fulminant ischemic colitis may require emergency colectomy. The disease must be differentiated from inflammatory bowel disease. Ischemia may be the cause of an elderly patient's first episode of colitis. Angiography may be helpful, but frequently does not detect arterial occlusion localized to the small blood vessels. Barium enema is most often unhelpful in this diagnosis.

Vascular Ectasias

Colonic angiodysplasias are reported with increasing frequency in the elderly. This lesion appears to be an ectasia of normal vasculature, rather than a malformation. Initially, the submucosal veins become dilated followed by dilation of the venules and capillaries [50]. These ectasias are usually multiple, occurring in the right colon and cecum. Boley and associates believe that these degenerative lesions are produced by chronic, partial, intermittent, and low-grade obstruction of the submucosal veins [50]. This occurs repeatedly over many years during intestinal contraction and distention. As the capillary rings dilate, the competency of the precapillary sphincters is diminished, resulting in an arteriovenous communication. This final structural change results in the angiographic picture of "early-filling veins." Whenever this condition is seen on arteriography, it must be remembered that some of these venous filling lesions will actually be vessels within colonic cancer. In this instance, the vessels will be tumor vessels, rather than vascular ectasias.

Vascular ectasias may sometimes be diagnosed at the time of colonoscopy, but in many cases angiography is necessary for determining the presence of these lesions. Boley and coworkers have suggested that when an elderly patient presents with active lower gastrointestinal bleeding and the site is not identifiable with nasogastric suctioning or with lower gastrointestinal hemorrhage, angiography should be done before barium enema or other studies [9]. In cases in which the bleeding has stopped, arteriography may be deferred until after contrast intestinal radiographic studies are done. These authors recommend right hemicolectomy in all patients who have had an episode of bleeding and who have angiographic evidence of vascular ectasia.

Vasculitis of the Colon

Vasculitis with extensive necrosis of the small and large intestine can occur as a complication of rheumatoid disease, systemic lupus erythematosus, and polyarteritis nodosa. With vasculitis, irreversible patchy gangrene of the bowel occurs. Resection is necessary for survival, and even then the results can be dismal.

RECTAL PROLAPSE

Rectal prolapse is most common in elderly and debilitated patients. Originally, it was thought that the disorder was a sliding hernia of the pouch of Douglas through a weakened and attenuated pelvic floor, and efforts were directed at repairing the pelvic floor defect. It is now recognized that this defect is secondary to the rectal prolapse rather than the cause. The anatomic defect is an unusually mobile rectum that moves freely into a vertical plane to form a straight tube in continuity with the rectosigmoid colon and anus. Increased abdominal pressure with the rectum in this position results in an intussusception that protrudes through the anus as a procidentia of the rectum [51].

Two types of operation are in current use for rectal prolapse: transabdominal rectopexy as popularized by Ripstein [52] and the one-stage perineal procedure with resection of the rectal prolapse and primary anastomosis and repair of the pelvic diaphragm as described by Altemeier [53]. Each procedure has its advocates.

Williams et al. [54] advocate perineal rectosigmoidectomy, especially in elderly, high-risk patients. They report a 10% recurrent rectal prolapse rate, but fecal incontinence was improved in all patients. The perineal operation is also advocated by Ramanujam and Venkatesh [55], who report a recurrence rate of only 4.8% and improvement in anal continence in 78% of patients. All 41 patients were elderly, and the majority had significant associated risk factors, but there was minimal morbidity and no mortality.

The Ripstein rectopexy is technically easier but requires a laparotomy. Some surgeons prefer to resect the redundant sigmoid colon, but most simply fix the rectum into the hollow of the sacrum with a plastic sling (Teflon, Marlex, Ivalon sponge) or suture without a fixation sling. The colorectal surgeons from Birmingham, England [56], prospectively assessed patients who had a Marlex mesh posterior rectopexy alone versus those who had sigmoidectomy with a sutured posterior rectopexy. They concluded that both procedures were equally safe and effective, but fewer patients were constipated after sigmoidectomy than following rectopexy alone.

The Lahey Clinic surgeons [57] reported their experience with 135 Ripstein operations with a median 41 months of follow-up. There was one postoperative death (0.7%). Recurrent prolapse occurred in 9.6% of patients and stricture at the site of the sling in three patients (2.2%). The Cleveland Clinic surgeons [58] reported their experience in 169 patients with the Ripstein procedure. Operative mortality was 0.6%. Median follow-up was 4.2 years. Recurrence of rectal prolapse was 8%. Fecal incontinence was improved in most patients, but persistence of prior constipation was more common after the Ripstein procedure than after resection rectopexy. In their opinion, the Ripstein procedure has been a safe operation with good anatomic repair of the prolapse and improvement of anal continence. These two clinics have had extensive experience managing patients with rectal prolapse. Both advocate the Ripstein procedure.

Surgeons in Finland [59] reported their experience with the Ripstein procedure in elderly patients (mean age, 74 years). There was no operative mortality in 17 patients. Prolapse recurred in 15%, with a mean follow-up of 3.5 years, but fecal incontinence improved. The procedure resulted in fecal impaction in these patients with prior severe constipation. They concluded that Ripstein rectopexy was useful in patients with rectal prolapse who are poor risks for more extensive operations such as sigmoidectomy.

For elderly patients with acute incarcerated prolapse, perineal excision is advised. Eight elderly patients were managed with this operation with no mortality and no recurrence of rectal prolapse [60].

The enthusiasm for minimally invasive surgery has extended to operations for rectal prolapse. Laparoscopic rectopexy for rectal prolapse has been reported in five women aged 64 to 84 years using fixation to the presacral fascia with Marlex mesh [61]. There was no recurrence of the prolapse in a follow-up of 4 to 27 months.

The Thiersch wire placed subcutaneously around the anal orifice is seldom used, but may be effective in severely debilitated patients with a life expectancy of only a few months who have recurrent massive rectal prolapse.

OGILVIE'S SYNDROME

Colonic pseudo-obstruction was recognized by Ogilvie in 1948. Various metabolic and pharmacologic causes have been reported, as well as spinal trauma and retroperitoneal hemorrhage. Jetmore and associates [62] found that patients with Ogilvie's syndrome were being treated with narcotics (56%), H_2 blockers (52%), phenothiazines (42%), calcium channel blockers (27%), corticosteroids (23%), tricyclic antidepressants (15%), and epidural analgesics (69%) at the time of their diagnoses. Electrolyte abnormalities included hypocalcemia (63%), hyponatremia (38%), hypokalemia (29%), hypomagnesia (21%), and hypophosphatemia (19%). In 52% of their 48 patients, the spine or retroperitoneum had been traumatized or manipulated.

Initial treatment consists of nasogastric suction and correction of fluid volume defects and electrolyte abnormalities. A short trial of this therapy is indicated for cecal diameters of 9 to 12 cm. The normal size of the cecum is up to 9 cm on a prone abdominal roentgenogram. Diameters of 12 to 14 cm are thought to be the threshold for perforation. If the cecal size reaches 12 cm, prompt colonoscopic decompression is indicated. Endoscopic decompression has been indicated since 1977 when Kukora and Dent [63] reported successful colonic decompression by colonoscopy.

Colonoscopy is now the treatment of choice for Ogilvie's syndrome [64]. Approximately one-third of patients require repeat colonoscopy for decompression. The average cecal diameter in patients with successful decompression was 12.4 cm [62].

If decompression is not successful in bringing the cecal distention to <12 cm, cecostomy is done. This may be performed under local anesthesia. Duh and Way [65] described a technique using laparoscopy-guided percutaneous cecostomy using a T-fastener to retract and anchor the cecum to the anterior abdominal wall and a Foley catheter as a cecostomy tube. Laparoscopic visualization of the cecum showed that it was not infarcted.

ACUTE APPENDICITIS

As the proportion of elderly individuals in the general population has increased, so has the percentage of elderly patients who have acute appendicitis. Peltokallio and Tykka found the proportion of their patients aged 60 and older with appendicitis had increased from 4.6% to 8.8% in the years between 1975 and 1980 [66]. Appendicitis in older individuals is more difficult to diagnose.

Abdominal pain in the elderly is usually present, but may be vague and not well localized. Anorexia, almost always present in younger individuals with appendicitis, may be absent in the elderly. Nausea and vomiting are less frequent. Fever occurs later. Leukocytosis is frequently absent [67].

Physical examination usually reveals abdominal tenderness. As in younger patients, localized abdominal tenderness is the single most important sign of appendicitis. Imaging studies may be helpful, including ultrasonography and limited computed tomographic scans of the abdomen. Early operation is advocated for suspected appendicitis. If acute appendicitis progresses to perforation and peritonitis, the morbidity and mortality increase. The mortality in elderly patients who have acute appendicitis is 4% compared with 1% in the general population [68].

The incidence of perforation is increased significantly within the older age group. In the study by Peltokallio and Tykka, the incidence of perforation in older patients increased from 32.8% to 43.7%. In younger patients, they found that the incidence of perforation had increased also, but to a lesser degree than that seen in the older age group [66]. Peltokallio and Tykka also found the duration of the symptoms of acute appendicitis to be approximately the same in both age groups [66]. The only significant difference in the symptoms of acute appendicitis between young and older individuals is that there seems to be a faster progression of the disease in the older patients. Peltokallio and Tykka suggest that this may be because of sclerotic arteries, atrophied mucous membranes, and scanty lymphatic tissue in the older appendix [66]. These changes, coupled with the older person's tendency to delay seeking medical attention and perhaps a hesitancy by the physician to risk surgical intervention in an older patient, are all probably reasons for the increased risk of perforation in these patients.

NEOPLASMS OF THE COLON AND RECTUM

Almost 150,000 people in the United States are diagnosed annually with colorectal cancer. It is estimated that 110,000 are >65 years of age. Unfortunately, the mortality from colorectal cancer has not improved significantly since the 1960s. The best hope for cure is early complete tumor excision, but almost 40% of patients have regional spread of their cancer at the time of diagnosis and 20% have distant metastases [69]. Early diagnosis is needed to improve survival rates.

Whenever the elderly patient has a complaint, history, signs, symptoms, or laboratory values, such as low hematocrit, that suggest a colon lesion, it should be investigated. Diarrhea, melena, anemia, frank rectal bleeding, abdominal pain, iron deficiency, guaiac-positive stools, and a change in bowel habits can result from a benign or malignant colon tumor. The discovery of a benign neoplasm, an atypical cell type adenoma, or a small Duke's A cancer of the rectum or colon in an elderly patient is tantamount to saving him or her from a life-threatening series of events. Any of the previously mentioned symptoms in a younger person would most likely lead to a thorough, exhaustive search, but in individuals from the age group in which most of these lesions are found, there has been a tendency to procrastinate.

A stool examination result that is positive for blood in an elderly patient on a meat-free diet for 5 days is due to neoplasm 50% of the time if an iron deficiency is also present. Rigid sigmoidoscopy reveals a polyp in 5% to 10% of elderly adults. The flexible fiberoptic scope allows the surgeon to visualize the rectum and sigmoid colon with an even higher yield of colorectal neoplasms.

The distribution of colonic polyps is more widespread through the colon than previously suspected. This is true not only of polyps, but is also true for cancer [66,70]. Bernstein

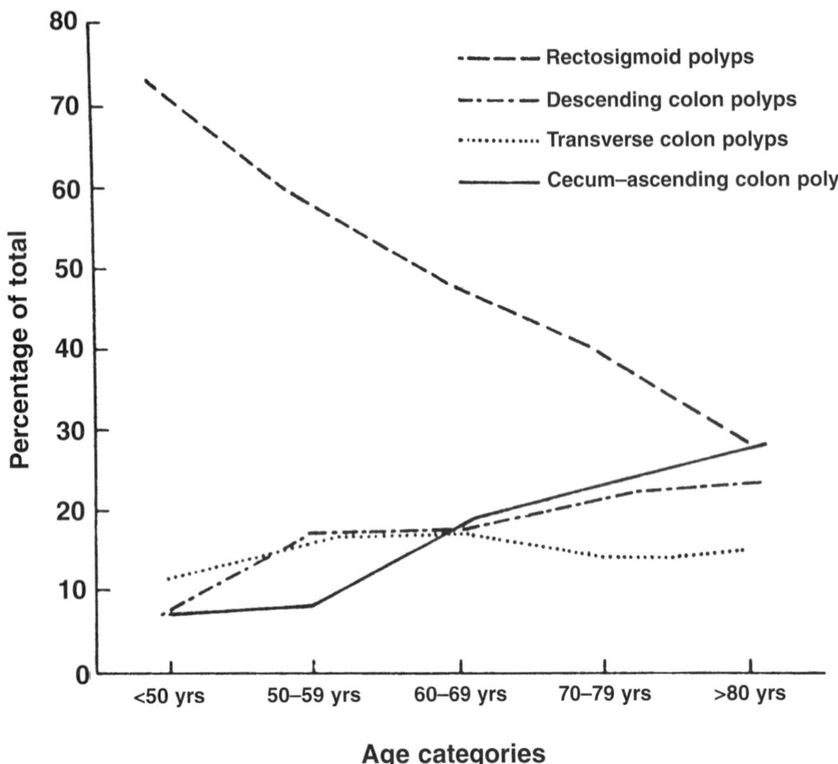

FIG. 27-3. Percentage distribution of polyps by age, illustrating the decreasing incidence of rectosigmoid lesions and increase in lesions of the cecum and ascending colon. (Reprinted with permission from Bernstein MA, Feczko PJ, Halpert RD, et al. Distribution of colonic polyps: increased incidence of proximal lesions in older patients. Radiology 1985;155:35–38.)

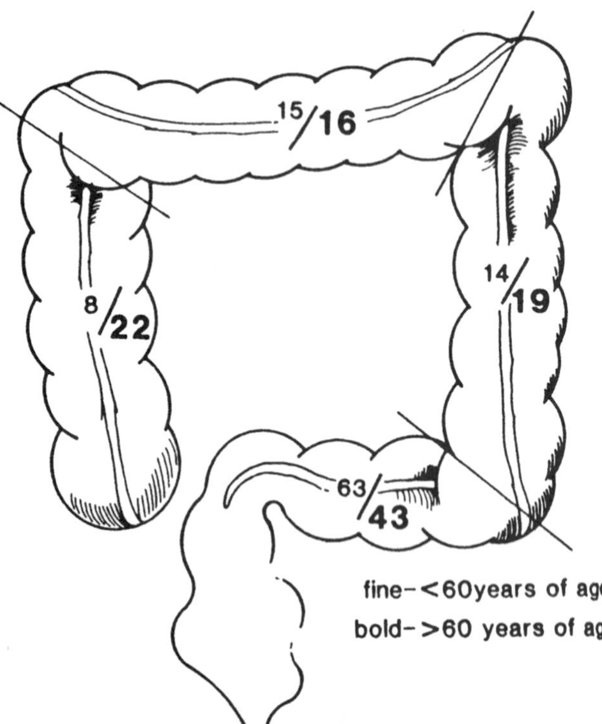

FIG. 27-4. Percentage of lesions before and after the age of 60. The marked increase in right-sided lesions and decrease in rectosigmoid lesions are statistically significant. (Reprinted with permission from Bernstein MA, Feczko PJ, Halpert RD, et al. Distribution of colonic polyps: increased incidence of proximal lesions in older patients. Radiology 1985;155:35–38.)

and his colleagues in 1985 reported on polyp distribution in the elderly [71]. They showed a marked tendency for a change in distribution from rectosigmoid in the young patient to a right colon location for lesions in the elderly (Figs. 27-3 and 27-4).

When a polyp, adenoma, area of ulceration, fungating lesion, or submucosal lesion is found, a biopsy or total removal of the lesion should be done. If a rectal polyp or benign lesion is found in the rectum or sigmoid colon, there is a 30% to 40% chance of another tumor being present elsewhere in the colon [72]. An air-contrast barium enema, colonoscopy, or both should then be done to rule out other lesions.

Colonoscopy is useful to confirm positive barium enema findings, look for other lesions, perform biopsies on lesions higher than the sigmoid, remove polyps, and confirm negative findings of barium enema. Once a cancer or benign polyp has been removed, colonoscopy or barium enema should be repeated in 1 year.

Benign Tumors

Polyps of the colon are the most common benign lesions. Ninety percent are hyperplastic and 10% neoplastic if all lesions <0.5 cm are examined. For lesions approximately 1 cm, 50% are neoplastic, and 1-cm polyps have a 10% chance of being malignant [73].

In elderly patients, the hyperplastic, inflammatory, and infectious polyps are the most frequently found benign lesions. An occasional lipoma, leiomyoma, or fibroma is

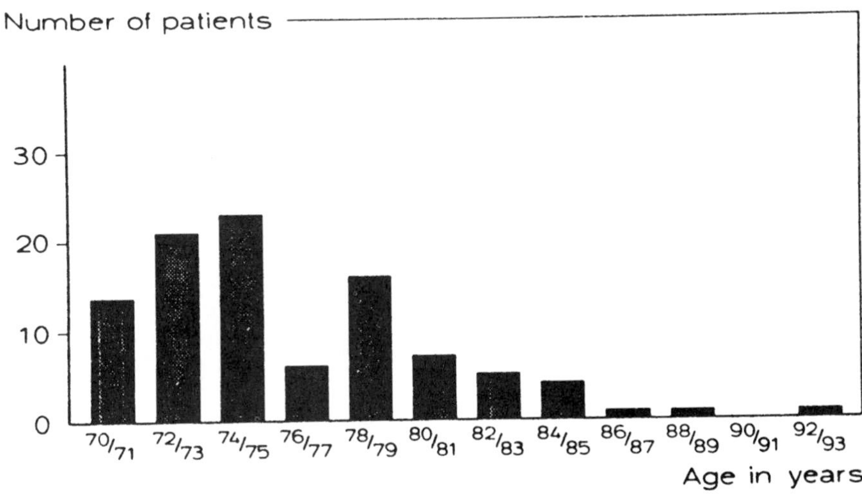

FIG. 27-5. Age distribution of carcinoma of the colon and rectum. (Reprinted with permission from Wobbes TH. Carcinoma of colon and rectum in geriatric patients. Age Ageing 1985;14:321–326.)

located [74,75]. The juvenile polyp is rare in adults, but occasionally a mixed juvenile-adenomatous polyp is seen in the elderly. Berg and coworkers emphasize that the true identity of all colon polyps must be made by histologic examination and that only then can their behavior be predicted [76]. This is an extremely important aspect of these lesions in the elderly in whom a large percentage of benign tumors may have undergone malignant change. All polypoid, sessile, or ulcerated lesions of the colon should be removed or biopsied through the sigmoidoscope or colonoscope. All benign tumors that are symptomatic, enlarging, bleeding, or of uncertain etiology should be removed even if this requires a laparotomy with colonic resection.

Malignant Tumors

The elderly patient is more apt to have a colon or rectal cancer than a younger person, with 25% of all cases of colon cancer occurring in patients over the age of 70 [77–79]. Of those cases occurring in persons >70 years of age, approximately 25% are in patients over age 80 (Figs. 27-5 and 27-6). In high-risk groups of elderly patients with anemia, melena, a history of colon cancer, a history of colon adenoma, ulcerative colitis, and Crohn's disease, patients should be studied every 6 months alternatively by barium enema and colonoscopy so that both studies are done each year until the patient is no longer classified as high risk. Once an adenoma is found, there is a 30% to 50% chance that another will appear. If adenomas are allowed to grow to >1 cm, the risk of cancer is increased. Adenomas that are 2 cm in diameter have a 35% to 45% rate of malignancy. The incidence of cancer increases from 40% to 60% in bilious adenomas [80]. In patients who have had a previous cancer of the colon, 3% to 5% have another cancer. Patients who have had previous breast cancer are at increased risk for the development of a colon cancer.

The distribution of cancer of the colon and rectum in the elderly is about the same as in the younger age group, with some groups reporting a higher incidence of cancer in the right colon in the elderly [81].

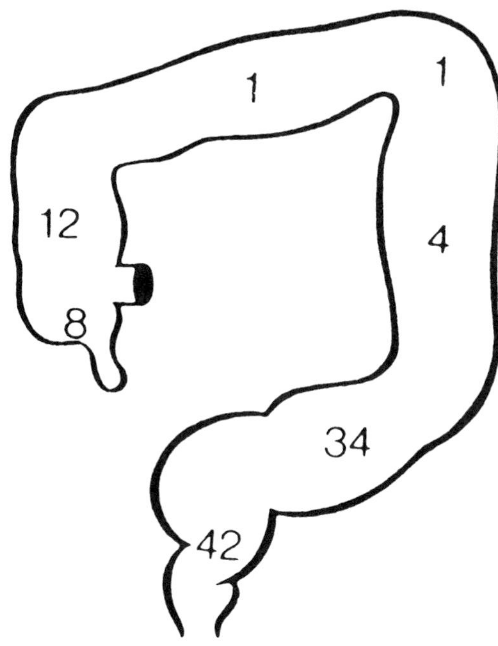

FIG. 27-6. Anatomic distribution of the tumors. (Reprinted with permission from Wobbes TH. Carcinoma of colon and rectum in geriatric patients. Age Ageing 1985;14:321–326.)

Treatment

The surgical treatment for cancer of the colon and rectum does not differ from accepted surgical procedures for younger individuals. Wide excision of the primary tumor and regional lymph nodes is the basis of surgical excision. Figure 27-7 shows the lymph node drainage from the rectum. Cohen et al. report a resectability rate of 84.9% in patients aged 70 years and over in a prospective series of patients with large bowel cancer [82].

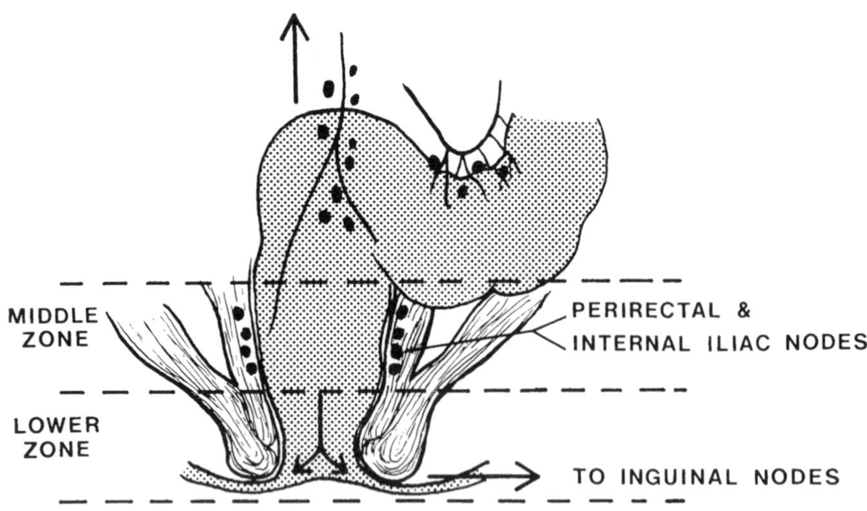

FIG. 27-7. Lymph node drainage from the anorectal area.

The Johns Hopkins group reviewed the results of colectomy in elderly patients with colon cancer from 1983 to 1985 [83]. Among 5,586 patients, the overall perioperative mortality was 5.0%, ranging from 3.3% in patients aged 66 to 69 years to 9.3% in patients aged 85 years and older. The overall survival rates at 1 and 2 years were 72% and 63%, respectively, decreasing with increasing age.

The St. Louis University Medical Center reported their results in high-risk elderly patients with advanced colorectal neoplasia [84]. Elderly high-risk patients (i.e., 70 years or older) with localized disease were compared with those with advanced disease. The mean age of all patients was 78.2 years. There was no difference in major morbidity between patients operated on for localized or advanced disease, which was defined as obstruction, perforation, hemorrhage, or metastatic disease. The mean actuarial 18-month survival was less for patients with advanced disease, but 83% of patients were alive at follow-up of 18 months. The authors concluded that morbidity and mortality associated with resection of colorectal neoplasia in high-risk elderly patients are acceptable even in the presence of advanced disease and that resection offers the best palliation and may improve quality of life in selected patients.

There has been a steady trend to treat rectal cancer with low anterior resection rather than abdominoperineal resection [85]. Low anterior resection for carcinoma has been associated with a low perioperative morbidity, satisfactory functional results, and acceptable recurrence rates.

Various local treatments may be tried for adenocarcinoma involving the distal rectum to preserve the anal sphincter. Full-thickness local excision or electrocoagulation was used in 40 patients at the Lahey Clinic with 75% survival for 5 years free of disease or free of disease at the time of death due to other causes [86].

Preoperative radiation for patients with rectal cancer has an increasing number of advocates, not only for initial treatment of unresectable cancer in an attempt to down-stage the lesion to facilitate resection [87], but also in all patients with rectal cancer. The results are not conclusive, but after a minimum 5-year follow-up, the local recurrence rate was statistically significantly lower after preoperative rather than postoperative radiotherapy, but there was no difference in overall survival [88].

Poor-risk patients and those unable to manage a colostomy may be better managed by irradiation, cryosurgery, or cauterization for rectal cancer [89].

Hobler compared a series of gastrointestinal patients aged 80 and over with a younger group of patients undergoing surgery for colon cancer [90]. There was no difference in the 3-year survival curves. The risk of mortality could be predicted by the stage of disease or type of operation required, but not by age group. The 80-years-and-older group had a median length of hospital stay of 18 days versus 15 days for the younger group.

Elderly patients with colorectal cancer have as good a prognosis as younger patients when compared with the same stage of disease. The elderly benefit from adjuvant therapy for node-positive colon cancer (stage II) and node-positive or node-negative rectal cancer (stage II or stage III). Adjuvant therapy can reduce recurrence and mortality and improve overall survival. Adjuvant chemotherapy with 5-fluorouracil and levamisole is given to patients with node-positive colonic cancer. Patients with stage II and III rectal cancers receive adjuvant therapy with radiotherapy and 5-fluorouracil. These therapies are estimated to reduce the incidence of recurrence by >30% [91].

Malignant Lesions of the Anus

The treatment for squamous cell carcinoma of the anus has changed from extended abdominoperineal resection to treatment by chemotherapy and radiation. Flam and associates reported that patients as old as 89 years with epidermoid carcinoma of the anus had complete regression of anal carcinoma following chemotherapy with 5-fluorouracil infusion and mitomycin C with simultaneous whole pelvic radiation to 30 to 45 Gy [92]. Six weeks after chemotherapy and radiation treatment, a biopsy is performed. If no residual cancer is found, repeat biopsies at 3, 6, and 12 months are recommended, and then annually. Abdominoperineal resection is used only for treatment failures, but has a poor prognosis in elderly patients [93].

Basal cell carcinoma and Paget's squamous cell carcinoma of the anus occur in the elderly and can usually be treated by wide excision and skin graft. Melanoma of the anus also tends to occur in older patients but has a poor prognosis [94,95].

Carcinoid Tumors of the Rectum

Treatment of rectal carcinoid tumors depends on the size of the lesion. For rectal carcinoid tumors <2 cm in diameter, local excision is sufficient. All tumors <2 cm in diameter, investigated by Shirouzu and associates [96] in a series of 24 patients, had no muscle layer invasion or lymph node metastasis except for an atypical carcinoid tumor that had both lymphatic and intramural metastases. Radical operation is necessary for tumors >2 cm in diameter and should be considered for the rare atypical carcinoid tumor regardless of size.

FECAL INCONTINENCE

Anal incontinence is frequently a problem in elderly, debilitated patients. Treatment depends on the cause of the condition. Fecal impaction should be checked in feeble, senile individuals and in bedridden patients. The diagnosis is readily made by digital rectal examination where a large hard mass is felt filling and distending the rectum while liquid feces come around the mass and out the anus, leading to incontinence. Only manual removal of the impacted fecal mass is effective. Enemas and cathartics will not accomplish this unpleasant task, which may require a general anesthetic. After relieving the impaction, a regimen of laxatives, suppositories, and enemas should be instituted to encourage regular bowel habits and avoid recurrence of impaction.

When incontinence is due to an old perineal injury, such as a third-degree obstetric laceration, treatment is surgical repair to reapproximate the anal sphincters. Neurogenic fecal incontinence may be improved by postanal repair [97] or total pelvic floor repair [98]. Muscle grafts or fascial slings are more successful in younger patients than in the elderly. The elderly patient with very lax anal sphincters and mucosal prolapse may benefit from Thiersch's operation, which is insertion of a silver wire or monofilament nylon placed subcutaneously around the anal orifice. A final resort when all else fails is to perform a divided sigmoid colostomy to improve nursing care of the patient. However, leakage of mucus through a patulous anus may remain a problem.

The Lahey Clinic [99] reported results from 76 operations for anal incontinence. In women with anterior sphincter defects, combining anoplasty skin closure and deep external sphincter plication gave better functional results than superficial reefing. The posterior proctopexy was useful in patients with intact external sphincters and incontinence without recognizable cause or after abdominal repair of rectal prolapse.

ANORECTAL FISTULAS

The treatment of anorectal fistulas depends on the nature or classification of the fistula. Approximately 80% of fistulas in the anal region are subcutaneous (57%) or low anal (75%). Low anal fistulas are also classified as low intersphincteric. These fistulas may be managed by laying open the fistula tract after passing a probe-pointed grove director through the external opening into the internal opening and exiting through the anus. The fistula track is laid open throughout its length by an incision onto the grove director. Fibers of the lower part of the internal and external anal sphincter muscles are cut, but this does not result in anal incontinence. The granulation tissue is scrapped off but the fibrous layer of the fistula is left intact. The sides of the wound are trimmed to remove overhanging skin and fat. The wound is then covered with a dressing.

High intersphincteric fistulas or intermuscular fistulas are more complicated. Goodsall's rule should be remembered [100]. If a transverses line is drawn across the midpoint of the anus, fistulas with their external openings anterior to this line usually run directly to the anal canal. Fistulas with external openings posterior to the transverse line tend to take a curved course terminating in an opening in the midline of the posterior wall of the anal canal. In treating these complicated fistulas, the surgeon must be aware of the anal sphincters and preserve anal continence. The anorectal ring must be identified and preserved. The greater part of both anal sphincters may be divided without loss of continence, but if the anorectal ring is divided, total loss of anal continence occurs [101].

The complicated anal fistulas may be managed by use of a seton. Pearl and associates, in a review of 116 patients, ranging up to 81 years in age, concluded that staged fistulotomy using a seton was a safe and effective method of treating high or complicated anorectal fistulas [102]. Williams and associates also advocate the use of seton treatment [103]. In 74 patients they found that high complex fistulas can be successfully treated with only minor loss of continence using different seton techniques. Horseshoe abscess fistulas may be managed by seton fistulotomy with counter drainage [104]. Anorectal fistulas complicated by rectovaginal fistula may be repaired by the endorectal advancement flap repair. This was successful in 93% of patients with complicated anorectal fistulas, avoiding fecal diversion and not injuring anal sphincter function [105].

SUMMARY

Chronologic age is less important than physiologic age in determining survival in patients undergoing colon resection. Mortality most often results from cardiopulmonary problems or sepsis. Preexisting disease and emergency procedures increase the morbidity and mortality in the elderly. Mortality may be decreased by performing early, elective operations in optimally prepared patients, rather than waiting until emergency laparotomy is necessary in the high-risk elderly patient. Elderly patients in good physiologic condition have operative risks similar to those of younger patients. Thorough preoperative determination of the elderly patient's physiologic condition is most important in determining the risk of operation. Age alone is a minor factor in determining operative risk if the patient's vital organs are physiologically intact and can handle the stress of a surgical procedure.

REFERENCES

1. Tucker JS. The ageing bowel. Practitioner 1981;225:1767–1771.
2. Pace JL. A detailed study of musculature of the human large intestine. PhD thesis, London, University of London, 1966.
3. Connell AM, Hilton C, Irvin G, et al. Variations in bowel habit in two population samples. BMJ 1965;2:1095–1099.
4. Milne JS, Williamson J. Bowel habits in older people. Gerontologia Clinica 1972;14:55–60.
5. Brocklehurst JC. Colonic disease in the elderly. Clin Gerontol 1985;14:725–747.
6. Avots-Avotins KV, Waugh DE. Colon volvulus and the geriatric patient. Surg Clin North Am 1982;62:249–260.
7. Morel P, Egeli RA, Wacht LS, et al. Results of operative treatment of gastrointestinal tract tumors in patients over 80 years of age. Arch Surg 1989;124:662–664.
8. Cathcart PM, Cathcart RS, Rambo WM. Management of massive lower gastrointestinal bleeding. Am Surg 1977;43:217–219.
9. Boley SJ, Dibose A, Brandt LJ, et al. Lower intestinal bleeding in the elderly. Am J Surg 1979;137:57–64.
10. Matolo NM, Link DP. Selective embolization for control of gastrointestinal hemorrhage. Am J Surg 1980;138:840–944.
11. Hanley PH, Hines MO. Analysis of two thousand consecutive proctologic examinations. South Med J 1956;49:475–484.
12. Lee HH, Spencer RJ, Beart RW Jr. Multiple hemorrhoidal bandings in a single session. Dis Colon Rectum 1994;37:37–41.
13. Alemdaroglv K, Vlualp KM. Single session ligation treatment of bleeding hemorrhoids. Surg Gynecol Obstet 1993;177:62–64.
14. Seow-Choen F, Ho YH, Ang HG, et al. Prospective, randomized trial comparing pain and clinical function after conventional scissors excision/ligation vs. diathermy excision without ligation for symptomatic prolapsed hemorrhoids. Dis Colon Rectum 1992;35:1165–1169.
15. Schuster MM. Disorders of the aging GI system. Hosp Pract 1976;11:95–103.
16. Shackleford RT, Zuidema GD. Surgery of the Alimentary Tract. Philadelphia: Saunders, 1982.
17. Parks TG. Natural history of diverticular disease of the colon. Clin Gastroenterol 1975;4:53–69.
18. Segal I, Solomon A, Hunt JA. Emergence of diverticular disease in the urban South African black. Gastroenterology 1977;72:215–219.
19. Whiteway J, Morson BC. Pathology of the ageing-diverticular disease. Clin Gastroenterol 1985;14:829–846.
20. Kyle J, Davidson AI. The changing pattern of hospital admission for diverticular disease of the colon. Br J Surg 1975;62:537–541.
21. Morson BC, Dawson IMP. Gastrointestinal Pathology (2nd ed). Oxford: Blackwell, 1979.
22. Almy TP, Howell DA. Diverticular disease of the colon. N Engl J Med 1980;302:324–331.
23. Stabile BE, Puccio E, van Sonnenberg E, et al. Preoperative percutaneous drainage of diverticular abscesses. Am J Surg 1990;159:99–104.
24. Levien DH, Mazier WP, Surrell JA, et al. Safe resection for diverticular disease of the colon. Dis Colon Rectum 1989;32:30–32.
25. Arnold GJ, Nance FC. Volvulus of the sigmoid colon. Ann Surg 1973; 177:527–537.
26. Peoples JB, McCafferty JC, Soher KS. Operative therapy for sigmoid volvulus. Identification of risk factors affecting outcome. Dis Colon Rectum 1990;33:643–646.
27. Thever C, Cheadle WG. Volvulus of the colon. Am Surg 1994;57: 145–150.
28. Subrahmanyam H. Mesosigmoidplasty as a definitive operation for sigmoid volvulus. Br J Surg 1992;79:683–684.
29. Bagarani M, Conde AS, Longo R, et al. Sigmoid volvulus in West Africa: a prospective study on surgical treatments. Dis Colon Rectum 1993;36:186–190.
30. Anderson MJ, Okike N, Spencer RJ. The colonoscopy in cecal volvulus. Dis Colon Rectum 1978;21:71–74.
31. Siroospour D, Berardi RS. Volvulus of the sigmoid colon: a ten-year history. Dis Colon Rectum 1976;19:535–541.
32. Starling JR. Initial treatment of sigmoid volvulus by colonoscopy. Ann Surg 1979;190:36–39.
33. Ballantyne GH, Brandner MD, Beart RW, et al. Volvulus of the colon, incidence and mortality. Ann Surg 1985;202:83–92.
34. Bak MP, Boley SJ. Sigmoid volvulus in elderly patients. Am J Surg 1986;151:71–75.
35. Crohn BB, Ginburg L, Oppenheimer GD. Regional ileitis: a pathologic and clinical entity. JAMA 1932;99:1323–1329.
36. Carr N, Schofield PF. Inflammatory bowel disease in the older patient. Br J Surg 1982;69:223–225.
37. De Dombal FT, Burton I, Goligher JC. Recurrence of Crohn's disease after primary excisional surgery. Gut 1971;12:519–527.
38. Nugent FW, Veidenheimer MC, Meissner WA, at al. Prognosis after colonic resection for Crohn's disease of the colon. Gastroenterology 1973;65:398–402.
39. Block GE, Moossa AR, Simonowitz D, et al. Emergency colectomy for inflammatory bowel disease. Surgery 1977;82:531–536.
40. Albrechtsen D, Bergan A, Nygaard K, et al. Urgent surgery for ulcerative colitis: early colectomy in 132 patients. World J Surg 1981; 5:607–615.
41. Reiss R, Deutsch AA. Emergency abdominal procedures in patients above 70. J Gastroenterol 1985;40:154–158.
42. Weedon DD, Shorter RG, Ilstrup DM, et al. Crohn's disease and cancer. N Engl J Med 1973;289:1099–1103.
43. Gyde SN, Prior P, Macartney JC, et al. Malignancy in Crohn's disease. Gut 1980;21:1024–1029.
44. Levinson JD, Wall AJ, Kirsner JB. The problem of carcinoma in inflammatory disease of the bowel: selective base experiences. South Med J 1972;65:209–214.
45. Lightdale CJ, Winawer SJ. Polyps and Tumours of the Large Intestine. In Hellemans J, Vantrappen G (eds), Gastro-Intestinal Tract Disorders in the Elderly. Edinburgh: Churchill Livingstone, 1984; 174–184.
46. Rosekrans PCM, Meijer CJLM, Vawal AM, et al. Allergic proctitis: a clinical and immunopathological entity. Gut 1980;21:1017–1023.
47. Ottinger J, Austen WG. A study of 136 patients with mesenteric infarction. Surg Gynecol Obstet 1967;124:251–261.
48. Holt PR. The small intestine. Clin Gastroenterol 1985;14:689–723.
49. Marston A. Ischemia. Clin Gastroenterol 1985;14:847–862.
50. Boley SJ, Sammartano R, Adams A, et al. On the nature and etiology of vascular ectasias of the colon, degenerative lesions of aging. Gastroenterology 1977;72:650–660.
51. Sawyers JL. Experience with the Ripstein procedure for massive rectal prolapse. South Med J 1970;63:639–641.
52. Ripstein CB. Procidentia: definitive corrective surgery. Dis Colon Rectum 1972;15:334–336.
53. Altemeier WA. One stage perineal surgery for complete rectal prolapse. Hosp Pract 1972;7:102–108.
54. Williams JG, Rothenberger DA, Madoff RD, et al. Treatment of rectal prolapse in the elderly by perineal rectosigmoidectomy. Dis Colon Rectum 1992;35:830–834.
55. Ramanujam PS, Venkatesh KS. Perineal excision of rectal prolapse with posterior levator ani repair in elderly high-risk patients. Dis Colon Rectum 1988;31:704–706.

56. Sayfon J, Pinho M, Alexander-Williams J, et al. Sutured posterior abdominal rectopexy with sigmoidectomy compared with Marlex rectopexy for rectal prolapse. Br J Surg 1990;77:143–145.
57. Roberts PL, Schoetz DJ Jr, Collier JA, et al. Ripstein procedure. Lahey experience: 1963–1985. Arch Surg 1988;123:554–557.
58. Tjandra JJ, Fazio VW, Church JM, et al. Ripstein procedure is an effective treatment for rectal prolapse without constipation. Dis Colon Rectum 1993;36:501–507.
59. Sainio AP, Halme LE, Husa AI. Anal encirclement with polypropylene mesh for rectal prolapse and incontinence. Dis Colon Rectum 1991;34:905–908.
60. Ramanujam PS, Venkatesh KS. Management of acute incarcerated rectal prolapse. Dis Colon Rectum 1992;35:1154–1156.
61. Cuschieri A, Shimi SM, Vander Velpen G, et al. Laparoscopic prosthesis fixation rectopexy for complete rectal prolapse. Br J Surg 1994;81:138–139.
62. Jetmore AB, Timmeke AE, Gathright JB Jr, et al. Ogilvie's syndrome: colonoscopic decompression and analysis of predisposing factors. Dis Colon Rectum 1992;35:1135–1142.
63. Kukora JS, Dent TL. Colonoscopic decompression of massive nonobstructive cecal dilation. Arch Surg 1977;112:512–517.
64. Martin FM, Robinson AM Jr, Thompson WR. Therapeutic colonoscopy in the treatment of colonic pseudo-obstruction. Am Surg 1988;54:519–522.
65. Duh QY, Way LW. Diagnostic laparoscopy and laparoscopic cecostomy for colonic pseudo-obstruction. Dis Colon Rectum 1993;36: 65–70.
66. Peltokallio P, Tykka H. Evolution of the age distribution and mortality of acute appendicitis. Arch Surg 1981;116:153–156.
67. Hall A, Wright TM. Acute appendicitis in the geriatric patient. Am Surg 1976;42:147–150.
68. Thorbjarnarson B, Loehr WJ. Appendicitis in patients over the age of 60. Surg Gynecol Obstet 1967;125:1277–1280.
69. Byrne A, Carney DN. Cancer in the elderly. Curr Probl Surg 1983;17: 182–183.
70. Maglinte DDT, Keller KJ, Miller RE, et al. Colon and rectal carcinoma: spatial distribution and detection. Radiology 1983;147:669–672.
71. Bernstein MA, Feczko PJ, Halpert RD, et al. Distribution of colonic polyps: increased incidence of proximal lesions in older patients. Radiology 1985;155:35–38.
72. Posner GL, Sharma DSN. Colon polyps: when are they malignant? Geriatrics 1981;36:57–60.
73. Lane N, Kaplan H, Pascal PR. Minute adenomatous and hyperplastic polyps of the colon: divergent patterns of epithelial growth with specific associated mesenchymal changes. Contrasting roles in the pathogenesis of carcinoma. Gastroenterology 1971;60:537–551.
74. Sweeney K, Petrelli N, Herrera L, et al. Cavernous hemangioma of the anus. J Surg Oncol 1984;27:286–288.
75. Fernandez MJ, Davis RP, Nora PF. Gastrointestinal lipomas. Arch Surg 1983;118:1081–1083.
76. Berg HK, Herrera L, Petrelli NJ, et al. Mixed juvenile-adenomatous polyp of the rectum in an elderly patient. J Surg Oncol 1985;29:40–42.
77. Wobbes TH. Carcinoma of the colon and rectum in geriatric patients. Age Ageing 1985;14:321–326.
78. Silverberg E. Cancer statistics 1983. CA Cancer J Clin 1983;33:9–25.
79. Hertz RE, Deddish MR, Day E. Value of periodic examination in detecting cancer of the rectum and colon. Postgrad Med 1960;27:290–294.
80. Khan AH. Colorectal carcinoma: risk factors, screening, early detection. Geriatrics 1984;39:42–47.
81. Adam YG, Calabrese C, Volk H. Colorectal cancer in patients over 80 years of age. Surg Clin North Am 1972;52:883–889.
82. Cohen JR, Theile DE, Holt J, et al. Carcinoma of the large bowel in patients aged 70 years and over. Aust N Z J Surg 1978;48:405–408.
83. Whittle J, Steinberg EP, Anderson, et al. Results of colectomy in elderly patients with colon cancer, based on Medicare claims data. Am J Surg 1992;163:572–576.
84. Fitzgerald SD, Longo WE, Daniel GL. Advanced colorectal neoplasm in the high-risk elderly patient: is surgical resection justified? Dis Colon Rectum 1993;36:161–166.
85. Kirwan WO, O'Riordain MG, Waldron R. Declining indications for abdominoperineal resection. Br J Surg 1989;76:1061–1063.
86. Stahl TJ, Murray JJ, Coller JA, et al. Sphincter-saving alternatives in the management of adenocarcinoma involving the distal rectum. 5-year follow-up results in 40 patients. Arch Surg 1993;128:545–549.
87. Whiting JF, Howes A, Osteen RT. Preoperative irradiation for unresectable carcinoma of the rectum. Surg Gynecol Obstet 1993;176: 203–207.
88. Frykholm GJ, Glimelius B, Pahlman L. Preoperative or postoperative irradiation in adenocarcinoma of the rectum: final treatment results of a randomized trial and an evaluation of late secondary effects. Dis Colon Rectum 1993;36:564–572.
89. Gingold BS. Local treatment (electrocoagulation) for carcinoma of the rectum in the elderly. J Am Geriatr Soc 1981;29:10–13.
90. Hobler KE. Colon surgery for cancer in the very elderly. Cost and 3-year survival. Ann Surg 1986;203:129–131.
91. Steele G Jr, Posner MR. Adjuvant treatment of colorectal adenocarcinoma. Curr Probl Cancer 1993;17:221–272.
92. Flam MS, John M, Lovalvo LJ, et al. Definitive nonsurgical therapy of epithelial malignancies of the anal canal. Cancer 1983;51:1378–1387.
93. Zelnick RS, Haas PA, Ajlovni M, et al. Results of abdominoperineal resection for failures after combination chemotherapy and radiation therapy for anal canal cancers. Dis Colon Rectum 1992;35:574–577.
94. Pyper PC, Parks TG. Melanoma of the anal canal. Br J Surg 1984; 71:671–672.
95. Wanebo HJ, Woodruff JM, Farr GH, et al. Anorectal melanoma. Cancer 1981;47:1891–1900.
96. Shirouzu K, Isomoto H, Kakegawa T, et al. Treatment of rectal carcinoid tumors. Am J Surg 1990;160:262–265.
97. Setticarroro P, Kamm MA, Nicholls RJ. Long-term results of postanal repair for neurogenic fecal incontinence. Br J Surg 1994;81:140–144.
98. Deen KI, Oya M, Ortiz J, et al. Randomized trial comparing three forms of pelvic floor repair for neuropathic fecal incontinence. Br J Surg 1993;80:794–798.
99. Stricker JW, Schoetz OJ Jr, Coller JA, et al. Surgical correction of anal incontinence. Dis Colon Rectum 1988;31:533–540.
100. Goodsall DH, Miles WE (eds). Disease of the Anus and Rectum. Part I. London: Longmans, 1900.
101. Goligher JC. Surgery of the Anus, Rectum and Colon (3rd ed). London: Baillière Tindall, 1980;179.
102. Pearl PK, Andrews JR, Orsay CP, et al. Role of the seton in the management of anorectal fistulas. Dis Colon Rectum 1993;36:574–577.
103. Williams JG, MacLeod CA, Rothenberger DA, et al. Seton treatment of high anal fistulae. Br J Surg 1991;78:1159–1161.
104. Vstynoski R, Rosen L, Stasik J, et al. Horseshoe abscess fistula. Seton treatment. Dis Colon Rectum 1990;33:602–605.
105. Kodner IJ, Mazor A, Shemesh EI, et al. Endorectal advancement flap repair of rectovaginal and other complicated anorectal fistulas. Surgery 1993;114:682–689.

Surgical Care for the Elderly, 2nd ed., edited by
R. Benton Adkins, Jr., and H. William Scott, Jr.
Lippincott–Raven Publishers, Philadelphia © 1998.

CHAPTER 28

Geriatric Urology

Pat O'Donnell

Elderly patients admitted for urologic surgery are among the highest percentage of patients admitted for any surgical specialty. The needs and attitudes about health care in older Americans are as apparent in urology as any specialty in medicine. For example, many urologic problems in older patients are routinely managed medically, whereas others require surgical intervention. Often surgical procedures in urology are necessary for the patient to survive, whereas other surgical procedures are performed for the specific purpose of improving the quality of life of the patient. Therefore, the clinical management decisions in urology routinely represent the entire spectrum of medical, surgical, personal, and social issues involved in health care of the elderly. Some of the common management decisions in urology involving older people are discussed in this chapter.

PROSTATE CANCER

Cancer of the prostate is the most commonly diagnosed malignancy in men and represents the second leading cause of cancer death in men [1]. Approximately 80% of men diagnosed with prostate cancer are >65 years of age. Between 1980 and the year 2000, a 37% increase in prostate cancer deaths and a 90% increase in the total number of prostate cancer cases is expected [2]. Prostate cancer clearly represents one of the greatest health care problems older men will face in the future (Fig. 28-1).

Early diagnosis is essential if the patient is to have treatment options that result in long-term survival. A prostate-specific antigen (PSA) level and a digital rectal examination (DRE) performed annually provide early detection for most patients. Patients who have a PSA of >4 ng/ml, an annual increase of >0.75 ng/ml, or an abnormal DRE should be considered for referral to a urologist for further evaluation. As older people assume more responsibility for their personal health, older men should be encouraged to remember their PSA values and be able to provide their last PSA level to any physician evaluating them.

Clinical Evaluation

Although older men with prostate cancer may present with voiding symptoms of frequency, urgency, and nocturia, most patients are asymptomatic in the early stages, which makes the annual PSA level and DRE extremely important for early diagnosis. If the PSA level or DRE is abnormal, multiple transrectal needle biopsies or transrectal ultrasound-guided biopsy may be done.

If the biopsy result is positive, clinical staging of the prostate cancer is done. A bone scan has traditionally been used to determine if metastasis has occurred. Computed tomography (CT) and magnetic resonance imaging (MRI) have been used by some clinicians to evaluate pelvic lymph nodes. Occasionally, a CT-guided biopsy of pelvic lymph nodes can avoid a staging operative procedure. Because a staging lymphadenectomy is a part of a radical retropubic prostatectomy, the CT and MRI can increase cost without significantly contributing to decision making about management in most patients. If radiation therapy is considered as the curative treatment, the imaging techniques represent the only nonsurgical assessment available for pelvic nodal disease. Laparoscopic pelvic lymphadenectomy may be used to determine the status of nodal disease in patients who elect radiation for curative treatment. For many patients, PSA values alone may prove adequate to indicate the stage of the disease for decisions about curative therapy.

Incidentally detected carcinoma of the prostate on simple prostatectomy specimens occurs in 10% to 20% of patients [3]. A clinically unsuspected low-grade (combined Gleason score <5) lesion that occupies 5% or less of the tissue resected by transurethral resection (TUR) or open prostatectomy is considered clinical stage A-1. Because only 15% of these patients can expect progression of their disease, either definitive therapy or follow-up with semiannual PSA level testing is considered appropriate treatment.

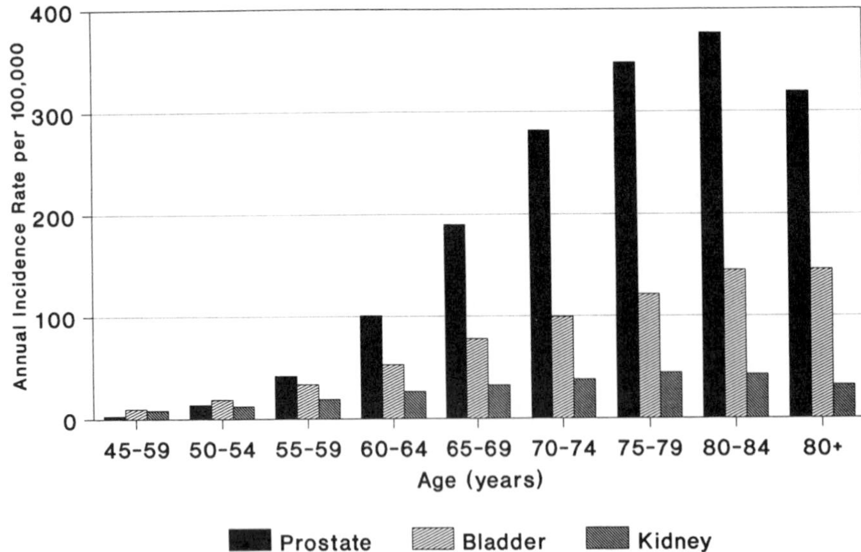

FIG. 28-1. The annual incidence of prostate, bladder, and kidney cancer in the United States. (Reprinted from National Institutes of Health Publication No. 89-2789, 1989.)

Treatment

Elderly men with clinically localized prostate cancer may elect to have a radical prostatectomy, radiation therapy, hormonal therapy alone, or no therapy at all. It was previously thought that older men typically had a less aggressive type of prostate cancer and would likely die of age-related diseases rather than prostate cancer. However, studies show that older men actually have a more aggressive, higher pathologic grade cancer than younger men [4]. In patients with prostate cancer, the relative survival rate (probability of not dying from prostate cancer) at 5 years is 51%, at 10 years 34%, and at 20 years 17% [5].

At age 65, the average man has a life expectancy of 14 years, at age 70 an additional 11 years, and at age 75 an additional 9 years [6]. Based on the survival rate of patients with prostate cancer and the expected survival in patients without prostate cancer, it appears likely that many older men with prostate cancer will actually die of prostate cancer rather than other causes related to advanced age. For organ-confined disease, the survival for radical prostatectomy ranges from 82% to 94% at 5 years, 63% to 78% at 10 years, and 27% to 60% at 15 years [1]. The survival rates for radiation therapy in organ-confined disease are 79% to 82% at 5 years, 59% to 63% at 10 years, and 36% at 15 years. Since 1980, the mortality and morbidity of radical prostatectomy has been reduced by significant improvements in operative techniques. With the continued increase in life expectancy and a continued decrease in the risk of a radical prostatectomy, surgery is being performed on increasingly older men, and it has become clinically unclear when an otherwise healthy patient is too old to be a candidate for surgery.

In patients with prostate cancer, the tumor grade, tumor stage, age of the patient, general health of the patient, and the patient's preference are all important factors in the selection of treatment. The multiple factors involved in the evaluation of treatment options emphasize the importance of early detection in older men, because without early detection, the complex clinical decisions involving all of these factors are not relevant as selection of curative-intent treatment by the patient and physician is not an option for the patient with advanced disease.

In older patients considered high risk for surgery or who prefer nonsurgical therapy, radiation therapy may be used [7]. The patient may select radiation therapy because of concern about the complications of impotence and incontinence following radical prostatectomy. However, radiation therapy has a 4% incontinence rate [8], a 45% impotence rate, as well as a 20% incidence of urinary complications including frequency, dysuria, and urethral stricture [9]. Following radical prostatectomy, incontinence occurs in 7% of all patients and 9% of patients >70 years of age [10]. Potency is preserved after radical prostatectomy in 80% of patients up to 60 years old, 57% of patients 60 to 69 years old, and 33% of patients 70 to 79 years old [11].

Patients who have clinical stage C prostate cancer may have pathologic stage B, stage C, or stage D-1 if a radical prostatectomy and pelvic lymphadenectomy are performed. Patients with stage C prostate cancer treated with hormonal therapy alone, radiation therapy alone, or surgery plus adjuvant hormonal therapy have a 5-year survival of approximately 50% to 64% and a 10-year survival of approximately 20% to 36% [1].

Approximately one-third of patients with prostate cancer have distant metastasis at the time of diagnosis. Because 80% of patients with prostate cancer are >65 years of age, a large number of new cases of prostate cancer will be elderly men with distant metastases. Prostate cancer remains refractory to conventional chemotherapeutic agents, and hormonal therapy remains the standard treatment for advanced disease. Bilateral orchiectomy results in a 95% reduction in circulating testosterone and ensures compliance with therapy. Medical therapy includes luteinizing hormone–releasing hormone analogues, diethylstilbestrol, and the antiandrogen flutamide. Combined medical therapy may have a therapeutic advantage, but it has not been well established.

In summary, prostate cancer is one of the most serious problems facing elderly men in the future. The disease has a complex and poorly understood natural history. Prostate cancer screening using PSA level and DRE has resulted in increased numbers of cases detected and diagnosis at earlier stages. The complex natural history of prostate cancer makes the assessment of risks and benefits of therapy especially difficult in the elderly patient. As men live longer, more are diagnosed with prostate cancer and more die of prostate cancer. Clinical management of older men should include screening programs that provide early detection that allows the patient and physician the choice of options that balance treatment risk, survival benefit, and long-term quality of life, specifically for the elderly patient.

BLADDER CANCER

Bladder cancer is rarely seen before age 50 and is five times more common in men than women [12]. The incidence of bladder cancer increases with advancing age, with >40% of all cases identified in patients over age 70 [13]. It is the fifth most common cancer diagnosed in the United States, with >50,000 new cases each year. Approximately 75% of all patients present with one or more low-grade, superficial papillary tumors. These tumors are usually treated initially by removal through a cystoscope. Superficial bladder cancer frequently recurs, often at a site distant from the initial tumor. Although recurrence of superficial bladder cancer is common, most patients are managed conservatively with periodic cystoscopic examinations because only 15% of these patients ultimately die of bladder cancer.

In contrast to superficial bladder cancer, approximately 25% of patients present with high-grade invasive bladder cancer, a very aggressive cancer that results in death from metastatic disease within 2 years of diagnosis if untreated. In patients with invasive bladder cancer, radical cystectomy and urinary diversion provide the best long-term results. Older people with invasive bladder cancer have a difficult management decision because the disease is rapidly fatal in most cases if untreated, and a radical cystectomy has a higher risk than most urologic procedures with a significant alteration in quality of life.

Clinical Evaluation

Gross, painless hematuria is the presenting symptom in approximately 85% of patients with bladder cancer. Additional patients are found to have microscopic hematuria on routine urinalysis. Elderly patients with gross or microscopic hematuria should have intravenous pyelography and cystoscopy. Patients who have hematuria associated with a urinary tract infection (UTI) should be followed for persistent hematuria, because the etiology of the hematuria may be an underlying bladder cancer.

Cystoscopy in older people is usually performed in the office using local anesthesia. If the intravenous pyelography result is abnormal, bilateral retrograde pyelography may be required to further evaluate the ureters and collecting system of the kidney. This can usually be performed in an outpatient surgery center using local anesthesia. Ultrasonography of the bladder and urine cytology are tests that can be helpful, but cannot replace cystoscopy.

If an abnormal area is seen in the bladder, a biopsy should be performed. Bladder tumor resection and biopsy are done endoscopically using general or regional anesthesia. The general medical condition of elderly patients rarely precludes TUR and biopsy of a bladder tumor. The most important information required to determine the prognosis of bladder cancer is the pathologic grade and depth of tumor invasion.

Treatment

Patients with low-grade superficial bladder tumors are not routinely evaluated for metastatic disease and are followed with office cystoscopy at 3-month intervals for the first year and at 6-month intervals for the next 2 years. Tumors with high recurrence rates during follow-up are at higher risk for progression to invasive bladder cancer and may be considered for intravesical therapy.

Older patients with invasive bladder cancer require careful assessment of the status of the disease, comorbid conditions, general health, and functional status, as well as the availability of family care givers. Radical cystectomy provides the best chance for cure, but can have a relatively high mortality and morbidity. The mortality and morbidity depend to some extent on the comorbid conditions of the patient and the environment in which the operation is performed. The environment includes the routine preoperative preparation, management of comorbid diseases by internal medicine staff, skill and experience of the surgeon with older patients, anesthesia, operating room conditions, and surgical intensive care unit conditions. With optimal conditions, the operative mortality is approximately 3% and the morbidity is 15% to 30%. Most surgeons are more comfortable using an ileal conduit for urinary diversion in high-risk older people. Continent diversion procedures should not be considered in elderly patients without complete evaluation of the functional status of the patient, because a higher level of cognitive function and dexterity is required for these procedures.

The primary alternative to radical cystectomy in older patients is radiation therapy. Patients are often advised to have radiation therapy because of comorbid conditions that increase the risk of radical surgery. The 5-year survival rates with radiation therapy are clearly inferior to radical cystectomy, with local recurrence rates of approximately 50%. Previous radiation therapy is frequently a determining factor for a surgeon's decision against the feasibility of radical surgery for invasive bladder cancer in high-risk elderly patients. If the risk of radical cystectomy in the high-risk patient can be reduced by optimizing the operating environment, initial surgical management offers the best chance for long-term survival of invasive bladder cancer.

In summary, most patients with bladder cancer present with gross, painless hematuria. Most have superficial bladder cancer that is managed with TUR and follow-up cystoscopy for evaluation of recurrence. Invasive bladder cancer must be treated aggressively. Radical cystectomy provides the best survival, but can have a high mortality and morbidity in older people if the operation and comorbid conditions are not managed carefully. Radiation therapy has a lower mortality, along with a considerably lower chance for cancer cure.

RENAL CANCER

Renal cell carcinoma (RCC) is the most common malignant tumor of the kidney. RCC occurs predominantly in the sixth and seventh decades of life [14]. Therefore, the incidence of RCC will increase as the median age of our population increases. Approximately one-third of patients present with advanced disease. Hematuria is a common presenting symptom, although RCC can present with diverse symptoms as well as paraneoplastic syndromes. CT scanning is the most useful study to assess the renal mass as well as other intra-abdominal organs and retroperitoneal lymph nodes. RCC in patients >age 70 tends to be smaller and appears to be somewhat less biologically active than in younger people. The most significant prognostic variable in patients with RCC is the stage of the tumor.

Surgical extirpation remains the only consistently curative modality for RCC. The operative mortality of radical nephrectomy has been reported between 2% and 5%. Reports on the operative mortality exclusively in the elderly could not be identified. Patients with a solitary metastatic focus have a 30% 5-year survival following an aggressive surgical approach. Except for the patient with a solitary metastatic focus, the 5-year survival for patients with metastatic RCC is only 13%, with a median survival of only 10 months. Radical surgery in these patients does not appear indicated. Also, traditional treatment modalities, cytotoxic chemotherapy, and radiotherapy have little impact on patients with metastatic RCC. Currently, promising experimental protocols are available to patients with advanced RCC and should be considered for any patient who is otherwise reasonably healthy.

BENIGN PROSTATIC HYPERPLASIA

The prevalence of benign prostatic hyperplasia (BPH) increases with age. Approximately 50% of men aged 51 to 60 years have BPH and >85% of men older than age 80 have histologic evidence of BPH [15]. The cumulative probability that a BPH-free 40-year-old man will develop BPH if he lives to age 80 is estimated at 78%. A 50-year-old man has a 25% chance of having a prostatectomy during his lifetime, and 29% of all men are expected to have a prostatectomy during their lifetimes [16,17]. Approximately 400,000 TURs of the prostate (TURPs) are performed each year in the United States [18].

The clinical significance of BPH is due to the symptoms that result from obstruction of the urinary bladder during voiding. Obstruction of the bladder not only results in a urinary stream that is small, slow to start, and intermittent, but also causes the bladder to become irritable, resulting in symptoms of frequency, urgency, and nocturia. Unrelieved bladder outlet obstruction results in irreversible changes in the bladder that cause persistent irritative voiding symptoms even after surgical treatment of bladder obstruction.

Clinical Evaluation

Patients with bladder outlet obstruction due to BPH usually present with symptoms of difficulty initiating voiding, a small urinary stream, decreased force of the urinary stream, and occasionally an intermittent stream. In addition, voiding symptoms usually include irritative bladder symptoms of frequency, urgency, and nocturia. Nocturia interferes with the quality of life of many patients and is usually a reliable symptom. Because patients may experience multiple symptoms in varying degrees of severity, a symptom score has been developed by the American Urological Association for clinical assessment of patients with BPH. Although the symptom score represents a standardized assessment of symptoms, the validity of the measurement is controversial [19].

As part of the initial evaluation, any patient who has symptoms of prostatism should have a PSA determination as well as a DRE to screen the patient for prostate cancer. The size of the prostate determined on rectal examination correlates poorly with symptoms of bladder outlet obstruction [20]. A small prostate gland may obstruct the bladder outlet whereas a large prostate gland may not.

A urinary flow rate is the most common test for evaluation of bladder outlet obstruction. It is a simple noninvasive test that can easily be performed in the office. The voided volume should be at least 150 ml for the test to be accurate. A maximum flow rate of <15 ml per second may indicate bladder outlet obstruction and should be further evaluated. Approximately 7% of patients with a maximum flow of >15 ml per second have outlet obstruction with an associated unusually high detrusor pressure.

Older patients frequently have voiding symptoms related to aging. Changes in bladder function associated with aging may produce symptoms similar to those seen with BPH. Therefore, any older man who is being considered for surgery for relief of bladder outlet obstruction should have a complete urodynamic evaluation to identify underlying bladder problems as well as to further characterize the obstruction. Surgery to relieve symptoms of bladder outlet obstruction is not likely be successful if obstruction does not exist.

Any patient being considered for surgery should have cystoscopy. However, cystoscopy cannot be used to determine the degree of obstruction. Only urodynamic evaluation with pressure-flow studies can determine the degree of bladder obstruction. It is preferable for the physician performing the cystoscopy to be the person performing the surgery. Cystoscopy provides the surgeon with insight into the anatomic characteristics of the prostate that are helpful in planning the operative procedure.

Treatment

TURP is the primary choice of treatment for bladder outlet obstruction. Over 80% of patients experience regression of symptoms after TURP [21]. The operative mortality of TURP is 0.2%. In older patients who are considered high risk for TURP, a transurethral incision of the prostate (TUIP) can usually be done. TUIP is a simple incision of the bladder neck and prostate that can be performed quickly. Even the high-risk elderly can usually tolerate this procedure. This procedure has excellent results when the prostate gland is small.

An open prostatectomy is recommended in patients with large prostate glands. Surgery in patients with large prostate glands is much more complicated regardless of whether done transurethrally or suprapubically. The decision to recommend an open prostatectomy rather than TURP is based on the surgeon's opinion of which procedure will result in the lowest risk to the patient.

Other surgical procedures include balloon dilation, prostatic hyperthermia, prostate stents, and laser therapy. To date, none of these match the high success rate and low complication rate of TURP. Pharmacotherapy of patients with symptomatic BPH is commonly used in younger patients, but side effects and efficacy remain problems for the elderly.

In summary, most men will develop BPH during their lifetimes if they live a normal life expectancy. Nearly one-third of all men will require surgical intervention during their lifetime for symptomatic BPH. TURP remains the most efficacious treatment with an extremely low mortality. As life expectancy increases, the occurrence of BPH will also increase, and treatment of this problem will require a major segment of our health care effort.

URINARY INCONTINENCE

Urinary incontinence is one of the most debilitating problems affecting older people. Approximately 40% of community-dwelling older women suffer from urinary incontinence. Of community-dwelling older men, approximately 20% suffer from incontinence. More than 55% of all chronic care patients have urinary incontinence. The annual cost for treatment of urinary incontinence in the United States is well over $10 billion. The annual cost of treatment of urinary incontinence is more than the combined costs of all coronary artery bypass surgery as well as all renal dialysis [22].

As women become older, the continence mechanism of the urethra becomes less effective. Therefore, when the patient coughs or strains, she is likely to leak urine. Unlike younger women who often have incontinence due to loss of urethral support that can be corrected by a urethral suspension procedure, elderly women often have a poorly functioning urethral mechanism that requires a urethral sling procedure to correct the incontinence.

The management of urinary incontinence in elderly women is extremely complex, and the treatment is based on a complete evaluation of bladder and urethral function. Complete urodynamic information on the anatomy and physiology of the bladder and urethra is necessary to successfully treat this group of patients. Incontinence due to a poorly functioning urethra in older women is called *intrinsic incontinence* or *intrinsic sphincter deficiency* (ISD) [23]. Incontinence due to loss of support of the urethra is called *anatomic incontinence.* Varying degrees of each abnormality may exist within the same patient. In addition, stress incontinence due to either intrinsic or anatomic incontinence can aggravate symptoms of urgency and produce urge incontinence. When a patient has symptoms of both stress incontinence and urge incontinence, it is called *mixed incontinence.* Mixed incontinence is common in older women [24].

The patient's statement that, "I leak when I cough," is typical of stress incontinence. The statement, "I have to hurry to the bathroom and I leak before I get there," is typical of urge incontinence. Older women with predominantly symptoms of urge incontinence should have complete evaluation of urethral function because coexisting stress incontinence is often present and overshadowed by symptoms of urge incontinence. Unlike younger women, urge incontinence in older women may occur abruptly without warning. This kind of urge incontinence is much more difficult to manage, especially if coexisting stress incontinence is present.

Clinical Evaluation

The incontinence history in older women is immensely important in characterizing the type and severity of incontinence. Complete urodynamic studies are essential to evaluate the bladder and urethral function in older women. A relatively common urodynamic finding in elderly women is detrusor instability. Detrusor instability is a spontaneous bladder contraction that the patient is unable to voluntarily inhibit. Detrusor instability is considered to be the etiology of incontinence by many physicians. However, detrusor instability is often seen in older patients who do not have incontinence, and many older people who have significant urge incontinence do not demonstrate detrusor instability on urodynamic evaluation. Among the most important urodynamic parameters in elderly women with urinary incontinence are maximum urinary flow rate, bladder capacity, bladder compliance, and urethral function studies, with particular emphasis on the leak point pressures.

Treatment

The treatment goal of any incontinence therapy is not only for the patient to be completely continent, but also for the patient to void normally. Although this treatment outcome is feasible in younger women, it may not be realistic for many elderly women with complicated incontinence and coexisting functional impairment. A reduction in frequency of incontinence episodes by 50% or more can significantly improve the quality of life of an elderly person. If a significant reduction in incontinence can be accomplished with minimal risk to the patient, it is successful in improving quality of life although incontinence may persist.

Behavioral therapy is often an initial treatment choice for elderly women because the risk of therapy is minimal [25]. Behavioral therapy programs are successful in improving bladder control in patients with a significant component of urge incontinence. Habit-training programs are among the most commonly used in elderly people and involve instruction of the patient in a timed voiding schedule using an interval of 2 hours. Bladder training programs use a voiding diary with the goal of gradually increasing the interval between voiding. This is primarily for patients with urge incontinence and associated voiding frequency. Pelvic muscle exercises involve a program of scheduled voluntary contractions of the pelvic muscles. Although the original technique described by Kegel has been modified many times, pelvic muscle exercises are often called Kegel exercises, even though the technique is somewhat different from the original description.

The most reliable and successful treatment involving pelvic muscle exercises is biofeedback therapy [26]. Although biofeedback therapy has excellent results in treatment of incontinence in older women, it involves the use of complex and expensive equipment and requires trained personnel to administer the therapy.

Pharmacologic therapy of incontinence in older women is aimed at decreasing bladder contractility and increasing outlet resistance [27]. One of the most commonly used drugs for decreasing bladder contractility in older patients is oxybutynin hydrochloride (Ditropan), a moderately potent anticholinergic agent with a strong independent musculotropic relaxant activity and local anesthetic activity as well. Phenylpropanolamine is one of the most commonly used medications in elderly women to increase bladder outlet resistance. Ditropan may produce side effects of confusion in some older people, and phenylpropanolamine may produce cardiovascular side effects such as hypertension.

The prevalence of ISD in elderly women limits the effectiveness of nonsurgical therapies because it does not appear that these therapies can correct intrinsic urethral incontinence. Patients who have ISD without loss of urethral support can be successfully treated with intraurethral injection. The most commonly used material is a bovine collagen derivative called *Contigen* (C.R. Bard, Inc., Covington, GA). Contigen is not indicated in elderly women with ISD and loss of urethral support. The only successful surgical option in these patients is a urethral sling procedure. In the absence of ISD, incontinence in older women due to a loss of urethral support responds to conventional urethral suspension procedures such as a Raz, Marshall-Marchetti-Krantz, or Burch procedure. Persistent urge incontinence following surgery in older women can be treated with behavioral therapy, pharmacologic therapy, or a combination regimen.

Unlike elderly women, stress incontinence due to urethral sphincteric incompetence is extremely rare in men who have not had previous prostate or pelvic surgery [28]. However, stress incontinence is not uncommon following a radical prostatectomy or colorectal surgery. The type of incontinence following radical prostatectomy is usually ISD, although bladder dysfunction may be involved. A complete evaluation of bladder function is required before any surgical treatment is considered. If the bladder capacity and compliance are normal, an artificial urinary sphincter is the most common procedure used to correct stress incontinence in men.

Incontinence in elderly men who have not had previous prostate or pelvic surgery is due to bladder hyperactivity. The bladder may contract periodically with no warning, resulting in an incontinence episode. Bladder hyperactivity may be caused or aggravated by bladder outlet obstruction in elderly men. Because BPH is common in older men, a complete urodynamic evaluation with emphasis on the pressure-flow study is essential in the evaluation of the etiology of incontinence in elderly men. If the etiology of urge incontinence in older men is bladder outlet obstruction, the symptom of incontinence should improve significantly following TURP.

Bladder hyperactivity is common after a stroke and may be the cause of incontinence in elderly men. If outlet obstruction also exists in these patients, TURP or TUIP should be considered, although incontinence is likely to persist due to residual bladder hyperactivity. If bladder hyperactivity exists without outlet obstruction, behavioral therapy, pharmacologic therapy, or combined therapy can be used. Unlike women, mixed incontinence is uncommon in men.

IMPOTENCE

Sexual function decreases with age. At age 40, only one man in 50 has erectile problems, whereas one man in four has erectile problems by age 65 [29]. It is important to realize that as men become older, sexual function can be more easily affected by experiences such as surgical procedures that may be relatively unrelated to the genitourinary system. Older people who are still sexually functional frequently have marginal sexual activity that can be significantly affected by any surgical procedure, especially if it has any psychological impact on the patient such as cancer surgery or cardiovascular surgery. Fortunately, clinical management of sexual function problems following surgery is relatively easy and successful in most patients. In patients who have impotence, a study of nocturnal erections using a RigiScan can be helpful in planning therapy. The frequency, duration, and rigidity of nocturnal erections are usually measured for three nights. Most patients have an excellent response to self-injection therapy. Vacuum erection devices are satisfactory for some patients. The high success rate of self-injection therapy has significantly reduced prosthetic implant surgery for impotence. However, for patients who find self-injection therapy unsatisfactory, prosthetic implant surgery has an excellent patient satisfaction rate.

URINARY TRACT INFECTION

UTI is one of the most common infections in the elderly [30]. The prevalence of UTIs in community-dwelling women over age 70 is 10%, and it increases in those over age 80 to 20%. By age 80, up to 10% of well men in the community have bacteriuria. The prevalence of bacteriuria in older people in chronic care is >50%. The majority of elderly people with bacteriuria is asymptomatic. Episodes of symptomatic infection occur infrequently. Asymptomatic bacteriuria does not appear to contribute directly to mortality in elderly subjects.

An important consideration in any surgical procedure in older people is that a UTI can be a significant source of postoperative complications. A negative urinalysis result at the time of preoperative testing may become positive if the interval between testing and surgery has been more than a few days. Patients with a negative urinalysis result may be catheterized in the perioperative period without recognizing that bacteriuria is present, potentially resulting in bacteremia. In addition, contamination of a wound at the time of surgery is possible. The urinalysis could be repeated on the date of surgery for elderly patients if the preoperative testing has been done more than a few days before surgery.

SUMMARY

Treatment of elderly patients with urologic problems must achieve the best quality of life possible. We must aggressively pursue ways to prolong survival without compromising quality of life. If high-risk surgery is the only way to prolong survival in elderly patients, we must find ways to reduce the risk of the operation. Complicated urologic procedures in older people require careful planning, careful operative technique, and aggressive postoperative management. A complicated operative procedure in older people usually consumes more resources and requires a longer hospital stay than a similar operation in a younger person. However, it is possible to perform complex operative procedures on community-dwelling elderly people and return those people to their previous living environment and preoperative functional status.

REFERENCES

1. Dreicer R, Williams RC. Management of Prostate Cancer. In O'Donnell PD (ed), Geriatric Urology. Boston: Little, Brown, 1994;125.
2. Carter HB, Coffey DS. The prostate: an increasing medical problem. Prostate 1990;16:39.
3. Brawer MK. The diagnosis of prostatic carcinoma. Cancer 1993;71 (3 Suppl):899.
4. Kerr LA, Zincke H. Radical retropubic prostatectomy for prostate cancer in the elderly and the young: complications and prognosis. Eur Urol 1994;25:305.
5. Adami HO, Norlen BJ, Malker B, Meirik O. Long-term survival in prostatic carcinoma, with special reference to age as a prognostic factor: a nationwide study. Scand J Urol Nephrol 1986;20:107.
6. U.S. Bureau of the Census. Statistical Abstract of the United States: 1987 (107th ed). Washington, DC: Government Printing Office, 1986.
7. Kaplan I, Bagshaw MA. Radiotherapy for Urologic Malignancies. In O'Donnell PD (ed), Geriatric Urology. Boston: Little, Brown, 1994;177.
8. Green N, Treible D, Wallack H. Prostate cancer: post-irradiation incontinence. J Urol 1990;144:307.
9. Zagars GK, von Eschenbach AC, Johnson DE. The role of radiation therapy in stages A-2 and B adenocarcinoma of the prostate. J Radiat Oncol Biol Phys 1988;14:701.
10. Igel TC, Barrett DM, Segura JW, et al. Perioperative complications from bilateral pelvic lymphadenectomy and radical retropubic prostatectomy. J Urol 1987;137:1189.
11. Catalona WJ, Bigg SW. Nerve sparing radical prostatectomy: evaluation of results after 250 patients. J Urol 1990;143:538.
12. Skinner EC, Skinner DG. Management of Bladder Cancer. In O'Donnell PD (ed), Geriatric Urology. Boston: Little, Brown, 1994;157.
13. Raghavan D. Management of advanced bladder cancer in the elderly. Urol Clin North Am 1992;19:797.
14. Danella JF, deKernion JB. Management of Kidney Cancer. In O'Donnell PD (ed), Geriatric Urology. Boston: Little, Brown, 1994;147.
15. Isaacs JT, Coffey DS. Etiology and disease process of benign prostatic hyperplasia. Prostate 1989;2(Suppl):33.
16. Glynn RJ, Campion EW, Bouchard GR, Silbert JE. The development of benign prostatic hyperplasia among volunteers in the normative aging study. Am J Epidemiol 1985;121:78.
17. Birkhoff JD. Natural History of Benign Prostatic Hypertrophy. In Hinman F (ed), Benign Prostatic Hyperplasia. New York: Springer-Verlag, 1983;5.
18. Reihmann M, Bruskewitz RC. Management of Bladder Outlet Obstruction in Elderly Men. In O'Donnell PD (ed), Geriatric Urology. Boston: Little, Brown, 1994;275.
19. Chai TC, Belville WD, McGuire EJ, Nyquist L. Specificity of the American Urological Association voiding symptom index: comparison of unselected and selected samples of both sexes. J Urol 1993;150:1710.
20. Andersen JT, Nordling J, Walter S. The correlation between symptoms, cystometric and urodynamic findings. Scand J Urol Nephrol 1979;13:229.
21. Lepor H, Rigaud G. The efficacy of transurethral resection of the prostate for benign prostatic hyperplasia. J Urol 1990;143:533.
22. O'Donnell PD. The pathophysiology of urinary incontinence in the elderly. Adv Urol 1991;4:129.
23. Kennelly M, McGuire EJ. Intrinsic Sphincter Deficiency. In O'Donnell PD (ed), Urinary Incontinence. St. Louis: Mosby–Year Book, 1997.
24. O'Donnell PD. Mixed Incontinence. In O'Donnell PD (ed), Urinary Incontinence. St. Louis: Mosby–Year Book, 1997.
25. O'Donnell PD. Behavioral Therapy for Incontinence. In O'Donnell PD (ed), Geriatric Urology. Boston: Little, Brown, 1994;301.
26. O'Donnell PD. Biofeedback Therapy. In Raz S (ed), Female Urology. Philadelphia: Saunders, 1996.
27. Broderick GA, Wein AJ. Pharmacologic Therapy for Incontinence. In O'Donnell PD (ed), Geriatric Urology. Boston: Little, Brown, 1994; 285.
28. O'Donnell PD. Pathophysiology of Incontinence in Elderly Men. In O'Donnell PD (ed), Geriatric Urology. Boston: Little, Brown, 1994; 229.
29. Donatucci CF, Lue TF. Management of Impotence. In O'Donnell PD (ed), Geriatric Urology. Boston: Little, Brown, 1994;345.
30. Nicolle LE. Urinary Tract Infection. In O'Donnell PD (ed), Geriatric Urology. Boston: Little, Brown, 1994;399.

Surgical Care for the Elderly, 2nd ed., edited by
R. Benton Adkins, Jr., and H. William Scott, Jr.
Lippincott–Raven Publishers, Philadelphia © 1998.

CHAPTER 29

Gynecologic Diseases

Howard W. Jones, III, and Lonnie S. Burnett

Gynecologic diseases in the elderly requiring surgical management are for the most part limited to neoplasms and genital organ prolapse secondary to pelvic support defects. Benign uterine leiomyomas, pelvic infections, endometriosis, and pelvic pain of uncertain etiology are common surgical problems in the premenopausal patient, but are rarely indications for surgery in the elderly. It is especially important to remember that benign uterine leiomyomas, occurring in 30% to 40% of adult women, can be expected to regress in the postmenopausal patient and rarely require surgical management. Although postmenopausal bleeding from benign causes is fairly common in the elderly, it is most often secondary to hormone replacement therapy. Diagnosis and management usually involve minor operative procedures such as endometrial biopsy, dilatation and curettage, and possibly hysteroscopy. Most often, these are performed in an office setting and are not discussed in this chapter.

Although the surgical techniques used for the treatment of genital prolapse and malignancies are essentially the same in the aged as in younger patients, the judgment required in selecting patients for a surgical versus a nonsurgical approach requires considerable experience and a thorough knowledge of treatment alternatives. In the patient who is a poor surgical candidate, alternative forms of therapy may be preferable, and the selection of the wrong candidate for surgical management may prove disastrous. On the other hand, we have seen many elderly women in whom a surgical procedure was not recommended only due to concerns for the patient's age. Several years later many of these women will still be alive and reasonably well, yet they continue to suffer even worse symptoms from their gynecologic problems. It is then that the patient and her doctors realize that it would have been better to have done the operation sooner.

The choice between surgical and nonsurgical treatment modalities for elderly patients is complicated by the relative lack of data examining age as a factor in gynecologic surgical outcomes. The aging female population will inevitably undergo surgery more frequently than in the past, however, and we can expect the accumulation and evaluation of age-specific data to follow this trend. Among more recent data, a large German study of 2,880 patients >80 years old indicated that advanced age alone does not preclude otherwise appropriate surgery [1].

GENITAL TRACT PROLAPSE

For most women, the basic anatomic defects ultimately leading to pelvic relaxation begin with damage to the supporting ligaments and fascia of the pelvis through the trauma of childbirth. Nevertheless, the development of many symptomatic relaxations as clinical entities requiring surgical intervention may not occur until years later, often when the patient is elderly and additional support is lost through attenuation and atrophy associated with aging. Pelvic neuropathies, especially those involving the pudendal nerves, may also be a contributing factor leading to genital organ prolapse through premature attenuation in the quality of both muscles and fascia supporting the pelvic viscera.

Any condition that increases intra-abdominal pressure (chronic cough, obesity, straining with defecation, lifting, vigorous exercises) results in an increased pressure on the pelvic floor and thereby an increased risk for prolapse, especially in the patient who already has earlier damage to supporting muscles, ligaments, and fascia through childbirth or pelvic neuropathy. Progressive pelvic relaxation, including total inversion of the vagina, may first become apparent in the elderly patient following an upper respiratory tract infection associated with intense coughing. Furthermore, increasing numbers of elderly women pursue active, healthy life-styles that include fast walking, aerobic exercises, and lifting exercises. The initiation of these programs by the elderly may be followed by the first evidence of uterine or vaginal descent, which may then be rapidly progressive unless the exercise programs are discontinued or modified. Often, the decision to pursue surgical intervention is based on the desire to continue an active life-style including exercise programs. Essentially all patients with prolapse, even when the prolapse is advanced, experience reduction of the prolapse and relief of symptoms in the supine or recumbent position. When symptoms are present, they are almost always made worse by the upright position, walking, lifting, and exercising.

Anatomic support of the uterus, vagina, urethra, bladder, and rectum is provided by the urogenital diaphragm, pubourethral ligaments, cardinal and uterosacral ligaments, endopelvic fascia, and levator ani muscles.

Urogenital Diaphragm

Arising from the inner surface of the descending pubic rami and located within the pubic arch, the urogenital diaphragm and its fascial layers provide support for the distal urethra and vagina and the vaginal outlet. Defects contribute to the formation of a urethrocele with posterior rotation of the urethra and vaginal outlet and attenuation of the perineum.

Pubourethral Ligaments

The posterior pubourethral ligaments arise from the superior surface of the urogenital diaphragm and its fascia, and from the posterior surface of the pubis and extend to the endopelvic fascia overlying the anterior vaginal wall in close proximity to the urethra. Damage to these ligaments contributes to the formation of a urethrocele.

Endopelvic Fascia

A well-defined layer of condensed endopelvic fascia surrounds the genital tract and its supporting structures and provides support to the vagina by its attachment to the pelvic wall in the region of the arcus tendineus extending from the pubis to the ischial spine. This fascia contributes to the formation of the cardinal ligaments, uterosacral ligaments, fascia overlying the vagina, and rectovaginal septum. Defects contribute to the formation of a wide variety of relaxation conditions, including cystourethrocele, uterovaginal prolapse, enterocele, and rectocele.

Cardinal Ligaments

The cardinal ligaments represent condensations of endopelvic fascia around vessels and nerves and extend bilaterally from the cervix to the pelvic side walls above the ischial spines. They become continuous with the endopelvic fascia overlying the anterior vaginal wall. Defects and attenuation contribute to uterovaginal prolapse.

Uterosacral Ligaments

The highly important uterosacral ligaments extend from the posterior lateral margin of the cervix and the upper vagina to the anterior surface of the sacrum on each side of the rectum and to the lateral pelvic side wall. They form the lateral boundaries of the cul-de-sac. Loss or attenuation of these strong supporting bands may result in prolapse of the uterus or the vaginal vault following hysterectomy.

Levator Muscles

The levator muscles originate from the arcus tendineus fascia overlying the obturator internus muscles and contribute to the formation of a muscular pelvic diaphragm providing support to both the vagina and rectum. The most caudal portion of this structure is represented by the puborectalis muscle and becomes the boundary of the pelvic hiatus. The urethra, vagina, and anal canal pass between the puborectalis muscles. These muscles originate from the posterior surface of the pubis and extend along the lateral wall of the vagina, where they join behind the upper portion of the anal canal and contribute to the direction of that structure and to fecal continence.

Pelvic relaxations may involve multiple clinical entities, including urethrocele, cystocele, uterovaginal prolapse, vaginal vault prolapse, enterocele, rectocele, relaxed vaginal outlet, and attenuation of the perineum and perineal body. Although it is convenient to discuss these entities separately, in most instances the patient will present with a combination of defects. When surgical repair is planned, it is important to identify each and every anatomic defect so that each may be corrected. Optimal surgical results and the avoidance of a high rate of recurrence require that each anatomic abnormality be corrected when feasible.

Cystourethrocele

Although urethrocele and cystocele may occur independently, they are more frequently seen as a combined defect, sometimes referred to as an *anterior compartment pelvic support defect. Urethrocele* refers to the sagging of the anterior vaginal wall and the underlying urethra and bladder neck. Because the external urethral orifice is moderately fixed at the vestibule, urethrocele results in a posterior rotation and descent of the urethrovesical junction from its normal position behind the symphysis. This is the anatomic defect commonly (but not always) associated with stress urinary incontinence.

Cystocele refers to the sagging of the anterior vaginal wall underlying the bladder and therefore characteristically involves the entire upper vagina. When a urethrocele and a cystocele occur together (cystourethrocele), the sagging involves the entire anterior vaginal wall from the urethral orifice to the cervix or to the vaginal apex if the uterus has been previously removed. Under these circumstances, the anterior wall may protrude well beyond the vaginal introitus (third degree). When a cystocele is present alone, especially with advanced degrees, urinary incontinence is rarely seen; in fact, the patient is more likely to experience incomplete bladder emptying and will sometimes have significant urinary retention.

Anterior compartment prolapse may result from loss of lateral pelvic support of the vagina and associated endopelvic fascia or from central defects in the endopelvic fascia overlying the vagina. For example, loss of support from the posterior pubourethral ligaments may contribute to posterior rotation of the urethra, and loss of vaginal and endopelvic fascial attachment to the arcus tendineus may contribute to cystocele. Central defects in the endopelvic fascia overlying the anterior vaginal wall may result in prolapse, even though lateral attachments may persist. Advanced cystourethrocele, beyond the vaginal introitus, is usually associated with descent of the cervix or the vaginal vault, indicating support defects at other sites.

Uterovaginal Prolapse

Descent of the uterus through the vaginal canal is preceded by loss of anterior or posterior flexion of the fundus, and both the cervix and vagina assume an axis similar to that of the vaginal canal. As the cervix descends beyond the middle third of the vaginal canal, symptoms of pressure and discomfort are common. Even more advanced prolapse brings the cervix beyond the vaginal introitus and may be followed by complete inversion of the vagina, a condition referred to as procidentia. With complete inversion, the bladder and distal ureters follow the anterior vaginal wall and are located outside of the pelvis. Acute urinary retention and significant distal ureteral obstruction may result but are usually corrected by replacement of the uterus into the pelvis.

Uterovaginal prolapse results from combined pelvic support defects, especially those associated with the uterosacral and cardinal ligaments. Advanced degrees of uterovaginal prolapse are always associated with other defects, such as cystourethrocele, enterocele, and rectocele.

Vaginal Vault Prolapse

Partial or complete prolapse of the vaginal vault is seen with increasing frequency among elderly women who have previously undergone abdominal or vaginal hysterectomy. The vaginal apex, corresponding to the site of vaginal transection occurring with hysterectomy, can usually be identified by remnants of the vaginal closure or by "dog ears" corresponding to the closure of the vaginal angles.

When advanced, the condition is always associated with other defects, especially cystourethrocele and enterocele. When the inversion is complete, the prolapse carries with it the urethra, bladder, and ureters and may be associated with both urethral and distal ureteral obstruction. A prolapsed vaginal vault, especially when advanced, becomes filled with loops of small bowel, resulting in a dependent bowel-filled sac that usually undergoes spontaneous reduction in the supine position, much like other nonincarcerated hernias. Incarceration of the small bowel rarely occurs.

Vaginal vault prolapse results from loss of support of both the uterosacral and cardinal ligaments, and when advanced is associated with the defects seen with a cystourethrocele.

Enterocele

A posterior enterocele results from extension and dissection of the cul-de-sac peritoneum through the fascia surrounding the posterior vaginal wall. The resulting hernia protrudes into the vaginal canal; it may extend to and beyond the vaginal introitus and is usually filled with small bowel and sometimes omentum when the patient is in an upright position. This condition may occur with a uterus still in place or following hysterectomy, in which case the hernia sac usually has an anterior margin that corresponds to the old vaginal apex where the vagina was previously closed.

Posterior enterocele frequently occurs along with other defects, especially uterovaginal or vaginal vault prolapse and rectocele. When occurring with a rectocele, the enterocele is always anterior, and both conditions can usually be appreciated by a careful rectovaginal examination.

Anterior enterocele is less common and usually is seen among women with a prior hysterectomy. The hernia sac lies anterior to the vaginal apex and in close proximity to the bladder. This condition is usually associated with defects at other sites, such as cystocele and vaginal vault prolapse.

Posterior enterocele is usually associated with a deep and exposed cul-de-sac and frequently with attenuated uterosacral ligaments. Any condition that displaces the vaginal axis anteriorly increases the risk of posterior enterocele. For example, retropubic urethrovaginal suspensions or vaginal vault suspensions to anterior supports such as the round ligaments significantly increase the risk of subsequent enterocele.

Rectocele

A rectocele is a protrusion or outpouching of the anterior rectal wall through a weakened or attenuated rectovaginal septum. Protrusion occurs into the vaginal lumen and may be large enough to extend outside the vaginal introitus. Some degree of rectocele is common among elderly women and most do not require surgical repair. Although the defect in most cases begins with damage resulting from childbirth, the progression and enlargement that occur in the elderly come not only from the attenuation of connective tissue through aging but also from long-standing poor bowel habits associated with chronic constipation, habitual laxative use, and straining during defecation. Advanced rectocele may be associated with difficulty in evacuating the rectal ampulla and may require reduction or counterpressure by a hand in the vagina during defecation. Rectocele is frequently associated with other defects, especially enterocele and a relaxed vaginal outlet (described in the following section). Differentiation between these conditions can usually be made by careful rectovaginal examination.

Relaxed Vaginal Outlet

Relaxed vaginal outlet refers to marked attenuation of the peritoneal body, usually preceded by tearing and stretching during childbirth. The perineal body is a pyramid-shaped body of tissue with its apex just inside the vagina corresponding to the junction of the anal canal and the rectal ampulla. This is also the site at which the puborectalis muscles pass lateral to the outer vagina and posterior to the upper anal canal. The base of the pyramidal perineal body is located at the perineum between the anus and the posterior vaginal fourchette, and these are usually separated by 3 to 4 cm. The perineal body includes the posterior aspect of the urogenital diaphragm and the conversion of the superficial and deep transverse perineal muscles with the bulbocavernosus muscles.

When the vaginal outlet shows marked attenuation, the distance between the anus and posterior fourchette is markedly reduced and the anal canal is in close proximity to the posterior vaginal wall. When damage to the perineal body is extensive, the external anal sphincter may be attenuated or divided, with possible incontinence of stool and gas.

Surgical Procedures for Pelvic Support Defects

The decision to pursue surgical treatment of pelvic support defects should be made after carefully considering the options, associated risks, and likely benefits. Pelvic prolapse, with few exceptions, is not life-threatening but may affect the quality of life and will often preclude a healthy life-style that includes physical activity such as walking or exercising. For the most part, pelvic support defects can be surgically repaired by the abdominal or vaginal route, except for repair of a rectocele and relaxed vaginal outlet, which must be performed vaginally. Laparoscopic approaches to pelvic support defect surgery are being performed with increasing frequency, but data are insufficient to judge long-term results. Especially for the elderly patient, a vaginal surgical approach is always preferable because of better tolerance and a shorter recovery period.

Goals of surgery for pelvic relaxation should be the correction of all significant defects with the restoration of normal genital tract anatomy: (1) the bladder neck should be in a normal retropubic position and should not be hypermobile with increases in intra-abdominal pressure, (2) the anterior vaginal wall beneath the bladder should be supported and should not move beyond the midplane of the vagina, (3) the apex of the vagina should be supported in the mid to posterior pelvis overlying the median raphe of the levator plate, (4) the vaginal length should be sufficient for normal sexual activity if desired by the patient, (5) the posterior vaginal wall should be supported by an intact rectovaginal septum without encroachment by an enterocele or rectocele, and (6) there should be a normal perineal body characterized by an anal canal of normal direction and length and a normal separation of the anus from the posterior fourchette.

Surgical Management of Cystourethrocele and Bladder Neck Hypermobility

Mild degrees of cystourethrocele are common in the elderly and most do not need surgical correction. The major indications for a surgical repair are symptoms that include stress urinary incontinence, discomfort associated with protrusion of a mass from the vaginal introitus, or recurring urinary retention. Uterovaginal prolapse frequently accompanies this condition, and the surgical correction most commonly used includes removal of the uterus.

Anterior Colporrhaphy

Anterior colporrhaphy is accomplished by the vaginal route and involves a midline incision in the anterior vaginal wall overlying the area of the defect. The vaginal wall is dissected away from the underlying urinary tract and endopelvic fascia, and the defect is corrected through plication of the endopelvic fascia to the midline and excision of the resulting excess vaginal wall. The operation is simple and brief, associated with minimal morbidity, and well tolerated, even in the elderly patient. The repair may extend to the urethral area, but if significant hypermobility of the bladder neck is present, other techniques are more likely to give long-lasting results.

Abdominal-Vaginal (Needle) Urethropexy

Pereyra, Stamey, and Raz have described needle urethropexy techniques designed to place the urethrovesical junction into a retropubic position and to correct hypermobility of the bladder neck [2]. The procedure begins vaginally with the exposure of the pubocervical or endopelvic fascia in the area of the bladder neck. Using monofilament, nonabsorbable suture, a ligature carrier, and a small suprapubic incision, bilateral suspending sutures are attached to the perivaginal fascia, passed through the retropubic space and tied over the fascia of the abdominal wall. The result is elevation of the urethrovesical junction to a retropubic position and correction of hypermobility associated with increases in intra-abdominal pressure. The procedure is brief, well tolerated in the elderly patient, and reported to be effective in approximately 90% of women. One special advantage is the option of carrying out other vaginal procedures when indicated without changing the patient's position on the operating table.

Retropubic Urethrovaginal Suspension

These procedures are carried out through the retropubic space and result in suspension of the vagina on either side of the urethra at the level of the bladder neck. The Marshall-Marquetti-Krantz procedure suspends the periurethral vagina to the symphysis pubis while the Burch procedure suspends the anterior vaginal wall to Cooper's ligament. Because these procedures change to some extent the vaginal axis, they are associated with some increased risk of subsequent enterocele.

Lateral Vaginal Repair

This technique aims at the restoration of normal anatomy through the reattachment of the perivaginal fascia to the arcuate line along the side wall of the pelvis. The arcus tendineus ligament represents the origin of the levator muscle from the fascia overlying the obturator internus muscle. When carried anteriorly, the technique is reported to restore the bladder neck to a retropubic position. The suspension ordinarily begins just anterior to the ischial spine and is aimed at correcting cystourethrocele caused by lateral vaginal defects.

Surgical Procedures for Vaginal Vault Prolapse and Enterocele

Vaginal McCall Culdoplasty

The vaginal McCall culdoplasty technique is used for the management of uterovaginal prolapse and associated enterocele. Following vaginal removal of the uterus, an incision is made along the midline of the posterior vaginal wall, and the enterocele sac is dissected free from the vagina and rectum. The sac is then ligated and excised, after which the uterosacral ligaments are plicated in the midline to create a shelf to which the vaginal vault is attached. The result is elimination of the enterocele and suspension of the vaginal vault. When the uterus has previously been removed, this procedure can frequently be used to suspend the vaginal vault and repair the enterocele, with the entire dissection being retroperitoneal with a vaginal approach.

Abdominal Colposacropexy

Advanced prolapse of the vaginal vault may be repaired abdominally by suspending the vagina to the anterior wall of the sacrum. The procedure usually requires the use of a graft such as Gore-Tex or Mersilene, which is attached to the sacrum at or below the promontory. The graft is then passed to the right side of the rectosigmoid and attached to the vaginal vault and covered by peritoneum. This technique gives excellent results but on occasion may be complicated by erosion of the graft into the vagina, which usually requires removal. It is especially useful when there are other indications for an abdominal approach such as a pelvic mass or when a short vagina may require lengthening for adequate sexual function.

Abdominal Enterocele Repair

An enterocele may be repaired abdominally by obliteration of the sac using several layers of circumferential sutures through the cul-de-sac peritoneum. Another technique involves the passage of permanent suture from one uterosacral ligament through the peritoneum of the cul-de-sac and then into the opposite ligament. When several such sutures are placed and tied, the floor of the pelvis is elevated by several centimeters and the cul-de-sac is obliterated. The result is a shelf along the floor of the pelvis made up of the uterosacral ligaments between the vaginal apex anteriorly and the rectosigmoid posteriorly. The shelf can also be used as a means of suspending the vaginal apex if needed.

Surgical Procedures for Repair of Rectocele and Relaxed Vaginal Outlet

The repair of rectocele and relaxed vaginal outlet is accomplished through a midline posterior vaginal wall incision that extends into the rectovaginal septum. The dissection extends superiorly to the uterosacral ligaments and inferiorly to the perineal body. The defect in the rectovaginal septum is repaired by multiple interrupted sutures, which may also include the fascia of the levator sling. Excess vaginal mucosa is then excised before closure of the posterior vaginal wall.

Repair of a relaxed vaginal outlet requires closure of the midline perineal defect. The puborectalis muscles are exposed and brought together in the midline to restore the apex of the perineal body. The remaining portion of the perineal body is reconstructed using interrupted sutures. The anal canal is then the proper length and in the proper direction and the reconstituted perineal body results in an appropriate separation of the anal canal from the vaginal fourchette.

Le Fort Procedure or Colpocleisis

When the patient's age and medical condition make the risk of a major operation unacceptable, the Le Fort procedure represents a compromise that may be acceptable, even though there is closure of the vagina and loss of sexual function. A rectangular strip of vaginal mucosa is excised from both the anterior and posterior vaginal wall beginning about 2 cm distal to the cervix. The opposing defects are sutured together with consecutive rows of absorbable sutures, resulting in closure of the vagina. A mucosa-lined tunnel on either side remains and permits the escape of cervical secretions or blood should the patient experience postmenopausal bleeding. The technique is generally quite effective but obscures the cervix from subsequent examination. Another significant disadvantage is the complication of induced stress urinary incontinence because of displacement of the bladder neck posteriorly.

Alternative to the Surgical Repair of Vaginal Prolapse

Pessaries are round, soft rubber devices of various shapes and sizes that may be inserted into the vagina for the correction of a prolapse, especially when it extends beyond the vaginal introitus. This alternative may be used by patients of any age, but is especially useful in the very elderly patient when medical problems increase the risk of a surgical procedure. The patient or, in some instances, a visiting nurse is instructed in the removal and replacement of the pessary at intervals of 7 to 10 days to prevent infection and vaginal ulceration. The device may be used indefinitely, but most patients ultimately find a surgical repair to be preferable.

MALIGNANT DISEASE

The common gynecologic malignancies show an increased age-specific incidence until the ninth decade. Although the number of patients in each of the older decades is smaller, a higher percentage of women in those decades develop malignant tumors.

Although alternatives to surgical therapy, such as radiation therapy, may provide similar results to surgical therapy in some diseases, the gynecologic surgeon should not be dissuaded from careful consideration of the surgical approach if this indeed provides the best chance of cure. Treatment alternatives should always be considered, but therapeutic compromises made with the idea that temporary palliation will suffice until the elderly patient succumbs to her other medical diseases all too often result in a different and difficult dilemma a few years later. At that time, the patient, who has still not yet died from old age, becomes increasingly symptomatic from her malignancy and is at this point even more of a risk for surgical treatment. Lichtinger and coworkers reviewed a series of 89 patients who were >75 years of age and who underwent major gynecologic operations for malignant tumors [3]. With modern surgical intensive care and multisystem monitoring now available, hospital mortality in this group was only 3.2%. Most of the surgical procedures were done for endometrial or vulvar carcinoma. When considering the management of gynecologic malignancy in the elderly patient with the double jeopardy of malignant disease and the general medical frailty of the usual aged patient, one may well decide that such a patient should be referred to a major medical center. At such a center the combined talents of multiple specialists who regularly deal with such problems will be available, and the success rate may well be improved.

The importance of a thorough and careful preoperative evaluation cannot be overemphasized. Not only does this evaluation allow the physician to identify potential problems and assess the risks of the surgical procedure or other treatment modalities, it also provides reassurance to the patient and her family that the surgeon and the consultants are approaching her situation with care and thoughtful deliberation. It is not unusual that the most difficult person to convince of the advisability of the operation is the patient herself. Too often, elderly women have seen their friends die from cancer, and they may feel that the outcome of the procedure will be a brief and painful period inevitably leading to death. They may resist all forms of therapeutic intervention. This attitude is also commonly expressed by family members of elderly patients and occasionally by the referring physician. It is most important to review the prognosis and natural history of the disease with the patient and her family. In many cases it is especially helpful if another elderly patient who has had the procedure 3 or 4 years previously can speak with the patient personally. Such a "living testimonial" carries far more weight than the physician's words ever can.

Despite increasing pressures to minimize hospitalization, elderly surgical patients may need preoperative admission for a bowel preparation, medical optimization, and hospital orientation. A study by Massad et al. [4] found that age and nutritional depletion, factors often associated with gynecologic malignancy, were also associated with increased length of stay after gynecologic surgery.

Endometrial Carcinoma

Adenocarcinoma of the endometrium is the most common invasive gynecologic malignancy in the United States. Most patients with this disease are postmenopausal, with an average age of 59 at the time of diagnosis. The most common presenting complaint of a patient with endometrial cancer is postmenopausal bleeding. This occurs in >90% of patients. High-risk factors for endometrial carcinoma include estrogen therapy, obesity, nulliparity, and a previous history of endometrial hyperplasia. Other causes for postmenopausal bleeding include hormonal therapy, atrophic vaginitis, endometrial polyps, and various types of endometrial hyperplasia.

Diagnosis and Staging

The techniques for evaluating postmenopausal bleeding have changed considerably in the past few years. If pelvic ultrasound is readily available, it may be used to measure endometrial thickness. When the uterus is well visualized and the total endometrial thickness (both front and back walls) is 5 mm or less, postmenopausal bleeding can be safely ascribed to atrophy with no risk of endometrial cancer. Patients with an endometrial thickness between 5 and 10 mm are at low risk for endometrial cancer, but an endometrial biopsy may be indicated in the older postmenopausal woman, especially if she is not on hormone therapy. If endometrial thickness is 10 mm or greater or if bleeding persists, a tissue specimen is indicated. This may be obtained by endometrial biopsy or dilatation and curettage. If an endometrial biopsy shows any significant degree of hyperplasia, formal dilatation and curettage is indicated to rule out invasive adenocarcinoma. The use of hysteroscopy is controversial, but it seems to be most helpful in identifying endometrial polyps [5]. In addition to endometrial hyperplasias, cancer, and polyps, hormonal therapy is a common

TABLE 29-1. *International Federation of Gynecology and Obstetrics (FIGO) staging for carcinoma of the corpus uteri*

Stage IA G123	Tumor limited to endometrium
Stage IB G123	Invasion to <one-half the myometrium
Stage IC G123	Invasion to >one-half the myometrium
Stage IIA G123	Endocervical glandular involvement only
Stage IIB G123	Cervical stromal invasion
Stage IIIA G123	Tumor invades serosa and/or adnexa, and/or positive peritoneal cytology result
Stage IIIB G123	Vaginal metastases
Stage IIIC G123	Metastases to pelvic or para-aortic lymph nodes or both
Stage IVA G123	Tumor invasion of bladder or bowel mucosa or both
Stage IVB	Distant metastases including intra-abdominal or inguinal lymph nodes or both

Histopathology: degree of differentiation

Cases of carcinoma of the corpus should be classified (or graded) according to the degree of histologic differentiation, as follows:

G1 5% or less of a nonsquamous or nonmorular solid growth pattern
G2 6–50% of a nonsquamous or nonmorular solid growth pattern
G3 >50% of a nonsquamous or nonmorular solid growth pattern

Notes on pathologic grading

1. Notable nuclear atypia, inappropriate for the architectural grade, raises the grade of a grade 1 or grade 2 tumor by 1.
2. In serous adenocarcinoma, clear cell adenocarcinomas, and squamous cell carcinomas, nuclear grading takes precedence.
3. Adenocarcinomas with squamous differentiation are graded according to the nuclear grade of the glandular component.

Rules related to staging

1. Because corpus cancer is now staged surgically, procedures previously used for determination of stages are no longer applicable, such as the findings from fractional dilatation and curettage to differentiate between stages I and II.
2. It is appreciated that there may be a small number of patients with corpus cancer who will be treated primarily with radiation therapy. If that is the case, the clinical staging adopted by FIGO in 1971 would still apply, but designation of that staging system would be noted.
3. Ideally, width of the myometrium should be measured along with the width of tumor invasion.

cause of postmenopausal bleeding, but mere discontinuation of the medication is not adequate management for postmenopausal bleeding. An ultrasound to measure endometrial thickness or an endometrial biopsy to sample the uterine contents is required. *The standard cervical Papanicolaou smear is not an adequate method of evaluating postmenopausal bleeding.* Various estimates suggest that Papanicolaou smear results will be positive in only 35% to 50% of all patients with endometrial carcinoma.

Once a diagnosis of endometrial adenocarcinoma has been made, the tumor must be staged for therapeutic, prognostic, and statistical purposes. The classification system for cancer of the uterus that is generally accepted throughout the world is the one proposed by the International Federation of Gynecology and Obstetrics shown in Table 29-1. This staging classification was changed in 1988 to a surgical staging system because most women with endometrial cancer undergo hysterectomy. Women unable to tolerate surgical staging may be classified by the older clinical staging system. Prognosis is related to tumor grade and depth of myometrial invasion so that these characteristics are included in the substages. In addition, although the vast majority of patients with endometrial carcinoma have typical endometrial adenocarcinoma, special note should be made of the histologic findings of adenosquamous carcinoma, clear cell, or papillary adenocarcinoma, all of which have a poor prognosis.

Therapy

Total abdominal hysterectomy with bilateral salpingo-oophorectomy is the cornerstone of treatment for patients with endometrial carcinoma [6]. Because the disease frequently occurs in elderly patients, often in association with obesity, diabetes, and hypertension, serious reservations concerning the surgical approach may be expressed by some elderly patients. Surgical removal of the uterus significantly improves survival in most patients with endometrial carcinoma, and every effort should be made to accomplish this goal if at all possible.

For patients with endometrial adenocarcinoma clinically confined to the uterus, most authorities in the United States would recommend initial total abdominal hysterectomy with bilateral salpingo-oophorectomy. This not only removes the primary cancer but also affords the opportunity for selective sampling of lymph nodes in the pelvic and aortic areas in women with poorly differentiated or deeply invasive tumors [7].

There is active disagreement about the place of adjunctive radiation therapy in patients with stage I endometrial carcinoma [8]. There is little evidence that postoperative pelvic radiation improves survival, although it may increase pelvic control in women with surgical stage I disease. In elderly patients at higher risk for radiation complications, adjunctive radiation may not be indicated.

TABLE 29-2. *Carcinoma of the corpus uteri from 1987 to 1989: distribution by stage and 5-year survival*

Stage	Patients treated	5-year survival (%)
I	9,430	86
II	1,852	66
III	1,277	44
IV	450	16

Source: Reprinted with permission from International Federation of Gynecology and Obstetrics. Annual Report on the Results of Treatment in Gynecological Cancer (Vol. 22). Stockholm: Radiumhemmet, 1994;75.

In patients with stage II disease, the incidence of pelvic node metastases is approximately 35%, and therefore, postoperative radiation is usually recommended. In most instances, hysterectomy is combined with both external pelvic radiation and intravaginal cesium. Lymph node biopsies may be done for prognostic reasons.

When the tumor has spread beyond the uterus in either stage III or IV disease, treatment is again individualized depending on the location and extent of the disease. However, total abdominal hysterectomy and bilateral salpingo-oophorectomy are recommended if the operation is technically feasible, if the patient has at least a 6-month life expectancy, and if she is otherwise a reasonable surgical candidate. The uterine bleeding associated with the progression of untreated tumor can be severe, and hysterectomy is thought to be extremely useful for palliation in these cases.

Laparoscopically assisted vaginal hysterectomy with bilateral salpingo-oophorectomy and appropriate laparoscopic lymph node sampling has become increasingly popular [9]. Clinical trials are now ongoing to evaluate the applicability and efficacy of this approach. Vaginal hysterectomy has been recommended for patients with stage I endometrial cancer if they are grossly obese or if a vaginal approach might offer a rapid surgical procedure with less morbidity [10]. This approach may be especially attractive in the elderly patient who will likely have some degree of pelvic relaxation and uterine prolapse and where simple vaginal hysterectomy (along with bilateral salpingo-oophorectomy if possible) would allow the skilled vaginal surgeon to complete the hysterectomy in 30 minutes or less. Radical abdominal hysterectomy and pelvic lymphadenectomy are rarely indicated in patients with endometrial carcinoma.

Alternatives to Surgical Therapy

In the elderly patient with significant associated medical conditions, the risk of a surgical procedure may be high, and alternative methods of therapy should be considered. Radiation therapy alone has been used rarely for the treatment of endometrial adenocarcinoma. Bickenbach and colleagues in a series of matched pairs of comparable cases clearly outlined that even patients with stage I cancers had a worse 5-year survival when hysterectomy was not part of their management [11].

Hormonal therapy with progestins has also been effective for palliation of endometrial carcinoma. This is usually not thought of as a curative treatment, although patients with well-differentiated tumors may respond well.

Results

The treatment results that can be expected for patients with endometrial adenocarcinoma are shown in Table 29-2. These data are collected from institutions throughout the world and reflect the excellent results obtainable in early stage disease [12]. A careful regression analysis demonstrated that increasing age was associated with decreasing survival. It is unclear whether this is due to less vigorous treatment of older women or to some other factor. In the management of endometrial carcinoma, hysterectomy plays such an important role that a patient's age in and of itself should not be a contraindication to a treatment plan that provides the best chance of cure.

Ovarian Cancer

Carcinoma of the ovary is the fourth leading cause of death from cancer among women in the United States [13]. The age-adjusted incidence shows a steady increase in ovarian carcinoma each year until age 85. More than one-third of patients with ovarian cancer are aged 65 or older.

One of the main reasons for the poor outcome in patients with ovarian carcinoma is the silent nature of this malignancy. Its intra-abdominal location makes it difficult to detect on examination, and three-fourths of all patients with ovarian carcinoma already have disease spread beyond the pelvis at the time of initial presentation. Until the disease has become widespread, symptoms are few and relatively nonspecific. Occasional vague pain, fullness, or bloating may be described. This vague pain is often transient and not too severe. Quite often, these symptoms are elicited only in retrospect, but in occasional patients these complaints elicit a thorough gastrointestinal workup that may be unrevealing. Serum CA-125 level is elevated >35 in 80% of epithelial ovarian cancer cases and may be a helpful diagnostic test along with pelvic ultrasound and computed tomography.

In a good review of data from the Surveillance, Epidemiology, and End Results Program of the National Cancer Institute, Yancik et al. [14] found that older patients with ovarian cancer had more advanced disease. The median age for ovarian cancer was 54 years for stage I and 62 years for stages III and IV. Seventy-three and one-half percent of patients over age 75 who had ovarian cancer had stages III and IV disease by the time the diagnosis was made, whereas only 47% of women under age 45 had such advanced dis-

TABLE 29-3. *Clinical staging of ovarian cancer*

Stage I	Growth limited to the ovaries
Stage Ia	Growth limited to one ovary; no ascites
(i)	No tumor on the external surface
(ii)	Tumor present on the external surface, capsule ruptured, or both
Stage Ib	Growth limited to both ovaries; no ascites
(i)	No tumor on the external surface; capsules intact
(ii)	Tumor present on the external surface, capsule(s) ruptured, or both
Stage Ic	Tumor either stage Ia or Ib, but with ascites* present or positive peritoneal washing results
Stage II	Growth involving one or both ovaries with pelvic extension
Stage IIa	Extension, metastases, or both to the uterus, tubes, or both
Stage IIb	Extension to other pelvic tissues
Stage IIc	Tumor either stage IIa or IIb, but with ascites present or positive peritoneal washing results
Stage III	Growth involving one or both ovaries with intraperitoneal metastases outside the pelvic, positive retroperitoneal nodes, or both; tumor limited to the true pelvis with histologically proven malignant extension to small bowel or omentum
Stage IV	Growth involving one or both ovaries with distant metastases; if pleural effusion is present there must be positive cytology to allot a case to stage IV; parenchymal liver metastases equals stage IV
Special category	Unexplored cases that are thought to be ovarian carcinoma

**Ascites* is peritoneal effusion that in the opinion of the surgeon is pathologic, clearly exceeds normal amounts, or both.
Source: Reprinted with permission from International Federation of Gynecology and Obstetrics. Annual Report on the Results of Treatment in Gynecological Cancer (Vol. 22). Stockholm: Radiumhemmet, 1994;39-40.

ease. Surgical stage and tumor grade are far more important prognostic variables than patient age.

Diagnosis and Staging

Ovarian cancer is a surgically staged disease because the diagnosis itself cannot be made with any certainty without a laparotomy [15]. The International Federation of Gynecology and Obstetrics staging system is shown in Table 29-3. Because ovarian carcinoma is a surgically staged disease, the need for an accurate evaluation of the extent of the disease at laparotomy should seem obvious. Patients with advanced disease present relatively little problem with staging and evaluation, but patients with stages I and II ovarian cancer may be inadequately staged unless a thorough evaluation of the abdomen is made, including washings for cytology, biopsy of the omentum, and careful inspection of the diaphragm, mesentery, and small bowel in addition to biopsy of the pelvic and aortic lymph nodes.

It is appropriate to consider who should do the surgical procedure for patients with ovarian cancer. In cases in which a small, mobile mass is present and the suspicion of ovarian cancer is low, any competent pelvic surgeon should be able to resect and properly stage the tumor to decide on the appropriate postoperative therapy. Nevertheless, Mayer et al. [16] compared the survival of patients with stages I and II disease who were originally operated on at Yale by gynecologic oncologists with a series of similar patients operated on by general gynecologists and other surgeons. All patients were treated postoperatively at Yale with platinum-based combination chemotherapy, and the patients originally operated by gynecologic oncologists had a statistically better survival rate. Thus, it seems reasonable to suggest that patients with a suspicion of ovarian cancer be referred to a gynecologic oncologist for primary surgery.

Alternatives to Surgical Therapy

Although the primary operative approach to ovarian carcinoma is important, occasionally patients have medical conditions or far advanced cancer that makes the surgical approach difficult or of questionable benefit. In patients with ascites or pleural effusion it is possible to make a presumptive diagnosis by cytologic examination of pleural or peritoneal fluid. Such patients may then be treated with several cycles of chemotherapy, with laparotomy being delayed to evaluate a response. If the effusions resolve and computed tomographic scans indicate a decrease in the size of the ovarian masses, resection may be reconsidered after several months. This is an acceptable approach for selected patients. Chemotherapy with a combination regimen including platinum, paclitaxel (Taxol), and cyclophosphamide are all highly effective. In general, thoracentesis before the initial operation reduces the risk of pulmonary complications, but the removal of ascites can usually be accomplished at the same time as the exploratory laparotomy and preoperative paracentesis is rarely necessary. Radiation therapy has a limited role in patients with ovarian cancer, and it is usually applicable only in patients with minimal or no residual disease after surgery.

Results

Surgical therapy alone is inadequate for ovarian carcinoma except for patients with stage Ia, grade 1 or 2 tumors who have undergone adequate staging evaluation. The 5-

TABLE 29-4. *Carcinoma of the ovary: actuarial 5-year survival by stage*

Stage	Number of patients	5-year survival (%)
Ia	845	83.5
Ib	188	79.3
Ic	606	73.1
Iia	140	64.6
Iib	272	54.2
Iic	336	61.3
IIIa	171	51.7
IIIb	366	29.2
IIIc	1,903	17.7
IV	1,291	14.3
Total	6,118	

Source: Reprinted with permission from International Federation of Gynecology and Obstetrics. Annual Report on the Results of Treatment in Gynecological Cancer (Vol. 22). Stockholm: Radiumhemmet, 1994;94.

year survival rates for patients with epithelial ovarian cancers are shown in Table 29-4. The overall survival rate for all patients is 39.1%. There is no doubt that newer combination chemotherapy has increased the length of survival, but the median survival for patients with stages III and IV disease is still only approximately 36 months. As noted previously, this is especially discouraging because the majority of patients with ovarian cancer already have stage III or IV disease at the time of diagnosis. Patient age alone, however, should not eliminate the potential benefits of aggressive management.

Cervical Cancer

Although radical hysterectomy and pelvic lymphadenectomy are frequently used in the treatment of patients with early stage cervical carcinoma [17], radiation therapy is probably equally effective and is an acceptable alternative in the older patient who is a poor surgical candidate. Occasionally, patients with recurrent cervical carcinoma are candidates for total pelvic exenteration. In the past, age >70 was a relative contraindication to this extensive surgical approach [18], but advances in perioperative management and medical therapy have made this contraindication less absolute. Patients with central pelvic recurrence after radiation therapy for cervical carcinoma who have no evidence of pelvic side wall or distant metastasis are potential candidates for pelvic exenteration. Such procedures require close cooperation between the anesthesiologist, surgeon, and nursing personnel and should be done only in major medical centers where adequate staffing and experience are available.

Carcinoma of the Vulva

Carcinoma of the vulva is one of the least common of all gynecologic malignancies, accounting for approximately 4% of female genital neoplasms. Surgical management with radical vulvectomy and bilateral inguinal-femoral lymphadenectomy continues to be the mainstay of treatment for vulvar carcinoma [19]. The average age of patients with this diagnosis is 72, and it is not uncommon to find patients in the ninth or tenth decades of life with this disease.

The presenting symptoms are frequently bleeding, pain, or a mass. Elderly patients often exhibit considerable denial about symptoms and may delay seeing the physician for months or even years despite persistent symptoms. Although experienced physicians may be able to recognize various vulvar lesions by inspection, when there is any question about the possibility of malignancy, a biopsy should always be done using a small 4-mm Keyes's biopsy punch with local anesthesia. There are several staging classifications used for vulvar carcinoma, but the clinical examination of tumor size and involvement of the vulva, vagina, and rectum is key. The presence or absence of palpably suspicious lymph nodes is also used in the clinical staging, but this is notoriously inaccurate, with approximately 30% false-positive and false-negative results.

Surgical Treatment

Despite the fact that this cancer commonly occurs in elderly patients, surgical therapy continues to be the main treatment modality and is usually well tolerated. Although radical vulvectomy with bilateral inguinal-femoral lymphadenectomy has been the treatment of choice for invasive vulvar carcinoma, various new approaches have been recommended for patients with minimal disease. Radical vulvectomy with unilateral inguinal lymphadenectomy has been widely adopted for patients with primary tumors <2 cm in diameter confined to one side of the vulva without involvement of any midline structures [20]. Pelvic radiation is now used in patients with inguinal lymph node metastases instead of pelvic lymphadenectomy.

Alternatives to Surgical Therapy

Most patients can tolerate the procedure to remove vulvar carcinoma. This can be done under regional or even local anesthesia if necessary. Radiation therapy is not well tolerated on the vulva and is used infrequently for the primary treatment of vulvar carcinoma. However, radical vulvectomy or even simple excision of the tumor mass followed by radiation therapy to the inguinal nodes is an effective alternative to lymphadenectomy. In most cases when the inguinal nodes are positive for cancer, whole pelvic irradiation therapy is given, rather than surgical pelvic lymphadenectomy. For women with very large vulvar cancers, including those with gross nodal metastases, a combination of preoperative external radiation given concomitantly with cisplatin and 5-fluorouracil chemotherapy has proved to be well tolerated and effective, at least with short-term follow-up.

TABLE 29-5. *Survival results for treatment of carcinoma of the vulva*

Stage	Number of patients	5-year survival (%)
I	578	83
II	574	60
III	515	51
IV	187	22
Total	1,854	

Source: Reprinted with permission from International Federation of Gynecology and Obstetrics. Annual Report on the Results of Treatment in Gynecological Cancer (Vol. 22). Stockholm: Radiumhemmet, 1994;102.

Results

Although surgery remains the mainstay of treatment, various combinations of therapy including preoperative radiation and chemotherapy plus radiation have been increasingly used to decrease the radicalness of the surgical procedure required. Survival results are shown in Table 29-5. The presence or absence of lymph node metastases is the single most important prognostic variable, but age is also an independent variable. As with other malignancies, older women tend to have a less favorable prognosis.

REFERENCES

1. Jaluvka V, Weitzel HK. Zur Altersgrenze in der operativen geriatrischen Gynaekologie. Zentralbl Gynakol 1995;117:233–236.
2. Richardson DA, Ostergard DR. Anterior Vaginal Repair Versus Retropubic Urethropexy: A Review of the Literature. In Ostergard DR (ed), Gynecologic Urology and Urodynamics. Baltimore: Williams & Wilkins, 1980;469–477.
3. Lichtinger M, Averett H, Penalver M, et al. Major surgical procedures for gynecologic malignancy in elderly women. South Med J 1986;79: 1506–1510.
4. Massad KS, Vogler G, Herzog TJ, Mutch DG. Correlates of length of stay in gynecologic oncology patients undergoing inpatient surgery. Gynecol Oncol 1993;51:214–218.
5. Cicinelli E, Romano F, Anastasio PS, et al. Sonohysterography versus hysterectomy in the diagnosis of endometrial polyps. Gynecol Obstet Invest 1994;38:266–271.
6. Lin HH, Chen CD, Chen CK, et al. Is total abdominal hysterectomy with bilateral salpingo-oophorectomy adequate for new FIGO stage I endometrial carcinoma? Br J Obstet Gynaecol 1995;102: 148–152.
7. Kilgore LC, Partridge EE, Alvarez RD, et al. Adenocarcinoma of the endometrium: survival comparisons of patients with and without pelvic node sampling. Gynecol Oncol 1995;56:29–33.
8. Carey MS, O'Connell GJ, Johanson CR, et al. Good outcome associated with a standardized treatment protocol using selective postoperative radiation in patients with clinical stage I adenocarcinoma of the endometrium. Gynecol Oncol 1995;57:138–144.
9. Childers JM. Operative laparoscopy in gynaecological oncology. Baillieres Clin Obstet Gynaecol 1994;8:831–849.
10. Peters WA, Andersen WA, Thornton WN, Morley GW. The selective use of vaginal hysterectomy in the management of adenocarcinoma of the endometrium. Am J Obstet Gynecol 1983;146:285–291.
11. Bichenbach W, Lochmuller H, Dirlich G, et al. Factor analysis of endometrial carcinoma in relation to treatment. Obstet Gynecol 1967; 29:632–636.
12. International Federation of Gynecology and Obstetrics. Annual Report on the Results of Treatment in Gynecological Cancer (Vol. 22). Stockholm: Radiumhemmet, 1994.
13. National Institutes of Health. Ovarian cancer: screening, treatment, and followup. NIH Consens Statement 1994;12(3):1–30.
14. Yancik R, Lies LG, Yates JW. Ovarian cancer in the elderly: an analysis of surveillance, epidemiology, and end results program data. Am J Obstet Gynecol 1986;154:639–647.
15. Hoskins WJ. Epithelial ovarian carcinoma: principles of primary surgery. Gynecol Oncol 1994;55(3 Pt 2):S91–S96.
16. Mayer AR, Chambers SK, Graves E, et al. Ovarian cancer staging: does it require a gynecologic oncologist? Gynecol Oncol 1992;47: 223–227.
17. Geisler JP, Geisler HE. Radical hysterectomy in patients 65 years of age and older. Gynecol Oncol 1994;53:208–211.
18. Matthews CM, Burke M, Morris TW, et al. Pelvic exenteration in the elderly. Obstet Gynecol 1992;79(5 Pt 1):773–777.
19. Franklin EW III, Weiser EB. Surgery for vulvar cancer. Surg Clin North Am 1991;71:911–925.
20. Hacker NJ, Van der Velden J. Conservative management of early vulvar cancer. Cancer 1993;71(Suppl 4):1673–1677.

Surgical Care for the Elderly, 2nd ed., edited by
R. Benton Adkins, Jr., and H. William Scott, Jr.
Lippincott–Raven Publishers, Philadelphia © 1998.

CHAPTER 30

Musculoskeletal Diseases

Ronald E. Rosenthal

Certain musculoskeletal disease processes are characteristically seen in elderly patients. Some are managed the same way as in younger patients, but many are not. Differences in functional capacity, life-style, mental status, and concomitant medical conditions may modify the management of a fracture, degenerative process, painful tendinitis, or inflammatory condition in an elderly patient. This chapter identifies and presents the management of some of the more common diseases due to skeletal demineralization, inflammatory arthritides, infections, degenerative conditions, neoplasms affecting the skeletal structures, and trauma. The latter category includes acute fractures and soft-tissue conditions, as well as chronic ligament and tendon pathology.

Elderly people may be active or sedentary, healthy or infirm, and their ultimate recovery may be more a function of their underlying health than of the treatment for a specific orthopedic condition. In general, the goal of treating the elderly is no different than in younger patients: restoration of function as rapidly and easily as possible. Many elderly patients live independently, and treatment must attempt to restore that independence. Elderly people unite their fractures as well as younger people, although the fracture union is of the same quality as the rest of the bone: an intertrochanteric fracture in a patient with severe osteoporosis will unite with the same osteoporotic bone that was there originally. A skeletal structure (or any other part of the body for that matter) is never restored to normal by an operation. Elderly people may have difficulty understanding and participating in their own rehabilitation programs. Realistic results must be anticipated from elective reconstructive surgery or from knee or shoulder arthroscopy following injury during recreational activity. Concomitant illness may make any surgery, except for a life-threatening emergency, too hazardous to consider. Family situations may simplify or complicate convalescence and rehabilitation after orthopedic surgery. Economic restrictions, mandated by government or managed care programs, may completely alter proposed treatment plans.

As is true in younger people, musculoskeletal conditions in the elderly are rarely life-threatening. Frequently, the surgeon has time to become acquainted with the patient and family, discuss various options, and be certain that the patient and family understand the expected result and the necessary participation by all concerned for a successful outcome. Successful orthopedic surgery in the elderly is highly gratifying to the patient and surgeon. A patient with a hip fracture can be returned to an ambulatory state; a patient with degenerative arthritis of the hip or knee can become pain free; a patient with rotator cuff shoulder pathology can resume playing golf and tennis; and a patient with metastatic carcinoma of a femur can become pain free and mobile, sometimes for several months.

Physicians are increasingly recognizing a subgroup of elderly patients called the *very elderly,* who are >80 years of age. These patients may require different approaches and treatment and have a different response than those 60 and 70 years old. Statistics and reports of treatment of the elderly that include all patients over age 60, for example, may be misleading if this group of very elderly is not considered separately. Orthopedic management of these patients may be different, as discussed under individual headings in this chapter. Age by itself is no contraindication to orthopedic surgical treatment [1].

FACTORS INFLUENCING ORTHOPEDIC TREATMENT

The single most important factor influencing decisions and outcomes in orthopedic surgery in an elderly patient is the patient's general health and functional state. Different functional patterns can be found among patients of the same age, particularly among the very elderly. Some patients are long-term nursing home residents, nonambulatory, and unable to communicate. Others are active, independent, alert, and functioning community members. Many elderly people have chronic but stable medical conditions such as controlled hypertension or mild cardiac decompensation. These conditions need not be contraindications to elective reconstructive surgery in an otherwise alert active person. Acute pulmonary edema, recent myocardial infarctions, and active pulmonary or urinary tract infections are contraindications to elective orthopedic surgery. Peripheral vascular disease, chronic pulmonary or renal disease, obesity, and diabetes may be relative contraindications to elective surgery, but may have to be accepted in urgent situations.

Skeletal demineralization, perhaps an indication of an inactive life-style, may modify different surgical procedures and alter projected outcomes. This is particularly true in fractures of the spine, wrist, or shoulder, where reduction cannot be maintained and residual deformity may be inevitable.

Concomitant illnesses, particularly those that require regular, potent medication, may profoundly influence the management of an orthopedic condition. Patients with iatrogenic hyperadrenalcorticalism secondary to prolonged corticosteroid treatment are at great risk following orthopedic procedures. Patients who require chronic anticoagulation must have anticoagulation evaluated and temporarily stopped before surgery. Patients taking long-term nonsteroidal anti-inflammatory drugs, with their potential for bleeding, should stop these medications before elective orthopedic surgery. Cigarette smoking, alcohol, and inactivity all are detrimental to the outcome of orthopedic surgery in elderly patients [2].

The patient's mental state is a major factor in decision making about proposed elective surgery. Many orthopedic procedures will fail without a vigorous, active rehabilitation program. A patient who cannot comprehend his or her role in the rehabilitation should not be considered for a major reconstructive procedure. Reconstructive procedures should be approached with great caution in patients who have had strokes or have spasticity or contractures.

Most patients will limp following major procedures on the lower extremities and will require a cane or even a walker, sometimes forever. Many may benefit from short-term inpatient rehabilitation before returning to their independent life. For many independent elderly people, restoration of their independence is their primary, and sometimes only, goal. Home care arrangements are frequently necessary, particularly for hip fracture patients, although current trends and cost-containment schemes may modify this arrangement considerably. Orthopedic patients should ideally become ambulatory rapidly after surgery, even with limited weight bearing. This allows maximal access to what may become dwindling resources for post-hospital rehabilitation. A few patients require long-term nursing home placement after orthopedic injuries. One study indicated that 25% of all hip fracture patients went into nursing homes. Other studies, however, have not confirmed this [3–5]. An acute injury may occur in the course of a medical catastrophe; the patient continues to deteriorate after surgical repair as part of the inexorable progression of the medical condition. Frequently, such a patient was barely living an independent life, and the family may have been contemplating nursing home placement when the event occurred and now must make that decision in a crisis. Social work services play a vital role in this situation.

OSTEOPOROSIS AND DEMINERALIZATION

Skeletal demineralization and its consequences are a major cause of disability in the elderly. Demineralization may be in the form of osteoporosis, osteomalacia, or both. For purposes of this chapter, the conditions are considered together. The exact incidence of osteoporosis is unknown, but it does afflict a majority of postmenopausal white women. Many etiologic causes have been proposed. Race, genetics, life-style, calcium deficiency, and early menopause have all been implicated. Two varieties of osteoporosis have been identified, one occurring in the perimenopausal period, and the other occurring years later. Inadequate dietary calcium has been increasingly implicated as a cause of diminished skeletal calcium, which then is further depleted by metabolic needs. Cigarette smoking has also been implicated in a variety of skeletal conditions, including demineralization and delayed or nonunion of fractures [6].

Osteoporosis does not involve all bones equally and has a predilection for the spine, wrist, and femur. Patients complain of pain and actual tenderness of the involved bones. Compression fractures, a form of pathologic fracture, occur even without obvious trauma, resulting in progressive thoracic kyphosis and loss of height. Even minor falls with injury to porotic bone may result in fractures about the shoulder, wrist, spine, and hip.

Identification of established osteoporosis is made on characteristic roentgenographic findings. The bone appears demineralized, the cortices of the affected long bones are thin, and the medullary canal is widened. The normal sclerotic appearance of the subchondral bone may be absent. Early osteoporosis is more subtle and may not be appreciated because of a technically poor roentgenographic study. Detailed densitometry studies, which require special equipment, are sometimes necessary.

To date there has been no effective treatment for all forms of skeletal demineralization. Exogenous estrogens can increase bone mass experimentally as can fluoride and calcitonin, but these two latter drugs cause profound side effects in patients. Sometimes an obvious correctable underlying cause such as hyperthyroidism is present, but more often a variety of factors are at work. Estrogens may be helpful in perimenopausal osteoporosis, particularly if other symptoms of menopause are present. The use of estrogens in older osteoporotic patients is controversial. Calcium intake should equal 1,600 mg per day, a figure that few elderly Americans achieve. Although calcium supplementation will not by itself rebuild bone mass, it can help prevent further demineralization, and most patients with osteoporosis should take calcium (with vitamin D) supplements. Fluoride, calcitonin, and other pharmacologic programs should be managed in specialized centers, often as part of a study protocol [7].

Weight-bearing, gravity-dependent activity is the key in management. Walking, with proper shoes and a cane, allows the body to be upright with positive gravity. Resumption and maintenance of an active life-style is also critical. Bracing of painful kyphosis has not been shown to be effective. Narcotic analgesia should be avoided even for painful conditions; dependence occurs in this age group.

Osteoporosis does not in itself constitute a contraindication to elective or urgent orthopedic surgery. However, the soft bone of the osteoporotic patient mandates certain alterations in standard surgical techniques. Different implants, more liberal use of methacrylate cement, and specific techniques are all part of the surgical management of these patients. Rapid mobilization of the affected part and of the entire patient is critical to the successful management of orthopedic conditions in patients with significant osteoporosis. Specific changes are presented later in this chapter.

INFLAMMATORY DISEASES AND INFECTIONS

Paget's Disease

Paget's disease (osteitis deformans) affects between 3% and 4% of all people over age 50. It may be monostotic or polyostotic. Approximately 20% to 40% of patients with Paget's disease have symptoms, some of them disabling. Symptomatic Paget's disease may be treated with calcitonin or etidronate.

Paget's disease may be a significant complicating factor in orthopedic surgery of the elderly. The surgeon treating Paget's disease must be aware of the variable and unpredictable nature of the disease. Pagetoid bone may be brittle, soft, vascular, or dense; long bones may be deformed; and articular surfaces may be distorted into symptomatic degenerative arthritis. Pathologic fractures may occur through pagetoid bone, unite readily after straightforward repair, or develop nonunion after complicated procedures. Arthroplasty for degenerated pagetoid joints can be routine or so complicated that the procedure must be abandoned. Even with these limitations, most fractures occurring in pagetoid bone are treated by internal fixation, and symptomatic degenerated joints secondary to Paget's disease may be successfully reconstructed with arthroplasties.

Malignant degeneration into osteogenic sarcoma or chondrosarcoma occurs in approximately 1% of all patients with this disease. The symptoms are increasing pain, mass, and sometimes pathologic fractures. These are highly malignant tumors; regardless of treatment the 5-year survival rate is <5% [8].

Crystal-Induced Arthropathy

Gout and calcium pyrophosphate arthropathy (pseudogout) may occur in the elderly. Acute exacerbations of gouty arthritis or pyrophosphate arthropathy may occur in any postoperative patient and present as an inflamed, reddened, painful joint mimicking acute septic arthritis. The knee and first metatarsophalangeal joint are common sites for acute exacerbations, which may follow biliary tract surgery.

The characteristic chondrocalcinosis of pyrophosphate arthropathy may be seen on roentgenography, whereas roentgenography of acute gout may be normal. The diagnosis is made on the results of laboratory studies of blood and synovial fluid. Crystals of urate or pyrophosphate, if present in a properly handled specimen, are diagnostic. Serum uric acid is elevated in gout but not in pyrophosphate arthropathy.

Treatment of acute crystal-induced arthritis is currently with indomethacin and a brief period of immobilization. The classic findings in long-standing gout—destroyed joints and urate deposits in facial cartilages—are rarely seen today. Severe degenerative disease may accompany pyrophosphate-induced arthritis, particularly in the shoulder [9].

Rheumatoid Arthritis

Rheumatoid arthritis in the elderly attacks men and women equally. Elderly rheumatoid patients are often chronically ill. They often take multiple medications, may have exogenous hyperadrenalcorticalism, are immunocompromised, and have limited stamina and activity patterns. Rheumatoid involvement of the cervical spine may result in C1–C2 subluxation, which, if unrecognized, may precipitate fatal spinal cord injury during intubation for elective surgery. Arthrodesis of C1–C2 is often necessary in rheumatoid patients.

Rheumatoid arthritis may present in the elderly as a nonspecific synovitis, without the characteristic fusiform swelling of the hands seen in younger people. The disease may have an indolent or rapidly aggressive course, resulting in profound joint destruction, and may take an active community-dwelling walker and put him or her in a wheelchair in a few months.

In spite of the increased risks of surgery in rheumatoid patients, many are helped by surgical reconstruction. The goals in the surgical management of this disease are to restore as much function and stability as possible. Arthrodeses, except in the spine and foot, are rarely performed in rheumatoid patients; the goal is maintenance of motion, and often partial correction of a deformity is satisfactory. Patients, particularly those with severe disabilities, may be happier than their surgeon with the result [10].

Total joint replacements have been described for the shoulder and elbow, and although these are uncommonly done except in specialized centers, they may be very successful in rheumatoid patients. Hand and wrist arthroplasties can also improve function and appearance. But the most gratifying results in rheumatoid patients are from reconstructive surgery to the lower extremities. Total knee or hip replacement may result in dramatic improvement in a patient's function and outlook. Total knee and hip replacements are discussed later in this chapter.

Specific characteristic deformities occur in the feet of rheumatoid patients. Enzymatic destruction of articular cartilage and supporting ligamentous structures results in hallux valgus deformity and dislocation of metatarsophalangeal joints of the lesser toes. Patients then develop painful plantar calluses and even ulcerations. These deformities cannot be corrected by bracing, and even custom made shoes ("space boots") do not always relieve pain. Surgical reconstruction of affected feet requires extensive bone resection. Arthrodesis of the first metatarsophalangeal joint and resection arthroplasties of the second through fifth metatarsophalangeal joints result in a well-aligned, although slightly shorter, foot that can allow the patient to wear a regular shoe and walk without pain [11]. The results of this procedure are the most gratifying this author has seen in 30 years' experience of operative orthopedic surgery.

Tendon ruptures may also occur in elderly rheumatoid feet, with progressive flat foot deformity. Soft-tissue procedures alone are inadequate treatment; only bony arthrodeses can correct these deformities. This extensive surgery may not be feasible in the elderly rheumatoid foot, and these patients may be treated palliatively with special shoes and molded inserts.

Surgical treatment does not affect the natural history of this disease, and rheumatoid patients need regular medical care, but well-timed surgical intervention may help such a patient resume an independent life with minimal assists.

Neurotrophic Arthritis

Classic neurotrophic arthritis and arthropathy were described by Charcot in the knees of patients with tertiary syphilis. Neurotrophic joints occur presumably secondary to impaired sensation and proprioception.

Neurotrophic arthropathy is seen today primarily in the feet of patients with diabetes mellitus. It may occur at any time in the course of the illness, but usually is seen in patients with long-standing diabetes, usually with other signs and symptoms of neuropathy. The foot becomes progressively painful, swollen, erythematous, and ultimately deformed. Initial roentgenography may be misinterpreted. Subtle fragmentation of a midfoot bone, often the navicular, is the first radiologic sign. Feet with early neurotrophy can be misdiagnosed as infected and treated vigorously with antibiotics before the correct diagnosis is made.

Treatment is frustrating; this is a manifestation of a progressive neurologic disorder. Initial treatment is with immobilization and non–weight bearing, for up to 3 months, until the fragments have consolidated. Progressive weight bearing in well-molded shoes, often with external support, is then begun. The elderly patient may have difficulty remaining active with a program of prolonged non–weight bearing. Progressive deformity and collapse of the midfoot may result in pressure ulcers, and ultimately require amputation for control [12,13].

Infections

Septic arthritis in the elderly is an ominous finding. Bacterial and fungal hematogenous septic arthritis in an elderly person often indicates an underlying disease with obvious or occult immunocompromise. Patients with metastatic malignancies, diabetes, or blood-forming organ diseases are at risk for developing septic arthritis. It may manifest with protean symptoms, such as aching pain, no fever, minimal leukocyte count elevation, and no obvious source, and may be confused with osteoarthritis or inflammatory arthritis. A characteristic late roentgenographic finding is destruction of the articular cartilage and excessive demineralization. The ultimate diagnosis is made with the results of the synovial fluid testing. A high leukocyte count, high synovial protein level, and low glucose level, and ideally, identification of an organism, are the diagnostic criteria. Treatment involves appropriate antibiotics and usually mechanical irrigation and debridement of the joint, followed by a brief period of immobilization, and then range-of-motion exercises. Most antibiotics readily cross the synovium, so that repeated aspirations and injections are not necessary. Surgical drainage and debridement are used to mechanically break up loculi and remove fibrinous plugs, so that systemic antibiotics may be effective. The underlying cause must be found and addressed. Infected joints, even if rapidly and successfully treated, usually show residual cartilage injury, stiffness, and deformity and may develop secondary degenerative joint disease.

Osteomyelitis, deep infection of bone, rarely occurs from hematogenous spread in elderly people. It usually follows open fractures or elective surgery, particularly when metal fixation or implants are used. The widespread use of prophylactic antibiotics in skeletal surgery has helped to decrease the incidence of postoperative infection [14]. Infection after fracture repair is usually treated by drainage and appropriate antibiotics. Fractures usually unite in the presence of infection as long as the fixation remains stable. Fixation is not usually removed until union has occurred. Infection following joint replacement usually cannot be corrected until the implant is removed. Following removal, antibiotic-impregnated methacrylate beads may be placed in the cavity for a period of several weeks, and then new implants replaced, with some measure of success. Osteomyelitis is not usually cured, even with radical treatment; a likelihood of recrudescence is always present.

Chronic osteomyelitis following open fractures in the elderly may be best treated by amputation, particularly if the lesion is distal to the knee. This treatment allows rapid mobilization and avoids prolonged repeated hospitalizations. Osteomyelitis may occur in the foot, usually associated with ischemic ulcers.

DEGENERATIVE JOINT DISEASES

Degenerative joint disease (degenerative arthritis, osteoarthritis) develops to some extent in most people with advancing age. It is often asymptomatic and is discovered as an incidental finding on roentgenography for some other purpose. Primary degenerative joint disease affects the spine, hips, knees, hands, and feet most commonly. Degenerative disease is rare in the ankle or upper-extremity joints unless there has been a previous fracture. Previous rotator cuff injury may predispose a shoulder to degenerative disease. Patients with disease in the hip may have a history of a hip condition in childhood; patients with disease in the knee may have a history of trauma or previous surgery (i.e., meniscectomy). However, most degenerative joint disease seen in the elderly is idiopathic. The natural history of this condition is usually unpredictable, characterized by exacerbations and remissions, often without any obvious inciting cause.

Conservative treatment includes moderate exercise and avoidance of those activities that are painful. Anti-inflammatory medication may relieve symptoms, but does not affect the natural course of the disease. Anti-inflammatory medication is often poorly tolerated by elderly people and may cause gastric upset, bleeding, fluid retention, and hypertension more commonly than in younger patients.

Certain conditions about the spine may be treated surgically, but for the most part, arthritis of the spine is managed nonoperatively. Degenerative disease in the hand usually affects the distal interphalangeal joints and, although cosmetically deforming, usually does not compromise hand function and is not treated.

Surgical treatment may benefit patients with disease of the hip, knee, or foot. Surgical treatment is the only effective way to modify the natural course of degenerative joint disease. Joint replacement arthroplasties of the hip and knee are among the most commonly performed orthopedic procedures in elderly patients. Patients who are otherwise in good health but whose life-style is compromised by a painful, deformed hip or knee may be dramatically helped by well-performed total joint replacement and vigorous rehabilitation and may be able to resume some sports and athletics [15]. Patients with leg claudication from spinal stenosis may benefit from surgical treatment, as may patients with deformed painful feet from hallux valgus and hammertoes.

Degenerative joint disease is rarely life-threatening. Major surgical procedures should be considered when the patient's life-style is significantly compromised, usually by pain. Preoperative evaluation must always include an honest discussion regarding the patient's role in the rehabilitation, and the expected goals. A patient should expect a stable, pain-free joint, while being aware that it is not usual, and that it may not last for his or her lifetime. A patient who cannot understand his or her own role in rehabilitation or who expects a miraculous cure is a poor candidate for reconstructive surgery.

Preoperative planning includes medical optimization and often correction of underlying bladder conditions before joint surgery. Patients treated with nonsteroidal anti-inflammatory medications, or any medications that alter coagulation, must discontinue those medications approximately 2 weeks before surgery. The use of autologous blood transfusions in major orthopedic elective surgery has been shown to be safe and cost-effective. This technique is widely practiced in most major centers [16].

Hip and Knee

Joint replacement has replaced all other forms of arthroplasty as the procedure of choice for the vast majority of patients with symptomatic degenerative joint disease of the hip and knee. Refinements in techniques of joint replacement from new knowledge of biomechanics and biomaterials are constantly being introduced, but the basic principles of arthroplasty, set forth by Sir John Charnley, have remained the same for over 35 years. The articular surfaces are resected and replaced with metal and polyethylene components that articulate with each other. The exact longevity of an implant depends on the age of the patient, the stresses to which the implant is subjected, and the technique used for implantation. There are a number of long-term follow-up studies indicating that some knee and hip replacements can remain functional for 20 years or more [17].

Literally thousands of joint replacements have been performed in the last 25 years. Yet neither the ideal materials, fixation, or surgical technique has been found. Cobalt-chrome alloys, titanium, and various metals all have their proponents. Interest has focused on ways to enhance bony ingrowth around the implant. Coating the implants with bone precursors and newer manufacturing techniques are being evaluated. Manufacturing process and thickness of the polyethylene acetabular and tibial components of total joints have received increased scrutiny. The exact role of methacrylate cement fixation is controversial [18,19].

Primary arthroplasties may fail over time due to loosening, breakage, settling, or infection. Increasing pain and deformity may be the first clue to loosening of an implant. Roentgenography demonstrates characteristic lucent areas, settling, and sometimes fracture or dislocation of one or more components. Revisions are becoming more common as the number of patients with preexisting primary arthroplasties continues to grow. Revision may require bone grafts, allografts, specialized components, and prolonged hospitalization and convalescence [20].

Complications of primary and revision arthroplasty may be life-threatening. The most serious and controversial is thromboembolic disease. The exact incidence of postoperative venous thrombi is controversial, but it is a well-described hazard. Most centers use a protocol to minimize the risk of thromboembolic complications, usually a combination of pharmacologic and mechanical means with aggressive mobilization. Studies have suggested that the anesthetic technique may play a role in postoperative thromboembolic complications and have recommended epidural rather than general anesthesia [21]. The usual protocol uses warfarin, beginning the night before surgery, and then titrated postoperatively to maintain the prothrombin level at 1.5 times normal. In the absence of any phlebitic or thrombotic complications, warfarin is usually stopped when the patient is fully mobilized. Some centers continue warfarin after discharge. This requires regular prothrombin tests, which must be arranged. Low-molecular-weight heparin (enoxaparin [Lovenox]) has been introduced as a substitute for warfarin. It must be given parenterally, but does not require daily prothrombin determinations and may be more cost-effective. Some studies have shown it to be effective in elective arthroplasty patients. Low-dose heparin has not been shown to be effective in orthopedic surgery; dextran has been abandoned by most centers [22–25].

Wound complications may occur. Antibiotic use and better surgical techniques have lowered the incidence of deep postoperative infection, but it still may occur and is catastrophic. Infection may present subtly, with no overt signs, except persistent pain. Characteristic roentgenographic findings may not develop for weeks. Implant dislocations and periprosthetic fractures can occur at any time. Loosening and settling of an implant may occur over time. Urinary retention and pneumonia can occur. These complications can often be forestalled by careful preoperative assessment, vigorous nursing care, and prompt mobilization.

The hybrid total hip replacement is commonly used, consisting of a cemented femoral component and a press-fit acetabular component with metal backing and an adjustable polyethylene liner. The patient is mobilized out of bed the day after surgery and bears weight progressively as tolerated. The greater trochanter is usually not detached. Most knee replacements are done in a similar hybrid fashion with a metal press-fit femoral component, a metal-backed polyethylene cemented tibial component, and a polyethylene cemented patellar component. Continuous passive motion is begun in the recovery room or the next day, and active range-of-motion exercises are instituted along with weight bearing as tolerated with a brief period of immobilization until quadriceps strength is restored. Successful rehabilitation after knee replacement cannot occur unless the knee is fully extended. Revision surgery often mandates variation of this protocol; a period of limited weight bearing may be necessary to allow healing of a reattached trochanter or ingrowth from a porous or coated femoral stem. Antibiotics are given intravenously perioperatively and usually discontinued at 24 to 48 hours postoperatively.

Foot

Degenerative disease in the foot is usually limited to the toes. At the first metatarsophalangeal joint, hallux valgus (bunion) may be part of the clinical picture; hammertoe deformities of the lesser toes commonly occur in the elderly. Metatarsal head callosities may accompany hammertoes. Even severely deformed toes may not be symptomatic as long as the patient can find a satisfactory shoe. Often, a well-padded large shoe with a wide toe box is adequate treatment. Patients often have grossly unrealistic expectations from foot surgery, fueled in part by newspaper and television advertisements. It is not uncommon to see a patient who has to be dissuaded from surgical treatment of a foot deformity and convinced of the advisability of conservative care.

However, symptomatic bunion or hammertoe deformities can only be corrected surgically. Contractures usually require excision of some bone for correction; soft-tissue procedures alone are rarely successful in the elderly. Underlying degenerative disease at the metatarsophalangeal joint is best managed by either excision (Keller-type procedure) or arthrodesis. Hammertoes can be corrected by a combination of metatarsophalangeal joint releases and interphalangeal joint excision. In those feet without significant degenerative joint disease, soft-tissue realignments of the first metatarsophalangeal joint and corrective osteotomy of the base of the first metatarsal may be indicated [26]. Overly aggressive surgery or rough handling of the tissues of an elderly foot may be catastrophic, with skin slough, persistent drainage, and gangrene. Patients with peripheral vascular disease, with a history of diabetes or heavy smoking, are often not candidates for elective foot surgery. All patients must be prepared for a convalescence of several months, and residual thickening of any toes surgically treated.

Foot deformities are commonly bilateral. I rarely treat bilateral foot deformities by simultaneous operations; a period of 6 to 12 weeks is allowed between procedures. Patients with multiple lower-extremity joint involvement considered for reconstructive surgery of the hip, knee, and foot should probably have the foot procedure done first.

Spine

Although most degenerative disease of the spine is relatively static, a particularly aggressive, florid form of hypertrophic osteoarthritis of the spine (disseminated idiopathic skeletal hyperostosis) resulting in bony ankylosis may develop in middle-aged and elderly men (Fig. 30-1). It may affect the entire spine, or a part of it. It is an inflammatory condition, and while it is developing patients have significant pain and usually require medication. Once the disease has run its course and ankylosis has developed, the pain usually disappears. These patients are at risk for fractures due to the limited motion. Disseminated idiopathic skeletal hyperostosis should not be confused with ankylosing spondylitis, a variation of rheumatoid arthritis that develops in younger men. Most degenerative disease of the spine is treated nonoperatively. Moderate, regular exercise, postural instruction, walking assists, and minimal analgesic medication are the mainstays of care.

Back pain occurring for the first time in an elderly patient may indicate metastatic or metabolic disease and may be the first indication of a serious underlying condition. Abdominal aortic aneurysm may present as back pain, as can prostatitis, or retroperitoneal malignancies. Back pain in younger patients is usually caused by disease in the spine and not referred from elsewhere. In the elderly, however, pancreatitis, gynecologic or retroperitoneal malignancies, or peptic ulcer disease can all refer pain to the back.

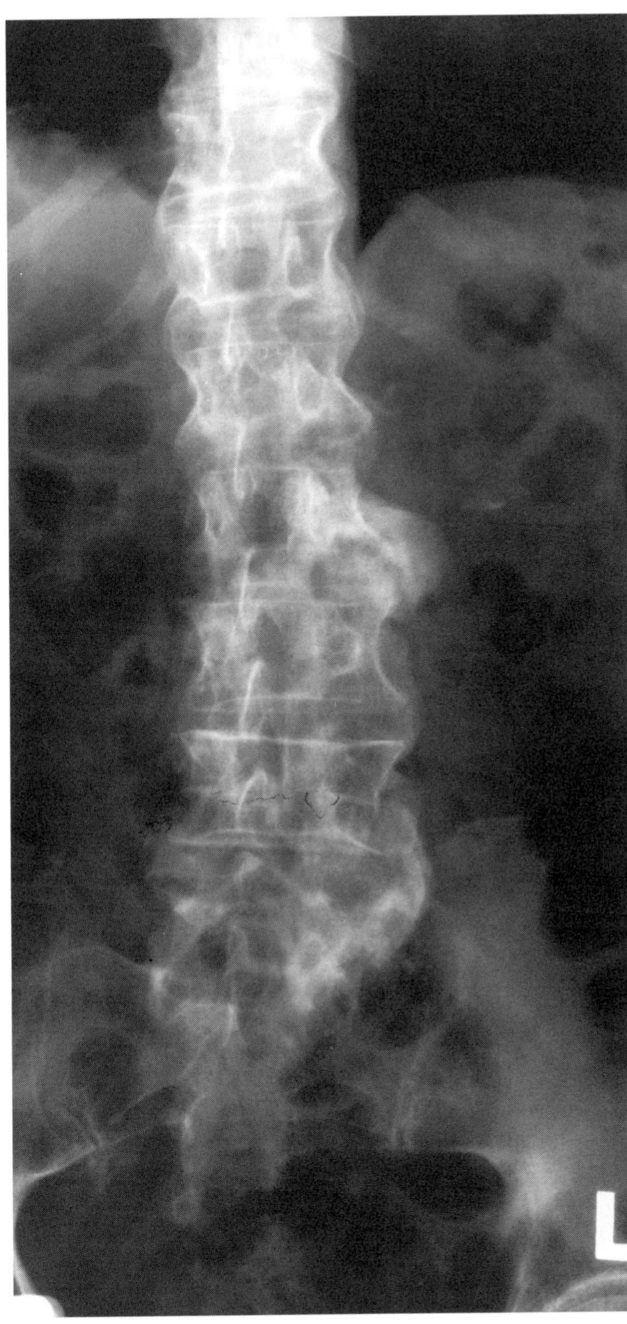

A

B

FIG. 30-1. Anteroposterior **(A)** and lateral **(B)** roentgenograms of a 70-year-old man with disseminated idiopathic skeletal hyperostosis and progressive back pain over 9 months. There is virtual complete osteophytic bridging of the intervertebral spaces, resulting in a fused spine.

Spinal stenosis is an accompaniment to degenerative joint disease, usually of the lumbar spine. Facet hypertrophy and disk degeneration, superimposed on a congenitally narrow canal from short, wide pedicles, results in intermittent pressure on the cauda equina and pain mimicking vascular claudication in the legs. Disabling symptoms may be relieved by decompressive laminectomy, with or without fusion. Patients with the characteristic radicular pain from a herniated lumbar or cervical disk may benefit from laminectomy. However, most patients with symptomatic degenerative joint disease, with or without stenosis or disk herniation, have a mechanical component to their pain pattern. Spinal surgery is most successful in relieving radicular, not mechanical symptoms; the latter may be worsened by ill-advised surgery [27].

Plain roentgenography is part of the initial evaluation. Patients with symptoms suggestive of spinal stenosis should have computed tomographic (CT) confirmation to identify the bony overgrowth of the canal. Herniated disks are better seen on magnetic resonance imaging (MRI). Radionuclide studies have little place in the evaluation of degenerative joint disease of the spine, because they will be abnormal if the plain films are abnormal. In general, CT scans are useful for identifying the three-dimensional bony anatomy, particularly of the axial skeleton, whereas MRI is more useful for

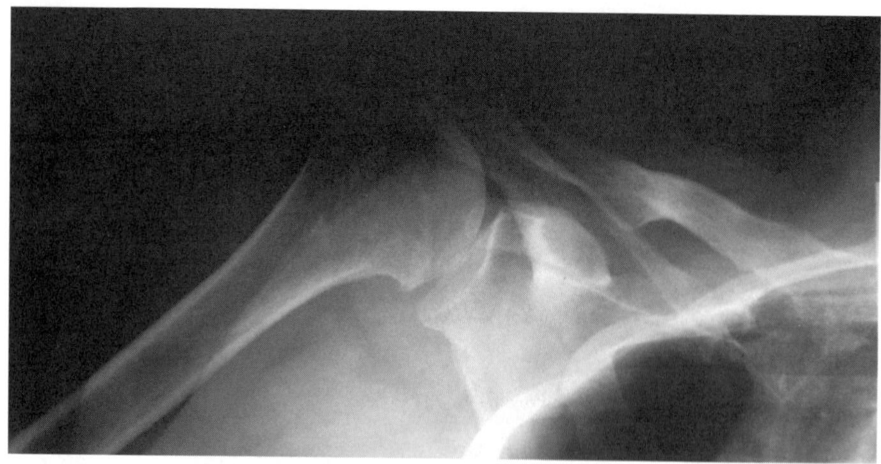

FIG. 30-2. Anteroposterior view of the shoulder of a 73-year-old woman with a chronic rotator cuff tear and shoulder pain that interfered with her golf game. The head of the humerus is displaced proximally, almost abutting the inferior border of the acromion. This patient was helped by an exercise program and continued to play golf.

identifying soft-tissue anatomy. Certain intramedullary lesions and even occult fractures can also be seen best with the MRI. Radionuclide bone scans are most useful for identifying lesions when the plain films are normal, and for identifying occult lesions as part of the evaluation for malignant disease of the skeleton. The latter is discussed elsewhere in this chapter.

RECREATIONAL INJURIES

Elderly people are often quite active; tennis, golf, jogging, and other competitive sports are played vigorously by an increasingly older patient population. Underlying degenerative joint disease or tendinitis may be present. Knee and shoulder symptoms may be superimposed on preexisting degenerative joint disease. Jogging may exacerbate underlying arthritis of the spine. Although an elderly person's recreational activity may sometimes have to be tailored to a preexisting condition, most patients can and should be treated to resume their recreational activity.

Shoulder injuries may be noted in golfers and tennis players. Underlying rotator cuff degeneration with or without tears is commonly present. Often, there is preexisting deformity of the acromion, and the disease process results from pressure of the overlying acromion against the rotator cuff. Patients characteristically complain of pain on overhead motion. Roentgenography may show a high-riding humeral head, indicative of rotator cuff tear (Fig. 30-2). Some patients benefit from arthroscopic debridement and repair. Rotator cuff repair, whether done arthroscopically or as an open procedure, requires a major rehabilitation effort. Patients unable or unwilling to undergo rehabilitation should not have the repair. For some of those patients, arthroscopic debridement alone, with its low morbidity, is satisfactory treatment [28].

Tendon ruptures may involve the biceps brachia, Achilles tendon, or gastrocnemius. Ruptures of the long head of the biceps brachia proximally usually are not treated, because the brachialis muscle can compensate. Surgical repair is only for cosmetic reasons; the distal stump of the biceps tendon is sutured into the intertubercular groove of the humerus, eliminating an unsightly mass on the flexor surface of the arm, but adding no strength to the biceps. Distal avulsions of the biceps from the proximal radius require repair to restore supination. Achilles tendon ruptures occur from sudden jumps, classically in tennis players. Surgical repair, except in a very elderly, minimally ambulatory patient, is recommended. Tears of the proximal gastrocnemius muscle may be dramatic: The patient feels and hears a snap, the calf swells, and ambulation is difficult. This condition, previously thought to be due to rupture of the plantaris muscle, now has been shown to be of the heads of the gastrocnemius. This condition heals spontaneously, requiring only protected weight bearing and reassurance. It may be confused with acute phlebitis, but a careful history can identify the correct diagnosis.

Knee injuries in the elderly may include meniscus tears, but often are superimposed on degenerative joint disease. Major ligament injuries are rare in elderly people. Loose bodies from prior injuries may cause mechanical locking. Evaluation may require diagnostic arthroscopy for definitive diagnosis. MRI evaluation of the elderly knee may be confusing; most patients >60 have MRI abnormalities of the menisci. Arthroscopic surgery is successful only when a surgically correctable lesion such as a bucket-handle or flap tear of a meniscus or a loose body is found. Rehabilitation in the form of range-of-motion and strengthening exercises is critical after knee injuries or surgery. The final result may be more dependent on the patient and the rehabilitation than on the surgeon.

FRACTURES

Fractures represent the major form of trauma in the elderly. The usual cause is a fall, but spontaneous fractures of the spine or femoral neck can occur in osteoporotic patients or those with skeletal malignancies. Patients usually fall in their own homes; they may trip on a rug or a cord, not see a wet spot on the floor, or become temporarily disori-

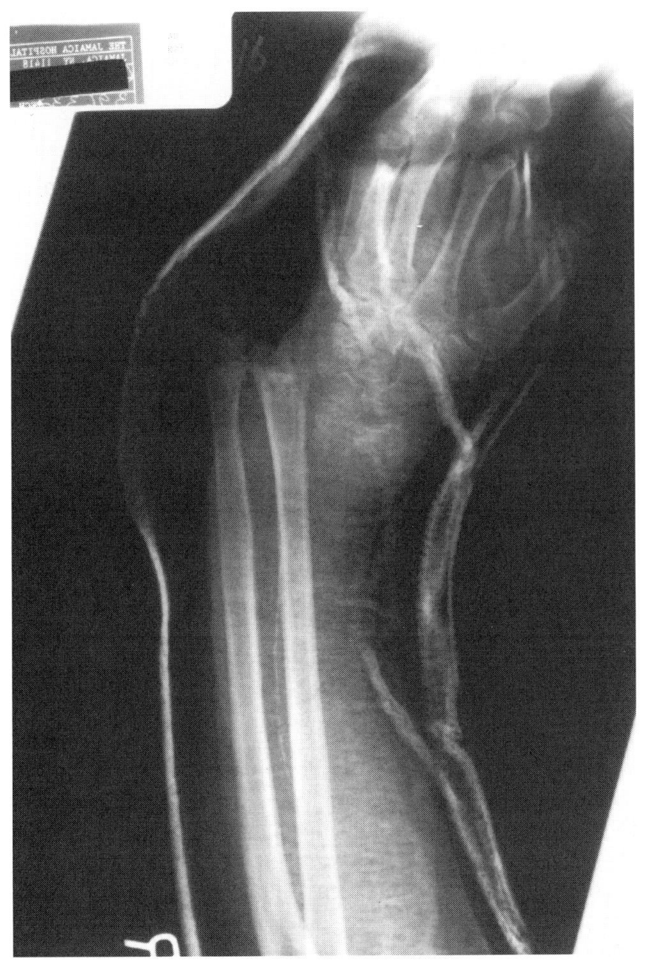

A

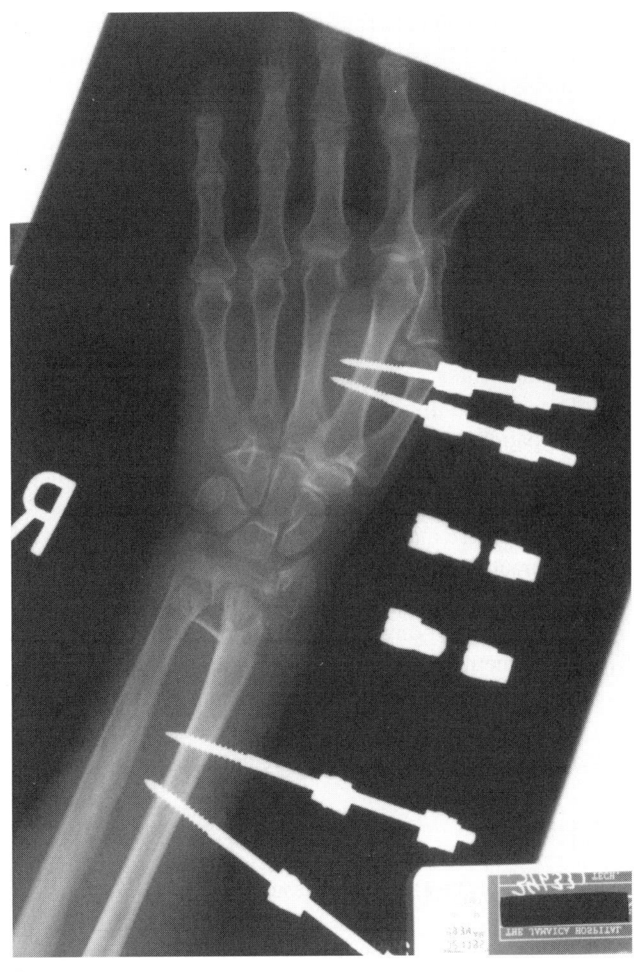

B

FIG. 30-3. Emergency department **(A)** and postoperative **(B)** roentgenograms of an 80-year-old woman who fell and sustained an open, severely displaced Colles' fracture of the distal radius. Note the almost complete dissociation of the distal radius. This was managed with debridement and an external fixator, with union of the fracture and a satisfactory result.

ented. Outdoors, patients may slip on ice or broken pavement, be hit by cars, assaulted, or tripped by their own pets. Elderly people can have auto accidents or fall while getting on or off buses. Injuries that would be trivial in a younger person may cause a major fracture in an older one [7,29].

This section considers the more common fractures seen in the elderly, with the exception of hip fractures, which are discussed in a subsequent section.

Fractures of the Wrist

These are the most common fractures seen in elderly people and occur from that most common of all mechanisms of fracture—a fall onto the outstretched hand. The Colles' fracture of the distal radius, described in 1814, is actually a spectrum of injuries, from an impacted, nondisplaced fracture of the distal radius to a comminuted, dorsally displaced fracture with an open wound, exposed ulnar styloid, and median or ulnar nerve injury (Fig. 30-3). Identification is usually not difficult; a characteristic "silver fork" deformity with shortening of the radial side of the wrist and hand and dorsal displacement is seen. These fractures can usually be readily reduced by closed manipulation under local or block anesthesia and casting, but frequently lose position due to compression of the porotic bone and comminution of the articular surface. Union of this fracture occurs readily, regardless of the form of treatment, and the end result is a reasonably functioning, although deformed wrist.

Attempts to restore and maintain normal alignment and allow early motion of wrist and more importantly the fingers have led to many different techniques over the years. The importance of restoring articular alignment and radial length has been emphasized, primarily in younger patients. External and internal fixation techniques and combinations of both have been described. Some currently available external fixators allow wrist motion while still in place. External fixation has the advantage of restoring and maintaining radial length without a cast. However, the distraction necessary to maintain reduction may cause stiffness, the pins may loosen or become superficially infected, and the entire apparatus is unsightly and often frightening to the patient. Internal fixation alone is rarely used in the elderly [30,31]. Regardless of treatment, some residual disability, stiffness, or deformity is inevitable following fractures about the wrist.

This author's preference is to manipulate the fracture closed and, if acceptable reduction is achieved, follow the patient closely as an outpatient. If significant slippage occurs in the first week, the fracture is remanipulated under anesthesia and a fixator is applied with two pins in the second and third metacarpals and two pins at the junction of the middle and distal third of the radius. The fixator is removed as an outpatient procedure at 6 weeks and vigorous exercises are begun. Open fractures, fractures with nerve involvement, and fractures with massive swelling that precludes the use of a circular cast are managed with a fixator primarily.

Other fractures of the wrist are managed similarly. Dislocations of the carpal bones must be recognized and reduced by open methods if anatomic reduction cannot be achieved by closed methods. Median and ulnar nerve injuries can exist with fractures of the wrist. Most of these resolve after reduction of the fracture, although carpal tunnel release may be necessary for some median nerve entrapment syndromes.

Fractures of the Elbow

Fractures of the elbow also result from a fall, usually on the outstretched hand. Radial head fractures may, if minimally displaced, be managed by sling and early motion. Supracondylar fractures may be extensively comminuted and may not be amenable to surgical fixation, so that splinting and encouragement to begin early motion are the best treatments. Despite severe deformity, very elderly patients may get useful function after this injury. In younger, healthier patients with reasonably good bone stock, good results may be expected from open reduction and internal fixation with a construct of dual plates and screws. This is a formidable procedure, requiring considerable experience as well as special equipment. Fractures of the olecranon can usually be treated by internal fixation, although comminuted fractures may be excised and the triceps tendon repaired to the proximal ulna, with good reported results [32].

Fractures of the Humerus

These fractures unite readily and can usually be managed nonoperatively as long as a patient can be ambulatory. The weight of the upper extremity acts as traction, allowing reasonable alignment. A sling and swathe, sling and cuff, hanging arm cast, and coaptation plaster splints are all used to manage these fractures. Wide displacement and angulation may be compatible with good function. Surgical fixation is generally reserved for open fractures, fractures in multiply injured people, or those who cannot be ambulatory. A few proximal fractures cannot be aligned by closed means and require fixation. Plates have been the mainstay of surgical treatment of humeral fractures, but newer intramedullary devices may have advantages in allowing insertion by a closed technique, minimizing surgical risks, and facilitating union. Nerve injuries, usually radial, may occur with fractures at the junction of the middle and distal thirds of the humerus. These are almost always neuropraxias and recover spontaneously. Surgical intervention is only indicated for nerve injuries when the injury occurs after or during closed treatment.

Fractures and Dislocations of the Shoulder

Fractures of the proximal humerus may be impacted or displaced. Impacted fractures usually do not displace, unite readily, and may be managed with a sling and early motion. Even widely displaced fractures about the shoulder may unite and result in good function. Most fractures that do not involve the anatomic neck unite readily. They can be managed with a sling and early pendulum exercises, with the expectation of a satisfactory result. Open reduction and internal fixation of proximal humerus fractures is difficult and may be precarious in severely demineralized bone.

The most severe shoulder injuries are fracture dislocations and those in which the articular surface is broken off at the anatomic neck. The articular fragment then is avascular and will not unite. These injuries are best treated with prosthetic hemiarthroplasty and early motion. Although a pain-free shoulder usually results, some residual stiffness remains [33,34].

Fractures that do not involve the articular surface, where the head is broken off at the surgical neck, may rotate into an unacceptable position. These can sometimes be managed by closed reduction and percutaneous pin fixation from the shaft into the head. The pins are then removed after 4 to 6 weeks and motion started. The rarely performed formal open reduction of a proximal humerus fracture usually requires a complex construct of plates, screws, or tension band wires. If fixation is sufficiently firm, early motion is begun.

Dislocations of the shoulder, without major fracture, can occur in elderly people. Usually they result from a fall, but may be seen following assault. The incidence of nerve injuries is higher in this group of patients. The axillary and median nerves are the most commonly involved. Careful initial examination to document nerve injury is mandatory.

Roentgenography for all shoulder injuries should include anteroposterior, trans-scapular (Y view), and axillary views. A posterior dislocation of the head may be missed in a complex four-part fracture if adequate roentgenographs are not obtained. Dislocations should be reduced promptly after roentgenograph is obtained. Prolonged immobilization is not necessary after dislocations; recurrence is rare in the elderly, and late stiffness is the major concern. As union occurs, serial roentgenography may show progressive distal subluxation of the humeral head, which is usually due to relaxation of the ligamentous structures and corrects itself with exercises.

Fractures of the Pelvis

Fractures of the pelvis in the elderly fall into two categories: high energy and low energy. High-energy injuries occur from automobile accidents and follow a pattern seen in younger patients. Major pelvic disruptions in the elderly usually accompany other injuries and are often fatal. These injuries are discussed in Chapter 33.

Displaced pelvic fractures may involve the acetabulum. The techniques used in younger patients for open reduction and fixation of these complex injuries may not be applicable due to porotic bone or associated injuries. These patients are often better managed by early mobilization and late total hip reconstruction.

Low-energy injuries usually result from a fall and tend to be lateral compression injuries. The pelvis, even in an elderly patient, possesses considerable elastic recoil, so that a buckling type fracture occurs in one or more pubic rami. The patient may complain of pain in the hip and groin and must also be evaluated for occult femoral neck fracture. Associated impaction fractures of the sacral ala may be present but not visible on anteroposterior roentgenography. Roentgenography should include inlet and outlet views to identify a possible sacral fracture, and if plain anteroposterior films show a possible fracture into the acetabulum, obturator oblique views should also be obtained. Most low-energy pelvic fractures are stable and are managed with early ambulation weight bearing as tolerated with a walker or cane. The presence of a sacral or acetabular fracture prolongs a patient's convalescence and rehabilitation. Prophylactic anticoagulation, using a protocol similar to that for arthroplasty, is often used as an adjunct in managing patients with pelvic fractures, particularly if there is a delay in mobilization.

Fractures of the Femur

Fractures of the femur may, like fractures of the pelvis, occur from high- or low-energy injuries. Management of femur fractures in the elderly is no different than in younger people, that is, internal fixation to allow mobilization. Available internal fixation devices now allow a wide spectrum of femur fractures to be treated surgically. Closed intramedullary nailing with proximal and distal interlocking is the procedure of choice for most fractures of the femoral shaft. Subtrochanteric and supracondylar fractures can also be managed with intramedullary nailing.

Intramedullary nailing of femur fractures in the elderly usually requires proximal and distal interlocking and is not sufficiently rigid to allow early weight bearing [35]. However, the rapidity of union with this technique is such that most patients can bear weight after 6 weeks. This procedure, even carried out closed, may be accompanied by significant blood loss from the medullary canal. Fat and thromboembolic phenomena and pulmonary, cardiac, and urinary tract complications can all occur. Studies have implicated intramedullary fat as a potential complication of reaming femoral fractures [36]. Comparisons of results for reamed and nonreamed nails are ongoing at several major centers, and preliminary reports seem to indicate that nonreamed, interlocked nails may be as effective as reamed nails and may have a lower incidence of postoperative pulmonary complications. However, at present, reamed, locked intramedullary nails are the gold standard for the treatment of the vast majority of fractures of the femoral shaft, particularly in the elderly (Fig. 30-4).

Plate fixation of femoral fractures may be indicated when intramedullary nailing is impossible due to preexisting joint replacement components about the knee or hip. Fractures may occur around or beyond implants. The management of these periprosthetic fractures is often complex. Fractures that occur through an implant usually result in loosening of that implant, so that fracture repair must include revision and replacement of the implant. Fractures occurring below an implant frequently do not disturb the implant, and the fracture can be managed without exchanging the implant.

Fractures and Dislocations of the Knee

Dislocations and major ligament injuries of the knee are rare in the elderly. The ligamentous structures are stronger than the underlying bone, and the usual patterns of injury are different than in younger patients. Knee injuries in the elderly commonly follow a fall, usually onto the flexed knee, whereas in younger people they occur more commonly from twisting or contact. Fractures may occur through the patella, supracondylar region of the femur, or tibial plateau(s).

The management of these fractures is to restore function. Nondisplaced patellar fractures are managed with immobilization and weight bearing. Displaced supracondylar and plateau fractures, in an otherwise healthy ambulator, are managed with open reduction and internal fixation. Constructs of plates and screws, sometimes with bone grafts, are used for both of these fractures. Indirect reduction of supracondylar fractures, where the plate is fixated to the major fragments and the comminuted segments are not dissected free and anatomically reduced, but spanned so that their blood supply attachments are left intact, results in less surgical morbidity and more rapid union than older techniques of anatomic reduction of all fragments [37]. Closed intramedullary nails introduced retrograde through the intercondylar notch have been described for managing supracondylar fractures in the elderly. This technique avoids extensive incisions and blood loss and often allows rapid union [38]. Postoperative continuous passive motion machines may be used in fractures of the knee if fixation has been firm enough to allow early motion.

Regardless of the treatment, fractures of the knee usually require 3 months of non–weight bearing until union. This may predispose the elderly patient to contractures and a

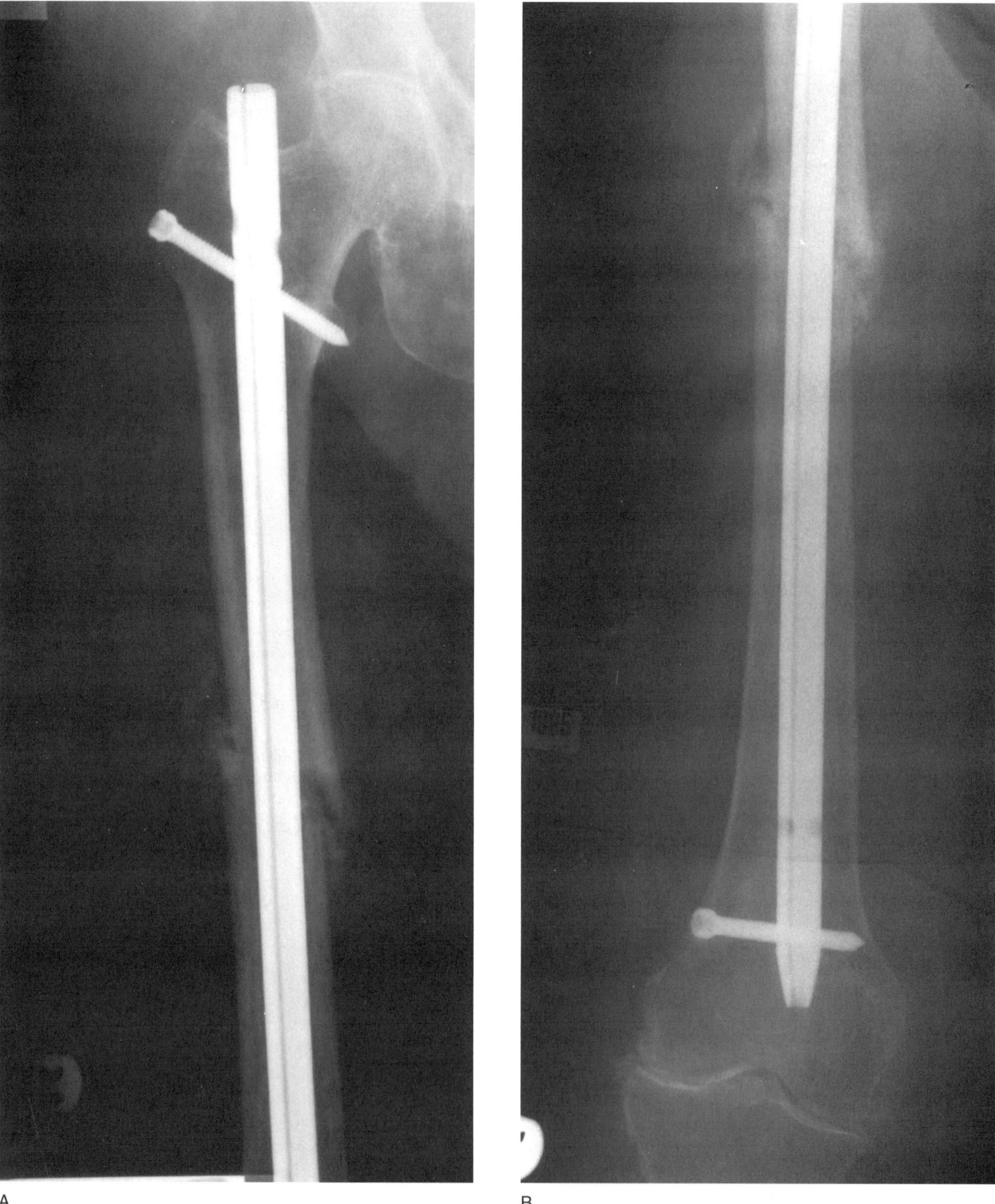

A B

FIG. 30-4. An 85-year-old woman fell at home, sustaining this femoral shaft fracture. It was treated with a closed, reamed, intramedullary nail, with proximal **(A)** and distal **(B)** locking. These radiographs made 6 weeks postoperatively show early callus, at which time she was allowed weight bearing. The fracture united.

slow rehabilitation period before the patient can resume his or her life-style.

Fractures of the knee also occur in very elderly, nonambulatory nursing home patients after trivial trauma. These should be managed simply, with a well-padded knee immobilizer and passive transfer activities, with the expectation that early union will occur in 6 weeks [35]. The rare open supracondylar fracture in a dependent, nonambulatory patient with porotic bone and poor tissue is best managed by primary amputation.

Fractures of the Tibia

These are relatively uncommon in the elderly, resulting from a severe fall or being hit by a car. The principles of management are the same as for any other weight-bearing bone fracture. Nondisplaced or minimally displaced fractures are managed in a well-padded cast and early weight bearing. More complex fractures require fixation. Surgical treatment must be carried out with great care. The skin over the elderly tibia is particularly fragile; wound complications can be catastrophic. Closed nailing in the tibia is the treatment of choice for most fractures that require internal fixation. Nail fixation is not always secure enough to preclude casting, but often is the best way to mobilize a patient and ensure a well-functioning extremity.

Plates have a limited role in tibial fractures in the elderly. They are mostly used in patients with preexisting knee replacements where intramedullary nails cannot be inserted or in complex fractures too proximal or distal to be stabilized adequately with a nail. Long bone plating requires non–weight bearing until complete union occurs, usually in 3 to 4 months. The porotic bone of the elderly patient does not support external fixators well, and mangling grade III open fractures, particularly if part of a polytrauma pattern, should be treated by primary amputation and early prosthetic fitting [39].

Fractures of the Ankle and Foot

Twisting injuries from falls and crush injuries are the major causes of fractures to the ankle and foot in the elderly. As in the knee, sprains and ligament injuries are relatively uncommon in this age group. Whereas in younger patients, open reduction and internal fixation is the preferred treatment for virtually any displaced fracture of the ankle, controversy exists about the wisdom of such treatment in the elderly. The porotic bone and fragile skin about the ankle may prevent firm fixation and result in skin slough. Closed treatment in a cast may achieve an adequate, although not anatomic reduction, with a satisfactory result without the risk of surgical complications [40]. However, reduction of an unstable fracture can be difficult to maintain in a cast; nonunion may result, and skin complications secondary to the cast can occur. External fixation may be successful for some fractures, but there is a high incidence of pin tract problems and loosening.

Widely displaced fractures and fracture dislocations may be open, often extensive wounds. The skin is usually torn or avulsed rather than lacerated, often having more severe underlying injury than is immediately apparent. Open ankle fractures require prompt surgery: irrigation, debridement, and reduction.

I prefer internal fixation using standard techniques, and immobilization with a lightweight cast for 6 weeks for displaced, unstable ankle fractures, open or closed, in elderly patients. The lateral malleolus is fixated with a posteriorly placed antiglide plate to allow for bicortical screw fixation, and the medial malleolus is fixated with one or two screws. With careful attention to skin and good fixation, results of treatment of ankle fractures in the elderly should approach the success of results seen in younger patients.

Fractures of the foot usually result from a direct blow or crush injury. These fractures may be massively swollen or so occult as to be overlooked. Good quality roentgenography usually demonstrates foot fractures. Minimally displaced fractures can be managed with minimal immobilization and weight bearing as tolerated; more displaced fractures may require fixation. Open fractures of the toes, often from lawnmower injuries, are best managed by primary amputation. Fractures of the calcaneus usually do not lend themselves to the surgical techniques advocated for younger patients, and are usually treated closed.

Foot injuries are sometimes overlooked, particularly in the presence of a more dramatic injury. Any swelling in a foot following trauma should prompt suspicion of a fracture and should be investigated.

Pathologic Fractures

Malignancies, either primary or metastatic, may weaken bone to the point at which pathologic fracture occurs. Multiple myeloma is the most common primary malignancy of bone. It may present as a solitary lytic area with no systemic signs or symptoms or as disseminated disease with the characteristic blood abnormalities. Carcinomas of the breast, lung, and prostate are the most common metastatic lesions to bone. Kidney, thyroid, and colon carcinomas are less common. Metastatic lesions of bone may be occult, but usually the patient has a history of dull, aching pain, along with systemic signs and symptoms of weight loss and anemia. Fractures may occur spontaneously or after trivial trauma. Metastatic disease characteristically involves the spine, pelvis, femur, and humerus. Metastatic involvement distal to the knee or elbow is rare.

Extensive workup to identify a primary cancer is often deferred until a fracture is stabilized. Preliminary workup need only identify other occult lesions that might interfere with fixation or anesthesia. The fracture itself may be managed with closed nailing and not be entered unless a tissue diagnosis has not been established or debulking the lesion is thought useful. Pathologic lesions may be vascular, particularly those from renal cell carcinomas, or they may be relatively avascular. Methacrylate cement is used as a filler where bone has been eroded, and as an adjunct to fixation with metal devices. Postoperatively, patients are mobilized rapidly, and any treatment indicated for the primary lesion is begun [41].

Vertebral body fractures and fractures about the hip and femur are the most common. Pathologic fractures tend to be inordinately painful and may prevent mobilization. Metastatic carcinomas tend to be radioresistant and unresponsive to chemotherapy. For these reasons pathologic fractures, except in terminal patients or where the bone is too extensively involved to support any kind of fixation, should be surgically stabilized. Modifications of standard fixation techniques, augmented with methacrylate cement, are usually used. The goal is to stabilize the fracture so that the patient can be mobilized pain free. Pathologic fracture implies progressive disease. Patients have a limited life span, and fracture union is not necessarily a goal of treatment. Union may nonetheless occur, even if postoperative radiation or chemotherapy is used.

Impending pathologic fractures can be identified about the femur and hip; involvement of the medial cortex, >one-third of the diameter of the shaft, and the subtrochanteric area all suggest the femur is at risk. Prophylactic fixation of these lesions is indicated, because ultimate fracture, if untreated, is inevitable.

Lesions of the femoral head or neck are treated by hemiarthroplasty, sometimes with a long-stem component, and cement augmentation. Lesions of the proximal femur may be treated with intramedullary nailing. Fixation into the head (Recon Nail, Smith & Nephew, Inc., Memphis, TN) is used with proximal lesions; more distal ones can be managed with standard interlocking nails. Impending or actual pathologic fractures of the humerus may be either managed with plates and cement or with interlocking humeral nails.

As with many other orthopedic surgical procedures, the natural course of the tumor is not altered by stabilizing a pathologic fracture. The precise temporal course of a patient with metastatic carcinoma may be unpredictable, although some reports indicated that a lesion of the proximal femur, particularly if from lung or breast, indicated an approaching terminal state [42]. Patients can usually be made pain free, often for several months, and returned to their homes. Aggressive surgical management of patients with metastatic disease to the skeleton is often the more conservative approach [43].

Multiple myeloma is often highly radiosensitive. Small lesions may not need surgical treatment, but larger lesions should be stabilized. Primary musculoskeletal tumors, although rare, occur in this age group. Many can be treated successfully with radical limb-sparing resections. These tumors should be managed by experienced surgeons in specialized centers. Chapter 6 discusses soft-tissue primary tumors.

Open Fractures

Open fractures in elderly patients often occur from less violent trauma than in younger patients. The principles of management are the same, however. Prompt wound debridement, fracture stabilization, and delayed closure or coverage are the treatment standards. Volume resuscitation must be carefully monitored in the elderly. Antibiotics are used until the wound is closed or covered. External fixation may be used in comminuted fractures, and bone grafting may be necessary. Elderly people do not tolerate multiple trips to the operating room or prolonged recumbency. Definitive surgical management must be concluded promptly. Severe open fractures about the lower leg, ankle, or foot may be best managed by early amputation and prosthetic fitting. Elderly patients can handle well-fit below-the-knee prostheses very well [42].

Fractures of the Hip

The term *hip fracture* includes fractures of the proximal femur, which are divided into intracapsular (femoral neck) and extracapsular (intertrochanteric or subtrochanteric) fractures. Dislocations and fracture dislocations of the hip or acetabulum are rare; nondisplaced acetabular fractures may accompany a fracture of the pelvis from a fall.

Fractures about the hip constitute the most important group of fractures in the elderly. The definitive management differs for intracapsular and extracapsular fractures, but there are several factors common to all. The usual mechanism of hip fracture in the elderly is a fall. Elderly patients usually fall in their own home, but may be injured in many different ways, indoors or outdoors. Elderly people tend to stay indoors during bad weather; falls on ice and snow are relatively uncommon. Scatter rugs, wet or slick floors, objects on the floor may not be seen by someone with impaired vision. People may be struck by cars, miss a curb, be victims of assault, or be tangled in the leash of their pet dog [7]. Those who drive may be involved in vehicular accidents. The patient with a hip fracture almost always cannot walk after the injury; people who live alone may wait for many hours before help comes.

A hip fracture is a potentially life-threatening situation in an elderly patient. The fracture cannot be adequately splinted, and the patient cannot be mobilized; in fact, any motion is painful. The goal of treatment of all hip fractures is rapid patient mobilization, and this can rarely be accomplished without surgical stabilization. A few impacted fractures, those that occur in terminally ill patients, or those in demented, nonambulatory patients with impaired pain sensation may be treated nonoperatively [44]. Acute myocardial infarction, pulmonary edema, and decubitus in the proposed surgical site may preclude surgical treatment. With those exceptions, patients with fractures about the hip should be treated surgically.

Hip fractures are becoming a problem in the very elderly as the American population ages. At this author's institution and the Geriatric Rehabilitation Center, Parker Jewish Geriatric Institute, New Hyde Park, NY, the average age of hip fracture patients is 82. Ninety-five percent are women, and 80% are independent-community ambulators. My oldest hip fracture patient was 104 years old. The potential costs of this injury to society cannot be calculated accurately, but run into billions of dollars annually.

Medical illnesses commonly found in this age group must be identified. Medical optimization of a patient can usually be accomplished within 24 hours, and surgery should proceed promptly. There is controversy regarding the ideal timing. Statistics indicate that the longer an elderly patient with a hip fracture waits for surgery, the higher the complication rate. This may be a function of intercurrent illness: Sicker patients take longer to be medically optimized. A hip fracture may be part of a progressive, inexorable medical decline, which cannot be identified as such preoperatively. Ideally, patients should be operated on within 24 hours of injury [45].

Most hip fracture repair is carried out under general or spinal or epidural anesthesia. Local or regional anesthesia is rarely satisfactory for hip fracture surgery. No anesthetic technique is ideal; there are advantages and disadvantages to each type. Most hospital anesthesia departments have a preference for one over the other, and the choice should be left in the anesthesiologist's hands. Anesthetic considerations in the elderly are more fully discussed in Chapter 5.

Postoperative mobilization is critical. Surgical stabilization should be sufficiently firm to allow chair mobilization, and ideally, prompt ambulation with weight bearing as tolerated. Pulmonary, urologic, skin, and psychiatric complications are minimized with early mobilization. Postoperative hemoglobin must be maintained; fracture and surgical blood loss may be more than initially calculated.

Thromboembolic complications occur in hip fracture patients as they do in elective arthroplasty patients. Some studies indicate that the thrombus forms at the time of injury and is already present at the time of surgery. The best mechanism of prophylaxis for thromboembolic complications in patients with hip fractures remains controversial. Lower-extremity venous thrombi arising from clinically silent foci are common in patients with hip fractures. Thromboembolic phenomena are a leading cause of postoperative death. Thigh and pelvic thrombi are more dangerous than calf thrombi. Most authors recommend a protocol combining pharmacologic and mechanical prophylaxis, similar to the protocols used for patients undergoing elective arthroplasty. However, patients with hip fractures tend to be older and more fragile than elective arthroplasty patients. Complications from anticoagulation include idiosyncratic reactions to warfarin, intraoperative bleeding from large fracture surfaces, wound hematoma, and systemic bleeding, which are more common in the hip fracture patient [22,46]. Anticoagulation must be carefully monitored. Our current protocol is to begin warfarin the night of surgery and follow the same protocol as for elective arthroplasty. Patients may continue to shower emboli even while anticoagulated. Those patients, and those who are at high risk for thromboembolic complications but cannot be anticoagulated, should be considered for a vena cava filter. Lovenox has not yet been shown to be effective in hip fracture patients in a controlled study. I use warfarin anticoagulation prophylaxis on all patients with hip fracture unless there is a specific contraindication.

Patients with acute fractures about the hip present with a characteristic clinical picture. There is a history of a fall and subsequent inability to move. There may be a history of a transient syncope, or the patient may tell you that he or she tripped on a rug. The involved lower extremity is shortened, externally rotated, and does not move actively. Any passive motion is painful. Neurovascular complications are rare with hip fracture patients, but underlying peripheral vascular disease may be present and can be identified without undue discomfort. Roentgenography in two planes may be necessary, and the diagnosis is usually made radiologically, ideally with roentgenography in two planes. Chest roentgenography, electrocardiographic studies, chemistry checks, and evaluations of preexisting illness are all performed.

A frank, positive discussion with the patient and family is in order. A patient with a hip fracture is expected to recover. Early involvement with social service and discharge planning should be started promptly. Once the fracture has been identified, plans can be made for treatment, which is carried out as soon as the patient is medically optimized.

Femoral Neck Fractures

Femoral neck fractures may result from a fall or from a sudden twisting injury. A patient may say that he or she turned suddenly, felt a snap in the hip, and then fell. The fracture is usually oblique rather than transverse, implying a rotary, rather than direct blow injury. Because these are intracapsular fractures, bleeding is minimal, and there may not be much shortening. These patients are reported to be younger than those with intertrochanteric fractures, but in this author's experience, hip fracture patients are the same age, regardless of the type of fracture.

A femoral neck fracture may not be displaced, but impacted as a result of a direct blow, or it may be occult. A patient has a history of a fall and is able to walk subsequently but with hip and groin pain with each step. The hip may not be shortened, and the patient may have active control. Careful physical examination and roentgenographic evaluation is necessary. Pain on passive internal and external rotation of the hip is a clue. A fracture line may be subtle and only seen on properly positioned anteroposterior roentgenography. MRI has been demonstrated to be the most sensitive, specific indicator of occult femoral neck fracture, and this should be carried out if there is still doubt about the diagnosis [47]. A patient may give a history of a fall 1 or 2 weeks previously, with residual pain in the groin, but not enough to prevent ambulation. The patient may have been evaluated in a hospital emergency department, where roentgenography was done, and no fracture was identified. Subsequently, a trivial incident may result in sudden collapse of the hip. Roentgenography now shows a displaced femoral neck fracture, often just below the head (subcapital). If the initial roentgenography films are now reviewed, the fracture either can be seen retrospectively or the roentgenography noted to be inadequate. Untreated impacted or occult

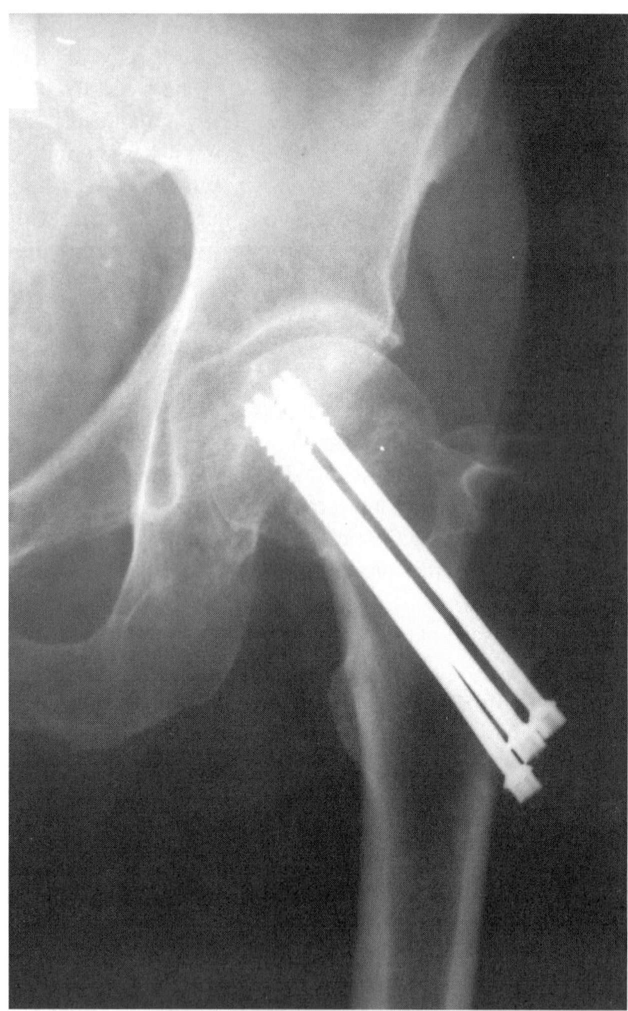

FIG. 30-5. A 78-year-old woman fell and sustained this impacted fracture of the femoral neck, which was managed with cannulated screws. Full weight bearing was allowed, and the fracture united after 4 months.

femoral neck fractures are likely to displace within 3 weeks of the initial injury.

Impacted or nondisplaced femoral neck fractures are commonly treated with in situ pin fixation. Current recommendations are for three parallel pins, placed under roentgenographic control, up the femoral neck into the subchondral bone of the head. This procedure results in little blood loss and minimal surgical morbidity, but does require a specialized fracture table, an operating room image intensification unit, and an experienced technician (Fig. 30-5).

The displaced femoral neck fracture is still the unsolved fracture. Internal fixation after manipulative reduction in the elderly may be precarious and fail. Good results in experienced hands with internal fixation in elderly, but not very elderly, patients have been shown [48]. In addition to minimal surgical morbidity, internal fixation has the advantage of maintaining the patient's own femoral head, resulting in a hip that is closer to normal. Nonetheless, major complications associated with attempted internal fixation, such as failure of fixation, deformity, prolonged non–weight bearing, reoperation, and avascular necrosis of the femoral head have led to widespread use of head resection and prosthetic hemiarthroplasty in elderly patients with femoral neck fractures. This technique is a relatively straightforward surgical procedure. It uses a regular operating room table. The hip joint capsule is opened posteriorly, the head extracted, and the implant fitted into place and driven down the femoral shaft. The construct is then reduced, tested for stability, and the wound closed. This is a more extensive procedure than closed reduction and pinning, but proceeds along relatively avascular planes; transfusion is rarely necessary. Primary hemiarthroplasty in an otherwise normal hip with a freshly displaced femoral neck fracture has been the most widely used procedure for more than 40 years.

Different implants are available for this operation. The intramedullary one-piece prosthesis as described by Moore in 1953 is still widely used. Concerns about acetabular erosion and stem loosening with this implant have led to the development of newer devices. The bipolar prosthesis features an anatomically designed stem as used in total hip replacements and a double-bearing articular surface in the form of a metal-backed polyethylene shell that articulates with the acetabulum and the prosthetic femoral head (Fig. 30-6). These may be cemented into the femur and require a slightly longer operating room time. Another unipolar concept uses a separate head and neck piece that is assembled onto the stem before reduction. This allows more precise tailoring of the components to the individual patient. There is some controversy as to whether the bipolar prosthesis really articulates at both femoral and acetabular surfaces, whether all the motion is between the acetabular component and the acetabulum so that the implant functions as a unipolar hemiarthroplasty, or whether all the motion is between the acetabular and femoral components and the device acts as a total hip [49].

There is as yet no study showing the superiority of one implant over the other in terms of longevity in the elderly patient. The surgical technique and postoperative regimen are essentially the same for all hemiarthroplasty patients. The cemented bipolar prosthesis, however, costs approximately three times as much as a unipolar implant.

Hemiarthroplasty is only satisfactory in the absence of preexisting hip disease. A patient with preexisting arthritis and a femoral neck fracture or a patient with failed internal fixation should have a primary total hip replacement.

Postoperatively, the regimen is essentially the same regardless of the implant used. The patient is mobilized rapidly, bearing full weight as tolerated. Patients have remarkably little pain, and their convalescence is usually rapid. Complications include iatrogenic fracture of the shaft or greater trochanter while inserting the implant, sciatic nerve injury, and postoperative dislocation. A patient who has had a hemiarthroplasty must follow the same precautions as a patient who has had a total hip replacement and must avoid bending beyond 90 degrees, excessive internal rotation, and adduction of the hip.

This operation should result in a strong, stable, painless but not normal hip. As with any implant in the body, over a period of time failure can occur, in the form of loosening, erosion, protrusion, with resulting pain and instability. The exact durability of any implant cannot be predicted, but is entirely satisfactory for an elderly patient with minimal functional needs and a limited life span. My current practice is to use internal fixation with three cannulated screws for impacted or nondisplaced fractures regardless of the patient's age, a cemented bipolar prosthesis in healthy patients under 70, and a modular uncemented implant in all others.

Intertrochanteric Fractures

Intertrochanteric fractures are the most common fractures about the hip. They almost always result from a fall, usually onto the side. Intertrochanteric fractures are almost always displaced and may be extensively comminuted, with considerable blood loss. However, these fractures unite readily and predictably following internal fixation. Roentgenography shows the characteristic fracture pattern. The preoperative evaluation is the same as with other fractures, except that provisions should be made for either preoperative or intraoperative transfusion.

Anesthesia is induced, the patient is placed on the fracture table, and the fracture manipulated under image control. Fracture reduction, particularly restoration of length and alignment, can usually be achieved this way. Extensively comminuted fractures may not be reduced by this closed technique, and formal exposure and surgical manipulation of the fragments may be necessary. Overcorrection of shortening may occur in patients who have had spinal anesthesia, with its greater relaxation. A long lateral incision is then made, and under image control, a guidewire is introduced into the lateral femoral shaft distal to the greater trochanter and drilled up the femoral neck into the head. The pin should be parallel to the long axis of the neck and either in the center or the inferior half of the neck, and within a few millimeters of the femoral head articular surface so it engages the harder subchondral bone. Accurate placement of the roentgenography unit is necessary to ensure reliable imaging. Once proper position of the pin has been achieved (it may require two or three attempts), a cannulated compression screw is inserted over the pin and attached to a side plate, which is then fixed to the femoral shaft with screws. If the fracture is reduced and not extensively comminuted, this procedure is accomplished without ever disturbing the fracture site. The screw and plate construct is then compressed by means of a set screw, roentgenography is used to check the repair, and the wound is closed (Fig. 30-7).

Comminuted fractures, where the greater and lesser trochanters are separate pieces, cannot always be anatomically reduced. Sometimes, direct fracture manipulation allows stable reduction, but sometimes the fragments are too comminuted. Stability may be achieved by allowing the proximal and distal fracture ends to impact on each other, essentially ignoring trochanteric fragments. This technique allows enough stability for weight bearing, although the extremity may be shortened and externally rotated because of the fracture of the greater trochanter, and the patient may have a marked Trendelenburg's limp. A properly placed hip

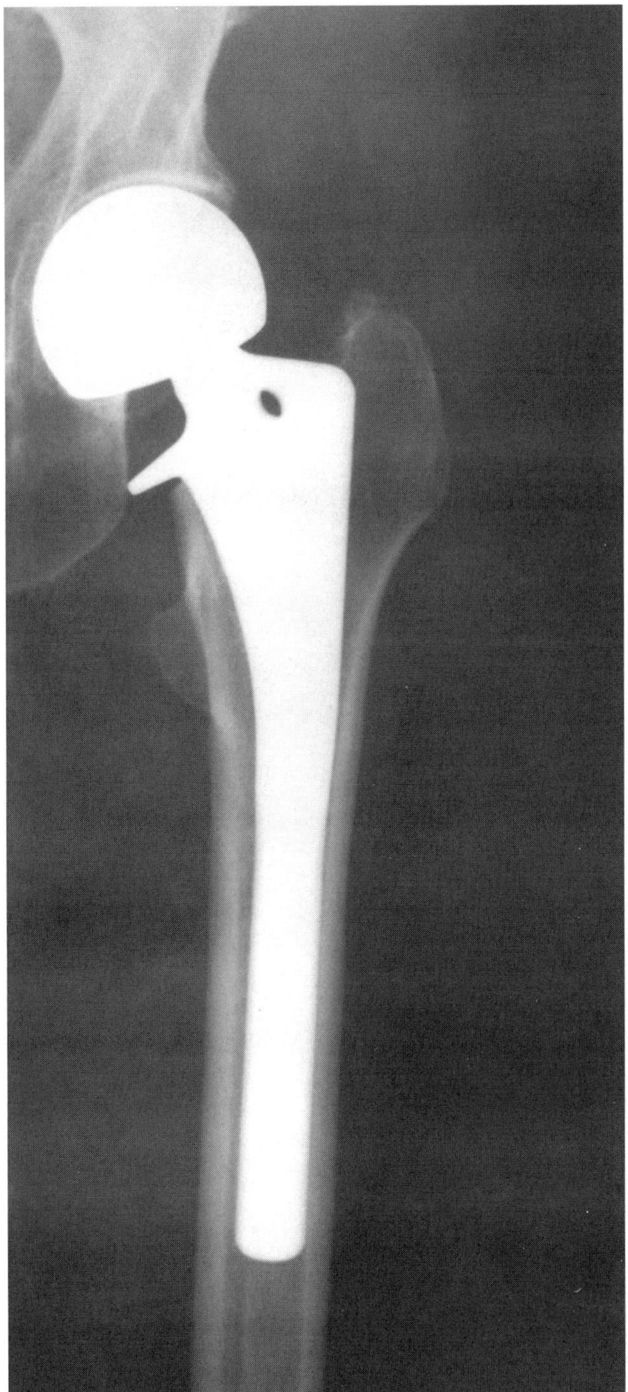

FIG. 30-6. A bipolar prosthesis was used to treat a displaced femoral neck fracture in a 68-year-old woman. This device, like other hemiarthroplasties, allows immediate weight bearing.

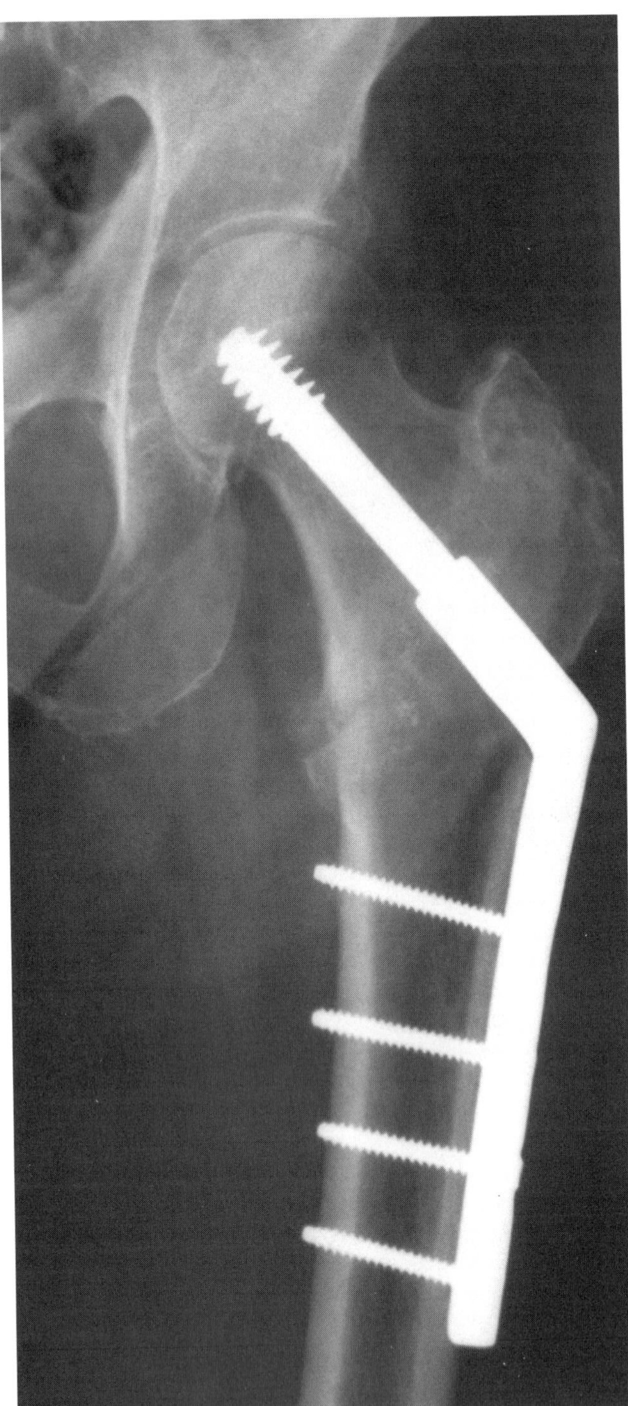

FIG. 30-7. An intertrochanteric fracture was reduced and fixated with this hip compression screw and four-hole plate in a 79-year-old man after a fall. This allowed immediate weight bearing and union in this position after 4 months.

compression screw construct allows controlled impaction and union, so that formal medial displacement osteotomy, described before the introduction of the hip compression screw, is often unnecessary [50]. Another technique to improve stability is to fixate the fracture in valgus, thus minimizing lateral forces (Fig. 30-8). I rarely perform displacement osteotomy, even in extensively comminuted fractures.

The success of closed intramedullary nailing for femoral shaft fractures has led to the development of similar devices for use in intertrochanteric fractures. The rationale for the use of the Gamma nail (Howmedica, Inc., Rutherford, NJ) and its clones is that the fracture is not directly exposed, the union rate is more rapid, and this semiclosed technique minimizes blood loss. Flexible, condylocephalic nails were proposed as a way of treating intertrochanteric fractures by a totally closed technique [51]. These devices have their proponents, but no study has yet shown their results to be superior to those with the hip compression screw, a technique introduced in 1959 and little changed since then [52].

Nonunion of an intertrochanteric fracture is rare, usually secondary to infection, metabolic disease, or incorrect placement of a compression screw. Actual implant failure is virtually unheard of using modern hip compression screws.

The postoperative regimen is the same as for femoral neck fractures: rapid mobilization. However, the surgical approach divides the vastus lateralis muscle, and patients may postoperatively mobilize more slowly after repair of intertrochanteric fractures. Regardless of the method of fixation, the patient should be allowed full weight bearing. The hemoglobin must be monitored, because bleeding from bone ends may continue for 1 or 2 days postoperatively. I routinely use suction drainage, removing the drains at 48 hours. Antibiotics and anticoagulation are used as they are in femoral neck fractures.

Fracture union routinely occurs within 4 months, but a patient may require a full year for convalescence. A permanent limp, often very slight, but sometimes marked, is virtually inevitable. I encourage patients to use a cane on the uninvolved side indefinitely.

Subtrochanteric Fractures

Subtrochanteric fractures are those distal to the lesser trochanter and proximal to the femoral isthmus. Except for those secondary to pathologic lesions, isolated subtrochanteric fractures are uncommon in elderly people. Most subtrochanteric fractures are combined intertrochanteric-subtrochanteric fractures, where a fracture line extends from the greater trochanter distal to the lesser trochanter. These fractures are considered separately because the surgical and postoperative management is different from intertrochanteric fractures.

Fractures with a small subtrochanteric component are managed surgically like intertrochanteric fractures, that is, with a hip compression screw. A longer side plate, to allow four screws through both cortices of the femur distal to the lowest fracture line, is used. This gives adequate stability for union, but does not allow early weight bearing. More distal fractures may be managed with an antegrade Recon intramedullary nail, with proximal screws directed into the femoral neck. This construct may allow early weight bearing, but it is a technically demanding procedure and often requires a prolonged anesthesia time.

Subtrochanteric fractures do not unite as rapidly or as readily as intertrochanteric fractures. Rehabilitation is markedly delayed if early weight bearing cannot be instituted. These fractures are usually best protected by a period of toe-touch (or foot-flat) weight bearing, whereby the extremity is allowed to rest on the floor during ambulation. The forces across the hip joint are greater during non–weight bearing because of the muscle pull necessary to hold the extremity off the floor than with resting the foot on the floor.

REHABILITATION

Rehabilitation of the elderly may be simple or complex. Discharge planning and rehabilitation plans should be in place before admission for patients undergoing elective procedures and begin on admission for patients undergoing emergency procedures. Current practices aimed at decreasing length of hospital stay have focused on rehabilitation centers or specialized rehabilitation departments in acute care hospitals. Patients can then get maximal therapy and be with others in similar situations while requiring minimal nursing care. Although the cost of acute hospital care is lowered, the overall cost is increased. Patients who live alone, however, benefit from such services and return to their preinjury environment more rapidly.

Patients with family members living at home may not require specialized centers, but may be rehabilitated with outpatient home care arrangements. A patient with a stable fracture or joint replacement, who is ambulatory and alert enough to participate in his or her own rehabilitation will do well at home with minimal assistance.

The changing economic environment may well completely alter the management and rehabilitation and home care phase of the care of the elderly. But the goal remains the same: restoration of an elderly, independent person to the independent life-style that he or she was living before the orthopedic illness or injury. This is a realistic goal for most elderly patients, regardless of their orthopedic disease or injury.

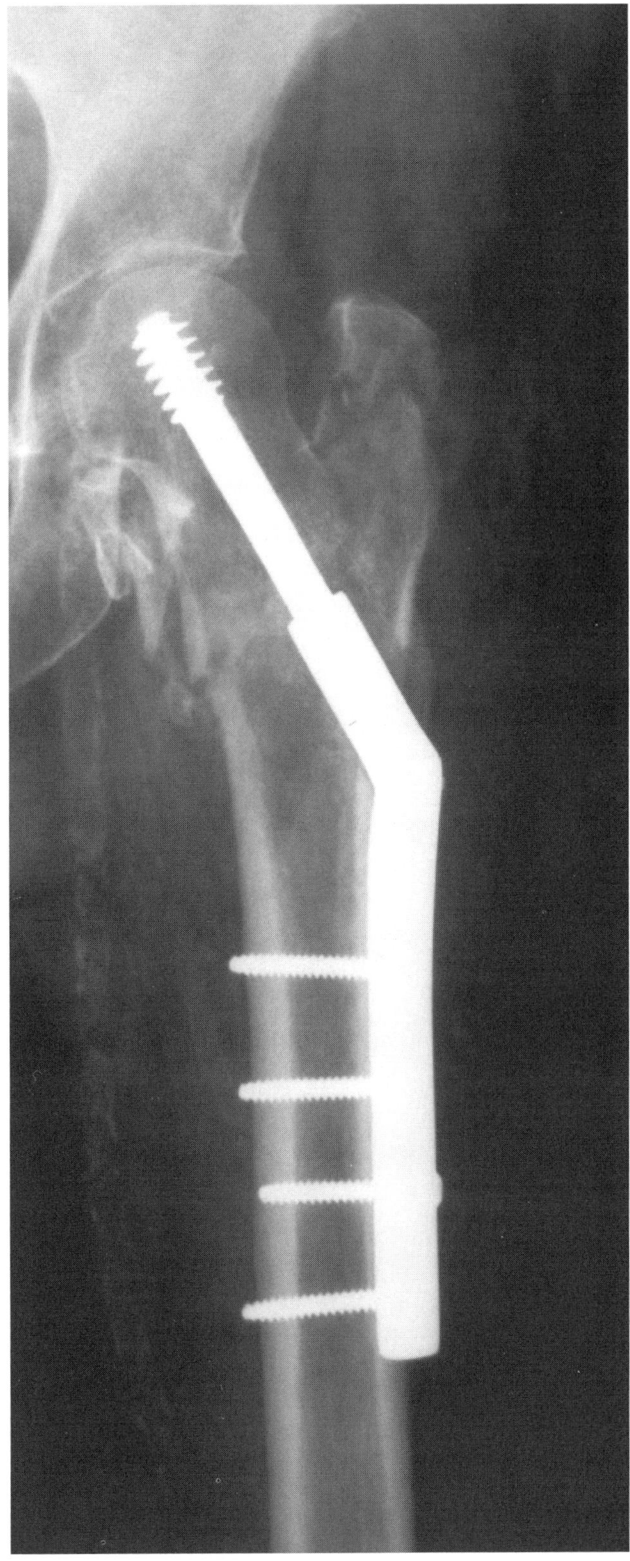

FIG. 30-8. A comminuted intertrochanteric fracture was sustained when this 72-year-old man was struck by a car. It was fixated in a valgus position to minimize the chances of shortening. Roentgenogram made 6 weeks postoperatively shows good alignment and early callus. Note the difference between this fracture and the one shown in Fig. 30-7.

REFERENCES

1. Adkins RB Jr, Scott HW Jr. Surgical procedures in patients aged 90 years and older. South Med J 1984;77:1357–1364.
2. Nelson HD, Nevitt MC, Scott JC, et al. Smoking, alcohol, and neuromuscular and physical function in older women. JAMA 1994;272:1825–1831.
3. Kenzora JE, McCarthy RE, Lowell JD, et al. Hip fracture mortality: relation to age, treatment, pre-operative illness, time of surgery and complications. Clin Orthop 1984;186:45–56.
4. Koval K, Zuckerman J. Functional recovery after hip fractures. J Bone Joint Surg Am 1994;76:751–754.
5. Ogilvie-Harris DJ, Botsford DJ, Hawker RW. Elderly patients with hip fractures: improved outcome with the use of care maps and with high-quality medical and nursing protocols. J Orthop Trauma 1993;7:428–437.

6. Burstein AH, Reilly DT, Martens M. Aging of bone tissue: mechanical properties. J Bone Joint Surg Am 1976;58:82–86.
7. Grisso JA, Kelsey JL, Strom BL, et al. Risk factors as a cause of hip fractures in women. N Engl J Med 1991;324:1326–1329.
8. Bockman RS, Weinerman SA. Medical treatment for Paget's disease of bone. Instr Course Lect 1993;42:425–433.
9. Ziminski CM. Treating joint inflammation in the elderly: an update. Geriatrics 1985;40:73–88.
10. Wells GA, Tugwell P, Kraag GR, et al. Minimum important differences between patients with rheumatoid arthritis: the patient's perspective. J Rheumatol 1993;20:557–560.
11. Mann RA, Coughlin MJ. The rheumatoid forefoot: a review of the literature and method of treatment. Orthop Rev 1979;8:105–114.
12. Brodsky JW. Management of Charcot joints of the foot and ankle in diabetes. Semin Arthrop 1992;3:58–62.
13. Brodsky JW. Amputations of the Foot and Ankle. In Mann RA, Coughlin MJ (eds), Surgery of the Foot and Ankle. St. Louis: Mosby, 1994;959–990.
14. Burnett JW, Gustilo RB, Williams DN, et al. Prophylactic antibiotics in hip fractures: a double-blind prospective study. J Bone Joint Surg Am 1980;62:457–462.
15. Mallon WJI, Callaghan JJ. Total knee arthroplasty in active golfers. J Arthroplasty 1993;8:299–306.
16. Goodnough LT, Shafron D, Marcus RE. Utilization and effectiveness of autologous blood donation for arthroplastic surgery. J Arthroplasty 1990;5:S89–S94.
17. Schulte KR, Callaghan JJ, Kelley SS, et al. The outcome of Charnley total hip arthroplasty with cement after a minimum twenty year follow-up: the results of one surgeon. J Bone Joint Surg Am 1993;75:961–975.
18. Maloney WJ, Harris WH. Comparison of a hybrid with an uncemented total hip replacement: a retrospective matched-pair study. J Bone Joint Surg Am 1990;72:1349–1352.
19. Rorabeck CH, Bourne RB, Lewis PL, et al. The Miller-Galante knee prosthesis for the treatment of osteoarthrosis: a comparison of the results of partial fixation with cement and fixation without any cement. J Bone Joint Surg Am 1993;75:402–408.
20. Allan DG, Lavoie GJ, McDonald S, et al. Proximal femoral allografts in revision hip arthroplasty. J Bone Joint Surg Br 1991;73:235–240.
21. Prins MH, Hirsh J. A comparison of general anesthesia and regional anesthesia as a risk factor for deep vein thrombosis following hip surgery: a critical review. Thromb Haemost 1990;64:497–500.
22. Woolson ST, McCrory DW, Walter JF, et al. B-mode ultrasound scanning in the detection of proximal venous thrombosis after total hip replacement. J Bone Joint Surg Am 1980;72:983–987.
23. Hall R, Raskob G, Pineo G, et al. A comparison of subcutaneous low molecular weight heparin with warfarin sodium for prophylaxis against deep-vein thrombosis after hip or knee implantation. N Engl J Med 1993;329:1370–1376.
24. Colwell CW, Spiro TE, Trowbridge AA, et al. Use of enoxapaparin, a low-molecular-weight heparin, and unfractionated heparin for the prevention of deep venous thrombosis after elective hip replacement. J Bone Joint Surg Am 1994;76:3–13.
25. Faino P, Suomalainen O, Rehmberg V, et al. Prophylaxis for the prevention of venous thromboembolism after total knee replacement. J Bone Joint Surg Am 1994;76:1814–1818.
26. Johnson KA. Bunion of the Great Toe: What and Why? In Johnson KA (ed), Surgery of the Foot and Ankle. New York: Raven, 1989;1–34.
27. Herno A, Airaksinin O, Saari T. Long-term results of surgical treatment of lumbar spinal stenosis. Spine 1993;18:1471–1474.
28. Esch JC, Ozerkis LR, Helgager JA, et al. Arthroscopic subacromial decompression: results according to the degree of rotator cuff tear. Arthroscopy 1988;4:241–244.
29. Barker SB, Harvey AH. Fall injuries in the elderly. Clin Geriatr Med 1985;1:501–512.
30. Howard PW, Stewart HD, Burke FD, et al. External fixator or plaster for severely displaced comminuted Colles fractures? J Bone Joint Surg Br 1989;71:68–73.
31. Seitz WH Jr, Putnam MD, Dick HM. Limited open surgical approach for external fixation of distal radius fractures. J Hand Surg [Am] 1990;15:288–293.
32. Gartsman GM, Sculco TP, Otis JC. Operative treatment for olecranon fractures—excision or open reduction with internal fixation. J Bone Joint Surg Am 1981;63:718–721.
33. Schegel TF, Hawkins RJ. Displaced proximal humeral fractures: evaluation and treatment. J Am Acad Orthop Surg 1994;2:54–66.
34. Hawkins RJ, Switlyk P. Acute prosthetic replacement for severe fractures of the proximal humerus. Clin Orthop 1993;289:156–160.
35. Rosenthal, RE. Problem fractures of the femur in the very elderly. Perspect Orthop Surg 1991;2:27–39.
36. Pell ACH, Christie J, Keating JF, et al. The detection of fat embolism by transoesophageal echocardiogram during reamed intramedullary nailing: a study of 24 patients with femoral and tibial fractures. J Bone Joint Surg Br 1993;75:921–925.
37. Bone LB. Indirect fracture reduction: a technique for minimizing surgical trauma. J Am Acad Orthop Surg 1994;2:247–254.
38. Lucas SE, Seligson D, Henry SL. Intramedullary supracondylar nailing of femoral fractures: a preliminary report of the GSH supracondylar nail. Clin Orthop 1993;296:200–206.
39. Georgiadis GM, Behrens FF, Joyce MJ, et al. Open tibial fractures with severe soft-tissue limb loss: limb salvage compared with below-knee amputation. J Bone Joint Surg Am 1993;75:1431–1441.
40. Beauchamp CG, Clay NR, Thexton PW. Displaced ankle fractures in patients over 50. J Bone Joint Surg Br 1983;65:329–332.
41. Behr JT, Dobozi WR, Badrinath K. The treatment of pathologic and impending pathologic fractures of the proximal femur in the elderly. Clin Orthop 1985;198:173–178.
42. Zickel RE, Mouradian WH. Intramedullary fixation of pathologic fractures and lesions of the subtrochanteric region of the femur. J Bone Joint Surg Am 1976;58:1061–1066.
43. Weiss GN, Gorton TN, Read CR, et al. Outcomes of lower extremity amputations. J Am Geriatr Soc 1990;38:877–883.
44. Sherk HH, Snape WJ, Loprett FL, et al. Internal fixation vs. non-treatment of hip fractures in senile patients. Clin Orthop 1979;141:196–198.
45. Sexson SB, Lehner JT. Factors affecting hip fracture mortality. J Orthop Trauma 1987;1:298–304.
46. Schlag G, Gandernak T, Pelinka H, et al. Thromboembolic prophylaxis in hip fractures. Acta Orthop Scand 1970;57:340–347.
47. Rizzo PF, Gould ES, Lyden JP, et al. Diagnosis of occult fractures about the hip: magnetic resonance imaging compared with bone-scanning. J Bone Joint Surg Am 1993;75:395–401.
48. Asnis SE, Wanick-Sgaglioni L. Femoral neck fractures treated with pins. J Bone Joint Surg Am 1994;76:1793–1803.
49. Bochner RM, Pellici PM, Lyden JP. Bipolar hemiarthroplasty of the femoral neck: clinical review with special emphasis on prosthetic motion. J Bone Joint Surg Am 1988;70:1001–1010.
50. Koval KJ, Zuckerman JD. Hip fractures: II. Evaluation and treatment of intertrochanteric fractures. J Am Acad Orthop Surg 1994;2:150–156.
51. Pankovich AM, Tarabishy IE. Ender nailing of intertrochanteric and subtrochanteric fractures. J Bone Joint Surg Am 1970;62:635–640.
52. Bridle SH, Patel AD, Bircher M, et al. Fixation of intertrochanteric fractures of the femur: a randomized prospective comparison of the Gamma nail and the Dynamic hip screw. J Bone Joint Surg Br 1991;73:330–334.

Surgical Care for the Elderly, 2nd ed., edited by
R. Benton Adkins, Jr., and H. William Scott, Jr.
Lippincott–Raven Publishers, Philadelphia © 1998.

CHAPTER 31

Neurosurgical Diseases

Byron Young and William F. Meacham

One of the many significant changes in clinical medicine since 1970 has been the altered concept of surgical management of disorders of the elderly. In the past, most surgical options were routinely dismissed for patients of advanced years because they were considered too old for surgery. In 1965, the point at which many patients were considered too old for elective surgery was 65 years of age; somewhat later, patients 75 to 80 years of age were considered surgical candidates. Today, patients in their late 80s are no longer considered too old for surgery.

A somewhat similar concept affected the treatment of the very young; many premature infants were also deprived of surgical attention by clinical decisions based on age alone, without consideration of the possibility of success. This clinical philosophy was based on the belief that the cardiovascular and pulmonary systems of the immature and the aged could not withstand the anesthetic and the surgical procedure with predictable success [1].

Along with the other disciplines of surgery, neurosurgery has gradually adopted a more progressive attitude toward intracranial and intraspinal procedures in patients generally regarded as elderly. Undoubtedly, this change in attitude has occurred because of an improved ability to ensure the maintenance of normal physiologic support during the operative procedure, improvement in anesthesia, improved control of vascular systems, an improved ability to obtain adequate hemostasis, and the availability of impeccable postoperative care. Today, an increasing number of senior citizens require the clinical care once given primarily to younger patients. The predictable life span of the healthy newborn is now >70 years; in 1945, it was only 40 years.

The neurosurgical disorders of older patients differ little from those in the mature groups of patients under the age of 65, although the frequency of their occurrence may change significantly as further aging takes place. For example, the elderly are more likely to develop metastatic intracranial tumors, rather than primary glial tumors and meningiomas [2].

This chapter describes the clinical problems of the nervous system that occur among the elderly, especially those conditions that may be treated surgically. The use of some of these treatment options for the elderly remains controversial, and no recipe-type therapeutic approach can be applied. This leaves many of the critical decisions about treatment to the surgeon and patient; the clinical condition of the patient and the patient's views about quality of life and acceptable risk are the most important factors in treatment decisions.

INFLAMMATORY DISEASES OF THE CENTRAL NERVOUS SYSTEM

Brain Abscess

Probably the most frequently occurring infectious disorder of the central nervous system requiring surgical treatment is brain abscess. In modern times, however, this is not a common lesion in the older age groups, to some degree because of the universal use of antibiotics for infections. The few elderly patients with brain abscesses often develop them as a contiguous infection from the paranasal sinuses into the frontal lobe area. Some abscesses spread from a middle ear or mastoid infection into the temporal lobe or cerebellum. The rare multiple brain abscesses occurring as the result of septic bacteremia are almost always fatal unless a prompt and specific response to antibiotic therapy is obtained. The solitary abscess should always be treated with an appropriate antibiotic, particularly in the early phase when meningitis and local cerebritis are present. However, this treatment ideal may be difficult to obtain with confused, disoriented, and stuporous senile patients. The diagnosis of brain abscess, once difficult, is now simple with the use of magnetic resonance imaging (MRI), which should be used in every instance of suspected intracranial pathology in the elderly.

Abscesses can generally be cured by needle tapping and aspiration, along with appropriate antibiotic treatment. The purpose of needle aspiration is not simply to remove purulent material, but also to relieve tension within the abscess cavity, which then enables the neovascular capsule to further its protective function and the antibiotic to gain access to the infectious wall. This relieves the tension that could lead to rupture into the ventricle or subarachnoid space, thereby creating a life-threatening complication. Occasionally, an abscess does not resolve and requires excision by open craniotomy.

The response of the elderly patient to successful brain abscess therapy is rewarding, and full recovery may occur if the accompanying cerebritis has not produced a serious neurologic deficit. All patients should probably be kept on protective antiseizure medication for a year or longer after the infection has cleared.

Subdural Empyema, Epidural Abscess, and Spinal Epidural Infection

Subdural empyema, epidural abscess, and spinal epidural infection occur rarely but are serious because they threaten survival and are associated with great functional loss after recovery. The diagnosis is made by MRI, and the appropriate treatment is obvious: surgical evacuation with appropriate systemic antibiotics. Spinal epidural abscess requires prompt evacuation to avoid the permanent paralysis occasioned by ischemic compression of the spinal cord and cauda equina. It is important to remember that a lumbar puncture done for diagnostic or myelographic purposes is hazardous under these conditions; if the needle passes into the subarachnoid space after traversing the epidural abscess, meningitis is assured. Slow advancement of the needle with constant aspiration during each stage secures purulent material from the epidural space, confirming the diagnosis and avoiding disastrous results. MRI is the fastest and most certain diagnostic test for epidural abscess.

INTRACRANIAL NEOPLASMS

It is unfortunate that the diagnosis of intracranial neoplasm in the elderly is often made at autopsy. The almost habitual tendency to attribute alterations of consciousness, personality changes, and focal neurologic deficits to cerebrovascular disease or senile dementia in elderly patients is a reflection of clinical practice of earlier times [3]. The ease of diagnosis with enhanced computed tomography (CT) and MRI now places the responsibility on every physician who assumes no neoplasm is present.

There is some concern that treatment of conditions requiring hospitalization is more costly for the elderly and that the elderly benefit less from the treatment than younger patients. Layon et al. [4], however, showed that there was no difference in the final outcome, quality of life, or hospital costs for treating brain tumor patients over the age of 65 years than for treating those under the age of 65. McGrail and Ojemann [5] reported excellent results for treating patients 70 years of age or older for benign intracranial tumors, including meningiomas and acoustic neuromas. Likewise, Macchiarini et al. [6] showed that age did not adversely affect survival for patients with resectable non–small cell lung cancers who also had a solitary brain metastasis and underwent combined excision of the lesions.

Intracranial tumors are more common among the elderly than the younger age group, although the types of neoplasms may vary considerably; the occurrence of glioblastoma, for instance, diminishes in frequency after patients reach the age of 65, whereas that of meningioma increases [7]. In our experience, the most common neoplasms among the elderly have been metastatic tumors, followed by malignant primary gliomas and finally by meningiomas. Acoustic neuromas and pituitary adenomas occur less frequently.

Craniotomy for resection of tumor has long been the preferred treatment for accessible malignant primary and metastatic brain tumors. Stereotactic radiosurgery, however, which has become more widely available, may become an acceptable, indeed preferred, treatment for metastatic tumor and small malignant gliomas. The procedure, which is noninvasive and performed without general anesthesia, destroys tumor cells by delivering focused high doses of radiation. This procedure has considerable potential advantages for treating both malignant and benign tumors of the elderly. Several articles reported favorable results for this procedure in treating acoustic neuromas, metastatic tumors, and even small malignant gliomas [8,9]. Flickinger et al. [10] showed that radiosurgery provides excellent control of solitary brain metastasis. In a review of a series of 116 patients, local control of the tumor was achieved in 85%; only 15% of the patients experienced tumor recurrence. Combining conventional fractionated radiotherapy and radiosurgery improved control of the tumor locally, but did not significantly influence the length of survival.

Metastatic Tumor

The aging patient with a metastatic intracranial tumor presents a therapeutic problem of considerable neurosurgical importance. To assume that the situation is untreatable is unwarranted. We have seen useful palliation extending for periods of several years for some patients with tumors; for others, however, all therapy failed. Virtually all metastatic cerebral lesions have an associated area of edema and swelling, and patients with these tumors benefit promptly from the oral administration of dexamethasone. Often, the improvement in symptoms is dramatic, giving the clinician and the patient time to consider the advisability of surgical removal of the lesion. If it is solitary and situated in an area from which it can be removed without predictable risk, and if the excision will result in useful palliation rather than crippling survival, craniotomy should be strongly recommended. This assumes that the patient's general systemic situation is appropriate for the surgical attempt and that the primary lesion is not an immediate hazard to survival. For lesions located deep within the hemisphere or in the basal ganglia, it is advisable to consider the continued use of corticosteroids and appropriate radiation therapy if possible.

Malignant Astrocytomas

Grades III and IV malignant astrocytomas occur frequently among geriatric patients, although not as often as in patients aged 40 to 65 years. We consider these two gliomas to be glioblastomas. Patients of any age with these tumors have a median survival of only approximately 1 year, even with surgery, radiation therapy, and chemotherapy. Patients harboring such neoplasms benefit from corticosteroid administration and should be considered for resection of the tumor only if the lesion can be removed with a low risk of worsening or causing a disabling neurologic deficit [11]. Lesions centered in the corpus callosum, parietal motor area, and speech areas are usually not surgically treated, but instead are treated with stereotactic radiosurgery or radiation therapy.

Meningiomas

The meningioma is a benign tumor occupying areas where clusters of arachnoidal granulations occur: the parasagittal area, sphenoid ridge, olfactory groove, tuberculum sellae, convexity, and torcular Herophili. In our experience, the most common sites for this tumor among older patients are the sphenoid, parasagittal, and pterional areas. Rarely, the meningioma may undergo a sarcomatous change and become highly invasive and virtually incurable. The meningioma is usually a slow-growing tumor that allows the brain to adapt to the encroaching, noninvasive mass and therefore may produce no symptoms of intracranial pressure for a long time. Usually, neither headache nor papilledema is present, and only transient sensory motor symptoms may be described and then dismissed as a transient ischemic attack [12]. Strangely, the meningioma often invades and penetrates the aura, skull, and scalp, but not the underlying brain, which may be only compressed. The diagnosis of meningioma is simplified by the protruding lump seen on the skull in the parasagittal, temporal, or convexity area. MRI is now an essential study for this condition.

Small areas of tumor may be left if necessary. If this is done, and if the meningioma is growing slowly, no clinical signs of recurrence will probably be seen in the elderly patient's lifetime. If, however, the tumor can be completely removed without risk to the brain or vascular structures, this should always be done [13]. Convexity meningiomas routinely lend themselves to complete removal, but the medially placed sphenoid ridge tumor or the tuberculum sellae tumor often involves other structures, and the surgeon must preserve the associated structures or the patient will suffer severely from crippling neurologic deficits. These residual lesions, when <3 cm in diameter, are better treated with stereotactic radiosurgery than with conventional surgery.

For the elderly patient, there is also some virtue in only following the course of a meningioma. This is true for tumors that have produced few if any symptoms, provided that the patient is neurologically intact and willing to cooperate in frequent periodic follow-up [14]. Many of the smaller tumors never show evidence of significant growth or the development of new symptoms. In contradistinction, however, some patients with residual tumor show signs of rapid recurrence within 6 to 12 months. Such tumors are almost always of the fibroangioblastic type. The psammomatous meningioma is virtually always slow and delinquent in its regrowth characteristics. Radiation therapy and stereotactic radiosurgery may have a salutary effect on the growth activity of meningiomas.

Neoplasms of the Posterior Fossa (Acoustic Neuromas)

Neoplasms of the posterior fossa are much less common among the elderly than among children and young adults, although the acoustic neuroma or eighth nerve tumor is seen with increasing frequency among older patients. Beginning as a small tumor within the porous acoustica interna, the acoustic neuroma may cause only annoying symptoms of tinnitus, hearing loss, and vertigo. However, as the tumor progressively enlarges, it extends out into the cerebellopontine angle and may then impair the function of cranial nerves V, IX, X, and XI. Further enlargement compresses the lateral cerebellum and pons, and it may then cause obstructive hydrocephalus that jeopardizes survival. The use of the operating microscope and microsurgical techniques have enabled surgeons to remove these tumors totally with preservation of the facial nerve, although the operative procedure may be lengthy.

Older patients who have developed obstructive hydrocephalus from the growth of the acoustic neuroma should undergo ventriculoperitoneal shunt placement; the operation for tumor removal should be delayed until the patient has shown a favorable, stable response from the decreased intracranial pressure. Intracapsular removal of tumors >3 cm in diameter is performed, leaving the capsule and the seventh nerve intact, but removing the capsule from the pontine and posterior surfaces as the tumor is gutted by piecemeal curettage and suction. This operation can be done easily and with reasonable safety, and it does not subject the elderly patient to a long operative procedure that may endanger facial nerve functions. No attempt is made to remove the nodule of tumor from the internal canal of the ear.

Similarly, those patients harboring only a small intracanalicular tumor are not subject to any operative procedure, but are followed up periodically to determine by repeat scanning whether the tumor is enlarging enough to justify its surgical removal [15]. This conservative approach to these tumors is appropriate for the elderly. When tumors <3 cm in diameter are proved to be increasing in size, stereotactic radiosurgery is usually a better option for elderly patients than surgical resection. Mendenhall et al. [16] showed that excellent results can be obtained by treating acoustic schwannomas with stereotactic radiosurgery. They reported a series of 19 patients, all of whom showed either signs of tumor regression or no change in the size of the tumor. No patient experienced any tumor resection in a 3-year follow-up.

Pituitary Tumors

Pituitary tumors have long been considered a rarity among older patients. However, autopsy studies have shown that pituitary adenomas are common among the aged [17]. Many of these tumors present with symptoms of hypopituitarism such as amenorrhea, decreased libido, or diminished energy levels. These symptoms are often interpreted as ordinary accompaniments of old age and do not trigger the medical evaluation that younger patients would undergo. Bitemporal hemianopia, a late sign of pituitary tumor, is often the reason elderly patients first seek medical evaluation. When these tumors secrete prolactin, treatment with bromocriptine is usually successful in decreasing them and decompressing the optic structures. When the tumor is not a prolactinoma, surgery is best performed by the transsphenoidal approach. Transsphenoidal surgery for large pituitary adenomas is preferred over transcranial surgery because the complication rate is lower. In the series by Black et al. [18], 81% of patients with preoperative visual-field deficits experienced postoperative improvement, 19% experienced no change, and none experienced significant worsening after transsphenoidal surgery. This procedure has revolutionized the safety and efficacy of pituitary tumor removal.

When surgery cannot be performed, radiation therapy frequently provides satisfactory long-term results. Hughes et al. [19] treated 108 patients with pituitary adenomas with radiotherapy alone. The 10-year progression-free survival rate was 60%, and tumor control was obtained in 77%. Grigsby et al. [20] showed that the only prognostic variable affecting the disease-free interval after surgery and postoperative radiation therapy for pituitary adenoma was irradiation dose. Age was not a significant variable.

Lesions that secrete growth hormone or adrenocorticotropic hormone are distinctly less common among elderly patients. These lesions are more refractory to radiation therapy, and if there are associated symptoms of diabetes and hypertension or shortening life span, surgical intervention is needed to provide the earliest possible control of these debilitating side effects. One or 2 years may be required after treatment with radiation therapy before secretion of these functional adenomas is attenuated.

NEUROSURGICAL DISORDERS OF THE SPINE

Metastatic Tumor

Unfortunately, the most common intraspinal neoplasm among aged patients is metastatic tumor, usually located in the thoracic area and secondary to malignancies of the prostate, lung, and breast or from unknown primary sites [21]. The progression of symptoms from spinal cord lesions is highly variable, ranging from insidious to very rapid. Common initial symptoms are localized spinal pain, weakness, radicular pain, ataxia, and urinary incontinence. MRI is the diagnostic study of choice, because it has a high sensitivity for early lesions and most clearly establishes the site and extent of neural involvement. The physician must be attentive and responsive to the appearance of back pain in an elderly patient harboring a primary malignant systemic neoplasm. Elderly patients with known primary cancer who develop significant back pain should undergo MRI to rule out a metastatic spinal tumor. Waiting for neurologic signs to develop before performing MRI too often results in permanent and devastating paraplegia or quadriplegia.

Metastatic spinal tumors that do not cause instability or neurologic deficit are treated with radiation therapy alone. It is unclear whether tumors that cause neurologic deficit are best treated with radiotherapy alone or with surgical decompression followed by radiotherapy. The authors usually use surgery and fixation, if necessary, plus radiotherapy.

Meningiomas

Clinically, the presence of Brown-Séquard syndrome (lateral cord compression) with ipsilateral motor loss and contralateral sensory loss is almost pathognomonic of intraspinal tumor. The most common benign spinal cord tumor of the elderly is clearly the meningioma. It usually occupies the thoracic spine and produces slowly progressing symptoms often diagnosed as vascular disorders or spondylitic disease. The cervical area is next most often involved with either meningioma or neurofibroma, but the lumbar area is exceptionally free of meningioma in favor of neurofibroma. The only effective therapy for these crippling tumors is to remove them surgically. Decompression of the spinal cord by tumor removal is well tolerated by the elderly patient, and excellent clinical recovery may be anticipated if the procedure is done carefully and before permanent capillary ischemia of the spinal cord has occurred.

Spondylosis

The disorder known as *spondylosis* results from spinal stenosis caused by disk degeneration, osteophyte formation, facet hypertrophy, and enlargement of the ligamenta flavum [22]. This condition may occur at any spinal level, but is most common in the midcervical and low lumbar areas. The symptoms may be dramatically relieved if an adequate laminectomy is done in conjunction with shaving of the facets to create a satisfactory enlargement of the canal. If pressure ischemia of the spinal cord, cauda equina, or nerve roots has progressed to an irreversible stage before the laminectomy is done, the degree of neurologic deficit may remain unchanged, although its progression may be halted by the decompression.

Intramedullary Tumors

Intramedullary tumors of the spinal cord are not common among older patients, although low-grade astrocytomas and metastatic lesions are occasionally found. The removal of such tumors requires great caution and skill on the part of the surgeon; one must avoid operative damage to the cord parenchyma that would increase the neurologic deficit. In some cases a limited biopsy followed by radiation therapy constitutes the procedure of choice [23].

INTRACTABLE PAIN

Trigeminal Neuralgia

The clinical entity known as *tic douloureux* or *trigeminal neuralgia* is almost totally confined to older patients. The precise cause of this disorder is not known, although evidence suggests that it may be vascular compression of the trigeminal posterior root. The diagnosis is made purely by history, because there is no reliable objective test or findings of value. MRI should be performed, however, to rule out a tumor of the posterior fossa as the cause of the pain. It should be emphasized that the painful attacks are brief and confined to the anatomic distribution of the trigeminal nerve, and that the pain is never constant, although the attacks may be so frequent that the patient complains of constant pain. Unless the patient has typical trigeminal neuralgia, no surgical procedures to relieve the pain should be performed; otherwise the development of anesthesia dolorosa may ensue, which will defy all therapeutic attempts to control it.

Typically, the appropriate therapy for tic douloureux is the most conservative method that is successful. The use of phenytoin (Dilantin), carbamazepine (Tegretol), and simple analgesics should be used and maintained if effective. Alcohol blocking of the peripheral nerve branches is useless except as a temporary measure. The same can be said for the section avulsion of the peripheral branches. If, on the other hand, conservative measures have failed and the patient's condition is favorable, a surgical procedure should be used. For patients >70 years of age, a percutaneous procedure, which can be performed in the radiographic suite, is preferred. The commonly used procedures are balloon compression, radiofrequency lesioning, and glycerol injection. We favor percutaneous balloon compression. Stereotactic radiosurgery has recently been introduced as another treatment for trigeminal neuralgia and appears to be as effective as other methods. The procedure may be proved to be particularly applicable for the elderly because of its relative safety [24]. Craniotomy for microvascular decompression is commonly used and preferred for younger patients, but it is not the authors' first choice for the elderly. In our community, the elderly patient with intractable tic pain desires one trip to the operating room for relief if conservative measures have been ineffective.

Glossopharyngeal Neuralgia (Tic Douloureux of the Nervus Intermedius)

Glossopharyngeal neuralgia is much less common than trigeminal neuralgia but is just as severe and cannot be tolerated when the attacks become frequent. The same medicinal controls should be tried. Tic douloureux of the nervus intermedius is extremely rare and may respond to Tegretol.

Metastatic Lesion

Intractable pain from metastatic lesions in older individuals should be tempered with the judicious use of narcotics in doses sufficient to control pain and to give a period of gratifying relief to the patient. It is foolhardy to insist on the use of such drugs on a 4- or 6-hour basis; the patient should have the drug when he or she needs it, not when the order requires or allows it. The concern that the patient will become addicted to the medication does not trouble the authors under these dismal and terminal circumstances. Surgical procedures for pain control are rarely indicated in these circumstances.

INTRACRANIAL ANEURYSMS

Unruptured Aneurysms

The appropriate therapy for unruptured aneurysms of the cerebral vascular system is of great clinical importance. It is estimated that only 2% of all intact cerebral aneurysms rupture in a year. For the elderly, this lends credence to the conservative philosophy of leaving such lesions undisturbed in favor of periodic observation to determine whether progressive enlargement has occurred [25]. If there is evidence that this has happened within a short time, it is probably wise to recommend an operative approach to contain the aneurysm. If the aneurysm is located where there is a reasonable chance of success without serious neurologic deficit resulting, it should be clipped.

Ruptured Aneurysms

Subarachnoid hemorrhage resulting from a ruptured intracranial aneurysm is treated in precisely the same manner as for younger patients. If the older patient survives this critical period without a permanent major neurologic deficit and has an alert mental state, the decision regarding surgical attack on the aneurysm must then be made. Inagawa et al. [26] showed that patients 70 years of age or older with ruptured aneurysms have a significantly poorer outcome than patients under the age of 70. The mortality for patients 70 years of age or older was 55%. Likewise, the operative outcome for patients in this age group was worse. Approximately one-third of patients 70 years of age or older are predicted to survive for 5 years. An aggressive surgical attack on the aneurysm is often well tolerated in the systemically healthy senior patient. It should be understood that no recipe-type therapy can apply to these hazardous lesions and that each case must be individually appraised and therapy decided on [27]. Endovascular treatment of aneurysm, which is becoming more widely used, will be particularly advantageous for the elderly.

Arteriovenous Malformations

Arteriovenous malformations are not a common problem among older patients. When such a lesion is discovered in a patient of advanced age, the decisions regarding the most appropriate treatment are difficult. Rarely, however, is surgical excision indicated, because the risk of death from hemorrhage over the expectedly limited life span of older patients is often less than the risk of surgery. Incidentally discovered arteriovenous malformations bleed at a 1% rate per year. Arteriovenous malformations discovered after a seizure bleed at about the same rate. The rebleeding rate for these lesions is 3% to 4% per year, with an annual morbidity of approximately 1%. After 2 to 3 years, the annual rebleeding rate is approximately 2%. In contrast to younger patients, the elderly rarely require treatment with radiosurgery; stereotactic radiosurgery provides no protection against rebleeding for 2 years after treatment.

HYDROCEPHALUS

Two forms of ventricular enlargement in the older patient are frequently encountered, the pathophysiology of which is not completely understood. A frequently seen aspect of the aging process is atrophy of the brain parenchyma through loss of nerve cells and of the glia (principally microglia). As a result, the subarachnoid pathways and ventricles show a compensatory increase in size. This has been called *hydrocephalus et vacuo,* a term that is widely used but probably incorrect. At any rate, CT or MRI can easily disclose the enlargement of the fluid-filled areas and the atrophy of the cortex. The same picture may be seen in Alzheimer's disease, but because there is no effective treatment for either of these disorders in the elderly, no surgical consideration is involved [1].

A possibly treatable form of hydrocephalus among the elderly is normal-pressure hydrocephalus, characterized by a triad of clinical problems consisting of dementia, gait disturbance, and urinary incontinence ("unwitting wetting"). This condition may be dramatically altered with ventricular decompression by means of a ventriculoperitoneal shunt. At this time there is no reliable method of determining the ideal surgical candidate for this procedure. It has been shown that patients who have significant reflux of radioactively labeled protein from the lumbar subarachnoid space into the ventricles are probably good surgical candidates [28]. In a review of our own series we found that the best results of surgical treatment occurred among those patients whose prime clinical problem was gait disturbance. The poorest results were among those patients whose primary symptom was dementia. The operative procedure is easily done under light anesthesia and is well tolerated by the aging patient. Unfortunately, a good clinical result cannot be predicted preoperatively with any degree of certainty.

NEUROSURGICAL ASPECTS OF TRAUMA

Injuries to the head and spine are probably the most common cause of life-threatening disorders of the nervous system in older persons. Age is a significant factor in predicting outcome from severe head injury. Although favorable outcome from such injuries is not very high among any age group, vegetative state or death are twice as likely for those >55 years of age as for those 35 to 45 years of age (approximately 80% vs. 40%) [29]. The treatment of severe head injury is the same for young adults and for the elderly, but secondary pulmonary and renal complications are common among the elderly.

Skull Fractures

As is true for younger patients, the elderly generally tolerate fractures of the skull quite well and require no treatment unless the fracture is compound, in which case it must be debrided and closed. In the case of basal skull fractures resulting in cerebral spinal fluid otorrhea, rhinorrhea, or both, recumbency is appropriate and necessary. Depressed fractures of the convexity of the skull may be left alone unless the depressed fracture is greater than the combined thickness of all of the layers of the skull, in which case the underlying cerebral cortex may be lacerated or compressed. The elevation or the actual removal of such an area of skull is thought by some to reduce the ultimate glial response and to minimize the likelihood of post-traumatic epilepsy. We suspect, however, that the result of this maneuver is principally one of cosmetic restoration, and this is usually not thought to be of prime importance for older patients.

Hematomas

The chronic subdural hematoma, a potentially curable condition that afflicts the elderly far more commonly than young adults, is easily diagnosed by CT or MRI. Failure to use these diagnostic tools because the clinical evidence suggests that the symptoms are from a vascular disorder or from a degenerative disease is inexcusable. The insidious development of the symptoms from the hematoma occurring after a fall or a mild bump on the head, often forgotten by the elderly, may well simulate those symptoms seen with a stroke or with the altered cerebration of a degenerative disorder. Enlargement of the hematoma by microhemorrhages from the neovascular membrane may finally produce brain compression incompatible with consciousness, and stupor and coma intervene. It is apparent that the virtually universal use of CT and MRI will tend to eliminate the likelihood of overlooking this disorder, and we can help eliminate its tragic effect if effective treatment then follows.

Surgical evacuation, by craniotomy, burr holes, or twist-drill craniotomy, is the preferred treatment for these lesions. When CT scan shows that the lesions are composed primarily of isodense or hypodense blood, twist-drill drainage, which can be performed with local anesthesia in the intensive care unit, is a particularly attractive option for treating the elderly patient. The possibility of bilateral subdural hematoma is always present, and when this situation is disclosed the two sides should be treated simultaneously and identically. It is well known that some subdural hematomas are spontaneously absorbed and can be watched closely by repeated scanning, but only if the patient shows no progressive deterioration. It remains true that the surgical approach ensures the best outcome even today [30–32].

The acute epidural hematoma constitutes the most dramatic of clinical conditions that may be rectified and for which a good outcome may be achieved. Only if prompt action is taken to recognize and decompress an acutely compromised brain is this possible. The classic history consists of a blow to the head with transient loss of consciousness, and then a lucid interval followed by confusion, headache, and alterations of consciousness along with other neurologic sequelae. Obviously, the sequence of events in the history may vary, and there may be no report of a lucid interval, but whenever rapid and progressive deterioration occurs after a head injury, medical staff should be alerted to the possibility of a hemorrhage from the middle meningeal artery. Therapeutic delay in this situation can be fatal, and the time-consuming and useless skull radiography and detailed neurologic examinations may result in the patient's unnecessary death. Currently, a hastily performed scan of the head may be permissible, but only if the patient's vital signs are stable and there is no indication of approaching respiratory paralysis.

Emergency burr openings should be made in the emergency room if rapid neurologic changes and respiratory arrest occur. If clotted blood issues, success is possible, and the control of bleeding and wound closure can be accomplished in a timely manner in the operating room. A tragedy seen many times by one of the authors is the arrival in the emergency room of a moribund patient with dilated, fixed pupils, profound coma, and decerebrate posturing, accompanied by detailed radiographs taken by a well-meaning clinician some 50 miles away who referred the patient with the findings of an obvious epidural hematoma. Fortunately, some epidural arterial injuries clot before a large mass of hematoma is present. The pitfall is that such clotting may give false assurance to the physician regarding the patient's safety. This lesion when clotted often has several small rebleeding episodes (the stuttering epidural) that may ultimately produce the same crisis described previously with untreated epidural hematoma.

Spinal Injuries

Injuries to the bony spine that are not unstable are well tolerated by elderly patients if there is no associated injury to the neural elements. Most elderly patients with vertebral compression fractures, however, do well if they are not confined to bed. It is well established that the elderly patient tolerates this type of confinement poorly, and it is almost a formal invitation to respiratory infection, confusion, and disorientation. Unless it is imperative that an operative procedure such as spinal fusion be performed, the older patient does well and usually better with simple braces and a short period of limited physical activity. Just as with younger patients, elderly patients with unstable fractures must be treated with fixation, fusion, or both. Bone fusion rates are lower among elderly patients than among adults in their 40s or 50s.

When damage to the spinal cord or cauda equina occurs, the prognosis becomes infinitely worse. The elderly person who suffers an acute quadriplegic or paraplegic injury becomes at once a candidate for a series of complications. Pneumonia, urinary tract infection (from an indwelling catheter), pressure sores, and deep vein thrombosis all contribute to shortened survival for this unfortunate elderly patient.

CAROTID ARTERY STENOSIS

Carotid artery stenosis is particularly common among those patients >70 years of age. Elderly patients with carotid stenosis >60% to 70%, whether symptomatic or asymptomatic, should be offered prophylactic carotid endarterectomy (CEA), assuming that they have an acceptable cardiac risk [33,34]. Few patients should be denied surgery. The standard for meeting cardiopulmonary criteria for CEA is no different for patients in their 60s than for those in their late 70s. The Asymptomatic Carotid Atherosclerosis Study, which showed that prophylactic CEA was beneficial for patients with high-grade asymptomatic carotid artery stenosis, included patients up to 79 years of age [34].

REFERENCES

1. Samorajski T. How the human responds to aging. J Am Geriatr Soc 1976;24:4–11.
2. Long DM. Aging in the nervous system. Neurosurgery 1985;17: 348–354.
3. Godfrey JB, Caird FJ. Intracranial tumors in the elderly: diagnosis and treatment. Age Ageing 1984;13:152–158.
4. Layon AJ, George BE, Hamby B, et al. Do elderly patients overutilize healthcare resources and benefit less from them than younger

patients? A study of patients who underwent craniotomy for treatment of neoplasm. Crit Care Med 1995;23:829–834.
5. McGrail KM, Ojemann RG. The surgical management of benign intracranial meningiomas and acoustic neuromas in patients 70 years of age and older. Surg Neurol 1994;42:2–7.
6. Macchiarini P, Buonaguidi R, Hardin M, et al. Results and prognostic factors of surgery in the management of non–small cell lung cancer with solitary brain metastasis. Cancer 1991;68:300–304.
7. Holmes FF. Aging and cancer. Recent results. Cancer Res 1983;87:1–75.
8. Somaza S, Kondziolka D, Lunsford LD, et al. Stereotactic radiosurgery for cerebral metastatic melanoma. J Neurosurg 1993;79:661–666.
9. Loeffler JS, Alexander E III, Shea WM, et al. Radiosurgery as part of the initial management of patients with malignant gliomas. J Clin Oncol 1992;10:1379–1385.
10. Flickinger JC, Kondziolka D, Lunsford LD, et al. A multi-institutional experience with stereotactic radiosurgery for solitary brain metastasis. Int J Radiat Oncol Biol Phys 1994;28:797–802.
11. Ransohoff J. Role of surgery in the treatment of malignant gliomas. Cancer Treat Rep 1976;60:717–718.
12. Salcman M. Brain tumors in elderly patients. Am Fam Physician 1983;27:137–143.
13. Salcman M. Brain tumors and the geriatrics patient. J Am Geriatr Soc 1982;30:501–508.
14. Tomita T, Raimondi AJ. Brain tumors in the elderly. JAMA 1981;246:53–55.
15. Silverstein H, McDaniel A, Norrell H, et al. Conservative management of acoustic neuroma in the elderly patient. Laryngoscope 1985;95:766–770.
16. Mendenhall WM, Friedman WA, Boom FJ. Linear accelerator–based stereotactic radiosurgery for acoustic schwannomas. Int J Radiat Oncol Biol Phys 1994;28:803–810.
17. Kovacs K, Ryan N, Horvath E, et al. Pituitary adenomas in old age. J Gerontol 1980;35:16–22.
18. Black PM, Zervas NT, Candia G. Management of large pituitary adenomas by transsphenoidal surgery. Surg Neurol 1988;29:443–447.
19. Hughes MN, Llamas KJ, Yelland ME, et al. Pituitary adenomas: long-term results for radiotherapy alone and postoperative radiotherapy. Int J Radiat Oncol Biol Phys 1993;27:1035–1043.
20. Grigsby PW, Simpson JR, Emami BN, et al. Prognostic factors and results of surgery and postoperative irradiation in the management of pituitary adenomas. Int J Radiat Oncol Biol Phys 1989;16:1411–1417.
21. Valenstein E. When to suspect spinal cord lesions in the elderly. Geriatrics 1979;34:80–95.
22. Fast A, Robin GC, Floman Y. Surgical treatment of lumbar spinal stenosis in the elderly. Arch Phys Med Rehabil 1985;66:149–151.
23. Huang CY, Matheson J. Spinal cord tumours in the elderly. Aust N Z J Med 1979;9:538–541.
24. Kondziolka D, Lunsford LD, Flickinger JC, et al. Stereotactic radiosurgery for trigeminal neuralgia: a multiinstitutional study using the gamma unit. J Neurosurg 1996;84:940–945.
25. Dacey RG Jr, Pitkethly D, Winn HR. Enlargement of an intracranial aneurysm in the eighth decade of life. J Neurosurg 1985;62: 600–602.
26. Inagawa T, Yamamoto M, Kamiya K, et al. Management of elderly patients with aneurysmal subarachnoid hemorrhage. J Neurosurg 1988;69:332–339.
27. Symon L, Vajda J. Surgical experiences with giant intracranial aneurysms. J Neurosurg 1984;61:1009–1028.
28. Petersen RC, Mokri B, Laws ER Jr. Surgical treatment of idiopathic hydrocephalus in elderly patients. Neurology 1985;35:307–311.
29. Marshall LF, Marshall SB. Outcome Prediction in Severe Head Injury. In Wilkins RH, Rengachary SS (eds), Neurosurgery (Vol. 11, 2nd ed). New York: McGraw-Hill, 1996;2717–2721.
30. Robinson RG. Chronic subdural hematoma: surgical management in 133 patients. J Neurosurg 1984;61:263–268.
31. Waga S, Sakakura M, Fujimoto K. Calcified subdural hematoma in the elderly. Surg Neurol 1979;11:51–52.
32. Samudrala S, Cooper PR. Traumatic Intracranial Hematomas. In Wilkins RH, Rengachary SS (eds), Neurosurgery (Vol. 11, 2nd ed). New York: McGraw-Hill, 1996;2797–2807.
33. North American Symptomatic Carotid Endarterectomy Trial Collaborators. Beneficial effect of carotid endarterectomy in symptomatic patients with high-grade carotid stenosis. N Engl J Med 1991;325: 445–453.
34. Executive Committee for the Asymptomatic Carotid Atherosclerosis Study. Endarterectomy for asymptomatic carotid artery stenosis. JAMA 1995;273:1421–1428.

Surgical Care for the Elderly, 2nd ed., edited by
R. Benton Adkins, Jr., and H. William Scott, Jr.
Lippincott–Raven Publishers, Philadelphia © 1998.

CHAPTER 32

Diseases of the Adrenal Glands: Surgical Aspects

Jon A. van Heerden and Clive S. Grant

Is there anything inherently different regarding surgical adrenal disease in the elderly, or is a discussion about diseases of the aged simply a reiteration of what is well known about adrenal gland disease in all age groups? What makes the elderly patient with adrenocortical and adrenal medullary problems special? There is little doubt that the symptoms and signs of endogenous hypercortisolism (Cushing's syndrome) in the elderly patient are quite similar to those seen in younger patients. However, the elderly patient is much more likely to have symptoms and signs of Cushing's syndrome secondary to exogenous hypercortisolism as a result of corticosteroid administration. This is true because of the many disease entities, such as rheumatoid arthritis, pulmonary disease, and renal diseases, that may be much more common in the older population. Similarly, the elderly patient might unwittingly develop exogenous hypercortisolism because of the chronic intake of self-administered "arthritis pills," which may, unbeknown to the consumer, contain corticosteroids. A particularly difficult diagnostic conundrum is the older patient with chronic renal failure, an entity that is more common at the latter stages of life [1]. Not only can hemodialysis modulate the diurnal variations in plasma cortisol secretion [2], but renal failure per se may result in poor gastrointestinal absorption of dexamethasone [3] (which, therefore, should be administered intravenously in this setting), spurious overestimation of plasma levels, abnormal cortisol binding, and abnormal response to dexamethasone administration. All of these factors may make the diagnosis of endogenous hypercortisolism extremely difficult in the elderly patient.

The clinical diagnosis of hypercortisolism may also be problematic because of the changes that occur in the elderly patient's habitus due to the normal aging process (Fig. 32-1), especially if there is chronic alcohol abuse as well. In this latter instance, the clinical picture of a flushed face, hyperglycemia, osteoporosis, cutaneous ecchymosis, and so forth can accurately mimic the picture found in patients with endogenous hypercortisolism. It should also be remembered that hypercortisolism in the elderly, even to a minor degree, may aggravate problems common in the elderly such as hypertension, depression, senile dementia, and osteoporosis.

Are there any distinct physiologic alterations of the neuroendocrine system that occur with the normal aging process?

1. Plasma noradrenaline concentrations appear to increase with advancing age. This may be as a result of reduced clearance of noradrenaline from the circulation in the aging population. When this is coupled with the increasing evidence of a diminished responsiveness of beta-adrenoceptor–mediated function in the elderly population, it is not surprising that plasma levels are elevated. Interestingly enough, there is little or no evidence to suggest that there is any alteration in the alpha-adrenoceptor mechanisms with increasing age. It has been postulated that the observed increase in norepinephrine levels in men, particularly over the age of 60 years, may be correlated with a marked decrease in stage IV sleep and more frequent periods of wakefulness. The decrease in receptor responsiveness may, theoretically, be an important mechanism for age-related decrease in tissue sensitivity to those hormones [4–6].
2. There appears to be a steady decrease in aldosterone secretion with advancing age. This has been shown to be the result of a definite decrease in aldosterone secretion by the adrenal cortex and not of alterations of the metabolic clearance of aldosterone, which remains unchanged with advancing age.
3. Similarly, plasma renin activity declines with increasing age and is most likely the primary cause of the lowered aldosterone value usually reported in older patients. This physiologic change perhaps has the greatest importance when one is considering the diagnosis of primary hyperaldosteronism in the elderly patient. It should be appreciated

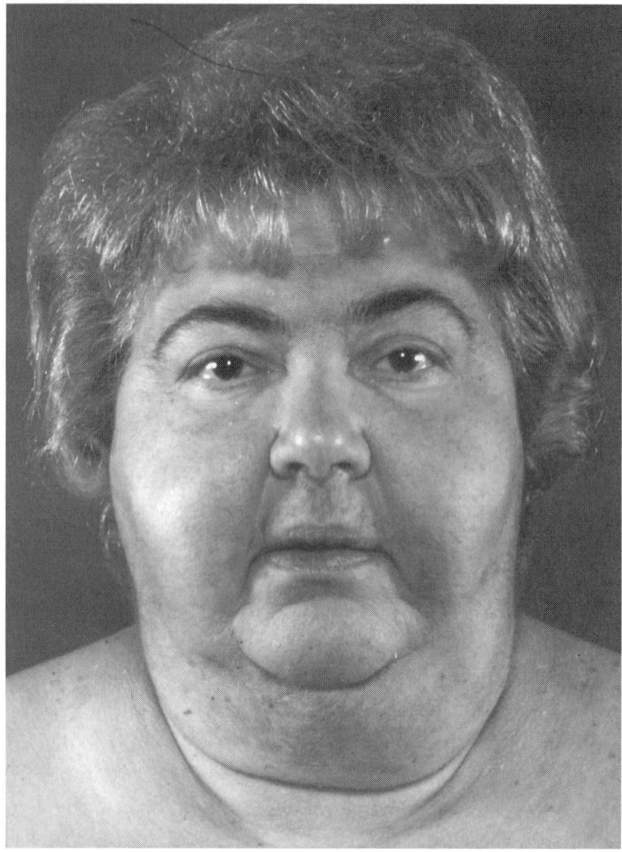

FIG. 32-1. Old age or hypercortisolism? The patient had Cushing's syndrome secondary to an adrenocortical carcinoma.

that the normal aldosterone values decrease as age increases [7,8]. Of interest is the fact that the adrenal circadian system appears to be totally unaffected by advancing age [9].

4. Extensive studies have been designed to evaluate the metabolic response to stress in the elderly. It has been clearly documented that plasma cortisol levels were significantly higher in the elderly than in the young controls, that the plasma renin response to stress was lower in the older age group, and that there was no change demonstrated in the renin-aldosterone and electrolyte response when older and younger patient groups were compared [10].

5. Similar studies have been performed to establish whether the immunoreactive corticotropin reserve was impaired in old age and whether a depletion of this reserve could account for the increased morbidity and mortality following operations in the elderly age group. These studies have shown that there is no decrease in the immunoreactive corticotropin reserve following various surgical procedures in the older age group [11].

Clinically, it should be remembered that the incidence of both adrenal hyperfunction and hypofunction is extremely low in the elderly population. Despite all of the physiologic changes enumerated previously, the essential clinical features of the surgical diseases of the adrenal glands do not basically differ from those found in younger patients. The postoperative complication rate for these surgical procedures should be anticipated to be higher in this senior population group because of the attending ravages of old age, that is, atherosclerosis, cardiovascular heart disease, hypertension, diabetes mellitus, renal failure, and so forth. In an attempt to obtain objective data in our own practice, we have analyzed our experience with all of our patients over the age of 65 years who underwent surgical treatment for Cushing's syndrome (14 patients), adrenocortical carcinoma (six patients), pheochromocytoma (nine patients), incidentaloma (16 patients), and primary hyperaldosteronism (14 patients) during the period 1989 through 1993.

TABLE 32-1. *American Society of Anesthesiologists' preoperative evaluation classification*

Class I	Normally healthy patient
Class II	Patient with mild systemic disease
Class III	Patient with severe systemic disease that is not incapacitating
Class IV	Patient with an incapacitating systemic disease that is a constant threat to life
Class V	Moribund patient who is not expected to survive for 24 hours with or without operation

Of cardinal importance before any surgeon recommends surgery is that the potential benefits of the surgical procedure be weighed against the risks of or alternatives to the operation. Multiple factors will and should influence that decision. They include differing factors such as the expertise of the entire medical and surgical team, the medical status of the patient, and the primary and secondary diseases present. To quantify numerically all ramifications of these categories and to produce a meaningful formula for universal application defies the current status of our sophisticated technology. Rather, this is the substance of individual surgical judgment. Careful, honest analysis of surgical results, one's own and those of others, is the cornerstone of this judgment.

Presuming that high-quality medical care is available, one can then focus on the patient and his or her particular disease. The chronologic, and more importantly, the physiologic age of the patient is of clearly recognized importance as a determinant of operative risk [12]. From an epidemiologic perspective, this issue deserves significant attention. Whereas there were 22 million people over the age of 65 in the United States in 1985, the same age group is projected to increase to an excess of 32 million by 1995 [13]. One must also be cognizant of the changing life expectancy of this elderly population. Nearly 90% of those aged 60 to 64 years, 75% of people aged 70 to 74, and 50% of those aged 80 will live another 5 years [13].

The objective assessment of operative risk accounting for age and other factors affecting physiologic status has been widely practiced by anesthesiologists in the United States for years (Table 32-1) [14]. Moreover, Del Guercio and

TABLE 32-2. *Multivariate index of cardiac risk in noncardiac surgical procedures*

	Preoperative factor	Points
1	S3 gallop, congestive heart failure	11
2	Myocardial infarction ≤6 months	10
3	Abnormal electrocardiographic rhythm other than atrial premature contractions	7
4	≥5 premature ventricular contractions per minute	7
5	Age >70 years	5
6	Intraperitoneal operations	3
7	Important valvular aortic stenosis	3
8	Poor general medical condition, for example, abnormal electrolyte levels, renal insufficiency, chronic liver disease, chronically bedridden patient	3

Source: Modified from Goldman L, Caldera DL, Nussbaum SR, et al. Multifactorial index of cardiac risk in noncardiac surgical procedures. N Engl J Med 1977;297:845–850.

TABLE 32-3. *Grading system for multivariate index of cardiac risk in noncardiac surgical procedures*

	Points	Life-threatening complication (%)	Cardiac deaths (%)
Class I	0–5	0.7	0.2
Class II	6–12	5	2
Class III	13–25	11	2
Class IV	26	22	56

Source: Modified from Goldman L, Caldera DL, Nussbaum SR, et al. Multifactorial index of cardiac risk in noncardiac surgical procedures. N Engl J Med 1977;297:845-850.

Cohn used preoperative invasive monitoring techniques to develop a more precise preoperative risk staging system. This has become a system that can optimize hemodynamic parameters and lessen the risk [15]. The American Society of Anesthesiologists (ASA) classification correlated well with these high-risk patients although the specific physiologic defect could be identified only by using the sophisticated invasive techniques. Because cardiac disease occurs frequently and is the most common cause of death in the elderly surgical patient, particular emphasis should be placed on yet another reported multifactorial assessment of cardiac risk (Tables 32-2 and 32-3) [12].

We included the assessment of the calculated operative risk using the ASA classification and the multifactorial cardiac risk scheme in reviewing patients who were 65 years of age or older and who underwent adrenalectomy at the Mayo Clinic between 1989 and 1993. These studies included all patients operated on for Cushing's syndrome (14 patients) and nonfunctioning adrenocortical adenomas (16 patients) (Tables 32-4 and 32-5). All of these particular operations were elective. Combined ASA classifications R and HI accounted for 93% of these patients, with two postoperative complications occurring in the ASA class II group and one in the ASA class IH group.

Categorized by the multifactorial scheme, there were five class I patients (17%), 14 class II patients (47%), 11 class III patients (36%), and no class IV patients. The operative mortality was a single ASA class II 80-year-old patient (3%) who died of a pulmonary embolus 26 days after postoperative excision of a 5.0-cm nonfunctioning incidentaloma.

CUSHING'S SYNDROME

During the period of study (1989 to 1993), 69 patients underwent adrenalectomy for hypercortisolism at our institution. Of these, 14 (20%) were in patients over the age of 65 years. To establish the diagnosis of Cushing's syndrome in this elderly group was no more difficult or complex than in younger patients. All patients presented with the characteristic stigmata of Cushing's syndrome, and the standard laboratory evaluation yielded the expected results [16,17].

TABLE 32-4. *Patients 65 years of age or older undergoing adrenalectomy for Cushing's syndrome (1989 to 1993)*

Age (yrs)/sex	Approach	Pathology (diameter in cm)	ASA class	Multifactor score	Multifactor class
76/F	Abdominal	Hyperplasia	2	8	2
65/F	Abdominal	Adenoma (2.5)	2	3	1
75/F	Posterior	Adenoma (3.5)	3	5	1
69/M	Abdominal	ACTH-producing pheochromocytoma	3	6	2
65/F	Posterior	Adenoma (2.5)	2	0	1
68/M	Posterior	Hyperplasia	3	0	1
74/F	Posterior	Adenoma (4.2)	3	5	1
69/F	Posterior	Adenoma (2.7, 4.0)	2	0	1
76/F	Posterior	Hyperplasia	3	8	2
66/F	Posterior	Adenoma (5.2)	3	7	2
71/M	Posterior	Hyperplasia	3	7	2
68/M	Posterior	Hyperplasia	3	3	1
69/F	Posterior	Hyperplasia	2	3	1
66/M	Posterior	Hyperplasia	2	0	1

ASA = American Society of Anesthesiologists; ACTH = adrenocorticotropic hormone.

TABLE 32-5. *Patients 65 years of age or older undergoing adrenalectomy for incidentalomas (1989 to 1993)*

Age (yrs)/sex	Approach	Size (cm)	Additional procedures	ASA class	Multifactor score	Multifactor class
80/F	Posterior	5.0	—	2	5	1
75/M	Anterior	5.0	Excision colonic adenoma	2	8	2
69/F	Anterior	4.0	—	1	3	1
69/F	Anterior	4.0	—	2	3	1
69/F	Anterior	4.5	Excision liposarcoma	1	3	1
75/F	Anterior	5.5	Excision gastric ulcer	3	8	2
66/M	Anterior	4.0	—	1	3	1
72/F	Posterior	4.3	—	2	5	1
69/M	Anterior	6.0	—	3	3	1
75/M	Anterior	3.0	Cholecystectomy, liver biopsy	3	10	2
70/M	Posterior	4.0	—	2	5	1
67/F	Posterior	6.0	—	1	0	1
65/M	Posterior	3.0	—	1	0	1
73/M	Posterior	4.5	—	2	12	2
69/F	Posterior	5.2	—	2	0	1
84/F	Anterior	5.9	—	2	8	2

ASA = American Society of Anesthesiologists.

Despite a decreased degree of adrenocortical responsiveness in our elderly patients, the correspondingly reduced clearance rate resulted in the usual cortisol values [18]. Secretion of adrenocorticotropic hormone (ACTH) continues to follow the typical circadian rhythm, with normal basal levels, brisk response to stress, and maintenance of the servo feedback mechanism of the ACTH-cortisol axis [11]. Abdominal computed tomography (CT) is especially valuable in imaging the adrenal glands, and by using this technique, virtually all Cushing's adrenal adenomas can be identified [19]. When combined with chest CT scan, ectopic ACTH-producing tumors can frequently be identified [20]. Classically, endogenous hypercortisolism may be classified as follows:

- I. ACTH-dependent
  - A. Pituitary
    - 1. Corticotrope adenoma
    - 2. Corticotrope multinodular hyperplasia
  - B. Ectopic
    - 1. Ectopic ACTH-secreting tumor
    - 2. Ectopic corticotropin-releasing hormone–secreting tumor
    - 3. Ectopic ACTH-secreting and corticotropin-releasing hormone–secreting tumor
- II. ACTH-independent
  - A. Unilateral adrenal disease
    - 1. Adenoma
    - 2. Carcinoma
  - B. Bilateral adrenal disease
    - 1. Macronodular hyperplasia
    - 2. Primary pigmented nodular adrenal disease (Fig. 32-2)

In this representative group of patients (see Table 32-4), there was no operative mortality. Postoperative morbidity was confined to a single 69-year-old patient (patient no. 4) who required postadrenalectomy abdominal exploration for control of hemorrhage from a duodenal ulcer. This was coincidentally the only patient in whom a concomitant procedure (cholecystectomy and excision of a gastric leiomyoma) was performed. This is in keeping with our overall experience during the period 1981 through 1991 in which we encountered an operative mortality of 2.6% with a concomitant morbidity of 4% [21]. Of the 13 patients in whom no concomitant abdominal operative procedure was planned, the adrenal glands were explored via the posterior approach in 11 patients. We continue to favor this approach and are impressed with the minimal postoperative morbidity that ensues and with the decrease in length of hospitalization. Although often more technically demanding, it is an approach that is "bad for the surgeon, but good for the patient." Our current indications for the posterior approach to the adrenal glands are (1) bilateral adrenocortical hyperplasia (Cushing's disease), (2) aldosterone-producing adenomata, and (3) small (<5.0 cm) nonfunctioning and functioning adenomata. In all of these instances, naturally, no concomitant abdominal procedures should be either planned or indicated.

Interest in laparoscopic adrenalectomy is steadily growing. Our experience to date has been limited and, as yet, we are unsure what the exact role of this new approach will be in the practice of adrenal surgery.

All patients with hypercortisolism undergoing adrenalectomy require supplemental corticosteroid administration. Patients who have undergone bilateral adrenalectomy are eventually tapered to a maintenance dosage of prednisone (7.5 mg in divided doses) and usually mineralocorticoid fludrocortisone acetate (Florinef, 0.1 mg/day). Unilaterally adrenalectomized patients should have gradual total withdrawal of exogenous corticosteroids. This slow withdrawal may require 6 to 12 months.

It should be stressed again that the surgical treatment of choice for Cushing's disease in patients of any age continues to be transsphenoidal hypophysectomy, which is performed with low mortality and, in most experienced neurosurgical centers, a cure rate of 80% to 85% [17]. In our

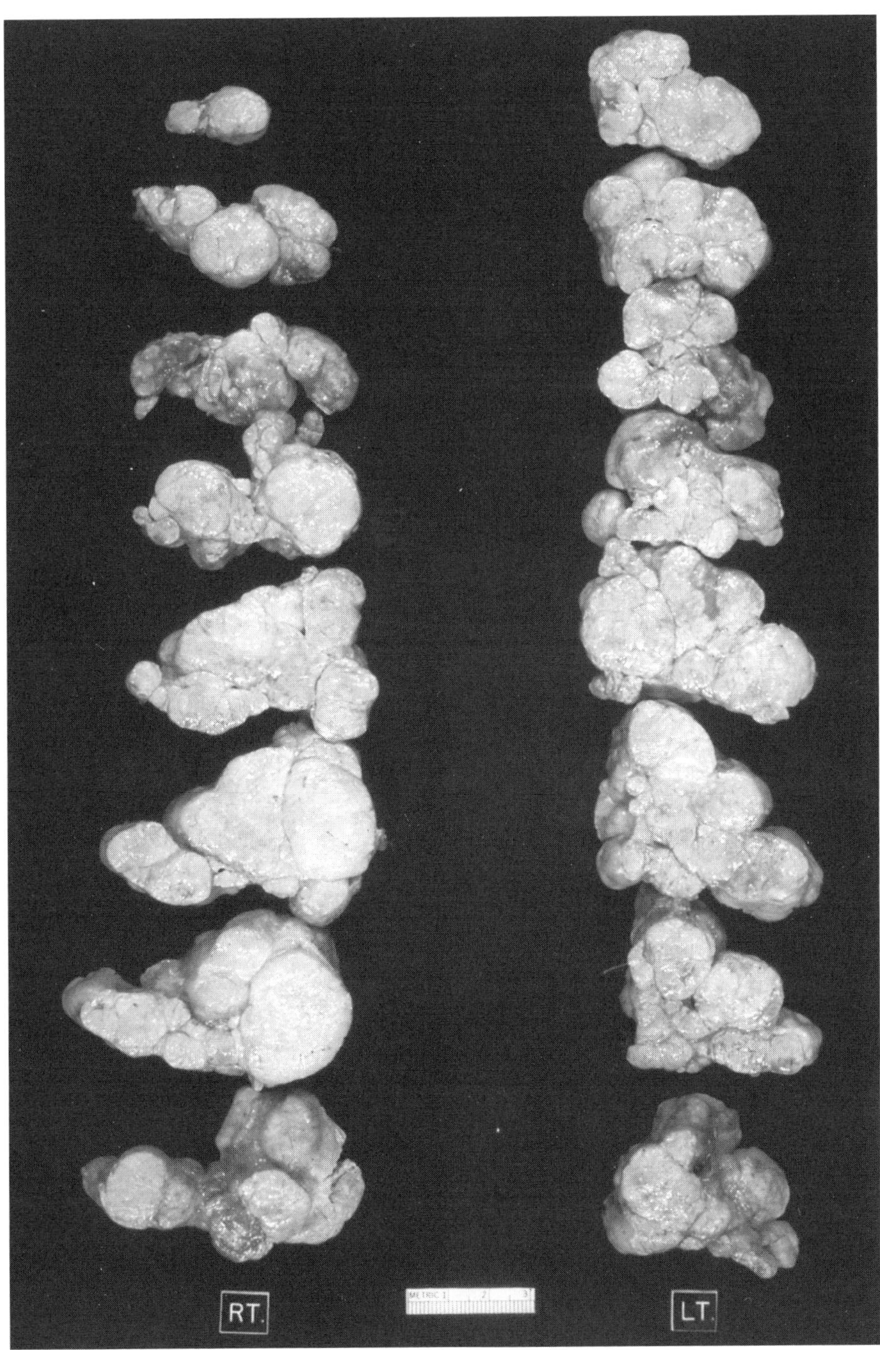

FIG. 32-2. Gross appearance bilateral microfollicular and macrofollicular non–adrenocorticotropic hormone-dependent adrenocortical hyperplasia.

opinion, the principal indicators for adrenalectomy in the patient with Cushing's disease are (1) when pituitary surgery fails, (2) when rapid and assured control of hypercortisolism is indicated, and (3) when concomitant abdominal operations are required.

INCIDENTALOMAS (NONFUNCTIONING ADRENOCORTICAL ADENOMAS)

During the period 1989 through 1993, 44 patients underwent excision of nonfunctioning adrenocortical adenomata at our institution. Of these, 14 (32%) were in patients over the age of 65 years. In contrast to the well-accepted agreement about the health benefits from and the value of adrenalectomy in the treatment of Cushing's syndrome, considerable controversy exists about the proper method of management for these nonfunctioning adrenal tumors. In 1974, some investigators considered all nonfunctioning adrenal tumors to be malignant [22]. However, this was before the advent of CT and subsequent radiologic discovery of more small, asymptomatic adrenal tumors (incidentalomas). Approximately 1% to 15% of normal individuals harbor these asymptomatic tumors as reported in autopsy series [23,24]. These

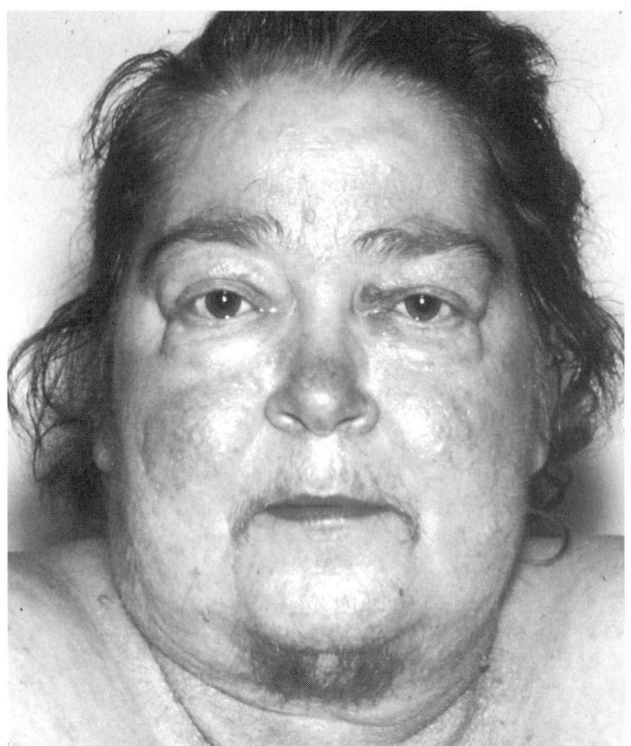

FIG. 32-3. Patient with adrenocortical carcinoma. Typical cushingoid appearance with additional features of virilization.

tumors seem to represent localized overgrowth of adrenocortical cells, may be considered a normal part of the aging process, and are more common in patients with hypertension, cardiovascular disease, and diabetes [25].

When such a nodule of the adrenal gland is discovered, particularly if the tumor is >1.0 cm in diameter, appropriate tests should always be performed to exclude the presence of abnormal hormonal activity because unsuspected pheochromocytomas have been uncovered in this manner [26]. As a minimum workup, all of these patients should have morning and evening cortisol levels, urinary metanephrines, and serum potassium determinations to exclude Cushing's syndrome, pheochromocytoma, and primary hyperaldosteronism, respectively. The principal dispute then revolves around whether these tumors should be excised or simply observed with serial CT scans. One report seriously questions the advisability of ever using the conservative approach when four of eight incidentally discovered tumors were found to be malignant [27]. With the real potential of incubating a cancer, caution is therefore emphasized when deciding to allow small tumors to enlarge. There is support for the aggressive approach to these lesions but most reports advise selective surgical excision [28–30]. We have taken a somewhat more aggressive approach than Copeland, who prefers to watch some tumors up to 6 cm [28]. Somewhat arbitrarily, we have advised adrenalectomy for the treatment of all nonfunctioning adrenal tumors >4.0 cm unless other medical contraindications exist [12,17,31]. Additionally, we are encouraged by the discriminatory power of magnetic resonance imaging (MRI), separating pheochromocytomas and adrenal metastases from primary cortical tumors [32,33]. Whether this modality will prove to be as valuable in distinguishing an adrenocortical carcinoma from a benign adenoma still remains to be seen.

As seen in Table 32-5, our incidentalomas varied in size from 3.0 to 6.0 cm and were benign adenomata in all instances. In four patients (25%), a concomitant abdominal procedure was planned. The operative mortality was confined to a single patient (6.2%) (patient no. 1), who died of a pulmonary embolus 26 days postadrenalectomy, whereas another 73-year-old man required a prostatectomy in the postoperative period because of urinary retention. Because the pathology was both benign and nonfunctional in all of these patients, the dilemma regarding the decision for or against surgical removal is thus readily evident. We believe that the indications for elective excision of incidentally discovered nonfunctional adenomas should be (1) tumors >4.0 cm in diameter, (2) tumors that have enlarged on serial CT, (3) the patient's desire (anxiety), and (4) occurrence in younger patients (<45 years).

ADRENAL CORTICAL CARCINOMA

Primary carcinoma of the adrenal cortex is an extremely rare malignancy, accounting for only an estimated 0.2% of all cancers. This is reflected in our own experience: During the years 1989 through 1993, we saw and operated on only 19 patients with adrenocortical carcinomas of whom six (32%) were over the age of 65. This rarity, by nature, leads to few centers and few individual surgeons who have had a large experience with these interesting, highly malignant tumors. It is both intriguing and depressing to deal with these patients, intriguing because the tumor presentation is often bizarre and depressing because the prognosis, regardless of the treatment used, is in most instances dismal.

Adrenocortical carcinoma should be suspected when one or a combination of several of the following occur:

1. A mixed hormonal picture is seen with adrenocortical carcinomas, which will often produce and secrete not only corticosteroids but mineralocorticoids and sex hormones as well (Fig. 32-3). Usually one of these hormones produced by the cancer will cause a dominant clinical presentation, for example, Cushing's syndrome. If carefully tested, most of these patients with adrenocortical carcinoma are found to have a mixed hormonal picture. This is in contrast to the pure, single hormonal production of both benign adenomas and adrenocortical hyperplasia.
2. Excessive urinary ketosteroid production is seen, usually measuring >30 to 40 mg/day.
3. A disproportionate ketosteroid elevation is common. These latter two features suggest that there is a rapid cell turnover and an immaturity of the ongoing biochemical process.

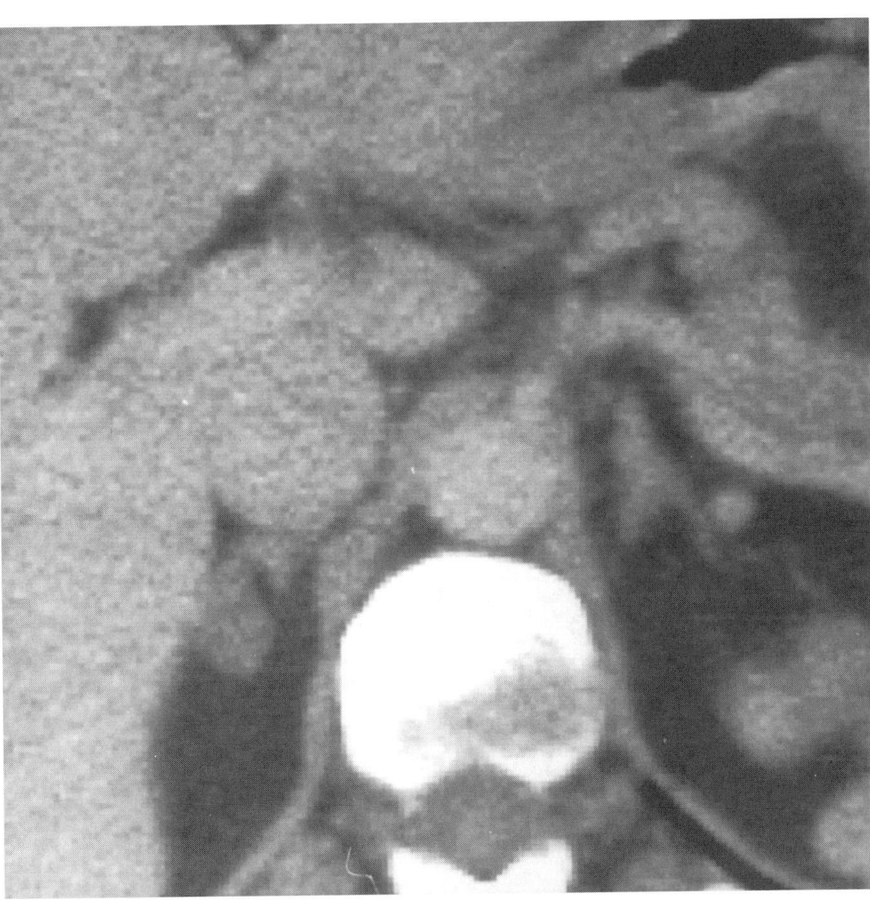

FIG. 32-4. Computed tomographic scan demonstrating a normal right adrenal gland and a 9.9-cm left pheochromocytoma.

4. Abdominal symptoms, in particular abdominal pain, and the finding of an abdominal mass suggest the diagnosis.
5. Rapid onset of this disease contrasts with that of Cushing's syndrome secondary to either adrenocortical or pituitary adenoma in which case the onset of the disease may be so insidious that the diagnosis may be missed for a long time.
6. Elevation of dehydroepiandrosterone level is another reflection of the immaturity of the biochemical process in the rapidly growing malignancy. The malignant cells are biochemically immature and inefficient, which in turn leads to a high level of 17-ketosteroids and a high urinary level of corticosteroid precursor metabolites.

Presentation

In a study from our institution, we found that 58% of adrenocortical carcinomas were functioning, whereas 42% were nonfunctioning [34]. Those that presented with hormonal function were divided into Cushing's syndrome (42%), a mixed syndrome (33%), mineralocorticoid excess (11%), and miscellaneous (14%). The 42% of patients who presented with nonfunctioning tumors were diagnosed and categorized according to their presenting findings as follows: pain (33%), fatigue (29%), abdominal mass (17%), unexplained weight loss (14%), and fever of unknown origin (7%).

Localization

The accurate localization of the side and exact site of adrenal tumors, in general, has been revolutionized since the advent of CT in the mid-1970s. CT remains the modality of choice for localizing adrenal tumors and cysts of all types. Experience with MRI is growing, and the early results are promising, particularly the possibility of differentiating between benign versus malignant and functioning versus nonfunctioning adrenal tumors. One of the benefits of CT is the ease with which the contralateral adrenal gland can be visualized. This obviates the unnecessary surgical exploration of the opposite gland in most instances, especially when a normal gland is clearly visualized by this study (Figs. 32-4 through 32-6).

Pathology

Most adrenocortical carcinomas are either grade 2 or 3 lesions (Broder's classification). Metastases are quite common. Usual sites of spread include local invasion (42%), followed by liver (22%), lung (23%), regional lymph nodes (5%), distal lymph nodes (3%), peritoneum (5%), bone (3%), and small bowel (2%). Most adrenocortical carcinomas are large, with most series reporting a mean diameter of 12 to 14 cm (Fig. 32-7). We have never encountered a

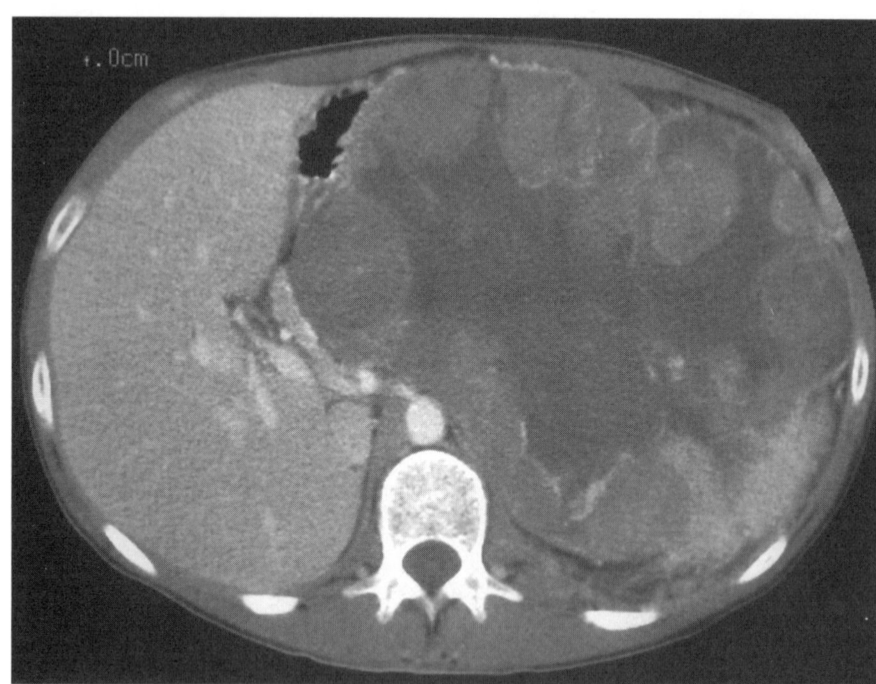

FIG. 32-5. Computed tomographic scan demonstrating a huge left adrenal tumor.

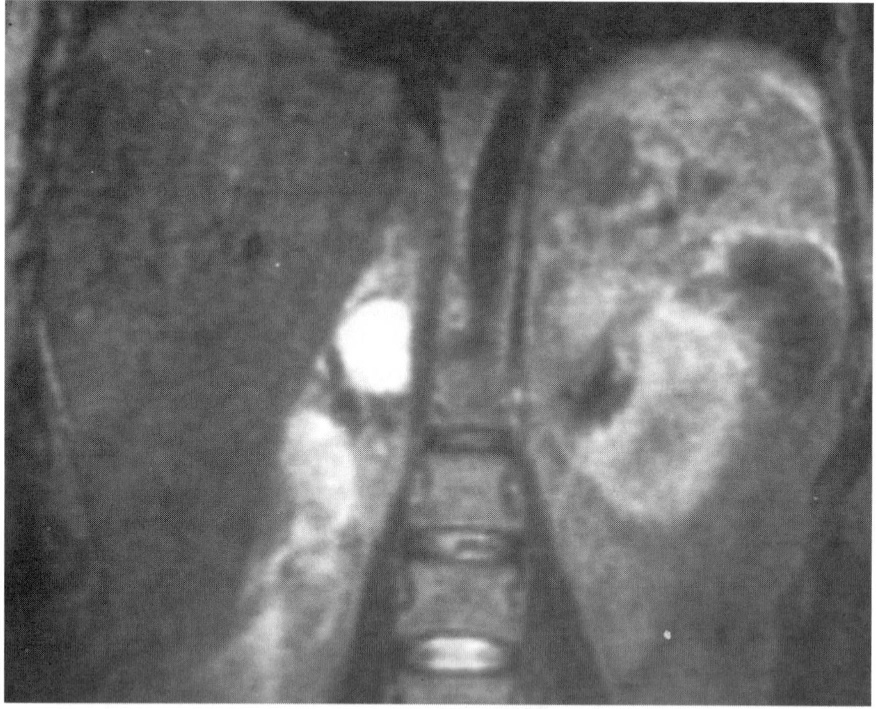

FIG. 32-6. Magnetic resonance image demonstrating functioning (pheochromocytoma) right adrenal tumor.

malignant adrenocortical tumor of <4.5 cm in diameter. As is true of most malignant endocrine tumors, the histologic diagnosis of adrenocortical carcinoma is difficult. This is particularly true if a needle biopsy or a small local surgical biopsy is performed. The surgeon can greatly aid the pathologist in establishing the exact diagnosis, particularly by identifying and removing suspected sites of extra-adrenal spread. All patients undergoing operation for adrenocortical carcinoma should be staged according to the criteria of McFarlane, subsequently modified by Sullivan (Table 32-6).

Operation

The treatment of choice for all malignant adrenocortical tumors is surgical extirpation. Unfortunately, this has been

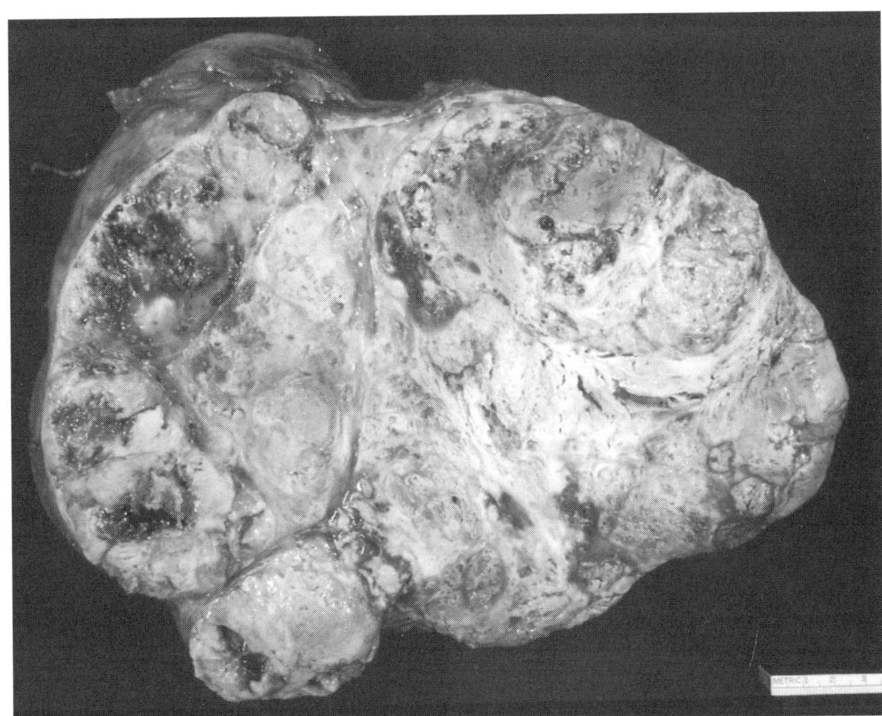

FIG. 32-7. Typical gross appearance of an adrenocortical carcinoma.

possible in our experience in only 50% of patients undergoing abdominal exploration. This has also been the experience of others. At the time of resection, great care should be taken to stage the patient accurately and greater care not to rupture the capsule of the tumor. Rupture and spillage of the tumor virtually ensures the possibility of local recurrence in the near future.

Adjuvant Therapy

Although a great variety of protocols for adjuvant therapy have been tried, the only chemotherapeutic modality that holds promise (albeit minimal) is that of a prolonged course of mitotane (Ortho'DDD), an adrenolytic agent. The drug dose is as follows:

1. Adrenolytic: Ortho'DDD, 1 to 2 g/day for 18 months.
2. Palliation: (a) Aminoglutethimide, 1 to 2 g/day (principally blocks the conversion of cholesterol to pregnenolone), and (b) metyrapone, 2 to 6 g/day (blocks the conversion of deoxycortisol to cortisol).

Approximately two-thirds of patients with nonresectable disease respond by showing evidence of corticosteroid suppression following initiation of Ortho'DDD therapy. Perhaps more exciting is the prospect of using this as adjuvant treatment in patients who have been resected for cure. Some of these patients are subsequently treated with an 18-month course of this chemotherapeutic agent. The best study supporting this concept is that by Steingart and his colleagues [35], although we have not been able to duplicate this favorable experience [36].

TABLE 32-6. *Staging criteria (McFarlane and Sullivan)*

T1	Tumor ≤5 cm, no invasion
T2	Tumor >5 cm, no invasion
T3	Tumor any size, locally invading, but not involving adjacent organs
T4	Tumor any size, locally invading adjacent organs
N0	No regional positive nodes
N1	Positive regional nodes
M0	No distant metastatic disease
M1	Distant metastatic disease
Stage I	T1N0M0
Stage II	T2N0M0
Stage III	T1 or T2N1M0, T3N0M0
Stage IV	Any T, any N, M1, T3N1, T4

Survival

The overall 5-year survival of patients with malignant adrenocortical tumors in our experience has been approximately 16%. This cure rate, however, increases to 32% in the subgroup of patients resected for cure. The mean survival for patients with stages I, II, III, and IV lesions is 25, 24, 28, and 12 months, respectively. In our study of patients undergoing palliative resection, we found that this exercise afforded no increased survival when compared to exploration with biopsy alone.

Summary of Data in Patients Over 65 Years of Age

Our experience with the six patients over the age of 65 with adrenocortical carcinoma is summarized in Table 32-7.

TABLE 32-7. *Summary of data in patients 65 years of age or older undergoing adrenalectomy for adrenocortical cancer (1989 to 1993)*

Age (yrs)/ sex	Presentation	Hypercortisolism	Hyperaldosteronism	Sex hormones	Size (cm)	Morbidity	Follow-up (mos)
76/F	Persistent edema	X	—	X	10.5	—	Died of tumor progression (6)
77/F	Elevated blood pressure	—	X	—	10.0	Died of sepsis (20 days)	—
71/F	Pain	—	—	—	10.0	Died of pulmonary embolism (30 days)	—
72/M	Abdominal swelling	X	—	—	9.5	—	Died of tumor progression (4)
66/M	Incidental	—	—	—	4.5	Died of myocardial infarction (21 days)	—
67/M	Weight loss	—	—	—	7.6	—	Died of pneumonia, with no evidence of disease recurrence (19)

They represent rather classically encountered features for patients of any age with this disease. In particular, the findings were as follows: (1) The correct preoperative diagnosis was seldom made. The modes of presentation, signs, and symptoms were vague and nonspecific in all patients. This led to delayed diagnosis. (2) The mean diameter of the tumors was approximately 9.0 cm. (3) The operative mortality was 50%. (4) The mean survival of the three surviving patients was 9.6 months.

PHEOCHROMOCYTOMA

> Although morphologically benign, it is physiologically malignant.
>
> —Epperson

1927 was a banner year for surgical endocrinology: The first insulinoma was operated on, as was the first pheochromocytoma in North America, both by Dr. C.H. Mayo in Rochester, MN. Earlier that year, the first pheochromocytoma in the world, however, had been resected in Lausanne, Switzerland, by Professor Roux of Roux-en-Y fame. Since that time, pheochromocytoma (the great mimicker) has intrigued all investigators, principally because of its fascinating and bizarre behavior and presentation. It remains one of the six causes for surgically remedial hypertension, the others being (1) coarctation of the aorta, (2) primary hyperaldosteronism, (3) Cushing's syndrome, (4) thyrotoxicosis, and (5) renal artery stenosis.

From 1989 to 1994, 54 patients underwent surgical exploration at our institution for proven pheochromocytomas; of these, nine (17%) were in patients over the age of 65.

Presentation

The classic presentation of a patient with a pheochromocytoma is bouts of paroxysmal hypertension. This occurred in 72% of 110 patients of all ages treated by us [37]. The investigator should be careful not to rule out the diagnosis of pheochromocytoma in a patient presenting with steadily sustained hypertension only. The classic spells of paroxysmal hypertension are characterized by cardiac awareness, tachycardia, occipital headaches, anxiety, flushing, sweating, nausea, and vomiting. During these spells, a systolic blood pressure of 160 to 260 mm Hg or more is usually obtained. Besides having the presentation of sustained and paroxysmal hypertension, the patient with a pheochromocytoma may also present with an abdominal mass. The presence of a pheochromocytoma may be found serendipitously during the investigation of patients from families with the multiple endocrine neoplasia type 2 syndrome.

Catecholamine Metabolism

There are three main catecholamines (dopamine, norepinephrine, and epinephrine) whose metabolic pathway (along with their degradation products) is depicted as in Fig. 32-8.

Diagnosis

Although the diagnosis may be clinically suspect, the definitive diagnosis of pheochromocytoma and of a catecholamine excess depends on the chemical demonstration of the same. This can be performed by measuring either the degradation products (metanephrines, vanillylmandelic acid, or homovanillic acid) or by direct measurement of the catecholamines themselves. The most reliable of all these measurements is the measurement of urinary fractionated catecholamines (dopamine, epinephrine, and norepinephrine) by high-pressure liquid chromatography. The measurement of 24-hour urinary metanephrines is a good screening test and the result is positive in approximately 96% of

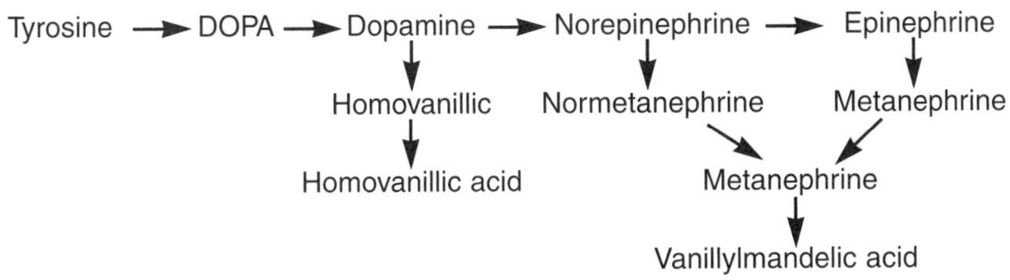

Tyrosine → DOPA → Dopamine → Norepinephrine → Epinephrine
Dopamine → Homovanillic → Homovanillic acid
Norepinephrine → Normetanephrine → Metanephrine
Epinephrine → Metanephrine → Metanephrine
Metanephrine → Vanillylmandelic acid

FIG. 32-8. The three main catecholamines (dopamine, norepinephrine, and epinephrine) and their metabolic pathways (along with their degradation products) are shown.

patients with a pheochromocytoma. Both false-positive and false-negative results may, however, be obtained if the patient has received intravenous radiographic contrast material within 48 hours of metanephrine determination.

Localizing Modalities

At the time of this writing, only three modalities for the localization of adrenal medullary tumors need to be discussed: CT, ^{131}I metaiodobenzylguanidine (MIBG), and MRI. These have supplanted all other localizing modalities. MIBG is of special interest because it is known to be concentrated only in an abnormal adrenal medulla (adrenal medullary hyperplasia or pheochromocytoma) or in a paraganglioma. When MIBG is administered, it is important to block iodine uptake by the thyroid gland by the administration of iodine 24 hours before and 7 days after the scan. We have found the MIBG scan to have a sensitivity of 79%, a specificity of 96%, and an overall accuracy of 88% (Fig. 32-9) [38]. The scan is of major benefit in a patient with either a suspected malignant or recurrent pheochromocytoma. Additionally, it may be of great help in a patient suspected of having multiple adrenal or extra-adrenal pheochromocytomas or paragangliomata, for example, the multiple endocrine neoplasia 2A and B syndromes, neurofibromatosis, Carney's triad (i.e., multiple paragangliomata, atrial myxomas, and gastric leiomyomas), and the von Hippel–Lindau disease.

Our experience with MRI for pheochromocytoma is steadily increasing; of particular importance is the seeming ability of MRI to differentiate between functioning and nonfunctioning medullary and cortical tumors (see Fig. 32-6). In our experience [37], the positive and negative predictive value for MRI is 90% and 50%, respectively.

Preoperative Preparation

We believe that all patients with pheochromocytomas require both alpha- and beta-blockade preoperatively. With this pharmacologic blockade, there is no need for intravenous volume expansion. The drugs we currently recommend are phenoxybenzamine (Dibenzyline), 30 to 90 mg per day for 7 to 10 days, and propranolol (Inderal), 30 mg per day for 3 days. This preoperative blockade requires careful monitoring in the older patient who may be less tolerant of induced changes in blood pressure. We aim for nasal stuffiness and postural hypotension as an end point, both being evidence of adequate alpha-blockade.

Operative Strategy

The secret to the successful outcome during resection of the pheochromocytoma is to "steal the tumor away from the patient." By this we mean that there will be minimal intraoperative tumor manipulation with early adrenal vein ligation whenever possible. In the past, we adhered to the recommendation that all pheochromocytomas should be approached transabdominally. The posterior approach, however, which has been suggested by others, may be used for tumors approximately ≤6 cm when excessive intraoperative tumor manipulation is not anticipated. This has been facilitated by adequate preoperative blockage, although the posterior approach must be viewed with great caution in the elderly patient.

A successful outcome is also predicated on the active participation of an anesthesiologist experienced in the management of hypertensive episodes. These intraoperative hypertensive episodes, which occur commonly during tumor manipulation despite adequate blockade, are best managed by the immediate infusion of sodium nitroprusside (Nipride). Both hypotension and cardiac arrhythmias (with the exception of sinus tachycardia) are uncommonly seen since the advent of preoperative pharmacologic blockade. Post–tumor removal hypotension is mild and occurs in approximately 20% to 25% of patients.

In patients with a history of cardiac disease and particularly in older patients (>55 years), we believe it is valuable to place a Swan-Ganz catheter. The postoperative course of the majority of our patients is totally uneventful—no unusual pharmacologic or fluid manipulation is necessary—a situation that is largely due to the routine institution of preoperative alpha- and beta-blockade.

Pathology

Pheochromocytomas are equally distributed between the right and left adrenal glands (Fig. 32-10). Extra-adrenal tumors (paragangliomata) and bilateral tumors occur in approximately 10% to 15% of patients and are more common in patients with multiple endocrine neoplasia type 2A or B syndromes (medullary thyroid carcinoma, pheochro-

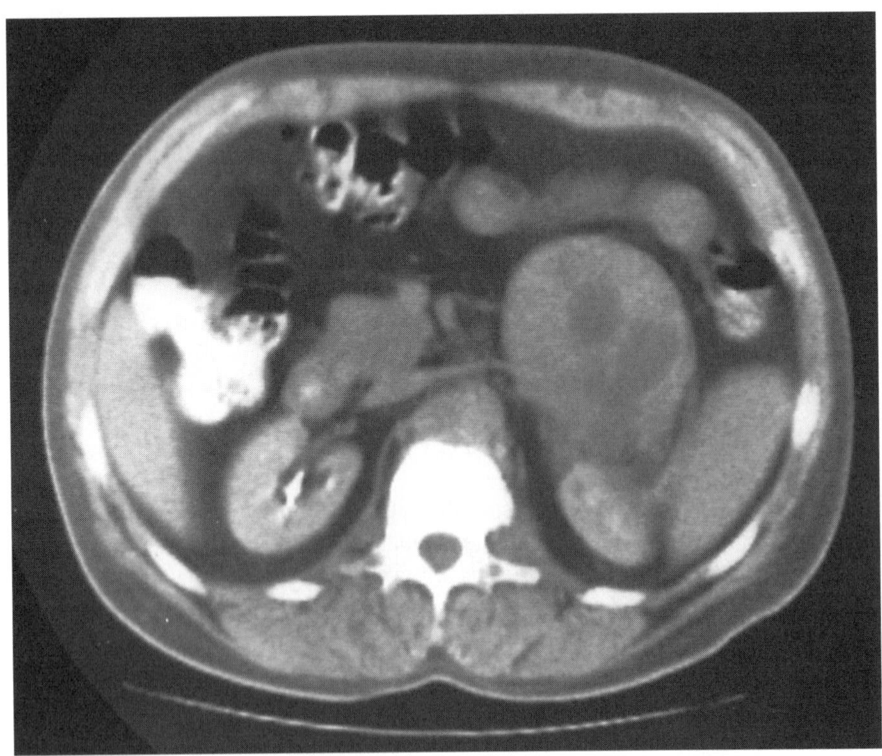

A

FIG. 32-9. (A) Computed tomographic scan demonstrating large, partly cystic left pheochromocytoma. **(B)** ^{131}I meta-iodobenzylguanidine scan confirming the pheochromocytoma.

mocytoma, normal [A] and abnormal [B] phenotype, and hyperparathyroidism) (Fig. 32-11) [39]. In these syndromes, the cellular pathology varies from the subtle changes of the precursor of pheochromocytoma (adrenal medullary hyperplasia) to frank bilateral tumor formation. These familial syndromes occur in approximately 10% of patients with pheochromocytoma. Approximately 10% of pheochromocytomas are malignant, with this incidence increasing to close to 50% in patients with extra-adrenal tumors (paragangliomata).

Prognosis

The operative mortality is 4% to 5% for patients undergoing tumor resection. In those patients with malignant pheochromocytomas, the 5-year survival is approximately 50%. Of importance to most patients, however, is the cure of the hypertension and the freedom from the severe paroxysmal attacks. If the preoperative hypertension was paroxysmal, almost all patients can be assured of a normotensive state postoperatively. In those patients who present with sustained hypertension, two-thirds should be rendered normotensive, with one-third requiring some form of antihypertensive medication postoperatively. Those patients with symptomatic metastatic pheochromocytoma can be well controlled with long-term phenoxybenzamine administration. In patients with benign disease, as documented by yearly urinary studies, the paroxysmal attacks cease.

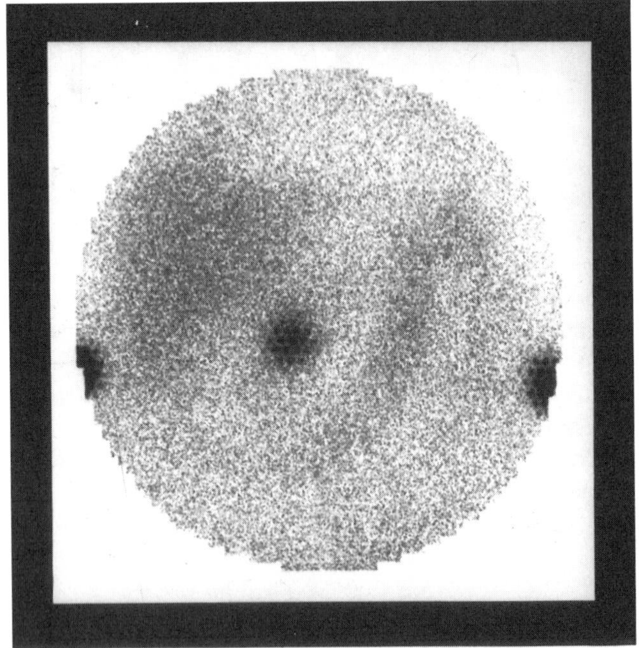

B

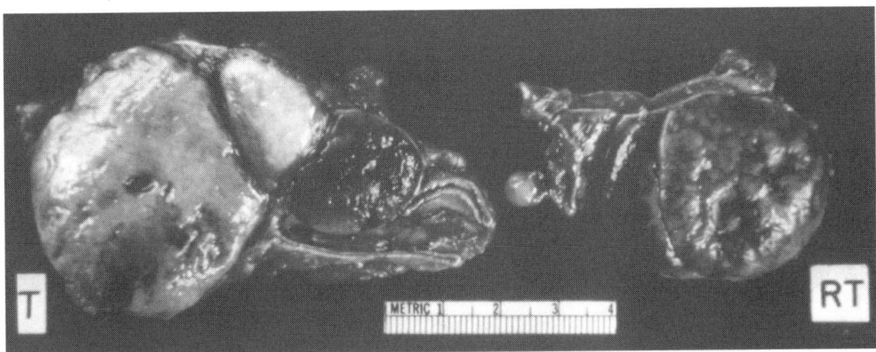

FIG. 32-10. Typical gross appearance of sporadic pheochromocytoma.

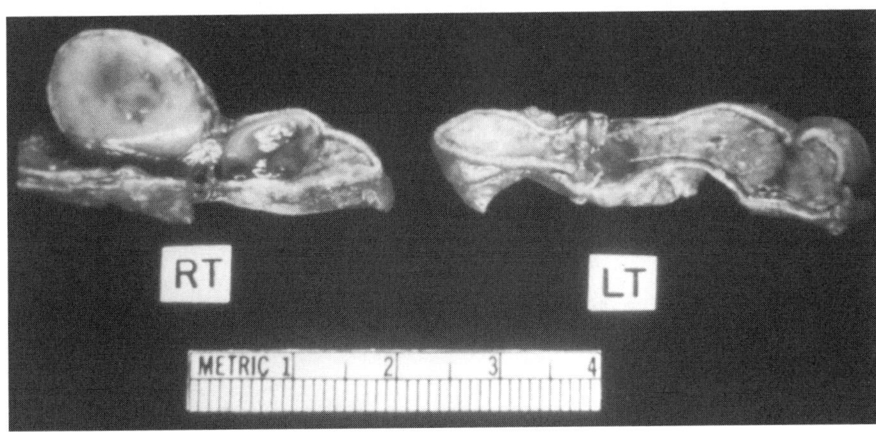

FIG. 32-11. Typical bilateral tumors with associated adrenal medullary hyperplasia in a patient with multiple endocrine neoplasia II.

TABLE 32-8. *Summary of data in patients 65 years of age or older undergoing adrenalectomy for pheochromocytoma (1989 to 1993)*

Age (yrs)/sex	Presentation	Catecholamines	Pathology (cm)	Follow-up (mos)
68/M	Acute hyperparathyroidism	Increased	Malignant (7.0)	Well (31)
81/F	Asymptomatic	Increased	Benign (3.0)	Well (17)
67/F	Asymptomatic	Normal	Benign (2.0)	Well (48)
71/F	Spells	Increased	Benign (5.0)	Well (33)
69/M	Arrhythmia	Increased	Benign (7.0)	Well (24)
78/M	Incidental	Increased	Benign (10.0)	Well (12)
65/M	Spells	Increased	Benign (3.0)	Well (36)
67/F	Spells	Increased	Benign (8.0)	Died (26)
67/F	Fatigue	Increased	Benign (2.6)	Well (12)

Summary of Data in Patients Over 65 Years of Age with Pheochromocytoma

Our experience with the nine patients of 65 years of age and older who had pheochromocytoma is summarized in Table 32-8. Several important features are worth noting:

1. Urinary catecholamine secretion was measured in all patients, being elevated in all but one, and affirming the accuracy of catecholamine determination.
2. The operative mortality was 0%, emphasizing that surgical resection of pheochromocytomas, a once feared undertaking, can today be performed by experienced endocrine surgeons and experienced support personnel with negligible morbidity and mortality.
3. The 11% incidence of malignancy is in keeping with most other reports.
4. At completion of this study, eight of the nine patients were alive, with the cause of death in the one patient being cerebral vascular accident.

PRIMARY ALDOSTERONISM

During the period 1989 through 1993, 46 patients underwent adrenalectomy for primary aldosteronism at our institution. Of these, 14 (30%) were 65 years of age or older. Primary aldosteronism has a prevalence of approximately 2% in the hypertensive population and is the result of renin-independent overproduction of aldosterone. Most patients with

TABLE 32-9. *Five subtypes and treatment of primary aldosteronism*

Subtype	Treatment
Unilateral aldosterone-producing adenoma	Adrenalectomy
Bilateral idiopathic hyperaldosteronism	Medical
Unilateral primary adrenal hyperplasia	Adrenalectomy
Glucocorticoid-remediable aldosteronism	Medical
Aldosterone-producing adrenocortical carcinoma	Adrenalectomy

primary aldosteronism are asymptomatic but manifest hypertension, which is often severe and recalcitrant to conventional antihypertensive therapy, hypokalemia (severe), low plasma renin activity, and increased secretion of aldosterone.

Five subtypes of primary aldosteronism are currently recognized; this subtype recognition is important because therapy differs markedly (Table 32-9). The screening and subtype evaluation can be accomplished accurately and in a cost-effective manner by following the schemata outlined by Young (Figs. 32-12 and 32-13) [40,41].

Summary of Data in Patients Over 65 Years of Age with Primary Aldosteronism

Review of Table 32-10 emphasizes the following:

1. The diagnosis was usually delayed. In the 14 patients, hypertension (which usually required treatment with multiple antihypertensive medications) had been present for, on the average, 18.8 years, which is quite remarkable.
2. The favored surgical approach was posterior. This approach resulted in no operative morbidity or mortality.
3. All patients became normotensive postadrenalectomy, although 11 of 14 required continued antihypertensive medication. This was most often single-drug therapy taken once daily, a considerable difference from the preoperative situation.

In closing, a reiteration of an earlier statement in this chapter is worthwhile: Careful, honest analysis of surgi-

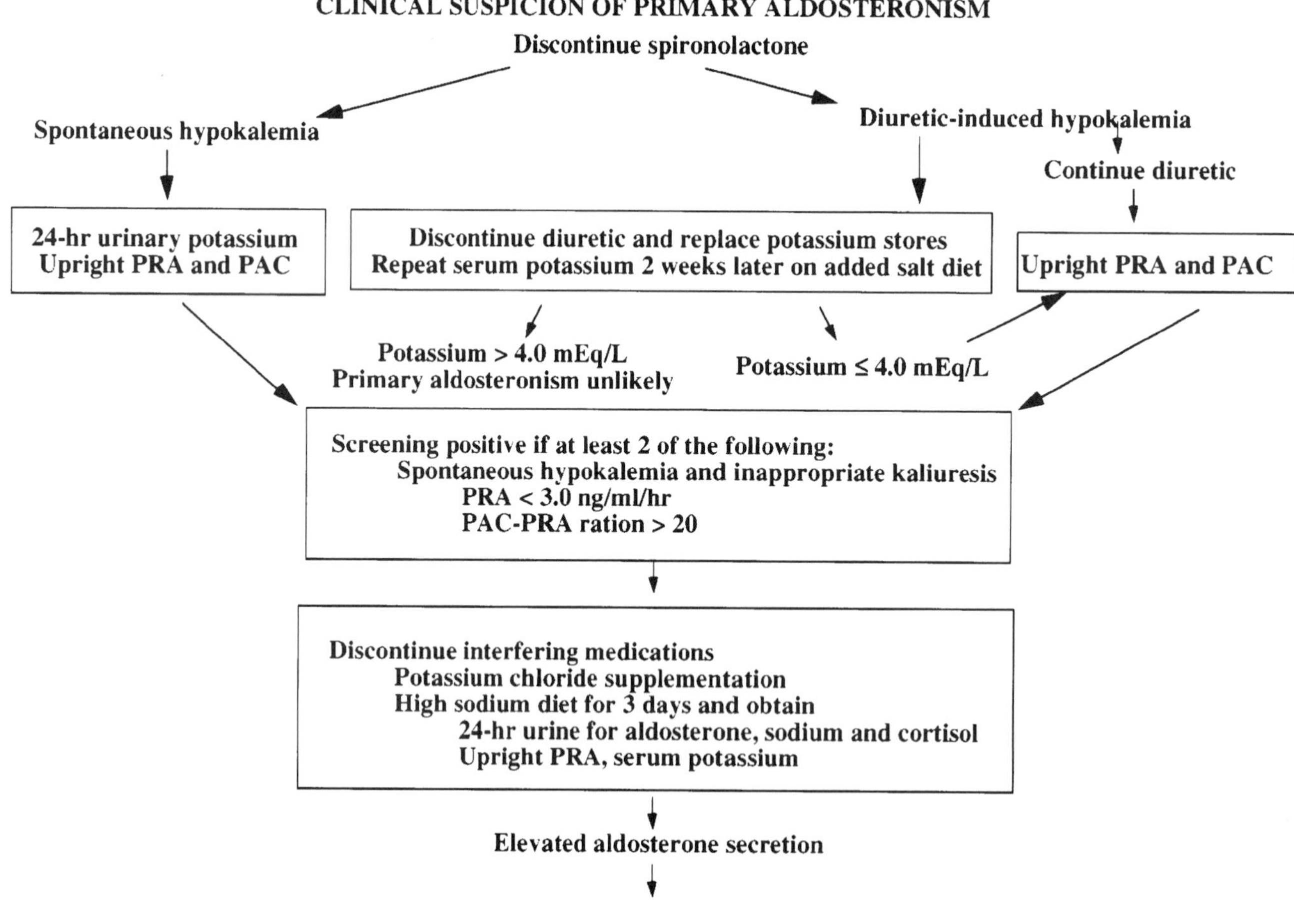

FIG. 32-12. Screening and confirmatory studies for primary aldosteronism. (PRA = plasma renin activity; PAC = plasma aldosterone concentration.) (Reprinted with permission from Young WF Jr, Hogan MJ, Klee GG, et al. Primary aldosteronism: diagnosis and treatment. Mayo Clin Proc 1990;65:96–110.)

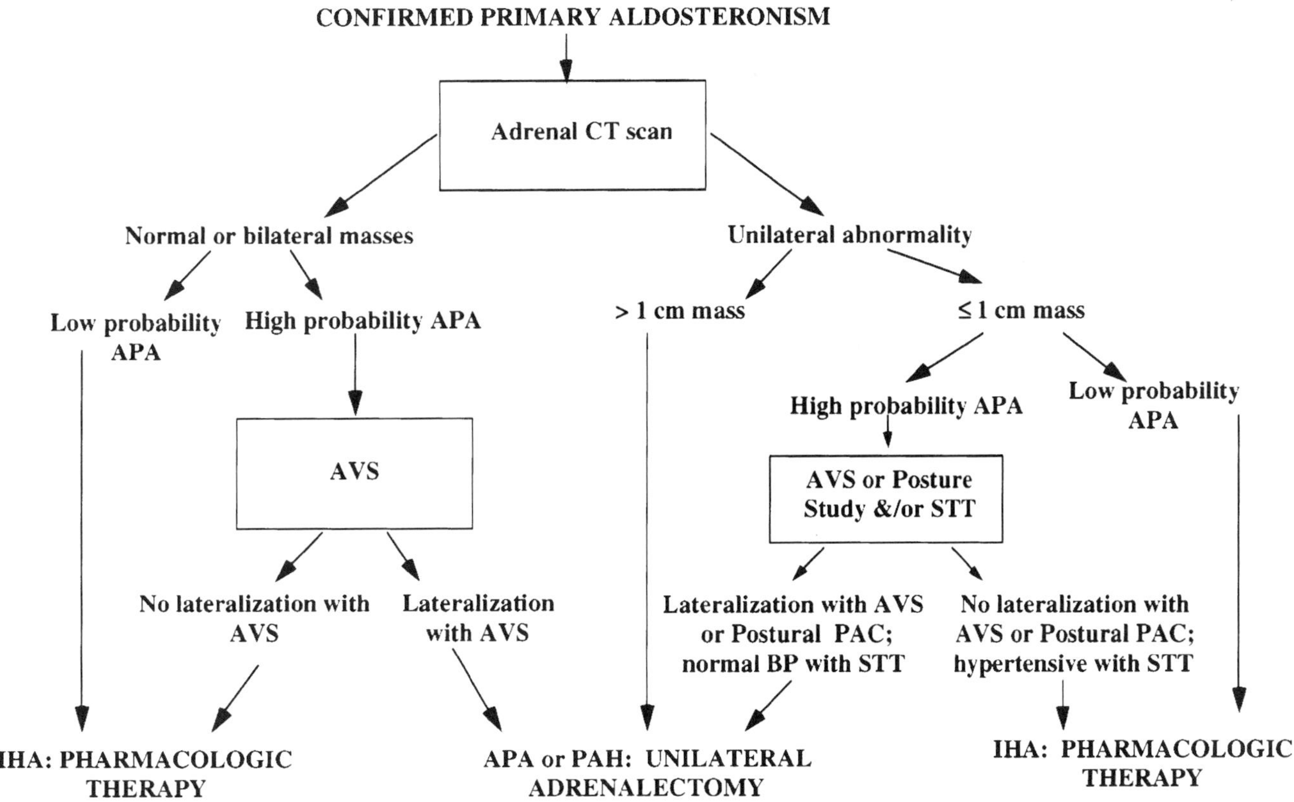

FIG. 32-13. Subtype evaluation of primary aldosteronism. (CT = computed tomography; APA = aldosterone-producing adenoma; PAC = plasma aldosterone concentration; AVS = adrenal venous sampling; STT = spironolactone treatment trial; PAC = plasma aldosterone concentration; BP = blood pressure; PAH = primary adrenal hyperplasia; IHA = idiopathic hyperaldosteronism.) (Reprinted with permission from Young WF Jr, Hogan MJ, Klee GG, et al. Primary aldosteronism: diagnosis and treatment. Mayo Clin Proc 1990;65:96–110.)

TABLE 32-10. *Summary of data in patients 65 years of age or older undergoing adrenalectomy for primary aldosteronism (1989 to 1993)*

Age(yrs)/ sex	Duration of hypertension (yrs)	Pathology (cm)	Approach	Normotensive	Antihypertensive medications	Follow-up (mos)
67/M	20	Adenoma (0.8)	Posterior	Yes	No	6
69/M	12	Hyperplasia	Posterior	Yes	Yes	8
66/M	5	Adenoma (1.0)	Posterior	Yes	Yes	54
69/M	30	Adenoma (1.2)	Posterior	Yes	Yes	48
68/M	20	Adenoma (2.0)	Posterior	Yes	Yes	40
71/M	23	Adenoma (0.9)	Laparoscopic	Yes	Yes	11
67/M	8	Adenoma (1.5)	Posterior	Yes	Yes	17
69/M	40	Adenoma (2.0)	Posterior	Yes	No	20
65/F	20	Hyperplasia	Posterior	Yes	Yes	9
69/M	20	Adenoma (1.5)	Anterior	Yes	Yes	55
67/M	20	Adenoma (0.9)	Posterior	Yes	No	12
70/M	20	Adenoma (1.1)	Posterior	Yes	Yes	36
65/F	25	Adenoma (1.0)	Posterior	Yes	Yes	13
66/F	25	Adenoma (2.0)	Posterior	Yes	Yes	18

cal results, one's own and those of others, is the cornerstone of individual surgical judgment. This judgment is of paramount importance in the care of all surgical patients, but particularly in the care of senior citizens in all of our practices.

REFERENCES

1. Sharp N, Devlin JT, Rinmer JM. Renal failure obfuscates the diagnosis of Cushing's disease. JAMA 1986;256:2564–2565.
2. Ramirez G, Gomez-Sanchez C, Meikle WA, Jubiz W. Evaluation of the hypothalamic hypophyseal adrenal axis in patients receiving

long-term hemodialysis. Arch Intern Med 1982;142:1448–1452.
3. Wallace EZ, Rosman P, Toshav N. Pituitary-adrenocortical function in chronic renal failure: studies of episodic secretion of cortisol and dexamethasone suppressibility. J Clin Endocrinol Metab 1980;50:46–51.
4. Kelly J, O'Malley K. Adrenoceptor function and aging. Clin Sci 1984;66:509–515.
5. Ziegler MG, Lake CR, Kopin IJ. Plasma noradrenalin increases with age. Nature 1976;261:333–335.
6. Lake CR, Ziegler MG, Coleman MD, Kopin U. Age adjusted plasma norepinephrine levels are similar in normotensive and hypertensive subjects. N Engl J Med 1977;296:208–209.
7. Hegstad R, Brown RE, Jiang NS, et al. Aging and aldosterone. Am J Med 1983;74:442–448.
8. Noth RH, Lassman MN, Tan SY, et al. Age and the renin aldosterone system. Arch Intern Med 1977;137:1414–1417.
9. Touitou Y, Sulon J, Bogden A, et al. Adrenal circadian system in young and elderly human subjects: a comparative study. J Endocrinol 1982;93:201–210.
10. Blichert-Toft M, Christensen V, Engquist A, et al. Influence of age on the endocrine-metabolic response to surgery. Ann Surg 1979;190:761–770.
11. Blichert-Toft M, Hammer L. Immunoreactive corticotropin reserve in old age in man during and after surgical stress. J Gerontol 1976;31:539–545.
12. Goldman L, Caldera DL, Nussbaum SR, et al. Multifactorial index of cardiac risk in noncardiac surgical procedures. N Engl J Med 1977;297:845–850.
13. Mason JH, Gau FC, Byme MP. General Surgery. In Steinberg FU (ed), Cowdry's The Care of the Geriatric Patient (5th ed). St. Louis: Mosby, 1976;299–325.
14. Dodd RB. Anesthesia. In Steinberg FU (ed), Cowdry's The Care of the Geriatric Patient (5th ed). St. Louis: Mosby, 1976;217–246.
15. Del Guercio LRM, Cohn JD. Monitoring operative risk in the elderly. JAMA 1980;243:1350–1355.
16. Edis AJ, Grant CS, Egdahl RH. Manual of Endocrine Surgery (2nd ed). New York: Springer, 1984;151–205.
17. Carpenter PC. Cushing's syndrome: update of diagnosis and management. Mayo Clin Proc 1986;61:49–58.
18. Ohashi M, Kato K, Nawata H, Ibayashi H. Adrenocortical responsiveness to graded ACTH infusions in normal young and elderly human subjects. Gerontology 1986;32:43–51.
19. Hattery RR, Sheedy PF, Stephens DH, van Heerden JA. Computed tomography of the adrenal gland. Semin Roentgenol 1981;16:290–300.
20. White FE, White MC, Drury PL, et al. Value of computed tomography of the abdomen and chest in investigation of Cushing's syndrome. BMJ 1982;284:770–774.
21. van Heerden JA, Young WF Jr, Grant CS, Carpenter PC. Adrenal surgery for hypercortisolism: surgical aspects. Surgery 1995;117:466–472.
22. Lewinsky BS, Grigor KM, Symington T, Neville A. The clinical and pathologic features of "non-hormonal" adrenocortical tumors. Cancer 1974;33:778–790.
23. Russi S, Blumenthal HT, Gray SH. Small adenomas of the adrenal cortex in hypertension and diabetes. Arch Intern Med 1945;76: 284–291.
24. Dobbie JW. Adrenocortical nodular hyperplasia: the aging adrenal. J Pathol 1969;99:1–18.
25. Neville AM. The nodular adrenal. Invest Cell Pathol 1978;1:99–111.
26. Prinz RA, Brooks MH, Churchill R, et al. Incidental asymptomatic adrenal masses detected by computed tomographic scanning: is operation required? JAMA 1982;248:701–704.
27. Seddon JM, Baranetsky N, VanBoxel PJ. Adrenal "incidentalomas:" need for surgery. Urology 1985;25:1–7.
28. Copeland PM. The incidentally discovered adrenal mass. Ann Intern Med 1983;98:940–945.
29. Glazer HS, Weyman PJ, Sagel SS, et al. Nonfunctioning adrenal masses: incidental discovery on computed tomography. AJR Am J Roentgenol 1982;139:81–85.
30. Mitnick JS, Bosniak MA, Megibow AJ, Naidich DP. Nonfunctioning adrenal adenomas discovered incidentally on computed tomography. Radiology 1983;148:495–499.
31. Herrera MF, Grant CS, van Heerden JA, et al. Incidentally discovered adrenal tumors: an institutional perspective. Surgery 1991;110: 1014–1021.
32. Reinig JW, Doppman JL, Dwyer AJ, et al. Adrenal masses differentiated by MR. Radiology 1986;158:81–84.
33. Glazer GM, Woolsey EJ, Borrello J, et al. Adrenal tissue characterization using MR imaging. Radiology 1986;158:73–79.
34. Henley DJ, van Heerden JA, Grant CS, et al. Adrenal cortical carcinoma—a continuing challenge. Surgery 1983;94:926–931.
35. Steingart DE, Motazdy A, Noonan RA, Thompson NW. Treatment of adrenal carcinoma. Arch Surg 1982;117:1142–1146.
36. van Heerden JA, Grant CS, Weaver AL. Primary carcinoma of the adrenal cortex: an institutional surgical perspective. Acta Chirurg Aust 1993;25:216–220.
37. Orchard T, Grant CS, van Heerden JA, Weaver A. Pheochromocytoma—continuing evolution of surgical therapy. Surgery 1993;114: 1153–1158.
38. Swenson SJ, Brown MJ, Sheps SG, et al. Use of 131-MIBG scintigraphy in the evaluation of suspected pheochromocytoma. Mayo Clin Proc 1985;60:299–304.
39. van Heerden JA, Sizemore GW, Carney JA, et al. Surgical management of the adrenal glands in multiple endocrine neoplasia type II syndrome. World J Surg 1984;8:612–621.
40. Young WF Jr, Hogan MJ, Klee GG, et al. Primary aldosteronism: diagnosis and treatment. Mayo Clin Proc 1990;65:96–110.
41. Young WF Jr. Primary Aldosteronism. In Rakel RE (ed), Conn's Current Therapy 1993. New York: Saunders, 1993;610–614.

Surgical Care for the Elderly, 2nd ed., edited by
R. Benton Adkins, Jr., and H. William Scott, Jr.
Lippincott–Raven Publishers, Philadelphia © 1998.

CHAPTER 33

Trauma

John A. Aucar and Kenneth L. Mattox

The successful management of the traumatized elderly patient is a clinical challenge that demands the firm appreciation of the basic principles encompassed in acute trauma care and the special demands imposed by advanced age. These demands result from structural and physiologic differences between elderly persons compared with those with greater physiologic reserve, in addition to those demands imposed by an increased incidence of underlying systemic disease. Thirty-six percent of trauma victims between 65 and 74 years old were found to have preexisting disease in a regional review of >27,000 trauma admissions [1]. This increased to 41% of those 75 years of age or older. Length of hospital stay was found to be significantly related to age, Injury Severity Score (ISS), and the presence of preexisting disease. Because the elderly represent an increasing proportion of the general population, and many elderly patients remain productive and active well past the age of 65, it is clear that the social and economic implications of trauma among the elderly are significant.

There is no precise definition of elderly; however, the age at which the elderly patient is commonly distinguished from the remainder of the population is somewhat arbitrarily designated at 65 years old. This seems to be the age at which the risk of death by falls begins to increase and correlates to an increasing incidence of strokes. The risk of death from cancer and heart disease begins to increase sharply at between 45 and 50 years of age [2]. Both chronologic and physiologic aging occur as a continuous spectrum, and "premature aging" is encountered relatively commonly. The single most important function of age distinction is to facilitate statistical analysis. Some perspectives regarding trauma care in the elderly stem from specific reviews of injuries encountered in this population, whereas others stem from extrapolation of principles encountered in the care of elderly patients with other surgical diseases. Principles learned from risk assessment in elective and emergency surgery should be applied to the trauma patient until specific data become available. Advanced age may carry an increased risk of morbidity or mortality for any major physiologic insult. This risk should not affect management decisions, except for the most elective of interventions, because the complications associated with missed or untreated injuries can be devastating to the elderly.

The nearly 31 million Americans over age 65 represented approximately 12.4% of the population in 1993 [2] compared with 11% in 1981 [3]. Although there was a slight increase in the number of accidental deaths, from 24,000 to 25,500, in this age group, accidents dropped from the fifth to the seventh leading cause of death. This represents approximately 1.7% of deaths among older Americans. The accidental death rates in patients 65 years old and older is greater than the average accidental death rate for all ages combined. However, it remains well below the accidental death rate in the group aged 15 to 24 years, where a peak of 44% of deaths are caused by accidents. Table 33-1 summarizes the mortality among major trauma victims by age, taken from analysis of 46,613 patients under the Major Trauma Outcomes Study of The American College of Surgeons. The peak mortality from trauma occurs in the group aged 75 to 84 years old (see Table 33-1) [4].

When examined from the standpoint of hospital admission for trauma, one must take into account the type of hospital and setting. The North Carolina trauma registry, which includes level I and II trauma centers statewide, recorded 17% of their 21,000 trauma admissions over a 3-year period to affect patients 65 years old or older [5]. Less than 6% of the nearly 8,700 trauma admissions for a 2-year period at the Ben Taub General Hospital in Houston, Texas, involved patients in that age group (Ben Taub Trauma Registry, 1993–1994). National data from 1985 indicates that although the elderly made up 12% of the population, they consumed 23% of the trauma volume and 28% of the cost of trauma care [6]. Although trauma predominately affects young people, any institution involved in the management of acute injuries must be attuned to the special needs of the elderly traumatized patient.

TABLE 33-1. *Overall mortality by age group*

Age (yrs)	Percent
14–24	8.9 (1,716/19,169)
25–34	9.8 (1,231/12,496)
35–44	9.8 (570/5,809)
45–54	10.6 (323/3,051)
55–64	14.4 (348/2,419)
65–74	15.6 (285/1,658)
75–84	20.1 (281/1,396)
85+	16.9 (104/615)

Source: Finnelli FC, Jonsson J, Champion HR, et al. A case control study for major trauma in geriatric patients. J Trauma 1989;29:541.

TABLE 33-2. *Mechanism of injury incidence and mortality*

	>65 years		<65 years	
Injury	Incidence (%)	Mortality (%)	Incidence (%)	Mortality (%)
Fall	46.0	11.7	11.0	6.0
Motor vehicle accident	28.2	20.7	33.5	9.0
Pedestrian hit	10.0	32.6	7.9	13.5
Stab wound	2.6	17.3	11.9	4.7
Gunshot wound	5.5	52.1	13.0	19.5
Motorcycle accident	0.4	11.8	7.7	11.9
Other	7.0	13.8	14.9	5.4
Unknown	0.3	19.0	0.1	9.8
Total	100	—	100	—

Source: Finnelli FC, Jonsson J, Champion HR, et al. A case control study for major trauma in geriatric patients. J Trauma 1989;29:541.

GENERAL CONSIDERATIONS IN ELDERLY TRAUMA

Trauma Scoring

There have been some organized attempts to identify the utility of trauma scoring systems in elderly patients. One of these, a retrospective study from the University of Tennessee, showed that a 10% probability of death was reached with an ISS of 17.3 in older patients compared with 23.9 in patients <65 years old [7]. The mortality was related to the cause and severity of trauma and the number of complications. There was an increased mortality for less severe injuries relative to a younger patient group. However, there did not seem to be an increased risk of mortality based on preexisting disease. A prospective British study found the Trauma and Injury Severity Score (TRISS) methodology to show correlation with the probability of survival, except for elderly patients with single orthopedic injuries in which there were major differences between the observed and expected outcomes [8]. Another British study found discrepancies between the outcomes and risk assessed by TRISS and reverse trauma score methods, suggesting that the TRISS makes inadequate allowances for the effects of age and that the ISS/age method is more reliable [9]. A Belgian study of 126 multiply injured patients 65 years old and older found no significant difference in age or ISS between survivors and nonsurvivors although they found the Glasgow Coma Scale had significant prognostic value for both survival and functional recovery [10]. In that series, 83% of the patients were still alive at 6 months and 78% of the survivors who lived at home before injury were able to return to their normal surroundings. Nine percent of the survivors had undergone prolonged endotracheal intubation. Based on the mixed results encountered in the literature, trauma scoring systems should be applied with caution in elderly patients until further refinements improve their reliability. The greatest value of scoring systems remains their ability to provide for the comparison of patient groups rather than to predict the survival of individual patients. Perhaps the clinical course in the early post-traumatic period will reflect a likelihood of long-term survival. Resource allocations notwithstanding, aggressive trauma care for the elderly is justified.

Injury Risk, Patterns, and Prevention

Elderly people lack many of the protective mechanisms that younger people take for granted. Impaired visual acuity, dark adaptation, accommodation, and peripheral vision, as well as decreased hearing, leave the elderly person vulnerable to environmental dangers, which might otherwise be avoided. These factors are frequently aggravated by the presence of cataracts, glaucoma, and vestibular degeneration. Weakness caused by declining muscle mass and aggravated by arthritic impairment and coordination difficulties can lead to slowed reaction times in the face of impending danger. Postural hypotension can be found in 10% of those over age 65 and may result from decreased cardiovascular adaptability or from accentuated side effects of commonly encountered medications [11]. These factors can turn a seemly benign and innocuous environment, such as the home, into a hazardous trauma trap.

Although the specific patterns of injury are related to the mechanism encountered in any given instance, the distribution of injuries is quite different between young and old populations. The relative incidence of various mechanisms of injury and their associated mortality in patients over and under 65 years of age is illustrated in Table 33-2 [4].

Falls are a relatively infrequent mechanism of injury in younger patients; however, falls are a common cause of death in the elderly. Falls contribute to approximately 1.5 times more traumatic deaths than motor vehicle accidents in the patients aged 75 and over [2]. Motor vehicle accidents are the most common mechanism of injury in patients aged 65 to 74 and second most common in those 75 and over. Among the 25 million licensed drivers aged 65 and older in the United States, there is a relatively low rate of fatal motor vehicle accidents per number of drivers, but a high rate per number of miles driven [2]. Ethanol intoxication is implicated as a contributing factor in motor vehicle accidents only one-fifth as often among elderly drivers compared with youths [12]. The elderly are involved in automobile-pedestrian accidents more commonly than any other age group, including children [13].

Burns are the third leading cause of death among elderly trauma victims. Advanced age significantly reduces the chance of surviving major burn injuries [14,15]. Major inhalation injuries are nearly uniformly fatal in elderly burn victims [15]. However, percent of total body surface area burned is still the most significant predictor of burn injury outcome [15,16]. Burns involving >10% of body surface area in the elderly should be considered serious and those involving >40% to 50% of body surface area are nearly always fatal [14,15].

Another important mechanism of injury, frequently overlooked and most likely under-reported, is elder abuse. Numerous misguided motives may lead the caregivers, often family members of elderly persons, to a variety of insults ranging from neglect to violent assault. When the instigator of a life-threatening injury happens to be the next of kin, also responsible for subsequent decisions regarding level of care, the managing physician may find himself or herself in a difficult social dilemma. In such cases it is appropriate to notify legal and administrative authorities immediately so that guardianship and proxy for medical affairs may be reassigned.

The most desirable method by which to minimize the morbidity and mortality of trauma among the elderly is prevention. Public awareness and education about the implications of trauma should be a part of any community health program. There are many overlooked opportunities to improve safety in the home, public places, and institutions devoted to the care of elderly persons. Table 33-3 lists a number of specific measures by which the environment can be modified to improve safety and reduce the risk of injury among the elderly [17].

TABLE 33-3. *Home safety checklist*

- Institutional setting
  - Check bed for proper height
  - Check floor for throw rugs
  - Check lighting in hallways and pathway to bathroom
  - Check bathroom tub and toilet for proper height
- House setting
  - Bathroom
    - Use rubber mats in tub
    - Install grab bars in tub or shower and by toilet
    - Take up floor mats when not in use
    - Adjust height of toilet seat
  - Outside
    - Provide adequate lighting in walkways
    - Repair uneven or cracked sidewalks
    - Install handrails on stairs and steps
    - Keep shrubbery trimmed on pathway to house
  - All living spaces
    - Check for adequate illumination
    - Eliminate toys and low-lying furniture
    - Secure carpet edges
    - Reduce clutter
    - Put light switches at top and bottom of stairs
    - Install night lights at outlets near stairs
    - Make sure steps are even and of the same size and height
    - Avoid waxing floors
    - Remove door thresholds
    - Remove throw rugs
    - Remove cords and wires from floor
    - Ensure phone is reachable from floor

Source: Reprinted with permission from Rubenstein LZ, Robbins AS, Schulman BL, et al. Falls and instability in the elderly. J Am Geriatr Soc 1988;36:266.

Metabolic Response to Injury

The physiologic changes by which trauma victims respond to their injuries have been well studied and include a hypermetabolic phase with an obligatory nitrogen and potassium loss and an increase in catecholamines, mineral corticoid, glucocorticoid, and antidiuretic hormone levels [18]. The stress response includes increased oxygen consumption and activation of leukocyte-produced inflammatory mediators. This complex metabolic response requires significant physiologic reserve and sometimes can even overwhelm the young and healthy, leading to a systemic sepsis syndrome. Elderly patients began at a disadvantage, frequently unable to compensate for the increased respiratory and cardiovascular demands, and often are unable to balance the physiologic demands imposed by injury with those inherent in resuscitation and treatment. A study from the Ben Taub General Hospital, suggested that early and aggressive fluid resuscitation in penetrating trauma is not as beneficial as previously thought and may be detrimental to patient outcome [19]. Whether these early findings will be applicable to blunt trauma and specifically to elderly trauma victims remains to be examined. The current belief is that the principles of trauma care should transgress any boundaries of age and should be applied more diligently and with less error in the elderly population.

Initial Evaluation

One of the basic principles of modern trauma care is that evaluation and management of the trauma victim must begin at the scene of injury. Recurrent controversies have arisen regarding the relative utility of initiating treatment in the field compared with immediate transport to a trauma center [20] and the relative value of various transportation modes. The use of air evacuation by helicopters had significant impact on the effective management of battlefield trauma in the Vietnam war [21]. However, its extrapolation to contemporary civilian settings has met with mixed reviews [22–24]. An efficient emergency medical ground transport system is not only more cost-effective, but superior to air transportation, with a possible exception of wilderness, high-rise, and off-shore rescues. Delay of transportation for the sake of initiating resuscitative measures is rarely indicated except perhaps for emergency airway management [25]. A prospective cohort study from Hartford Hospital compared the resource use between a group of trauma patients transported directly from the scene to a trauma center, with those subsequently referred to a trauma center after initial care at another hospital [25]. They found that the average length of stay for patients transported directly to a trauma center was much shorter than that for patients received by interhospital transfers. That study recognized that elderly patients use more resources than younger patients matched for severity of injury and advocated the direct transport of severely injured patients to a trauma center for definitive care. The primary consideration of any field intervention is to prevent the patient's deterioration or aggravation of injuries during transportation for definitive care.

Elderly patients remain more vulnerable to aggravation of their injuries during initial management, due to many of the same factors that originally predisposed them to injury. Limited homeostatic reserve makes it imperative that they be protected from excessive exposure, which could rapidly lead to hypothermia. Thin and fragile skin may avulse due to shearing forces applied while simply trying to move or reposition the patient. Immobilization, when appropriate, is important to protect against the occurrence or aggravation of orthopedic injuries due to brittle bones. However, immobilization of the elderly trauma victim exposes them to cutaneous pressure ulcerations, as well as stiff joints, over a relatively short period. Venous thrombosis and subsequent pulmonary embolism may also develop rapidly due to immobilization and override the most effective trauma resuscitation.

Once in the emergency department, elderly trauma victims should be managed with the same organized approach as their younger counterparts using the advanced trauma life support protocols recommended by the American College of Surgeons Committee on Trauma [26]. These patients, however, not only have a lower tolerance for exposure, but they may not tolerate the pain-induced catecholamine response that frequently accompanies severe trauma. Manipulation of injured sites should be kept to a minimum during workup. Impaired sensation, including vision and hearing, can limit communication and aggravate the patient's anxiety. During the primary survey, the airway must be established and protected while maintaining careful protection of the cervical spine. Topical anesthesia in the hypopharynx of an awake patient about to be intubated can greatly reduce the threat of inducing tachycardia from laryngeal stimulation. Breathing should be assessed frequently and consideration given to the limited respiratory reserve frequently encountered in elderly patients. Rib cage fragility and underlying chronic lung disease make the elderly especially prone to rib fractures and pneumothorax. Traumatic intubation can precipitate pneumothorax and, if unrecognized, can be devastating. Careful assessment of circulatory and volume status is essential. Naturally decreased skin turgor can lead to a mistaken assumption of hypovolemia. Any concern for fluid intolerance makes measurement of the central venous pressure or pulmonary artery pressure advisable in the early period. Urinary catheterization is also advisable but may require special techniques due to the high incidence of hyperprostatism in elderly men. Familiarity with the use of coudé catheters and filiform followers should limit the need for suprapubic catheterization to cases involving urethral injuries. Elderly patients in apparent hemorrhagic shock should have no delay in the administration of blood combined with rapid surgical control of the bleeding site. Atherosclerosis, frequently encountered in the elderly, may aggravate preexisting circulatory compromise. This can occur by limiting vascular contraction, which is normally a protective mechanism against bleeding. In addition, it can promote intravascular thrombosis during low flow states, near or away from the site of injury, including the coronary circulation. These considerations emphasize the need for rapid, careful, and effective management of the elderly trauma victim during the early postinjury phase.

During the secondary survey, it is imperative to use all available information, including that obtained during the prehospital period and primary survey. A detailed past medical history is essential, including medication use, allergies, and an assessment of baseline functional status. Because these histories are often complex, contact with the patient's primary physician and review of previous records can be extremely helpful. A detailed assessment of preexisting conditions and the patient's physiologic reserve requires careful evaluation of cardiovascular, pulmonary, musculoskeletal, and underlying central nervous system disease. With these issues addressed, detailed examination should follow, including careful exposure and inspection of injured areas, with rapid recovering to prevent hypothermia. Consideration of specific injuries should then be pursued.

ELDERLY TRAUMA BY BODILY SYSTEM

Head Injury

Head injuries in elderly patients show similar manifestations to those in the younger population. The manifestations include altered mentation, focal sensory or motor deficits, and altered hemodynamic responses. Some elderly patients, however, may have significant underlying chronic neurologic deficits, making the separation of acute and chronic symptoms problematic. Dementia, sensory deficits, and generalized weakness may make the neurologic examination difficult to interpret. In addition, ocular disease may confound funduscopy, an important part of the neurologic examination, limiting its usefulness. Although numerous studies show a correlation between the Glasgow Coma Scale at the time of presentation with eventual neurologic recovery and survival after severe injuries, some studies show an increased reliability of that scale when evaluated at presentation and at least 6 hours after presentation [27,28]. The number of computed tomographic (CT) scan abnormalities encountered in patients with severe head injuries appears to correlate inversely with the likelihood of survival and seems to overshadow the effect of age [27]. One series of 195 elderly patients with severe head injuries showed that all patients remaining comatose at least 72 hours after injury died within 6 months and that patients with an intracranial pressure >20 mm Hg had a higher mortality at both 72 hours and 6 months after injury [29]. This study suggests that consideration be given to the level of consciousness and increased intracranial pressure when counseling families about the likelihood of recovery after major head injuries. Because there is no reliable indicator or group of indicators that accurately predicts survival or recovery from severe head injury when evaluated immediately postinjury, aggressive therapy in the early phase is justified. The standard approach of monitoring, controlled ventilation, reduction of cerebral edema, and early drainage of intracranial mass lesions are applicable to the elderly victim of head injury. Hypotension must be avoided or treated aggressively to maintain cerebral perfusion.

Musculoskeletal Injuries

Osteoporosis and skeletal muscle atrophy leave the elderly trauma victim susceptible to more severe injuries from equivalent or lesser impact than are their younger counterparts. Head injury may be associated with cervical spine injuries; these can be particularly difficult to diagnose due to associated arthritic changes. Unstable pelvic fracture usually involves injury at two locations on the pelvic ring. One of these may be ligamentous, such as sacroiliac or pubic symphyseal disruption. When pelvic fractures occur in association with motor vehicle accidents, they can be severe, with a propensity for extensive hemorrhage. Such fractures are frequently associated with intra-abdominal injuries and are usually devastating to the elderly patient. Posterior pelvic ring fractures are associated with injury to vascular structures, hemodynamic instability, and high transfusion requirements and are frequently fatal [30]. Unstable pelvic fracture are associated with a higher complication rate irrespective of age, mechanism, or anatomic location [31].

Fractures of the pubic and ischial rami secondary to falls are relatively common. These are generally stable, often do not require surgical intervention, and allow for good functional recovery. Femoral shaft and neck fractures are common in elderly patients, and are best treated by early surgical stabilization [32]. Severely injured patients (ISS >15) showed decreased mortality and hospitalization length when repair was performed at 2 to 4 days after injury. Nonsurgical treatment is often practiced in patients with overriding contraindications to surgery. These patients have a higher associated mortality and often have prolonged hospitalization. Frequently, they succumb to the complications of bed rest, including deep venous thrombosis, pulmonary embolism, pneumonia, and cutaneous pressure ulcers. Multicenter studies have established the significant reduction in mortality by early fixation of fractures associated with multiple injuries in both younger and older age groups [33]. Prophylactic anticoagulation has been used with increasing frequency in the perioperative management of orthopedic injuries. Prophylactic placement of an inferior vena cava filter is becoming increasingly popular and may reduce the risk of pulmonary embolism from occult deep vein thrombi, facilitating early mobilization. Noninvasive evaluation including duplex ultrasonography is useful for detecting the presence of preoperative and postoperative deep venous thrombosis, which should be treated by anticoagulation or caval filter placement [34]. If noninvasive means are inconclusive, venography should be performed. Early ambulation of the elderly trauma victim is of the highest importance to prevent the potentially devastating complications associated with bed rest and inactivity.

Another orthopedic injury frequently encountered in elderly patients is a Colles' fracture, resulting from a fall on the outstretched, dorsiflexed hand. This results in fracture of the distal radius in the metaphyseal area, usually accompanied by a fracture at the base of the ulnar styloid process. This can be managed by immobilization for 6 to 8 weeks. Internal or external fixation may be required in the presence of comminution or instability [35]. Fractures of the humerus frequently occur at the surgical neck and are usually characterized by pain, tenderness, and ecchymosis in the shoulder or upper arm. Impacted fractures with <1 cm displacement and <45 degree angulation can usually be treated with a shoulder sling and progressive range of motion. Disimpacted fractures generally require hospitalization and surgical fixation [36]. Patients with comminuted proximal humeral fractures may require prosthetic shoulder replacement to relieve pain and restore function [35]. Elderly patients with complex limb injuries should be considered for early amputation if associated injuries, preexisting disease, and debilitation make prolonged surgical reconstruction exceedingly risky. Age alone, however, should not be a contraindication to limb salvage. A fairly good salvage rate for type III tibial fractures with associated vascular injuries has been demonstrated in patients >60 years of age [37].

Thoracic Trauma

Chest injuries in the elderly population can be particularly devastating. Blunt chest trauma carries three times the mortality in patients >65 compared with any other age groups (Table 33-4) [38]. Although elderly patients with blunt chest trauma seem to present with a lower incidence of shock, the incidence of cardiopulmonary arrest at arrival is higher. Fractures of the bony thorax represent the most common

TABLE 33-4. *Mortality in 515 cases of blunt chest trauma by age group**

	Teens	20–40 years	41–64 years	Elderly
Deaths (%)	18	13	12	37
Survival (%)	82	87	88	63

*$p = 0.0002$.
Source: Shorr RM, Rodriguez A, Indeck MC, et al. Blunt chest trauma in the elderly. J Trauma 1989;29:234–237.

thoracic injury. Rib fractures may be associated with clavicular, scapular, or sternal fractures. Lung lacerations with subsequent pneumothorax, hemothorax, or parenchymal hemorrhage must be recognized and treated immediately. Most often, tube thoracostomy or observation is the only treatment required. Careful and continuous monitoring is essential to identify patients who initially appear stable but may require subsequent thoracotomy for persistent bleeding. A clotted hemothorax results when bleeding has stopped but the chest is inadequately drained. This can lead to lung entrapment and should be treated by operative evacuation within 3 to 5 days to optimize respiratory function and reduce the need for subsequent decortication [39]. Evacuation of clotted hemothorax should especially be considered if there is loss of 25% of lung volume on chest roentgenography and in the presence of an air-fluid level, fever, or leukocytosis.

Significant thoracic injuries can occur in the absence of fractures of the bony thorax; however, this is less common among the elderly compared with the general trauma population (13% vs. 26%) [38]. This observation is probably related to decreased chest wall compliance. Contrary to the effect of restraint systems on younger motor vehicle accident victims, lap and shoulder belts do not reduce and may increase the severity of thoracic injuries in elderly motorists [40]. Limited pulmonary reserve, reduced alveolar surface, and decreased patency of small airways can magnify the effects of chest wall injuries. Patients with underlying congestive heart failure or chronic pulmonary disease are particularly susceptible to chest injury, and even simple rib fractures can be devastating.

It is important to administer adequate analgesia by oral, parenteral, or epidural routes to optimize respiratory dynamics and minimize splinting. Mild-to-moderate degrees of flail chest usually require ventilatory assistance in patients >65, whereas an equivalent injury may be managed without a ventilator in younger patients. Arterial blood gases and pulse oximetry should be obtained for a baseline measurement and to follow the status of pulmonary injury. When contusions occur, the resulting hypoxia can be severely aggravated by excessive fluid administration. The need for ventilatory assistance should be anticipated and instituted early rather than awaiting overt respiratory failure [41].

Blunt injury to the heart can be accompanied by arrhythmias, with electrocardiographic changes and myocardial enzyme elevation. Most blunt cardiac injuries are thought to be clinically insignificant. Controversy exists about the need for prolonged monitoring and diagnostic evaluation in the absence of profound dysrhythmia [42]. Echocardiography has been recommended to evaluate wall motion abnormalities and to detect pericardial effusions. In severe cases, cardiac rupture can occur, which leads to immediate death. More commonly, the physician evaluating elderly trauma patients must attempt to distinguish a blunt myocardial injury from ischemic heart symptoms due to underlying disease. The possibility that an ischemic cardiac event precipitated the trauma must be considered. Unfortunately, measurement of fractional creatine phosphokinase is not sensitive or specific for predicting complications of blunt myocardial injury [43]. When emergency surgery is required to address traumatic injuries, it should not be delayed due to the presence of blunt myocardial trauma [44]. Invasive monitoring may improve the outcome in elderly patients with significant injuries and associated blunt myocardial injury complicated by rhythm or motion abnormalities [45]. Hemodynamic support with intra-aortic counterpulsation may benefit selected patients; however, this remains to be established in the trauma setting.

Traumatic rupture of the aorta is a serious injury in the old or young trauma victim. Five of 114 cases reported in one series affected patients >60 years old [46]. Shorr et al. reported a 75-year-old survivor of traumatic aortic rupture associated with multiple injuries [38]. Loss of elasticity and atherosclerotic plaques of the great vessels may predispose elderly patients to disruption of the vascular intima and media due to shearing forces associated with rapid deceleration. Unless the adventitia or parietal pleura remains intact, the injury is immediately lethal [47]. It is estimated that only 10% to 20% of patients with this injury reach the hospital alive. Unless the lesion is recognized and repaired, delayed rupture results in progressive mortality of approximately 1% per hour. The injury should be suspected in the presence of a suggestive mechanism or with any of the suggestive radiographic findings listed in Table 33-5 [48].

Contrast aortography has been the gold standard by which the injury is identified. Transesophageal ultrasound examination may prove to be of significant benefit. The role of dynamic sequential CT scanning is not yet defined. When encountered, it is important that the patient's blood pressure be maintained at or below normal levels to reduce the risk of delayed rupture while awaiting surgical correction.

Abdominal Injuries

Evaluation and management of abdominal injuries in elderly trauma victims pose special problems. As with inflammatory conditions, the classic signs of peritoneal irritation may not be present. However, due to impaired compensatory mechanisms, they may show signs of hypovolemic shock with relatively little blood loss. Impaired communication, associated injuries, and the use of corticosteroids can contribute to catastrophic delays in the recognition of intra-abdominal injuries. The same applies to the recognition of post-traumatic abdominal sepsis. Although elderly patients are less tolerant of surgery, they are also less tolerant of missed injury. These patients may succumb rapidly to cardiopulmonary and septic complications of untreated injuries and, therefore, an aggressive diagnostic and interventional approach is warranted. Up to 35% of elderly patients with multiple trauma have significant abdominal injuries [49]. Such injuries can have a mortality 4.7 times higher among older patients compared with young trauma victims [4]. In the absence of associated injuries or other debilitating factors, negative laparotomy results are generally well tolerated. However, in the presence of such factors, negative laparotomy results may contribute to a disastrous delay in the recognition and treatment of otherwise salvageable conditions. This leaves little margin for error in the evaluation of the elderly trauma patient. Diagnostic peritoneal lavage and CT both contribute significantly to the identification or exclusion of operable abdominal injuries [50]. Diagnostic peritoneal lavage is rapid and less costly than CT and is advocated among many high-volume trauma centers. It may be particularly helpful in elderly patients who are more likely to exhibit hypotension in the absence of intra-abdominal bleeding. A nasogastric tube and Foley catheter are essential prerequisites for performing diagnostic peritoneal lavage. CT scanning should only be considered in hemodynamically stable patients. It should include both the abdomen and pelvis and has the advantage of being able to evaluate the retroperitoneum, as well as identifying low-grade solid organ injuries that may be considered for nonoperative management. Its sensitivity is improved by the use of intravenous and upper gastrointestinal contrast. However, if a CT scan of the head is to be performed to rule out acute head injury, intravenous contrast should be withheld until completion of that study. Bolus intravenous contrast infusion can produce nausea and vomiting, making continuous airway monitoring imperative. Any patient suspected of having significant abdominal injury and undergoing CT scan should have a nasogastric tube placed. Dilute barium placed through the nasogastric tube can help delineate the duodenum and pancreas. The contrast should be evacuated immediately following the scan. Waiting for the contrast to fill the small bowel is *not* an objective in the evaluation of trauma and can lead to serious consequences.

Once operable abdominal injuries are detected, prompt surgical intervention is imperative. Further evaluation and resuscitation is usually best performed in the operating room or postoperatively. Injuries that are not life threatening can be managed once the patient's condition has been stabilized. The use of damage control laparotomy, addressing hemorrhage by ligation and packing, with subsequent staged reoperation for definitive repair, is a useful approach for major abdominal trauma [51–53]. It requires significant physiologic reserve, and elderly patients unable to tolerate abbreviated laparotomy are unlikely to survive complex injuries treated by prolonged operative intervention. With less severe injuries, it may be advisable to perform the most expeditious and definitive procedure, such as splenectomy, rather than assume the risk of continued bleeding and the need for reoperation due to a failed splenorrhaphy.

TABLE 33-5. *Plain chest radiographic clues suggestive of blunt injury to the descending thoracic aorta*

Loss of aortic knob contour
Widened mediastinum (>8 cm)
Depressed left mainstem bronchus (>140 degrees)
Lateral tracheal deviation
Left pleural apex hematoma (cap)
Deviation of nasogastric tube in esophagus from midline
First, second, or both rib fractures
Loss of left paraspinal pleural strip
Calcium layering at aortic knob
Massive left rib fractures
Obvious false aneurysm at aortic isthmus
Massive left hemothorax
Fracture of clavicle or scapula
Fracture or dislocation of thoracic spine
Loss of aorto-pulmonary window
Anterior displacement of trachea
Fracture of sternum

Source: Mattox KL, Wall MJ. Traumatic aneurysm of the thoracic aorta. Chest Surg Clin North Am 1992;1:413–421.

PERIOPERATIVE CONSIDERATIONS

Monitoring

Because of limited physiologic reserve, a high incidence of underlying systemic disease, and intolerance of traumatic stress, elderly patients are frequently monitored in an intensive care unit. This is appropriate even in association with moderate mechanisms of injury. Cardiac monitoring with careful observation of the respiratory status and intermittent or preferably continuous pulse oximetry is a minimal requirement for the moderately or severely injured elderly person. Cautious fluid administration is advised to prevent fluid overload. In cases of hemodynamic instability or severe underlying cardiac or pulmonary disease, invasive hemodynamic monitoring, including the use of an indwelling arterial catheter, and pulmonary artery catheter is recommended [45]. Line sepsis, the most common complication of invasive monitoring, must be considered and treated promptly by catheter site rotation. Prophylactic use of an antiarrhythmic medication, such as lidocaine, during insertion of central venous and pulmonary artery catheters should be considered. Balloon inflation within the pulmonary artery should be kept to minimum to avoid the infrequent but devastating complication of pulmonary artery rupture. Institutions equipped with intermediate care or step-down units may find these appropriate for observing elderly patients with mild or moderate trauma.

TABLE 33-6. *Immune defense parameters and case examples*

Decreased
IgM levels
Immunoglobulin activity
Interferon-alpha and interferon-gamma levels
Thymic hormone levels
Neutrophil chemotaxis, phagocytosis, oxygen radical production
Delayed hypersensitivity reaction
T-lymphocyte mitogen-induced proliferation
Langerhans' cell number and function
Normal (N) or unknown (U) change
IgG and IgA levels (N)
Complement levels (N)
B-lymphocyte number (N)
T-lymphocyte number (N)
T-lymphocyte subpopulation (U)
Monocyte number (N)
Neutrophil number (N)
Tissue macrophage function (U)
Interleukin 1 and 2 levels (N)

Source: Plewa MC. Altered host response and special infections in the elderly. Emerg Med Clin North Am 1990;8:193–206.

Fluid Management and Nutrition

Fluid management in the elderly can be problematic. Management of the volume status within narrow perimeters must balance the risk of hypovolemia against that of congestive heart failure. Impaired renal function may be present, even with normal laboratory values. The serum creatinine concentration may be misleadingly low in elderly patients with impaired protein metabolism. Creatinine clearance calculations based on serum creatinine are only reliable in the steady state and may underestimate the degree of renal impairment during the acute phase of injury. Tissue necrosis from crush injury, burns, or gangrene can precipitate acute renal failure and release myoglobin and free hemoglobin, as well as elevation of the serum potassium level [54].

In addition to active management of the patient's injuries and the resulting complications, it is important to provide support for any preexisting disease. Contact with the patient's primary physician is extremely valuable in assessing the baseline status and obtaining an accurate listing of current medications. The relative need for each of those medications must be reassessed in the light of acute trauma, understanding that sudden withdrawal of certain medications, such as corticosteroids, antihypertensives, and diuretics, may be devastating to the patient's physiology.

Malnutrition is relatively common among the elderly population. Despite a lower basal metabolic rate, they still require a continuous fuel source to maintain their metabolic functions. The implementation of early postoperative or post-traumatic feeding is thus a desirable goal. This often requires parenteral or enteral tube feeding [55]. Nutritional assessment should be based on a combination of anthropometric, biochemical, and clinical information as well as dietary history [56]. Total parenteral nutrition should be instituted cautiously in elderly patients, especially if there is concomitant hepatic, renal, or cardiac disease due to potential fluid intolerance [57]. Protein intolerance can result from or aggravate limited hepatic or renal reserve. Carbohydrates may be poorly tolerated due to occult diabetes and an osmotic diuresis may confuse fluid management. The high respiratory quotient that results from carbohydrate metabolism may lead to carbon dioxide accumulation and make ventilator weaning difficult. Lipid intolerance can lead to rapid accumulation resulting in fatty liver. There is some evidence that total parenteral nutrition promotes bacterial translocation from the gut [58]. Enteral feeding has become the method of choice for nutritional support [59]. Enteral feeding promotes normal gastrointestinal motility, maintains intestinal villous integrity, and decreases bacterial translocation. Enteral feeding should only be used, however, in hemodynamically stable patients who are not dependent on inotropic or vasopressor support. They must be carefully observed for any signs of gastrointestinal insufficiency, which may reflect a relative mesenteric ischemia. The physician should have a low threshold for placement of a feeding jejunostomy tube in elderly patients undergoing laparotomy for trauma. Gastrostomy likewise provides reliable gastrointestinal access for decompression or feeding, without the untoward effects of nasogastric intubation.

Infections

Infection is the most common complication encountered in trauma victims who survive their initial injury and occurred in 14.5% of 456 elderly trauma patients reviewed at the University of Tennessee [7]. Pneumonia is the most commonly encountered infectious complication; however, urinary tract infection, line sepsis, phlebitis, and cellulitis of lacerations, burns, and surgical wounds are common. Acute sinusitis can be caused by prolonged nasotracheal or nasogastric intubation. Elderly patients are known to have impairment of various immunologic mechanisms with preservation of others (Table 33-6) [60]. Frequently, fever and white blood cell responses are diminished, especially in the presence of compromised nutrition. Infections may become well established before they are recognized. Mental status changes are sometimes reflective of early sepsis and may be followed by septic shock, with a short intervening diagnostic opportunity.

Prophylactic antibiotics are useful in trauma surgery for periods <24 hours. Treatment for longer periods should be considered empiric therapy or preferably be directed by culture results. Elderly patients may be particularly vulnerable to antibiotic toxicity and bone marrow suppression. Nephrotoxic agents should be used with extreme caution. If aminoglycosides are used, once daily dosing to achieve high peak levels and allow complete clearance of the drug from the circulation is as effective as other dosing regimens with less incidence of toxicity [61,62]. Injudicious use of antibiotics is also known to promote bacterial resistance, which can be devastating in the elderly population. Pneumococcal vaccination may not be as effective following splenectomy in older patients due to impaired antibody responses. Many elderly patients lack protective immunity from tetanus and the judicious use of both active and passive immunization may help prevent this potentially lethal infection [60].

Activity

Early mobilization of the elderly trauma patient is a high priority. Inability to ambulate may result from weakness; pain due to fractures, contusions, or surgical incisions; or joint stiffness due to post-traumatic immobility. Patients with preexisting arthritis and limited ability to ambulate before trauma are likely to pose the greatest rehabilitative challenge. Reluctance to ambulate may stem from a fear of falling, especially if this was the mechanism of the patient's original injury. Patients hospitalized for falls are discharged to a nursing home more than three times more frequently than those hospitalized for other mechanisms [63]. Tethering the patient with an oxygen line, intravenous line, drains, Foley catheter, nasogastric tube, and cardiac monitors further discourages activity. It is important that these modalities be used only when their benefits outweigh their risks.

If a patient cannot ambulate, passive and active range-of-motion exercise in bed is essential to prevent further muscle atrophy and joint stiffness. Frequent turning and good nutrition are both essential to prevent or heal pressure ulcerations. Specialized beds are a useful adjunct but not a substitute for mobility in bed. An overhead trapeze can be a tremendous aid to bedridden elderly patients and provides satisfaction by allowing them to contribute to their own mobility. Any elderly trauma victim suspected of having a lower-extremity deep venous thrombosis should have a duplex venous scan. If thrombus is encountered, a vena caval filter and early ambulation is preferable to continued bed rest. Anticoagulation may still be relatively indicated to minimize the postphlebitic sequelae. Patients who must remain in bed sometimes require restraints to prevent unsuccessful ambulation or dislodgment of essential lines. Modern hospital policies require that specific indications and time limits accompany restraint orders. Restrained patients are vulnerable to a variety of restraint-related complications and are unable to protect themselves from the well-meaning but misguided interventions of their doctor or nurse.

Recovery

Elderly trauma patients by virtue of their special physiologic, psychological, and sociologic needs provide a special challenge. A coordinated effort on the part of physicians, hospital nurses, home health care nurses, physical therapists, and social workers will often be required to optimize the chances for a favorable outcome. Nurses experienced in adult medical, surgical, and intensive care units are usually well aware of these needs and often are required to provide total nursing care including repositioning, feeding, and bathing. The development of bed sores, generally thought to result from a combination of pressure and poor nutrition, can be devastating and often accounts for prolonged hospitalization after recovery from the initial traumatic insult. Elderly patients who were independent and living at home at the time of their injuries stand the best chance for rehabilitation in an independent living environment. Such rehabilitation is often a long and painstaking process. Initiating range-of-motion physical therapy helps reduce joint stiffness, which can occur even in the absence of musculoskeletal injuries. The sooner such therapy is begun, the better. Physical therapy must often be continued on an outpatient basis, and many of these patients benefit from temporary placement in rehabilitation hospitals or assisted living environments. The overall goal of therapy is to establish some element of independence and self-sufficiency for daily living. In many elderly patients the potential remains for economic productivity.

MEDICOSOCIAL ISSUES

The allocation of medical resources is a socially and politically sensitive issue. A large proportion of medical resources are currently consumed by the elderly in their last days or weeks of life. This occurs in the treatment of disease and trauma. The more severe the injury, the more likely the patient will consume advanced and expensive technological interventions. Advances in medical care have led to an increase in life expectancy and a decrease in premature death. These trends are partly responsible for the increasing proportion of elderly people in the population. However, these trends will likely reach their limit, resulting in a rectangularization of the life expectancy curve. It is likely that in the near future resource allocations will become increasingly important and consideration of age and underlying disease will lead to an economic triage, which may be unfavorable for potentially salvageable elderly trauma victims. The final effects of the current trend of managed care and capitation of health care spending are yet to be seen. We are in the midst of a changing social perspective regarding the use of "do not resuscitate" orders. The decision to withdraw or withhold care is often influenced by cultural differences, as well as the individual perspectives of physicians, patients, patients' families, administrators, and society. The principles of benevolence and comfort care are becoming increasingly accepted. Another issue in evolution involves the use of practice guidelines in trauma, whereby an algorithmic approach to the evaluation and management of injuries or injury patterns may be imposed by system design. The rigidity with which such guidelines should be used is still a matter of debate and whether these guidelines should be modified based on the patient's age will surely be a matter of debate. For such guidelines to be successful, they must be based on sound physiologic principles that are likely to transgress the consideration of age and have at least an annual mandated re-evaluation.

FUTURE PERSPECTIVES

A number of current trends will improve the ability to categorize, evaluate, and treat elderly trauma victims. Database registries will help clarify the role of trauma scoring systems and shed light on the changing epidemiology of trauma. Improvements in general care and advancing treatment technologies will, it is hoped, improve outcomes, lower mortality, and provide better functional recovery. Further study of inflammatory mediators and their role in the septic response, as well as their relation to other homeostatic mechanisms such as the coagulation cascade, will likewise also improve the odds for trauma victims of any age. More remote technology such as artificial tissues and organs may become practical in the treatment of trauma once the systemic response to injury comes under control. The development and refinement of such technologies will depend on a societal commitment to medical and surgical research and a continued interest in trauma care from a variety of medical and surgical disciplines.

REFERENCES

1. MacKenzie EJ, Morris JA, Edelstein SL. Effect of preexisting disease on length of hospital stay in trauma patients. J Trauma 1989;29: 757–765.
2. National Safety Council. Accident Facts (1993 ed). Itasca, IL: National Safety Council, 1993.
3. National Safety Council. Accident Facts (1981 ed). Itasca, IL: National Safety Council, 1981.
4. Finnelli FC, Jonsson J, Champion HR, et al. A case control study for major trauma in geriatric patients. J Trauma 1989;29:541–548.
5. Covington DL, Maxwell JG, Clancy TVC. Hospital resources used to treat the injured elderly at North Carolina trauma centers. J Am Geriatr Soc 1993;41:847–852.
6. MacKenzie EJ, Morris JA, Smith GS, Fahey M. Acute hospital costs of trauma in the United States: implications for regionalized systems of care. J Trauma 1990;30:1096–1103.
7. Smith DP, Enderson BL, Maull KI. Trauma in the elderly: determinants of outcome. South Med J 1990;83:171–177.
8. Wardrope J, Cross SF, Fothergill DJ. One year's experience of major trauma outcome study methodology. BMJ 1990;301:156–159.
9. Bull JP, Dickson GR. Injury scoring by TRISS and ISS/age. Injury 1991;22:127–131.
10 Broos PL, D'Hoore A, Vanderschot P, et al. Multiple trauma in elderly patients. Factors influencing outcome: importance of aggressive care. Injury 1993;24:365–368.
11. Martin RE, Teberian G. Multiple trauma and the elderly patient. Emerg Med Clin North Am 1990;8:411–420.
12. Wolf ME, Rivara FP. Nonfall injuries in older adults. Annu Rev Public Health 1992;13:509–528.
13. Santora TA, Schinco MA, Trooskin SZ. Management of trauma in the elderly patient. Surg Clin North Am 1994;74:163–186.
14. Banerjee C. Burns in elderly patients. J Indian Med Assoc 1993;91: 206–207.
15. Hunt JL, Purdue GF. The elderly burn patient. Am J Surg 1992;164: 472–476.
16. Bhatia AS, Mukherjee BN. Predicting survival in burned patients. Burns 1992;18:368–372.
17. Rubenstein LZ, Robbins AS, Schulman BL, et al. Falls and instability in the elderly. J Am Geriatr Soc 1988;36:266–278.
18. Sabiston DC Jr (ed). Textbook of Surgery: The Biological Basis of Modern Surgical Practice (14th ed). Philadelphia: Saunders, 1991.
19. Bickell WH, Wall MJ, Pepe PE, et al. Immediate versus delayed fluid resuscitation for hypotensive patients with penetrating torso injuries. N Engl J Med 1994;331:1105–1109.
20. Trunkey DD. Is ALS necessary for pre-hospital trauma care? J Trauma 1984;24:86–87.
21. Neel S. Army aeromedical evacuation procedures in Vietnam: implications for rural America. JAMA 1968;204:309–313.
22. Cocanour CS, Ursic CM, Fischer RP. Are scene flights for penetrating trauma justified [abstract]? J Trauma 1995;39:166.
23. Schiller WR, Knox R, Zinnecker H, et al. Effect of helicopter transport of trauma victims on survival in an urban trauma center. J Trauma 1988;28:1127–1134.
24. Baxt WG, Moody P. The impact of a rotorcraft aeromedical emergency care service on trauma mortality. JAMA 1983;249:3047–3051.
25. Schwartz RJ, Jacobs LM, Yaezel D. Impact of pre-trauma center care on length of stay and hospital charges. J Trauma 1989;29:1611–1615.
26. Alexander RH, Proctor HJ. Advanced Trauma Life Support Program for Physicians (5th ed). Chicago: American College of Surgeons, 1993;19–37.
27. Waxman K, Sundine MJ, Young RF. Is early prediction of outcome in severe head injury possible? Arch Surg 1991;126:1237–1242.
28. Pal J, Brown R, Fleiszer D. The value of the Glasgow Coma Scale and Injury Severity Score: predicting outcome in multiple trauma patients with head injury. J Trauma 1989;29:746–748.
29. Ross AM, Pitts LH, Kobayashi S. Prognosticators of outcome after major head injury in the elderly. J Neurosci Nurs 1992;24:88–93.
30. Klein SR, Saroyan RM, Baumgartner F, Bongard FS. Management strategy of vascular injuries associated with pelvic fractures. J Cardiovasc Surg 1992;33:349–357.
31. Poole GV, Ward EF, Griswold JA, et al. Complications of pelvic fractures from blunt trauma. Am Surg 1992;58:225–231.
32. Fakhry SM, Rutledge R, Dahners LE, Kessler D. Incidence, management, and outcome of femoral shaft fracture: a statewide population-based analysis of 2805 adult patients in a rural state. J Trauma 1994; 37:255–261.
33. Bone LB, McNamara K, Shine B, Border J. Mortality in multiple trauma patients with fractures. J Trauma 1994;37:262–265.
34. Fishmann AJ, Greeno RA, Brooks LR, Matta JM. Prevention of deep vein thrombosis and pulmonary embolism in acetabular and pelvic fracture surgery. Clin Orthop 1994;305:133–137.
35. Kerns RJ, Gartsman GM. Upper Extremity Fractures and Dislocations. In Mattox KL, Moore EE, Feliciano DV (eds), Trauma (2nd ed). Norwalk, CT: Appleton & Lange, 1988;597–605.
36. Neer CS II. Displaced proximal humeral fractures: classification and evaluation. J Bone Joint Surg Am 1970;52:1077–1089.
37. Ritchie AJ, Small JO, Hart NB, Mollan RAB. Type III tibial fractures in the elderly: results of 23 fractures in 20 patients. Injury 1991;22: 267–270.
38. Shorr RM, Rodriguez A, Indeck MC, et al. Blunt chest trauma in the elderly. J Trauma 1989;29:234–237.
39. Eddy AC, Carrico JC, Rusch VW. Injury to the Lung and Pleura. In Mattox KL, Moore EE, Feliciano DV (eds), Trauma (2nd ed). Norwalk, CT: Appleton & Lange, 1988;357–371.
40. Martinez R, Sharieff G, Hooper J. Three-point restraints as a risk factor for chest injury in the elderly. J Trauma 1994;37:980–984.
41. Levy DB, Hanlon DP, Townsend RN. Geriatric trauma. Clin Geriatr Med 1993;9:601–620.
42. Mattox KL, Fline LM, Carrico CJ, et al. Blunt cardiac injury. J Trauma 1992;33:649–650.
43. Fabian TC, Cicala RS, Croce MA, et al. A prospective evaluation of myocardial contusion: correlation of significant arrhythmias and cardiac output with CPK-MK measurements. J Trauma 1991;31:653–659.
44. Fabian TC, Mangiante EC, Patterson CR, et al. Myocardial contusion in blunt trauma: clinical characteristics, means of diagnosis, and implications for patient management. J Trauma 1988;28:50–56.
45. Scalea TM, Simon HM, Duncan AO, et al. Geriatric blunt multiple trauma: improved survival with early invasive monitoring. J Trauma 1990;30:129–134.
46. Cowley RA, Turney SZ, Hankins JR, et al. Rupture of thoracic aorta caused by blunt trauma. J Thorac Cardiovasc Surg 1990;100:652–661.

47. Duhaylongsgod FG, Glower DD, Wolfe WG. Acute traumatic aortic aneurysm. J Vasc Surg 1992;15:331–343.
48. Mattox KL, Wall MJ. Traumatic aneurysm of the thoracic aorta. Chest Surg Clin N Am 1992;1:413–421.
49. Oresckovich MR, Howard JD, Copass MK. Geriatric trauma: injury patterns and outcome. J Trauma 1984;24:565–572.
50. Meyer DM, Thal ER, Weigelt JA, Redman HC. Evaluation of computed tomography and diagnostic peritoneal lavage in blunt abdominal trauma. J Trauma 1989;29:1168–1172.
51. Hirshberg A, Mattox KL. Damage control in trauma surgery. Br J Surg 1993;80:1501–1502.
52. Burch JM, Ortiz VB, Richardson RJ, et al. Abbreviated laparotomy and planned reoperation for critically injured patients. Ann Surg 1992;215:476–484.
53. Hirshberg A, Wall MJ, Mattox KL. Planned reoperation for trauma: a two year experience with 124 consecutive patients. J Trauma 1994; 37:1–5.
54. Olivero JJ. Postsurgical acute renal failure: which patients are at greatest risk. J Crit Ill 1994;9:673–685.
55. Rolandelli RH, Ullrich JR. Nutritional support in the frail elderly surgical patient. Surg Clin North Am 1994;74:79–92.
56. Dwyer JT, Gallo JJ, Reichel W. Assessing nutritional status in elderly patients. Am Fam Physician 1993;47:613–620.
57. Dean RE. Total Parenteral Nutrition (2nd ed). Chicago: Precept, 1990; 80–81.
58. Alverdy JC, Aoys E, Moss GS. Total parenteral nutrition promotes bacterial translocation from the gut. Surgery 1988;104:185–190.
59. Pingleton SK. Enteral nutrition and infection in the intensive care unit. Semin Respir Infect 1990;5:185–190.
60. Plewa MC. Altered host response and special infections in the elderly. Emerg Med Clin North Am 1990;8:193–206.
61. Gleckman R, Hibert D. Afebrile bacteremia. A phenomenon in geriatric patients. JAMA 1982;248:1478–1481.
62. Greenfield RA. Symposium on antimicrobial therapy. VI. The aminoglycosides. J Okla State Med Assoc 1993;86:119–123.
63. Alexander BH, Rivara FP, Wolf ME. The cost and frequency of hospitalization for fall-related injuries in older adults. Am J Public Health 1992;82:1020–1023.

Surgical Care for the Elderly, 2nd ed., edited by
R. Benton Adkins, Jr., and H. William Scott, Jr.
Lippincott–Raven Publishers, Philadelphia © 1998.

CHAPTER 34

Thermal Injuries

David T. Harrington and Basil A. Pruitt, Jr.

BURNS IN THE ELDERLY IN THE UNITED STATES

Who are the elderly? Retirement often begins at 60 years of age and Medicare eligibility usually begins at 62 years of age. When this chapter was written for the first edition, the elderly were defined as patients who were >50 years old. As this group ages, yet remains an active and vital part of the community, this breakpoint of 50 appears dated. However, when one examines the mortality for any given burn size, burn mortality begins to increase dramatically in the fifth decade. Our definition of elderly as >50 years old, therefore, reflects not an arbitrary cutoff, but an age that we and many authors have found an effect of age on mortality statistics (Fig. 34-1) [1].

The population of the United States is aging. In 1985, approximately 11.5% of the U.S. population was >65 years old, by 2025 this number is projected to be 20% [2]. Death rates at all ages are decreasing, most dramatically in the "old, old," the population aged >80. This group is the fastest growing segment of the population. Their numbers should double by the year 2000 [2]. This demographic change poses tremendous challenges politically, socially, and medically.

BURNS IN THE ELDERLY AT THE U.S. ARMY INSTITUTE OF SURGICAL RESEARCH

In general, the elderly tolerate trauma poorly, that is, given the same level of injury, the elderly have a higher mortality than younger patients [3]. This has also been our experience with the elderly who suffer thermal injuries. The Baux Index was developed in 1961 to predict the outcome after thermal injury. It was simply age plus burn size. Patients with an index >75 were considered to have severe injury and patients whose index was >100 were thought to have an invariably fatal injury [4]. Survival after thermal injury, however, has been increasing. The burn size at which there is 50% mortality (LD_{50}) has increased for both the young adult and the older patient. The LD_{50} for the group aged 15 to 40 years old has increased from 43% body surface area (BSA) burn in the period 1945 to 1957 to 75.6% BSA from 1985 to 1989. Patients >41 years of age have seen an increase in their LD_{50} from 23% BSA to 44% BSA during the same period (Table 34-1) [5].

An analysis of variables for thermally injured patients at U.S. Army Institute of Surgical Research (USAISR) shows that the strongest prognostic variables for survival are age and burn size [6]. An equation developed to predict survival has been based on these two variables:

$$\text{Predicted mortality} = \frac{F}{F+1}$$

$$F = \exp\left(-5.427 + (0.08823*\text{TBSA}) - (0.1689*A) + (0.4639*A*A/100) - [0.2383*A*A*(A/10{,}000)]\right)$$

where A is age and TBSA is total body surface area burn.

Other variables can affect survival following burn injury. Inhalational injury can add up to 20% to the mortality after thermal injury [7]. Other authors have found that high 24-hour fluid requirements and an increasing number of complications during the hospital course also correlate with mortality [1]. Age, burn size, and inhalational injury, which quantify the stress placed on the patient by the injury and which are easily obtained within hours of injury, are our preferred prognostic determinants. These factors are so strong statistically that premorbid illnesses do not enter our or other centers' analyses of predicted mortality [1,4,7]. This finding is not unexpected. In all types of trauma, survival for the elderly patient correlates with Injury Severity Score (ISS), type of trauma, and complications, rather than preexisting diseases [3]. Burns from which young adults would survive are associated with an increased mortality as age increases. A 30% BSA burn has a negligent mortality, <5%, in the young adult population (20 to 40 years old), yet in the

The opinions or assertions contained herein are the private views of the authors and are not to be construed as official or as reflecting the views of the U.S. Army or the Department of Defense.

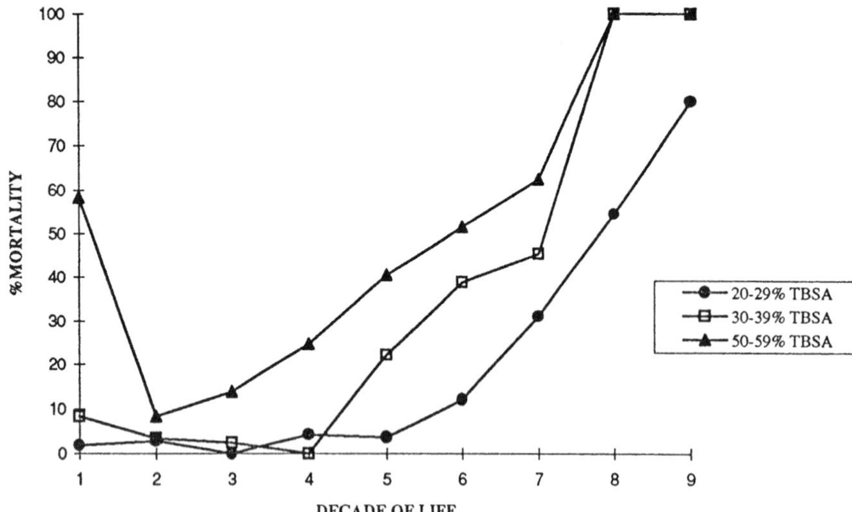

FIG. 34-1. Increases in mortality with increasing age and extent of burn for 1983 to 1994. (TBSA = total body surface area.)

sixth decade that rate is 38.9%, and by the eighth decade that rate is 100% (see Fig. 34-1).

The records of all patients over the age of 50 admitted to the USAISR between January 1986 and December 1994 were collected and reviewed. Three hundred fifteen elderly patients were identified, with a mean burn size of 21.8%, a mean full-thickness component to the injury of 11.5%, and an overall survival of 76.2%. The most common etiologies of thermal injury were ignition of gasoline or other combustible substance in 27% of admissions, scald injury from hot water or grease in 21.8%, and structure fire in 19%. Electrical contact, chemical injury, contact with hot metal, and burns related to cigarettes made up the rest of the burn population. In our general burn population, the overall mortality from thermal injury, despite similar distributions of age and burn size, decreased from 27.1% in 1979 to 8.5% during the period 1987 to 1991 [6]. This trend has extended to the elderly burn patient. The elderly population from 1964 to 1972 had a mean burn size of 31% with a 15% full-thickness component. The mortality in that period was 44% [8]. The elderly in the period from 1976 to 1985, with similar extent of total and full-thickness burns, continued to have high rates of mortality, with 48% of that population dying after thermal injury [9]. In the period from 1986 to 1994, the average burn size decreased to 21.8%, and the mortality declined even more rapidly to 23.8% of elderly admissions.

TABLE 34-1. *Improving survival in thermally injured patients from 1945 to 1957 and 1985 to 1989*

Age (yrs)	LD_{50} 1945–1957	LD_{50} 1985–1989
0–14	51	53
15–40	43	76
>41	23	44

LD_{50} = extent of burn (% of total body surface area) associated with 50% mortality.

Source: Data from Pruitt BA Jr, McManus AT. The changing epidemiology of infection in burn patients. World J Surg 1992;16:57–67.

GENERAL CONSIDERATIONS

Physiology of Aging

Proper functioning of an aging organ system is dependent on two factors. The first is the status of the organ in the face of the gradual deterioration of age and disease. Second, function depends on the level of performance required. With aging, the epidermis and dermis change. In the epidermis the number of proliferating basal keratinocytes decreases, resulting in a reduced proliferative reserve of the skin, and the rete ridges become effaced. The number of Langerhans' cells decreases by 50%, with an associated reduction in their antigen presentation function [10–12]. The dermis thins, loses hyaluronic acid and dermatan sulfate (glycosaminoglycans), and becomes less vascular. A pronounced regression and disorganization of capillary loops in the papillary dermis result in impaired wound healing. The dermis is also less cellular, with fibroblasts, macrophages, and mast cells all decreasing in number. Finally, these changes in the dermis are accentuated with a history of sun damage [10,12]. The elderly manifest these deficiencies by their increasing difficulty in healing donor sites in each successive decade of life. Despite a uniform method of harvesting skin at 10/1,000ths of an inch, delayed donor site healing was noted to occur in 4.1% of the population aged 50 to 59 years of age, but increased to 38.8% in the group aged 80 to 89 years of age.

The elderly, who are less able to withstand the stress that thermal injury demands, are also more susceptible to thermal injury because of their decreased ability to perceive danger and react appropriately. Between the ages of 20 and 90, the number of pacinian (pressure) and Meissner's

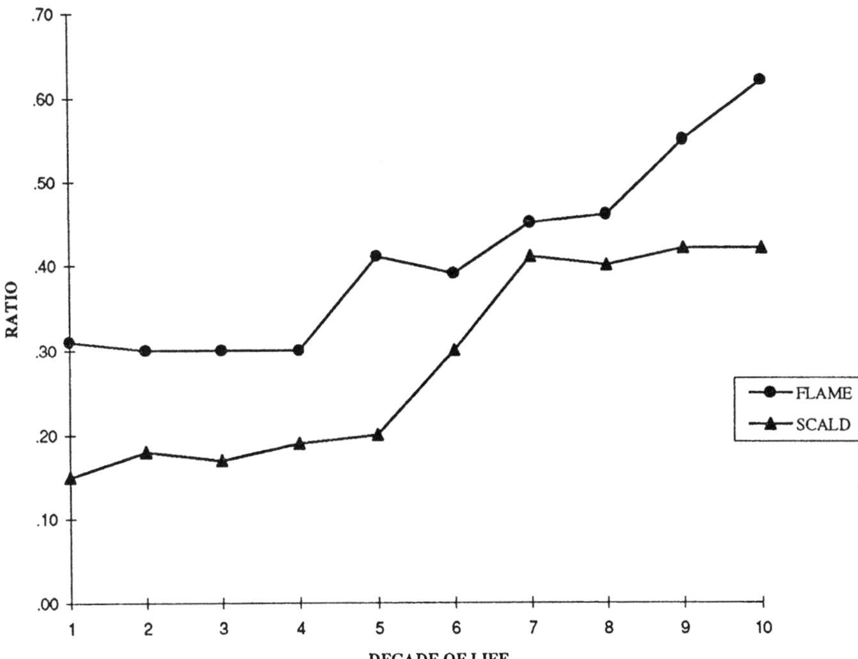

FIG. 34-2. The ratio of full-thickness burn size to total burn size increases with age for scald and flame injuries. (TBSA = total body surface area.)

(touch) corpuscles decrease nearly 75%. This reduction results in less pain acuity. As the pain threshold is increased, the elderly are less able to perceive and therefore to sense and react to danger [10,12]. The cumulative effect of aging on mobility and overall neurologic function leads to impaired judgment and decreased ability to get away from offending insults [1]. These deficiencies are manifested by a 15% increase in the rate of inhalational injury in those >70 years when compared with their younger counterparts aged 50 to 69 years.

With decreased sensation, perception, and mobility, burn injury can occur quickly. Exposure to 55°C (130°F), the upper limit of suggested tap water temperature, causes discomfort in 2 to 3 seconds, partial-thickness burns at approximately 30 seconds, and full-thickness burns only at exposures >5 minutes. Yet exposure to 70°C (158°F) temperatures causes discomfort in <1 second, partial-thickness burns in 1 second, and full-thickness burns in approximately 10 seconds [13,14]. A national review of fatal tap water burns from 1979 to 1986 revealed 459 occurrences (57 deaths per year). Nineteen percent occurred in patients <11 years old, and 50.8% occurred in patients >74 years old. Although these data did not control for burn size, this problem is significant, with death rates from scald injury increasing after the age of 50 years and dramatically increasing after 75 years of age [15]. The cumulative effects of poorly vascularized skin, decreased sensation, and impaired mobility appear to make the elderly more prone to full-thickness injury. For both flame and scald injuries, the elderly have an increased proportion of their injury that is full thickness as compared with younger patients (Fig. 34-2).

In addition to changes in the skin, there are age-related changes in immune function. Although B-cell function shows little change with age, both helper T and killer T cells have a dramatic decline in their functional ability. Many T cells appear normal morphologically, and although some respond to an antigen challenge, the percentage of T cells that respond normally declines with age [16,17]. Cell cultures of mononuclear cells reveal that older patients (>60 vs. <40 years old) have decreased induction of interleukin 2 (IL-2) and IL-2R messenger RNA, decreased IL-2 secretion, reduced percentage of IL-2R–positive cells, and decreased density of IL-2 receptors after phytohemagglutinin stimulation [18]. Antigen-presenting cell lines, macrophages, and dendritic cells appear to have normal function [16].

The endocrine system undergoes varied changes with aging. Levels of circulating antidiuretic hormone are elevated, reflecting a new osmotic set point in the elderly. Due to a decreased catecholamine level and increased somatostatin stimulation of the hypothalamus, the elderly have lower basal levels and diurnal peaks of growth hormone with subsequently lower circulating insulin-like growth factor [19]. The incidence of glucose intolerance and frank diabetes mellitus, with its attendant increased risk of cardiovascular complications, increases with age secondary to post-receptor insulin resistance [20]. With aging, however, the integrity of the pituitary and thyroid hormone axes are generally preserved. Although secretion of thyroid hormone declines with aging, homeostasis is maintained by a decreased clearance, resulting in normal levels of thyroid hormone and thyroid-stimulating hormone. Basal levels of circulating cortisol are normal in the elderly, although an exaggerated and prolonged cortisol response to stress occurs due to insensitivity of the hypothalamus and pituitary gland to feedback inhibition [19,21]. In sum, perturbations of the hormonal milieu occur in the elderly, yet the circulating levels of the essential thyroid and adrenal hormones are preserved.

The function of the renal system also declines, with age-related changes evident in both the glomeruli and tubules. For the population as a whole there is a 30% loss of the kidney mass between the ages of 50 and 90. Glomerular filtration rate declines gradually after the age of 30, and between 50 and 90 it shows a 30% decrease in its rate. Serum creatinine levels in the elderly are often normal, reflecting a depleted lean body mass, not a preservation of creatinine clearance. The renal tubules show signs of tubular shortening, changes in the basement membrane, and associated interstitial fibrosis. Functionally, the kidneys show decreased ability to both excrete, in cases of hypervolemia, and retain, in the face of hypovolemia, salt and water [22]. These changes translate into a higher incidence of resuscitation-related fluid overload in the elderly burn population. Although this decline in function is true for the elderly population as a whole, the elderly are in actuality quite a heterogenous population. Acute medical care for this population demands individualizing treatment because many elderly maintain high levels of function in their organ systems such as the kidney, whereas others show dramatic declines [23,24]. The decrease in glomerular filtration rate and tubular function leaves less physiologic reserve such that ischemic injuries or exposures to nephrotoxic drugs are poorly tolerated. This diminished reserve of the aged renal system is shown by an increasing rate of acute renal failure in our patients with both increasing age and extent of burn. Acute renal failure in our elderly population carries an 85% mortality.

Given these changes in the renal system, antibiotic use should be carefully considered and closely monitored. Empiric therapy of suspected infections, except in the most critically ill patient, should be avoided. Once an infection is documented, medications that are predominately eliminated by the kidney, such as vancomycin and the aminoglycosides, should be dosed according to age and closely monitored by serum levels. Serum levels of these drugs, even when dosed appropriately for age and renal function, can vary widely in both burned and nonburned critically ill patients [25,26]. When the microbial sensitivities of the infecting organism are known, consideration should be given to reducing the reliance on nephrotoxic medications. Preoperative prophylactic antibiotic regimens should also take into account the renal function of the patient. The authors' standard preoperative prophylactic regimen of vancomycin and an aminoglycoside has increasingly been replaced by vancomycin and either a cephalosporin or aztreonam in our elderly patients.

Blood levels of therapeutic drugs depend not just on renal clearance but on absorption, volume of distribution, protein binding in the serum, and the individual's sensitivity to the medication. The elderly lose lean body mass, increase their level of body fat, and have decreased total body water with advancing age. Liver blood flow is reduced by 35% between the ages of 40 and 65 years. Drugs such as diazepam and midazolam, which are primarily cleared by the liver and are lipid soluble, have been shown to have increased half-lives in the elderly [27,28]. Water-soluble drugs such as cimetidine and digoxin have a reduced volume of distribution with resultant high initial blood levels and decreased half-lives [27]. Although the elderly often have decreased levels of albumin and alpha$_1$-acid glycoprotein, common drug carriers in the serum, the resultant higher free drug serum levels are thought to have little clinical importance [28].

Decreased cognitive function, much like the age-related decrements in kidney function, occurs at different rates for each person. A majority of the elderly show no debility, yet, with increasing age, a significant minority of the elderly show signs of dementia. Dementia is most commonly caused by Alzheimer's disease or multiple cerebrovascular accidents, although post-traumatic and other less common primary neurologic disorders can also cause this disorder. It is estimated that approximately 1% to 5% of the elderly between the ages of 50 and 70, and 20% to 50% of the elderly >70 years meet the criteria for dementia [29–31]. Dementia can be a profoundly debilitating disease. One population-based study revealed that patients of the same age with documented dementia had a higher 3-year mortality than those without the diagnosis of dementia [30]. Four percent of our study population carried this diagnosis. These patients had on average a more extensive and deeper burn, a greater incidence of inhalational injury, and higher rates of pneumonia. Forty-four percent of all patients between the ages of 50 and 70 years with >30% BSA burn survived, yet of the five patients in this group who carried the diagnosis of dementia, none survived. Unfortunately, no specific treatment for this condition and its common side effect of agitation are available, other than eliminating the confounding presence of hypoxia, hypoglycemia, or infection, creating a supportive environment, and judiciously using neuroleptics and benzodiazepines [32].

Local and Systemic Response to Thermal Injury

The body's response to thermal injury begins with the inflammatory reaction in the burn wound. Thermal injury can cause areas of full-thickness injury, called the zone of coagulation, where proteins are denatured and no viable cellular elements remain. The injury can also create areas of marginal injury, the zone of stasis. In this zone, the potential for repair and return to normal function exists if further damage, in the form of reperfusion injury or infection, are avoided. Yet in these areas of marginal burn injury, the body responds by edema and the margination and recruitment of white cells. Leukocytes have been recognized as central mediators in local microvascular injury in the burn wound. In an animal model of the zone of stasis, monoclonal antibodies to the leukocyte antigen complex CD18 and its vascular endothelial ligand, intercellular adhesion molecule-1 (ICAM-1), were able to preserve perfusion in this critical zone. This was true whether the antibodies were given preinjury or 30 minutes postinjury. This gives credence to the role of neutrophils in the pathogenesis of burn wound progression and stimulates the search for therapies to protect this critical zone [33].

Thermal injury induces release of a host of mediators and cytokines. Oxidants, elaborated by white cells in the zone of injury; prostaglandins; and leukotrienes all contribute to the local edema and inflammatory response after thermal injury. Cytokines, which are suppressed in nonstressed individuals, are also elaborated after burn injury. IL-1 is produced by monocytes and macrophages primarily. IL-2, which augments cell-mediated immunity and cytotoxic T-cell killing, is produced by T-lymphocytes. IL-6 can be elaborated by many cell lines including macrophages, neutrophils, and fibroblasts. Tumor necrosis factor (TNF), produced by macrophages, endothelial cells, neutrophils, and lymphocytes, is also elevated after thermal injury. The production of these cytokines depends on the status of the reticuloendothelial system. A primed system—one that has been primarily stimulated by the burn injury and then secondarily by circulating endotoxin from the burn wound or the gut—produces an exaggerated response to further stimulation. This system is without normal negative feedback loops and therefore within this system there is the potential for a self-perpetuating inflammatory process, even in the absence of infection [34].

Circulating levels of cytokines are markers of the body's stress response, with some cytokines elevated proportionately to the severity of the injury and others increased in the presence of infection. When circulating levels of IL-6, IL-1β, and TNF-α were measured in 27 burn patients and compared with controls, several observations were made. The IL-1β level, which induces T-cell proliferation and modulates production of other cytokines (IL-6), is highest during the first postburn week and declines over time. Elevations of IL-1β levels were noted to correlate with increasing burn size and to return to normal as the hypermetabolic response to the burn waned. IL-6, which is involved in T-cell activation, induction of hepatic acute phase protein synthesis, and stimulation of hematopoiesis, is highest during the first postburn week and declines over time. High levels of IL-6, correlated with mortality: Nonsurvivors had significantly higher IL-6 levels. TNF-α did not correlate with burn size or outcome [35]. In septic patients and in patients who sustained mechanical trauma, other authors have corroborated this correlation between levels of IL-6 and mortality and further have shown that these levels correlate to both the presence and severity of infection [36,37]. Although these cytokines may just be markers of the body's response to injury, IL-1β and IL-6 may themselves influence the host immune system and the metabolic response in the first 2 to 3 weeks postburn.

Criteria for Burn Center Admission

Many burns can be cared for outside of a burn center. Burns that involve >20% BSA, burns that involve highly functional or cosmetic areas such as the face, hands, feet, genitalia, and perineum, full-thickness burns with a >5% BSA, or thermal injury with associated inhalational injury should be referred to a burn center for care. Patients at the extremes of age, <10 years old and >50 years old, have been identified as groups that benefit by burn center attention at lower TBSA burns. Thermal injury involving >10% of the BSA is considered a criterion for burn center admission in these age groups [38] (Table 34-2).

TABLE 34-2. *Criteria for burn center referral*

Total body surface area (second and third) >10% in patient <10 and >50 years old
Total body surface area (second and third) >20% in patient 11–49 years old
Burns of highly functional or cosmetic areas: face, hands, feet, genitalia, perineum, major joints
Third-degree burns >5% in all ages
Inhalation injury associated with burn
Circumferential burns of extremities or trunk
Electrical burns
Chemical burns involving highly functional or cosmetic areas
Burns in patient with significant preexisting illness that would complicate burn care
Burns with other trauma in which the burn is the greatest threat to the patient
Hospitals without qualified personnel or adequate equipment

Source: Data from Gillespie RW, Dimick AR, Gillespie PW, et al. Initial Assessment and Management. In Advanced Burn Life Support Course: Instructor's Manual. Lincoln, NE: Nebraska Burn Institute, 1994.

INITIAL ASSESSMENT AND TREATMENT

Airway and Respiratory Concerns

Inhalational injury increases burn mortality in an age-related and burn size–related fashion. Mortality of a patient with thermal injury is increased by a maximum of 20% if inhalational injury has occurred. Subsequent pneumonia after these injuries increase mortality by an additional 40%. The increase in mortality is most pronounced in the midsize burns. Patients with small burns do not have their mortality increased significantly by inhalational injury, and patients with large burns do not have an appreciable increase in their already dismal mortality [7]. In the elderly population from 1976 to 1985, 36% suffered an inhalational injury, with 62% of these patients developing pneumonia and 72% eventually succumbing to their injuries [9]. From 1986 to 1994, 25% of the patients had inhalational injury diagnosed by bronchoscopy or xenon scanning. Only 41% of these patients developed pneumonia, with an associated mortality of 51%.

Inhalational injury to the upper airway or the lower airway and lung parenchyma accompanies burn injury in up to 35% of patients [7,39]. Inhalational injury can be both thermal and chemical. Thermal injury is usually confined to the upper airway because of the capacity of the glottis for efficient heat exchange. Occasionally a steam injury, because of the higher thermal capacity of steam, can overwhelm the glottis and result in direct thermal injury to the trachea and bronchi. Chemical injury of the airway can be caused by fine particles with adherent irritants or cytotoxic chemicals or by aerosolized cytotoxic chemicals. Generally, these toxic inhalants are deposited in the airways such that the largest particles and those inhalants with the greatest irritant properties and greatest water solubility are found more proximally in the airways [40]. Both injuries can pose challenges in the acute care of a thermally injured patient.

The history of the event and physical examination of the patient are poor predictors of those patients who have suffered inhalational injury. Although a significant majority of patients with inhalational injury have a history of being in a confined space and have facial burns on physical examination (73% and 93%, respectively), 21% of patients confined to a closed space and 52% of patients with facial burns do not have an inhalational injury on thorough evaluation [7]. A chest radiograph is also a poor screening test for this injury. At the USAISR, inhalational injury is evaluated by early bronchoscopy and, if necessary with a normal bronchoscopy result, by ^{133}xenon ventilation-perfusion lung scanning. These modalities have >90% accuracy in detecting inhalational injury [40].

Management of the upper airway is a critical first step in the care of a thermally injured patient. Upper airway edema is usually maximal 12 to 24 hours postburn. Early bronchoscopy and observation in an intensive care setting of patients thought to be at risk for inhalational injury is warranted [40]. Any sign of impending airway obstruction, such as stridor noted on physical examination or significant edema at the time of bronchoscopy, warrants prophylactic intubation. Performing bronchoscopy over an endotracheal tube allows assessment of the airway and direct visualization of the endotracheal tube placement beyond the glottis if intubation is elected. At the USAISR we prefer nasotracheal intubation because of patient comfort and the stability of this airway over the orotracheal route.

The respiratory mucosa is very sensitive to injury. Even a short duration of exposure to irritants can result in loss of cilia and superficial epithelial erosions. More prolonged exposure results in epithelial necrosis and sloughing. After local injury the inflammatory cascade is activated, and within 2 hours there are histologic inflammatory changes present in the respiratory mucosa. Release of vasoactive substances after inhalational injury results in pulmonary hypertension and bronchospasm. The cumulative effect of this injury leaves the lung with a decreased compliance, sloughing epithelium, impaired cilia, and an inflammatory infiltrate. These changes can lead to cast formation, obstruction of bronchioles, and atelectasis, which are accompanied by worsening oxygenation and ventilation [40]. This injury has significant impact on burn survival, particularly in the elderly patient in whom aging has reduced lung elasticity and ciliary activity in association with a decrease in vital capacity and a diminished cough reflex [22,41].

Therapy for inhalational injury is primarily supportive, because if barotrauma is minimized and there is no intervening infection, the acute epithelial sloughing and inflammatory exudate resolve in 12 to 14 days [7,42]. Bronchospasm should be treated aggressively with inhaled bronchodilators. Corticosteroids in the acute phase are to be avoided [42,43]. Barotrauma can be minimized by ventilating at the lowest peak airway pressure and rate that adequately ventilate the patient. High peak airway pressures and high ventilator rates translate into higher mean airway pressures. These pressures may even decrease tracheobronchial mucosal blood flow [40]. Experimental models of inhalational injury have shown that higher levels of barotrauma (rate pressure product) result in significantly increased histologic damage to the lung parenchyma [44]. Use of permissive hypercapnia, with blood pH ≥7.32, is well tolerated and may minimize barotrauma. High levels of positive end-expiratory pressure, which also increase mean airway pressure, should not be used to drive the oxygen saturation >93%, a level of saturation that is well tolerated [40].

In patients with respiratory mucosa damaged by inhalational injury, the ideal ventilator would ventilate at low peak airway pressures, facilitate clearance of sloughed mucosa and secretions, and recruit collapsed airways. A ventilator that has these abilities is the Volume Diffusive Respirator (VDR, available from Percussionaire Corp., Sandpoint, ID), a high-frequency flow-interrupter ventilator that superimposes oscillatory airflow on a pressure-control generated tidal volume. We have used it for burn patients with inhalational injury since the mid-1980s. In a primate model, the VDR ventilator could attain the same level of ventilation and oxygenation as conventional volume ventilation with less barotrauma (rate pressure product), less histologic evidence of injury at necropsy, and lower bronchoalveolar lavage elastase levels (a marker of granulocyte activation) [44]. A retrospective analysis of our use of the VDR ventilator revealed decreased rates of pneumonia (29% vs. 52.3%) and mortality (16.4% vs. 42.7%) when using the VDR versus conventional ventilation. Using the USAISR predictor of survival, these differences in survivorship between the conventional and VDR ventilation groups were shown to reflect not only overall improved survival during the study period but also a beneficial effect of the VDR ventilator [39].

Another concern with victims suspected of having inhalational injury is carbon monoxide poisoning. Carbon monoxide binds to hemoglobin 220 times more avidly than oxygen and has also been shown to have affinity for cytochrome oxidase. In the presence of carbon monoxide, therefore, oxidative metabolism is inhibited at three levels. The first is a decreased oxygen-carrying capacity and subsequent oxygen delivery because of carbon monoxide displacing oxygen from its normal binding site on the hemoglobin molecule. Second, carbon monoxide, in binding to hemoglobin, interferes with normal oxygen-hemoglobin dissociation in the tissues [40]. Last, the limited oxygen delivered to the cellular oxidative apparatus in the cell might not be used efficiently, if at all, because of the binding of carbon monoxide to cytochrome oxidase [45,46]. For these reasons, any patient suspected of inhalational injury should receive 100% oxygen until carbon monoxide poisoning is ruled out and carboxyhemoglobin is <10%. The half-life of carboxyhemoglobin is dependent on the percent oxygen delivered (FIO_2). When a patient is breathing room air, the half-life of carboxyhemoglobin is 250 minutes, on 100% FIO_2 it is 40 to 50 minutes, and when breathing oxygen at 2 atm it is 27 minutes. Although this 20-minute advantage appears to justify the use of hyperbaric oxygen for carbon monoxide poisoning, one study demonstrated a surprising number of side effects that complicated burn care and there are no data confirming a long-term benefit [47]. We have reserved this treatment modality for those rare symptomatic patients suffering coma, seizures, or respiratory failure. We believe that transporting a patient for a marginally efficacious therapy in the face of ongoing resuscitation is potentially dangerous [40].

The burn eschar can also impair ventilation. If the burn injury to the trunk is full thickness and circumferential, it may restrict chest wall expansion, resulting in a decreased lung compliance and the need for higher airway pressures to attain the same level of ventilation. In this setting, chest wall escharotomies can be life-saving. Escharotomies can be performed at the bedside due to the insensate nature of third-degree burns and are carried through the burn and superficial fascia only to the depth that will permit the cut edges of the eschar to separate. Deeper incisions into viable tissue are avoided. The escharotomy incisions are placed in the anterior axillary lines and, if the eschar extends onto the anterior abdominal wall and restricts chest wall motion, they are connected transversely across the chest by a costal margin escharotomy incision.

The development of new clinical therapies and ongoing laboratory investigations promise improvements in the treatment of inhalational injury. One therapy addresses severe inhalational injury that denudes the airway, leading to the formation of bloody casts consisting of inspissated mucus and hemorrhagic plugs that can obstruct the airway. In this setting, aerosolized heparin, 10,000 U given as a nebulized treatment every 6 hours, can reduce the catastrophic complication of occluded airways and respiratory decompensation [48,49]. Another area of interest is the use of pharmacologic agents to modify the pulmonary response to inhalational injury. Pentoxifylline, through its hemorheologic and antithrombotic effects, may improve the microcirculation. Moreover, its inhibitory effect on cytokine release and leukocyte activation has been shown to decrease leukocytosis, polymorphonuclear neutrophil counts, and total protein content in pulmonary lavage fluid after inhalational injury. Treatment with pentoxifylline has been shown to decrease pulmonary hypertension and extravascular lung water and improve pulmonary compliance after inhalational injury [50]. Finally, platelet-activating factor antagonists, free radical scavengers such as dimethyl sulfoxide, and surfactant replacement are all being studied [40].

Fluid Resuscitation and Circulation

Edema forms in both burned and unburned tissues after thermal injury. Many factors contribute to its formation. Increases in endothelial permeability and deviations from the normal Starling's forces such as increases in intravascular hydrostatic pressure and decreases in intravascular oncotic pressure and interstitial hydrostatic pressure, have been invoked to explain edema formation. The direct effect of heat, the release of complement and inflammatory mediators, and the elaboration of cytokines in the burn wound creates a local and a generalized endothelial leak. This leak is maximal in the first 6 to 8 hours postburn, then declines for the remainder of the 24 hours postburn. The large endothelial pores, whose radii are increased to 40 nm after thermal injury, are also increased in number and appear to account for the increase in permeability. A gap of this magnitude renders the oncotic effect of molecules such as albumin, dextran, and pentafraction insignificant [51,52]. Although the increased permeability and loss of intravascular oncotic pressure are contributors to edema formation, they cannot explain all the increases in tissue edema after thermal injury. Studies of a canine hindpaw burn model revealed that over the first 3 hours postburn, when most burn edema forms, 47% of edema was secondary to permeability changes, and 53% was due to increases in increased capillary hydrostatic pressure. The increased capillary hydrostatic pressure was attributed to a decrease in precapillary resistance occurring simultaneously with normal arterial pressure and postcapillary resistance [51]. Finally, a previously unrecognized contributor to burn wound edema is the development of negative interstitial pressure. By measuring the change in electrical conductance at the end of a glass micropipette, negative interstitial pressures as low as 40 mm Hg have been documented in the burn wound for the first 2 hours after injury [53].

With increased vascular permeability and edema formation, crystalloid resuscitation in the first 24 hours is based on the modified Brooke formula (Table 34-3). This formula is used for patients with burns of >20% BSA, and the fluids are given intravenously. Due to the high incidence of ileus after thermal injury of this extent, oral resuscitation should not be used. One-half the volume estimated for the first 24 hours is given over the first 8 hours and the second half is given over the subsequent 16 hours. It should be emphasized that this formula, and other fluid-resuscitation formulas, are meant to be starting points for volume infusion. After setting the initial rate, the infusion is titrated to maintain adequate tissue perfusion manifested by a urine output of 0.5 ml/kg per hour. In the second 24 hours, after the leak in the vascular endothelium has mostly sealed, the patient is placed on a 5% albumin infusion commensurate with the patient's total burn size and 5% dextrose in water to maintain an adequate urine output.

The elderly pose a special problem for the burn surgeon in the resuscitation phase: They have a reduced cardiac index at

TABLE 34-3. *Modified Brooke formula for fluid resuscitation after thermal injury*

0–24 Hours postburn	2 ml/kg body weight/% BSA burned lactated Ringer's solution: One-half given over the first 8 hrs Second half given over the subsequent 16 hrs
24–48 Hours postburn	5% albumin infusion: 0.3 ml/kg/% BSA burn for 30–50% BSA burns 0.4 ml/kg/% BSA burn for 50–70% BSA burns 0.5 ml/kg/% BSA burn for >70% BSA burns D5W infusion: to maintain urine output >0.5 ml/kg/hr

BSA = body surface area; D5W = 5% dextrose in water.

rest and, once stressed, have a reduced capacity to increase their cardiac output and heart rate [41]. Furthermore, the aged heart is less responsive to catecholamine stimulation and relies on ventricular dilation, increased preload, and stroke volume to augment cardiac output in response to stress. Between 1986 and 1994, 22% of the elderly patients admitted to our center carried a diagnosis of coronary artery disease. Twelve percent of patients had severe cardiac disease, with a history of myocardial infarction or coronary artery bypass grafting or a prior episode of congestive heart failure. The elderly also have more abnormal renal glomeruli, a decreased creatinine clearance, and a decrease in renal blood flow even under normal conditions [41]. The aged kidney is less able to respond to hypovolemia because of an inefficient conservation of water and salt and to hypervolemia due to its inability to excrete an acute increase in intravascular salt and water [54]. A review of elderly burn patients revealed, not surprisingly, that the survivors were younger, had smaller burns, and had a decreased incidence of inhalational injury than nonsurvivors. Hemodynamic monitoring of these patients over the first 4 days postburn revealed that although all patients were resuscitated to the same urine output (30 to 50 ml per hour) the survivors showed lower mean pulmonary artery pressures, lower right atrial pressures, lower pulmonary capillary wedge pressures, higher cardiac indexes, and higher stroke indexes than nonsurvivors [55]. These findings reveal how aged organ systems, when asked to function at a level higher than baseline, often cannot meet the task. This decompensation can contribute to the increased mortality of elderly burn patients.

A small percentage of burn patients with massive injury never attain hemodynamic or respiratory stability. This population is referred to as *failures of resuscitation*. In the general burn population treated at the USAISR from 1987 to 1991, 12 of 1,094 admissions (1.1%) met this definition [6]. The elderly would appear to be at increased risk for this outcome. From 1986 to 1994, 2.6% of the study population met this definition and died within 48 hours of their injury. These patients were older than the rest of the study population, with a mean age of 75 years (vs. 65 years), and had massive injuries, with a mean TBSA burn of 54% and a rate of inhalational injury of 60%. From 1976 to 1985, 36.6% of elderly burn patients never attained sufficient hemodynamic or respiratory stability to undergo operative debridement or grafting. This rate has dropped to 8.6% in the current study period although this may reflect in part the decrease in mean TBSA between the two periods (34% vs. 21.8%) [9]. A comparison of elderly patients with burns of >20% BSA who were treated during 1986 to 1988 with those treated during 1992 to 1994 revealed no significant change (15.7% vs. 17.6%) in the percentage of the elderly who could not be adequately stabilized for operative intervention.

Abnormalities in the cardiac and renal systems and the high rate of early mortality in the elderly burn population demand intensive management of these patients. The elderly are less able than younger patients to increase oxygen delivery in the face of increased oxygen demands. Maintaining the patient's hematocrit >30 to augment the oxygen-carrying capacity of the blood is therefore necessary. During periods of rapid fluid shifts, such as the resuscitation phase or the perioperative period, patients with extensive burns and those with a history of cardiac disease should be monitored by means of a pulmonary artery catheter. From 1986 to 1994, more than one-half the patients who had burns involving >20% of the BSA or were >70 years of age required invasive monitoring at least once during their hospital course. In patients with known cardiac disease more than one-half the patients with burns of >10% BSA or who were >60 had invasive monitoring (Fig. 34-3). After optimizing oxygen delivery every effort should be made to decrease oxygen consumption. Reducing exposure to hypothermic temperatures, adequately relieving pain, and avoiding inadequate ventilatory support can all reduce oxygen consumption [54]. Despite the most meticulous care, a high mortality in the elderly burn patient still occurs. New therapies need to be developed if improved survival in these severely stressed elderly patients is to be attained.

Part of the resuscitation phase includes monitoring the patient for evidence of decreased peripheral perfusion. A circumferential full-thickness extremity wound can act as a constricting tourniquet as the edema-generated increase in tissue pressure beneath the unyielding eschar first exceeds venous pressure and then overcomes capillary perfusion pressure. These events produce a compartment syndrome of the limb that can lead to tissue ischemia and necrosis if unrecognized. Assessment of distal perfusion can be done by physical examination looking for cyanosis, delayed capillary refilling (>5 seconds), and progressive, unrelenting paresthesias. The burn itself may cause swelling, pallor, coolness to the touch, and even lesser sensory changes that can make the physical examination unreliable [56]. Because measurements of compartment pressures in burned limbs have shown that muscle compartment pressures usually increase over the first 24 hours postinjury, then stabilize or return to normal, some authors recommend invasive pres-

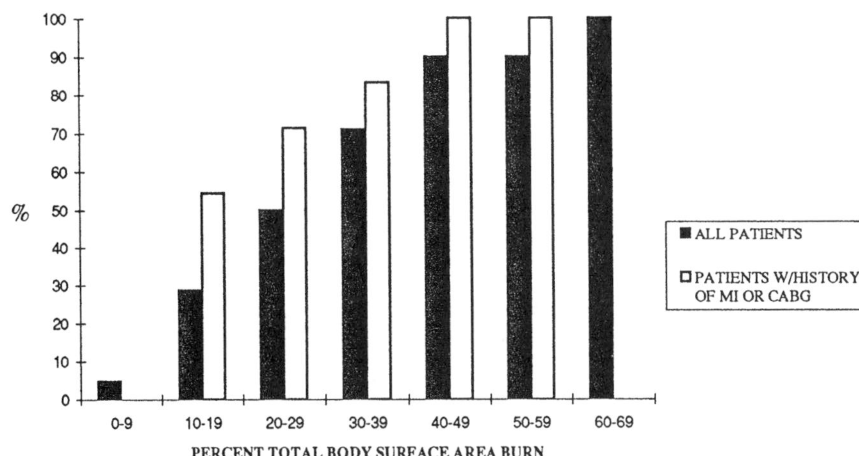

FIG. 34-3. The use of pulmonary artery catheters increases with increasing burn size and in the presence of a cardiac history. (MI = myocardial infarction; CABG = coronary artery bypass grafting.)

sure monitoring. In normal patients, compartment pressures are usually <9 mm Hg, yet in patients with circumferential limb burns 90.3% have pressures >9 mm Hg. Intervention, by means of escharotomy, is used when pressure within the compartment exceeds 30 mm Hg. This pressure is considered the threshold of tissue ischemia [57]. One drawback of this method is the potential of seeding the deep muscle compartments with bacteria from the burn wound. The authors recommend elevating burned extremities with additional active exercise for 5 minutes of each hour to decrease tissue edema. The limbs are evaluated by Doppler flow probe at the distal vessels, that is, digital or palmar arch in hands and pedal pulses in feet. Loss of these pulses as assessed by the Doppler flow probe necessitates escharotomy in the involved limb. Relying on the Doppler flow probe rather than physical examination saves up to 40% of patients unnecessary escharotomies and does not appear to put any tissue at risk for necrosis [56]. Escharotomies are performed using an electrocautery device or a scalpel at the bedside. Because these incisions are placed through full-thickness burns, which are insensate, general or local anesthesia is unnecessary. The incision is placed in the full-thickness burn in the mid-lateral or mid-medial line of the limb. Continuing the escharotomy across joints is important, because they are common sites of tight constriction to blood flow. The incision is carried only through the burn eschar and superficial fascia, not deeper into viable tissue. In such an incision, bleeding is minimal and readily controlled by pressure or electrocoagulation.

Beginning in the resuscitation phase and continuing through the elderly patient's hospital stay, hypothermia should be rigorously prevented. The elderly have a decreased ability to maintain body temperature in response to a cold environment and, once cold, have a diminished ability to rewarm themselves [58–60]. Hypothermia is thought to contribute to perioperative cardiac morbidity in elderly patients and is a known contributor to coagulopathy by inhibition of the enzymatic reactions of the coagulation cascade [58,61,62]. Preoperative skin warming, forced–heated air devices, and higher ambient operating room temperatures have been shown to conserve body heat during the perioperative period. Forced–heated air devices have also been shown to decrease postoperative forearm to fingertip skin surface temperature gradient, a measure of vasoconstriction, and circulating norepinephrine levels [58,61,63]. The thermally injured patient should be protected from the stress of hypothermia. The ambient temperatures in patient rooms and the operative suite in our burn center are maintained at 31 to 32°C (88 to 90°F). During transportation of patients to the operative suite or diagnostic studies, they should be covered with a heat reflective blanket. Heating lamps are used to rewarm any patient who develops a core temperature <36°C.

LATER CARE

Wound Care

Goals in the care of the burn wound are twofold. The first goal is to control microbial colonization, thereby preventing the wound from being a source of sepsis. The second is to excise areas of deep partial and full-thickness burns to promote return of maximal function and to ensure the best cosmetic result. Effective topical antimicrobials, isolation techniques, wound biopsy histology to diagnose invasive infection, and early excision and grafting of the burn wound are some of the innovations used to meet these goals. These advances in burn care are thought to have contributed to the recent increases in the survival of burn patients.

An ideal topical agent should penetrate the eschar, have good activity against the colonizing organisms, should not interfere with wound healing, and have minimal systemic absorption and toxicity. No one agent can meet all these criteria and the choice of a topical agent is a balance of relative advantages and disadvantages. The problem lies in the burn wound. It is an avascular layer made of denatured protein, which provides a rich culture media for proliferating microorganisms. Initially, the eschar is populated by sparse gram-

TABLE 34-4. *Histologic classification of burn wound colonization and invasion*

Stage	Level	Histology
Colonization	1a, superficial	Sparse microbial population on burn wound surface
	1b, penetration	Microorganisms in variable thickness of eschar
	1c, proliferation	Dense organisms at viable–nonviable interface
Invasion	2a, microinvasion	Organisms immediately subjacent to subeschar space
	2b, generalized	Widespread penetration into viable tissues
	2c, microvascular	Involvement of lymphatics and microvasculature

Source: Data from Pruitt BA Jr, McManus AT. The changing epidemiology of infection in burn patients. World J Surg 1992;16:57–67.

positive organisms, but after the third to fifth postburn day these organisms are replaced by a dense gram-negative bacterial flora and later by fungal organisms [5].

Sulfamylon burn cream is an 11.1% suspension of the acetate salt of mafenide, an N' unsubstituted sulfonamide. Mafenide acetate is water soluble, penetrates the eschar well, and has good activity against gram-positive and gram-negative organisms, especially *Pseudomonas aeruginosa.* The drawbacks of this agent are that it is temporarily painful when applied to partial-thickness wounds and, because it is absorbed from the burn wound and is a carbonic anhydrase inhibitor, bicarbonate is lost in the urine, which may result in a metabolic acidosis in patients who cannot compensate by ventilatory mechanisms. Five percent of patients develop a maculopapular rash due to the agent. Silvadene burn cream, the most frequently used topical antimicrobial, is a 1% suspension of silver sulfadiazine in a water-soluble cream. Its broad spectrum of activity (*Staphylococcus aureus, Escherichia coli, Enterobacter*, and, claimed by some, *Candida*) is due to its two active components, the sulfadiazine and silver ions. Its application is painless to the patient. Its disadvantages are a frequently occurring transient leukopenia, atopy as manifested by a rash (<5%), and the development of resistant strains of *Enterobacter cloacae* and *P. aeruginosa.* Silver nitrate solution (0.5%) is also an effective antimicrobial because of the infrequent development of silver-resistant organisms. Due to its minimal penetration of the eschar however, it has little role in the treatment of large or full-thickness injuries in which a heavy microbial population has been established before topical therapy has been instituted. Because of the solubility characteristics of the silver salts, silver nitrate solution is prepared in distilled water, resulting in a very hypotonic solution. The resultant absorption of water and the leaching of sodium, potassium, and chloride into the dressings necessitates scheduled monitoring of fluid and electrolyte balance and correction of identified imbalances. These dressings should be wetted frequently to ensure that the silver concentration at the wound surface does not exceed 2% to 3% [5,64].

The authors currently use mafenide acetate and silver sulfadiazine burn creams in an alternating fashion. After the morning bedside bath or shower using chlorhexidine solution for cleansing, the burn wound is covered with mafenide acetate burn cream. Silver sulfadiazine burn cream is applied 12 hours later. The wounds are left open. Use of both creams in an alternating manner delivers the superior intraeschar antimicrobial control of mafenide acetate and the greater breadth of action of silver sulfadiazine, without the painful application of mafenide before sleep and a marked reduction of the risk of a significant metabolic acidosis associated with twice a day application of mafenide. Burns of special areas are treated differently. Burns of the face are treated solely with silver sulfadiazine, and the ears, because of the risk of chondritis, are treated with a twice a day application of mafenide.

Controlling the microbial density of the burn wound needs to be accompanied by an effective protocol to limit cross contamination of patients with resistant strains of organisms. Vigorous enforcement of an infection control program has been shown to be capable of eliminating endogenous strains of resistant organisms and their comorbid effect [5,65–67]. Scheduled culturing of sputum, urine, and the wound (three times per week) enables one to assess the effectiveness of patient isolation techniques and provides information about predominant endemic organisms and the flora colonizing individual patients. Strict adherence to environmental control procedures is followed: All nurses, physicians, technicians, and visitors wear masks, gowns, and gloves when they are in a patient's room. Hands are washed on entry and exit.

The care of the burn wound also demands daily inspection by a physician to monitor for signs of infection. A change in the appearance of the wound—dark brown discoloration, areas of rapid eschar separation, hemorrhagic discoloration of subeschar tissue, or edema and erythema of unburned skin at the margins of the wound—should prompt biopsies of suspicious areas. These biopsies can be assessed by quantitative culture or wound histology. Quantitative culture is useful only in a negative sense, that is, there is a 96.1% correlation of low counts with negative histology results, but only 36% of quantitative cultures showing growth of $>10^5$ organisms per gram of tissue had evidence of invasion by histologic examination. Quantitative cultures are best used as an adjunct to histology by providing species identification and antibiotic sensitivities [68]. Histologic examination of a burn wound biopsy is the only reliable means of making a diagnosis of burn wound infection, differentiating microbial colonization from invasion, and identifying the depth and extent of microbial penetration (Table 34-4). Wound histology has the additional advantage of rapidity of diagnosis;

the results are available within 45 minutes when the frozen section technique is used and within 4 hours when the permanent section technique is used.

Wound Closure

The definitive treatment of the burn wound is excision and grafting. In 1947 Cope recommended early excision of the burn wound to reduce the incidence of wound infection, but even limited studies of excision failed to identify an increase in survival. However, the need for early excision is based not only on survival, but also on cosmetic and functional results. Wounds requiring >2 to 3 weeks to heal typically have an unstable epithelium and develop hypertrophic scarring. This hypertrophic scarring has both cosmetic and functional ramifications [69]. Patients with deep dermal burns who undergo early excision spend less time as inpatients, have decreased hospital and physician costs, miss fewer workdays, and most importantly, require less regrafting [70]. Deep partial-thickness wounds that take >2 to 3 weeks to close spontaneously and full-thickness wounds should be grafted.

The elderly should not be denied early excision. Despite the perception that the elderly may be too frail to undergo operative therapy, the elderly tolerate early excision and grafting well [1,71]. Nonoperative management of small burns in functionally unimportant areas can result in less morbidity and mortality and similar functional outcomes, but this is at the expense of prolonged healing of the open wounds. In one study on this topic, the average time to wound closure in the nonoperative group was 3.2 months as compared with 1.5 months in the operative group [72]. In recent years the authors have steadily reduced the average postburn day of first operation in the elderly. In 1976 the day of first grafting was the thirty-second postburn day, in 1985 it was the eighteenth postburn day, and in 1994 it was the ninth postburn day [9]. The average postburn day of complete wound healing decreased from 49.3 days in the years between 1986 and 1989 to 38.0 days in the 3 years beginning in 1992. This change predominately reflects the decrease in our average extent of burn, for postburn days to healing as a percent of TBSA burn changed little from 1992 to 1995. From 1992 to 1994, patients who did not undergo operative intervention healed their wounds by postburn day 16 on average. Deeper burns, of a deep dermal and full-thickness nature, were grafted. Nonoperative management of thermal injuries in the elderly should be limited to unequivocally superficial burns and, in the frail patient, to deeper burns of little functional importance.

The approach to burn wound excision and grafting should be individualized on the basis of the extent and location of the burn and the physiologic state of the patient. Tangential excision of the burn wound, which involves removal of successive thin layers of the burn wound with a guarded knife or dermatome to the level of viability, offers the advantage of preserving body contours and, if the burn is superficial, the possibility of grafting on the deep dermal layer. Although the use of tourniquets for the excision of the eschar on burned limbs can reduce operative hemorrhage, performing tangential excision often causes significant blood loss in amounts equal to or exceeding the circulating blood volume. Excision of the burn wound with a scalpel or electrocautery device at the level of the investing fascia can be done with less blood loss than tangential excision, theoretically decreasing the physiologic stress of the surgery. Generally, a wound bed excised to fascia has an increased rate of engraftment in comparison with a wound bed of adipose tissue, but may result in greater disfigurement. The elderly all too often have deep burns, because as previously noted, the ratio of full-thickness burn to TBSA burn increases with each decade of life. The authors prefer tangential excision and reserve fascial excision for those patients with a large component of full-thickness burn, a burn with a high associated mortality, or poor cardiac or respiratory reserve. Because of the loss of dermal thickness and vascularity with aging, and therefore concerns over donor site healing, split-thickness skin for grafting is harvested at a moderately thin level of 0.010 in. [10,12]. The harvested site is dressed with fine mesh gauze or an occlusive synthetic covering, which may decrease patient discomfort and hasten donor site epithelialization. If the same donor sites need to be harvested multiple times, consideration should be given to the subcutaneous administration of growth hormone (0.2 mg/kg per day) to reap the potential benefit of augmented donor site healing as documented in burned children [73,74].

In treating patients with thermal injury with an associated mortality of <50%, priority is given to autografting areas of high cosmetic or functional importance such as the hands, feet, face, and joints. In those patients with higher expected mortality, priority is given to excision and grafting of large flat surfaces to reduce the extent of the burn wound as rapidly as possible. Split-thickness grafts can be applied as intact sheets or can be expanded by means of a mesh dermatome to ratios of 1.5:1, 2:1, 3:1, 4:1, 6:1, and 9:1. The face and hands are preferentially covered with sheet autograft and treated with an open technique postoperatively to monitor for signs of seroma or hematoma formation. Other areas are covered with grafts meshed to ratios of 1.5:1 to 4:1 as dictated by the availability of donor sites and are dressed with a nonadherent inner layer of material that reduces shearing and is held in place by coarse mesh gauze wetted every 4 to 6 hours with 0.5% silver nitrate or 5% mafenide acetate solution. Higher ratios of expansion are avoided because of the prolonged time required for closure of the interstices and increased scar formation [75].

The elderly, because of their difficulty in healing donor sites, and patients with massive burn wounds and limited donor sites, would appear to be the ideal candidates for the use of cultured epithelial autografts. Initial reports using sheets of cultured autologous keratinocytes were encouraging, with a

40% to 60% engraftment of such tissue. These early reports noted that engraftment was better on patients <18 years of age and in beds prepared with allograft versus exposed wounds filled with granulation tissue [76,77]. Our results in 16 patients, with BSA burns of >40%, showed initial engraftment of 64.4%. This declined to 46% engraftment by the time of discharge. More discouraging was the actual percentage of the body surfaces covered. It was a mere 4.7% on average, with a mean cost of $43,705 per patient. Decreased engraftment occurred when the cultured cells were applied to fascia as compared with deep dermis and when they were applied to patients with burns of >70% of the body surface. Unfortunately, cultured epidermis fails where it is most needed, in the elderly and on patients with large, deep burns [78]. The fragility of the cells, which lack a supporting dermis and anchoring fibrils, is postulated as the cause of these poor results. It is hoped that techniques of grafting on previously placed and well-vascularized allodermis or commercially prepared nonantigenic allodermis will increase the longevity and durability of cultured epithelial autografts.

To prevent shearing of split-thickness skin grafts and to ensure their vascularization, the grafted area is immobilized for 5 to 7 days postoperatively. In the elderly this period of immobilization is usually well tolerated but associated with certain risks. Aspiration, atelectasis, and pneumonia; the development of decubitus ulcers; and increased joint stiffness, demanding more extensive postoperative rehabilitation, are all potential drawbacks of immobilization. In young patients with small burns of the feet, early ambulation with an Unna's paste boot, even 4 hours postoperatively, has been shown not to compromise graft take [79]. If this can be proven to be efficacious in the elderly population some postoperative morbidity might be avoided.

Nutrition

Thermal injury provokes a hypermetabolic response in the host. High levels of circulating epinephrine and norepinephrine result in a catabolic state [80]. This increase in metabolic rate is proportionate to the size of burn and decreases as wound closure is realized. In burns of 20% to 40% and burns of >75%, resting energy expenditure returns to normal approximately 100 to 150 and 250 days postburn, respectively [81]. Formulas to estimate the caloric needs of these highly stressed individuals can be quite inaccurate. In one study using indirect calorimetry to measure energy expenditure, the Harris-Benedict formula was found to underestimate caloric needs by an average of 23% and the Curreri formula to overestimate needs by 58% [82]. In the authors' institution, indirect calorimetry measurements have been used to develop a formula to predict nutritional needs based on age, sex, and burn size. The formula is used in the first 30 days postburn after which indirect calorimetry measurements are made to establish caloric needs [81].

The increased metabolic demands of injury are often imposed on an elderly patient who is already malnourished. In surveys of chronic care facilities, the rate of malnutrition in the residents ranges from 30% to 85%; however, malnutrition is not confined to the institutionalized elderly. The community-based elderly are also at risk and should be assessed for signs of malnutrition when they are admitted to a burn center. The rate of malnutrition in the ambulatory elderly is poorly documented in the United States, but studies from Great Britain identified an incidence of between 6% and 12%. Physical limitations such as poor dentition and dysphagia, medical conditions such as chronic obstructive lung disease, congestive heart failure, neurologic impairments, and depression, and financial constraints can all contribute to the poor nutritional status of the elderly. Physicians may contribute to a patient's malnutrition by imposing dietary restrictions that are needed to treat medical conditions [83,84]. Populations with chronic medical conditions, such as renal failure requiring chronic peritoneal dialysis and chronic obstructive lung disease necessitating hospitalization, are at even higher risk of malnutrition, with 40% and 60% of these populations, respectively, being malnourished [85,86]. Preexisting malnutrition can affect morbidity and mortality. Malnourished patients with chronic obstructive lung disease have significantly greater requirements for mechanical ventilation and show a trend toward higher mortality [86].

Soon after admission, patients should be assessed both for their underlying nutritional status and their ability to support themselves nutritionally during hospitalization. Patients with burns of >30% of the body surface can rarely meet their caloric needs by spontaneous intake and failure to meet the burn-induced increased metabolic demand results in the erosion of lean body mass. Such patients should be supported by enteral tube feedings. Most commercial enteral formulas suffice, but because of the increased incidence of lactose intolerance with aging, a lactose-free formulation should be considered. Within the first week postburn, a feeding tube should be placed per nares beyond the ligament of Treitz or into the fourth portion of the duodenum under fluoroscopic guidance. Distal placement allows continuous feeding perioperatively and intraoperatively with minimal risk of aspiration [87]. Using this protocol, the need for parenteral nutrition, with its attendant risks of line sepsis and pneumothorax, has been strikingly reduced in our center over 4 years.

Enteral feedings in the elderly burn patient demand close monitoring. Calcium, magnesium, phosphorus, and potassium often rapidly shift into the intracellular compartment at the initiation of feeding, necessitating careful monitoring of these electrolytes [83]. The elderly are known to tolerate glucose loads poorly as compared with their younger counterparts, both in a nonstressed and stressed environment. Intolerance to glucose loads are thought to be secondary to a decreased peripheral sensitivity to insulin, although one study documented additional deficiencies of lower insulin and C-peptide levels in response to glucose loading. By means of a hyperglycemic glucose clamp study, younger trauma patients were shown to metabolize their exogenous

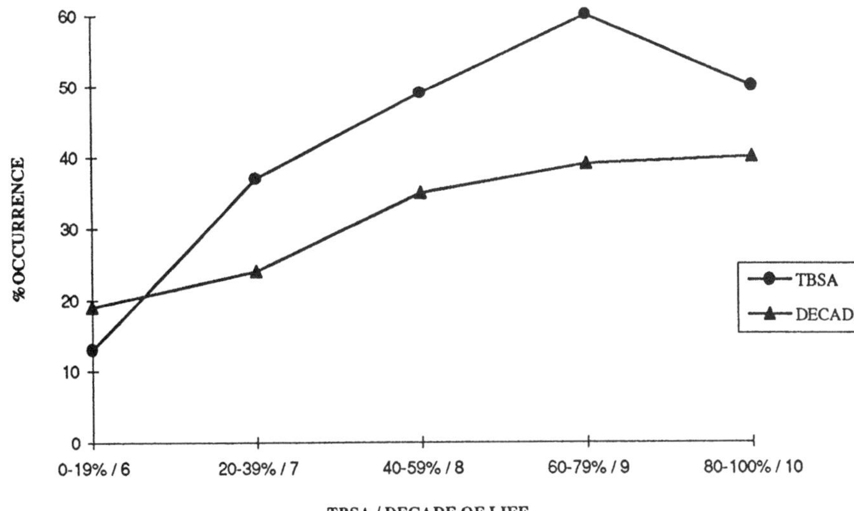

FIG. 34-4. The risk of pneumonia increases with age and extent of burn. (TBSA = total body surface area.)

glucose load at a rate of 5.4 mg/kg per minute (±1.8), as compared with 3.6 mg/kg per minute (±1.0) in the elderly trauma patient [88,89]. During nutritional supplementation in the elderly, the clinician should therefore be cognizant of exogenous glucose loading and endeavor to maintain blood glucose <250 mg/dl. This approach has been shown to improve both collagen metabolism and the function of neutrophils. Hypoglycemia, because of the often impaired ability of the elderly to respond to low blood sugars, should also be avoided [90].

COMPLICATIONS

Pneumonia

Infection as the primary cause of mortality in burn patients decreased in the 1980s from 64% to 42%. During this period, the site of infection causing mortality also changed such that lung-related infection as the cause of mortality increased from 59.6% to 79.8% [6]. The risk of developing pneumonia without evidence of inhalational injury is 8.8%. With inhalational injury diagnosed by xenon scan only, the incidence of pneumonia increases to 19.5%, and with bronchoscopic evidence of inhalational injury, the risk climbs to 45.8%. Increased burn size also correlates with increased rates of pneumonia [7]. The diagnosis of pneumonia is made on the basis of sputum leukocytosis (>25 neutrophils and <25 squamous cells per high power field), fever, change in the character and volume of the sputum, and radiographic evidence of a pulmonary infiltrate. Tracheobronchitis presents similarly to pneumonia but without a radiographic infiltrate. Once the diagnosis of pneumonia is made, antibiotic therapy, directed at the predominant organism in the sputum culture, is begun. Unless dictated by the culture and sensitivities of the infecting organism, antibiotics with a broad spectrum of activity are avoided. In the elderly patients admitted to the unit from 1986 to 1994, 30.8% developed evidence of pneumonia and tracheobronchitis (24.8% and 12.1%, respectively). The group of patients who developed pneumonia had more extensive burns (mean extent of burn, 34.5% vs. 17.6%) and had a higher incidence of inhalational injury (41% vs. 20%) than those who did not develop pneumonia. During this period, pneumonia had an associated mortality of 53.8%. In this elderly population the risk of pneumonia increased with increasing burn size and with each successive decade of life (Fig. 34-4).

From 1981 to 1982, up to 20% of all admissions to U.S. Army Burn Center required endotracheal intubation or tracheostomy for airway control and ventilatory assistance [91]. Tracheostomy has been reported to be required in 3% of burn patients. The indication for tracheostomy is usually the need for prolonged ventilatory assistance and, less commonly, acute loss of airway patency. Twenty-eight percent of patients with tracheostomies are reported to develop major late upper-airway sequelae, such as tracheal stenosis, tracheoesophageal fistula, and tracheoarterial fistula [92]. The need for mechanical ventilation is greater in the elderly than in younger patients, with 40.4% requiring more than a few days on the ventilator. From 1986 to 1994, 13.7% of the elderly burn patients required tracheostomy for prolonged ventilatory assistance.

Gastrointestinal Bleeding

Before the institution of routine antacid prophylaxis for upper gastrointestinal hemorrhage, such bleeding was a common and lethal condition. In patients with a >35% BSA burn, mucosal ulcerations could be found in up to 90% of patients by endoscopy. One-fourth of these patients with mucosal ulcerations developed clinically significant bleeding (requiring >3 U over a 24-hour period), with half that group requiring surgical intervention (13% of patients). These bleeding episodes were associated with a 50% to 70% mortality [93].

Therapy today is directed at prevention of stress ulcer complications. Patients at risk for gastrointestinal hemorrhage, those patients with a >30% BSA burn, receive intermittent intravenous cimetidine and instillation of antacids through their nasogastric tube every 1 to 2 hours to maintain their gastric pH >4.5. This protocol has nearly eliminated this condition in our unit (<2% of patients). In our elderly population, <1% developed symptoms of upper gastrointestinal bleeding from 1986 to 1994.

Concern about a possible relationship between intragastric buffering and nosocomial pneumonia prompted a prospective study of sucralfate antiulcer prophylaxis in thermally injured patients. Although three bleeding events occurred in the sucralfate group and none in our standard prophylaxis group, this difference in the rate of gastrointestinal bleeding was not statistically significant. Although sucralfate did decrease the recovery of gram-negative bacteria in gastric aspirates (48% vs. 60%), no difference in the rate of recovery of gram-negative organisms in the sputum was noted (70%). Patients in the sucralfate group who required mechanical ventilation actually had an increased rate of pneumonia as compared with the group treated with cimetidine and antacids (42.8% vs. 17.9%). When this finding was analyzed by a stepwise logistic regression analysis, age, burn size, and the need for intubation were predictive for the development of pneumonia, but inhalational injury and type of stress ulceration prophylaxis were not [94].

Venous Thrombosis

Deep venous thrombosis is believed to be an uncommon occurrence in burn patients. From 1980 to 1989 at the USAISR, only 0.9% of all thermally injured patients had clinical evidence of a deep venous thrombosis. During that period, only 1.2% of burn patients had a clinically significant pulmonary embolism. Because of the low incidence of these complications and because of the associated risk of bleeding, heparin prophylaxis has not been routinely used [95,96]. The low risk of venous thromboembolism in burn patients has been attributed to the arteriovenous shunting in the burn wound resulting in augmented venous flow rates and the hyperdynamic state of the burn patient with its high cardiac output. However, a retrospective review of the incidence of deep venous thrombosis in our center from 1990 to 1994 revealed that its incidence has increased to 2.2% of admissions and that the elderly burn patient may be at an increased risk. During the period encompassing these two reviews, the detection of deep venous thrombosis was dependent on the physician's clinical suspicion and subsequent confirmation by venography or duplex ultrasonography. This increased incidence, therefore, might be real or simply represent a higher rate of detection. A prospective study using duplex ultrasonographic screening in all burned patients is ongoing to determine the true incidence of deep vein thrombosis in burn patients and to evaluate if the elderly burn patient is at an increased risk.

Suppurative thrombophlebitis is also a well-recognized complication of thermal injury. Fewer than 50% of burn patients with suppurative phlebitis manifest local signs of infection. This absence of physical signs is the danger of suppurative thrombophlebitis. Hematogenous pneumonia or an unexplained, repeated recovery of a single organism from blood culture may be the only indication that there is a suppurative vein. Once this diagnosis is entertained, all previously cannulated veins need to be evaluated. A peripheral vein site requires surgical exploration and central vein sites should be evaluated by duplex ultrasonography. Identification of a suppurative peripheral vein requires institution of antibiotic therapy and excision of the vein. The excision should extend to a level where there is unequivocally normal vein wall and free back bleeding to avoid overlooking an area of intraluminal suppuration. The wound is left open with a light packing that is changed twice daily. When the wound bed is clean and without signs of infection, it is closed secondarily or by skin graft. Prevention of suppuration should be the primary form of therapy. Strict limitations (72 hours) on the time an intravenous cannula, peripheral or central, can be left in place and effective control of the microbial density of the burn wound have decreased the incidence of suppurative thrombophlebitis in our burn patients. The incidence of suppurative phlebitis has decreased from 6.9% of admissions in 1969 to 0.71% more recently (Fig. 34-5) [5,97]. The elderly have also shown a decreased incidence of this condition from 9.3% in the period from 1964 to 1972 to 0.3% more recently [8].

Invasive Burn Wound Infection

The advent of effective topical antimicrobials, rigid infection control procedures, and early burn wound excision have dramatically decreased the overall incidence of invasive burn wound infection. Patients at risk for bacterial and fungal invasive infections have extensive burns (54.4% BSA and 62.5% BSA, respectively), a high incidence of inhalational injury (51% and 47%, respectively), and high mortality (70.6% and 74.5%, respectively). Subdividing invasive infection into bacterial and fungal invasion between the years 1980 and 1989 revealed that although the incidence of bacterial wound invasion dramatically decreased, from 8.9% to 1.1% of admissions, fungal wound invasion remained constant, between 5% and 10% of admissions. The explanation for the persistence of fungal invasion is unclear but appears secondary to the lack of effective topical creams against the filamentous fungi, *Aspergillus*, and mucormycosis.

Detection of invasive wound infection requires prompt action. In the case of bacterial invasion, treatment includes clysis of the burn wound with a broad-spectrum penicillin every 8 to 12 hours, administration of a broad-spectrum penicillin and an aminoglycoside intravenously, and wound

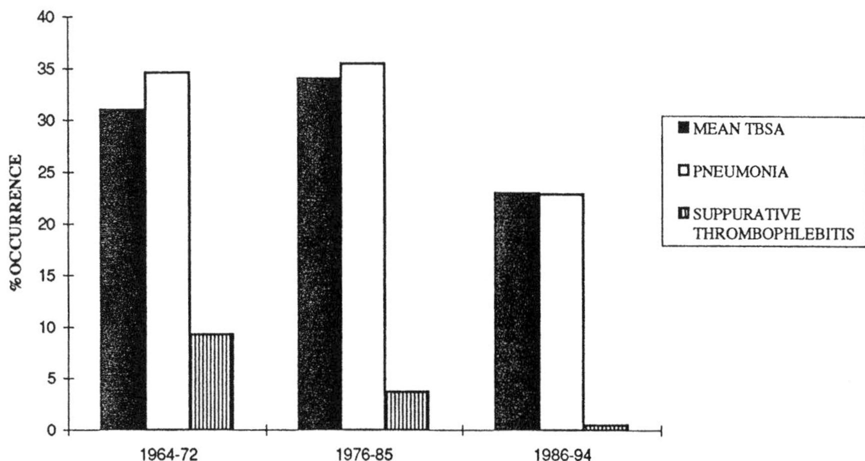

FIG. 34-5. A decrease in mean burn size (mean total body surface area [TBSA]) over time has been associated with lower rates of infectious complications. (USAISR = U.S. Army Institute of Surgical Research.) (Data modified from Pruitt BA Jr, Mason AD, Hunt JL. Burn Injury in the Aged or High-Risk Patient. In Siegel JH, Chodoff PD [eds], The Aged and High Risk Surgical Patient. New York: Grune & Stratton, 1976; and Missavage AE, Pruitt BA Jr. Thermal Injuries in the Elderly. In Adkins RB, Scott HW [eds], Surgical Care for the Elderly. Baltimore: Williams & Wilkins, 1988.)

excision as soon as the patient can tolerate operative intervention. The wound is treated with a gauze dressing or biological dressing after excision. Fungal invasion requires intravenous amphotericin B, topical clotrimazole cream, and wide excision to include amputation if the organisms have extensively invaded the muscles of a limb, as soon as the patient can be stabilized for the operating room [98].

Decubitus Ulcers

Decubitus ulcers occur in all hospitalized patients. It is estimated that 4.7% of all hospitalized patients develop a pressure decubitus. The elderly are at higher risk, because of their poorly vascularized skin and decreased sensation as well as preexisting wasting; the elderly develop this complication in the hospital at a rate of 10% to 20% [99]. Elderly burn patients, because of weight loss secondary to the hypermetabolism of burn injury and the need for prolonged immobilization after grafting, are at a still greater risk for developing pressure ulceration. Scar contraction after spontaneous healing and split-thickness skin grafting can also result in increased stiffness of joints and further loss of mobility in the elderly population. The stiffness and loss of mobility after thermal injury are additive to premorbid functional deficits of the patient. Simple maneuvers such as frequent turning from side to side and repositioning of the limbs are the most effective preventive measures. Physical and occupational therapies need to be used early to encourage elderly patients to be active participants in their rehabilitation [8].

Suppurative Chondritis

Suppurative chondritis of the ear can be a disfiguring complication of thermal injury. The diagnosis is suggested by ear pain (often refractory to narcotics), an erythematous and edematous appearance to the ear, and an increase or obliteration in the auriculocephalic angle. Much like suppurative thrombophlebitis and decubitus ulcers, prevention is the preferred treatment of suppurative chondritis [100]. This is accomplished by twice daily application of Sulfamylon cream and absolute avoidance of pressure on the burned ear. By following these principles, the incidence of suppurative chondritis in patients with ear burns in our unit decreased from 20% in 1967 to 3% in 1984. Once an infection occurs, treatment involves prompt local debridement, if early enough in the course, or aggressive debridement, which may necessitate a bivalve of the ear and resection of all necrotic tissue [101].

PREVENTION OF BURNS

Given the debility and often fatal outcome of thermal injury in the elderly, it is unfortunate that many of these injuries could have been prevented. The cessation of smoking could decrease the incidence of thermal injury. Seventeen (5.4% of admissions during the study period) of the burns were due to smoking accidents in which the victim's clothes or bedding caught fire. Hot water scald burns (9.2% of admissions during the study period) could be limited by simply setting home water heaters <55°C (130°F). Water at this temperature needs >5 minutes of contact to cause a full-thickness injury [13,14]. Finally, the most common etiology for thermal injuries during the period was flame resulting from ignition of a flammable liquid. All too often these substances were used carelessly to burn brush, prime carburetors, or start outdoor barbecues. These preventable injuries tragically accounted for 41.6% of admissions.

ECONOMIC FACTORS

The percentage of elderly in the population is expanding and with it the cost of their health care. In 1970, Medicare and Medicaid expenses for people over the age of 65 were $10 billion annually; by 1985, due to inflation, increased enrollees, and increased aggressiveness of medical care, this had increased to $85 billion [102]. Many authors have reported financial losses for their institutions from Diagnosis-Related Groups reimbursements because many elderly burns cannot be classified in the higher reimbursement category of major burns (full-thickness component >20%). These categories do not take into account that a 20% TBSA burn in an elderly patient is a major burn [1,4].

Future attempts at cost containment in medical expenses might target the elderly burn patient. A universal finding after thermal injury is that nonsurvivors commonly incur expenses at two to three times the rate of survivors. As a group, nonsurvivors are older and have larger percentage BSA burns. The concern of many burn surgeons is that economic pressures will be brought to bear on burn centers to withhold therapy in those elderly patients who can be "predicted" to have a poor outcome [1,4].

Inpatient hospital costs should not be allowed to determine the care or noncare of the elderly burn patient. The ability to return elderly patients to the original home environment with a reasonable level of function should be the endpoint to determine aggressiveness of medical care. Eighty percent to 90% of surviving patients under the age of 75 return to the home environment after thermal injury [1,103]. However, in the >75 group, a significant proportion, between 25% and 35%, require placement in nursing homes and extended care facilities [1,4]. Our experience with burn injury >20% shows that patients >65 years of age have a 61.5% mortality, yet 45% of the survivors returned to the home environment. Patients over the age of 75 with a >20% BSA burn had 84.2% mortality. No survivors returned to the home environment directly on discharge.

The chance of surviving a burn injury has consistently improved, and this improvement has not been denied to the elderly. From 1985 to 1986, 84.4% of patients over the age of 65 with burns of >20% BSA died. Cost-containment advocates might have targeted this group of patients for noncare and allowed them to expire from their injuries. In this group the mortality between 1992 and 1994 was still high, but had fallen to 57.9%. There is still room for progress in the care of the elderly burn patient. Modulation of the inflammatory response, development of durable cultured epidermal-dermal matrixes, and innovations in the treatment of inhalational injury promise breakthroughs in the care of the thermally injured. Economic pressures and the expanding legions of the elderly will prompt difficult decisions in the years to come. A consistent improvement in outcome after thermal injury should not be sacrificed.

REFERENCES

1. Saffle JR, Larson CM, Sullivan J, et al. The continuing challenge of burn care in the elderly. Surgery 1990;108:534–543.
2. Cassell CK, Brody JA. Demography, Epidemiology, and Aging. In Cassell CK, Riesenber DE, Sorensen LB, et al. (eds), Geriatric Medicine (2nd ed). New York: Springer, 1990.
3. Smith DP, Enderson BL, Maull KI. Trauma in the elderly: determinants of outcome. South Med J 1990;83:171–177.
4. Hammond J, Ward CG. Burns in octogenarians. South Med J 1991;84:1316–1319.
5. Pruitt BA Jr, McManus AT. The changing epidemiology of infection in burn patients. World J Surg 1992;16:57–67.
6. Cioffi WG, Kim SH, Pruitt BA Jr, et al. Cause of Mortality in Thermally Injured Patients. In Lorenz S, Zellner PR (eds), Die Infektion beim Brandverletzten. Darmstadt: Steinkopff, 1993.
7. Shirani KZ, Pruitt BA Jr, Mason AD Jr. The influence of inhalation injury and pneumonia on burn mortality. Ann Surg 1987;205:82–87.
8. Pruitt BA Jr, Mason AD, Hunt JL. Burn Injury in the Aged or High-Risk Patient. In Siegel JH, Chodoff PD (eds), The Aged and High Risk Surgical Patient. New York: Grune & Stratton, 1976.
9. Missavage AE, Pruitt BA Jr. Thermal Injuries in the Elderly. In Adkins RB, Scott HW (eds), Surgical Care for the Elderly (1st ed). Baltimore: Williams & Wilkins, 1988.
10. Balin AK. Skin Disease. In Evans JG, Williams TF (eds), Oxford Textbook of Geriatric Medicine. Oxford: Oxford University Press, 1992.
11. Goldfarb MT, Ellis CN, Voorhees JJ. Dermatology. In Cassell CK, Riesenberg DE, Sorensen LB, et al (eds), Geriatric Medicine (2nd ed). New York: Springer, 1990.
12. Fenske NA, Lober CW. Structural and functional changes of normal aging skin. J Am Acad Dermatol 1986;15:571–585.
13. Lawrence JC, Bull JP. Thermal conditions which cause burns. Engineer Med 1976;5:61–63.
14. Bull JP. Burns. Postgrad Med J 1963;39:717–723.
15. Walker AR. Fatal tapwater scald burns in the USA, 1979–86. Burns 1990;16:49–52.
16. Fox RA. Immunology and Ageing. In Evans JG, Williams TF (eds), Oxford Textbook of Geriatric Medicine. Oxford: Oxford University Press, 1992.
17. Miller RA. Minireview: the cell biology of aging: immunological models. J Gerontol 1989;44:B4–B8.
18. Nagel JE, Chopra RK, Chrest FJ, et al. Decreased proliferation, interleukin 2 synthesis, and interleukin 2 receptor expression are accompanied by decreased mRNA expression in phytohemagglutinin-stimulated cells from elderly donors. J Clin Invest 1988;8:1096–1102.
19. Harman SM, Blackman MR. The Hypothalamic-Pituitary Axes. In Evans JG, Williams TF (eds), Oxford Textbook of Geriatric Medicine. Oxford: Oxford University Press, 1992.
20. Morrow LA, Herman WH, Halter JB. Diabetes Mellitus. In Evans JG, Williams TF (eds), Oxford Textbook of Geriatric Medicine. Oxford: Oxford University Press, 1992.
21. Mooradian AD. Normal age-related changes in thyroid hormone economy. Clin Geriatr Med 1995;11:159–169.
22. Evers BM, Townsend CM, Thompson JC. Organ physiology of aging. Surg Clin North Am 1994;74:25–39.
23. Gurwitz JH, Avorn J. The ambiguous relation between aging and adverse drug reactions. Ann Intern Med 1991;114:956–965.
24. Lindeman RD, Tobin J, Shock NW. Longitudinal studies on the rate of decline in renal function with age. J Am Geriatr Soc 1985;33: 278–285.
25. Zaske DE, Chin T, Kohls PR, et al. Initial dosage regimens of gentamicin in patients with burns. J Burn Care Rehabil 1991;12:46–50.
26. Zaske DE, Strate RG, Kohls PR. Amikacin pharmacokinetics: wide interpatient variation in 98 patients. J Clin Pharmacol 1991;31:158–163.
27. Williams L, Lowenthal DT. Drug therapy in the elderly. South Med J 1992;85:127–131.
28. Schenker S, Bay M. Drug disposition and hepatotoxicity in the elderly. J Clin Gastroenterol 1994;18:232–237.
29. Rossor MN. Management of neurological disorders: dementia. J Neurol Neurosurg Psychiatry 1994;57:1451–1456.
30. Skoog I, Nilsson L, Palmertz B, et al. A population-based study of dementia in 85-year-olds. N Engl J Med 1993;328:153–158.
31. Evans DA, Funkenstein HH, Albert MS, et al. Prevalence of Alzheimer's disease in a community population of older persons: higher than previously reported. JAMA 1989;262:2551–2556.
32. Kunik ME, Yudofsky SC, Silver JM, et al. Pharmacologic approach to management of agitation associated with dementia. J Clin Psychiatry 1994;55(Suppl):13–17.
33. Mileski W, Borgstrom D, Lightfoot E, et al. Inhibition of leukocyte-endothelial adherence following thermal injury. J Surg Res 1992;52: 334–339.

34. Youn YK, LaLonde C, Demling R. The role of mediators in the response to thermal injury. World J Surg 1992;16:30–36.
35. Drost AC, Burleson DG, Cioffi WG, et al. Plasma cytokines following thermal injury and their relationship with patient mortality, burn size, and time postburn. J Trauma 1993;35:335–339.
36. Hack CE, DeGroot ER, Felt-Bersma RJ, et al. Increased plasma levels of interleukin-6 in sepsis. Blood 1989;74:1704–1710.
37. Ertel W, Faist E, Nestle C, et al. Kinetics of interleukin-2 and interleukin-6 synthesis following major mechanical trauma. J Surg Res 1990;48:622–628.
38. Gillespie RW, Dimick AR, Gillespie PW, et al. Initial Assessment and Management. In Advanced Burn Life Support Course: Instructor's Manual. Lincoln, NE:Nebraska Burn Institute, 1994.
39. Rue LW, Cioffi WG, Mason AD, et al. Improved survival of burned patients with inhalation injury. Arch Surg 1993;128:772–780.
40. Fitzpatrick JC, Cioffi WG Jr. Inhalation injury. Trauma Q 1994;11:114–126.
41. Kane RL, Ouslander JG, Abrass IB. Clinical Implications of the Aging Process. In Kane RL, Ouslander JG, Abrass IB (eds), Essentials of Clinical Geriatrics (3rd ed). New York: McGraw-Hill, 1994.
42. Walker HL, McCleod CG Jr, McManus WF. Experimental inhalation injury in the goat. J Trauma 1981;21:962–964.
43. Levine BA, Petroff PA, Slade CL, et al. Prospective trials of dexamethasone and aerosolized gentamicin in the treatment of inhalation injury in the burned patient. J Trauma 1978;18:188–193.
44. Cioffi WG, DeLemos RA, Coalson JJ, et al. Decreased pulmonary damage in primates with inhalation injury treated with high-frequency ventilation. Ann Surg 1993;218:328–337.
45. Goldbaum LR, Orellano T, Dergal E. Mechanism of the toxic action of carbon monoxide. Ann Clin Lab Sci 1976;6:372–376.
46. Fiamingo FG, Jung DW, Alben JO. Structural perturbation of the a3–CuB site in mitochondrial cytochrome C oxidase by alcohol solvents. Biochemistry 1990;29:4627–4633.
47. Grube BJ, Marvin JA, Heimbach DM. Therapeutic hyperbaric oxygen: help or hindrance in burn patients with carbon monoxide poisoning. J Burn Care Rehabil 1988;9:249–252.
48. Cox CS Jr, Zwischenberger JB, Traber DL, et al. Heparin improves oxygenation and minimizes barotrauma after severe smoke inhalation in an ovine model. Surg Gynecol Obstet 1993;174:339–349.
49. Brown M, Desai M, Traber LD, et al. Dimethylsulfoxide with heparin in the treatment of smoke inhalation. J Burn Care Rehabil 1988;9:22–25.
50. Ogura H, Cioffi WG, Okerberg CV, et al. The effects of pentoxifylline on pulmonary function following smoke inhalation. J Surg Res 1994;56:242–250.
51. Pitt RM, Parker JC, Jurkovich GJ, et al. Analysis of altered capillary pressure and permeability after thermal injury. J Surg Res 1987;42:693–702.
52. Ferrara JJ, Dyess DL, Collins JN, et al. Effects of pentafraction administration on microvascular permeability alterations induced by graded thermal injury. Surgery 1994;115:182–189.
53. Lund T, Onarheim H, Reed RK. Pathogenesis of edema formation in burn injuries. World J Surg 1992;16:2–9.
54. Watters JM, Bessey PQ. Critical care for the elderly patient. Surg Clin North Am 1994;74:187–197.
55. Agarwal N, Petro J, Salisbury RE. Physiologic profile monitoring in burned patients. J Trauma 1983;23:577–583.
56. Moylan JA, Inge WI, Pruitt BA Jr. Circulatory changes following circumferential extremity burns evaluated by the ultrasonic flowmeter: an analysis of 60 thermally injured limbs. J Trauma 1971;11:763–770.
57. Saffle JR, Zeluff GR, Warden GD. Intramuscular pressure in the burned arm: measurement and response to escharotomy. Am J Surg 1980;140:825–831.
58. Frank SM, Beattie C, Christopherson R, et al. Epidural versus general anesthesia, ambient operating room temperature, and patient age as predictors of inadvertent hypothermia. Anesthesiology 1992;77:252–257.
59. Wagner JA, Robinson S, Marino RP. Age and temperature regulation of humans in neutral and cold environments. J Appl Physiol 1974;37:562–565.
60. Hind M. An investigation into factors that affect oesophageal temperature during abdominal surgery. J Adv Nurs 1994;19:457–464.
61. Frank SM, Higgins MS, Breslow MJ, et al. The catecholamine, cortisol, and hemodynamic responses to mild perioperative hypothermia. Anesthesiology 1995;82:83–93.
62. Gubler KD, Gentilello LM, Hassantash SA, et al. The impact of hypothermia on dilutional coagulopathy. J Trauma 1994;36:847–851.
63. Just B, Trevien V, Delva E, et al. Prevention of intraoperative hypothermia by preoperative skin-surface warming. Anesthesiology 1993;79:214–218.
64. Monafo WW, Freedman B. Topical therapy for burns. Surg Clin North Am 1987;67:133–145.
65. Mason AD Jr, McManus AT, Pruitt BA Jr. Association of burn mortality and bacteremia: a 25-year review. Arch Surg 1986;121:1027–1031.
66. McManus AT, McManus WF, Mason AD Jr, et al. Microbial colonization in a new intensive care burn unit. Arch Surg 1985;120:217–223.
67. McManus AT, Mason AD Jr, McManus WF, et al. A decade of reduced gram-negative infections and mortality associated with improved isolation of burned patients. Arch Surg 1994;129:1306–1309.
68. McManus AT, Kim SH, McManus WF, et al. Comparison of quantitative microbiology and histopathology in divided burn-wound biopsy specimens. Arch Surg 1987;122:74–76.
69. Deitch EA, Wheelahan TM, Rose MP, et al. Hypertrophic burn scars: analysis of variables. J Trauma 1983;23:895–898.
70. Engrav LH, Heimbach DM, Reus JL, et al. Early excision and grafting vs. nonoperative treatment of burns of indeterminate depth: a randomized prospective study. J Trauma 1983;23:1001–1004.
71. Deitch EA. A policy of early excision and grafting in elderly burn patients shortens the hospital stay and improves survival. Burns 1985;12:109–114.
72. Housinger T, Saffle J, Ward S, et al. Conservative approach to the elderly patient with burns. Am J Surg 1984;148:817–820.
73. Herndon DN, Barrow RE, Kunkle KR, et al. Effects of recombinant human growth hormone on donor site healing in severely burned children. Ann Surg 1990;212:424–431.
74. Fleming RYD, Rutan RL, Jahoor F, et al. Effect of recombinant human growth hormone on catabolic hormones and free fatty acids following thermal injury. J Trauma 1992;32:698–703.
75. Pruitt BA Jr, Goodwin CW Jr, Pruitt SK. Burns. In Sabiston DC Jr (ed), Textbook of Surgery: The Biological Basis of Modern Surgical Practice (14th ed). Philadelphia: Saunders, 1991.
76. Teepe RG, Kreis RW, Koebrugge EJ, et al. The use of cultured autologous epidermis in the treatment of extensive burn wounds. J Trauma 1990;30:269–275.
77. Deluca M, Albanese E, Bondanza S, et al. Multicentre experience in the treatment of burns with autologous and allogenic cultured epithelium fresh or preserved in a frozen state. Burns 1989;15:303–319.
78. Rue LW, Cioffi WG, McManus WF, et al. Wound closure and outcome in extensively burned patients treated with cultured autologous keratinocytes. J Trauma 1993;34:662–668.
79. Grube BJ, Engrav LH, Heimbach, DM. Early ambulation and discharge in 100 patients with burns of the foot treated by grafts. J Trauma 1992;33:662–664.
80. Wilmore DW, Long JM, Mason AD Jr, et al. Catecholamines: mediator of the hypermetabolic response to thermal injury. Ann Surg 1974;180:653–669.
81. Milner EA, Cioffi WG, Mason AD, et al. A longitudinal study of resting energy expenditure in thermally injured patients. J Trauma 1994;37:167–170.
82. Turner WW, Ireton CS, Hunt JL, et al. Predicting energy expenditures in burned patients. J Trauma 1985;25:11–16.
83. Rolandelli RH, Ullrich JR. Nutritional support in the frail elderly surgical patient. Surg Clin North Am 1994;74:79–93.
84. Buckler DA, Kelber ST, Goodwin JS. The use of dietary restrictions in malnourished nursing home patients. J Am Geriatr Soc 1994; 42:1100–1102.
85. Jones MR. Etiology of severe malnutrition: results of an international cross-sectional study in continuous ambulatory peritoneal dialysis patients. Am J Kidney Dis 1994;23:412–420.
86. Laaban JP, Kouchakji E, Dore MF, et al. Nutritional status of patients with chronic obstructive pulmonary disease. Chest 1993;103:1362–1368.
87. Buescher TM. Perioperative Enteral Feedings. In Proceedings of the 45th Anniversary Symposium, USAISR. Washington, DC: US Government Printing Office, 1992.
88. Katz MS, Lowenthal DT. Influences of age and exercise on glucose metabolism: implications for management of older diabetics. South Med J 1994;87:S70–S73.
89. Watters JM, Moulton SB, Clancey SM, et al. Aging exaggerates glucose intolerance following injury. J Trauma 1994;37:786–791.

90. McMurray JF. Wound healing with diabetes mellitus: better glucose control for better wound healing in diabetics. Surg Clin North Am 1984;64:769–778.
91. Lund T, Goodwin CW, McManus WF, et al. Upper airway sequelae in burn patients requiring endotracheal intubation or tracheostomy. Ann Surg 1985;201:374–382.
92. Jones WG, Madden M, Finkelstein, et al. Tracheostomies in burn patients. Ann Surg 1989;209:471–474.
93. McElwee HP, Sirinek KR, Levine BA. Cimetidine affords protection equal to antacids in prevention of stress ulceration following thermal injury. Surgery 1979;86:620–626.
94. Cioffi WG, McManus AT, Rue LW, et al. Comparison of acid neutralizing and non-acid neutralizing stress ulcer prophylaxis in thermally injured patients. J Trauma 1994;36:541–547.
95. Rue LW, Cioffi WG Jr, Rush R, et al. Thromboembolic complications in thermally injured patients. World J Surg 1992;16:1151–1155.
96. Purdue GF, Hunt JL. Pulmonary emboli in burned patients. J Trauma 1988;28:218–219.
97. Pruitt BA Jr, McManus WF, Kim SH, et al. Diagnosis and treatment of cannula-related intravenous sepsis in burn patients. Ann Surg 1980;191:546–554.
98. Becker WK, Cioffi WG, McManus AT, et al. Fungal burn wound infection. Arch Surg 1991;126:44–48.
99. Cooney TG, Reuler JB. Pressure Sores. In Cassell CK, Riesenberg DE, Sorensen LB, et al. (eds), Geriatric Medicine (2nd ed). New York: Springer, 1990.
100. Purdue GF, Hunt JL. Chondritis of the burned ear: a preventable complication. Am J Surg 1986;152:257–259.
101. Mills DC, Roberts LW, Mason AD Jr, et al. Suppurative chondritis: its incidence, prevention, and treatment in burn patients. Plast Reconstr Surg 1988;82:267–276.
102. Pawlson LG. Health Care Implication of an Aging Population. In Hazzard WR, Andres R, Bierman EL, et al. (eds), Principles of Geriatric Medicine and Gerontology (2nd ed). New York: McGraw-Hill, 1990.
103. Larson CM, Saffle JR, Sullivan J. Lifestyle adjustments in elderly patients after burn injury. J Burn Care Rehabil 1992;13:48–52.

Surgical Care for the Elderly, 2nd ed., edited by
R. Benton Adkins, Jr., and H. William Scott, Jr.
Lippincott–Raven Publishers, Philadelphia © 1998.

CHAPTER 35

Head and Neck Cancer

John M. Castle and Riley Rees

Elderly patients, defined as 65 years and older, account for >50% of all cancer cases and two-thirds of all cancer deaths in the United States [1]. These patients have 10 times the risk of developing cancer than a person <65. This problem will only intensify as our mean population age continues to increase.

Intraoral head and neck carcinomas account for 5% of all malignancies. The American Cancer Society estimates more than 41,000 new cases and 12,000 deaths from head and neck cancer in 1997 [2]. Squamous cell carcinoma makes up approximately 95% of these neoplasms. Men are affected more than women; however, this ratio has been decreasing as more women continue smoking.

The etiology of high head and neck cancer rates in the elderly appears to be multifactorial. Certainly, long-term exposure to carcinogens predisposes the elderly to cancer. Alcohol and tobacco use have been strongly associated with head and neck cancer [3–5]. The form of tobacco—smoked (e.g., cigarette, cigar, pipe) or smokeless (e.g., snuff, dip, chew)—appears to carry the same danger [6]. Cutaneous basal cell and squamous cell carcinomas are directly related to sun exposure. Nickel and chromium in the workplace have been related to sinus and nasopharyngeal cancer [7]. Chronic inflammation and trauma from dentures or poor oral hygiene may also serve as inciting agents. Viral infection from the Epstein-Barr virus has been associated with nasopharyngeal cancer in Asia. At a cellular level, the elderly may be more susceptible to carcinogens because of impaired DNA repair, defective tumor suppressor genes, or enhanced oncogene expression [8]. There also may be an age-related decrease in immune function. Immunosuppressed patients such as transplant and human immunodeficiency virus patients are known to suffer a higher incidence of neoplasms.

Several prejudices are reflected in the treatment of cancer in the elderly [9]. Many elderly people share misconceptions and fears about cancer. As a result, they participate in fewer cancer detection programs. Early cancer symptoms are often missed or attributed to aging. When they finally present, the disease is in a more advanced stage, limiting the treatment options. With such advanced disease, treatment options are sought to avoid the pain and suffering from more aggressive protocols. The goal of therapy is often palliation and not cure. In addition, there is an age bias among health care professionals, with the elderly receiving less aggressive screening, diagnosis, and treatment. The elderly are often excluded from clinical trials for these reasons.

ANATOMY

A thorough understanding of head and neck anatomy is important in identifying, staging, and treating any head and neck neoplasm. The oral cavity is bounded by the lips, hard palate, and anterior two-thirds of the tongue. The buccal mucosa, alveolar ridges, and retromolar trigone are also included in this space.

The oropharynx is composed of the posterior and lateral pharyngeal walls. It contains the base of the tongue, soft palate, and tonsils. The nasopharynx is that portion of the pharynx that lies superior to the soft palate. The hypopharynx is that portion of the pharynx from the base of the tongue to the cricopharyngeus. It is posterior to the larynx and includes the pyriform sinuses.

The larynx is composed of three parts. The glottis contains the true vocal cords. The supraglottic region extends from above the true cords cephalad to the epiglottis including the false cords, ventricular wall, and arytenoepiglottic folds. The subglottic region contains the larynx below the true cords. The lymphatic drainage has been grouped into five levels as shown in Fig. 35-1.

Patterns of cervical node metastases have been mapped and provide the keys to accurate diagnosis [10]. Oral cavity neoplasms tend to spread to levels I, II, and III. Tumors of the larynx, oropharynx, and hypopharynx usually spread to levels II, III, and IV. Isolated level IV tumor is more commonly seen from metastatic disease originating below the clavicles. Nasopharyngeal lesions often go to level V.

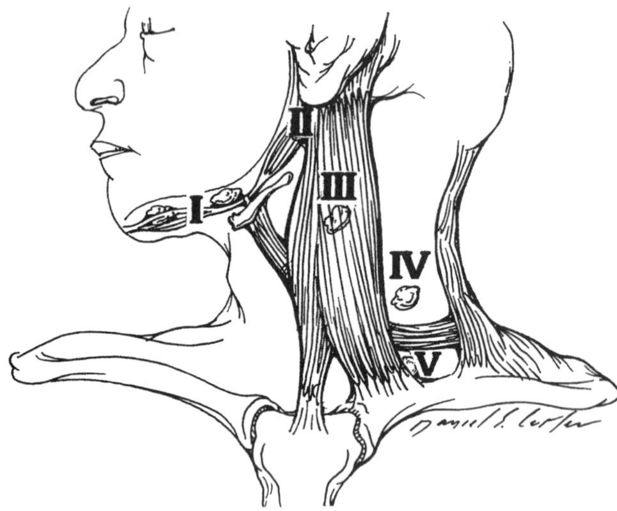

FIG. 35-1. Cervical lymph node levels: level I, submandibular; level II, upper jugular; level III, midjugular; level IV, lower jugular; and level V, posterior cervical.

TABLE 35-1. *Staging of head and neck cancers*

Site	Stage	Description
Oral cavity and oropharynx (based on tumor size)		
	T1	Tumor ≤2 cm (greatest diameter)
	T2	Tumor >2 cm, but not >4 cm
	T3	Tumor >4 cm
	T4	Tumor >4 cm with invasion of adjacent tissue
Larynx		
Supraglottis		
	T1	Tumor confined to one subsite
	T2	Tumor involves more than one subsite without cord fixation
	T3	Tumor confined to larynx with cord fixation
	T4	Massive tumor extending beyond larynx
Glottis		
	T1a	Tumor limited to one vocal cord
	T1b	Tumor involves both vocal cords
	T2	Tumor extends to supraglottis or subglottis
	T3	Tumor limited to larynx, fixed vocal cords
	T4	Massive tumor extending beyond larynx
Subglottis		
	T1	Tumor limited to subglottis
	T2	Tumor extends to vocal cords
	T3	Tumor limited to larynx, fixed vocal cords
	T4	Massive tumor extending beyond larynx

DIAGNOSIS

The diagnosis of head and neck cancer begins with a thorough history and physical examination. A history of alcohol and tobacco use places the patient at high risk for aerodigestive neoplasms. Any mass in the head or neck of an elderly person should be considered cancer until proven otherwise. Nonhealing oral sores, bleeding, or trismus may be signs of oral cancer. A history of speckled patches (leukoplakia) or red patches (erythroplasia) in the oral cavity may signal a premalignant lesion that demands further workup. Malignant transformation is noted in up to 5% of leukoplakia and in as many as 65% with erythroplasia [11,12]. Bloody, foul-smelling nasal discharge or recurrent sinusitis can be seen with nasopharyngeal cancer. Hoarseness, stridor, persistent coughing, or otalgia often suggest laryngeal tumors. Odynophagia and dysphagia may be seen with oropharyngeal and hypopharyngeal tumors and are usually a late finding in elderly patients. Facial paralysis or weakness may be a sign of parotid tumor with facial nerve invasion.

The mainstay of the head and neck examination is visualization and palpation. A complete examination can be easily done in the office with a headlight or reflecting mirror, dental mirror, and a flexible nasal endoscope. First, the head and neck are inspected and palpated for any asymmetry or mass. The same is done for the oral cavity. A speculum examination of the nasal cavity is performed. The pharynx and larynx are inspected with a dental mirror. Thereafter, nasal endoscopy complements the mirror examination. A mass in the neck should undergo fine-needle aspiration. Fine-needle aspiration has >90% accuracy for squamous cell carcinoma when an adequate sample is obtained [13]. The needle tract does not seed tumor cells. Visible nasal or oral mucosal lesions should be directly biopsied using local anesthesia.

The basic radiologic studies are a chest x-ray and a neck computed tomographic (CT) scan. The chest x-ray can identify lesions in the lung fields, the most common site of metastatic spread. It can also provide information on the cardiopulmonary status of the patient, which is important in elderly patients, many of whom are smokers. Lung parenchyma, pulmonary vascular status, and heart size can be evaluated. CT scan of the neck is important to define the extent of the primary lesion and provide information on nodal status [14].

Examination under anesthesia is carried out on all patients before definitive therapy. More extensive palpation of the oral cavity and pharynx can be performed. Next, direct laryngoscopy is done to visualize the larynx and hypopharynx, with biopsy specimens taken as needed. Bronchoscopy is indicated in patients with signs and symptoms of upper airway disease. Likewise, esophagoscopy should be performed on patients with dysphagia or odynophagia. A thorough examination of the upper aerodigestive tract is important because of the 10% to 15% incidence of synchronous neoplasms [15]. The incidence of metachronous tumors is 15% to 25%, with most diagnosed within 3 years of the primary tumor [16].

STAGING

The staging of head and neck cancer is important for defining treatment and prognosis. The American Joint Committee for Cancer Staging TNM system (revised in 1992) is currently in use [17]. The primary tumor's size and local extent is represented by the letter *T* (Table 35-1). The larynx tumor staging is based on tumor extension and fixation of

TABLE 35-2. *Staging of cervical nodes*

Cervical node categories	
N0	Clinically negative nodes
N1	Single homolateral node <3 cm
N2a	Single homolateral node 3–6 cm
N2b	Multiple homolateral nodes <6 cm
N2c	Bilateral/contralateral nodes <6 cm
N3	Node >6 cm
Staging	
Stage I	T1 N0 M0
Stage II	T2 N0 M0
Stage III	T3 N0 M0, T1/T2/T3 N1 M0
Stage IV	Any T4, any N2/N3, any M0

the vocal cords. The hypopharynx has a similar staging system. Tumor size is the main determinant in the oral cavity and oropharynx.

The cervical node staging is represented by the letter *N* (Table 35-2). Cervical node disease is present in 30% of patients at diagnosis and subsequently develops in another 20% (Fig. 35-2). The number of lymph nodes positive for cancer and the presence of extranodal disease are related to the incidence of tumor recurrence and distant metastases [18,19].

Distant metastases are based on their presence (Ml) or absence (M0). One study demonstrated distant metastases in 11% of patients with head and neck cancer [20]. As expected, distant metastases were more commonly seen with large primary tumors and extensive cervical node disease. Lung (83%) was the most common site, followed by bone (31%) and liver (6%). Survival is poor, with most patients living <1 year.

By combining T, N, and M, a staging system for head and neck cancer is constructed. The general 5-year cure rate for overall head and neck cancer is >75% for stage I, 50% to 75% for stage II, 25% to 50% for stage III, and <25% for stage IV [21].

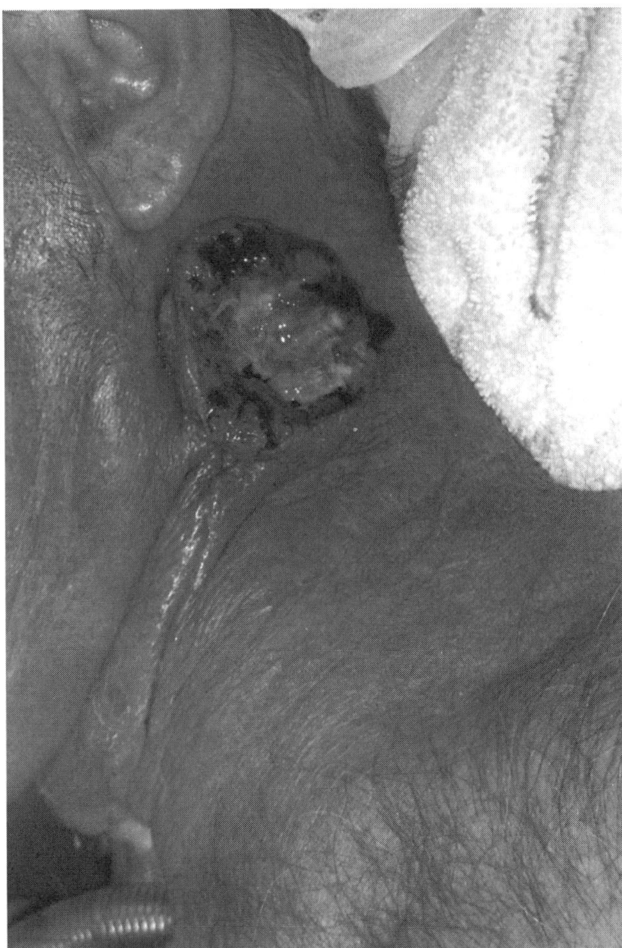

FIG. 35-2. Ulcerated cervical lymph node.

TREATMENT

Pretreatment diagnostic evaluation is important in the elderly because of associated comorbidities. Cardiac status should be evaluated by electrocardiography with further workup as needed. Patients with angina require stress testing. Cardiac disease can be treated medically and special perioperative monitoring can be used. Pulmonary disease is common in this population. Pulmonary function tests along with a chest x-ray should be obtained. Many patients benefit from bronchodilators and other medical therapy because pulmonary complications are formidable after head and neck surgery. Malnutrition with significant weight loss is commonly seen. This has been associated with increased postoperative complications and longer hospitalizations [22]. Nutritional supplementation either enteral or parenteral is often needed before, during, and after treatment. Weight and nutritional parameters should be monitored during treatment. Albumin, prealbumin, or transferrin measurements can be used to follow nutritional status. Malnutrition from heavy alcohol use should alert the physician to possible liver disease and potential alcohol withdrawal symptoms at the time of treatment. Attempts should be made to identify these high-risk patients [23].

Surgery, radiation, and chemotherapy are the treatment modalities of head and neck cancer. Small tumors (T1, T2) can be treated with surgery or radiation therapy alone. Currently, surgery followed by radiation is the mainstay for most advanced head and neck neoplasms. The goal of surgery is removal of the entire tumor and a 2-cm margin of tumor-free tissue. Surgery is indicated for large tumors, tumors invading into adjacent structures such as bone or cartilage, and cervical node disease. Surgery is indicated for those patients who are noncompliant or unable to travel for radiation treatments. Salvage surgery may represent the only treatment option after patients have failed radiation or combined chemoradiation. Palliative surgery has a role in local wound control for end-stage head and neck disease.

There are several disadvantages with surgery. First, vital structures are often sacrificed to fully excise tumors, leaving deficits in breathing, speech, swallowing, and mastication. Frequently, these patients already feed poorly and have underlying malnutrition. Microscopic disease at the wound margin or lymph nodes beyond the resection can be overlooked. Extensive resections of the head and neck are associated with significant functional morbidity. However, several clinical studies have shown that if comorbidities are controlled, surgical complications and survival are similar between the elderly and younger groups [24,25].

Radiotherapy is an important modality for treating head and neck neoplasms either as primary treatment or to control local disease. Radiation alone is equally effective in treating most small tumors (T1, T2). This avoids speech, swallowing, and cosmetic deformities. Unfortunately, as tumor mass increases or cervical lymphatics are involved, radiotherapy becomes less effective. For advanced stage III and IV neck disease, postoperative radiation is usually started 6 weeks after ablative surgery. It is important that the wound is fully healed prior to radiotherapy. Local and regional control is improved by treating potential microscopic disease in the area. Radiotherapy may also be useful for unresectable disease or positive margins. Pain from end-stage or metastatic disease may be treated with radiotherapy. Hyperfractionated radiation given twice daily, 4 to 6 hours apart, appears to be effective treatment for squamous cell carcinoma of the head and neck [26].

There are also several disadvantages to radiotherapy. Radiation alone is not effective against bulky tumors or tumors that have invaded adjacent structures such as bone. Preoperative radiotherapy is associated with a higher surgical complication rate due to problems with wound healing. Adjacent normal tissue may be injured, resulting in osteoradionecrosis, dry mouth, or wound dehiscence with fistula formation [27].

Chemotherapy has been useful for stages III and IV head and neck cancer. The use of platinum compounds such as cisplatin or carboplatin combined with 5-fluorouracil has produced initial response rates of 85% to 95% [28,29]. The use of cisplatin alone has produced partial response rates of 68% [30]. Combining chemotherapy with radiotherapy produces complete responses in some patients. Chemotherapeutic agents such as platinum compounds induce radiation sensitization of the tumor and make radiotherapy more effective [31,32]. Induction chemotherapy prior to radiation has demonstrated response rates similar to surgical resection for advanced laryngeal cancer, although survival is unaffected [33]. The advantage of induction chemotherapy is organ preservation and treatment of metastatic disease. Unfortunately, the elderly are more sensitive to chemotherapy. Myelotoxicity, mucositis, cardiotoxicity, and central nervous system toxicity may be more severe in older patients [34]. Reduced renal clearance requires dose adjustments. The combined effect of chemotherapy and radiation is variable in these patients.

Cervical node disease has traditionally required surgical treatment. The radical neck dissection (RND) introduced by Crile in 1906 and popularized by Martin et al. has been the primary treatment of neck disease [35,36]. Classic RND involves cervical lymph node removal from the clavicle to the base of the skull including the sternocleidomastoid muscle, internal jugular vein, and spinal accessory nerve. Preferred treatment requires nodal tissue removed en bloc with the primary tumor to ensure removal of all intervening lymphatics.

RND often produces functional deficits. A major complication is shoulder weakness resulting from transection of the spinal accessory nerve. Facial swelling can be a significant problem, especially if bilateral RNDs are performed. The carotid artery, repositioned beneath the skin, is at risk of rupture if wound breakdown occurs. A modified RND preserves either the sternocleidomastoid muscle, jugular vein, spinal accessory nerve, or a combination of these structures. Bocca et al. describe the functional neck dissection, which spares the sternocleidomastoid, the internal jugular vein, and the spinal accessory nerve [37]. In their review of 843 cases, functional neck dissection had comparable survival and recurrence rates with RND for node-negative necks and mobile cervical node disease with a lower morbidity. Functional neck dissection is contraindicated for fixed lymph node disease or recurrent neck disease. An uninvolved spinal accessory nerve can be spared even in a neck with grossly positive results without reduction in survival or control of neck disease [38]. Selective neck dissections remove only specific lymphatic areas and include the supraomohyoid (levels I, II, and III) and the jugular (levels III, IV, and V) dissections. Radiation therapy is often added postoperatively for advanced cervical disease. Radiotherapy appears to reduce local recurrence but does not improve survival [39].

Cervical metastasis from an unknown primary cancer is seen in 5% of patients and deserves special attention. Squamous cell metastases found above the clavicle are usually from a head and neck source, although they can occur from lung, breast, and stomach neoplasms. Triple endoscopy (i.e., laryngoscopy, bronchoscopy, and esophagoscopy) should be performed and biopsies of the tonsils, base of tongue, nasopharynx, and pyriform sinuses should be obtained. Treatment requires neck dissection and continued postoperative surveillance for a primary lesion. Postoperative radiation is useful for nasopharyngeal lesions, but may not influence survival [40].

Head and neck cancer with N0 necks should undergo the appropriate neck dissection if the size, site, and grade of the primary tumor make it high risk for metastases. Selective neck dissection (supraomohyoid or jugular) is appropriate in some cases and may be expanded intraoperatively if nodal disease is found.

ORAL CAVITY

Carcinoma of the lip is a disease of elderly men. More than 90% of lower lip lesions are squamous cell carcinomas. These tumors are usually well differentiated and grow slowly, presenting as an ulcer that fails to heal. Lip cancer is associated with sun exposure, with a higher incidence among fair-skinned individuals, people with outdoor occupations, and people who live in the southern United States. Cigarette and pipe smoking are risk factors. The lymph drainage is to submental and submandibular nodes. This may be bilateral if the tumor is in the midline. Cervical metastases occur in only 5% to 10% of patients. Because these lesions are visible, they usually come to medical attention at an early stage and are easily biopsied for a pathologic diagnosis. Aggressive, advanced lip cancer is uncommon in the elderly unless it is neglected.

Equally effective is surgical excision or radiotherapy in T1 and T2 lesions. In the elderly, surgery is preferred to avoid the lip atrophy and dryness after radiation [41]. Treatment with a shield excision is the preferred treatment. Primary closure is possible if one-third or less of the lip is involved. There is great laxity of the lower lip in elderly patients. Larger defects can be closed using lip advancement or lip-sharing techniques [42]. Neck dissection is indicated for cervical disease. Supraomohyoid dissection may be an acceptable alternative in node-negative necks with large primary tumors. Postoperative radiation is important for larger lesions (T2–T4). Five-year survival rates are between 70% and 90% unless there is cervical node disease [43].

Carcinoma of the tongue is predominantly squamous cell carcinoma occurring in elderly individuals. Most lesions are painful ulcerations that occur along the edge of the anterior two-thirds of the tongue. Alcohol, tobacco, and poor oral hygiene contribute to the development of this tumor. Lymph node drainage is to level I, II, and III nodes. Metastatic potential is great, with 20% to 60% of patients with positive nodes at presentation, and bilateral node spread is frequent [44]. Elderly patients are dependent on their tongue for speech and swallowing. Loss of tongue function is devastating. Great care must be taken to avoid impairing tongue mobility and sensation. Therefore, tongue flaps are poor reconstructive choices for oral defects in the elderly.

Treatment is controversial for tongue cancer. Surgery with preservation of maximal tongue function is preferred for lesions of the anterior two-thirds [45]. Wide excision of the primary tumor along with RND is indicated for cancer-positive nodes. Supraomohyoid neck dissection may be substituted for node-negative disease. Speech and swallowing usually return to normal after resection of anterior tongue lesions. Radiation therapy is more appropriate for posterior one-third tongue lesions because wide excision can cause severe impairment of speech and swallowing. Five-year survival rates are 71% to 85% for negative nodes and 26% to 38% for positive nodes [46].

The floor of the mouth is a frequent site of oral cancer. A painful mass or ulcer is the usual presentation. These tumors are aggressive, with a high incidence (50%) of distant metastases [47]. Tumor thickness >7 mm and perineural invasion are poor prognostic factors [48]. Early stage disease is effectively treated with surgery. Advanced stage disease is treated with surgery followed by radiation therapy.

OROPHARYNX

The oropharynx produces higher grade and more aggressive tumors than the oral cavity [49]. These tumors are often occult until they are large with extensive nodal spread. Often, cervical node metastasis is the presenting sign. The tonsillar region is the most common site of lesions. Palatine tumors are often multicentric and associated with synchronous tumors of the head and neck. They are frequently found sooner because of their location beneath dentures and their propensity to bleed.

The success of treatment of small lesions (T1 and most T2) is equivalent between surgery and radiotherapy. Radiation is usually chosen in the elderly because it preserves function and avoids surgical morbidity. However, osteoradionecrosis is a significant problem when it occurs. Advanced lesions are treated with a combination of wide excision, neck dissection, and postoperative radiation. Aspiration is a problem if the resection extends into the vallecula. Palatal surgery requires the use of palatal obturators, which must be frequently adjusted to ensure a secure fit.

LARYNX

Laryngeal carcinoma is the second most common site of cancer in the head and neck. The larynx is divided into three regions: supraglottic, glottic, and subglottic. Glottic tumors are the most common (60%), followed by supraglottic tumors (40%), and subglottic (1% to 4%). Glottic lesions produce hoarseness whereas supraglottic lesions often remain occult until they reach an advanced stage. The lymphatic drainage of the vocal cord region is poor, with little cervical spread until advanced disease of stages T3 (22%) and T4 (41%) [50]. Therefore, glottic tumors rarely metastasize. The supraglottic region has a rich lymphatic system and a much higher rate of nodal disease. Tumors of the supraglottic region commonly spread along the aryteno-epiglottic fold or into the pyriform sinus.

The treatment of glottic lesions depends on the stage of disease. T1 and most T2 lesions are treated equally successfully by surgery or radiation with 5-year survival rates >90% and 65%, respectively [51]. Radiotherapy is usually recommended, especially in the elderly, because voice function is preserved. Endoscopic excision and CO_2 laser ablation have been effective in treating T1 and some T2 glottic disease [52]. Surgical salvage rates of 80% have been achieved for radiation failures [53]. Conservative laryngeal surgery with vertical partial laryngectomy and subtotal laryngectomy have been used with good success in selected patients. Unfortunately, many elderly patients do not have the pulmonary reserve for these procedures. Advanced glottic cancers (T3 and T4) are treated with total laryngectomy, neck dissection, and postoperative radiotherapy. In an effort to preserve the larynx, combination chemotherapy and radiation has been used for advanced glottic lesions with limited success.

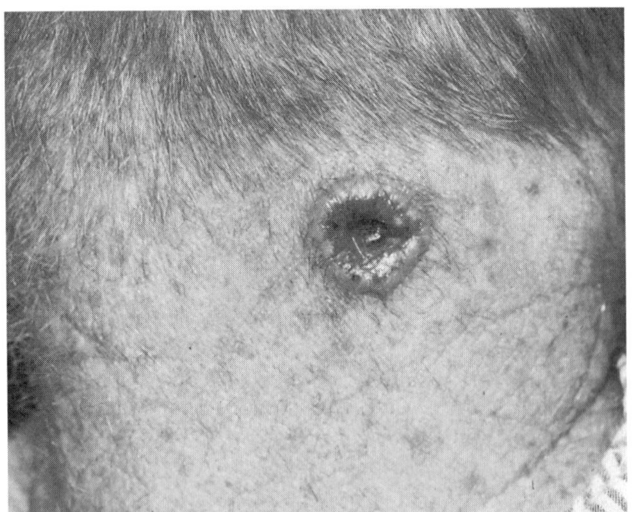

FIG. 35-3. Squamous cell carcinoma of neck.

Treatment of supraglottic cancer is more aggressive. Most early lesions (T1 and T2) have similar 5-year survival with radiotherapy or surgical excision [54]. Supraglottic and subtotal laryngectomy have been advocated for small lesions [55]. However, they have been associated with a high incidence of aspiration and are not indicated for patients with underlying pulmonary disease. Stages III and IV supraglottic lesions are treated by total laryngectomy, neck dissection, and postoperative radiation therapy. Five-year survival rates are 69% to 88% for stage I, 73% to 78% for stage II, 50% to 68% for stage III, and 10% to 50% for stage IV [56].

SALIVARY GLAND

The major salivary glands are the parotid, submandibular gland, and sublingual gland. There are also minor salivary glands in the mucous membranes of the oral cavity. The vast majority of salivary tumors occur in the parotid gland, followed distantly by the submandibular gland and minor salivary glands. More than 75% of parotid tumors are benign pleomorphic adenomas [57]. Warthin's tumor is the next most common benign tumor of the parotid gland. Mucoepidermoid carcinoma is the most common malignant tumor of the parotid gland followed by malignant mixed tumors [58]. Acinic cell carcinoma, adenocarcinoma, adenoid cystic carcinoma, and squamous cell carcinoma are less common. High-grade mucoepidermoid and squamous cell carcinoma are the most aggressive types. Submandibular gland and minor salivary lesions account for 10% of salivary tumors, of which 90% are malignant [59].

Facial nerve paralysis is an ominous sign suggesting tumor infiltration and has a grim prognosis. Clinically positive lymph nodes are seen in 14% of malignant major salivary gland tumors, whereas an additional 12% are found at the time of pathologic examination [60]. Large tumor size and high histologic grade are associated with nodal spread.

Surgery is the treatment of salivary tumors. In the parotid gland, most benign lesions can be removed by superficial parotidectomy alone [61]. Parotid malignancies should be treated with total parotidectomy. Aggressive malignancies are treated by radical parotidectomy, which includes facial nerve resection. Neck dissection is required for cervical nodes testing positive for cancer and high-risk node-negative necks. Tumors invading neck structures require RND. Postoperative radiotherapy is indicated for high-grade mucoepidermoid, malignant mixed, adenoid cystic, adenocarcinoma, and squamous cell carcinoma. Treatment of the other salivary glands involves resection of the gland to achieve negative margins. Local recurrence is an important predictor of patient survival. The 10-year survival for malignant salivary tumors is 74% for stage I, 56% for stage II, 32% for stage III, and 10% for stage IV [62]. When analyzed by histologic grade, the 5-year survival was 94% for low-grade tumors and 26% for high-grade tumors.

NONMELANOMA SKIN CANCER

Basal cell and squamous cell skin tumors are the most common form of cancer in the United States, accounting for >700,000 new cases a year [2]. The vast majority of these lesions are found on the sun-exposed head and neck (Fig. 35-3). This disease is most common among the elderly. Certain sunlight exposure in the ultraviolet (UV) B range (290 to 320 nm) is associated with the development of skin cancer [63]. There is a linear correlation between UV light exposure and skin cancer. With each 8- to 10-degree decline in latitude the incidence of cutaneous squamous carcinoma doubles. The incidence of UV-induced skin tumors appears to be inversely related to skin melanocyte content [64]. Those individuals who are fair-skinned, blue-eyed, sunburn readily, or tan poorly are at higher risk. Arsenic, psoralens, nitrogen mustard, and radiation exposure are all associated with skin cancer [65]. The relationship to radiation is dose dependent, with a latency period up to 20 years. Marjolin's ulcer is cutaneous squamous cell carcinoma arising from a burn, chronic inflammation, or chronic infection. Actinic keratosis may be a premalignant skin lesion, especially in the elderly, that presents as a rough, raised pigmented lesion. The malignant transformation rate is <10% [66]. After one skin cancer, the risk of developing a second skin tumor in 5 years is 50% [67]. Usually these tumors are phenotypically the same.

Basal cell carcinoma is the most common form of skin cancer and is four times more common than squamous cell carcinoma. These tumors arise from the basal layer of the epidermis. They classically present as a slow-growing, elevated, pearly white lesion (Fig. 35-4). These tumors rarely metastasize, but can locally invade aggressively by shelving and skating. Eighty-five percent occur on the head and neck, with 25% to 30% on the nose, where they have the highest rate of recurrence [68].

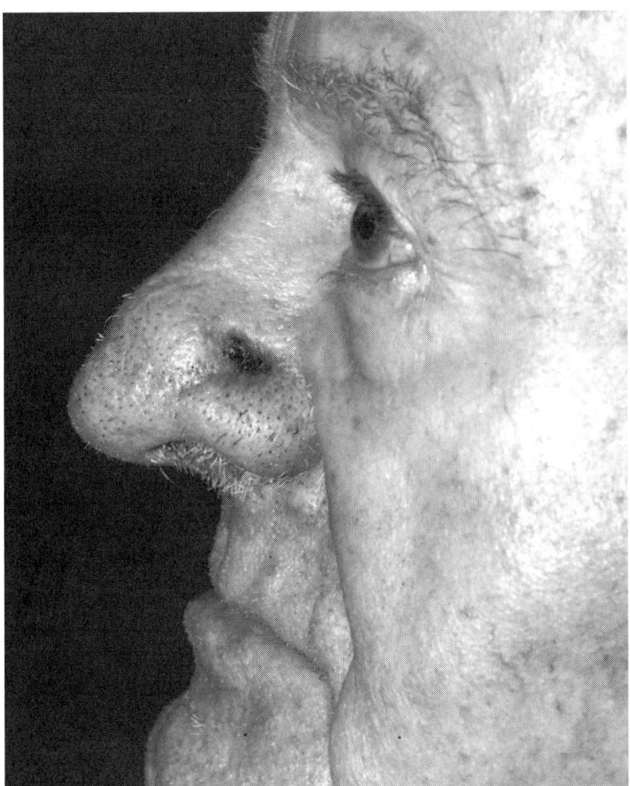

FIG. 35-4. Basal cell carcinoma.

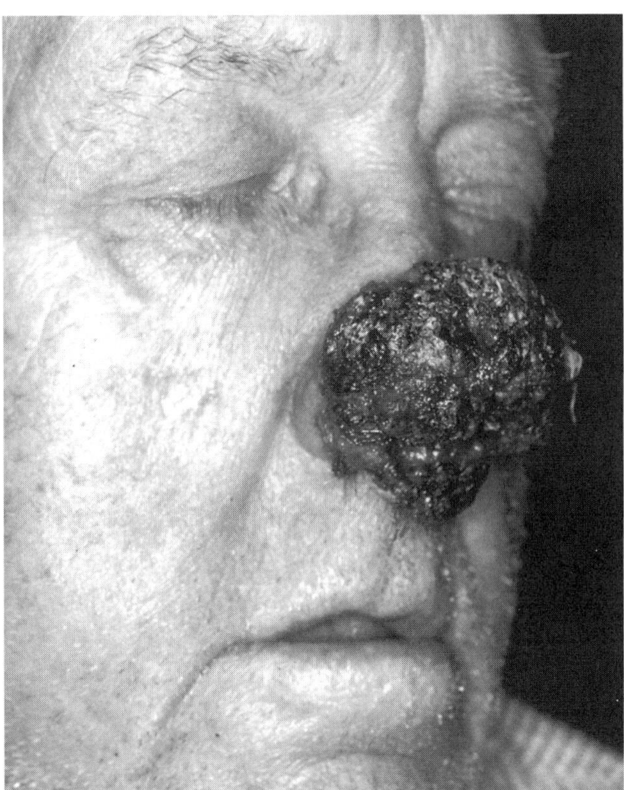

FIG. 35-5. Squamous cell carcinoma of the nose.

Basal cell carcinoma can be divided into several clinical types: nodular (50%), superficial (10%), pigmented (6%), and morpheaform or sclerosing (2%) [69]. The nodular form usually presents as a pearly colored nodule and progresses to a central ulcer with rolled borders. The superficial form is often scaly and erythematous with a threadlike border and is often confused for eczema or a fungal infection. Pigmented basal cell carcinoma is often confused with malignant melanoma. The morpheaform lesion is often described as a healing scar and has a histologically aggressive growth pattern.

Surgery is the primary therapy for basal cell carcinoma. Surgical excision is highly effective, with a 95% cure rate [70]. A 5-mm margin is generally adequate for most small lesions. Larger and histologically aggressive tumors such as morpheaform and infiltrative types require at least 1-cm margins for cure.

Mohs' micrographic surgery is preferred to conventional surgical therapy in certain cases. This treatment involves excising multiple thin layers of tissue until all pathologic evidence of tumor is gone. Mohs' surgery is indicated for lesions adjacent to the eye, ear, and nose. Recurrent, large, histologically aggressive, or previously irradiated tumors can be effectively treated by this method. Radiation is usually reserved for eyelid lesions or as an adjunct to surgery.

Cutaneous squamous cell carcinoma grows rapidly and has a greater metastatic potential than basal cell carcinoma. It arises from epidermal keratinocytes and is thought to follow the initiation and promotion theory of cancer. Regional lymphatic spread occurs in addition to local invasion and distant metastasis. The classic lesion appears as a translucent nodule on sun-damaged skin that may have crusts of skin and ulcerated areas (Fig. 35-5). The most common site in the head and neck of the elderly patient is the ear (Fig. 35-6). Although exceedingly rare in the elderly, xeroderma pigmentosum and albinism are associated with an increased risk of squamous cell carcinoma of the skin. Bowen's disease is squamous cell carcinoma in situ that presents as a sharply demarcated, scaly plaque. The plaque often heals, flakes, and then recurs. It may in time degenerate to malignancy so surgical excision is recommended.

Keratoacanthoma is a benign lesion with a histologic appearance similar to ulcerative squamous cell carcinoma (Fig. 35-7). It presents as a rapidly growing, firm, raised lesion with a keratin plug that grows rapidly over several months and resolves over a similar period. The biopsy specimen must include both edges. The clinical behavior is often locally aggressive.

Surgery is the preferred treatment option. The 5-year recurrence rate for each method has been reported as 8% for surgical excision, 3% for Mohs' excision, and 10% for radiotherapy [71]. Recurrence rates are higher for tumors on the lip and ear. Excising surgical margins of 1 cm with frozen sections to confirm margins is a useful approach to treatment. Larger margins are indicated for large, deep, or recurrent tumors. The indications for Mohs' surgery are similar to those mentioned for basal cell carcinoma. Initial ablation is

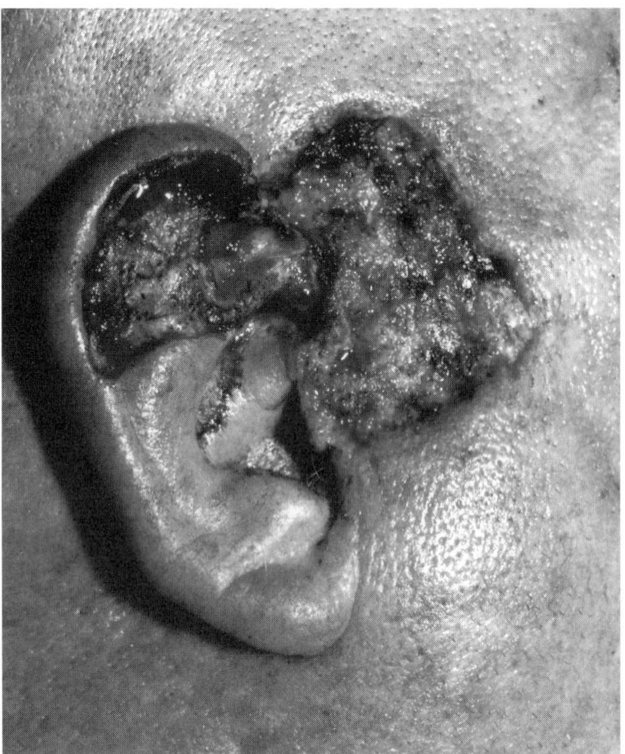

FIG. 35-6. Squamous cell carcinoma of the ear.

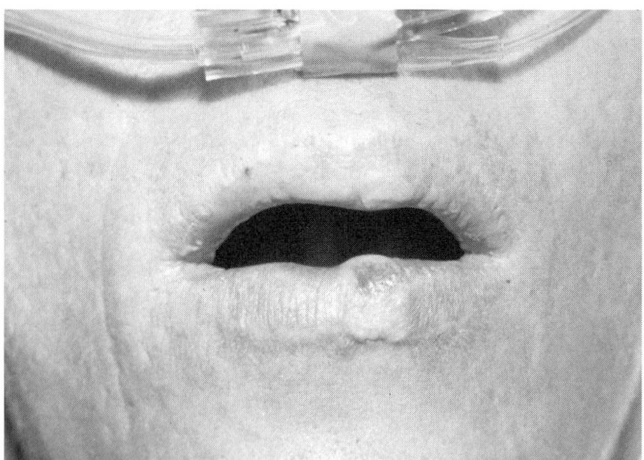

FIG. 35-7. Keratoacanthoma of the lip.

important because recurrent tumors are harder to control and have a higher rate of regional lymphatic spread.

SUMMARY

The elderly bear the greatest burden of head and neck cancer. Despite this liability, prevention and early detection in screening programs are useful approaches. Unfortunately, they often present with more advanced disease, which translates into a worse outcome. A greater awareness of smoking, alcohol, and sun-exposure risks is needed as this will affect the elderly of tomorrow. The elderly deserve the same aggressive treatments as younger patients. Where equivalent therapeutic options are available, preservation of function is critical. If cure cannot be achieved, then palliative intervention should be considered. Unfortunately, the elderly are often left out of new experimental treatment protocols. As the population ages, these issues will become even more important.

REFERENCES

1. Yancik R, Ries L. Cancer in older persons. Cancer 1994;74(Suppl): 1995–2003.
2. Parker SL, Tong T, Bolden, S, Wingo PA. Cancer statistics, 1997. CA Cancer J Clin 1997;47:5–27.
3. Mashberg A, Boffett P, Winkelman R, Garfinkel L. Tobacco smoking, alcohol drinking, and cancer of the oral cavity and oropharynx among US veterans. Cancer 1993;72:1369–1375.
4. Blot W, McLaughlin J, Winn D, et al. Smoking and drinking in relation to oral and pharyngeal cancer. Cancer Res 1988;48:3282–3287.
5. Elwood J, Pearson J, Skippen D, Jackson S. Alcohol, smoking, social and occupational factors in the aetiology of cancer of the oral cavity, pharynx, and larynx. Int J Cancer 1984;34:603–612.
6. Lione L. The smokeless habit. Cancer News Autumn, 1985.
7. Pedersen E, Hogetveit A, Anderson A. Cancer of the respiratory organs among workers at a nickel refinery in Norway. Int J Cancer 1973;12:32–41.
8. Cohen H. Biology of aging as related to cancer. Cancer 1994; 74(Suppl):2092–2100.
9. Berkman B, Rohan B, Sampson S. Myths and biases related to cancer in the elderly. Cancer 1994;74(Suppl):2004–2008.
10. Shah J. Patterns of cervical lymph node metastasis from squamous carcinomas of the upper aerodigestive tract. Am J Surg 1990;160:405–409.
11. Waldron C, Shafer W. Leukoplakia revisited. A clinicopathologic study of 3256 oral leukoplakias. Cancer 1975;36:1386–1392.
12. Mashberg A, Feldman L. Clinical criteria for identifying early oral and oropharyngeal carcinoma: erythrodysplasia revisited. Am J Surg 1988;156:273–275.
13. Schwarz R, Chan N. Fine needle aspiration cytology in the evaluation of head and neck masses. Am J Surg 1990;159:482–485.
14. Schindler E, Reck R. Value and limits of computer-assisted tomography. Head Neck Surg 1980;2:287–292.
15. Hordijk G, Bruggink T, Ravasz L. Panendoscopy, a valuable procedure? Otolaryngol Head Neck Surg 1989;101:426–428.
16. Shaha A, Hoover E, Mitrani M, et al. Synchronicity, multicentricity, and metachronicity of head and neck cancer. Head Neck Surg 1988;10:225–228.
17. Beahrs O, Henson D, Hutter R, Kennedy B (eds). Staging of Cancer (4th ed). Philadelphia: Lippincott, 1992.
18. Leemans C, Tiwari R, Natuta J, et al. Recurrence at the primary site in head and neck cancer and the significance of neck lymph node metastases as a prognostic factor. Cancer 1994;73:187–190.
19. Leemans C, Tiwari R, Natuta J, et al. Regional lymph node involvement and its significance in the development of distant metastases in head and neck carcinoma. Cancer 1993;71:452–456.
20. Calhoun K, Fulmer P, Weiss R, Hokanson J. Distant metastases from head and neck squamous cell carcinomas. Laryngoscope 1994;104: 1199–1205.
21. Ariyan S. Cancer of the Upper Aerodigestive System. In McCarthy J (ed), Plastic Surgery (Vol. 5). Philadelphia: Saunders, 1990;3412–3477.
22. Linn B, Robinson D, Klimas N. Effects of age and nutritional status on surgical outcomes in head and neck cancer. Ann Surg 1988;207:267–273.
23. Pelczar B, Weed G, Schuller D. Identifying high-risk patients before head and neck oncologic surgery. Arch Otolaryngol Head Neck Surg 1993;119:861–864.
24. Kowalski L, Alcantara P, Magrin J, Parise O. A case-control study on complications and survival in elderly patients undergoing major head and neck surgery. Am J Surg 1994;168:485–490.
25. Sarkar S, Mehta S, Tiwari J, et al. Complications following surgery for cancer of the larynx and pyriform fossa. J Surg Oncol 1990; 43:245–249.

26. Wendt CD, Peters LJ, Ang KK, et al. Hyperfractionated radiotherapy in the treatment of squamous cell carcinomas of the supraglottic larynx. Int J Radiat Oncol Biol Phys 1989;17:1057–1062.
27. Larson D, Lindberg R, Lane E, Goepfert H. Major complications of radiotherapy in cancer of the oral cavity and oropharynx. A 10 year retrospective study. Am J Surg 1983;146:531–536.
28. Chang T. Induction chemotherapy for advanced head and neck cancers, a literature review. Head Neck Surg 1988;10:150–159.
29. Jacobs MC, Eisenberger M, Oh MC, et al. Carboplatin (CBDCA) and radiotherapy for stage IV carcinoma of the head and neck: a phase I–II study. Int J Radiat Oncol Biol Phys 1989;17:361–363.
30. Frustaci S, Barzan L, Tumolo S, et al. Intra-arterial continuous infusion of cisadiamminedichloroplatinum in untreated head and neck cancer patients. Cancer 1986;57:1118–1123.
31. Eisenberger M, Jacobs M. Simultaneous treatment with single agent chemotherapy and radiation for locally advanced cancer of the head and neck. Semin Oncol 1992;19(Suppl 11):41–46.
32. Weissler M, Melin S, Sailer S, et al. Simultaneous chemoradiation in the treatment of advanced head and neck cancer. Arch Otolaryngol Head Neck Surg 1992;118:806–810.
33. Wolf G (Department of Veteran Affairs Laryngeal Cancer Study Group). Induction chemotherapy plus radiation compared with surgery plus radiation in patients with advanced laryngeal cancer. N Engl J Med 1991;324:1685–1690.
34. McKenna R. Clinical aspects of cancer in the elderly. Cancer 1994; 74(Suppl):2107–2117.
35. Crile G. Excision of cancer of the head and neck with special reference to the plan of dissection based on 132 operations. JAMA 1906;47:1780–1786.
36. Martin H, Del Valle B, Ehrlich H, Cahan W. Neck dissection. Cancer 1951;4:441–499.
37. Bocca E, Pignataro O, Oldini C, Cappa C. Functional neck dissection: an evaluation and review of 843 cases. Laryngoscope 1984;94:942–945.
38. Anderson P, Shah J, Cambronero E, Spiro R. The role of comprehensive neck dissection with preservation of the spinal accessory nerve in the clinically positive neck. Am J Surg 1994;168:499–502.
39. O'Brien C, Smith J, Soong S, et al. Neck dissection with and without radiotherapy. Am J Surg 1986;152:456–463.
40. Davidson B, Spiro R, Patel S, et al. Cervical metastases of occult origin: the impact of combined modality therapy. Am J Surg 1994;168:395–399.
41. Wilson J, Walker E. Reconstruction of the lower lip. Head Neck Surg 1981;4:29–44.
42. Tittle B, Rohrich R. Lip, cheek, and scalp reconstruction and hair replacement. Select Reading Plast Surg 1994;7:1–37.
43. Petrovich Z, Kuisk H, Tobochnik N, et al. Carcinoma of the lip. Arch Otolaryngol 1979;105:187–191.
44. White D, Byers R. What is the preferred initial method of treatment for squamous carcinoma of the tongue? Am J Surg 1980;140:553–555.
45. Mendelson B, Woods J, Beahrs O. Neck dissection in the treatment of carcinoma of the anterior two-thirds of the tongue. Surg Gynecol Obstet 1976;14:375–380.
46. Whitehurst J, Droulias C. Surgical treatment of squamous cell carcinoma of the oral tongue. Arch Otolaryngol 1977;103:212–215.
47. Zelefsky MJ, Harrison LB, Fass DE, et al. Postoperative radiotherapy for oral cavity cancers: impact of anatomic subsite on treatment outcome. Head Neck 1990;12:470–475.
48. Brown B, Barnes L, Mazariegos J, et al. Prognostic factors in mobile tongue and floor of mouth carcinoma. Cancer 1989;64:1195–1202.
49. Barrs D, DeSanto L, O'Fallon W. Squamous cell carcinoma of the tonsil and tongue-base region. Arch Otolaryngol 1979;105:479–485.
50. Johnson J, Myers E, Hao S, Wagner R. Outcome of open surgical therapy for glottic carcinoma. Ann Otol Rhinol Laryngol 1993;102: 752–755.
51. Howell-Burke D, Peters L, Goepfert H, Oswald M. T2 glottic cancer. Arch Otolaryngol Head Neck Surg 1990;116:830–835.
52. Davis R, Kelly S, Parkin J, et al. Selective management of early glottic cancer. Laryngoscope 1990;100:1306–1309.
53. Schwaab G, Mamelle G, Lartigau E, et al. Surgical salvage treatment of TI/T2 glottic carcinoma after failure of radiotherapy. Am J Surg 1994;168:474–475.
54. Desanto L. Early supraglottic cancer. Ann Otol Rhinol Laryngol 1990;99:593–597.
55. Chevalier D, Piquet J. Subtotal laryngectomy with cricohyoidopexy for supraglottic carcinoma: review of 61 cases. Am J Surg 1994;168:472–473.
56. Fu K, Eisenberg L, Dedo H, Phillips T. Results of integrated management of supraglottic carcinoma. Cancer 1977;40:2874–2881.
57. Friedman M, Levin B, Grybauskas V, et al. Malignant tumors of the major salivary glands. Otolaryngol Clin North Am 1986;19:625–636.
58. O'Brien J. Head and neck I: tumors. Select Reading Plast Surg 1995;8(9):1–49.
59. Campbell J, Morgan D, Oates J, Pearman K. Tumors of the minor salivary glands. Ear Nose Throat J 1989;68:137–140.
60. Armstrong JG, Harrison LB, Thaler HT, et al. The indications for elective treatment of the neck in cancer of the major salivary glands. Cancer 1992;69:615–619.
61. Woods J. Parotidectomy versus limited resection for benign parotid masses. Am J Surg 1985;149:749–750.
62. O'Brien C, Soong S, Herrera G, et al. Malignant salivary tumors—analysis of prognostic factors and survival. Head Neck Surg 1986;9:82–92.
63. Johnson T, Rowe D, Nelson B, Swanson N. Squamous cell carcinoma of the skin. J Am Acad Dermatol 1992;26:467–480.
64. Urbach F. Geographic distribution of skin cancer. J Surg Oncol 1971; 3:219–234.
65. Cottel W. Skin tumors I: basal cell and squamous cell carcinoma. Select Reading Plast Surg 1992;7:1–34.
66. Marks R, Rennie G, Selwood T. Malignant transformation of solar keratoses to squamous cell carcinoma. Lancet 1988;1:795–797.
67. Karagas M, Stukel T, Greenberg R, et al. Risk of subsequent basal cell carcinoma and squamous cell carcinoma of the skin among patients with prior skin cancer. JAMA 1992;267:3305–3310.
68. Roenigk R, Ratz JL, Bailin PL, Wheeland RG. Trends in the presentation and treatment of basal cell carcinomas. J Dermatol Surg Oncol 1986;12:860–865.
69. Silverman M, Kopf A, Bart R, et al. Recurrence rates of treated basal cell carcinoma. Part 3: surgical excision. J Dermatol Surg Oncol 1992;18:471–476.
70. Freeman R, Knox J. Treatment of skin cancer. Recent Results Cancer Res 1967;1:1.
71. Rowe D, Carroll R, Day C. Prognostic factors for local recurrence, metastasis, and survival rates in squamous cell carcinoma of the skin, ear, and lip. J Am Acad Dermatol 1992;26:976–990.

Surgical Care for the Elderly, 2nd ed., edited by
R. Benton Adkins, Jr., and H. William Scott, Jr.
Lippincott–Raven Publishers, Philadelphia © 1998.

CHAPTER 36

Plastic and Reconstructive Care

John B. Lynch and R. Bruce Shack

Plastic surgery in the elderly may be required for a wide variety of benign or malignant conditions and may be aesthetic, reconstructive, or both. Because the major malignant conditions affecting the elderly, such as melanoma, parotid tumors, and other head and neck surgery, are amply covered in other chapters of this book, this presentation is limited to skin lesions and common benign and functional reconstruction required by elderly patients.

Age alone is never a contraindication to surgical therapy in and of itself [1], but we continue to see many patients with nonemergent conditions who have been discouraged from having elective surgical procedures by their primary physician when, in fact, the burden of their problem may be worse by virtue of their advancing years and the benefit to be achieved by an elective procedure is much greater. For example, one 75-year-old patient with symptomatic mammary hypertrophy had been discouraged for 10 years from undergoing surgical correction of this condition based on her age alone. Although this condition may be quite symptomatic in a younger patient, in this patient the symptoms were further aggravated by osteoarthritis of the cervical spine. Following reduction mammoplasty, the symptomatic improvement achieved was even greater than in an otherwise healthy, younger patient.

SKIN LESIONS

One of the most frequent reasons that patients seek plastic surgical consultation is for the evaluation of skin lesions. Many skin lesions are benign degenerative changes characterized by localized areas of hyperpigmentation. They may cause the patient to be concerned about melanoma. Although dozens of lesions, both benign and malignant, develop in the elderly patient, by far the most frequently encountered are cysts, seborrheic keratosis, actinic keratosis, basal cell carcinoma, and squamous cell carcinoma. A variety of lesions arising in the skin and mucosa, which are not in themselves neoplastic, give rise to carcinoma with sufficient frequency that they are properly termed *precancerous.* These include (1) keratoses—actinic, localized (cutaneous horn), and arsenical; (2) occupational dermatosis (from tar products); (3) radiographic or radiation dermatitis; (4) xeroderma pigmentosum; and (5) leukoplakia.

Cysts

Cystic lesions of epithelial origin cause frequent tumorlike formations in the skin, varying in size from a few millimeters to several centimeters. Within the cyst is a cheesy substance composed of keratinized material, desquamated partially cornified cells, and granular debris. The walls of the cyst are lined by epithelium, and there may be skin appendages as well. Once established, they tend to enlarge slowly and are exposed to trauma and recurrent infection and always require total surgical removal for cure.

Seborrheic Keratosis

Seborrheic keratosis is a pigmented papilloma, most commonly on the trunk, but also on the arms, neck, and face. Clinically, the lesion is black, brown, or tan; is flat to polypoid in profile; and can be mistaken for melanoma. Microscopically, the lesion consists of a thickened epidermis with cystic areas containing keratin. The cells in the lesion usually resemble basal cells, and the cysts appear to form from invaginations of the horny layer. Melanin present in the cells of the tumor give it its characteristic pigmentation. These lesions are quite superficial, involving only the epidermis. If a punch biopsy is done to establish the diagnosis, no further treatment is required because these lesions have no malignant potential. However, they may be locally irritated or aesthetically displeasing, so their removal is often recommended. Discrete lesions respond well to surgical excision. Because of their superficial nature, they also can be adequately treated by cautery, curettage, or application of other destructive agents, such as liquid nitrogen, all with minimal scarring.

Actinic Keratosis

Actinic keratoses are precancerous lesions characterized by hyperkeratosis and thickening of the outer cornified layers of the epithelium. Clinically, these present as small plaque-like lesions that are frequently ulcerated and tend to produce itching and other minor symptoms. Often the hyperkeratotic plaque peels off, and the lesion appears to be healed, only to recur within a few weeks. Histologically, these lesions exhibit atrophy in the deeper portions of the skin. A striking feature is the presence of atypia in the cells of the lower layers of the epidermis. Sunlight appears to be the primary causative factor, and if untreated, progression to carcinoma occurs in a high percentage of these lesions. Although localized lesions responded well to excisional biopsy, the extent of these skin changes in some patients may be so extensive and diffuse as to defy surgical treatment. In patients with extensive disease, multiple biopsies are frequently required to establish the diagnosis of actinic keratosis. Then the application of topical 5-fluorouracil on a daily basis for 3 to 6 weeks is an effective method of treatment. During the course of treatment, the reaction of 5-fluorouracil in the areas of abnormal skin is intense: It produces a marked degree of hyperemia, frequently with blistering and superficial ulceration. After the drug is discontinued, the lesions crust and heal. When extensive areas are treated and some localized areas of abnormality persist, repeat biopsy and surgical excision are indicated.

Basal Cell Carcinoma

Basal cell carcinoma is the most frequent type of skin cancer, appearing most commonly on the exposed surfaces of the body and particularly frequently on the upper two-thirds of the face, about the nose and eyelids. Basal cell carcinoma is a tumor characterized by slow growth, and it essentially never metastasizes. Clinically, the lesion presents as (1) nodular, (2) ulcerating, or (3) morpheaform. The nodular form is a localized discrete lesion with sharp borders, is small in its early stages, and responds well to total surgical excision. As time goes by and the lesion enlarges, central ulceration occurs, the borders tend to become more irregular and indistinct, and wider excision is required. In the morpheaform type of basal cell carcinoma, the tumor is characterized by the formation of fibrous tissue, which produces a serpiginous irregular lesion that exhibits multiple small ulcerations with indistinct borders. In this type of basal cell carcinoma, the nests of tumor cells are interspersed in a dense fibrous stroma. Total surgical excision of these lesions may require resection of extensive areas, and skin grafting or flaps may be required for coverage.

Although basal cell carcinomas are radiosensitive, the use of radiation therapy can require a protracted course of treatment and generally should be avoided because of the additional damage to the skin and surrounding tissue that may result from the irradiation. In certain recurrent lesions, particularly in important anatomic areas, such as the medial canthus of the eyelid, where the borders of the lesion are clinically indistinct, Mohs' chemosurgery has been used increasingly in recent years [2]. This technique originally involved fixing the normal tissue in situ with zinc chloride. This was followed by removing sections of the lesion for histologic examination and continuing to remove serial sections of the tissue until histologically clear margins had been obtained [3]. Currently, fresh tissue techniques with frozen sections accomplish the same result. By Mohs' chemosurgery, tumors that are difficult to evaluate may show much more extensive tissue involvement than can be appreciated clinically. This technique is extremely tedious and time-consuming and often results in significant defects requiring plastic surgery closure. Although helpful in difficult cases, Mohs' micrographic excision should be reserved for the occasional lesion. It is most useful for recurrent lesions that have indistinct borders that cannot be clearly identified clinically or where excessive resection of tissue is undesirable. The overwhelming majority of basal cell carcinomas can be more expeditiously treated by total surgical excision and closure as required.

Squamous Cell Carcinoma

Squamous cell carcinoma, as is basal cell carcinoma, is most commonly seen in persons after the fifth decade. It is sometimes related to chronic injury or irritation but most often is the result of sun damage. This tumor may present as a nodular mass or a verrucous or ulcerating lesion. Growth tends to be more rapid than in the basal cell carcinoma, and metastasis to regional lymph nodes ultimately occurs in inadequately treated lesions. Distant metastasis is rare and usually occurs as a terminal event in patients with uncontrolled tumors. In certain types of chronic irritation, such as old unstable burn scars or long-standing cutaneous ulceration from any cause, there is a progressive histologic change in the epidermis consisting of pseudoepitheliomatous hyperplasia that may imitate the appearance of squamous cell carcinoma, and differentiation may be difficult [4]. In this reactive hyperplasia, the epidermal cells are usually limited by a definite membrane, and there is less irregularity of cells and only minor architectural derangement. Eventually, usually after a lag time of 15 to 20 years, invasive malignancy may develop.

In these lesions, incisional or excisional biopsy should establish the diagnosis. After the diagnosis has been established, total surgical extirpation is the treatment of choice. Because of the ultimate propensity for lymph node involvement if not totally removed, questionable surgical margins are always an indication for re-excision. In advanced lesions involving underlying muscles or bone, a combination of resection and irradiation may be the preferable method of treatment. Regional node dissection is indicated when the regional lymph nodes become involved. The chemotherapeutic agents available for treatment of uncontrollable squamous cell carcinoma tend to produce irregular remissions of short duration and, until better drugs are developed, are of limited clinical usefulness.

Lentigo Maligna

Lentigo maligna is frequently seen in elderly patients and usually occurs about the face [5]. Clinically, it presents as an irregular pigmented lesion that varies in size from quite small to several centimeters in diameter. It tends to be smooth and flat with uneven borders. The degree of pigmentation may vary from light brown to dark black. Histologically, at this stage the lesion consists of intraepithelial melanoma in situ and is often referred to as *Hutchinson's freckle*. Although it may wax and wane, if untreated, the natural evolution is the development of invasive melanoma within this lesion, and it should be totally extirpated [6,7].

BREAST PROCEDURES

A variety of breast conditions in the elderly may require plastic surgical techniques. The most common indications, by far, are reconstruction of the breast after mastectomy and reduction mammoplasty.

Breast Reconstruction After Mastectomy

Breast cancer continues to be a disease of the older patient, but it is being diagnosed earlier in younger patients with increasing frequency. As a result, requests for breast reconstruction after mastectomy have increased exponentially in recent years. The objectives of breast reconstruction are (1) restoration of the breast mound to eliminate the need for an external prosthesis, (2) achievement of breast symmetry (usually requiring some modification of the remaining breast), and (3) reconstruction of the nipple-areolar complex if the patient desires. The current ablative techniques for treatment of breast cancer are more conservative, with preservation of more skin and the pectoralis major and minor muscle. In patients in whom adequate skin is present, the insertion of a breast prosthesis, usually beneath the muscle, and any required modification of the remaining breast, such as ptosis correction or reduction, are sufficient to achieve restoration of the breast mound and symmetry at the first procedure. After approximately 3 months, any required adjustment to the breast reconstruction can be performed and reconstruction of the nipple-areolar complex accomplished (Fig. 36-1). In patients in whom the remaining skin is marginal, the use of a tissue expander has increased in recent years. This in an inflatable device that can be placed either beneath the skin or beneath skin and muscle. It contains a small valve or reservoir that can be injected percutaneously with saline at intervals of a few days until the desired degree of skin stretching has been achieved. Following a period of time to allow for tissue accommodation, the temporary device is then replaced with a permanent prosthesis and nipple areolar reconstruction performed.

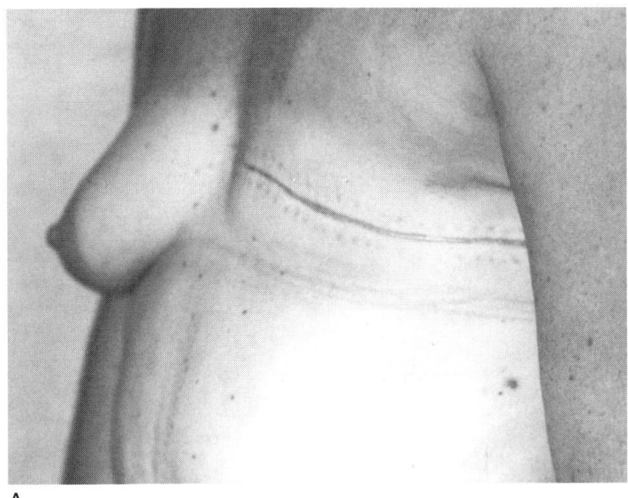

A

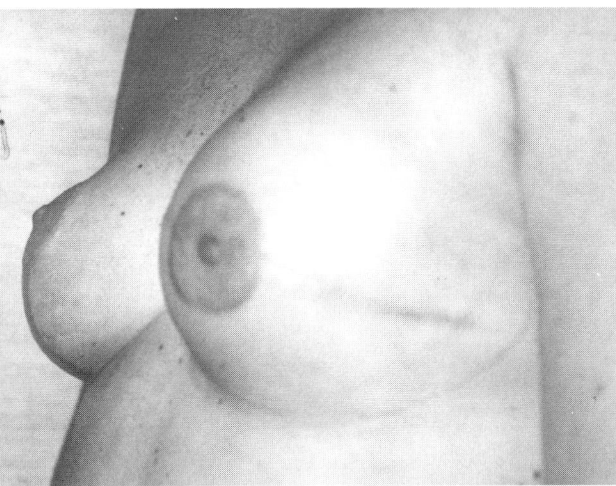

B

FIG. 36-1. (A) A 58-year-old woman with the typical sequelae of a left modified radical mastectomy. **(B)** Result following left breast reconstruction with tissue expander technique, nipple areolar reconstruction, and mastopexy of the opposite breast for symmetry.

In patients in whom the available skin is inadequate for reconstruction, either from irradiation or because more extensive initial surgery was required, soft-tissue replacement becomes a necessary part of the reconstruction. In the past, the latissimus dorsi musculocutaneous flap with an implant was extensively used [8–10]. However, the texture of the skin from the back is thicker and stiffer than normal breast skin and does not make an ideal replacement. In addition, the scar on the back is objectionable to some patients. For this reason, there has been increasing use of the transverse rectus abdominis musculocutaneous flap, which pro-

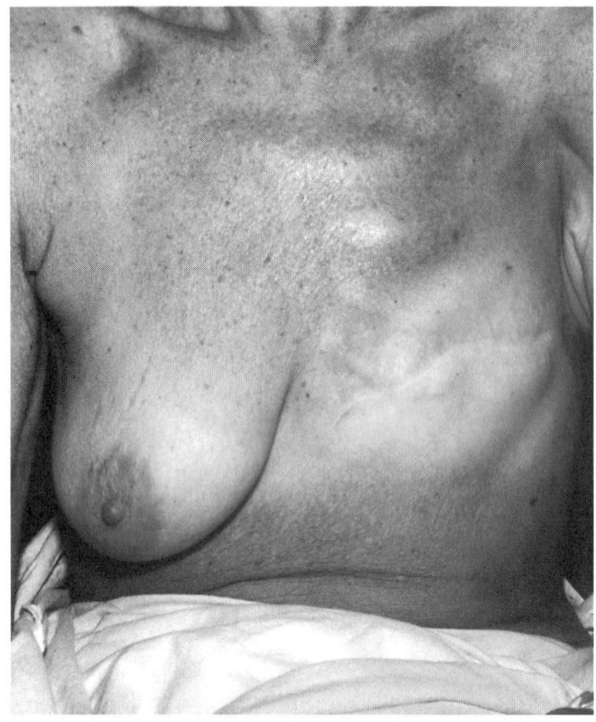

A

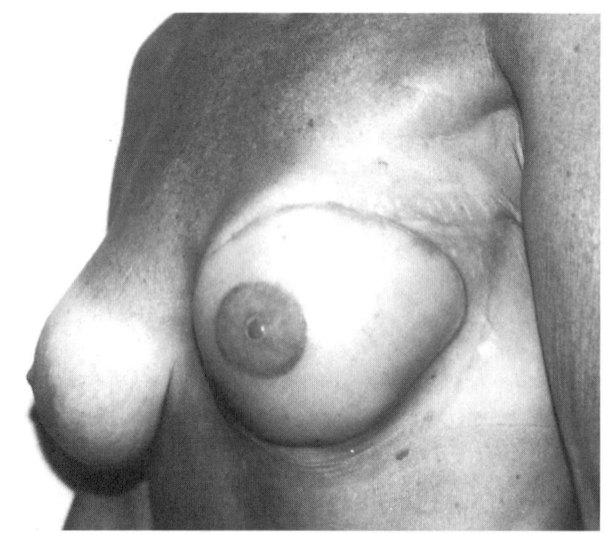

B

FIG. 36-2. (A) A 60-year-old woman with sequelae of left radical mastectomy. **(B)** Result following reconstruction with transverse rectus abdominis musculocutaneous flap.

vides ample skin and enough soft tissue to eliminate the necessity of a prosthesis [11–13] (Fig. 36-2).

Most breast reconstructions are performed in two stages. The morbidity is low, the complication rate is acceptable, and these procedures are well tolerated by the elderly patient. The timing of breast reconstruction is important, because, to defer reconstruction arbitrarily for a set period such as 1 year, may deprive the patient of the benefit of reconstruction at the time it is most important to her. The breast reconstruction techniques currently available do not interfere with subsequent chemotherapy or irradiation if this is indicated. A survey by the American Society of Plastic and Reconstructive Surgeons of its membership in 1995 indicated that in patients having breast reconstruction, 38% undergo some initial reconstruction at the time of mastectomy and 62% of reconstructions are delayed until the wound is healed. In selected patients, the insertion of a prosthesis or tissue expander at the time of initial mastectomy may have great psychological benefits. Others are candidates for most extensive reconstructive procedures that can be performed immediately at the time of mastectomy. These include the transverse rectus abdominis musculocutaneous flap and the latissimus dorsi flap with or without an implant.

Reduction Mammoplasty

Although mammary hypertrophy in an occasional patient may be associated with endocrine abnormalities, the overwhelming majority of patients develop this condition without any associated underlying pathology. In younger patients this can be a source of embarrassment and self-consciousness, as well as of physical symptoms. Depending on the degree, mammary hypertrophy may produce symptoms of pressure and heaviness. In more advanced cases, chronic pressure from the bra straps produces pain and discomfort in the shoulders, back, and neck, and brachial plexus symptoms can result from the continuous constriction of bra straps over the shoulder. Postural changes caused by the large, heavy breasts also contribute to back and neck pain. Although many of these patients tend to be somewhat overweight, weight reduction alone does not have a significant influence on the volume of the breast tissue itself. With advancing years, the nuisance and chronic symptoms may become more severe, particularly if aggravated by osteoporosis or osteoarthritis of the upper spine and shoulders. The surgical procedures available for reduction mammoplasty are meticulous, tedious, and time consuming, but because no major cavities are entered and the normal body physiology is not disturbed, these procedures are well tolerated by elderly patients and the morbidity is minimal.

Most of the surgical techniques for reduction mammoplasty are based on designing a pattern of skin incisions that permits removal of excess skin and parenchyma to accomplish a satisfactory reduction of the breast while repositioning the nipple more superiorly based on a dermoparenchymal pedicle [14,15]. An occasional patient is still seen for whom the most expeditious course, because of massive hypertrophy, may be partial amputation of the breast and transfer of the nipple as a free skin graft [16]. The use of a pedicle transfer is applicable to most patients and the results are generally better. In properly selected patients, the relief of symptoms is so predictable that as a group these patients tend to have a high level of patient satisfaction (Fig. 36-3).

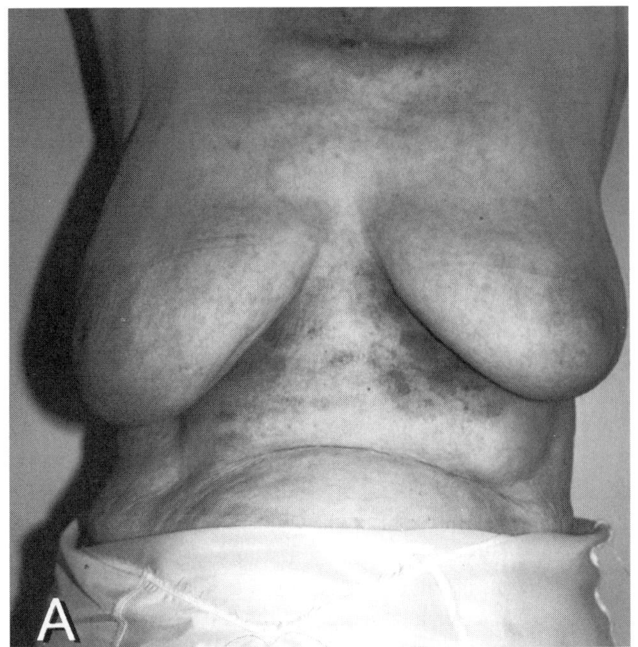

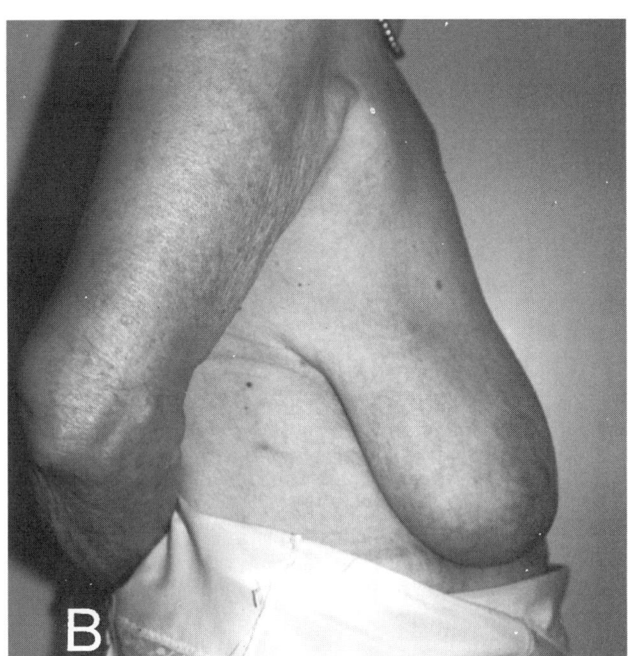

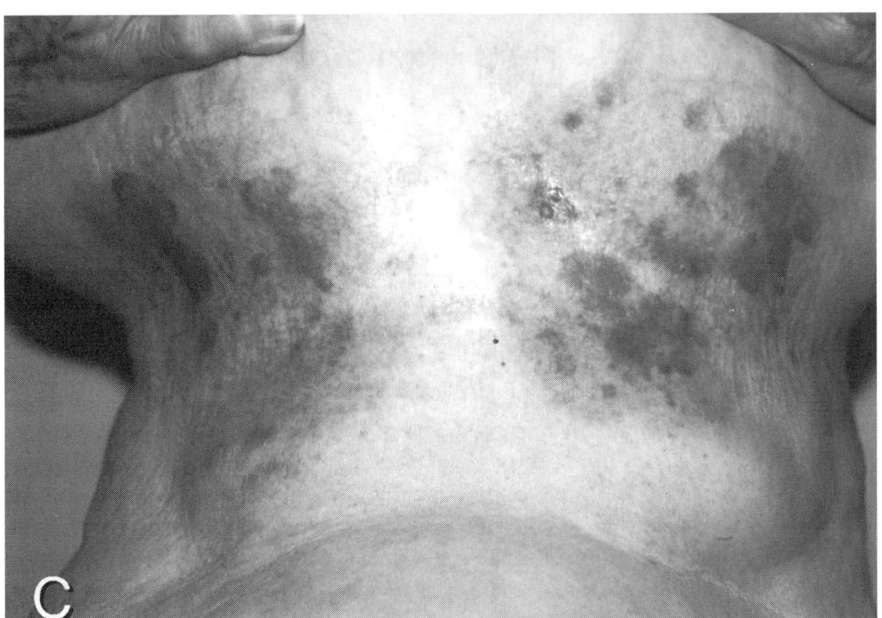

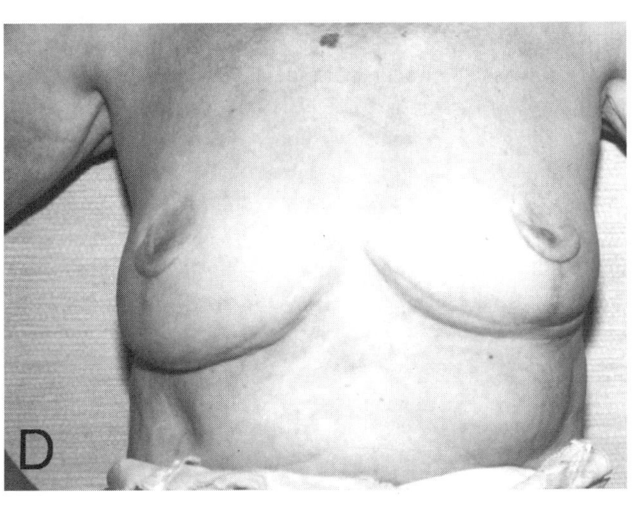

FIG. 36-3. **(A)** A 76-year-old woman with heavy ptotic breasts and severe intertriginous changes refractory to medical treatment for 4 years. **(B)** Lateral view. **(C)** Close-up of the severe intertrigo of the inframammary fold. **(D)** Postoperative result showing complete resolution of the skin problem.

TABLE 36-1. *Muscles used most frequently for muscle flap or musculocutaneous flap reconstruction*

Head and neck
Temporalis
Sternocleidomastoideus
Platysma
Trapezius
Pectoralis major
Latissimus dorsi
Trunk and perineum
Pectoralis major
Latissimus dorsi
Rectus abdominis
Gluteus maximus
Biceps femoris
Gracilis
Tensor fascia lata
Lower extremity and foot
Tensor fascia lata
Rectus femoris
Vastus lateralis
Vastus medialis
Gastrocnemius
Soleus
Extensor digitorum communis
Flexor digitorum brevis

The complications that can result from this procedure include wound infection, hematoma or seroma formation, localized areas of delayed healing, areas of tissue necrosis that in extreme cases can include the nipple, and some temporary loss of sensation in the surgical area with a variable degree of recovery over time. The incidence of major complications of this type is low, and the morbidity of the procedure is small compared with the symptomatic improvement achieved. One occurrence that must be kept in mind is that as a result of the extensive surgical dissection required, it is not uncommon for small localized areas of fat necrosis to develop, which may not be apparent until several weeks to a few months following the procedure. These areas of fat necrosis usually present as a localized area of tenderness and mild pain associated with a palpable, firm, hard nodule that is clinically suspicious of carcinoma. When this fat necrosis develops during the early postoperative period, if the mammogram shows no calcifications suggestive of malignancy and if the pathology report of the tissue removed at operation shows no proliferative or other precancerous change, it is safe to defer biopsy and keep these patients under observation for a period of time with the expectation that the fat necrosis will resolve spontaneously.

One other complication that occurs occasionally is Mondor's disease, an inflammatory process of the veins in the anterior chest wall and inferior surface of the breast. It presents clinically as vertical, linear bands immediately beneath the breast or on the inferior surface of the breast. The exact etiology is unknown, but it can occur after any type of breast surgery. It is a completely benign, self-limiting condition that resolves spontaneously over a few weeks and requires only symptomatic treatment and patient reassurance.

Difficult Reconstructive Problems

In recent years, reconstructive techniques have developed that enable one-stage correction of difficult problems that formerly required multiple stages over a prolonged period of time or for which no good solution was present. These include the use of (1) muscle flap transfers on their vascular pedicle with application of skin grafts; (2) transfer of musculocutaneous flap units as a one-stage procedure on the muscles' vascular pedicle; and (3) free transfer of muscle flaps, musculocutaneous flaps, skin flaps, and other tissue including bone and bowel as a free transfer using microvascular anastomoses. A list of the more commonly used musculocutaneous flaps is provided in Table 36-1.

Despite the presence of associated medical disease, such as diabetes, and the increasing frequency of peripheral vascular arteriosclerotic disease in elderly patients, the muscle flaps, musculocutaneous flaps (Fig. 36-4), or free microvascular flaps (Fig. 36-5) offer the potential of one-stage reconstruction with a minimum of morbidity.

AESTHETIC SURGERY

In addition to functional reconstructive problems encountered in the elderly, one of the more frequent reasons for plastic surgical consultation by older patients is a request for aesthetic surgery, primarily facial rejuvenation. With our society's emphasis on physical appearance and physical fitness, many elderly patients are interested in achieving improvement in their appearance.

Preoperative evaluation of patients seeking cosmetic surgery is of paramount importance. In stable, well-adjusted individuals who are seeking some physical improvement in their appearance for their own satisfaction and who have anatomic changes that can be reasonably improved, the results are good and the patients tend to be very satisfied. If, on the other hand, patients are seeking cosmetic surgery in a vain attempt to regain their lost youth, from a sense of uselessness as they approach retirement, or from a sense of loss after the death of a spouse, great caution should be exercised. The most commonly requested procedures are for face-lifts, eyelid surgery, and forehead or brow lift, but requests for evaluation include a wide variety of other procedures, such as rhinoplasty, facial peel, collagen injections, suction-assisted lipectomy, and correction of excess tissue folds about the arms, breasts, abdomen, and thighs.

Face-Lift

Patients seeking consultation for face-lifts are usually most concerned about tissue relaxation and sagging that

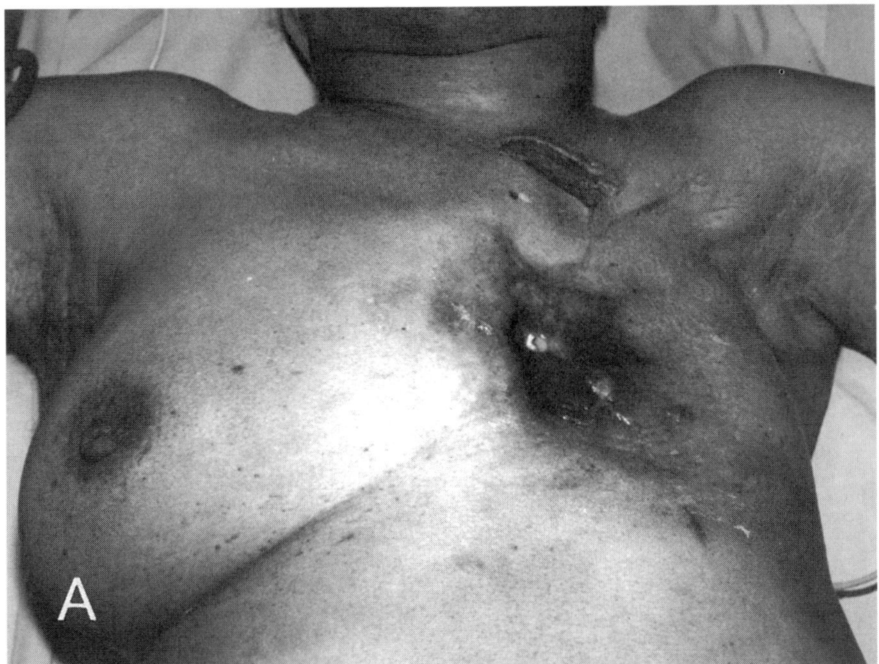

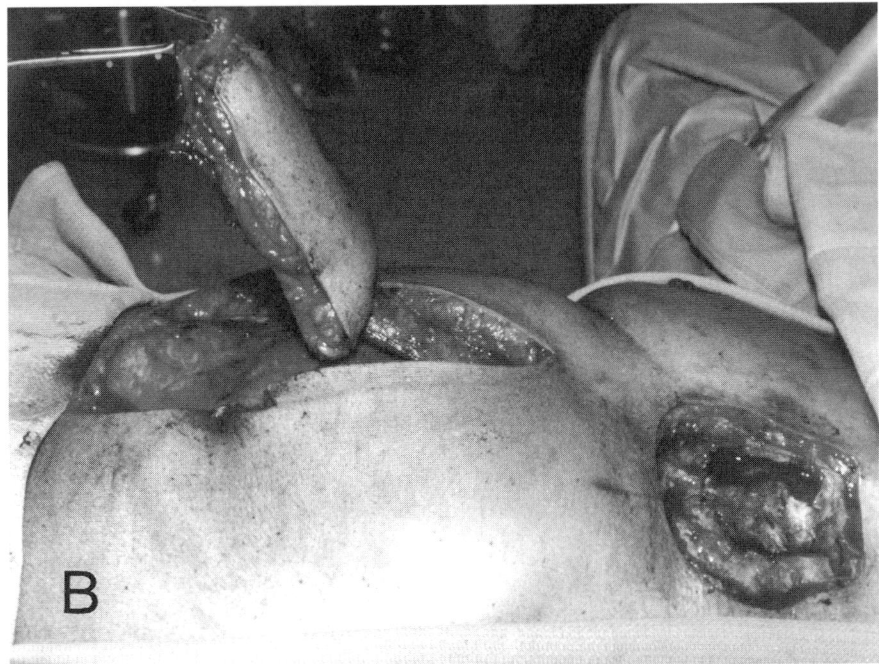

FIG. 36-4. (A) An 82-year-old woman following mastectomy and radiation with severe radiation ulcer of the anterior chest wall. **(B)** Intraoperative photograph showing full-thickness resection of the chest wall to remove the ulcer and elevate a rectus abdominus musculocutaneous unit for reconstruction.

involve the nasal labial crease, jaw line, and neck, with or without the presence of vertical bands. The surgical approach in suitable patients consists of an incision in the temple that extends down the preauricular area and behind the ears. Through this incision, a skin flap of the face and neck is undermined, and the skin is advanced, trimmed, and sutured into position. A variety of ancillary procedures tailored to the individual patient's requirements are currently incorporated as part of the face-lift procedure. These include plication, advancement, and other tissue manipulations; flaps using the superficial musculoaponeurotic system over the parotid and upper neck region; surgical correction of the vertical bands caused by the leading edge of the platysma; use of platysma flaps; and suction lipectomy of the submental area. These procedures can be performed under local or general anesthesia and are usually performed as outpatient procedures. The morbidity includes bruising and swelling and temporary sensory changes in the undermined skin of the face and neck. Major complications of infection, hematoma, tissue necrosis, and nerve injury are infrequent and collectively are found in <5% of the patients undergoing this procedure.

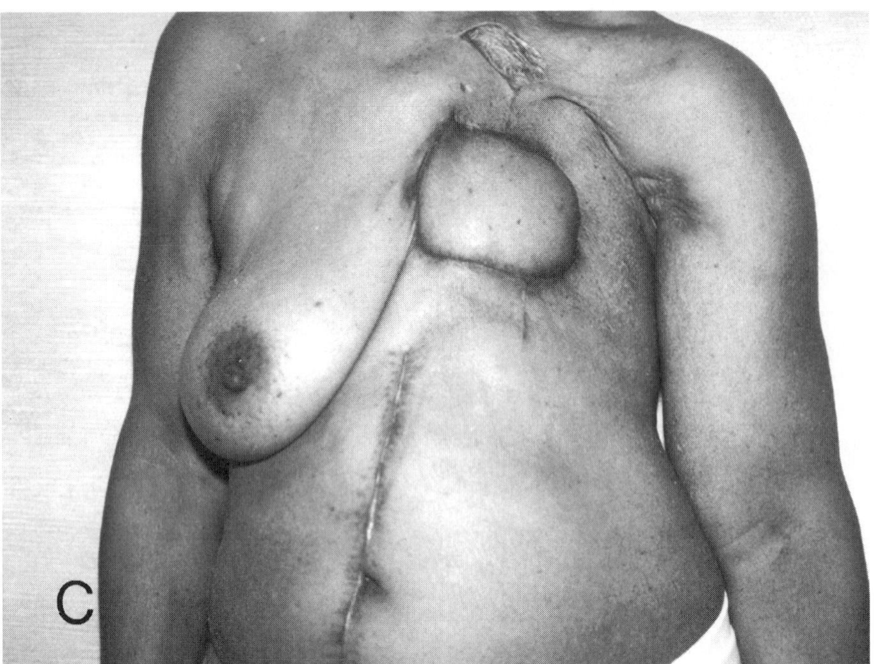

FIG. 36-4. *continued* **(C)** Postoperative results showing stable, healed wound.

Eyelids

Patients frequently seek correction of excessive fullness in the upper and lower eyelids. This fullness may be simply skin redundancy and, in the upper lid, can be sufficiently severe to partially obstruct lateral vision. In addition to the skin redundancy, there is often bulging of the orbital fat to produce the characteristic baggy eyelids. These fat pads tend to retain edema and give a puffy appearance to the eyelid tissue. Careful preoperative evaluation in these patients is required, not only of visual acuity but also of associated problems of brow ptosis, ptosis of the lacrimal gland, atony of the lower eyelid that predisposes to postoperative ectropion, and other associated abnormalities. The most common procedure for correction of upper and lower eyelid problems is a local anesthetic procedure usually performed as an outpatient procedure: skin is removed from the upper eyelid, and the incision is deepened if necessary through the orbicularis oculi muscle and the septum orbitale to remove the bulging fat pads that usually present in the central and medial portion of the upper eyelid. In the lower eyelid, the skin excision must be conservative to avoid over-resection with resulting ectropion. Again, the incision is deepened if required to remove the fat bulges in the lower eyelid, which are three in number as compared with two in the upper eyelid.

Facial peeling addresses the fine crepelike wrinkles (e.g., crow's feet) that are not corrected by blepharoplasty or facelift. The peels can be superficial, involving only the epidermis, or deeper peels that remove the upper layers of the dermis as well. Superficial peels are usually performed as an office procedure without anesthesia using one of the alphahydroxy acids such as glycolic or lactic acid. They cause only erythema without blistering or ulceration so the patient can resume normal makeup routines within 48 to 72 hours. These peels require repeated application, usually on a weekly basis for 6 to 8 weeks, to achieve maximum improvement.

Deeper peels are performed with either phenol or trichloroacetic acid or increasingly with ultra-pulsed CO_2 laser techniques. These deeper peels require sedation in most patients and cause superficial ulceration of the skin surface with crusting and scabbing that requires 7 to 10 days to heal. The results obtained are much more pronounced than those with epidermal peels. However, the erythema that results lasts approximately 3 months and the risk of scarring, although low, is increased. Careful patient selection is critical to good results.

These facial peeling procedures can be performed independently or in conjunction with other facial operations as indicated by the patient's needs and desires.

SUMMARY

In summary, all the procedures used in younger patients may be used in the elderly. These include repair of all forms of trauma, such as wounds, lacerations, facial fractures, burns, and so forth. Precancerous and malignant lesions tend to be encountered more frequently in older patients, as are a variety of degenerative skin changes. Aesthetic surgical procedures are increasingly requested by elderly patients, and the majority of these can be safely performed as outpatient procedures with minimum morbidity and good results. As previously stated, all the techniques used in aesthetic and reconstructive surgery in younger patients are equally applicable to the elderly patient, and the ones most frequently used in this group have been briefly reviewed.

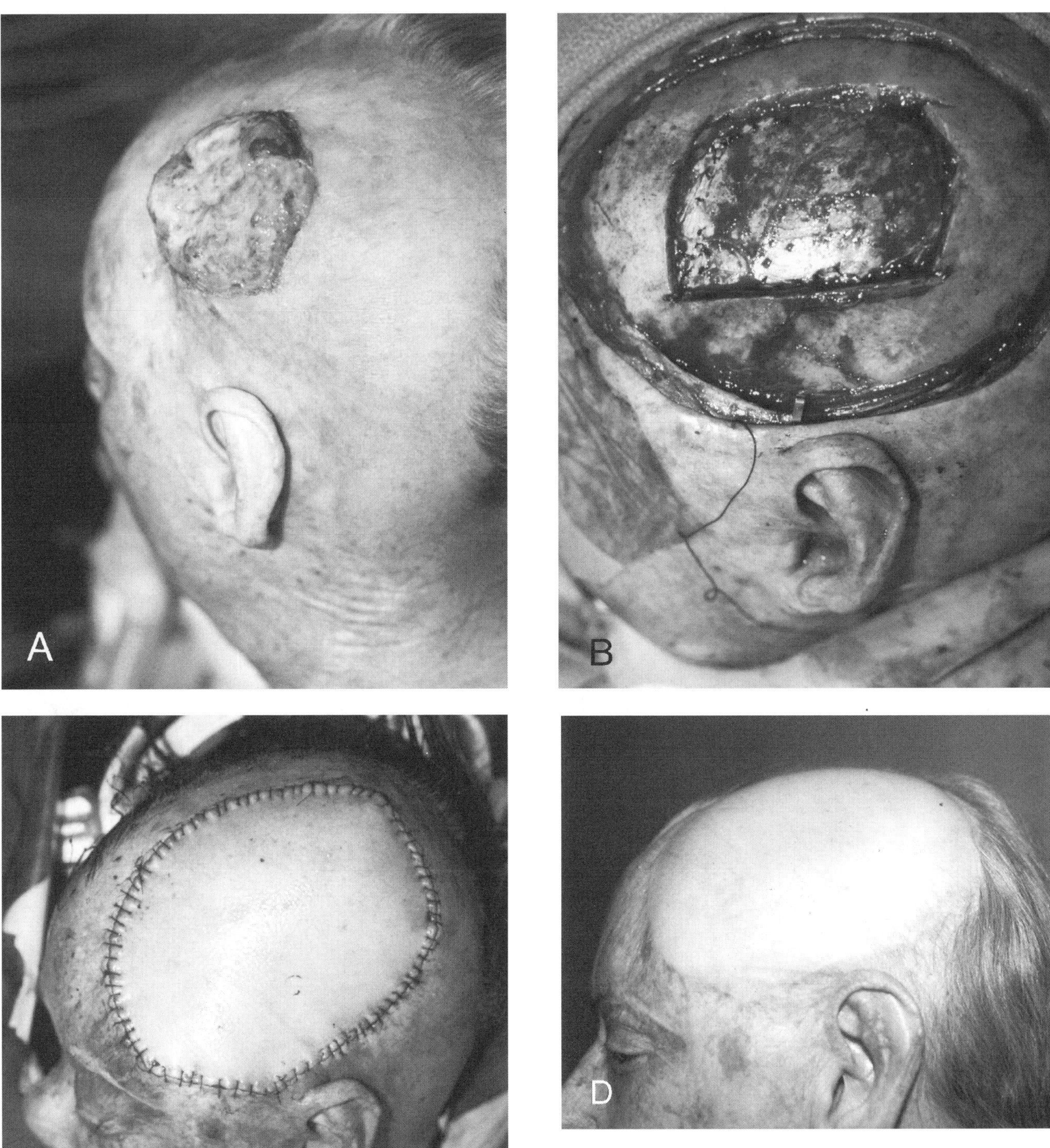

FIG. 36-5. **(A)** A 73-year-old woman with large, invasive squamous cell carcinoma of the scalp arising in an old burn scar from a burn in infancy. **(B)** Defect of the scalp and calvarium following full-thickness resection down to dura. **(C)** Immediate postoperative result following reconstruction of the defect with a free latissimus dorsi musculocutaneous flap. **(D)** Healed, stable wound 6 months after ablation and reconstruction.

REFERENCES

1. Brown LL. Anesthesia in the geriatric patient. Clin Plast Surg 1985; 12:51–60.
2. Mohs FE. Chemotherapy for microscopically controlled excision of skin cancer. J Surg Oncol 1971;3:257–267.
3. Tromovitch TA, Stegman SJ. Microscopic-controlled excision of cutaneous tumors: chemosurgery, fresh tissue technique. Cancer 1978;41: 653–658.
4. Arons MS, Rodin AE, Lynch JB, et al. Scar tissue carcinoma—an experimental study with special reference to burn scar carcinoma. Ann Surg 1966;163:445–460.
5. Davis J, Pack GT, Higgins GK. Melanotic freckle of Hutchinson. Am J Surg 1967;113:457–463.
6. Franklin JD, Reynolds VH, Bowers DG, Lynch JB. Cutaneous melanoma of the head and neck. Clin Plast Surg 1976;3:413–427.
7. Shelley WB, Shelley ED. The ten major problems of aging skin. Geriatrics 1982;37:107–113.
8. Bostwick J. Aesthetic and Reconstructive Breast Surgery. St. Louis: Mosby, 1983.
9. Mathes SJ, Nahai F. Clinical Applications for Muscle and Musculocutaneous Flaps. St. Louis: Mosby, 1982.
10. McCraw JB, Penix JO, Baker JW. Repair of major defects of the chest wall and spine with the latissimus dorsi myocutaneous flap. Plast Reconstr Surg 1978;62:197–206.
11. Robbins TH. Rectus abdominus myocutaneous flap for breast reconstruction. Aust N Z J Surg 1978;49:527–530.
12. Drever JM. Total breast reconstruction. Ann Plast Surg 1981;7:54–61.
13. Hartrampf CR, Scheflan M, Black PW. Breast reconstruction with a transverse abdominal island flap. Plast Reconstr Surg 1982;69: 216–225.
14. Strombeck JO. Mammoplasty: report of a new technique based on the two-pedicle procedure. Br J Plast Surg 1960;13:79–90.
15. McKissock PK. Reduction mammoplasty with a vertical dermal flap. Plast Reconstr Surg 1972;49:245–252.
16. Conway H, Smith J. Breast plastic surgery: reduction mammoplasty, mastopexy, augmentation mammoplasty, and mammary construction: analysis of 245 cases. Plast Reconstr Surg 1958;21:8–19.

Surgical Care for the Elderly, 2nd ed., edited by
R. Benton Adkins, Jr., and H. William Scott, Jr.
Lippincott–Raven Publishers, Philadelphia © 1998.

CHAPTER 37

Solid Organ Transplantation

Robert E. Richie, Richard N. Pierson, III, Mark Fox, Michael L. Cheatham, and C. Wright Pinson

Advanced age, once considered a serious relative contraindication to solid organ transplantation, has become less of a concern as the field of transplantation has progressed scientifically and clinically with improved overall results. Upper age limits at individual transplant programs are generally increasing, and there is much more concern about an individual patient's physiologic status than the patient's absolute age in years. This is important because, as life expectancy increases, so does the proportion of our elderly population.

Several encouraging points about transplantation in the elderly exist. In general, data in most areas of organ transplantation demonstrate comparably good results in older patients, although it is important to note that in most reports, these patients have been very carefully selected. Older patients are reported to suffer fewer episodes of organ rejection and decreased severity of rejection. The maturity of this group of patients generally ensures excellent compliance with medical regimens. Finally, society views the contributions of individuals in this age bracket to our social and professional fabric with great value and that, coupled with extended life expectancy, supports the application of solid organ transplantation to this population.

On balance, concerns do exist about solid organ transplantation in the elderly. In some authors' views, survival rates are somewhat inferior in the elderly, and there is some question as to whether older patients regularly return to a good quality of life [1–3]. Elderly patients have more comorbidities, especially cardiovascular disease, that can contribute to poor outcomes. Additionally, older patients have a relatively poor tolerance to serious infection and, in general, have a decreased immune response. Thus, again, it is important to emphasize careful patient selection and avoidance of patients with unacceptable surgical risks. Some authors are concerned about the limited life expectancy of older patients compared with that of younger patients, about appropriate application of health care resources, and especially about the scarcity of donor organs. These issues raise significant ethical debate.

RENAL TRANSPLANTATION

Robert E. Richie

Renal transplantation as a method of treatment of end-stage renal disease has gained widespread acceptance throughout the world. Current data show that the 1-year graft survival rate is 81% and the 3-year graft survival rate is 69%; the patient survival rates are 93% at 1 year and 87% at 3 years for those recipients receiving cadaver allografts [4].* In the case of living donors, the results are even better, with graft survival rates of 91% at 1 year and 84% at 3 years; the patient survival rates are 97% at 1 year and 94% at 3 years. Such was not always the case, however; in the early experience with this mode of therapy, the graft survival rate was <60%, and the patient survival rate was 62% at 1 year [5–7]. As a result, only the best risk candidates were offered the opportunity to receive a transplant, and patients considered at high risk were advised to continue dialysis as a form of therapy. Patients in the older age group were thought to be in the higher risk group, not only because they more frequently had other concomitant diseases such as cardiovascular disease, pulmonary disease, and diabetes, but also because with advancing age immunocompetence is diminished [8]. There was a reluctance to further compromise the immune system by giving immunosuppressive medication. Because of the shortage of donor organs, another issue that was raised concerned the ethics of giving a cadaver kidney to a high-risk patient whose long-term survival might be diminished [9].

*The data and analyses reported in the 1995 Annual Report of the U.S. Scientific Registry of Transplant Recipients and Organ Procurement and Transplantation Network have been supplied by the United Network for Organ Sharing. The authors alone are responsible for the reporting and interpretation of these data.

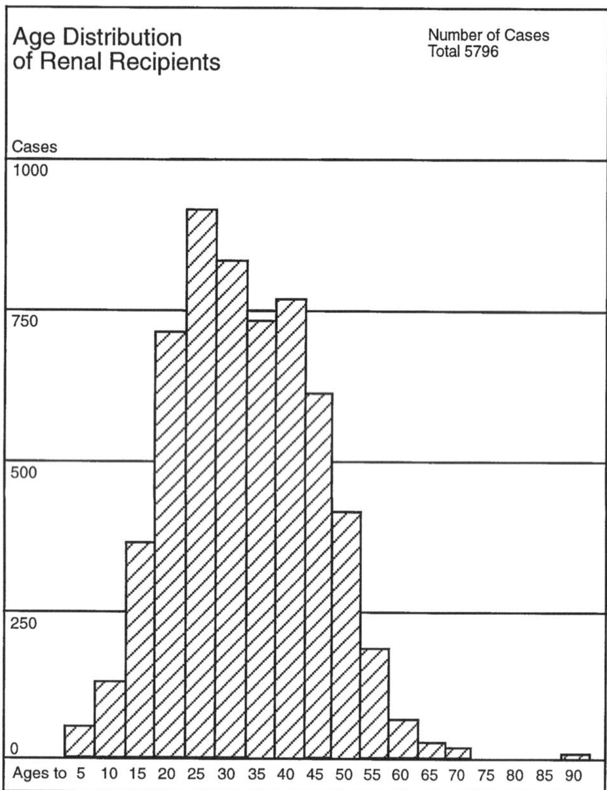

FIG. 37-1. Distribution of ages of kidney recipients reported to Human Renal Transplant Registry between 1953 and 1971. (Reprinted with permission from the Ninth Report of the Human Renal Transplant Registry. JAMA 1972;220:253–260.)

Review of the Literature

In 1971, Simmons et al. [10] examined a group of patients considered at high risk, either due to complicating factors such as diabetes, abnormal lower urinary tracts, severe myocardial disease, previous gastrointestinal ulceration with bleeding, lupus erythematosus or polyarteritis, psychiatric disturbances, or other conditions such as cystinosis and tuberculosis, as well as extremes of age such as children <16 and adults >45 years of age. The reason these patients were considered at high risk was that there was an increased chance that the kidney would fail either from the preexisting disease or that the patient would not tolerate the stresses of the procedure or the immunosuppression. Of 18 adults aged 45 years or older, eight received kidneys from living related donors (either siblings or children). At the time of the report, seven of the eight were alive and well. On the other hand, 10 of the 18 older patients received cadaver transplants; in this group, only two (20%) had a functioning kidney at 1 year and six (60%) died within 1 year. Four died with good renal function and two died after rejection. From this study, it was thought that the older patient did not tolerate the immunosuppressive medication as well and frequently died from infectious complications. These authors' conclusion was that patients >45 years of age were at too great a risk to be considered for a transplant with a cadaver kidney, and unless there was a potential living donor, they should not be advised to undergo a transplant. It was recommended that they stay on chronic maintenance dialysis.

Based on this report and others, many programs were reluctant to offer transplantation to older patients [11]. In 1972, the Ninth Report of the Human Renal Transplant Registry summarized data on 5,432 patients [12]. Few patients over the age of 60 years (Fig. 37-1) had received a renal transplant. Of this small group, two patients over the age of 80 years had received a renal graft, and neither survived. In 1973, the National Transplant Registry reported that of a total of 16,023 transplants, only 80 (0.49%) were in recipients aged 61 years or older [13].

In 1975, Delmonico et al. [13] reviewed their results with transplants with the older age group, defined as patients >51 years of age. Of a series of 26 patients, six were 60 years or older, the oldest was 69 years of age. All six received cadaver allografts, and at the time of the report, five of the six had functioning grafts. In 1980, Ost et al. [7] in Sweden reviewed the results in 34 patients aged 60 years or older (mean age, 63 years) receiving transplants between 1971 and 1977 and compared this series with a group of younger patients aged 16 to 49 years. Data showed that there was poorer length of survival for both patients and grafts for the older age group. Complications were more numerous, but there was less irreversible rejection. Thus, they recommended that the dose of prednisolone be reduced in the older age group and that these patients continue to be offered transplantation.

In the early 1980s, cyclosporine was added to the immunosuppressive regimen, with dramatic improvements in both patient and graft survival rates [14–16]. In 1989, Pirsch et al. [17] reported on the use of quadruple immunosuppression (Minnesota antilymphoblast globulin, cyclosporine, prednisone, and azathioprine) in patients >60 years of age (N = 34): The 3-year actuarial patient and graft survival rates were 91% and 74%, respectively. Surgical complications and rejection episodes were seen less frequently than in younger patients. Medical complications such as infection, on the other hand, were seen more frequently but were easily managed. The authors concluded that transplantation was no longer contraindicated in the elderly patient. Others reported similar results [18–22].

Reports from Europe echoed the results achieved in this country, with Tapson et al. [23] from the United Kingdom reporting on a group of 13 patients with a mean age of 64 years (range, 62 to 67 years) who underwent cadaveric renal transplantation. One graft never functioned, and the patient returned to peritoneal dialysis. Eight patients were still alive with a functioning graft. The remaining patients died an average of 11 months after the transplant (range, 1 to 33 months). All had a functioning graft at the time of death. Causes of death were acute pancreatitis, vascular hemorrhage, cerebrovascular accident, and myocardial infarction. Although the results of renal transplantation were generally good, and by questionnaire 60% of dialysis patients were interested in having a transplant, there was little chance of their receiving one in Britain. Most of the elderly patients with end-stage renal disease did not have a suitable living donor, and cadaver organs were given preferentially to younger recipients. This study also showed that the elderly patient with end-stage renal disease who was accepted for dialysis could expect a 5-year survival rate of only 53%. Therefore, this group concluded that elderly people do well with renal replacement therapy, having a good length of survival and quality of life, and that patients over the age of 60 years should not be denied treatment of their renal disease solely because of their age.

Hestin et al. [24] from France analyzed data from 337 renal transplants performed between January 1, 1987, and November 30, 1992. Immunosuppression consisted of antilymphocyte globulin, cyclosporine, prednisone, and azathioprine. Thirty-two (10%) of the patients were 60 years of age or older at the time of transplantation (mean age, 64 years; range, 60 to 71 years) and 305 patients were 12 to 59 years of age (mean age, 41 years). The two groups were compared, and there were no significant differences noted in either patient or graft survival rate at 36 months (84% and 76%, respectively, in the older group compared with 96% and 83%, respectively, in the younger group). In the older group, all grafts lost were the result of patient death (two of five) or transplant nephrectomy (three of five), with two of the latter from arterial thrombosis and one from lymphoproliferative disease. In the younger age group, chronic rejection accounted for the majority of grafts lost (23 of 43). In the elderly group, acute rejection occurred in only 16% of the patients. Although, in general, the two most common causes of end-stage renal failure in an elderly population are nephrosclerosis and diabetes [25], in this group of elderly patients, nephrosclerosis and polycystic kidney disease were the most frequent causes of renal failure. This was thought to be due to the fact that patients with diabetes frequently have complicating medical conditions, and transplantation is therefore contraindicated. This group concluded that renal transplantation was an acceptable form of therapy for end-stage renal disease in the older patient if there were no obvious contraindications. As transplantation is less costly than dialysis, they recommended that this treatment alternative be proposed to motivated patients. Their only reservations were related to issues of compliance in patients taking their immunosuppressive medications, returning for post-transplant follow-up visits, and the ethical dilemma of giving an allograft to an older patient instead of a younger one because there is a shortage of donor organs.

Albrechtsen et al. [26] from Norway looked at 126 older patients ranging in age from 70 to 83 years (mean, 73 years) who received transplants between 1983 and 1993. Twenty patients received grafts from living donors. All grafts from living donors functioned, but 2% of the grafts from cadaver donors never functioned. Patient survival rates at 1 and 5 years were 80% and 74%, respectively, for living donor transplants and 80% and 54%, respectively, for cadaver donor transplants. Graft survival rates at 1 and 5 years were 80% and 74%, respectively, for living donor transplants and 78% and 52%, respectively, for cadaver allografts. Fifty-three grafts (83%) were lost due to patient death (graft was functioning), 15% from rejection, and 2% from recurrent disease. In their series, 91% of patients with end-stage renal disease >70 years of age were candidates for renal transplant, but only 45% of patients >70 years were candidates. Transplantation was provided to 81% of patients <70 years of age, but to only 53% of patients >70 years of age. In part, this was because there were fewer living donors available for the older patients, and many died while awaiting a cadaver kidney. Sixteen percent of the older patients received a living donor graft compared with 32% of the younger patients. This group's conclusions were that kidney transplants could be performed in the older age group with a favorable outcome and that there were no data to support the use of age alone in the selection of recipients for renal transplantation.

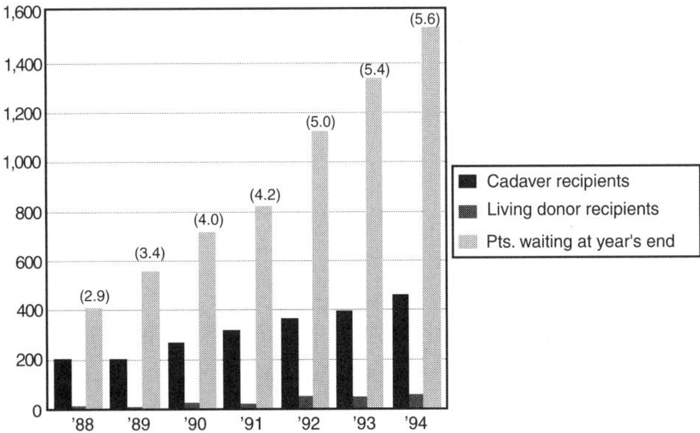

FIG. 37-2. This graph shows the total number of patients 65 years and older, who received a kidney transplant either from a cadaver or living donor for each of the years listed. Also shown is the total number of patients 65 years and older who were waiting for cadaver kidneys at the end of each year listed. The numbers in parentheses represents the percent of patients of all ages waiting for each of these years. (From United Network for Organ Sharing; Division of Organ Transplantation, Bureau of Health Resources Development, Health Resources and Services Administration. 1995 Annual Report of the U.S. Scientific Registry for Transplant Recipients and the Organ Procurement and Transplantation Network—Transplant Data: 1988–1994. Rockville, MD: U.S. Department of Health and Human Services, 1995.)

In the 1990s, we have seen an increase not only in the number of elderly (>65 years) renal transplant recipients, but also in the number of elderly patients waiting for a cadaver kidney (Fig. 37-2) [4]. This is because with cyclosporine for immunosuppression, it has been demonstrated that older patients do as well as or better than many of their younger counterparts. In addition, as the age of the population shifts, the number of older patients with renal failure has increased. In the U.S. Renal Data Systems 1991

Annual Report [27],* 50% of new patients who enter therapy for end-stage renal disease are >61 years of age. Nevertheless, because there is a shortage of cadaver organs, the question of whether organs should be allocated to this group with a limited life expectancy (and the accompanying ethical concerns) is valid [28]. In the United States, the average life expectancy after age 59 is an additional 20 years, whereas if one develops end-stage renal disease, this is reduced to 4.2 years [27]. In 1995, Schaubel et al. [29], using data from the Canadian Organ Replacement Registry, did a controlled comparison of transplantation and dialysis in the elderly with respect to patient survival. This study looked at 6,400 patients aged 60 years or older registered with the Canadian Organ Replacement Registry between 1987 and 1993. They picked this time frame because renal transplantation was uncommon in this age group before 1983. The results of this study showed that the 5-year survival for patients who received a renal transplant was 81% compared with 51% for the dialysis group (P <0.0001). They concluded that these results support the potential advantage of transplantation in the elderly with regard to patient survival.

Evaluation and Selection of the Elderly Transplant Recipient

An older patient with end-stage renal disease who wants to be considered for a renal transplant undergoes an extensive evaluation. Most of the evaluation can be done on an outpatient basis. A complete history is taken and a physical examination is done. A video presentation about transplantation is given to the patient. This is followed by a thorough counseling session, usually conducted by a transplant surgeon, at which time the potential complications, risks, and expected outcome are discussed in detail. Unless there are absolute contraindications to transplantation and the candidate still wishes to be considered for a transplant, the in-depth evaluation is begun. Laboratory evaluation includes complete blood count, electrolytes, blood urea nitrogen, creatinine, cholesterol, serum proteins, albumin, liver function studies, and serologies to include human immunodeficiency virus, cytomegalovirus, and hepatitis B and C viruses. Blood is drawn for histocompatibility matching, and serum is saved to be used for cytotoxic crossmatching once a matching kidney has been identified. Skin tests are placed to check for a prior exposure to tuberculosis. Routine chest radiography and electrocardiography are performed.

If there is a history of smoking, pulmonary function tests are done. If the pulmonary function test results are abnormal, then consideration for a transplant is deferred until the patient has ceased smoking for at least 3 months and improvement is shown in the pulmonary function test results. A pulmonologist may be consulted. In the older patient, routine cardiac evaluation includes a dobutamine echocardiography or exercise right ventriculography. If these test results are positive or there is a history of diabetes, a cardiac catheterization is done. Based on the patient's history and findings at physical examination, evaluation of the carotid arteries or the peripheral vasculature may be necessary. Evaluation of the gastrointestinal tract includes routine gallbladder ultrasonography for all diabetics or any patient with a history suggestive of gallbladder disease. If gallstones are present, a cholecystectomy is advised in the older patient before transplantation. A history of peptic ulcer disease warrants investigation by endoscopy. If ulcer disease is present, this will need to be treated, with healing documented by repeat endoscopy before the patient is placed on the transplant list. Also, these individuals will need to be placed on H_2 blockers in the post-transplant period.

Because the incidence of diverticulosis and diverticulitis increases with age [30], and one of the most lethal complications after transplantation is colonic perforation, some programs have advocated routine pretransplant barium enemas to ascertain the presence of diverticula in older recipients [31]. Based on data that showed the inability to predict which patients are at risk for colonic complications as well as on data on those patients who had such a complication (i.e., the long amount of time between occurrence and transplant) [32], we no longer perform a routine barium enema, but rather do this only in those patients with a history of prior difficulty. If the barium enema shows diverticulosis and there is a history of repeated episodes of diverticulitis, a colonoscopic examination is done, and a colonic resection may be advised before transplant because of the high mortality associated with perforation in the post-transplant period [33]. A history of pancreatitis deserves careful evaluation because of the high morbidity and mortality associated with the development of pancreatitis and associated complications in the immunosuppressed patient [34,35].

Because obesity is associated with increased complications and decreased graft survival, our recommendation is to defer consideration for transplantation until the body mass index is 30 or less [36–38]. If there is a history of a malignancy, consideration for transplantation should be deferred until there is at least a 2-year interval with no evidence of disease [39]. Exceptions to this rule are renal cell carcinomas discovered incidentally, in situ carcinomas, low-grade bladder cancers, and basal cell skin cancers, in which case a waiting period is unnecessary. A waiting period of >2 years may be necessary for malignant melanomas, breast carcinomas, and colorectal cancer [39]. All older male recipients should have a prostate-specific antigen test and older female recipients should have mammography performed as part of the pretransplant evaluation.

On completion of the previously mentioned studies, the candidate is presented to an evaluation committee whose members include transplant surgeons, transplant nephrologists, nurses, immunologists, social workers, nutritionists, a psychiatrist, and a urologist.

If the patient is accepted as a candidate, the source of the donor organ must be determined. Are there any potential liv-

*The data reported here have been supplied by The United States Renal Data System (USRDS). The interpretation and reporting of these data are the responsibility of the author(s) and in no way should be seen as an official policy or interpretation of the USRDS.

ing donors either related or unrelated? Sibling donors are preferred, but the siblings of older recipients are also older and often have medical contraindications. Progeny as donors are favored because of the excellent proven results, although if there are no suitable living donors, patients are still considered for inclusion on a list for a cadaver donor. Nevertheless, this is an area of debate because of the shortage of cadaver donors.

Perioperative and Postoperative Management

The perioperative management of the older patient differs little from the routine care of any transplant recipient. Once a donor organ has been identified and the cytotoxic crossmatch has been reported as being negative, the transplant procedure is carried out. A triple-lumen central venous catheter is placed to monitor the central venous pressure and to give intravenous fluids. An arterial line for monitoring arterial pressure and a pulmonary artery catheter are not placed routinely but may be warranted in selected cases. The standard immunosuppression regimen consists of corticosteroids and azathioprine intraoperatively and in the post-transplant period. Polyclonal antithymocyte serum is given until cyclosporine is started and has achieved therapeutic blood levels. Prednisone and azathioprine are continued, and the patient is discharged on cyclosporine, prednisone, and azathioprine. The patient is evaluated at weekly intervals on an outpatient basis. Should the patient have a suspected rejection episode, a biopsy is performed. If there is histologic evidence of rejection, treatment is given, consisting of antithymocyte serum and bolus corticosteroids.

Vanderbilt Experience

Between April 1962 and March 1996, 2,184 renal transplants were performed at the Nashville Veterans Affairs and Vanderbilt Medical Centers. Forty-two of these recipients have been between 60 and 67 years of age, with an average age of 63 years. Thirty patients received cadaver kidneys and 12 received kidneys from living donors. Half of the living donors were siblings and the other half were progeny of the recipient. Twenty-four were men and 18 were women. Thirty-seven were white and five were black. Forty-one received primary grafts and one had received two previous transplants. The most common reasons for failure of the native kidneys were chronic glomerulonephritis, polycystic kidney disease, and diabetes mellitus.

The graft survival for these 42 patients at 1, 2, and 3 years was 89%, 77%, and 71%, respectively. The patient survival at the same time interval was 92%, 87%, and 79%, respectively. Of these 42 patients, there have been 10 deaths ranging from 3 weeks to 21.8 years post-transplant. Importantly, seven (70%) of the 10 patients who died had a functioning graft at the time of death. The other three patients lost their graft and were returned to dialysis prior to death. Twenty-nine of the 42 (69%) were still alive with a functioning kidney from 1 month to 9.6 years (average, 37.5 months). Three of the 42 patients lost their kidney to rejection and are still alive on dialysis. Eight patients experienced major complications after the transplant such as bleeding ruptured aortic aneurysm, perforated colonic diverticulum, and strangulated hernia requiring bowel resection.

The following case report is but one example of the benefits elderly patients can receive from a successful renal transplant.

Case Report

A 63-year-old woman, a retired nurse, with end-stage renal disease due to polycystic kidney disease received a cadaver kidney transplant in November 1971. She had been on chronic hemodialysis for 3 years. There was immediate function of the transplanted kidney, and she was discharged 18 days after the transplant. Immunosuppression consisted of prednisone and azathioprine. The serum creatinine level was 2.1 at the time of discharge. She was hospitalized 6 weeks after the transplant and treated for a rejection episode with bolus corticosteroids. Nine years after the transplant, she had a repair of an epigastric hernia. Two years after this, she developed an umbilical hernia that was repaired. At this admission, she had a blood urea nitrogen level of 16 and a creatinine level of 0.9. She continued to be followed as an outpatient and maintained excellent renal function. She died in September 1993, 2 months before her eighty-fifth birthday, at home from a presumed myocardial infarction. During the 21 years after her cadaver transplant, she was able to lead a normal life (Fig. 37-3). She saw her grandson graduate from medical school and enjoyed the birth of her great-grandson.

Conclusions

At the time that renal transplantation was being developed, advanced age was considered to be a relative if not absolute contraindication, because if pharmacologic immunosuppression was added to the already suppressed immune status seen with the natural aging process, it was believed that this would pose too great a risk to the individual's life. Subsequent data did not support this, and with the addition of cyclosporine to the immunosuppressive regime, it was seen that older patients immunologically did as well if not better than their younger counterparts. Concomitant with the increase in age of the dialysis population, we have seen an increase in the number of older recipients waiting for a kidney transplant. The only issue to be debated is an ethical one: Should an "old old" individual (>70 to 75 years) [40], whose natural life expectancy without renal disease is limited, have access to a scarce resource (cadaver kidneys)? One approach to this ethical dilemma is to transplant kidneys from older cadaver donors into older recipients [41]. Even though the life expectancy on dialysis may be less than that with a functioning renal transplant, some nephrologists contend that this is the preferred method of treatment. Philosophically, it seems reasonable to consider renal transplantation in older recipients if there is a potential living donor

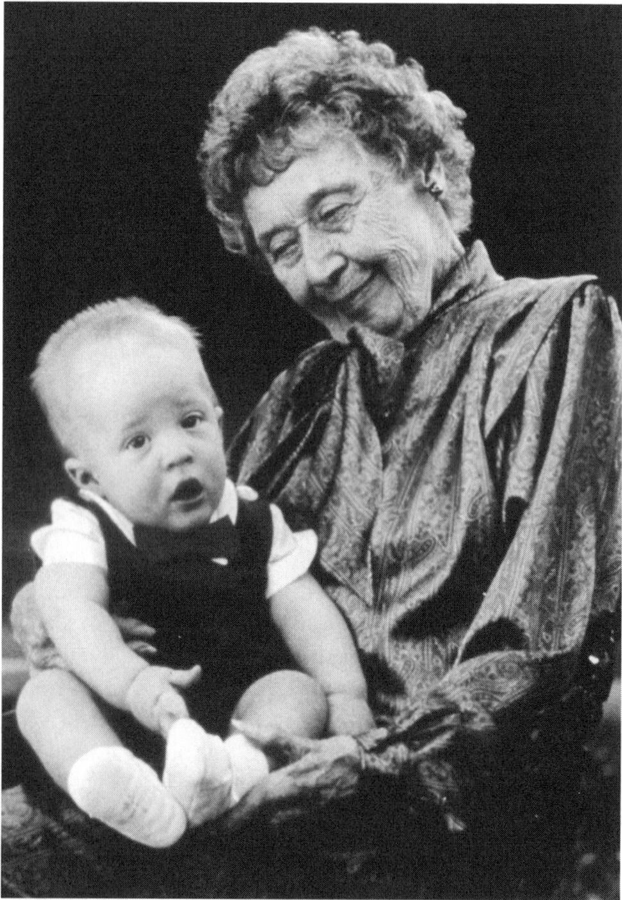

FIG. 37-3. Elderly woman with great-grandson. She lived an additional 21 years of a normal life after receiving a kidney transplant at the age of 63.

who gives informed consent and is willing to be a donor. Under these circumstances, the recipient could reasonably expect to live out a normal life span.

LIVER TRANSPLANTATION

Michael L. Cheatham and C. Wright Pinson

Liver transplantation in the elderly patient is becoming more commonplace, as statistics from the United Network for Organ Sharing (UNOS) database demonstrate (Table 37-1) [4]. With experience, improved antirejection drugs, and refined operative techniques, transplant surgeons have repeatedly brought down the age limits they have set regarding eligibility for hepatic transplantation [42,43]. There is currently no recommended absolute age limit with respect to who may receive a liver transplant; each patient is considered individually to determine that individual's suitability for transplantation. This has resulted in successful transplantation in patients >80 years of age [4].

In the past, it was argued that elderly recipients would not tolerate liver transplantation as well as younger recipients, would have increased morbidity and mortality, and would represent an inefficient use of scarce donor organs. These concerns have been negated by statistics from both the UNOS database and multiple individual studies that demonstrate similar survival and complication rates when elderly recipients are compared with younger recipients (Table 37-2) [27,42–48]. In part, this success may be due to careful selection of those elderly patients most likely to benefit from liver transplantation. Such patient selection, however, is prudent, given the current scarcity of donor organs and the steadily increasing size of the transplant waiting list as well as the cost of a complicated transplantation procedure.

Review of the Literature

In 1991, Stieber et al. [48], at the University of Pittsburgh, reported the largest series of elderly orthotopic liver transplant patients. They performed transplants in 156 patients >60 years of age, four of whom were >70 years of age. Of note, 45 (29%) of these patients were classified as being of the then more-advanced acuity UNOS status 3 or 4. Actuarial 1-year survival for the elderly patients was 71% compared with 78% for patients between 18 and 60 years of age. The survival rate after retransplantation was also similar. A trend toward fewer episodes of rejection and a decreased requirement for immunosuppression were noted in the elderly subgroup. This study concluded that "physiological age is vastly more important than the chronological age" with respect to length of survival following liver transplantation and that advanced age was therefore not a contraindication to liver transplantation [48].

In 1991, Pirsch et al. [44,45] at the University of Wisconsin, reported liver transplantation in 23 patients who were 60 years of age or older. These patients were retrospectively compared with 84 demographically similar patients who were between 18 and 59 years of age. Although not statistically significant, elderly patients were less likely to develop rejection than were younger patients (52% vs. 69%) and had fewer episodes of rejection per patient (0.78 vs. 1.13). Infection rates were similar. A common (20%) postoperative complication in the elderly group was spinal compression fracture due to hepatic osteodystrophy. Length of hospital stay was similar. Actuarial 1-year patient survival was 85% for the elderly group versus 81% for the younger group. Interestingly, elderly recipients were very compliant with their follow-up. These authors concluded that age alone should not be a contraindication to liver transplantation.

In 1993, Emre et al. [46], at the Mount Sinai School of Medicine, retrospectively analyzed 39 transplant patients over the age of 60 and compared them with 163 patients between the ages of 18 and 60 years. They further subdivided each group by pretransplant UNOS status at that time (1, functional at home; 2, requiring home care; 3, in the hospital; 4, in the intensive care unit on life support). Twenty (51%) of the elderly patients and 56 (34%) of the younger

TABLE 37-1. *Liver transplantation by year*

	1988	1989	1990	1991	1992	1993	1994
All ages	1,713	2,201	2,690	2,954	3,064	3,440	3,652
Age ≥65 years	29	46	90	144	155	181	192
Percent of total	1.7	2.1	3.3	4.9	5.1	5.3	5.3

Source: United Network for Organ Sharing; Division of Organ Transplantation, Bureau of Health Resources Development, Health Resources and Services Administration. 1995 Annual Report of the U.S. Scientific Registry for Transplant Recipients and the Organ Procurement and Transplantation Network—Transplant Data: 1988–1994. Rockville, MD: U.S. Department of Health and Human Services, 1995.

patients were either of UNOS status 3 or 4, denoting an increased acuity for transplantation. Preexisting cardiovascular disease and diabetes mellitus were more common in the elderly group, although not significantly so, and the two groups were otherwise similar with respect to demographics and indications for transplantation. Age was not found to be a significant predictive variable for incidence of rejection, postoperative renal failure, length of stay in the hospital, surgical complications, or infection. One-year actuarial survival was similar for the elderly and younger patient groups for both UNOS status 1 and 2 patients (84% vs. 87%, respectively) and status 3 and 4 patients (75% vs. 66%, respectively). These authors concluded that age >60 years was not a contraindication in properly selected patients.

In a 1994 report, Bromley et al. [47], at King's College Hospital, reported on transplants in 40 patients who were 60 years of age or older, 60% of whom received transplants for primary biliary cirrhosis. These patients were compared with 40 case control patients between 18 and 60 years of age matched by disease process, Child-Pugh score, intraoperative blood loss, and date of transplantation. Although elderly patients tended to have more preexisting cardiovascular and pulmonary disease than did their younger controls, there were no differences between the two groups with respect to intraoperative interventions required, infections, incidence of surgical complications, or length of survival. As in the findings of Pirsch et al. [44,45], graft rejection was less likely to occur in the elderly group but did not reach statistical significance. The only significant finding was a slightly longer hospital stay in the elderly group (24 vs. 20 days; $P < 0.03$). They concluded that age >60 years should not preclude liver transplantation and noted that >10% of liver transplant recipients in the United Kingdom in 1992 were >60 years of age.

Evaluation and Selection of the Elderly Liver Transplant Recipient

Elderly liver transplant recipients differ from their younger counterparts in several important respects. These differences must be kept in mind if transplantation in the elderly is to be successful. A significant difference is the inherent decrease in immune response that occurs with aging [48]. This immunologic change can be both beneficial

TABLE 37-2. *Survival rates after liver transplantation*

	1 Year (%)	2 Years (%)	3 Years (%)
All ages	79.2 ± 0.3	75.4 ± 0.4	72.7 ± 0.4
Age ≥65 years	73.4 ± 1.8	68.0 ± 2.0	64.2 ± 2.2

Source: United Network for Organ Sharing; Division of Organ Transplantation, Bureau of Health Resources Development, Health Resources and Services Administration. 1995 Annual Report of the U.S. Scientific Registry for Transplant Recipients and the Organ Procurement and Transplantation Network—Transplant Data: 1988–1994. Rockville, MD: U.S. Department of Health and Human Services, 1995.

and detrimental to the elderly recipient's outcome. With a reduction in immune surveillance, the elderly patient appears to have a lower incidence of rejection and a decreased requirement for immunosuppressive medications such as corticosteroids, azathioprine, and the calcineurin phosphatase inhibitors cyclosporine and tacrolimus. Rejection episodes, when they do occur, tend to be less severe. This decreased immunologic sensitivity, however, also places the elderly recipient at an increased risk for post-transplant bacterial, viral (herpesvirus, cytomegalovirus, Epstein-Barr virus), and fungal (*Candida, Aspergillus, Legionella, Nocardia, Cryptococcus*) infections, as well as for malignancy (squamous cell carcinoma, non-Hodgkin's lymphoma, soft-tissue sarcoma).

Perhaps the most important difference in the elderly transplant recipient is the prevalence of other preexisting medical problems in addition to the underlying hepatic disease. Whereas younger recipients tend to be fairly healthy apart from their hepatic dysfunction, elderly recipients frequently present with long-standing cardiac, pulmonary, renal, or metabolic disease. Cardiovascular disease and infection are the two most common causes of death after solid organ transplantation. As the elderly population is at an increased risk for these complications, both of these factors must be carefully anticipated in the preoperative evaluation if transplantation is to be successful.

Carey et al. [49] studied the prevalence of coronary artery disease in patients over the age of 50 years who were being considered for hepatic transplantation and found that 27% had moderate-to-severe coronary artery disease by angiography. Diabetes mellitus was the most predictive risk factor for the presence of coronary artery disease in this group of patients, but male sex and family history were also important considerations. Diabetes, although not an absolute contraindication to transplantation, is a significant risk factor for increased perioperative morbidity and mortality. Hyperglycemia is well known to be associated with decreased wound healing and impaired neutrophil function. Trail et al. [50] analyzed the impact of diabetes mellitus on the outcome of hepatic transplantation and found no difference in overall graft or patient survival rate. Diabetic patients were, however, more likely to develop minor bacterial, fungal, and viral infections, such as wound infections. Major bacterial infections, such as sepsis, positive blood culture results, or both, were more common in the diabetic group but did not reach statistical significance. The presence of diabetes, therefore, coupled with the necessity of chronic immunosuppression to prevent graft rejection and the decreased responsiveness of the immune system, make the elderly patient even more likely to develop infectious complications in the peritransplant period. Elderly diabetic patients undergoing transplant evaluation therefore require special consideration, given their increased risk for both cardiac and infectious complications.

Elderly patients are also more likely to have preexisting chronic pulmonary disease due to tobacco abuse or environmental exposure than are their younger counterparts. Their baseline pulmonary function is therefore frequently diminished and they are more likely to require oxygen therapy and bronchodilators to maintain adequate pulmonary physiology. Elderly patients are thus more likely to require prolonged postoperative ventilator support and are more difficult to wean from mechanical ventilation [51].

Renal function characteristically diminishes with age. This becomes an important consideration in the elderly patient with regard to dosing of antibiotics, H_2 blockers, and antirejection medications such as cyclosporine and tacrolimus, all of which can contribute to renal dysfunction. These toxicities are aggravated by intravascular volume depletion, which must be carefully avoided. The elderly recipient may also need adjustment in prescribed doses of other medications. Narcotics, benzodiazepines, and other drugs that have central nervous system or respiratory depressant side effects may need to be administered at reduced doses in the elderly to avoid oversedation or toxicity.

Metabolic diseases such as hepatic osteodystrophy are more common in the elderly recipient, especially in postmenopausal women with cholestatic liver disease. These patients may present with or develop evidence of pathologic fractures secondary to bone resorption as a result of their chronic liver disease. This condition is exacerbated by the decreased mobility associated with the early posttransplant period as well as by the use of corticosteroid immunosuppression. It is managed most effectively with calcium supplementation, early mobilization of the patient postoperatively, and minimization of immunosuppressant drugs.

Preoperative Evaluation

At the Vanderbilt Transplant Center, we have pursued a multidisciplinary approach to the preoperative evaluation of liver transplant candidates, especially the elderly recipient, who is more likely to have preexisting medical conditions, involving transplant hepatology and surgery, cardiology, pulmonology, anesthesiology, infectious disease, hematology, psychiatry, nutrition, social work, medical ethics, and pastoral care. Representatives of each of these services are also integrally involved in the pretransplant, peritransplant, and post-transplant care of each recipient.

By virtue of their age, elderly recipients are at a higher risk for perioperative cardiac complications during liver transplantation. This necessitates a careful preoperative cardiac evaluation of each patient being considered for transplantation. All patients over the age of 50 years are evaluated by a transplant cardiologist and undergo echocardiography to assess left ventricular function and rule out valvular heart disease or pulmonary hypertension. Exercise stress testing is performed to identify asymptomatic coronary artery disease that might become significant in the peritransplant period. If warranted by cardiac history or if dysfunction is identified, coronary angiography, right-sided heart catheterization, or both are performed to evaluate the severity of coronary artery disease and pulmonary hypertension.

In addition to routine chest radiography, all patients have pulmonary function testing with spirometry and baseline arterial blood gas determinations. Evidence of pulmonary dysfunction on these studies mandates evaluation by a transplant pulmonologist. Therapeutic interventions such as pulmonary bronchodilators and the cessation of tobacco use are instituted in an attempt to maximize preoperative pulmonary function. Radiographic evidence that suggests the presence of a pulmonary or mediastinal abnormality is an indication for computed tomography (CT) of the chest to rule out the presence of infection and occult primary or metastatic malignancy. Routine skin testing for tuberculosis is performed.

The risk for development of malignancy increases with age. The elderly transplant patient must therefore be evaluated carefully for the presence of not only hepatic malignancies such as hepatocellular carcinoma or cholangiocarcinoma, but also for extrahepatic malignancies, including breast, cervical, colon, and skin cancer. The routine abdominal CT scan obtained for all patients assists in this evaluation. Female patients routinely have mammography performed to rule out breast cancer and Papanicolaou's smear to assess for cervical carcinoma. Esophagoduodenoscopy and colonoscopy are performed as indicated by the patient's past medical history and review of systems if the possibility of gastrointestinal malignancy exists.

Evidence accumulated over the past decade has emphasized the importance of a patient's nutritional status in reducing the risk of surgical complications such as infection and multiple system organ failure. Adequate preoperative nutrition is important in preventing bacterial translocation in the perioperative period. This is especially true in the elderly patient population, in whom nutrition has frequently suffered as a result of long-standing medical illnesses. Registered dietitians perform a careful nutritional evaluation on each patient and assist in maximizing the patient's preoperative nutritional status.

Perioperative Management

Intraoperative and postoperative management of the elderly liver recipient is similar to that for any other recipient, with a few exceptions. All patients are invasively monitored with a pulmonary artery catheter and arterial line. Meticulous attention to the elderly patient's intravascular volume status and coagulation profile is essential. The use of intraoperative thromboelastography can greatly facilitate the identification of coagulation disorders and guide therapy to correct coagulopathies that occur. Due to the prevalence of preexisting cardiopulmonary disease in the elderly patient population, invasive hemodynamic monitoring is even more important in these patients than in the younger transplant population. In addition to providing information about the patient's intravascular volume status, such monitoring also provides an assessment of the elderly patient's frequently diminished ventricular function and response to pharmacologic support. This monitoring may also be useful in the preoperative setting to facilitate hemodynamic optimization of the elderly UNOS status 1 or 2 patient whose cardiac dysfunction may be significant.

In contrast to younger transplant recipients, the elderly patient may require a longer period of postoperative mechanical ventilation due to preexisting pulmonary disease or to the diminished pulmonary function associated with aging. Nevertheless, active attempts should be made to extubate patients and discontinue mechanical ventilation as soon as physiologically feasible, given the increased risk for pneumonia associated with prolonged intubation.

We routinely use venovenous bypass in the elderly transplant patient. Unlike younger patients, who with good cardiac physiology may be able to tolerate the anhepatic phase and not require bypass, the elderly transplant recipient is less able to tolerate the physiologic demands associated with crossclamping of the portal vein and inferior vena cava. The use of venovenous bypass tends to decrease the development of mesenteric congestion and edema and provides for a more stable physiologic course during and after the anhepatic phase of transplantation.

In the longer term, we advise careful monitoring for the elderly recipient as for all recipients. We place additional emphasis on cancer screening, dietary monitoring, calcium supplementation, infection surveillance, and cardiovascular monitoring of the elderly transplant recipient.

Conclusions

The past decade has seen a continual re-evaluation of the age limit for liver transplantation. Multiple studies have now demonstrated that the elderly patient can undergo transplantation with survival rates comparable to those of younger patients and with similar complication rates. Elderly transplant recipients appear to undergo fewer episodes of rejection, require less immunosuppression, and tend to be more compliant with post-transplant follow-up than their younger counterparts. Careful preoperative evaluation and intraoperative and postoperative management of elderly transplant recipients are essential to achieve successful transplantation due to the increased incidence of preexisting cardiopulmonary disease and risk for infection seen in the elderly population. Liver transplantation should not be withheld from patients based on their chronologic age; patients should be carefully considered for transplantation based on their individual status and the presence of coexisting medical problems.

HEART AND LUNG TRANSPLANTATION

Richard N. Pierson, III, and Mark Fox

Considerable experience with transplantation of thoracic organs for elderly patients has been accumulated. As for other solid organ transplants, advanced patient age has evolved from an absolute to a relative contraindication to thoracic transplantation. Current exclusion criteria based on a prospective recipient's chronologic age vary among centers in the United States and among different countries, but arbitrary cutoffs for heart (65 years), lung (60 years), and heart-lung or double-lung (45 years) transplantation are prevalent. These generally accepted guidelines are based primarily on considerations of appropriate allocation of scarce donor organs and increasingly convincing evidence that, despite careful candidate selection, both short-term and intermediate-term outcomes are slightly worse for older recipients. Use of older (and therefore "marginal") donors for older recipients is a concept that has been proposed to reconcile the critical shortage of donor organs with the clinical needs of elderly patients, but this approach has important adverse consequences for recipients of such organs. Because current age criteria and survival rates differ substantially for heart, single- or double-lung, and heart-lung transplantation, each category of thoracic transplantation is considered separately.

Heart Transplantation

With the advent of cyclosporine, results of heart transplantation in patients <55 years of age improved dramatically, emboldening thoracic transplant teams to extend therapy to older patients. Only 2% of heart transplants performed before 1983 were in patients >55 years of age; however, the proportion of recipients in this age group increased to 25% in 1986 [52] and 39% between 1990 and 1994. The percentage of patients over the age of 65 years who received transplants increased from 1.9% to 2.9% between 1987 and 1994. These trends demonstrate that heart transplant programs are increasingly willing to accept older patients as candidates.

TABLE 37-3. *Percentage of heart recipients receiving older donor hearts by recipient age at transplantation*

Recipient age (yrs)	Recipients having donor >45 years of age (%)	Recipients having donor >60 years of age (%)
<35	7.8	0.2
35–44	9.7	0.4
45–60	13.8	0.5
>60	16.3	1.3

Source: Data and statistics from International Society for Heart and Lung Transplantation database for all primary thoracic transplants performed from 1990 through 1994, stratified by recipient and donor age, and analyzed by multivariate logistic regression analysis (Pierson R, unpublished data).

Early reports from Spain and Italy suggested that outcomes for patients over the age of 60 years were similar to those for younger patients [53,54]. The International Society for Heart and Lung Transplantation (ISHLT) registry statistics document a statistically significant trend toward worse survival rates with increasing recipient age, however [1,2].* In patients >65 years of age, operative mortality is 5% higher than in younger patients (88% vs. 93% survival at 30 days); the difference in length of survival between older and younger patients increases steadily through intermediate-term follow-up, reaching a 9% differential (71% vs. 80%) at 2 years. A more rapid decline in length of survival over time after transplant is also evident for those recipients between 60 and 65 years of age relative to those <60 years of age. Importantly, the relative risk of advanced recipient age is evident even when other risk factors (such as increased donor age and prior transplant) are excluded. Beyond 3 years, survival curves for patients <60 years of age and those over this age are essentially parallel [1,2], suggesting that the added actuarial risk for older recipients may be balanced by a higher incidence of other lethal factors (e.g., chronic rejection) in the younger cohort in long-term follow-up (>2 years). Thus, results of heart transplantation in the elderly are slightly but significantly (P <0.02) worse than in younger patients, and age at operation not only influences perioperative survival but is also associated with increased mortality during the intermediate term.

Several factors contribute to higher mortality in older patients. Fabbri et al. [55] reviewed results in 206 patients, 46 of whom were over the age of 55 years, receiving heart transplants using a consistent immunosuppressive regimen at a single institution. Ninety-day mortality was 22% in the older group compared with 11% in younger patients. Although the incidence of infection was similar in both groups, death from infection accounted for most of the increased mortality in older recipients, implying an important difference in the consequences of therapeutic immunosuppression to the older host. Rejection rates were comparable between the groups, but death as a consequence of rejection also occurred more commonly in older patients. These findings suggest that no important decrease in immunoresponsiveness to the heart graft is conferred in older recipients (when considered as a group), and further suggest that older patients were not overimmunosuppressed. It seems likely that the well-documented reduction in physiologic resilience associated with advanced age, in the context of common complications such as infection or rejection, is an important independent contributor to worse outcomes among older heart transplant recipients [3]. Data on cause of death from ISHLT registry statistics support this interpretation [1,2]. Operative mortality is approximately 7% for patients <60 years of age versus approximately 10% for older patients. Deaths attributed to immediate or early cardiac failure (both preservation related and immunologically mediated) occur with similar frequency across all age groups. Death due to cerebrovascular accidents (stroke, intracerebral hemorrhage) and multisystem organ failure also occur with similar frequencies, suggesting that current screening practices successfully prevent an otherwise expected higher incidence of these complications in elderly patients. Nevertheless, infection-related mortality, particularly that due to bacterial infection, is higher in older patients (8% to 13% for those over the age of 50 years vs. 5% for those <50 years).

Based on the rational but untested assumption that the longevity and physiologic characteristics of an older donor heart are suitable for an older recipient, coupled with the perceived appropriateness of allocating older donors to older patients, older recipients are more likely to receive an organ from an older donor (Table 37-3). Donor age has an important influence on perioperative and intermediate-term survival, however. Registry data (excluding retransplants and patients receiving transplants before 1990) reveal that for recipients of any age, increasing donor age has a significant adverse influence on outcome; the increased relative risk of poor outcome associated with an older donor is independent of recipient age (Table 37-4). Indeed, donor age >60 years was the most important individual risk factor for poor outcome for primary heart transplant patients in the 1995 ISHLT review (relative risk, 3.49) [2]. One intriguing observation, that increased donor age persists as an important independent risk factor for increased mortality for up to 2 years, remains unexplained. The survival rates at 2 years for recipients of hearts from donors aged 45 to 60 years and from those >60 years of age are lower by 10% and 20%, respectively, compared with the survival rate of recipients whose donors were <35 years of age.

A component of the donor age effect is attributable to the context in which use of older donors is considered: Older donors may be used only in desperation for critically ill recipients, thereby biasing the result against older donors. Although relative acuity of recipient illness has not been

*Data and statistics are obtained from the ISHLT database for all primary thoracic transplants performed from 1990 through 1994, stratified by recipient and donor age, and analyzed by multivariate logistic regression analysis (R Pierson, unpublished data). Results reported in this chapter that are not otherwise cited were derived from this ongoing analysis.

TABLE 37-4. *Relative risk of recipient death over time after heart transplant*

Donor age (yrs)	1 Month	3 Months	1 Year	2 Years
<35	1.0	1.0	1.0	1.0
35–44*	1.4	1.3	1.3	1.4
45–60*	2.0	1.8	1.8	1.7

*P <0.02.

Source: Data and statistics from International Society for Heart and Lung Transplantation database for all primary thoracic transplants performed from 1990 through 1994, stratified by recipient and donor age, and analyzed by multivariate logistic regression analysis (Pierson R, unpublished data).

independently controlled for in available analyses of registry statistics, its influence might be expected to be restricted to short-term (1- and 3-month) follow-up. Thus, it is probable that a component of the donor effect apparent at 1 month (9% survival difference between donors <35 years of age [94%] and >60 years of age [85%]) may be due to recipient factors. Nevertheless, the older donor effect continues to increase, as indicated by a persistent increased relative risk of death and the associated growing disparity in survival up to 2 years. This unexpected observation may be explained by reviewing the causes of death segregated by time after transplant and stratified by recipient age; such an analysis has not yet been performed. Importantly, if factors that can be screened for at donor evaluation or reversed with early detection and intervention are identified, this analysis might result in improved results with older donors and consequent safe expansion of the heart donor pool.

Thus, both donor and recipient factors contribute to the observed survival difference between patients under and over the age of 60. Why are results as good as they are? Speculatively, selection bias, to exclude comorbidity and in favor of younger physiologic age, almost certainly contributes to relatively good outcomes. These highly selected patients may be more compliant with medication regimens than their younger counterparts; theoretically, older recipients may have a less vigorous immune response to their graft and, consequently, may be less likely to develop chronic rejection. The relevance and relative importance of these factors are unknown.

In summary, transplanting hearts into patients >60 years of age is slightly less successful than is the case for younger patients. Approximately 3% to 5% of the added operative mortality in elderly recipients is attributable to recipient factors such as the reduced resilience and greater susceptibility to bacterial infection that accompany older age. Additional higher risks of similar magnitude are associated with use of older donors, a risk currently borne disproportionately by older recipients. Although the outcome is slightly worse for the elderly (>60 or 65 years of age), and elderly recipients continue to suffer higher attrition during intermediate-term follow-up, overall outcomes are still quite acceptable by historical standards and compared with results with other organs. In this context, 2-year survival rates >70% may be viewed as validation of current practice.

Lung Transplantation

Before 1988, perioperative mortality was 20% for single- and double-lung recipients [1,2]. By 1993, operative mortality had decreased to approximately 10%, likely due to improvements in patient selection, advances in surgical approaches, and an expanded arsenal of agents with which to treat infection and rejection. Despite these advances, the survival rate after lung transplantation is approximately 50% at 3 years, reflecting the substantial immunologic and technical difficulties associated with transplanting this organ. Because of the more acute shortage of appropriate donor organs and relatively disappointing outcomes even in younger recipients, current practice at most transplant centers is to exclude patients >60 years of age from consideration.

Interestingly, ISHLT registry statistics from 1990 through 1994 indicate that early rates of survival for single-lung transplants are similar for the first 3 months (88% at 1 month, 83% at 3 months), regardless of recipient age. Historically, patients over the age of 60 years had significantly higher operative mortality and a worse survival rate (60% vs. 70%) at 1 year; however, since 1990, the survival rate at 1 year has improved to 70% in the 60- to 65-year age range, although results in patients <60 years of age improved only slightly, to 73%. At 2-year follow-up, 57% of the 147 patients (of 2,142 lung recipients who have received transplants since 1990) in the 60- to 65-year age group were living, compared with 64% of younger patients. Few patients over the age of 65 years (19 of 2,142) have received single-lung transplants. Despite comparable 10.1% mortality at 1 month, recipients over the age of 65 years had significantly worse survival rates at 1 (52%) and 2 years (42%). Thus, elderly recipients of single-lung transplants have poorer outcome than younger patients, and the difference is particularly dramatic for those over the age of 65 years. In contrast to results with older donor hearts, there is no adverse consequence to using older lungs for recipients of any age group.

For bilateral sequential single-lung (double-lung) transplant patients, operative mortality over the age of 45 years is 20%, compared with 10% for patients <45 years of age. Insufficient data are available from the UNOS/ISHLT registry to identify specific causes of death, which might be helpful in improving patient selection and anticipating and perhaps preventing lethal complications in this young elderly population. We speculate that the rigors of double-lung transplantation may unmask subclinically impaired cardiovascular fitness and immunologic resilience, which, in turn, may account for the higher observed mortality.

Heart-Lung Transplantation

Historically, heart-lung transplantation carried an operative mortality between 20% and 25%; this did not improve between 1990 and 1995, although individual high-volume centers have mortality under 10%. Despite similar operative and 3-month survival rates (81% and 77%, respectively) heart-lung recipients over the age of 40 years have approximately 1.7 times the relative risk of death within the first year, resulting in 1-year survival rates of 66% (vs. 72% in younger patients). Important additional attrition (approximately 12%) occurs in all age groups between 1 and 2 years, but is similar for both younger (<40 years) and older patients.

Many programs exclude patients >45 years of age from consideration for heart-lung transplantation due to the shortage of donor organs and the accurate perception of increased risk associated with this operation. Only 36 of 211 (17%) heart-lung transplants reported to the ISHLT between 1990 and 1994 were in patients over the age of 45 years, and follow-up beyond 3 months is available in only 15 patients. The operative survival rate, at 70%, is 14% lower in patients over the age of 50 years, and 1- and 2-year survival rates are significantly lower, by 18% and 24%, respectively, in this group than in patients <45 years of age: Only 36% of heart-lung recipients >50 years of age were living 2 years after transplantation. Relatively poor operative results combined with high attrition over subsequent follow-up argue strongly that heart-lung transplantation is usually not an appropriate intervention even for highly selected patients over the age of 50 years. In our view, this procedure should be regarded as excessively hazardous to a potential recipient in this age group and an inappropriate use of scarce donor organs until better results are achieved in younger recipients.

Ethical Considerations in Thoracic Transplantation

Heart and lung transplantation in the elderly places all the most difficult ethical issues in transplantation in sharp focus. Although cumulative survival is worse for the elderly compared with that for younger patients, the majority of elderly heart transplant recipients benefit dramatically, and outcomes for the elderly are generally quite acceptable by historical standards. An elderly patient's probability of survival is far better with transplantation than without. In addition, outcomes in carefully selected elderly patients are comparable with those in younger patients who are in extremis or have significant comorbidity. Thus, we conclude that transplantation of hearts or lungs in the elderly (60 to 65 years of age) is reasonable for the individual patient.

The difficulty for transplant professionals lies in achieving an appropriate balance between promoting optimal outcomes for the group of potential recipients and the physician's fundamental responsibility to be each individual patient's advocate. In terms of social utility, the fate of any particular patient is secondary to the overall good to be achieved for society. To maximize efficacy for the population of patients with end-stage cardiopulmonary failure, organs should be allocated to those patients for whom a successful outcome is most likely, and thus away from the elderly and most critically ill. Nevertheless, decisions to transplant are made on a case-by-case basis, where benefit (utility) for the individual patient is paramount.

Establishing programmatic criteria such as an arbitrary patient age above which transplantation will not be considered, is an objective way to establish limits and permits a reasonable balance to exist between the limited supply of, and overwhelming demand for, this potentially life-saving resource. Such arbitrary guidelines, if rigidly applied, however, eliminate physician judgment from the decision-making process—a high price to pay, and one that may result in exclusion of physiologically appropriate elderly candidates.

Conclusions

Heart transplant results in elderly (>60 years) patients, although slightly worse than in younger cohorts, support application of this life-saving therapy in physiologically appropriate individual candidates; the primary constraint is the shortage of suitable donor organs. Lower operative mortality has recently improved the risk to benefit equation for lung transplantation in the elderly. Nevertheless, survival rates of 50% at 3 years even in younger patients are discouraging with regard to possible extension of this modality to patients >65 years of age. Whether improved short- and long-term outcomes can be achieved for older thoracic organ recipients and, in particular, for double-lung and heart-lung patients is not clear but might be facilitated by restricting application of this modality to institutions with a large and ongoing experience, because improved outcomes with other complex surgical procedures and in high-risk patients have been demonstrated to correlate well with high volume and accumulated institutional experience.

Diversion of donor organs to recipients >65 years of age is a controversial subject that continues to be debated within the thoracic transplant community. The shortage of available donor lungs is even more severe than for hearts, and no long-term mechanical support alternative exists at present, resulting in a 30% mortality for those patients listed for lung transplantation. Until a solution to the critical donor organ shortage is found, we believe that acceptance of patients over the age of 65 years for hearts, over the age of 60 years for single-lung transplantation, and over the age of 45 years for double-lung or heart-lung transplantation should remain exceptional. Expansion of the human donor pool is unlikely to resolve the problem of donor scarcity; if successful, permanent implantable mechanical assistance devices and xenotransplantation may greatly alter the equation.

SUMMARY

Throughout this chapter, we have documented the literature demonstrating increasingly satisfactory results for solid organ transplantation over time in the elderly. One may reasonably expect improved results with further experience with lung and heart-lung transplantation in the elderly as well. It is important to emphasize that these good clinical results in the elderly population are a reflection of very careful patient selection. Individuals who represent high surgical risks with significant comorbidities, especially cardiac or vascular problems, need to be viewed with great caution. Nevertheless, absolute age is clearly less of a concern than it has been in the past. This is important, given the relative increase in the proportion of our population that we would term elderly.

The major debate that remains in some minds revolves around limitations of resources and especially scarcity of donor organs. Along with many other authors, we have concluded that performing solid organ transplants for elderly patients certainly does not constitute a waste of donor organs based on outcomes. Whether in the evolving U.S. health care environment, payers and society will be willing to bear the substantial financial costs associated with transplantation for the elderly remains to be seen. Just and efficacious allocation of scarce resources must balance the best interests of an individual patient against those of the entire population of potential recipients. Thus, an important ethical issue posed by the allocation of scarce donor organs revolves around the concerns of justice and utility as they apply to the conflicting interest of the individual patient and a larger group of potential recipients. Should the gift of life be extended to those who have already had a long life if, as is presently the case, other younger patients will die as a consequence? This question, although easily answered in the abstract, loses relevance at the bedside of an individual patient at any age whose length of survival without transplantation may be measured in months or days and whose outcome after transplant is similarly unknowable. In the face of these uncertainties, justice does not require that every patient be treated the same, regardless of age; rather, the practitioner seeks to be consistent and fair and to balance the likely benefits and burdens among the populations of patients with end-stage organ failure. In the final analysis, transplant physicians and surgeons must consider the risks associated with the candidate's physiologic age in light of these difficult and perhaps unanswerable ethical questions. Ultimately, the physicians caring for an individual patient now must make their best judgment regarding consideration of the patient as a candidate for transplantation and, at the same time, abide by the programmatic guidelines that serve the best interest of the overall population of potential organ recipients.

REFERENCES

1. Hosenpud JD, Novick RJ, Breen TJ, et al. The Registry of the International Society for Heart and Lung Transplantation: eleventh official report—1994. J Heart Lung Transplant 1994;13:561–570.
2. Hosenpud JD, Novick RJ, Breen TJ, et al. The Registry of the International Society for Heart and Lung Transplantation: twelfth official report—1995. J Heart Lung Transplant 1995;14:805–815.
3. Kern L. The elderly heart surgery patient. Crit Care Nurs Clin North Am 1991;3:749–756.
4. United Network for Organ Sharing; Division of Organ Transplantation, Bureau of Health Resources Development, Health Resources and Services Administration. 1995 Annual Report of the U.S. Scientific Registry for Transplant Recipients and the Organ Procurement and Transplantation Network—Transplant Data: 1988–1994. Rockville, MD: U.S. Department of Health and Human Services, 1995.
5. Wedel N, Brynger H, Blohme I. Kidney transplantation in patients 60 years and older. Scand J Urol Nephrol Suppl 1980;54:106–108.
6. Kock B, Kuhlback B, Ahonen J. Kidney transplantation in patients over 60 years of age. Scand J Urol Nephrol Suppl 1980;54:203–205.
7. Ost L, Groth CG, Lindholm B, et al. Cadaveric renal transplantation in patients of 60 years and above. Transplantation 1980;30:339–340.
8. Weigle WO. Effects of aging on the immune system. Hosp Pract 1989;15:112–119.
9. Evans RW. A cost-outcome analysis of retransplantation: the need for accountability. Transplantation Rev 1993;7:163–175.
10. Simmons RL, Kjellstrand CM, Buselmeier TJ, et al. Renal transplantation in high risk patients. Arch Surg 1971;103:290–298.
11. Najarian JS, Kjellstrand CM, Simmons RL. High-risk patients in renal transplantation. Transplant Proc 1977;9:107–111.
12. Anonymous. The ninth report of the Human Renal Transplant Registry. JAMA 1972;220:253–260.
13. Delmonico FL, Cosimi AB, Russell PS. Renal transplantation in the older age group. Arch Surg 1975;110:1107–1109.
14. Morris PJ. Cyclosporin A—overview. Transplantation 1981;2:349–354.
15. Borel JF, Feurer C, Gubler HB, et al. Biological effects of cyclosporine A: a new antilymphatic agent. Agents Actions 1976;6:465–475.
16. Calne RY, White DJG, Thiru S, et al. Cyclosporine A in patients receiving renal allografts from cadaver donors. Lancet 1978;2:1323–1327.
17. Pirsch JD, Stratta RJ, Armbrust MJ, et al. Cadaveric renal transplantation with cyclosporine in patients more than 60 years of age. Transplantation 1989;47:259–261.
18. Vivas CA, Hickey DP, Jordan ML, et al. Renal transplantation in patients 65 years old or older. J Urol 1992;147:990–993.
19. Roza AM, Gallagher-Lepak S, Adams MB. Renal transplantation in patients more than 65 years old. Transplantation 1989;48:689–725.
20. Tesi RJ, Elkhammas EA, Davies EA, et al. Renal transplantation in older people. Lancet 1994;1:462–464.
21. Shah B, First MR, Munda R, et al. Current experience with renal transplantation in older patients. Am J Kidney Dis 1988;12:516–523.
22. Schulak JA, Mayes JT, Johnston KH, et al. Kidney transplantation in patients aged sixty and older. Surgery 1990;108:726–733.
23. Tapson JS, Rodger RSC, Mansy H, et al. Renal replacement therapy in patients aged over 60 years. Postgrad Med J 1987;63:1071–1077.
24. Hestin D, Frimat L, Hubert J, et al. Renal transplantation in patients over sixty years of age. Clin Nephrol 1994;42:232–236.
25. Porush GF, Faubert PF. Chronic Renal Failure. In Porush GF, Faubert PF (eds), Renal Disease in the Aged. Boston: Little, Brown, 1991;285.
26. Albrechtsen D, Leivestad T, Sodal G, et al. Kidney transplantation in patients older than 70 years of age. Transplant Proc 1995;27:986–988.
27. National Institutes of Health, National Institutes of Diabetes and Digestive and Kidney Diseases. U.S. Renal Data System, 1991 Annual Data Report. Bethesda, MD: National Institutes of Health, 1991.
28. Ismail N, Hakim RM, Helderman JH. Renal replacement therapies in the elderly. Part II: renal transplantation. Am J Kidney Dis 1994;23:1–15.
29. Schaubel D, Desmeules M, Mao Y, et al. Survival experience among elderly end-stage renal disease patients—a controlled comparison of transplantation and dialysis. Transplantation 1995;60:1389–1394.
30. Colcock BP. Recent experience in the surgical treatment of diverticulitis. Surg Gynecol Obstet 1965;121:63–69.

31. Sawyer OI, Garvin PJ, Codd JE, et al. Colorectal complications of renal allograft transplantation. Arch Surg 1978;113:84–86.
32. McCune TR, Nylander WA, Van Buren DH, et al. Colonic screening prior to renal transplantation and its impact on post-transplant colonic complications. Clin Transpl 1992;6:91–96.
33. Church M, Braun WE, Novick AC, et al. Perforation of the colon in renal homograft recipients. A report of 11 cases and a review of the literature. Ann Surg 1986;203:69–76.
34. Chapman WC, Nylander WA, Williams LF Jr, et al. Pancreatic pseudocyst formation following renal transplantation: a lethal development. Clin Transpl 1991;5:86–89.
35. Taft PM, Jones AC, Collins GM, et al. Acute pancreatitis following renal allotransplantation: a lethal complication. Dig Dis 1978; 23:541–544.
36. Holley JL, Shapiro R, Lopatin WB, et al. Obesity as a risk factor following cadaveric renal transplantation. Transplantation 1990;49:387–389.
37. Pirsch JD, Armbrust MJ, Knechtle SJ, et al. Obesity as a risk factor following renal transplantation. Transplantation 1995;59:631–647.
38. Halme L, Eklung B, Salmela K. Obesity and renal transplantation. Transplant Proc 1995;27:3444–3445.
39. Penn I. The effect of immunosuppression on pre-existing cancers. Transplantation 1993;55:742–747.
40. Neugarten B. Age groups in American society and the rise of the young-old. Ann Am Acad Political Social Sci 1974;415:187–198.
41. Cecka JM, Terasaka PI. Optimal use of older donor kidneys: older recipients. Transplant Proc 1995;27:801–802.
42. Starzl TE, Todo S, Gordon R, et al. Liver transplantation in older patients. N Engl J Med 1987;316:484–485.
43. Shaw BW. Transplantation in the elderly patient. Surg Clin North Am 1994;74:389–400.
44. Pirsch JD, Kalayoglu M, D'Alessandro AM, et al. Orthotopic liver transplantation in patients 60 years of age or older. Transplantation 1991;51:431–433.
45. Pirsch JD, Kalayoglu M, D'Alessandro AM, et al. Orthotopic liver transplantation in patients over 60 years of age. Transplant Proc 1991;23:1456–1457.
46. Emre S, Mor E, Schwartz ME, et al. Liver transplantation in patients beyond age 60. Transplant Proc 1993;25:1075–1076.
47. Bromley PN, Hilmi I, Tan KC, et al. Orthotopic liver transplantation in patients over 60 years old. Transplantation 1994;58:800–803.
48. Stieber AC, Gordon RD, Todo S, et al. Liver transplantation in patients over sixty years of age. Transplantation 1991;51:271–273.
49. Carey WD, Dumot JA, Pimentel RR, et al. The prevalence of coronary artery disease in liver transplant candidates over age 50. Transplantation 1995;6:859–864.
50. Trail KC, Stratta RJ, Larsen JL, et al. Results of liver transplantation in diabetic recipients. Surgery 1993;114:650–658.
51. Evers BM, Townsend CM, Thompson JC. Organ physiology of aging. Surg Clin North Am 1994;74:23–39.
52. Miller LW, Vitale-Noedel N, Pennington DG, et al. Heart transplantation in patients over age fifty-five years. J Heart Transplant 1988;7:254–257.
53. Anguita M, Arizon JM. Heart transplantation in Spain: the Spanish National Registry of Heart Transplantation (1984–1992). J Heart Lung Transplant 1994;13:950–957.
54. Liv U, Milan A, Bortolotti U, et al. Results of heart transplantation by extending recipient selection criteria. J Cardiovasc Surg 1994;35: 377–382.
55. Fabbri A, Sharples LD, Mullins P, et al. Heart transplantation in patients over 54 years of age with triple-drug therapy immunosuppression. J Heart Lung Transplant 1992;11:929–932.

SECTION IV

Italian and British Experience and Future of Surgery in the Elderly

Surgical Care for the Elderly, 2nd ed., edited by
R. Benton Adkins, Jr., and H. William Scott, Jr.
Lippincott–Raven Publishers, Philadelphia © 1998.

CHAPTER 38

History and Current Status of Surgical Care for the Elderly in Italy

Giorgio Gaggiotti, Massimo Mengani, Giovanni Lamura, Claudia Giammarchi, Roberto Ghiselli, and Vittorio Saba

Surgical care for the elderly is an evolved specialty in Italy. Some factors contributing to this evolution are the high level of societal esteem for the elderly, a political climate favorable to health care in general and to health care for the elderly in particular, and advances in surgical care for elderly patients resulting from studies on the treatment of this patient population as a specialty.

DEMOGRAPHICS OF THE ITALIAN POPULATION, WITH EMPHASIS ON THE ELDERLY

Evolution of the Italian Population

Since the unification of Italy over 130 years ago, the Italian population has more than doubled, growing from 26 million in 1861 to over 57 million (Table 38-1). This increase occurred mainly at the end of the last century and in the first three-fourths of the present one, slowing down considerably after the mid-1970s. At present, the growth rate is only slightly positive, and according to forecasts, it is going to decrease even further in the near future, dropping to negative values and resulting in a demographic contraction for the first time ever in this country.

Breaking down the demographic evolution in Italy into its two components, natural and migratory (Table 38-2), it can be seen that the trend toward demographic contraction derives exclusively from the first component, that is, the difference between births and deaths. As a matter of fact, this difference became negative for the first time in 1993, and only an increase in immigration from abroad prevented the overall population level from decreasing. Furthermore, population contraction attributable to the natural component is due to a significant and steady drop in the birth rate, which has plummeted after World War II along with the death rate.

This set of circumstances, along with the progressive increase in life expectancy (Table 38-3), has led to a steady increase in the number of elderly in Italy. Currently, Italy is one of the first countries in the world where the population >60 years of age, nearly 12.5 million people and equal to 22% of the total population, is outgrowing the population <20 years of age (Table 38-4) [1]. However, this phenomenon is not evenly distributed throughout the country: In the northern regions, the population >60 years of age represents on average 20% to 25% of the overall population (with a high of 28% in the region of Liguria), whereas in the south the same group accounts for 15% to 18% of the total (with a low of 15% in the region of Campania) [2].

Major Consequences of Aging in the Italian Population

To properly plan health services for the elderly, the increase in life expectancy must be analyzed to determine whether this increase is characterized by acceptable health levels or if it is instead marked by degenerative diseases and disability. No consolidated body of literature exists at present that identifies a system of laws that explains the interrelations between aging and disease. The genetic theory that attempts to link the speed of the aging process to exogenous (i.e., environmental) and endogenous (i.e., genetic) factors is an example of a theory that fails to identify these laws. Therefore, the most pressing objective is to create the theoretical framework needed to delay to the furthest extent possible the onset of the most devastating effects, both psychophysical and social, of degenerative diseases. This is accomplished not only by preventing the disease itself but also by delaying its onset. Prevalence and incidence data on chronic, degenerative pathologies in old age play a fundamental role in this endeavor, espe-

TABLE 38-1. *Evolution of Italian population from 1861 to 1994*

Year	Population (thousands)	Average annual increase (%)
1861	26,328	—
1871	28,151	6.7
1881	29,791	5.7
1901	33,778	6.6
1911	36,921	8.6
1921	37,856	2.4
1931	41,043	8.6
1936	42,399	6.5
1951	47,516	7.4
1961	50,624	6.4
1971	54,137	6.7
1981	56,557	4.4
1991	56,778	0.4
1994	57,269	2.3
2003 (projected)	57,455	0.0
2013 (projected)	55,665	–0.3

Sources: Modified from Italian National Institute of Statistics. Conoscere l'Italia—Introducing Italy (English-Italian Edition). Rome: Istituto Nazionale di Statistica, 1995; and Italian National Institute of Statistics. Bollettino Mensile di Statistical N. II. Rome: Istituto Nazionale di Statistica, 1995.

cially in terms of recognizing the dimension that problems regarding health and social care will assume as a consequence of the great demographic changes we are witnessing today [3].

Socioeconomic Aspects

The well-being of the elderly person is closely linked to a series of factors of which health is only the most immediate: others, not necessarily less important, are the economic, psychological, and social factors that affect old age. Economic possibilities and social support networks may in fact favor or heavily condition the independence, life-style, and health conditions of an elderly person, and therefore the need for medical care and rehabilitation.

In Italy, as in other countries, the phenomenon of aging is characterized by a strong feminization [4], as a result of the longer life span of women, who at the age of 65 have a life expectancy that is 4 years longer than that of their male peers (18.5 vs. 14.7 years) [5]. In the final stages of life, this difference becomes all the more evident, so that among the population >75 years old women represent nearly two-thirds of the total. This phenomenon and the fact that men are usually older than women when they get married explain why widowhood affects most elderly women but rarely men [2].

Up to the present, the family has been the principal source of social support for the elderly population in Italy, a situation that is typical of most Mediterranean countries. The changes now taking place in the structure of the Italian family (especially the lower propensity to get married and have children) are contributing greatly to the progressive reduction in the size of the family unit and of extended family net-

TABLE 38-2. *Components of the evolution of Italian population from 1861 to 1994 (yearly average increase rates per 1,000 inhabitants)*

Years	Total increase[a]	Natural rate[b]	Birth rate	Mortality	Net migration rate
1861–1870	—	—	37.6	30.3	—
1871–1880	6.7	—	36.9	29.9	—
1881–1890	5.7	—	37.8	27.3	—
1891–1900	6.6	—	35.0	24.2	—
1901–1910	8.6	11.1	32.7	21.6	—
1911–1920	2.4	6.6	27.2	20.6	—
1921–1930	8.6	11.6	28.2	16.6	–3.0
1931–1940	6.5	9.7	23.6	13.9	–0.2
1941–1950	7.4	7.8	20.5	12.7	–2.2
1951–1960	6.4	8.2	17.8	9.6	–3.3
1961–1970	6.7	8.4	18.1	9.7	–1.5
1971–1975	5.1	6.2	15.9	9.7	–0.1
1976–1980	3.2	2.9	12.6	9.7	0.2
1981–1985	0.1	1.0	10.6	9.6	–0.1
1986–1990	0.0	0.5	9.8	9.3	–0.5
1991	0.0	0.1	9.9	9.8	–0.1
1992	3.6	0.5	9.9	9.5	3.0
1993	3.1	–0.0	9.4	9.5	3.2
1994	2.3	–0.4	9.2	9.6	2.6

[a] Total increase rate is the sum of natural rate and net migration rate.
[b] Natural rate is the sum of birth rate and mortality rate.
Sources: Italian National Institute of Statistics. Conoscere l'Italia—Introducing Italy (English-Italian Edition). Rome: Istituto Nazionale di Statistica, 1995; Italian National Institute of Statistics. Bollettino Mensile di Statistical N. II. Rome: Istituto Nazionale di Statistica, 1995; Italian National Institute of Statistics. Le Regioni in Cifre. Edizione 1995. Rome: Istituto Nazionale di Statistica, 1995; and Italian National Institute of Statistics. Le Regioni in Cifre. Edizioni 1994. Rome: Istituto Nazionale di Statistica, 1994.

TABLE 38-3. *Evolution of life expectancy in the Italian population by gender at birth, 20 years of age, and 60 years of age*

	At birth (yrs)		At 20 (yrs)		At 60 (yrs)	
Years	Males	Females	Males	Females	Males	Females
1899–1902	42.6	43.0	43.0	43.1	13.5	13.6
1930–1932	53.8	56.0	46.8	48.5	15.2	16.1
1960–1962	67.2	72.3	51.7	56.1	16.7	19.3
1991	73.5	80.2	54.6	61.0	18.4	23.0

Sources: Italian National Institute of Statistics. Conoscere l'Italia—Introducing Italy (English-Italian Edition). Rome: Istituto Nazionale di Statistica, 1995; and Italian National Institute of Statistics. Bollettino Mensile di Statistical N. II. Rome: Istituto Nazionale di Statistica, 1995.

TABLE 38-4. *Percent of total Italian population by age group from 1951 to 1994*

Age (yrs)	1951	1961	1971	1981	1991	1994
<20	34.6	32.0	31.6	29.8	23.5	22.1
20–39	30.3	30.7	27.9	27.4	30.1	30.7
39–59	23.0	23.4	23.9	25.4	25.3	25.4
≥60	12.1	13.9	16.6	17.4	21.1	21.8
Total	100.0	100.0	100.0	100.0	100.0	100.0

Source: Italian National Institute of Statistics. Conoscere l'Italia—Introducing Italy (English-Italian Edition). Rome: Istituto Nazionale di Statistica, 1995.

works; this, in turn, reduces the likelihood that the elderly person will live with one of the members of the nuclear family unit or of the extended family. A national survey conducted in 1989 and 1990 showed that >60% of the elderly live as couples and 25% as singles, but the latter group reaches a high of 37% in the 65- to 85-year age bracket, dropping again in older age groups [6]. This phenomenon probably results from a combination of factors (the intensification of health problems is one of the most prevalent among them) that make living alone more difficult. Finally, it must be pointed out that among elderly singles, women are an overwhelming majority, a fact that must be explained not only by the demographic factors mentioned previously, but also by cultural factors, such as the greater willingness on the part of men to create a new family.

These considerations must be viewed in light of the fact that it is mostly women, wives or daughters, who care for the frailer members of the family, especially the elderly, looking after their personal needs (e.g., bathing and washing), doing the housework, and cooking the meals. Male members of the family participate only when external activities are concerned, such as going shopping or accompanying the elderly to medical examinations [7]. A survey carried out in 1992 by the Italian Institute for Studies on Social Services brought to light how often middle-aged women act as the main informal care givers [8]. By dedicating most of their time and energy to satisfying the needs of younger family members (children or grandchildren), husbands, and elderly members of the household (parents), middle-aged women suffer the consequences of the inefficient and insufficient care provided by the formal health care systems, both private and public [9].

As far as economic aspects are concerned, empiric evidence shows that the average income of elderly families (in which the head of the household is >65 years of age) is lower than that of the rest of the population [10]. This phenomenon is often associated with, and sometimes a reason for, lower levels of education, especially among the elderly and in the southern regions of the country [2]. Furthermore, income conditions are particularly unfavorable for women: Not only do they have lower monthly pensions than men, but they often receive only a social pension (a monetary integration granted to individuals with a low income). Women represent 84% of all social pension beneficiaries [11]. The result of this situation is that among all families living below the poverty line (where the poverty line is one-half the income of the national average as defined by International Standards of Poverty Line), 55% of those heads of households are women [12].

Socio-Health Aspects

Given the existing relationship between economic conditions and health, it is not surprising that the highest levels of disability [5], sickness, and need for health care services [13] have been documented among the elderly, as shown, for instance, by the level of expenses for health aids and services, which increases considerably after the age of 70.

Although the health conditions of the elderly, as well as that of the population in general, cannot be easily quantified, senile mortality constitutes an invaluable source of information. The current mortality in Italy for the female population >75 years is rather low at 7,856 deaths per 100,000 inhabi-

TABLE 38-5. *Mortality in the Italian population aged 75 years and older by sex, cause of death, and geographic area per 1,000 inhabitants in 1989*

	Northwest		Northeast		Central		South and islands	
Cause of death	Males	Females	Males	Females	Males	Females	Males	Females
Total	97.8	72.4	93.4	67.6	94.1	71.8	89.8	75.5
Tumors	23.9	12.6	24.5	12.2	22.8	11.7	16.2	8.7
Diabetes	2.0	2.8	1.9	2.8	2.7	3.4	2.9	4.6
Circulatory system	47.1	40.5	44.5	37.5	45.4	40.6	45.8	45.1
Respiratory apparatus	9.6	4.1	8.7	3.9	8.9	3.9	10.8	4.8
Digestive apparatus	4.4	3.0	4.1	2.9	4.4	3.0	4.7	3.2
Unclear symptoms	2.3	2.6	1.7	1.8	2.2	2.4	3.2	3.7
Accidents	3.1	2.8	3.1	2.4	3.0	3.0	2.2	2.2

Source: Farchi G, Buiatti E. La Speranza di Vita e la Mortalita Negli Anziani in Italia e in Europa. In Geddes M (ed), La Salute Degli Italiani—Rapporto 1993. Rome: Nuova Italia Scientifica, 1994;217–227.

TABLE 38-6. *Population over age 65 with at least one chronic disease by sex from 1986 to 1987*

	Males (%)	Females (%)
Elderly who suffer from at least one chronic disease	69.7	72.3
Prevalence of main chronic diseases		
Arthrosis and arthritis	34.3	48.2
Arterial hypertension	19.2	26.2
Heart diseases (excluded infarction)	12.0	14.1
Diabetes	10.4	13.2
Chronic bronchitis	22.4	11.5
Nervous disorders	6.4	9.2
Liver calculosis	3.0	5.4
Gastric and duodenal ulcer	7.6	3.9
Myocardial infarction	5.4	2.4

Source: Verdecchia A, Egidi V, Golini A. Popolazione Anziana, Invecchiamento Demografico e Condizioni di Salute. In Geddes M (ed), La Salute Degli Italiani—Rapporto 1993. Rome: Nuova Italia Scientifica, 1994;193–216.

tants, whereas for men it increases to 10,393 per 100,000 (standardized values for European population) [14]. When these data are analyzed in terms of pathologies, the statistics reveal that 58% of women die from diseases of the cardiocirculatory system and 15% from tumors, whereas the percentage of men who die of cardiocirculatory diseases is lower at 50%, but higher for tumors at 22%.

When the data are distributed according to the four main geographic areas in Italy (Table 38-5), it becomes apparent that the mortality for women in the South is due in large part to diabetes, cirrhosis, and circulatory diseases. This high mortality could be reduced, in part, by suitable prevention, early diagnosis, and therapy, especially where diabetes and associated complications are concerned. This lack of intervention mirrors the territorial imbalance between North and South in terms of the quality of the health care available.

Indicators that characterize health conditions as well as the intensity of health care use among the general population can be helpful informational sources. Several such indicators are the average number of chronic, degenerative diseases per capita, the average number of days of illness, or the number of days of confinement in bed. These indicators show that women are relatively disadvantaged compared with their male peers, even if not to a large degree. Table 38-6 presents data on chronic diseases that confirm that only for diabetes, liver calculosis, and gastric as well as duodenal ulcer do men have higher prevalence rates than women, of whom almost one-half suffer from arthrosis, arthritis, or both, as compared with only one-fourth of men [15].

As far as indicators of the intensity of health care use are concerned, an analysis of hospital admission rates indicates that men are hospitalized more often than women, because 20% of all men >65 years of age were hospitalized at least once in 1991, compared with 17% for women in the same age group. However, the average length of the hospital stay is slightly higher for women (27.5 vs. 24.5 days), although it leads less often to surgical intervention (28% vs. 32%) [15].

The aforementioned data reveal that, although women have a greater life expectancy, their longer life is often characterized by the presence of diseases that are seriously disabling, even if generally not immediately fatal. Among these disabling effects, immobility, as mentioned by Isaacs, represents one of the most inhibiting factors in terms of the independence for the elderly, both in their domestic life and in external social contacts [16]. Apart from psychological and environmental factors, the main causes of immobility are due to physical disease and complications such as fractures, pain in the hip or knee, angina, and limping.

The importance of fractures (especially those caused by falls) has often been stressed by epidemiologic studies, particularly in subjects with osteoporosis and vision problems that debilitate the natural defenses of the individual. This phenomenon is closely related not only to age, but also gender, as demonstrated by the fact that the average ratio between women and men who have suffered fractures is 2:1. The incidence, however, varies greatly between one country and another, with higher values being recorded in developed

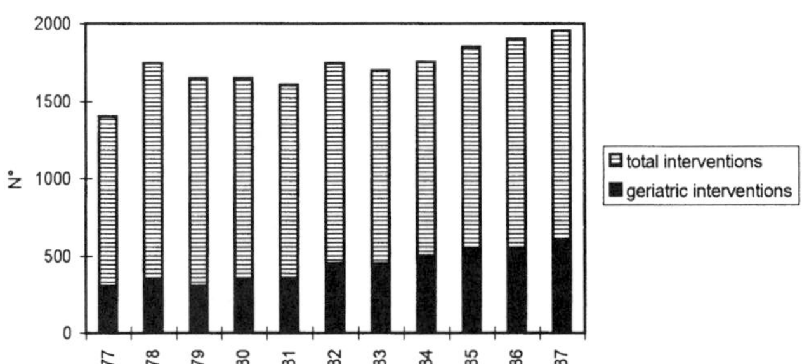

FIG. 38-1. Relationship between general and geriatric surgery between 1977 and 1987.

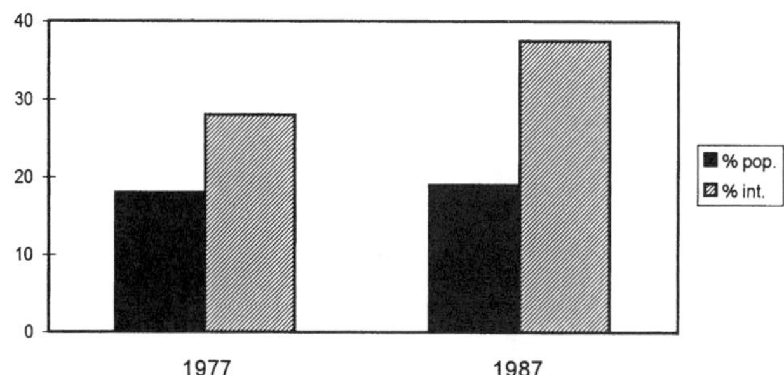

FIG. 38-2. Relationship between population growth and geriatric surgery between 1977 and 1987. (pop. = population; int. = intervention.)

nations. This tendency seems to be growing, as national surveys suggest. Moreover, projections at the global level, proposed by Cooper et al., estimate that in Europe the number of fractures is likely to increase by >50% in the next 30 years, from 407,223 in 1990 to 651,417 in 2025 [17].

In spite of the scarce data on this topic in Italy, it can be assumed that in Italy in 1981 to 1982 the number of hospital admissions for fractures was between 25,000 and 44,000, of which 40% were for fractures of the collum femoris. These fractures are prevalent in women and seem to grow exponentially with age, particularly after 75 years of age [18].

These data demonstrate how, as subjects grow older, their state of health can be affected by events that partially or totally reduce functional independence. Activities of daily living and instrumental activities of daily living are two of the most famous indexes used to assess the degree of disability of the subject. A recent national survey based on such indexes estimated that from 1987 to 1991 approximately 800,000 individuals over the age of 74 (almost one-fourth of the corresponding age group) were completely nonself-sufficient, that is, dependent on others for their most basic survival activities. An additional 1,300,000 elderly were unable to carry out some fundamental self-care and grooming activities on their own, namely taking a bath or shower, and needed periodic help to perform them. A striking result of this survey was the finding that of the 600,000 disabled persons (of all ages) living on their own, 82% were >64 years old and 70% women. Assuming that the prevalence coefficients for disability do not change over time (they are currently estimated at approximately 20% to 22% of the population >65 years of age) [19], it seems likely that the next few years will see a rapid growth in the number of disabled elderly, with a consequent increase in the demand for health care.

The empiric evidence from local sample surveys indicates that for lack of valid alternative solutions, many disabled persons continue to live in their own homes. This can be deduced in particular from the fact that among the population >65 years of age, the percentage of bedridden elderly does not vary greatly between those living in their own homes, approximately 4%, and those who live in institutions, approximately 6% to 7% [20].

COMMON SURGICAL DISEASES OF THE ELDERLY ITALIAN

Among the epidemiologic studies published on the incidence of geriatric surgery in Italy, without a doubt the most comprehensive research has been done by the Italian National Research Centres on Aging (INRCA) Center for Surgical Research in cooperation with the Anziano Operato Biancalana–Masera Foundation [21]. The research performed by the Fellows of the Foundation has played a defining role in bringing INRCA's research into being because of the methodologies used, the extensive nature of the research, and the type of analysis.

Twenty-four surgical centers distributed uniformly throughout Italy participated in the study, and the data collected has made it possible to evaluate the incidence of geriatric surgery with respect to general surgery in terms of the 180,000 patients operated on during the period from 1977 to 1987.

If old age is defined as beginning at age 60, one-third of the patients who underwent surgery in the sample group were elderly. An analysis of the 10-year period in question shows that geriatric surgery increased progressively from 26.4% in 1977 to 33.2% in 1987 (Fig. 38-1). When comparing this increase with the demographic statistics from the same period (Fig. 38-2), the percentage increase in surgical operations is considerably greater than the demographic change during the period in question. In fact, the relationship between the two indexes indicates that the intensity of geriatric surgical intervention rose from 1.53 to 1.76 (taking 100 as the mean index for the number of surgical interventions for the population on the whole, the frequency of geriatric surgery was 153 in 1977 and 176 in 1987). If the sample population is divided into two groups (Fig. 38-3), a 60- to 70-year-old group (seventh decade) and a 70 and older group (eighth decade), and then compared with the population as a whole, it can be seen that the increase in geriatric surgery is attributable for the most part to surgical interventions in the group aged 70 and older (24.3%). An analysis of how the pathologies are distributed shows that out of 20,000 patients who underwent surgery in the periods from 1977 to 1979 and 1976 to 1978 (outer limits of the period analyzed previously) hernias and hepatobiliary dis-

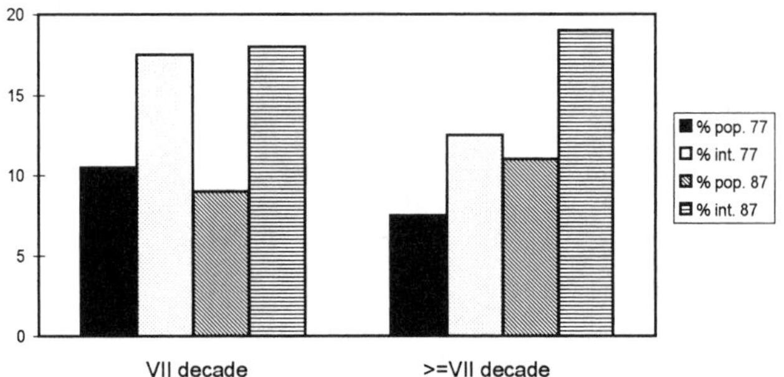

FIG. 38-3. Relationship between population growth and geriatric surgery between 1977 and 1987 subdivided by age group. (pop. = population; int. = intervention.)

eases appear most frequently, nearly 20% (if the comparison between the two sub-groups is maintained). This percentage increases slightly for the group aged 60 years (Fig. 38-4). As far as neoplastic pathologies are concerned for the group aged 70 and older, the predominant diseases are stomach and duodenum disorders (Fig. 38-5A). The frequency of breast, rectal, and left colon disorders follow in descending order with values of approximately 6%, without any differences existing between the two age groups.

When comparing the data for the two groups for the first 3-year period, the most evident differences appear in terms of gastroduodenal disease, where there is a considerable reduction in the frequency of surgical intervention between the 60-year-old and the 70-and-older groups, dropping from 13.2% to 6.9%. The data from this research show not only how classic geriatric surgery, urogenital and gynecologic, is still the most prevalent, but also how surgery on the upper abdomen is no longer age related.

An examination of the frequency of neoplasms reveals a 40% incidence of neoplastic disorders in the 60-year-old group and a 50% incidence in the 70-and-older group for those who underwent surgery.

It is obvious that the total incidence of neoplasms among the elderly would be statistically much higher were all the inoperable forms of the disorder taken into consideration. Out of all the patients, the highest percentage of neoplastic disorders in the stomach and duodenum was found in the patients who were 70 and older at 18.5%, whereas the percentage was 14% for the group aged 60 years. A comparison of the two 3-year periods shows that the percentage of thoracic interventions increased from 80% to 90% in the first subgroup and from 58% to 80% in the second. A comparison with the first 3-year period shows a clear increase in surgical interventions

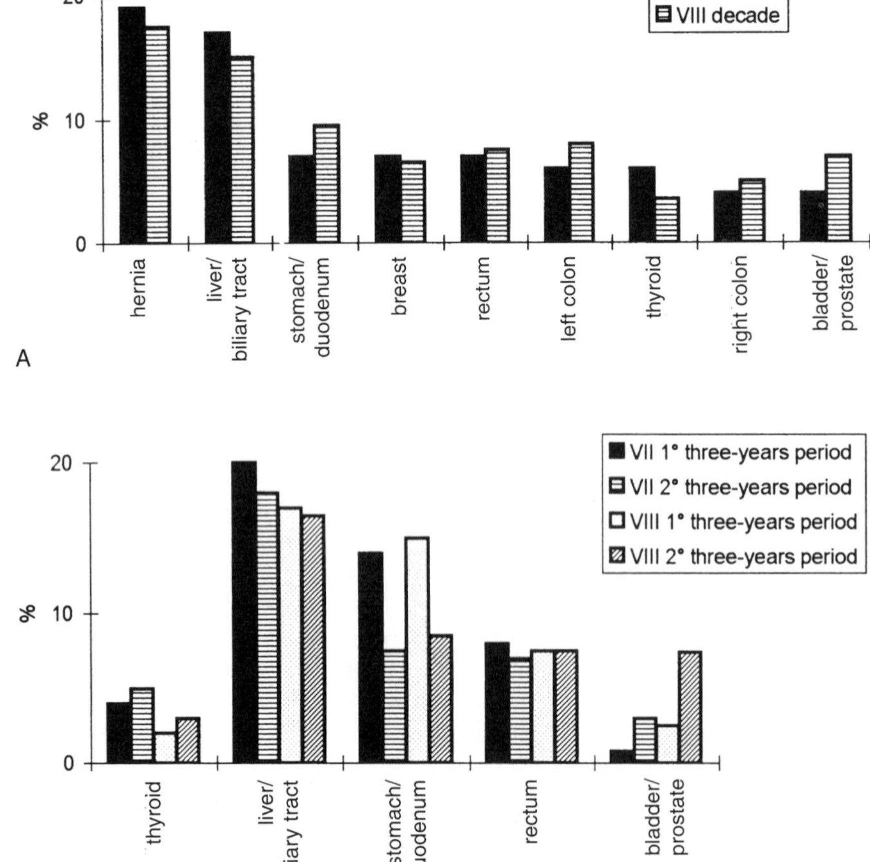

FIG. 38-4. (A) Incidence of surgical pathology between 1968 and 1988 in the two age groups. **(B)** A comparison of the most relevant pathologies in the two 3-year periods broken down by age group.

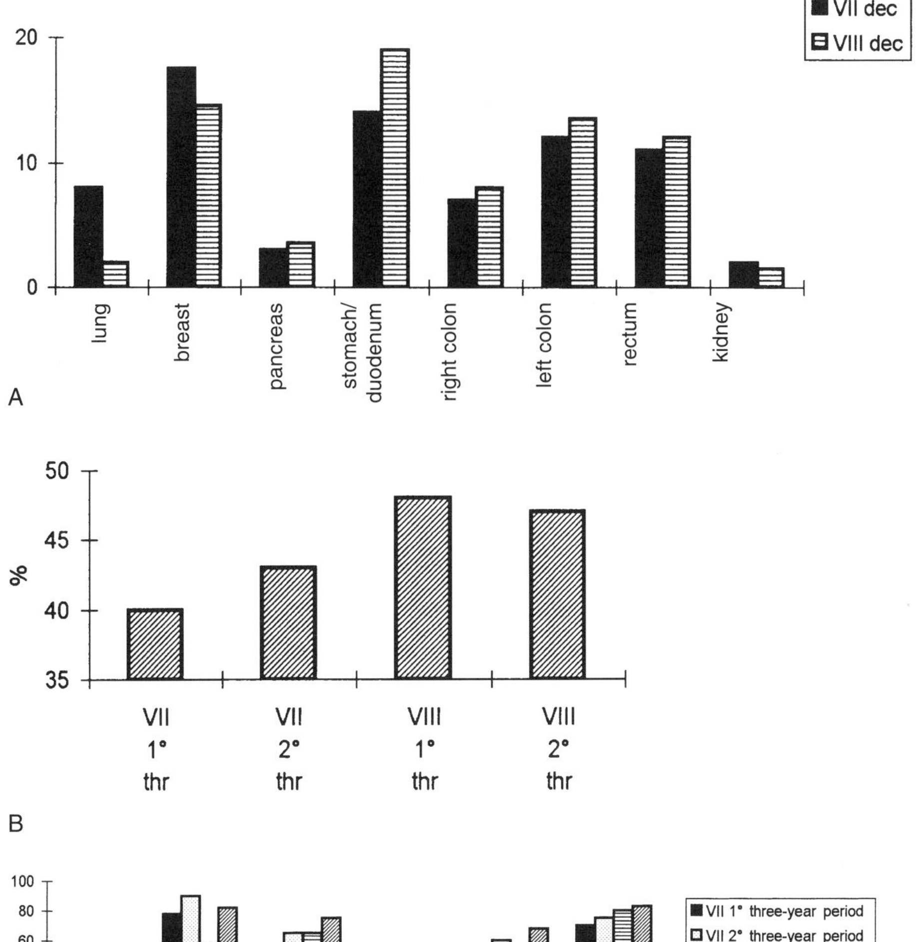

FIG. 38-5. (A) The absolute incidence of neoplasm. **(B)** A comparison between the first and second 3-year periods in absolute values. **(C)** A comparison subdivided into the various organs.

for malignant neoplasms in the right colon, increasing from 40% to 60% in the group aged 60 years and from 42% to 70% in the group aged 70 and older (Fig. 38-5B and C).

ECONOMIC AND POLITICAL CONSIDERATIONS

When defining the status of health care policies for the elderly in Italy, it is important to realize that there are two prevalent types of services in our country [22]: the nursing home and the family, which is a source not only of affection and solidarity, but above all compensates for the lack of public services. This is clearly represented in Table 38-7, where Italy shows the lowest percentage of institutionalized elderly among Western European countries [23].

Since 1975, the United States, following the reduction in the number of hospital beds for patients with acute conditions, has had to increase the number of nursing homes, which in 1987 cared for 5% of the population >65. In Italy, the allocation of hospital beds for long-term residents was already provided for with Law no. 132 in 1968. Law no. 595 in 1985 and no. 67 in 1988 reconfirmed the need to increase the number of beds for dependent elderly, the first reserving one bed per 1,000 inhabitants for rehabilitation, the other creating 140,000 beds in facilities for nonself-sufficient elderly.

The nursing home was and continues to be the main structure of the institutional care-giving system in Italy, a structure that until now had difficulty evolving toward more efficient models able to meet the needs of a population with care requirements that are diverse depending on psychophysical characteristics and age. Presently, nursing homes offer mainly a hotel and care-giving type of service for both self-sufficient and dependent elderly. The latest statistical data, relative to 1990, show that of the 2,807 nursing homes in Italy, approxi-

TABLE 38-7. *Population over 65 years of age living in residential institutions in western European countries*

Country (year)	Percent of population >65 years
Belgium (1981)	4.0
Denmark (1990)	5.0
France (1984)	4.5
Germany (1989)	5.9
Greece (1989)	0.6
Ireland (1986)	8.6
Italy (1990)	1.5
The Netherlands (1989)	7.8
Portugal (1989)	1.5
Spain (1988)	2.5
United Kingdom (1990)	5.0

Source: Glendinning C, McLaughlin E. Paying for Care: Lessons from Europe. London, Her Majesty's Stationery Office, 1993.

mately 8% (corresponding to 10% of the 158,032 total beds available) are reserved for dependent elderly, 38% (representing 24% of the total beds available) are for self-sufficient elderly, while the majority (53% of nursing homes and 66% of the beds available) have mixed users.

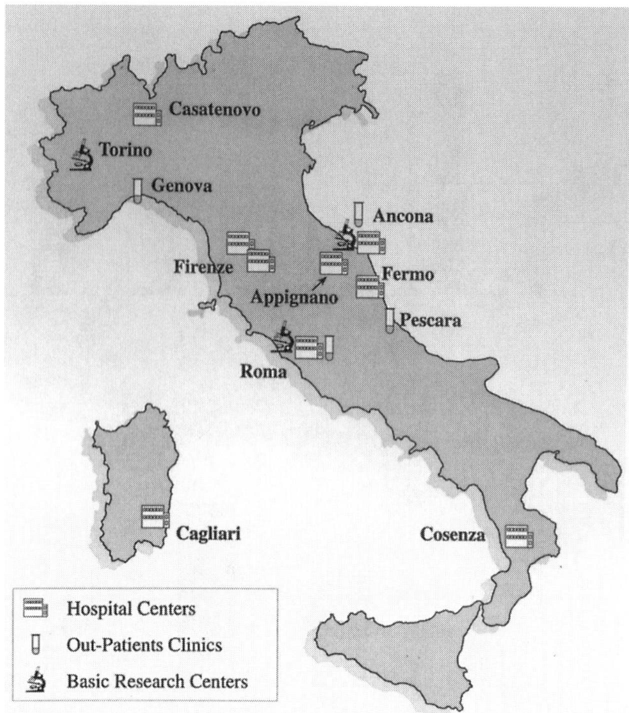

FIG. 38-6. Distribution of Italian National Research Centres on Aging throughout Italy.

Evolution of Substitutive Monetary Transfers

In Italy, special attention has always been given to the economic protection of the weaker members, and measures have been taken to keep the elderly in their original family by providing financial support to disabled persons. Since 1980, persons who are totally disabled and need constant care due to their inability to walk without permanent help from others, or to carry out daily living activities, are entitled to an "accompanying allowance." Most of them are elderly: In 1987, this figure stood at 217,347, equal to 2.7% of the total Italian resident population aged 65 and over. It increased to 428,318 (5.1%) in 1991, and reached 584,887 in 1994, or 6.4% of the total elderly population. In the case of total disability, the accompanying allowance does not in any way depend on income because it is believed that the costs of health care for maintaining an invalid in the family are high, whatever the individual economic situation.

IMPETUS FOR BEGINNING AND DEVELOPING THE ITALIAN NATIONAL RESEARCH CENTRES ON AGING INSTITUTE

Institutional Aims

The Institute's work focuses on aging, an extremely important phenomenon in our country. The gerontologic and geriatric problems associated with age are being met scientifically through clinical, epidemiologic, and socioeconomic studies that enhance the care-giving activities carried out in the various centers of the Institute: Ancona, Appignano, Cagliari, Casatenovo, Cosenza, Fermo, Florence, Genoa, and Rome.

Research carried out by the Institute aims at improving the quality of life of the elderly population and can be divided into three different interconnected areas: (1) baseline research, which identifies early signs of aging or age-related diseases (Gerontology Department); (2) applied clinical research, which deals with diagnosis and surgical therapy for age-related diseases and rehabilitation (Geriatric Hospitals); and (3) socioeconomic research, which analyzes the needs of both the elderly and their families, focusing on situations related to hospitalization (Socio-Economic Department). The Institute's activities are interdisciplinary and integrate applied and baseline research, focusing primarily on the connection between hospitalization and treatment and scientific research (Fig. 38-6).

One of the aims of the Institute is to work closely with other institutions, both at a national and international level, to promote the diffusion of research and information. It also promotes medical education and the training and updating of scientific and technical staff.

From a historical point of view, the INRCA Institute was founded as a hospice for the indigent elderly for the purposes of limiting the discomfort of old age and the psychological anguish brought on by solitude in the absence of the traditional support networks provided by the nuclear family. In a certain sense, the Institute attempts to replace the values of the typically patriarchal Italian family where the elderly are protected, both socially and emotionally, and in which disability and disease are not the subject of scorn or indifference.

With the development of modern medicine, and the consequent movement beyond the fatalistic approach to the diseases that affect the elderly, more specialized and targeted care is available. And in this context, INRCA has grown beyond its institutional role as a mere shelter, becoming an Institute for the Care of the Elderly with the establishment of new centers in various Italian cities. Thus, the Institute has assumed a well-defined role on the national level as a hospital specialized in various branches of medicine where treatments are studied, tested, and made available to the National Health Care Services. In this context of global health care for the elderly, surgery has developed into a rehabilitative treatment for the purposes of not only offering specific medical care, but also guaranteeing maximum autonomy after the surgical intervention and assistance outside the hospital environment.

Brief History of the Institute

The Institute was founded in 1844. On November 24 of that year a Poor People's Home was opened in Ancona by the Assembly of Merchants and Artisans. In the following years the Home was incorporated in the Charitable Congregation, later changed to a Municipal Board of Care. The Home regained its independent management in 1938. The events that shaped the present Institute began in 1955. In 1961, following the DPR (Presidential Decree), the Poor People's Home in Ancona was named the Vittorio Emanuele II Institute for the Rest and Care of the Elderly–INRCA, which in 1963 became the Istituto Nazionale per il Ricovero e Cura a Carattere Scientifico–INRCA. In light of the results achieved in the field of gerontology, in terms of research and application, the Ministry of Health in 1968, together with the Ministry of Public Education, awarded the Institute the title of Research Institute to INRCA.

Important Events

- 1962, opening of the Tambroni Boarding House in Ancona
- 1964, opening of the U. Sestilli Geriatric Institute in Ancona
- 1964, opening of the Geriatric Center in Rome
- 1964, opening of the Geriatric Center in Genoa
- 1967, renovation and transformation of the Boarding House into the Montagnola Hospital in Ancona
- 1968, opening of the Gerontological and Geriatric Research Department in Ancona
- 1968, legislation defined the role of the Institute within the sphere of public health care services and among the Institutes defined which should give health care assistance
- 1968, opening of the Geriatric Center in Turin
- 1969, opening of the "Poggiosecco" and "Fraticini" Hospitals in Florence
- 1969, opening of the Geriatric Center in Cagliari
- 1969, opening of the Geriatric Center in Cosenza
- 1970, opening of the Hospital in Fermo
- 1970, opening of the Hospital in Casatenovo
- 1974, opening of the Geriatric Center in Pescara
- 1974, opening of the Hospital in Rome
- 1974, opening of the Hospital in Cosenza
- 1996, assignment of the Hospital in Via Farinelli to the Local Health Board of Turin

NINO MASERA'S CONTRIBUTION TO THE DEVELOPMENT OF GERIATRIC SURGERY

The birth of geriatric surgery in Italy was initially characterized by a cultural approach that attempted to integrate the experience of the gerontologist with surgical evaluation. Geriatric surgery was officially recognized in the scientific community in 1967 on the occasion of the Conference of the Italian Association of Surgeons and subsequently affirmed through the study of geriatric surgery at the university level. In 1987 the Italian Society for Geriatric Surgery was founded and is currently part of the European Society for Geriatric Surgery. At present more than 20 hospital and university centers are involved in the study and development of surgical care for the elderly. The development of this branch of medicine in Italy is unequivocally tied to the fundamental contributions made by Professor Nino Masera.

Professor Masera, who is now deceased, was the son of a surgeon, and, like his father, was first a surgical pathologist before becoming involved in surgery. He gained invaluable experience in the field of surgery at the University of Pavia and Turin where he was primarily involved in thoracic surgery. His contributions to surgical care for the elderly began when he came to Ancona in 1969 as a member of INRCA. Here, he became the head of the surgical staff and authored a number of publications of fundamental importance to the field of geriatric surgery [24–28]. He played an instrumental role in creating a Center for Experimental Surgery in the Research Department at the Institute itself.

In 1981, he created the Biancalana-Masera Foundation for the postoperative study and care of the elderly, which was developed to help resolve the multiple problems related to geriatric surgery. One of the main goals of the Foundation is to promote interest in the problems the elderly face during operative and postoperative care, as well as to help make young doctors and nurses more sensitive to these problems, training them to resolve problems practically at the care level.

From a practical point of view, these objectives were reached through the institution of fellowships (with stipends) from the Institution; the clinical activities of the Fellows at the Foundation are not limited to the hospital stay of the patients, but also include a period in which the postoperative patients are monitored through visits to the home. In the last years of his life, Professor Masera dedicated the better part of his time and energy to the Foundation, which now awards 30 such fellowships annually throughout Italy.

The work of the Foundation's Fellows has helped conduct important studies on epidemiology and the quality of life.

PROJECTIONS FOR THE FUTURE CARE OF THE AGING POPULATION

The first proposals of the National Health Plan 1994–1996 aimed at substantial changes in the organization of the country's health care services through a restructuring of the hospital system and, more generally, of health care through modifying how the services are subsidized and evaluated. The incentives linked to the methods of subsidizing hospitals for acute patients, which is based on the Diagnosis-Related Groups system, lead almost automatically to an increase in the number of hospital admissions and to a simultaneous reduction in the length of the average hospital stay. Therefore, a reduction in hospitalization is likely to occur in the near future, with the earlier discharge of patients. This will probably lead to an increase in the need for additional health care in the home, in rehabilitation structures, as well as in nursing homes. These additional needs will only be met if further subsidies are made available to strengthen the role and effectiveness of these services.

The National Health Care Plan has proposed the following measures for 1997 and 1998:

- Reduction of the number of beds for acute patients from 297,165 to 257,123
- Transformation of 40,042 beds into rehabilitation and long-term beds for postacute patients
- Creation of 3,744 beds in the postacute sectors of rehabilitation and in long-term wards
- Conversion of 23,258 beds for outpatient rehabilitation in residential or semiresidential homes

The program to restructure and subsidize rehabilitation anticipates the creation of residential and semiresidential centers to ensure the greatest possible functional recovery, reach and maintain functional stability, prevent involutional processes, and remove and limit obstacles of a social nature. To achieve these aims, medical, psychological, pedagogic, and social intervention will be necessary.

The development of criteria to determine how health care will be subsidized will also aid in defining how the centers will be classified, according to the aims, types of service provided, and condition of patients admitted. This will also lead to a diversification of care, according to the age of the users, the previously treated disease, the intensity of treatment and the type of services offered, length of treatment, and whether care services are residential, semiresidential, or outpatient services.

REFERENCES

1. Lamura G, Mengani M. Elderly Women, Social Change and Care Patterns in Italy. Paper Presented at the III European Congress of Gerontology. In Knook DL, Dittmann-Kohli F, Duursma SA, et al. (eds), Ageing in a Changing Europe. Utrecht: Netherlands Institute of Gerontology, 1995.
2. Italian National Institute of Statistics. Le Regioni in Cifre. Edizioni 1994. Rome: Istituto Nazionale di Statistica, 1994.
3. Geddes M. La Salute Degli Italiani—Rapporto 1993. Rome: Nuova Italia Scientifica, 1994.
4. Mengani M, Gagliardi C. Older Women in the European Community: Social and Economical Conditions—Italian Report. Copenhagen: Dane Age Association, 1993.
5. Italian National Institute of Statistics. Alcuni Aspetti Demografici e Sociali Degli Anziani in Italia. Rome: Istituto Nazionale di Statistica, 1993.
6. Ricci M. Gli Anziani Che Vivono Soli in Italia: Dati e Riflessioni. In La Rosa M. (ed.), Autonomie Locali e Servizi Sociali, Serie XVIII, Vol. 2. Bologna, Italy: Mulino, 1995;233–236.
7. Dooghe G. The Ageing of the Population in Europe: Socioeconomic Characteristics of the Elderly Population. Brussels: Centrum voor Bevolkings-en Gezinsstudies, 1991.
8. Istituto per gli Studi sui Servizi Sociali. La Famiglia Anziana. Rome: Ministero dell'Intemo (Direzione generale dei servizi civili), 1995.
9. Mengani M, Lamura G. Elderly Women, Family Structure and Care Patterns in Italy. In Dooghe G, Appleton N (eds), Elderly Women in Europe. Brussels: Centrum voor Bevolkings-en Gezinsstudies, 1995;121–142.
10. Mirabile ML. Gli Anziani Poveri. In Paci M (ed), Le Dimensioni Della Disuguaglianza. Bologna, Italy: Mulino, 1993;288–292.
11. Ascoli U. Le Disuguaglianze Tra i Pensionati. In Paci M (ed), Le Dimensioni Della Disuguaglianza. Bologna, Italy: Mulino, 1993;454–465.
12. Sgritta GB, Innocenzi G. La Poverta. In Paci M (ed), Le Dimensioni Della Disuguaglianza. Bologna, Italy: Mulino, 1993;261–288.
13. Italian National Institute of Statistics. Indagine Multiscopo sulle Famiglie—Anni 1987–91. Volume 10: Condizione di Salute e Ricorso ai Servizi Sanitari. Rome: Istituto Nazionale di Statistica, 1994.
14. Farchi G, Buiatti E. La Speranza di Vita e la Mortalita negli Anziani in Italia e in Europa. In Geddes M (ed), La Salute Degli Italiani—Rapporto 1993. Rome: Nuova Italia Scientifica, 1994;217–227.
15. Verdecchia A, Egidi V, Golini A. Popolazione Anziana, Invecchiamento Demografico e Condizioni di Salute. In Geddes M (ed), La Salute Degli Italiani—Rapporto 1993. Rome: Nuova Italia Scientifica, 1994;193–216.
16. Isaacs B. The Giants of Geriatrics. Birmingham, AL: University of Birmingham, 1975.
17. Cooper C, Campion G, Melton LJ III. Hip fractures in the elderly: a world-wide projection. Osteoporos Int 1992;2:285–289.
18. Ferrucci L, Baroni A. Lo Stato di Salute Negli Anziani. In Geddes M (ed), La Salute Degli Italiani—Rapporto 1993. Rome: Nuova Italia Scientifica, 1994;229–252.
19. Consiglio Sanitario Nazionale. Le Residence Sanitaire Assistenziali Peranziani ed Anziani non Autosufficienti. Atti del Seminario di Trieste del 29–30 ottobre 1990. Roma, 1991.
20. Mengani M, Giammarchi C. Aspetti Quantitative Della Disabilita Nella Popolazione Anziana. Rassegna Geriatrica/Gerontechnology (XXXI) (Vol. 1). Ancona, Italy: INRCA, 1995;67–76.
21. Masera N, Esposito M. Epidemiologia in chirurgia geriatfica: studio policentrico nazionale nei reparti di chirurgia generate. Rassegna Geriatrica 1990;26:273–287.
22. Mengani M, Gagliardi C, Lamura G, et al. The Italian Case. In Kosberg JI (ed), International Handbook on Services for the Elderly. Westport/London: Greenwood, 1994;213–226.
23. Glendinning C, McLaughlin E. Paying for Care: Lessons from Europe. London: Her Majesty's Stationery Office, 1993.
24. Masera N. Il Rischio in Chirurgia Geriatrica. Padova, Italy: Piccin, 1987.
25. Masera N, Gaggiotti G. Guida all'Assistenza del Paziente Chirurgico Geriatrico. Napoli, Italy: Idelson, 1989.
26. Masera N, Ferrara I, Nano M. Chirurgia Geriatrica. Torino, Italy: Minerva Medica, 1990.
27. Masera N. Introduction: Quality of Life after Geriatric Surgery. Atti II World Week of Professional Updating in Surgery, Milan, Italy, July 15–22, 1990.
28. Masera N, Vowles KJ. The quality of life after operation on the elderly. Adv Surg 1991;84:199–200.

Surgical Care for the Elderly, 2nd ed., edited by
R. Benton Adkins, Jr., and H. William Scott, Jr.
Lippincott–Raven Publishers, Philadelphia © 1998.

CHAPTER 39

Surgical Care for the Elderly in the United Kingdom

David L. Crosby

In the United Kingdom, as in most Western countries, the number of aging patients benefiting from surgical procedures is increasing every year. The additional needs of such patients and the skills required to address them successfully are widely recognized and are dealt with elsewhere in this book. As with most areas of clinical practice, a multidisciplinary and holistic approach is necessary if the best possible results are to be obtained.

In common with the United States, the most striking aspect of this subject is the extent to which major operative procedures are now undertaken in octogenarians and nonagenarians, which would scarcely have seemed possible or even appropriate a few decades ago. The resection of aortic aneurysms, major gastrointestinal resections, and major joint replacements are no longer exceptional. This was highlighted in this country when Queen Elizabeth, the Queen Mother, underwent a successful total hip replacement in 1995 at the age of 96.

Undoubtedly, all this has been made possible by advances in anesthesia, metabolic and critical care, and improved clinical techniques, both diagnostic and therapeutic. However, what is required most by those caring for such patients is recognition, understanding, and acceptance of the special needs of the elderly population.

In elderly patients, the objectives of surgical treatment are frequently more limited than those in younger age groups. Although the prolongation of an active, enjoyable, and worthwhile life is the prime objective, the successful return to strenuous employment or vigorous leisure pursuits is seldom necessary. Although it is important not to deny any patient the possible surgical cure or palliation of a particular disease, it is also important to avoid surgery from which the patient can derive no real benefit.

DEMOGRAPHY

A 1989 World Health Organization report pointed out that by the year 2000 there will be 600 million people over the age of 60 in the world [1]. Two-thirds of these will be living in developing countries as compared with only 50% in 1960. The World Health Organization report also estimated that in China and India alone the number of people over age 60 will increase by 270 million between 1980 and 2020. Over the same period, the population of those over age 60 in the United States is expected to increase by just 30 million, with a similar increase expected in the former Soviet Union.

In comparison with these estimates, the increases in the elderly population of Europe (where the process of population aging began much earlier) superficially appears modest. The anticipated changes for Great Britain are shown in Fig. 39-1 and Tables 39-1 and 39-2. As can be seen, the major increases are predicted to occur in men and women >85 years of age and in men aged 75 to 84. Thus, by 2011, 18% of British women are expected to be 65 years or older and 3% will be 85 years or older. The corresponding percentages for men are 14% and 1.4%, respectively. Although the absolute numbers in the oldest age groups are not large compared with the whole population, patients >75 years are high consumers of medical and surgical resources, and these anticipated population changes will have a major impact on the future provision of surgical services.

The challenges are wide ranging. Not only will adequate resources be required, attitudes will also need to change. Elderly patients in surgical wards can no longer be regarded as inevitable but unwelcome intruders interfering with the surgical treatment of younger patients. The center of gravity of medicine and surgery has shifted toward the middle aged and elderly. Many of these patients have special anesthetic, surgi-

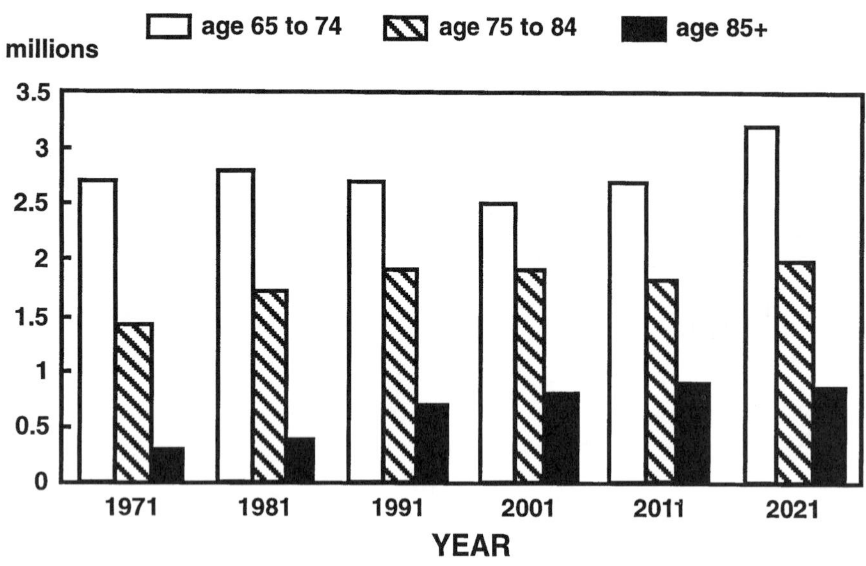

FIG. 39-1. Population of elderly women in Great Britain from 1971 to 2021. (From the Office of Population Censuses and Surveys. Series PP2, Number 16. London: Her Majesty's Stationery Office, 1987.)

TABLE 39-1. *Age-structure of the population (in millions) of Great Britain from 1971 to 2021*

Age (yrs)	1971	1981	1991	2001	2011	2021
Females						
0–64	23.4	23.0	23.4	24.1	24.2	23.9
65–74	2.7	2.8	2.7	2.5	2.7	3.2
75–84	1.4	1.7	1.9	1.9	1.8	2.0
85+	0.3	0.4	0.7	0.8	0.9	0.9
All ages	27.8	27.9	28.7	29.3	29.6	30.0
Males						
0–64	23.6	23.1	23.8	24.6	24.7	24.7
65–74	1.9	2.2	2.2	2.2	2.4	2.8
75–84	0.7	0.9	1.1	1.2	1.3	1.4
85+	0.1	0.1	0.2	0.3	0.4	0.4
All ages	26.3	26.3	27.3	28.3	28.8	29.3

Source: Data after 1987 is based on population projections from 1987 to 2027. Office of Population Censuses and Surveys. Population Projections. Series PP2, Number 16. London: Her Majesty's Stationery Office, 1987.

TABLE 39-2. *Population trends in Great Britain from 1987 to 2021*

Age (yrs)	1987	1991*	2001	2011	2021
Females					
0–64	99	100	103	104	103
65–74	102	100	93	99	117
75–84	98	100	100	94	102
85+	86	100	126	136	131
All ages	99	100	102	103	105
Males					
0–64	99	100	103	104	103
65–74	99	100	98	107	126
75–84	95	100	111	113	128
85+	83	100	145	183	196
All ages	99	100	103	105	107

*For purposes of comparison, age groups in 1991 are taken as equal to 100.

Source: Data after 1987 is based on population projections from 1987 to 2027. Office of Population Censuses and Surveys. Population Projections. Series PP2, Number 16. London: Her Majesty's Stationery Office.

cal nursing, rehabilitation, and social needs, and these needs must be fulfilled as a standard part of a surgical ward's work.

PRESENT USE OF SURGICAL FACILITIES BY AGING PATIENTS

Table 39-3 shows the age pattern of admissions to various surgical specialties in Britain using the available hospital inpatient inquiry data. When all surgical specialties are considered, patients aged 65 and over account for approximately one-fifth of admissions, although this underestimates the total number of beds occupied by the aged because older patients tend to stay longer in the hospital. In departments of trauma and orthopedics, approximately one-fourth of admitted patients are already over 65, whereas in general surgery the proportion is approximately one-third. In ophthalmology and urology over one-half of all patients admitted are currently aged 65 years or over.

TABLE 39-3. *Age and percentage of admissions to surgical specialties in England in 1985*

Specialty	0–14 yrs	15–64 yrs	65–74 yrs	75–84 yrs	85+ yrs	Total
All surgical specialties	12.9	69.1	9.7	6.9	1.4	100
Orthopedics and trauma	15.2	57.4	11.6	11.1	4.7	100
General surgery	10.6	57.5	16.6	12.6	2.8	100
Urology	5.4	44.4	26.6	20.4	3.3	100
Ophthalmology	15.7	32.4	22.4	23.8	5.8	100

Source: Based on Hospital In-Patient Enquiry, England. Main Tables, Series MB4, Number 27. London: Her Majesty's Stationery Office, 1985.

All these numbers are likely to increase. The physicians, nurses, and paramedical staff caring for elderly patients with medical problems will find increasingly that surgery will be beneficial for many of their patients. Davenport has estimated that of those people currently aged 65, one-half will require surgery at some time in their remaining lifetime [2]. Surgical care in the aging patient is important now and will become increasingly important in the future.

ORIGINS AND EVOLUTION OF THE NATIONAL HEALTH SERVICE IN THE UNITED KINGDOM

The National Health Service (NHS) is now almost 50 years old. It came into being on July 5, 1948, having been preceded by an Act of Parliament 2 years earlier [3]. It was a great personal achievement by a prominent left wing politician, Aneurin Bevan, against determined opposition by the medical profession of the day, as well as many political opponents. It was the culmination of many years of recurrent national concern at the state of the public health, including such issues as the control of infectious disease, neonatal and maternal mortality, and the poor physical state of recruits for the armed forces. An earlier report by Lord Beveridge [4] during the war years discussed the reform and extension of the social security system, together with proposals for a free NHS. The NHS was, therefore, embedded within wide-ranging postwar social reforms and a central component of what became known as the *welfare state*. As such, it was viewed by many as socialized medicine, both within the United Kingdom and abroad, and as unjustified governmental control of the delivery of health care.

However, even at the birth of the NHS, Bevan had to make significant concessions. Notably, hospital specialists were allowed to retain access to private practice, and general practitioners were allowed to retain independent contractor status and were not required to provide a salaried service. Despite many reorganizations and much evolution, the NHS currently retains the original principles that health care should be provided free at the point of need to all those who need it and funded out of general taxation. Most physicians and surgeons working in the NHS also undertake private practice in their own time.

However, within a short period of its establishment it became apparent, with the benefit of hindsight, that a major and naive miscalculation had been made. Whereas it was originally believed that successfully addressing the backlog of disease and deprivation would result in a health service that cost less each year, exactly the reverse occurred. This became explicit in the early 1960s with the advent of resource-intensive advances, such as cardiac surgery, dialysis, organ transplantation, and joint replacement. The subsequent history of the NHS has been one of escalating cost and attempts at containment by improvements in efficiency and effectiveness. Long waiting lists for treatment of nonurgent conditions have been a near constant feature, although standards of treatment of urgencies and emergencies have remained generally high.

PRESENT NATIONAL HEALTH SERVICE POSITION

The most recent reforms of the NHS were implemented (again with considerable opposition by the medical profession and political opponents) by the Thatcher government in 1990 [5], and have been the most far reaching since its inception. They have included wide-ranging changes including a separation between purchasing health authorities and providers such as self-governing Trust Hospitals, delegation of budgets and financial control to general practitioners, audit requirements, and managed competition between providers. These changes were largely based on ideas originally propounded by Alain Einthoven [6]. Supporters of the reforms claim that they have led to improved efficiency, better service for patients, and reduced waiting lists for treatment. Opponents insist that much money has been wasted on additional bureaucracy that should have been spent on patient care.

Of particular controversy since 1993 has been the implementation of "care in the community" for vulnerable groups such as the frail elderly. Whereas previously many of these patients might remain in hospital beds indefinitely, their care in the community, either in their own homes or in residential homes, became the responsibility of state-funded local authority social services. Moreover, such community care was means tested, so that those with modest savings have been required to contribute financially to their own care.

This separation between health care that remains free at the point of need, and social care that has to be paid for by those with sufficient money, has been bitterly resented by many who see it as a betrayal of the original promise of the NHS, namely, "free care from the cradle to the grave."

Whatever its difficulties have been, the NHS continues to enjoy wide public affection. All political parties compete in their avowed intention to both preserve and improve it, because to do otherwise would be political suicide. It certainly remains very efficient compared with most other Western countries, consuming only approximately 6.5% of the gross domestic product, a little more than one-half the present level in the United States.

EVOLUTION OF SPECIALTY GERIATRICS IN THE UNITED KINGDOM

Geriatric medicine (clinical gerontology) has been defined by Sir Fergus Anderson as "the branch of general medicine concerned with the health and the clinical, social, preventive and remedial aspects of illness in the elderly" [7]. This branch of medicine, which addresses the cluster of medical and social problems relevant to the aging population, flourished as a separate specialty during the 1950s and 1960s and now has a secure status within the NHS. However, there has been no parallel development in the surgical specialties. Most surgeons (with the obvious exceptions of neonatal and pediatric surgeons) recognize that a substantial component of their practice, whether gastrointestinal, orthopedic, cardiovascular, urologic, ophthalmic, or gynecologic, are increasingly concerned with patients of advancing years. Most surgeons now find themselves working closely with referring geriatricians and are dependent on their support in regard to rehabilitation services as an integral part of postoperative care.

Segregation of older patients into geriatric "care of the elderly" hospital wards, or even separate hospitals, has now markedly diminished in the NHS. Also, when such segregation does occur, it is not based on chronologic age but rather on problem-oriented needs—for example, Elderly Mentally Infirm (EMI) wards and respite care of elderly patients, to provide short periods of relief for caring relatives. Nearly all acute District General Hospitals—that is, those serving catchment populations of approximately 250,000 to 400,000—now provide specialist services for the elderly.

The great preponderance of health care for the elderly continues to be provided under the auspices of the NHS. The loading of premiums by private health insurance companies is such that few elderly citizens find them within their reach. Also, private health care companies in the United Kingdom are not disposed to insure for chronic mental or physical disease. Nevertheless, a significant proportion, perhaps 10%, of those delayed in receiving specific treatment, such as cataract extraction or total hip replacement by the NHS, currently purchase these procedures in private hospitals from private resources.

The academic development of geriatric medicine has evolved steadily, and all of the 25 medical schools in the United Kingdom have relevant academic departments.

AGEISM

Undoubtedly, negative attitudes in regard to the provision of all aspects of health care to elderly patients continue to exist. This is not least because so many old people see themselves as "too old to bother about." It is often the case that surgical innovations tend to be made available initially to young patients, and only later do older patients start to benefit. Similar differences can be observed between countries. In the United States, cardiac surgery in the very elderly has clearly become commonplace, while the realization of the potential benefits of this treatment has been much slower in Britain [8]. There seems little doubt that similar attitudes exist in relation to other treatments such as organ transplantation and dialysis [9]. At various times in the United Kingdom, geriatrics has been dubbed a "Cinderella specialty."

These inferences are drawn from observations of reduced access by elderly patients to facilities such as intensive care units, and segregation to geriatric hospital wards where investigations and treatment (including resuscitation) are pursued with less energy and enthusiasm. No doubt such negative attitudes have been fostered by erroneous beliefs that the outcomes of treatment for elderly patients are generally poor. To some extent, systems such as quality-adjusted life years advocated for prioritization of limited health care resources are biased against the elderly because of their limited life expectancies [10].

These concepts are morally unjustifiable. Older people have generally contributed more to the society in which they live than the young. Also, elderly patients should enjoy greater access to available health care, if only because they are likely to benefit from it for a larger proportion of their remaining life span. Increasing numbers of older people in the population should be seen as a resource and the result of successful policies, and not as some kind of looming disaster.

ORGANIZATION OF SURGICAL SERVICES FOR ELDERLY PATIENTS

Preoperative Assessment

The discovery of a disease that may be amenable to surgical treatment is no more than an indication for a full and detailed assessment of the patient concerned. Only when this has been done can a responsible opinion be given as to whether a surgical procedure is appropriate. Although not separated in practice, there are two principal aims: (1) to obtain a precise preoperative diagnosis, and (2) to discover concomitant disorders.

A precise preoperative diagnosis is necessary so that the requirements of the relevant operation can be assessed and properly planned. Thus, in obstructive jaundice, a knowledge of the exact cause of the obstruction usually facilitates the speed and ease with which the operation can be performed, thereby improving its safety. Accurate diagnosis of the extent of the disease is also of the greatest importance because operations unlikely to help the patient can be avoided—for example, the discovery of metastatic disease or the spread of disease to such an extent that the patient would be unable to withstand the magnitude of the operation required. At the same time, it is important not to advise unpleasant invasive, costly, and sometimes hazardous investigations, unless the information they can provide will affect the clinical decision that has to be made.

Only when concomitant disorders are known can the risks of any procedure be properly assessed. Thus, cardiorespiratory, renal, and metabolic disorders must be sought and the nutritional status of the patient assessed. To this end, all patients should have chest radiography, electrocardiography, full blood count, electrolyte and urea estimates, and examination of urine, especially for glucose. Sputum culture and pulmonary function tests including blood gas levels may also be appropriate. As much as possible, all deviations from normal should be corrected preoperatively, particularly cardiac failure, chest infection, hypovolemia, and electrolyte imbalance.

Preoperative evaluation of the mental status and psychological attitude of the patient is also important when advising a major surgical procedure, because it clearly has a bearing on the difficulties of postoperative management. Anxiety, agitation, and confusion may be due to correctable organic causes such as metabolic disturbance, drug therapy, and hypoxia. It is self-evident that the active and willing cooperation of the patient who accepts and understands the nature of the proposed operation should result in an improved chance of recovering from it.

The relationship between preoperative risk factors and postoperative outcome in elderly general surgical patients was examined by Seymour and Vaz [11,12]. Although increasing age had an influence on postoperative morbidity and mortality, the relationship between preoperative illness and postoperative outcome was more dramatic. In particular, it was noted that elderly patients with no preoperative medical problems had favorable patterns of postoperative morbidity and mortality. Data of this type and numerous other examples show the importance of preoperative assessment in the elderly. Elderly patients who are medically fit before surgery have little more to fear from modern surgical techniques than their younger counterparts, except perhaps in situations where multiple surgical complications and sepsis put such severe strain on physiologic systems that the reduced homeostatic reserve of the older patient becomes a critical factor.

Surgical Technique

There is no fundamental difference in the requirements for safe surgical technique in elderly patients compared with those necessary in younger age groups. Whatever the patient's age, surgical procedures should only be undertaken by the adequately skilled and experienced. Nevertheless, operations on elderly people are commonly more challenging for well-known reasons. Compensatory homeostatic and cardiorespiratory mechanisms are often impaired so that reduced blood loss is desirable and prolonged procedures are best avoided. Blood vessels are often more rigid, bones are more brittle, and soft tissues are more easily damaged and slower to heal. Manual dexterity and skill are clearly advantageous in reducing technical surgical errors, the consequences of which are likely to be magnified in frail elderly people, who may already be contending with adverse pathophysiologic disorders.

In addition, pathologic changes needing surgical attention are frequently more advanced, while the need for emergency procedures is increased. In emergency procedures there is less time to make crucial decisions about the indication and timing of the operation and less diagnostic information available on which to base such decisions. The discovery of unexpected findings at the time of the operation, the difficult decisions regarding what action should be taken, and whether additional and extensive procedures are justifiable must be based on considerable previous experience.

Therefore, the main aspects of the surgical care of older patients should be undertaken by fully trained and experienced surgeons. This indeed was one of the main recommendations of the Confidential Enquiry into Perioperative Deaths (CEPOD) report (see following discussion).

Advice, Consent, and Indemnity

The decision to advise or withhold surgical treatment for any patient can only be made after a full assessment of the situation. In offering an opinion the surgeon must allow time and opportunity for the patient to comprehend the risks and implications of having or not having the relevant surgical procedure. Often it is appropriate for the surgeon to return after sufficient time has been allowed for the patient to assimilate the advice that has been given. Although many patients will readily accept what is offered and may even prefer not to discuss any details, others will wish to cross-examine the surgeon about the risks of the operation, the procedures involved, and the chance of success. When the offer of surgical treatment is declined, the possible effects of refusal or delay should be explained but on no account should a reluctant patient be hectored or seduced into agreement. It should be stressed that it is the patient's decision that is of most importance, and that the decision can be changed without prejudice at a later time.

Not infrequently patients may be keen to undergo a procedure that the surgeon is unwilling to perform because of its risks and poor chance of success. This can be a difficult situation and one in which a second opinion is often appropriate.

It is often the case that elderly surgical patients wish their relatives to be involved in decisions about whether they should have surgery. Also, relatives sometimes express strong and uninvited views. In general, it should be stressed that provided the patient is mentally competent, it is the patient's own views and opinions that must be paramount. In legal terms, in the United Kingdom relatives normally have no power or obligation in this regard. Some patients may be temporarily confused because of the illness for which an operation is indicated. In these instances the decision must be the ultimate responsibility of the clinicians involved.

The problem of consent in the demented patient obviously poses special difficulties. In these situations, major procedures will usually be limited to surgery that will either relieve pain or distress or that will make the situation easier for those caring for the patient. Thus, for example, the excision of an ulcerating tumor, amputation of a gangrenous limb, or relief of intestinal obstruction are operations that will relieve suffering. On the other hand, elective procedures for extensive nonobstructive malignant disease are less easy to recommend in a demented patient. Hard and fast rules cannot and should not be laid down, and all patients must be considered individually.

As yet the full implications of the doctrine of informed consent are not known in the United Kingdom. The landmark legal cases are known by abbreviation as Bolam [13] and Sidaway [14]. In the 1957 Bolam case, a schizophrenic patient sustained bone fractures after electroconvulsive therapy, and in the 1984 Sidaway case, a patient suffered paralysis after a pain-relieving operation on the cervical spine. The patients had not been warned about the possibility of these non-negligent complications. In Bolam, the judge summed up that ". . . a doctor is not negligent if he is acting in accordance with a procedure accepted as proper by a responsible body of medical men skilled in that particular art, merely because there is a body of such opinion that takes a contrary view." This opinion was upheld in the Sidaway case by the majority of law lords at an appeal to the House of Lords. These judgments are now widely seen as "doctor friendly." Nevertheless, at present an exhaustive list of possible adverse consequences that may result from a therapeutic procedure need not all be disclosed to a patient, if the doctor concerned believes that this will cause undue distress, and if a body of responsible opinion of his or her peers is in agreement with his or her practice.

Indemnity for medical negligence suits brought by NHS patients is provided for all its employees by the NHS itself from a central fund. In regard to private patients, indemnity must be obtained by individual doctors and others by insurance with independent medical defense organizations. Sliding scales exist according to specialty and income but have yet to reach the levels that now exist in the United States. Thus, for an average United Kingdom orthopedic or vascular surgeon undertaking private practice this is currently approximately $7,500 to $10,000 per year.

Timing of Surgery

The timing of surgical procedures has to be balanced between the risks of delay and the possible improvement in the patient's condition that can be obtained by preoperative measures. The final decision is a matter of clinical judgment by the surgeon in consultation with the anesthetist and other colleagues and depends on balancing the chances of success, the risk of failure, and the likely course if an operation is not performed.

These factors must be assessed against the background knowledge and expertise of the surgical team concerned. Thus, it is the obligation of any clinician active in geriatric surgery to audit mortality and morbidity engendered in the surgical management of various disorders in relation to advancing age. The course of the untreated disease is more speculative because in many instances properly controlled clinical trials are ethically difficult to justify, for example, those involving the treatment of nonobstructive intra-abdominal malignancy. Therefore, for various reasons, a surgeon often has to make decisions on evidence that is necessarily incomplete.

It seems reasonable in comparing surgical results to classify surgical interventions as follows:

- Emergency: a life-saving operation in which resuscitation accompanies surgery
- Urgent: a life-saving operation preceded by resuscitation
- Scheduled: an operation performed usually within a few days or weeks of diagnosis
- Elective: an operation performed at a time convenient to the patient and surgical team

Facilities

Because elderly surgical patients often possess multiple risk factors, their postoperative care should be closely supervised so that any complications can be identified early and appropriate treatment given. Consequently, their interests are often best served by admission to a high dependency unit, where close observation and detailed monitoring of vital functions can be undertaken during critical periods of care. Also, effective methods of postoperative pain relief such as epidural analgesia can be given more safely in such units. This in turn implies acceptance of the concept of progressive patient care so that available resources are allocated most effectively and efficiently [15]. Although it is difficult to prove that mortality and

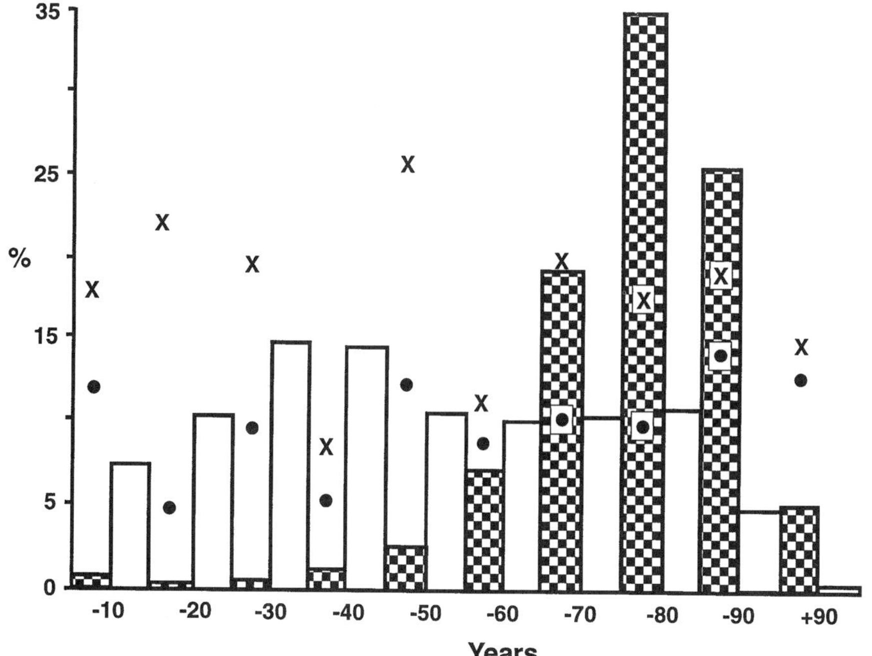

FIG. 39-2. Confidential Enquiry into Perioperative Deaths report. The histogram shows the operating rates (clear columns) by decade of age derived from the Hospital In-Patient Enquiry. (hatched columns = all the deaths reported to the Confidential Enquiry into Perioperative Deaths; • = proportion of deaths assessed by anesthetists to be associated with anesthesia; X = proportions of deaths assessed by surgeons to have avoidable factors.) (These are not precise definitions.) (Reprinted with permission from Buck M, Devlin HB, Lunn JN. Report of a Confidential Enquiry into Perioperative Deaths. London: Nuffield Provincial Hospital Trust and Kings Fund for Hospitals, 1987.)

morbidity are thereby reduced, there can be little doubt that the quality of care is improved and that patients appreciate the constant attendance of well-trained nurses in the early postoperative period.

Patients in need of support of vital functions, for example, artificial ventilation, may need admission to an intensive care unit where such facilities for critical care are constantly available.

Audit

The CEPOD [16] was a landmark in the United Kingdom: It represented the first collaboration of British anesthetists and surgeons in a widespread audit exercise, and, although it dealt with deaths in all surgical patients, two-thirds of all such deaths occurred in patients who were 65 or over. One of the main concerns raised by CEPOD was that a distressingly large number of the deaths that occurred were of very elderly patients who had been operated on during off hours by relatively junior staff. It was pointed out that a proportion of such deaths might have been avoided if anesthetic and surgical services had been better organized. Such conclusions have major implications for surgical training, the number of surgeons required for a given population, and the level of surgical and anesthetic care considered acceptable for elderly patients. The central importance of large-scale audits such as CEPOD is that they allow such questions to be asked. The concept of day-to-day self-audit is also growing within surgery and medicine, and in Britain surgeons and anesthetists have taken the lead. Because of their high mortality and multiplicity of medical and surgical problems, elderly patients potentially have the most to gain from systems of clinical self-audit. In the actual study it was found that 67% of the 30-day hospital mortality happened in patients aged 70 years or older. The surgeon assessors stated that the delivery of surgical care (i.e., decision to operate, actual operation, experience of surgeon) was deficient in approximately 13% of deaths. Anesthetist assessors stated that the delivery of anesthesia (i.e., agreement to anesthetize, actual anesthetic, experience of anesthetist) was deficient in approximately 14% of deaths. There was considerable commonality between these assessments, particularly in relation to deficiencies in resuscitation before operation and the involvement of experienced staff. The performance of nonemergency procedures on elderly people during unsocial hours was criticized in the report (Fig. 39-2).

Day Surgery

The rapid changes occurring in the provision of health care, with increasing emphasis on cost containment and individual patient needs, has resulted in a considerable growth of day surgery. This change has so far been less marked in the United Kingdom than in other countries [17]. Until recently, day surgical centers dealt with minor operations in patients whose physical status was American Society of Anesthesiologists (ASA) grades 1 and 2, but now patients graded ASA 3 are being presented for surgical treatment, including many elderly patients.

The advantages of day surgery for the elderly are convenience and less disruption to routine. Separation from family and friends is minimized, and there is an early return to home and familiar surroundings. This is not only socially desirable but medically advantageous [18]. Thus far the mortality of day surgery has remained low, and in the United Kingdom CEPOD study [16] there were no reported deaths associated with day surgery. The most common procedure carried out in day surgical facilities in the United Kingdom at present is cataract extraction, but with increasing expertise and experience, the range of surgical procedures is undoubtedly expanding.

OUTCOMES

There is little dispute that age-associated disease, rather than age per se, is the important determinant of outcome. Although it is true that on average an older patient will have more disease than a younger patient, every aged surgical patient deserves an individual assessment. When this is done, it will be found that approximately one-fifth of general surgical patients aged 65 years and older will have no detectable medical disease of any sort, and here the surgical outcome is usually satisfactory whatever their age [12]. Even in the remaining four-fifths of patients, many of the diseases encountered will be minor or treatable or it will be possible to mitigate some of their effects by careful perioperative management.

Nevertheless, the mortality for most surgical conditions increases with age, and at first sight the number of deaths following surgical procedures appears to be a totally objective means of measuring outcome and comparing the performance of different surgical units. In fact, numerous problems arise when death rates are used as the basis of a surgical audit, and these problems are particularly evident when elderly surgical patients are involved.

The first problem encountered when reading the literature on postoperative mortality is the lack of standardization of follow-up times. Some studies have confined their attention to the first 48 hours, whereas others report over a 10-year period. Because it is easy to collect, the mortality in the hospital is often recorded, but the duration of hospital stay is influenced by a number of administrative as well as medical factors, and the availability of facilities for rehabilitation, convalescence, or terminal care tends to introduce artifacts into the data. Much better, but more difficult to collect, is the mortality within a fixed period after the surgical operation. The exact time period chosen will depend on the aims of the given study. Thus, 1 month is a reasonable period for assessing many surgical conditions, but the mortality pattern following hip fracture, for example, is best studied for 6 to 12 months, and even longer periods of follow-up are necessary when the long-term effects of cancer therapy are being evaluated. In elderly patients, particularly when follow-up periods are long, it is necessary to calculate what the expected survival rate would have been in age-matched patients without any surgical problem.

A more fundamental problem when using mortality as a measure of outcome is the fact that death is often an inappropriate end point for judging surgical results, for example, a palliative procedure to relieve esophageal or bowel obstruction in a patient with inoperable malignancy. A high early mortality after such procedures is likely, but the surgeon who achieved better mortality figures by avoiding such palliative procedures would not necessarily be acting in the best interests of his or her patients. At the opposite end of the spectrum are operations such as the removal of cataracts under local anesthesia where mortality is very low and where the postoperative death rate is a totally inappropriate measure of surgical success. In operations for hip replacement the aim is to relieve pain or to improve function.

Mortality is, therefore, an inappropriate outcome measure in these situations, although it is relevant when the risks and benefits of a procedure are being considered, and when decisions are being made about policy matters such as the use of prophylaxis against thromboembolism or sepsis.

Despite these problems there are circumstances where mortality can give useful insights into the effectiveness of a surgical unit. However, to extract the most information from such statistics, a single overall mortality estimate is rarely of value. Rather it is better to go into more detail and to collect information on the broad causes of death, for example, underlying surgical or medical disease, anesthetic problems, postoperative medical or surgical implications, the aims of the procedure, whether or not death could have been potentially prevented, and the death rate in patients who were treated conservatively or judged to be too ill for surgery. Much work therefore remains to be done on the proper evaluation of outcome both for those patients who have undergone surgical interventions and those who have not.

CONCLUSION

The burgeoning numbers of those in the population >65 years old in the United Kingdom is mainly a consequence of better public health measures in the late nineteenth and early twentieth century rather than any critical improvements in the delivery of health care by the NHS during the last 50 years. However, the great improvement in the quality of survival of this population in the last few decades is attributable to a considerable extent to the universal availability of the NHS and not least to the accessibility of surgical treatment for common diseases. As for the future, it is now well established that modern medical technology has as much to offer the old as well as the young. Its future availability to all who can benefit may depend more on national economic success as well as social concern for the dignity and importance of its senior citizens than anything else.

REFERENCES

1. World Health Organization. Health of the Elderly. Report of a WHO Expert Committee. World Health Organization Technical Report Series. Geneva: World Health Organization, 1989;779:14–31.
2. Davenport HT. Anaesthesia in the Elderly. London: Heinemann, 1986.

3. The National Health Service Act, 1966.
4. The Beveridge Report on Social Insurance and Allied Services, 1942.
5. NHS and Community Care Bill, 1990.
6. Einthoven A. Reflections on the Management of the NHS. London: Nuffield Provincial Hospitals Trust, 1985.
7. Anderson F. An Historical Overview of Geriatric Medicine: Definition and Aims. In Pathy MSJ (ed), Principles and Practice of Geriatric Medicine. Chichester, NY: Wiley, 1985;7.
8. Elder AT, Cameron EW. Cardiac surgery in the elderly. BMJ 1989;299: 140–141.
9. Lawrance J. Dialysis shortfall kills hundreds. Times, London. January 22, 1996.
10. Smith A. Qualms about QALYs. Lancet 1987;1:1134–1136.
11. Vaz FG, Seymour DG. A prospective study of general surgical patients. I. Preoperative medical problems. Age Ageing 1989;18: 309–315.
12. Seymour DG, Vaz FG. A prospective study of general surgical patients. II. Post operative complications. Age Ageing 1989;18:316–326.
13. Bolam v Friern Hospital Management Committee (1957). 1 WLR 582.
14. Sidaway v Board of Governors of the Bethlehem Royal Hospital (1984). 1 All ER 1018 (CA) (1985) AC 871 (1985) 1AllER643 (HL)
15. The Royal College of Anaesthetists and the Royal College of Surgeons of England. Report of the Joint Working Party on Graduated Patient Care. London: The Royal College of Anaesthetists and the Royal College of Surgeons of England, January 1996.
16. Buck M, Devlin HB, Lunn JN. Report of a Confidential Enquiry into Perioperative Deaths. London: Nuffield Provincial Hospital Trust and Kings Fund for Hospitals, 1987.
17. Audit Commission. A Short Cut to Better Services: Day Surgery in England and Wales 1990. London: Her Majesty's Stationery Office, 1990.
18. Wetchler BV (ed). Anaesthesia for Out Patients (2nd ed). Philadelphia: Churchill Livingstone, 1990.

Surgical Care for the Elderly, 2nd ed., edited by
R. Benton Adkins, Jr., and H. William Scott, Jr.
Lippincott–Raven Publishers, Philadelphia © 1998.

CHAPTER 40

The Challenging Future

Robert W. Youngblood and R. Benton Adkins, Jr.

The future of surgical care for the elderly depends on a number of diverse factors, some of which are predictable, others are difficult to predict, and some defy the imagination. The direction of the demographic population shift seems obvious, but ethical issues evolving from social mores, public attitudes, and moral and religious beliefs tend to change slowly. As evidenced by the development of laparoscopic surgery, genetic alteration of cellular biology, and recent events in the fields of immunology, scientific and technological changes occur more rapidly. Alteration of environmental factors, disease processes such as seen with the acquired immunodeficiency syndrome virus, and cataclysmic, natural, or man-made phenomena are entirely unpredictable.

The role of surgery and the interaction of the surgeon of the twenty-first century with the elderly patient must be viewed through the unpredictable kaleidoscope of biopolitical and social change involving health care financing, population shifts, and alterations of public attitudes toward both surgical care and the elderly.

DEMOGRAPHICS

Recent population studies consistently show that more individuals are living into the eighth and ninth decades, which has resulted in an increasing proportion of elderly in the population, despite little change in the upper limits of longevity. This, plus the high birth rate after World War II, will result in an unprecedented plurality of elderly citizens in the second and third decades of the twenty-first century. From 1990 to 2050, the combined effect will result in an estimated fivefold increase in the 85-year-old and older population and a twofold estimated increase in the number of centenarians, while the overall population will grow by 53% [1].

These projections demand that the generation of gerontologists, physicians, and surgeons during this period of changing population patterns study the physical tolerances and adaptive abilities of the elderly and research methods for improving them. A team approach to care of the elderly, including shared outcomes data and multidisciplinary treatment protocols, would result in more comprehensive, yet efficient care [2]. Residency training for surgeons of all specialty groups should begin to prepare the surgeons of the next generation to care for this population segment. Research should also be intensified in the fields of political science and sociology so that changes in political power and social pressures can be anticipated. Certainly sensitivity to the special needs and lower tolerances so often associated with the surgical care of this population segment can only improve surgical care in general by making it more individualized.

POLITICAL TRENDS

Since 1965, when the federal government undertook, through its Medicare program, to underwrite health care for those who were over age 65, there have been significant changes in life expectancy, the ratio of workers to retirees, and the number of persons covered by Medicare, including the disabled and those with renal failure. Population shifts, increasing medical costs, and the fiscal policies of the Medicare program have threatened the viability of the entire system.

Because those involved represent so large a voting block, the legislature has avoided any significant alteration of the status quo. However, the declining ratio of supporters to recipients foreshadowed by this demographic shift will mandate drastic changes, if not complete revamping [3].

Although the administration and financing of the entire health care system in the United States is currently the largest role assumed by the federal government, there are many other new factors in the legislative area affecting the medical profession. If the role of government decreases and that of managed care increases, other political issues affecting the care of the elderly may assume increasing importance. These areas include regulations regarding managed care, laws covering malpractice reform, rulings regarding the pharmaceutical industry, and right-to-life issues. As significant demographic changes take place, issues of generational equity may affect and be affected by the political process at the national level. States that have refused to pay the coinsurance portion of the Medicare bills for the indigent elderly under the Medicaid provision of federal law are being faced with class action lawsuits by several state medical societies.

TECHNICAL ADVANCES

The advent of laparoscopy, thoracoscopy, and other minimally invasive procedures is already changing indications, risks, and attitudes regarding surgery. The progressive expansion of this technology combined with robotics and the techniques of virtual reality will continue to affect the surgical specialties of the twenty-first century, especially for the elderly and poor-risk patient.

Research into cellular biology, genetic alterations, cytokine reactions, nitrous oxide production with its effect on vascular endothelium, and immunologic responses and their control will alter the morbidity and mortality of surgical management in the elderly. As these basic phenomena are clarified, surgical care for the elderly may turn more toward the alleviation of functional disabilities with increased use of tissue and organ transplantation. Improved preoperative assessments, better monitoring of vital functions at the cellular level, and new anesthetic techniques will lessen the risk of many procedures, even in advanced age groups [4].

We must look at surgical therapy from the perspective of the elderly patient. Just because a procedure is technically feasible does not mean that it is desirable for the elderly unless it adds to comfort or improves quality of life. The surgeon should increasingly consider the decision regarding operative treatment from the viewpoint of the patient considering his or her life situation, functional independence, social issues, suffering, and prognosis. We must also consider the cost of a surgical procedure for possible cure and weigh this against the cost of long-term care for a patient with an uncorrected high-maintenance condition.

ETHICAL ASPECTS OF CARE

One of the most volatile and sensitive aspects of the care of the elderly involves dilemmas and decisions in the management of surgical diseases. Any decisions regarding surgical therapy based on the age of the patient should be determined by physiologic rather than chronologic age. However, because the ever-increasing population segment represents a disproportionately large number of mentally or physically compromised individuals requiring complex procedures, these issues become more complex. The health care industry and governmental issues of generational equity are likely to arise. On the more personal level, quality-of-life issues become paramount to the elderly patient and his or her family.

Difficult decisions regarding the final stages of life must be made with recognition of the patient's wishes, through advance directives, and the autonomy and self-determination of that process must be preserved as long as the individual is capable of participation in the decision-making process. Too often, in these days of sophisticated medical technology, patient autonomy is lost, and a process of physician paternalism supersedes patient choice [5]. We must preserve the dignity of the individual, alleviate suffering, respect and try to satisfy the patient's wishes, and prevent guilt and frustration on the part of the family. These heart-rending decisions, because of the multiplicity of factors and the vagaries of individual situations and personalities, must be made on an individual basis [6]. It is for the best if this interaction between the physician and the patient is not encumbered by medicolegal intrusion.

RESEARCH

Continuing research in a wide variety of areas, ranging from the enzymatic regulation of cellular activity to patient outcomes, is essential [7]. Such studies are now being threatened as funding for research and advanced medical specialty training is curtailed by current short-sighted cost contingencies. The United States, having long been a leader in basic scientific research and medical education, must not let this leadership be thwarted by political maneuvering and budgetary negotiations. We must learn from our past experiences and from other countries' experience, and we must solve the research funding problem soon.

CONCLUSION

We must be ever mindful of the apprehensions, aspirations, and desires of the elderly in using our surgical skills for their benefit and comfort. Because our success is accretive and always vulnerable, our care must be as mindful of the individual patient as it is of the whole health care environment. We, as surgeons, must continue to look to and plan for the opportunities and challenges of the future while we labor at resolving the problems of today.

REFERENCES

1. Seltzer MM. The Impact of Increasing Life Expectancy. New York: Springer, 1995.
2. Bull CN. Aging in Rural America. Newbury Park, CA: Sage, 1993.
3. Satin DG. The Clinical Care of the Aged Person. New York: Oxford University Press, 1994.
4. Crosby DL, Rees CAD, Semour DC. The Aging Surgical Patient. New York: Wiley, 1992.
5. Moody HR. Ethics in an Aging Society. Baltimore: Johns Hopkins University Press, 1992.
6. Meakins JL, McClaran JC. Surgical Care of the Elderly. Chicago: Year Book, 1988.
7. Katlic MR (ed). Geriatric Surgery: Comprehensive Care of the Elderly Patient. Baltimore: Urban & Schwarzenberg, 1990.

Subject Index

Note: Page numbers followed by f indicate figures; page numbers followed by t indicate tables.

D

R